# The Pathobiology of Neoplasia

# The Pathobiology of Neoplasia

Edited by

## Alphonse E. Sirica

*Medical College of Virginia*
*Virginia Commonwealth University*
*Richmond, Virginia*

*Plenum Press • New York and London*

Library of Congress Cataloging in Publication Data

The Pathobiology of neoplasia / edited by Alphonse E. Sirica.
    p.    cm.
  Includes bibliographies and index.
  ISBN-13: 978-1-4684-5525-0        e-ISBN-13: 978-1-4684-5523-6
  DOI:  10.1007/978-1-4684-5523-6
  1. Cancer cells. 2. Carcinogenesis. 3. Cancer invasiveness. I. Sirica, Alphonse E.
  [DNLM: 1. Cell Transformation, Neoplastic. 2. Neoplasms — etiology. 3. Neoplasms
— pathology. 4. Neoplasms, Experimental.] RC269.P38    1988
616.99′2071 — dc19
DNLM/DLC                                                        88-29012
for Library of Congress                                             CIP

© 1989 Plenum Press, New York
Softcover reprint of the hardcover 1st edition  1989
A Division of Plenum Publishing Corporation
233 Spring Street, New York, N.Y. 10013

# Contributors

**Marshall W. Anderson** • Laboratory of Biochemical Risk Analysis, National Institute of Environmental Health Sciences, Research Triangle Park, North Carolina 27709

**Frederick A. Beland** • National Center for Toxicological Research, Jefferson, Arkansas 72079

**Peter M. Blumberg** • Molecular Mechanisms of Tumor Promotion Section, Laboratory of Cellular Carcinogenesis and Tumor Promotion, National Cancer Institute, National Institutes of Health, Bethesda, Maryland 20892

**Anthony Cutry** • Biological Chemistry Division, Roswell Park Memorial Institute, Buffalo, New York 14263

**Patricia A. D'Amore** • Laboratory of Surgical Research and Department of Pathology, Children's Hospital and Harvard Medical School, Boston, Massachusetts 02115

**John DiGiovanni** • The University of Texas System Cancer Center, Science Park, Research Division, Smithville, Texas 78957

**Bhalchandra A. Diwan** • Biological Carcinogenesis Development, Program Resources, Inc., Frederick Cancer Research Facility, National Cancer Institute, Frederick, Maryland 21701

**Steven L. Dresler** • Department of Pathology, Washington University School of Medicine, St. Louis, Missouri 63110

**Mario R. Escobar** • Department of Pathology, Medical College of Virginia, Virginia Commonwealth University, Richmond, Virginia 23298

**I. J. Fidler** • Department of Cell Biology, M.D. Anderson Hospital and Tumor Institute, University of Texas System Cancer Center, Houston, Texas 77030

**Joseph V. Formica** • Department of Microbiology and Immunology, School of Basic Health Sciences, Virginia Commonwealth University, Richmond, Virginia 23298

**Barbara K. Hecht** • The Genetics Center and The Cancer Center, Southwest Biomedical Research Institute, Scottsdale, Arizona 85251

**Frederick Hecht** • The Genetics Center and The Cancer Center, Southwest Biomedical Research Institute, Scottsdale, Arizona 85251

**Arco Y. Jeng** • Research Department, Pharmaceuticals Division, Ciba-Geigy Corporation, Summit, New Jersey 07901

**Carol A. Jones** • Biological, Environmental, and Medical Research Division, Argonne National Laboratory, Argonne, Illinois 60439

*Michael Klagsbrun* • Laboratory of Surgical Research and Department of Biological Chemistry, Children's Hospital and Harvard Medical School, Boston, Massachusetts 02115

*Lance A. Liotta* • Laboratory of Pathology, National Cancer Institute, National Institutes of Health, Bethesda, Maryland 20892

*Robert G. McKinnell* • Department of Genetics and Cell Biology, University of Minnesota, St. Paul, Minnesota 55108-1095

*George K. Michalopoulos* • Department of Pathology, Duke University Medical Center, Durham, North Carolina 27710

*D. James Morré* • Department of Medicinal Chemistry and Pharmacognosy, Purdue University, West Lafayette, Indiana 47907

*R. Timothy Mulcahy* • Department of Human Oncology, University of Wisconsin–Madison, Madison, Wisconsin 53792

*Carl Peraino* • Biological, Environmental, and Medical Research Division, Argonne National Laboratory, Argonne, Illinois 60439

*Miriam C. Poirier* • National Cancer Institute, National Institutes of Health, Bethesda, Maryland 20892

*Sambasiva M. Rao* • Department of Pathology, Northwestern University Medical School, Chicago, Illinois 60611

*Janardan K. Reddy* • Department of Pathology, Northwestern University Medical School, Chicago, Illinois 60611

*Steven H. Reynolds* • Laboratory of Biochemical Risk Analysis, National Institute of Environmental Health Sciences, Research Triangle Park, North Carolina 27709

*Jerry M. Rice* • Laboratory of Comparative Carcinogenesis, Frederick Cancer Research Facility, National Cancer Institute, Frederick, Maryland 21701-1013

*David P. Rose* • Division of Nutrition and Endocrinology, American Health Foundation, Valhalla, New York 10595

*Avery A. Sandberg* • The Genetics Center and The Cancer Center, Southwest Biomedical Research Institute, Scottsdale, Arizona 85251

*Dante G. Scarpelli* • Department of Pathology, Northwestern University Medical School, Chicago, Illinois 60611

*Elliott Schiffmann* • Laboratory of Pathology, National Cancer Institute, National Institutes of Health, Bethesda, Maryland 20892

*Alphonse E. Sirica* • Department of Pathology, Medical College of Virginia, Virginia Commonwealth University, Richmond, Virginia 23298

*Mary L. Stracke* • Laboratory of Pathology, National Cancer Institute, National Institutes of Health, Bethesda, Maryland 20892

*James E. Talmadge* • Smith Kline & French Laboratories, Research and Development Division, Immunology and Antiinfectives Therapy, King of Prussia, Pennsylvania 19406

*Snorri S. Thorgeirsson* • Laboratory of Experimental Carcinogenesis, National Cancer Institute, National Institutes of Health, Bethesda, Maryland 20892

*Elizabeth K. Weisburger* • Division of Cancer Etiology, National Cancer Institute, National Institutes of Health, Bethesda, Maryland 20892

*Charles E. Wenner* • Biological Chemistry Division, Roswell Park Memorial Institute, Buffalo, New York 14263

*Eric H. Westin* • Department of Medicine, Division of Hematology/Oncology, Medical College of Virginia, Virginia Commonwealth University, Richmond, Virginia 23298

*Ulla M. Wewer* • Laboratory of Pathology, National Cancer Institute, National Institutes of Health, Bethesda, Maryland 20892; *present address:* University Institute of Pathologic Anatomy, 2100 Copenhagen, Denmark

*Peter J. Wirth* • Laboratory of Experimental Carcinogenesis, National Cancer Institute, National Institutes of Health, Bethesda, Maryland 20892

*James D. Yager* • Department of Anatomy, Dartmouth Medical School, Hanover, New Hampshire 03756

*Joanne Zurlo* • Department of Pharmacology and Toxicology, Dartmouth Medical School, Hanover, New Hampshire 03756

# Preface

This book is directed primarily to advanced graduate and medical students, postdoctoral trainees, and established investigators having basic research interests in neoplasia. Its content is based in part on the lecture outlines and selected histopathology laboratory components of an advanced course entitled The Pathobiology of Experimental Animal and Human Neoplasia, developed by me for the Experimental Pathology Curriculum of the Department of Pathology at the Medical College of Virginia. In this regard, an effort has been made to integrate pathology with carcinogenesis, genetics, biochemistry, and cellular and molecular biology in order to present a comprehensive and current view of the neoplastic process. For focus, emphasis is mainly being placed on the neoplastic cells themselves, and not on associated host-mediated responses. It is hoped that this book will accomplish its purpose of providing students and researchers who already possess strong but diverse basic science backgrounds with unifying concepts in tumor pathobiology, so as to stimulate new research aimed at furthering our understanding of neoplastic disease.

I wish to express my appreciation and heartfelt thanks to the authors, whose individual ranges of expertise and research experience clearly bring to their respective chapters unique perspectives that easily transcend any redundancy that may be present. In addition, I am grateful to Drs. George Vennart, Saul Kay, and Fred Meier, and to Ms. Connie Wilkerson of the Department of Pathology at MCV, for their helpful comments and their review of some of the material. I also want to thank Ms. Mary Phillips Born, Senior Editor with Plenum Publishing Corporation, for her most helpful suggestions and advice; Ms. Linda Sylte Wilson, Ms. Jennifer Lynn Ogren, and Ms. Hattie M. Wyche for typing portions of this work; and Ms. Charlotte Phillips for her valuable help in preparing the subject index. I further wish to acknowledge Dr. Henry C. Pitot, a good friend and advisor, and Director of the McArdle Laboratory for Cancer Research at the University of Wisconsin, who greatly influenced my interests in the pathobiology of neoplasia. Finally, I would like to dedicate this book to my wife Annette—whose caring, patience, and sense of humor, not to mention her much appreciated assistance in helping to resolve a number of key conflicts related to grammar and spelling, combined to make my editorial task easier—and to my little daughter Gabrielle and my infant son Nicholas—who are for me constant sources of wonderment.

Alphonse E. Sirica

*Richmond, Virginia*

# Contents

## Chapter 6. The Multistage Concept of Carcinogenesis ................... 131

*Carl Peraino and Carol A. Jones*

## Chapter 7. Organ and Species Specificity in Chemical Carcinogenesis and Tumor Promotion ............................................... 149

*Bhalchandra A. Diwan and Jerry M. Rice*

## Chapter 12. Genetics of Susceptibility to Mouse Skin Tumor Promotion

### John DiGiovanni

## Chapter 18. Biochemical Mechanisms of Action of the Phorbol Ester Class of Tumor Promoters ........................................................... 371

*Arco Y. Jeng and Peter M. Blumberg*

## Chapter 19. Biochemical Marker Alterations in Hepatic Preneoplasia and Neoplasia ..................................................................... 385

*Snorri S. Thorgeirsson and Peter J. Wirth*

## Chapter 28. Phenotypic Heterogeneity and Metastasis ................. 547

*James E. Talmadge and I. J. Fidler*

# Introduction

# Chronology of Significant Events in the Study of Neoplasia

## Alphonse E. Sirica

The purpose of this chronology is to provide both an historic and a current perspective related to the subject matter detailed in this book. No doubt, some omissions have been made, partly due to oversight, but mostly as a result of limited space. For a more detailed account of many of the earlier discoveries listed here, the reader is referred to the excellent work of Michael B. Shimkin, 1977, *Contrary to Nature*, U.S. Department of Health, Education and Welfare Publication, Washington, D. C., as well as to the specific references cited for each event.

| Year | Event | References |
|------|-------|-----------|
| Circa 1600 BC | The Edwin Smith Papyrus of ancient Egypt provides one of the earliest known references to clinical neoplasms in humans. | 1 |
| Circa 1550 BC | The Ebers Papyrus represents the first major collection of medical observations made on human neoplasms. | 2 |
| 460–375 BC | Hippocrates of Cos coined from the Greek word meaning crab the terms *karkinos* and *karkinōma*. Karkinos referred to lesions that included benign neoplasms, while karkinōma was used to describe solid malignant neoplasms. | 3 |
| AD 131–201 | Galen classified tumors as those "according to nature," those "exceeding nature," and those "contrary to nature." All true neoplasms, both benign and malignant, were placed in the last category. Galen also provided some insight as to the possible basis for choosing the crab (in Latin, *cancerum*) to symbolize malignant neoplasms when he stated "As a crab is furnished with claws on both sides of the body, so in this disease (probably carcinoma of the breast) the veins which extend from the tumor represent with it a figure much like that of a crab." Later, it was | 4 |

*Alphonse E. Sirica* • Department of Pathology, Medical College of Virginia, Virginia Commonwealth University, Richmond, Virginia 23298.

| Year | Event | References |
|------|-------|-----------|
| | also reported by Paul of Aegina (625–690 AD) that "some say that cancer is so called because it adheres with such obstinacy to the part it seizes that, like the crab, it cannot be separated from it without great difficulty." | |
| 1632 | Marco Aurelio Severino made the distinction for the first time between benign and malignant neoplasms of the breast. | 5 |
| 1700 | Bernardino Ramazzini focused attention on the fact that malignant neoplasms may arise as a result of occupational factors when he observed a higher incidence of breast cancer in nuns than in any other women. However, he also recognized correctly that this was related more to their celibate life than to their actual occupation. | 6,7 |
| 1757 | Henri François Le Dran pointed out that in its earliest stages, a malignant neoplasm is a local lesion, that it can spread to regional lymph nodes, and that it tends to recur. | 4,8 |
| 1761 | John Hill suggested that the use of tobacco in the form of snuff may result in the development of nasal cancers. | 9 |
| 1775 | Percival Pott related the high incidence of scrotal cancer in chimney sweeps to their extensive exposure to the carcinogenic effects of "soot." | 10 |
| 1801 | Marie-François-Xavier Bichat was the first to recognize malignant neoplasia as representing abnormal tissue; he made the distinction between the stroma and parenchyma of tumors. | 11 |
| 1829 | Joseph C. A. Récamier described invasion of veins by malignant neoplastic cells and introduced the term *metastases*, which he applied to a nodule in the brain that developed secondary to a primary carcinoma of the breast. | 12 |
| 1838 | Johannes Müller described the histologic features of a variety of neoplastic tissues and observed that they, like normal tissues of the body, are composed of cells, albeit abnormal ones. | 13 |
| 1863 | Rudolf Virchow expanded the classification and histologic descriptions of malignant neoplasms and extended his aphorism *omnis cellula e cellula* to include cancer cells. | 14 |
| 1865 | Karl Thiersch showed that epithelial neoplasms actually have their origin in epithelia. | 15 |
| 1876–1889 | Mistislav A. Novinsky performed in 1876 the first successful transplantation of malignant neoplastic tissue in dogs. This was also repeated by Wehr in 1888. Arthur Hanau in 1889 was the first to transplant an epidermoid cancer in rats. | 16 |

| Year | Event | References |
|------|-------|-----------|
| 1879 | F. H. Härting and W. Hesse described lung cancer in uranium mine workers. This represented the first unequivocal report of an internal neoplasm being linked to exposures to an environmental carcinogenic factor(s). | 17 |
| 1893–1896 | William B. Coley reported the first description of tumor necrosis in human malignant neoplasms. | 18,19 |
| 1895 | Ludwig Rehn provided the first report indicating a causal relationship between exposures of dye manufacturing workers to synthetic aniline dyes and their subsequent development of carcinoma of the urinary bladder. | 20 |
| 1896 | George T. Beatson was the first to demonstrate the hormonal dependence of advanced mammary carcinomas in premenopausal women by observing regression of the tumors following bilateral ovariectomy and the administration of thyroid extract. | 21 |
| 1902–1903 | The first X-ray-induced skin cancers were recognized in humans. | 22 |
| 1903–1907 | Amédée Borrel was the first to hypothesize without direct experimental evidence a viral etiology for cancer. | 23 |
| 1907 | Erwin F. Smith and C. O. Townsend found that the bacterium *Agrobacterium tumefaciens* was involved in the production of crown gall neoplasms in plants. | 24 |
| 1908 | Vilhelm Ellermann and Oluf Bang transmitted erythroblastic leukemia in chickens using a cell-free filtrate, which they postulated contained a virus. | 25 |
| 1910 | Pierre Edouard Jean Clunet reported the first experimentally induced malignant neoplasm in a rat that was previously exposed to X-irradiation. | 26 |
| 1911 | Peyton Rous produced sarcomas in chickens with a cell-free filtrate (virus) prepared from transplantable sarcoma cells. | 27 |
| 1912 | J. Schottlaender and F. Kermauner introduced the term carcinoma *in situ*. | 28 |
| 1913 | Ernest E. Tyzzer, using transplantable mouse tumors, developed one of the first experimental animal models for investigating metastasis and provided evidence supporting the role of mechanical forces or trauma in metastasis formation. | 29 |
| 1914 | Theodor Boveri proposed that malignant neoplasms developed from single cells that acquired a certain abnormality in their chromosomal constitution. This became known as the *somatic mutation theory of cancer* and suggested the clonal origin of neoplasms. | 30 |

| Year | Event | References |
|------|-------|------------|
| 1915 | Katsusaburo Yamagiwa and Koichi Ichikawa succeeded in producing epidermal carcinomas by chronically applying coal tar to the ears of rabbits. This discovery marked the beginning of experimental chemical carcinogenesis. | 31 |
| 1925–1932 | Ernest L. Kennaway and his associates identified a number of polycyclic aromatic hydrocarbons in coal tar, some of which were demonstrated to be carcinogenic in experimental animals. | 32,33 |
| 1926–1930 | Otto Warburg published the first major work on the biochemistry of neoplasms, entitled *The Metabolism of Tumors*. In this book, he described the glycolysis of a wide variety of benign and malignant neoplasms from both the human and experimental animals. Later studies, however, demonstrated exceptions to Warburg's generalization that malignant neoplastic cells are characterized by impaired respiration. | 34 |
| 1928 | George M. Findlay reported the production of skin cancer in mice that were exposed to ultraviolet (UV) light for long periods of time. | 35 |
| 1929 | Harrison S. Martland and R. E. Humphries related osteogenic sarcomas which developed in workers who painted watch dials to chronic exposures to radium. | 36 |
| 1932 | Antoine Lacassagne demonstrated the induction of mammary carcinomas in male mice following injections of estrogen. | 37 |
| 1933 | Richard E. Shope found that papillomas on the skin of rabbits were caused by a filterable infectious agent (virus). This was the first evidence relating the development of a mammalian neoplasm to a virus. | 38 |
| 1933–1935 | Tomizu Yoshida induced hepatocellular carcinomas in rats with the chronic feeding of the azo dye, o-aminoazotoluene. | 39,40 |
| 1934–1938 | Baldwin Lucké described a renal carcinoma in leopard frogs, which he concluded was caused by a virus. | 41 |
| 1936 | R. Kinosita identified 4-dimethylaminoazobenzene as being a more active hepatocarcinogen in rats than o-aminoazotoluene. | 42 |
| 1936 | John J. Bittner, by means of a cross-suckling experiment using high- and low-tumor strain mice, demonstrated that mammary carcinomas produced in these animals were caused in part by a milk factor (virus). | 43 |
| 1938 | Wilhelm C. Heuper produced bladder cancers in dogs by the administration of β-naphthylamide. | 44 |

| Year | Event | References |
|------|-------|-----------|
| 1938 | Alexander Haddow first observed a resistance of malignant neoplastic cells to the toxic and growth inhibitory effects of chemical carcinogens. | 45 |
| 1941 | Robert H. Wilson, Floyd DeEds, and Alvin J. Cox demonstrated 2-acetylaminofluorene, a candidate for pesticide use, to be a potent chemical carcinogen in rats. | 46 |
| 1941 | Harold P. Rusch and his associates identified the carcinogenic wavelength of UV light. | 47 |
| 1941 | Isaac Berenblum, using croton oil, provided the first evidence for the chemical enhancement of skin carcinogenesis in the mouse. | 48 |
| 1941–1944 | Peyton Rous and associates were the first to report the enhancing effect of irritation on the development of skin neoplasms in rabbit ears. In addition, they were the first to use the terms *initiation* and *promotion* in relationship to defining particular steps in skin carcinogenesis. | 49,50 |
| 1942 | Philip R. White and Armin C. Braun demonstrated that bacteria-free crown gall was truly an autonomous neoplasm of plants. | 51 |
| 1943 | Wilton R. Earle demonstrated spontaneous malignant cell transformation in cell culture. | 52 |
| 1944 | J. C. Mottram pioneered the two-stage model of skin carcinogenesis in the mouse by demonstrating that a single low dose of benzpyrene followed by multiple applications of croton oil could induce a large number of skin neoplasms. | 53 |
| 1944 | Dale Rex Coman demonstrated that squamous cell carcinoma cells exhibit decreased mutual adhesiveness for one another. This represented the first direct physical evidence suggesting an alteration in the cell surface of malignant neoplastic cells. | 54 |
| 1947 | Issac Berenblum and Philippe Shubik conducted studies that extended the findings of Mottram and that clearly demonstrated the stages of initiation and promotion in mouse skin carcinogenesis. | 55,56 |
| 1947 | Elizabeth C. Miller and James A. Miller demonstrated that hepatocarcinogenic aminoazo dyes bound covalently to liver proteins, focusing attention on interactions between reactive carcinogenic chemicals and cell macromolecules. | 57 |
| 1947–1949 | George O. Gey also observed spontaneous transformation of rat fibroblasts in tissue culture. | 58,59 |
| 1949 | Leslie Foulds generalized the concept of neoplastic progression and defined important principles governing this phenomenon. | 60,61 |

| Year | Event | References |
|------|-------|------------|
| 1950–1959 | Epidemiologic studies demonstrated a major association between lung cancer and cigarette smoking in humans. | 62–65 |
| 1951 | Ludwig Gross provided the first evidence for an etiologic role of viruses in mouse leukemia. | 66 |
| 1952 | An increase in leukemia was reported for the first time in Japanese survivors of the atomic bomb blasts in Hiroshima and Nagasaki. | 67 |
| 1953 | E. J. Foley provided the first clear evidence for the existence of a tumor-associated transplantation antigen in methylcholanthrene-induced mouse sarcomas. | 68 |
| 1954 | Jesse P. Greenstein authored his *Biochemistry of Cancer*, which appeared in its expanded form in 1954. In this monograph, Greenstein proposed his *convergence hypothesis*, which held that the biochemical enzymatic phenotypes of malignant neoplasms tended to converge toward a common pattern. While this hypothesis is no longer valid, Greenstein's work served as an important stimulus for subsequent biochemical studies on malignant neoplastic cells and tissues. | 69 |
| 1956 | Peter N. Magee and John M. Barnes demonstrated dimethylnitrosamine to be a hepatocarcinogen in the rat. | 70 |
| 1956 | Urethan (ethyl carbamate) was demonstrated by Isaac Berenblum and Nechama Haran-Ghera to act in the mouse as an tumor-initiating agent for skin carcinogenesis and as a complete carcinogen for lung carcinogenesis. Urethane has also been shown to be a complete liver carcinogen in rodents. | 71,72 |
| 1958 | Sarah E. Stewart and Bernice Eddy discovered the polyoma DNA tumor virus. | 73,74 |
| 1958–1964 | Important contributions were made by James and Elizabeth Miller and by John and Elizabeth Weisburger toward understanding the chemistry and metabolism of 2-acetylaminofluorene, 2-fluorenamine, and related compounds. In 1960, the Millers and John Cramer discovered in rats the important metabolic process of N-hydroxylation as the initial carcinogen-activation step for 2-acetylaminofluorene. | 75–77 |
| 1959–1960 | Direct experimental evidence for terminal differentiation of malignant neoplastic cells to benign cell types was demonstrated by G. Barry Pierce and associates for malignant embryonal carcinoma cells of a mouse teratocarcinoma, and by Armin C. Braun with single-cell clones derived from the crown gall tumor of plants. | 78–80 |
| 1960 | Peter C. Nowell and David A. Hungerford first described a specific chromosomal abnormality, now known as the | 81,82 |

| Year | Event | References |
|------|-------|------------|
| | Philadelphia chromosome, in human chronic granulocytic leukemia. | |
| 1960–1961 | Neoplastic transformation by an oncogenic DNA virus of cultured mouse and hamster embryo fibroblasts was first reported. | 83–86 |
| 1960–1964 | Howard M. Temin proposed his Provirus Hypothesis in 1960, followed in 1964 by his *DNA provirus hypothesis.* These served as the basis for future understanding of retroviral replication and tumor causation. | 87 |
| 1960–1965 | The development in humans of mesothelioma, an uncommon malignant neoplasm, was clearly linked to exposures to asbestos. | 88,89 |
| 1960–1965 | T. J. King, R. G. McKinnell, and M. A. DiBerardino demonstrated that when the nuclei of Lucké renal adenocarcinoma cells were implanted into activated but enucleated normal frog eggs, abnormal early-stage tadpoles were able to develop without showing any evidence of benign or malignant neoplastic change. | 90–92 |
| 1960–1968 | Harold P. Morris established a spectrum of transplantable rat hepatocellular carcinomas, known collectively as the Morris Hepatomas. The enzymology of these malignant liver neoplasms was extensively studied in the laboratories of Van R. Potter, George Weber, and Sidney Weinhouse. These latter studies eloquently demonstrated phenotypic heterogeneity in the various hepatoma enzyme and isozyme patterns, which were related in many instances to the state of neoplastic progression of each liver tumor. | 93–96 |
| 1960–1968 | Evidence for the existence of tumor-associated transplantation antigens was greatly extended by the studies of George and Eva Kline, Richmond T. Prehn, H. O. Sjögren, and I. Hellström. | 97–100 |
| ~1960–1969 | Direct demonstrations of ectopic hormone production by nonendocrine malignant neoplasms and the development of the APUD (*a*mine content, amine *p*recursor *u*ptake, amino acid *d*ecarboxylation) cell concept occurred. | 101–103 |
| ~1960–1969 | Significant findings related to alterations in plasma membrane composition and function were first reported for malignant neoplastic and transformed mammalian cells. These included altered cell-surface contact control of cell movement and proliferation, increased anodic electrophoretic mobilities, enhanced cell surface binding of certain lectins (e.g., wheat germ agglutinin and concanavalin A), defective intercellular communication, along with decreased or impaired gap junctions, and altered plasma membrane glycoprotein, glycolipid, and enzyme composition. | 104 |

| Year | Event | References |
|------|-------|------------|
| 1961 | Widespread outbreaks of hepatotoxicity and deaths among turkey poults and ducklings in England during 1960 led to the discovery of the aflatoxins derived from the common fungus *Aspergillus flavus*. This, in turn, resulted in the subsequent identification of the extremely potent chemical hepatocarcinogen, aflatoxin $B_1$. | 105–108 |
| 1962 | Stanley Cohen first isolated epidermal growth factor from the submaxillary glands of adult male mice. | 109 |
| 1962–1968 | DNA and RNA were first shown to be important macromolecular targets for the persistent binding of carcinogenic chemical metabolites. | 110 |
| 1963–1964 | G. I. Abelev and associates in 1963 identified $\alpha$-fetoprotein (AFP) in experimental hepatocellular carcinomas, and Phil Gold and Samuel O. Freedman in 1964 identified carcinoembryonic antigen (CEA) in human colon carcinomas. | 111,112 |
| 1964 | R. K. Boutwell first proposed that the stage of tumor promotion in mouse skin carcinogenesis could be further subdivided into two separate phases which he called *conversion* and *propagation*. | 113 |
| 1965 | Yoheved Berwald and Leo Sachs clearly demonstrated for the first time the neoplastic transformation of mammalian embryo cells in cell culture by carcinogenic chemicals. | 114 |
| 1965 | Baruch S. Blumberg and associates discovered the hepatitis B surface antigen (Australia antigen). | 115 |
| 1965–1968 | Erich Hecker and Benjamin L. Van Duuren and their co-workers independently succeeded in isolating and identifying the active tumor promoting phorbol diesters from croton oil. The most potent of these in the two-stage mouse model of skin carcinogenesis was found to be 12-*O*-tetradecanoyl phorbol-13-acetate (TPA). | 116–118 |
| 1968–1969 | James E. Cleaver demonstrated a defect in DNA repair in skin fibroblasts from patients with xeroderma pigmentosum (XP), an autosomal-recessive disease in which affected persons are susceptible to the development of sunlight-induced skin cancers. Shortly thereafter, Richard B. Setlow and his associates showed XP cells to be defective in the excision repair of pyrimidine dimers resulting from UV light exposure. | 119–121 |
| 1969 | Robert J. Huebner and George J. Todaro first proposed the *viral oncogene hypothesis*. | 122,123 |
| 1970 | David Baltimore as well as Howard M. Temin and Satoshi Mizutani simultaneously reported the discovery of viral RNA-dependent DNA polymerase (reverse transcriptase). | 124,125 |

| Year | Event | References |
|------|-------|-----------|
| 1970–1971 | The first reports appeared describing the development of adenocarcinoma of the vagina in young women whose mothers were treated with diethylstilbestrol (DES) during their pregnancy.* | 126,127 |
| 1970–1973 | The first viral oncogene, the *src* gene of Rous sarcoma virus, was elucidated by analyses of *src*-deletion mutants. | 130–132 |
| 1971 | Judah Folkman and his associates reported the isolation of tumor angiogenesis factor (TAF) from Walker 256 carcinoma cells. | 133 |
| 1971 | Charlotte Friend and co-workers demonstrated for the first time the stimulation of erythroid differentiation by dimethyl sulfoxide in a cloned cell line of murine virus-induced erythroleukemic cells. Subsequently, other cell lines of murine and human myeloid leukemic cells were developed in which the induction of differentiation by various agents was shown. | 134–137 |
| 1971–1981 | Carl Peraino and associates during 1971–1975 were the first to present evidence indicating that hepatocarcinogenesis in the rat could be separated into the stages of tumor initiation and promotion in a manner similar to that originally described for mouse skin carcinogenesis. Subsequently, Emmanuel Farber, Henry C. Pitot, and Peraino and co-workers independently developed new rat models of hepatocarcinogenesis important for use in defining the sequential cellular events that characterize multistage neoplastic development in liver. Experimental evidence for multistage carcinogenesis has been extended to include tumor development in a variety of epithelial tissues and organs other than those of epidermis and liver. | 72,138–141 |
| 1971–1983 | S. D. Balk in 1971 first postulated the existence of a platelet-derived growth factor. In 1974, Russell Ross and associates and Nancy Kohler and A. Lipton independently presented evidence directly indicating platelets to be a source of cell growth-promoting activity. During the ensuing 9 years, Harry N. Antoniades and co-workers isolated and characterized human platelet-derived growth factor (PDGF). | 142–147 |

*McFarlane et al.[128] recently questioned the validity of earlier studies suggesting a cause-and-effect relationship between diethylstilbestrol (DES) and clear cell adenocarcinoma of the vagina. However, Melnick et al.[129] have also recently found in a review of 519 cases of clear cell adenocarcinoma of the vagina and cervix that in 60% of all cases, the patient's mother had received DES during pregnancy and that 91% of the tumors were diagnosed when the patient was between 15 and 27 years of age. These investigators further determined the risk of developing clear cell adenocarcinoma of the vagina or cervix in females exposed *in utero* to DES to be one case per 1000 women from birth through age 34 and suggested that some other factor may also be involved in the pathogenesis of this rare type of malignant neoplasm.

| Year | Event | References |
|------|-------|-----------|
| 1973 | J. K. Baum and co-workers first reported the association between the development of hepatic adenomas in women and their use of oral contraceptives. | 148 |
| 1973–1975 | Bruce N. Ames and associates developed the *Salmonella*/liver microsome assay for identifying chemical carcinogens as mutagens. | 149,150 |
| ~1973–1981 | J. Michael Bishop and Harold E. Varmus and colleagues, investigating the *src* gene, pioneered the work on oncogenes associated with retroviruses. In this regard, they provided the first conclusive proof that viral oncogenes are acquired by transduction. Additional studies by these workers and others during this time clearly demonstrated that the oncogenes of retroviruses (viral oncogenes) are miscreant copies of normal cellular genes or proto-oncogenes that are highly conserved in evolution. | 151–155 |
| 1974 | The first cases of angiosarcoma of the liver in workers exposed to vinyl chloride were described. | 156 |
| 1974 | Philip J. Fialkow presented detailed studies with cell markers on the clonal origins of human benign and malignant neoplasms. | 157 |
| 1975 | G. Köhler and C. Milstein developed hybridoma technology for producing monoclonal antibodies. This, in turn, represented a significant development for the fields of tumor pathobiology and immunology. | 158 |
| 1975 | Beatrice Mintz, Karl Illmensee, and J. D. Gearhart demonstrated that when highly malignant mouse embryonal carcinoma cells were microinjected into genetically different blastocysts, these cells lost their neoplastic properties in the embryonic environment and participated in the normal development of the resulting chimeric mice as differentiated cell components of virtually all their major adult tissues. | 159,160 |
| 1975–1984 | Evidence for causal associations between viruses and specific human malignant neoplasms greatly increased. Such associations include those between hepatitis B virus and hepatocellular carcinoma, Epstein–Barr virus and Burkitt lymphoma and nasopharyngeal carcinoma, and more recently, papilloma virus and cervical carcinoma. Important animal models (Eastern woodchuck, Beechey ground squirrel, and Peking duck) for hepatitis B-like virus infections were also discovered. | 161–168 |
| 1975–1986 | E. A. Carswell and co-workers reported in 1975 the isolation of tumor necrosis factor. Bruce Beutler and Anthony Cerami and associates described in 1985 the purification of the macrophage factor, cachectin, and shortly thereafter | 169–171 |

| Year | Event | References |
|------|-------|-----------|
| | provided evidence that cachectin and tumor necrosis factor are homologous proteins. | |
| 1976 | Harold B. Hewitt and associates reported that in contrast to chemically and virally induced tumors, spontaneous murine neoplasms were poorly immunogenic in mice. | 172 |
| 1977 | Isaiah J. Fidler and Margaret L. Kripke provided the first direct evidence that metastasis results from preexisting variant subpopulations of cells within a primary malignant neoplasm. | 173 |
| 1977 | Lance A. Liotta and co-workers demonstrated *in vitro* the degradation of basement membrane by malignant neoplastic cells from a highly metastatic fibrosarcoma. This study provided the first direct indication of tumor enzymes capable of catalyzing the breakdown of basement membrane substrate and further suggested that metastatic neoplastic cells may be distinct from other tumor cells with regard to their invasive potential. | 174 |
| 1977–1980 | R. L. Erikson and associates first identified the oncogene protein product (p60 *src*) of Rous sarcoma virus-infected cells and demonstrated it to display protein kinase activity. Tony Hunter and Bartholomew M. Sefton, as well as Marc S. Collett and Erikson then showed this protein to function as a tyrosine-specific protein kinase. This work, in turn, served as the paradigm for other oncogenes encoding for tyrosine-specific protein kinases. | 175–178 |
| 1977–1983 | Specific mammalian cell-surface receptors were identified for epidermal growth factor (EGF) and for platelet-derived growth factor (PDGF), respectively. These receptors, along with those for insulin, insulinlike growth factor 1, and somatomedin-C were further shown to be associated with tyrosine-specific protein kinase activity. | 179–189 |
| 1978–1983 | Transforming growth factors were identified. | 190–193 |
| 1979 | Robert Gallo and associates provided the first conclusive demonstration of a retrovirus (HTLV) associated with a human malignant neoplasm, adult T-cell leukemia. | 194 |
| 1979 | Tumor promoting agents were first shown to inhibit intercellular communication (metabolic cooperation) between cultured mammalian cells. | 195–196 |
| 1979–1983 | Robert A. Weinberg, Geoffrey M. Cooper, Mariano Barbacid, and Michael H. Wigler and their associates independently demonstrated the presence of activated oncogenes in the DNA of various experimental animal and human malignant neoplastic cells, and/or of cells transformed by chemical carcinogens, which on being introduced by transfection into NIH 3T3 mouse fibroblasts, caused their malignant transformation. | 197–203 |

| Year | Event | References |
|------|-------|-----------|
| 1979–1984 | Thomas Y. Shih and Edward M. Scolnick and co-workers first identified the p21 polypeptide products of the ras group of oncogenes. Subsequently, p21 was shown to bind guanine nucleotides, to be oncogenic following particular amino acid substitutions and to possess a guanosine triphosphatase activity that was shown to be impaired following activation of the oncogenic potential of p21. | 204–209 |
| 1980–1982 | Peter Blumberg and Paul E. Driedger in 1980 presented the first evidence for a specific cellular receptor for phorbol diester tumor promoters. In 1982, Monique Castagna, as a visiting scientist in Yasutomi Nishizuka's laboratory, reported that phorbol diesters directly activate protein kinase C and hypothesized that protein kinase C may be the membrane target of these tumor-promoting agents. Shortly thereafter, in 1983, James Niedel and co-workers reported that the phorbol diester receptor of rat brain copurifies with protein kinase C. | 210–212 |
| 1980–1985 | Michael B. Sporn and George J. Todaro in 1980 first proposed the *autocrine-secretion hypothesis* to explain the relative autonomous growth of malignant neoplastic cells. In 1985, Sporn and Anita B. Roberts reiterated and revised this hypothesis to include the concept that malignant transformation may be the result not only of excessive production, expression, and action of positive autocrine growth factors, but also of the failure of cells to synthesize, express, or respond to specific negative growth factor chemicals. | 213,214 |
| 1982–1983 | Activation of proto-oncogenes was first shown to occur by either point mutation, chromosomal translocation, or gene amplification. | 202,215 |
| 1983–1984 | Evidence was first presented to establish the human retinoblastoma gene as a prototype for a class of tumor-suppressor genes. | 216,217 |
| 1983–1985 | Specific proto-oncogenes were first demonstrated to encode for particular growth factors, growth factor receptors, and nuclear proteins that can affect transcription. | 214,218–223 |
| 1983–1985 | Proto-oncogene expression was demonstrated during such nonneoplastic growth conditions as liver regeneration and embryonic development. | 224–227 |
| 1984–1985 | Transgenic mice containing various oncogenes or transforming genes were first used to demonstrate the relationship of these genes to the accelerated development of specific types of malignant neoplasms in these animals. | 228–230 |
| 1985 | Bert L. Vallee and associates isolated and characterized angiogenin, which is the first angiogenic protein to be obtained from human carcinoma cells. | 231 |

| Year | Event | References |
|------|-------|-----------|
| 1985 | Lance A. Liotta and his associates provided evidence suggesting that the metastatic capacity of NIH 3T3 fibroblasts transfected with Harvey ras was related to the activation of this oncogene and to the presence of a second component that is present in these cells, but not in C127 murine epithelioid cell transformants. | 232 |
| 1986 | Report of the isolation of human cDNA segment that detects a chromosomal segment having the properties of the gene that predisposes to retinoblastoma and osteosarcoma. | 233 |
| 1986 | Carlo Croce and associates described a common mechanism of chromosomal translocation in T- and B-cell neoplasia. | 234 |
| 1987 | Thorgeirsson and his colleagues demonstrated expression of the multidrug-resistant gene in preneoplastic and neoplastic liver nodules and in regenerating liver of the rat. | 235 |
| 1987 | The genetic locus of multiple endocrine neoplasia type 2A (MEN2A), an autosomal dominantly inherited human cancer syndrome characterized by medullary carcinoma of the thyroid, phaeochromocytoma and/or parathyroid adenomas, has been simultaneously reported by Mathew *et al.* and by Simpson *et al.* to be linked to at least two markers on chromosome 10; the D10S5 locus and the interstitial retinol-binding protein (IRBP) gene. | 236,237 |
| 1987 | Bodmer *et al.* localized the gene for familial polyposis coli (FAP gene) to chromosome 5. Solomon *et al.* at the same time reported that a relatively high proportion of sporadic human colorectal adenocarcinomas exhibit chromosome-5 allele loss, suggesting that becoming recessive for the FAP gene may be an important factor in the progression of many colorectal cancers. These findings add support to a hypothesis put forth by Alfred Knudson, Jr., in 1971, which holds that sporadic and inherited forms of particular types of cancer could be related to mutations in the same gene. | 238–240 |
| 1987 | Reynolds *et al.* provided data to suggest that B6C3F1 mouse liver may provide a sensitive assay to detect classes of proto-oncogenes susceptible to activation by chemical carcinogens. | 241 |
| 1987 | Nerenberg *et al.* demonstrated that the tat gene of human T-lymphotropic virus type 1 (HTLV-1), associated with human lymphoid malignancies, encodes an oncogenic protein that induces mesenchymal tumors in transgenic mice. Hinrichs *et al.* showed these tumors to be neurofibromas, indicating a close resemblance to human neurofibromatosis (von Recklinghausen disease). | 242–243 |

| Year | Event | References |
|------|-------|------------|
| 1987 | Vogelstein and co-workers provided data supporting a monoclonal origin for human colorectal neoplasms, by means of restriction fragment length polymorphisms. Their results further suggested that the loss of a gene on the short arm of chromosome 17 may be associated with the progression of benign colorectal adenomas to adenocarcinomas. | 244 |
| 1987 | Greenberg and associates reported that transformation of NIH 3T3 fibroblasts by a structurally divergent group of oncogenes encoding either tyrosine or serine/threonine kinases induces the metastatic phenotype in these cells. | 245 |
| 1987 | Liu and Bishop, and associates described mutations of the Ki-*ras* proto-oncogene in bone marrow cells from some patients with preleukemia (myelodysplastic syndrome). In one patient, a novel mutation in codon 13 of this gene was detected in marrow cells obtained 1.5 years before the clinical appearance of acute leukemia. | 246 |
| 1987 | Jimenez and Yunis provided experimental evidence to suggest that the rejection of chloroleukemia cells in the rat can occur through the process of terminal differentiation induced by treatments with appropriate levels of a differentiation factor (DF) that is found in rat lung-conditioned medium. | 247 |
| 1987 | Velu *et al.* used a retrovirus vector to introduce the human epidermal growth factor receptor gene (EGFR) into NIH 3T3 cells and demonstrated that overproduction of such receptors in these cells conferred a transformed phenotype that was dependent on the presence of epidermal growth factor. | 248 |
| 1987 | Leppert *et al.* mapped the gene for familial polyposis coli to the long arm of chromosome 5. | 249 |
| 1987 | Collard *et al.*, using T-cell hybridomas developed by fusing noninvasive nonmetastatic mouse BW5147 T-lymphoma cells with either invasive activated normal human peripheral blood lymphocytes or leukemic T-lymphoblasts, provided evidence that genes on human chromosome 7 may be involved in maintaining T-cell invasiveness and metastatic potential. | 250 |
| 1987–1988 | AP-1, a 44- to 45-K protein purified from HeLa cells was found to function as a mammalian cell transcriptional activator as well as an enhancer binding factor that mediates gene induction by phorbol ester tumor promotors. Peter Angel and his associates have also shown that the oncogene *jun* encodes an oncoprotein that is a sequence-specific transcriptional activator similar to AP-1. | 251–255 |

| Year | Event | References |
|------|-------|-----------|
| 1988 | Members of the carcinoembryonic antigen (CEA) gene family were localized to the short and to the long arm of human chromosome 19. | 256 |

## REFERENCES

1. Breasted, J. H., 1930, *The Edwin Smith Surgical Papyrus*, University of Chicago Press, Chicago.
2. Ebbell, B. 1937, *The Papyrus Ebers: The Greatest Egyptian Medical Document*, Levin and Munksgaard, Copenhagen.
3. Diamandopoulos, G. T., and Meissner, W. A., 1985, Neoplasia, in: *Anderson's Pathology*, Vol. 1 (J. M. Kissane, ed.), pp. 514–559, C. V. Mosby, St. Louis.
4. Bett, W. R., 1957, Historical aspects of cancer, in: *Cancer*, Vol. 1 (R. W. Raven, ed.), pp. 1–5, Butterworth, London.
5. Willis, R. A., 1960, *Pathology of Tumors*, 3rd ed., Butterworth, Washington, D.C.
6. Wright, W. C., 1940, *De Morbis Artificum by Bernardino Ramazzini, The Latin Text of 1713*, University of Chicago Press, Chicago.
7. Wright, W. C., 1964, *Ramazzini, B: De Morbis Artificum Diatriba*, Hafner, New York.
8. LeDran, H. F., 1757, Memoire avec un précis de plusieurs observations sur le cancer, *Mem. Acad. R. Chir.* **3**:1–54.
9. Redmond, D. E., Jr., 1970, Tobacco and cancer: The first clinical report, 1761, *N. Engl. J. Med.* **282**:18–23.
10. Pott, P., 1775, *Chirurgical Observations Relative to the Cataract, the Polypus of the Nose, the Cancer of the Scrotum, the Different Kinds of Ruptures, and the Mortification of the Toes and Feet*, Hawes, Clark and Collins, London.
11. Bichat, X., 1801, *Anatomie générale appliquée à la physiologic et à la médecine*, Brosson, Gabon et Cie, Paris.
12. Récamier, J. C. A., 1829, *Recherches sur le traitement du cancer, par la compression méthodique simple ou combinée et sur l'histoire générale de la même maladie*, Vol. 2, Gabon, Paris.
13. Müller, J., 1838, *Ueber den feinern Bau and die Formen der krankhaften Geschwülste*, G. Reimer, Berlin.
14. Virchow, R., 1863, *Die Krankhaften Geschwülste*, August Hirschwald, Berlin.
15. Thiersch, C. 1865, *Der Epitheliakrebs namentlich der Haut*, Engelmann, Leipzig.
16. Shimkin, M. B., 1955, A note on the history of transplantation of tumors, *Cancer* **8**:653–655.
17. Härting, G. H., and Hesse, W., 1879, Der Lungenkrebs, die Bergkrankheit in den Schneeberger Gruben, *Vrtljschr. Gerlichtl. Med.* **30**:296–309.
18. Coley, W. B., 1893, The treatment of malignant tumors by repeated inoculations of erysipelas: With a report of ten original cases, *Am. J. Med. Sci.* **105**:447–511.
19. Coley, W. B., 1896, The therapeutic value of the mixed toxins of the streptococcus of erysipelas and bacillus prodigiosus in the treatment of inoperable malignant tumors, with a report of one hundred and sixty cases, *Am. J. Med. Sci.* **112**:251–281.
20. Rehn, L., 1895, Blasengeschwülste bei Fuchsin-Arbeitern, *Arch. Klin. Chir.* **50**:588–600.
21. Beatson, G. T., 1896, On the treatment of inoperable cases of carcinoma of the mamma: Suggestions for a new method of treatment with illustrative cases, *Lancet* **2**:104–107.
22. Clifton, K. H., 1893, Ionizing radiation carcinogenesis in man, in: *Concepts in Cancer Medicine* (S. B. Kahn, R. R. Love, C. Sherman, Jr., and R. Chakravorty, eds.), pp. 67–88, Grune & Stratton, New York.
23. Borrel, A., 1907, Le problème du cancer, *Bull. Inst. Pasteur* **5**:497–512.
24. Smith, E. F., and Townsend, C. O., 1907, A plant tumor of bacterial origin, *Science* **25**:671–673.
25. Ellermann, V., and Bang, O., 1908, Experimentelle Leukämie bie Hühnern, *Centralbl. Bakteriol.* **46**:595–609.
26. Clunet, J., 1910, *Recherches expérimentales sur les tumeurs malignés*, Steinheil, Paris.
27. Rous, P., 1911, A sarcoma of the fowl transmissible by an agent separable from the tumor cells, *J. Exp. Med.* **13**:397–411.
28. Schottlaender, J., and Kermauner, F., 1912, *Zur Kenntnis des Uterus Karzinoms; monographische Studie über Morphologie, Entwicklung, Wachstum, nebst Beitragen zur Klinik der Erkrankung*, Karger, Berlin.

29. Tyzzer, E. E., 1913, Factors in the production and growth of tumor metastases, *J. Med. Res.* **28**:309–332.
30. Boveri, T., 1914, *Zur Frage der Entstehung maligner Tumoren*, Gustav Fisher, Jena.
31. Yamagiwa, K., and Ichikawa, K., 1918, Experimental study of the pathogenesis of carcinoma, *J. Cancer Res.* **3**:1–29.
32. Kennaway, E. L., and Hieger, I., 1930, Carcinogenic substances and their fluorescence spectra, *Br. Med. J.* **1**:1044–1046.
33. Cook, J. W., Hieger, I., Kennaway, E. L., and Mayneord, W. V., 1932, The production of cancer by pure hydrocarbons. Part 1, *Proc. R. Soc. B* **3**:455–484.
34. Warburg, O., 1930, *The Metabolism of Tumors* (translated by F. Dickens) Arnold Constable, London.
35. Findlay, G. M., 1928, Ultra-violet light and skin cancer, *Lancet* **2**:1070–1073.
36. Martland, H. S., and Humphries, R. E., 1929, Osteogenic sarcoma in dial painters using luminous paint, *Arch. Pathol. Lab. Med.* **7**:406–417.
37. Lacassagne, A., 1932, Apparition de cancers de la mamelle chez la souris mâle soumise à des injections de folliculine, *C. R. Acad. Sci.* **195**:630–632.
38. Shope, R. E., 1933, Infectious papillomatosis of rabbits, *J. Exp. Med.* **58**:607–624.
39. Yoshida, T., 1933, Uber die serienweise Verfolgung der Veränderungen der Leber bei der experimentellen Hepatomerzeugung durch *o*-Aminoazotoluol, *Trans. Jpn. Pathol. Soc.* **23**:636–638.
40. Sasaki, T., and Yoshida, T., 1935, Experimentelle Erzeugung des Leber karcinoms durch Fütterung mit *o*-Aminoazotoluol, *Virchows Arch. Pathol. Anat.* **295**:175–200.
41. Lucké, B., 1938, Carcinoma in the leopard frog. Its probable causation by a virus, *J. Exp. Med.* **68**:457–468.
42. Kinosita, R., 1936, Research on the carcinogenesis of the various chemical substances, *Gann* **30**:423–426.
43. Dmochowski, L., 1957, The part played by viruses in the origin of tumors, in *Cancer*, Vol. 1 (R. W. Raven, ed.), pp. 214–305, Butterworth, London.
44. Heuper, W. C., Wiley, F. H., and Wolfe, H. D., 1938, Experimental production of bladder tumors in dogs by administration of beta-naphthylamine, *J. Indust. Hyg. Toxicol.* **20**:46–84.
45. Haddow, A., 1938, The influence of carcinogenic substances on sarcomata induced by the same and other compounds, *J. Pathol.* **47**:581–591.
46. Wilson, R. H., DeEds, F., and Cox, A. J., 1941, Toxicity and carcinogenic activity of 2-acetaminofluorene, *Cancer Res.* **1**:595–608.
47. Rusch, H. P., Kline, B. E., and Baumann, C. A., 1941, Carcinogenesis by ultraviolet rays with reference to wavelength and energy, *Arch. Pathol. Lab. Med.* **31**:135–146.
48. Berenblum, I., 1941, The cocarcinogenic action of croton resin, *Cancer Res.* **1**:44–50.
49. Rous, P., and Kidd, J. G., 1941, Conditional neoplasms and subthreshold neoplastic states. A study of the tar tumors of rabbits, *J. Exp. Med.* **73**:365–389.
50. Friedewald, W. F., and Rous, P., 1944, The initiating and promoting elements in tumor production. An analysis of the effects of tar, benzpyrene, and methylcholanthrene on rabbit skin, *J. Exp. Med.* **80**:101–130.
51. White, P. R., and Braun, A. C., 1942, A cancerous neoplasm of plants—Autonomous bacterial-free crown-gall tissue, *Cancer Res.* **2**:597–617.
52. Earle, W. R., 1943, Production of malignancy *in vitro*, *J. Natl. Cancer Inst.* **4**:131–248.
53. Mottram, J. C., 1944, A developing factor in experimental blastogenesis, *J. Path* **56**:181–187.
54. Coman, D. R., 1944, Decreased mutual adhesiveness, a property of cells from squamous cell carcinomas, *Cancer Res.* **4**:625–629.
55. Berenblum, I., and Shubik, P., 1947, The role of croton oil applications associated with a single painting of a carcinogen in tumour induction of the mouse's skin, *Br. J. Cancer* **1**:379–382.
56. Berenblum, I., and Shubik, P., 1947, A new, quantitative, approach to the study of the stages of chemical carcinogenesis in the mouse's skin, *Br. J. Cancer* **1**:383–391.
57. Miller, E. C., and Miller, J. A., 1947, The presence and significance of bound aminoazo dyes in the livers of rats fed *p*-dimethylaminoazobenzene, *Cancer Res.* **7**:468–480.
58. Gey, G. O., Gey, M. K., Frior, W. M., and Self, W. O., 1949, Cultural and cytologic studies on autologous normal and malignant cells of specific *in vitro* origin. Conversion of normal into malignant cells, *Acta Univ. Int. Contra. Cancrum* **6**:706–712.
59. Gey, G. O., 1954–55, Some aspects of the constitution and behavior of normal and malignant cells maintained in continuous culture, *Harvey Lect.* **50**:154–229.
60. Foulds, L., 1949, Mammary tumours in hybrid mice: Growth and progression of spontaneous tumours, *Br. J. Cancer* **3**:345–375.
61. Foulds, L., 1965, Multiple etiologic factors in neoplastic development, *Cancer Res.* **25**:1339–1347.

62. Wynder, E. L., and Graham, E. A., 1950, Tobacco smoking as a possible etiologic factor in bronchiogenic carcinoma. A study of six hundred and eighty-four proved cases, *JAMA* **143:**329–336.
63. Doll, R., and Hill, A. B., 1956, Lung cancer and other causes of death in relation to smoking, *Br. Med. J.* **2:**1071–1081.
64. Hammond, E. C., and Horn, D., 1958, Smoking and death rates—Report of forty-four months of follow up of 187,783 men, *JAMA* **166:**1159–1172.
65. Dorn, H. F., 1959, Tobacco consumption and mortality from cancer and other diseases, *Publ. Health Rep. USA* **74:**581–593.
66. Gross, L., 1951, Spontaneous leukemia developing in C3H mice following inoculation, in infancy, with AK-leukemic extracts, or AK-embryos, *Proc. Soc. Exp. Biol. Med.* **76:**27–32.
67. Folley, J. H., Borges, W., and Yamawaki, T., 1952, Incidence of leukemia in survivors of the atomic bomb in Hiroshima and Nagasaki, Japan, *Am. J. Med.* **13:**311–321.
68. Foley, E. J., 1953, Antigenic properties of methylcholanthrene-induced tumors in mice of the strain of origin, *Cancer Res.* **13:**835–837.
69. Greenstein, J. P., 1954, *Biochemistry of Cancer*, 2nd ed., Academic, New York.
70. Magee, P. N., and Barnes, J. M., 1956, The production of malignant primary hepatic tumors in the rat by feeding dimethylnitrosamine, *Br. J. Cancer* **10:**114–122.
71. Berenblum, I., and Haran-Ghera, N., 1957, A quantitative study of the systemic initiating action of urethane (ethyl carbamate) in mouse skin carcinogenesis, *Br. J. Cancer* **11:**77–84.
72. Pitot, H. C., and Sirica, A. E., 1980, The stages of initiation and promotion in hepatocarcinogenesis, *Biochim. Biophys. Acta* **605:**191–215.
73. Stewart, S. E., Eddy, B. E., and Borgese, N. G., 1958, Neoplasms in mice inoculated with a tumor agent carried in tissue culture, *J. Natl. Cancer Inst.* **20:**1223–1243.
74. Eddy, B. E., Stewart, S. E., and Berkeley, W., 1958, Cytopathogenicity in tissue cultures by a tumor virus from mice, *Proc. Soc. Exp. Biol. Med.* **98:**848–851.
75. Weisburger, E. K., and Weisburger, J. H., 1958, Chemistry, carcinogenicity, and metabolism of 2-fluorenamine and related compounds, *Adv. Cancer Res.* **5:**331–431.
76. Miller, J. A., Cramer, J. W., and Miller, E. C., 1960, The N- and ring-hydroxylation of 2-acetylaminofluorene during carcinogenesis in the rat, *Cancer Res.* **20:**950–962.
77. Cramer, J. W., Miller, J. A., and Miller, E. C., 1960, N-hydroxylation: A new metabolic reaction observed in the rat with the carcinogen 2-acetylaminofluorene, *J. Biol. Chem.* **235:**885–888.
78. Braun, A. C., 1959, A demonstration of the recovery of the crown-gall tumor cell with the use of complex tumors of single-cell origin, *Proc. Natl. Acad. Sci. USA* **45:**932–938.
79. Pierce, G. B., Dixon, F. J., and Verney, E. L., 1960, Teratocarcinogenic and tissue forming potentials of the cell types comprising embryoid bodies, *Lab Invest.* **9:**583–602.
80. Braun, A. C., 1974, *The Biology of Cancer*, Addison-Wesley, Reading, Massachusetts.
81. Nowell, P. C., and Hungerford, D. A., 1960, Chromosome studies on normal and leukemic human leukocytes, *J. Natl. Cancer Inst.* **25:**85–109.
82. Nowell, P. C., and Hungerford, D. A., 1960, A minute chromosome in human chronic granulocytic leukemia, *Science* **132:**1497.
83. Vogt, M., and Dulbecco, R., 1960, Virus–cell interaction with a tumor-producing virus, *Proc. Natl. Acad. Sci. USA* **46:**365–370.
84. Dulbecco, R., and Vogt, M., 1960, Significance of continued virus production in tissue cultures rendered neoplastic by polyoma virus, *Proc. Natl. Acad. Sci. USA* **46:**1617–1632.
85. Sachs, L., and Medina, D., 1961, In vitro transformation of normal cells by polyoma virus, *Nature (Lond.)* **189:**457–458.
86. Stoker, M., and MacPherson, I., 1961, Studies on the transformation of hamster cells by polyoma virus in vitro, *Virology* **14:**359–370.
87. Temin, H. M., 1976, The DNA provirus hypothesis, *Science* **192:**1075–1080.
88. Wagner, J. C., Sleggs, C. A., and Marchand, P., 1960, Diffuse pleural mesothelioma and asbestos exposure in the north western cape province, *Br. J. Indust. Med.* **17:**260–271.
89. Newhouse, M. L., and Thomson, H., 1965, Mesothelioma of pleura and peritoneum following exposure to asbestos in the London area, *Br. J. Indust. Med.* **22:**261–269.
90. King, T. J., and McKinnell, R. G., 1960, An attempt to determine the developmental potentialities of the cancer cell nucleus by means of transplantation, in: *Cell Physiology of Neoplasia*, pp. 591–671, University of Texas Press, Austin.
91. King, T. J., and DiBerardino, M. A., 1965, Transplantation of nuclei from frog renal adenocarcinoma. I. Development of tumor-nuclear-transplant embryos, *Ann. NY Acad. Sci.* **126:**115–126.
92. DiBerardino, M. A., and Hoffner, N. J., 1980, The current status of cloning and nuclear reprograming in

amphibian eggs, in: *Differentation and Neoplasia* (R. G. McKinnell, M. A. DiBerardino, M. Blumenfeld, and R. D. Bergad, eds.), pp. 53–64, Springer-Verlag, Berlin.

93. Morris, H. P., and Wagner, B. P., 1968, Induction and transplantation of rat hepatomas with different growth rate (including "minimal deviation" hepatomas), in: *Methods in Cancer Research,* Vol. 4 (H. Busch, ed.), pp. 125–152, Academic, New York.

94. Potter, V. R., Watanabe, M., Pitot, H. C., and Morris, H. P., 1969, Systematic oscillations in metabolic activity in rat liver and hepatomas. Survey of normal diploid and other hepatoma lines, *Cancer Res.* **29:**55–78.

95. Weinhouse, S., 1972, Glycolysis, respiration, and anomalous gene expression in experimental hepatomas: G.H.A. Clowes Memorial Lecture, *Cancer Res.* **32:**2007–2016.

96. Weber, G., 1983, Biochemical strategy of cancer cells and the design of chemotherapy: G.H.A. Clowes Memorial Lecture, *Cancer Res.* **43:**3466–3492.

97. Prehn, R. T., 1960, Tumor-specific immunity to transplanted dibenz(a,h)anthracene-induced sarcomas, *Cancer Res.* **20:**1614–1617.

98. Sjögren, H. O., 1965, Transplantation methods as a tool for the detection of tumor-specific antigens, *Prog. Exp. Tumor. Res.* **6:**289–322.

99. Hellström, I., and Sjögren, H. O., 1966, Demonstration of common specific antigens in mouse and hamster polyoma tumors, *Int. J. Cancer* **1:**481–489.

100. Klein, G., 1968, Tumor-specific transplantation antigens, *Cancer Res.* **28:**625–635.

101. Gellhorn, A., 1969, Ectopic hormone production in cancer and its implications for basic research on abnormal growth, *Adv. Intern. Med.* **15:**299–316.

102. Pearse, A. G. E., 1969, The cytochemistry and ultrastructure of polypeptide hormone-producing cells of the APUD series and the embryologic, physiologic and pathologic implications of the concept, *J. Histochem Cytochem.* **17:**303–313.

103. Smith, L. H., 1976, The APUD cell concept, *J. Surg. Oncol.* **8:**137–142.

104. Wallach, D. F., 1972, *The Plasma Membrane: Dynamic Perspectives, Genetics and Pathology,* The English Universities Press, London.

105. Lancaster, M. C., Jenkins, F. P., and McL. Phip, J., 1961, Toxicity associated with certain samples of ground nuts, *Nature (Lond.)* **192:**1095–1096.

106. Sargeant, K., Sheridan, A., O'Kelly, J., and Carnaghan, R. B. A., 1961, Toxicity associated with certain samples of ground nuts, *Nature (Lond.)* **192:**1096–1097.

107. Newberne, P. M., and Butler, W. H., 1969, Effects of aflatoxin on the liver of domestic and laboratory animals: A review, *Cancer Res.* **29:**236–250.

108. Alpert, M. E., Hutt, M. S. R., Wogan, G. N., and Davidson, C. S., 1971, Association between aflatoxin content of food and hepatoma frequency in Uganda, *Cancer* **28:**253–260.

109. Cohen, S., 1962, Isolation of a mouse submaxillary gland protein accelerating incisor eruption and eyelid opening in the new-born animal, *J. Biol Chem.* **237:**1555–1562.

110. Miller, E. C., and Miller, J. A., 1966, Mechanisms of chemical carcinogenesis: Nature of proximate carcinogens and interactions with macromolecules, *Pharmacol. Rev.* **18:**805–838.

111. Abelev, G. I., 1971, Alpha-fetoprotein in oncogenesis and its association with malignant tumors, *Adv. Cancer Res.* **14:**295–358.

112. Gold, P., and Freedman, S. O., 1965, Demonstration of tumor-specific antigens in human colonic carcinomata by immunological tolerance and absorption techniques, *J. Exp. Med.* **121:**439–462.

113. Boutwell, R. K., 1964, Some biological aspects of skin carcinogenesis, *Prog. Exp. Tumor Res.* **4:**207–250.

114. Berwald, Y., and Sachs, L., 1965, In vitro transformation of normal cells to tumor cells by carcinogenic hydrocarbons, *J. Natl. Cancer Inst.* **35:**641–661.

115. Blumberg, B. S., Alter, H. J., and Visnich, S., 1965, A new antigen in leukemia sera, *JAMA* **191:**541–546.

116. Van Duuren, B. L., and Orris, L., 1965, The tumor-enhancing principles of *Croton tiglium* L., *Cancer Res.* **25:**1871–1875.

117. Hecker, E., 1968, Cocarcinogenic principles from the seed oil of *Croton tiglium* and from other Euphorbiaceae, *Cancer Res.* **28:**2338–2349.

118. Van Duuren, B. L., 1969, Tumor-promoting agents in two-stage carcinogenesis. *Prog. Exp. Tumor Res.* **11:**31–68.

119. Cleaver, J. E., 1968, Defective repair replication of DNA in xeroderma pigmentosum, *Nature (Lond.)* **218:**652–656.

120. Cleaver, J. E., 1969, Xeroderma pigmentosum: a human disease in which an initial stage of DNA repair is defective, *Proc. Natl. Acad. Sci. USA* **63:**428–435.

121. Setlow, R. B., Regan, J. D., German, J., and Carrier, W. L., 1969, Evidence that xeroderma pigmentosum cells do not perform the first step in the repair of ultraviolet damage to their DNA, *Proc. Natl. Acad. Sci. USA* **64:**1035–1041.

122. Huebner, R. J., and Todaro, G. J., 1969, Oncogenes of RNA tumor viruses as determinants of cancer, *Proc. Natl. Acad. Sci. USA* **64:**1087–1094.

123. Huebner, R. J., and Todaro, G. J., 1972, The viral oncogene hypothesis: New evidence, *Proc. Natl. Acad. Sci. USA* **69:**1009–1015.

124. Baltimore, D., 1970, Viral RNA-dependent DNA polymerase in virions of RNA tumour viruses, *Nature (Lond.)* **226:**1209–1211.

125. Temin, H. M., and Mizutani, S., 1970, RNA-dependent DNA polymerase in virions of Rous sarcoma virus, *Nature (Lond.)* **226:**1211–1213.

126. Herbst, A. L., and Scully, R. E., 1970, Adenocarcinoma of the vagina in adolescence, *Cancer* **25:**745–757.

127. Herbst, A. L., Ulfelder, H., and Poskanzer, D. C., 1971, Adenocarcinoma of the vagina. Association of maternal stilbestrol therapy with tumor appearance in young women, *N. Engl. J. Med.* **284:**878–881.

128. McFarlane, M. J., Feinstein, A. R., and Horwitz, R. I., 1986, Diethylstilbestrol and clear cell vaginal carcinoma—Reappraisal of the epidemiologic evidence, *Am. J. Med.* **81:**855–863.

129. Melnick, S., Cole, P., Anderson, D., and Herbst, A., 1987, Rates and risks of diethylstilbestrol-related clear-cell adenocarcinoma of the vagina and cervix. An update, *N. Engl. J. Med.* **316:**514–516.

130. Martin, G. S., 1970, Rous sarcoma virus: A function required for the maintenance of the transformed state, *Nature (Lond.)* **227:**1021–1023.

131. Vogt, P. K., 1971, Spontaneous segregation of nontransforming viruses from cloned sarcoma viruses, *Virology,* **46:**939–951.

132. Duesberg, P. H., 1983, Retroviral transforming genes in normal cells? *Nature (Lond.)* **304:**219–226.

133. Folkman, J., Merler, E., Abernathy, C., and Williams, G., 1971, Isolation of a tumor factor responsible for angiogenesis, *J. Exp. Med.* **133:**275–288.

134. Friend, C., Scher, W., Holland, J. G., and Sato, T., 1971, Hemoglobin synthesis in murine virus-induced leukemic cells in vitro: Stimulation of erythroid differentiation by dimethyl sulfoxide, *Proc. Natl. Acad. Sci. USA* **68:**378–382.

135. Collins, S. J., Ruscetti, F. W., Gallagher, R. E., and Gallo, R. C., 1978, Terminal differentiation of human promyelocytic leukemia cells induced by dimethyl sulfoxide and other polar compounds, *Proc. Natl. Acad. Sci. USA* **75:**2458–2462.

136. Breitman, T. R., Selonick, S. E., and Collins, S. J., 1980, Induction of differentiation of the human promyelocytic leukemia cell line (HL-60) by retinoic acid, *Proc. Natl. Acad. Sci. USA* **77:**2936–2940.

137. Sachs, L., 1980, Activation of normal differentiation genes and the origin and development of myeloid leukemia, in: *Differentiation and Neoplasia* (R. G. McKinnell, M. A. DiBerardino, M. Blumenfeld, and R. D. Bergad, eds.), pp. 212–216, Springer-Verlag, Berlin.

138. Peraino, C., Fry, R. J. M., and Staffeldt, E., 1971, Reduction and enhancement by phenobarbital and hepatocarcinogenesis induced in the rat by 2-acetylaminofluorene, *Cancer Res.* **31:**1506–1512.

139. Solt, D., and Farber, E., 1976, New principle for the analysis of chemical carcinogenesis, *Nature (Lond.)* **263:**701–703.

140. Pitot, H. C., Barsness, L., Goldsworthy, T., and Kitagawa, T., 1978, Biochemical characterization of hepatocarcinogenesis after a single dose of diethylnitrosamine, *Nature (Lond.)* **271:**456–458.

141. Peraino, C., Staffeldt, E. F., and Ludeman, V. A., 1981, Early appearance of histochemically altered hepatocyte foci and liver tumors in female rats treated with carcinogens one day after birth, *Carcinogenesis* **2:**463–465.

142. Balk, S. D., 1971, Calcium as a regulator of the proliferation of normal but not of transformed, chicken fibroblasts in a plasma-containing medium, *Proc. Natl. Acad. Sci. USA* **68:**271–275.

143. Ross, R., Glomset, J., Kariya, B., and Harker, L., 1974, A platelet-dependent serum factor that stimulates the proliferation of arterial smooth muscle cells in vitro, *Proc. Natl. Acad. Sci. USA* **71:**1207–1210.

144. Kohler, N., and Lipton, A., 1974, Platelets as a source of fibroblast growth-promoting activity, *Exp. Cell Res.* **87:**297–301.

145. Antoniades, H. N., Stathakos, D., and Scher, C. D., 1975, Isolation of a cationic polypeptide from human serum that stimulates proliferation of 3T3 cells, *Proc. Natl. Acad. Sci. USA* **72:**2635–2639.

146. Antoniades, H. N., Scher, C. D., and Stiles, C. D., 1979, Purification of human platelet-derived growth factor, *Proc. Natl. Acad. Sci. USA* **76:**1809–1813.

147. Antoniades, H. N., and Hunkapiller, M. W., 1983, Human platelet-derived growth factor (PDGF): Amino-terminal amino acid sequence, *Science* **220:**963–965.

148. Baum, J. K., Holtz, F., Bookstein, J. J., and Klein, E. W., 1973, Possible association between benign hepatomas and oral contraceptives, *Lancet* 2:926–929.

149. Ames, B. N., Durston, W. E., Yamasaki, E., and Lee, F. D., 1973, Carcinogens as mutagens: A simple test system combining liver homogenates for activation and bacteria for detection, *Proc. Natl. Acad. Sci. USA* 70:2281–2285.

150. McCann, J., Choi, E., Yamasaki, E., and Ames, B. N., 1975, Detection of carcinogens as mutagens in the Salmonella/microsome test: Assay of 300 chemicals, *Proc. Natl. Acad. Sci. USA* 72:5135–5139.

151. Stehelin, D., Varmus, H. E., Bishop, J. M., and Vogt, P. K., 1976, DNA related to the transforming gene(s) of avian sarcoma viruses is present in normal avian DNA, *Nature (Lond.)* 260:170–173.

152. Spector, D. H., Baker, B., Varmus, H. E., and Bishop, J. M., 1978, Characteristics of cellular RNA related to the transforming gene of avian sarcoma virus, *Cell* 13:381–386.

153. Bishop, J. M., 1981, Enemies within: The genesis of retrovirus oncogenes, *Cell* 23:5–6.

154. Bishop, J. M., 1983, Cancer genes come of age, *Cell* 32:1018–1020.

155. Bishop, J. M., 1985, Viral oncogenes, *Cell* 42:23–38.

156. Creech, J. L., Jr., and Johnson, M. N., 1974, Angiosarcoma of the liver in manufacture of polyvinyl chloride, *J. Occup. Med.* 16:150–151.

157. Fialkow, P. J., 1974, The origin and development of human tumors studied with cell markers, *N. Engl. J. Med.* 291:26–35.

158. Köhler, G., and Milstein, C., 1975, Continuous cultures of fused cells secreting antibody of predefined specificity, *Nature (Lond.)* 256:495–497.

159. Mintz, B., Illmensee, K., and Gearhart, J. D., 1975, Development and experimental potentialities of mouse teratocarcinoma cells from embryoid body cores, in: *Teratomas and Differentiation* (M. I. Sherman and D. Solter, eds.), pp. 59–82, Academic, New York.

160. Mintz, B., and Illmensee, K., 1975, Normal genetically mosaic mice produced from teratocarcinoma cells, *Proc. Natl. Acad. Sci. USA* 72:3585–3589.

161. Blumberg, B. S., Larouze, B., London, W. T., Werner, B., Hesser, J. E., Millman, I., Saimot, G., and Payet, M., 1975, The relation of infection with hepatitis B agent to primary hepatic carcinoma, *Am. J. Pathol.* 81:669–682.

162. Szmuness, W., 1978, Hepatocellular carcinoma and hepatitis B virus: Evidence for a causal association, *Prog. Med. Virol.* 24:40–69.

163. de-Thé, G., Geser, A., Day, N. E., Tukei, P. M., Williams, E. H., Beri, D. P., Smith, P. G., Dean, A. G., Bornkamm, G. W., Feorino, P., and Henle, W., 1978, Epidemiological evidence for causal relationship between Epstein-Barr virus and Burkitt's lymphoma from Ugandan prospective study, *Nature (Lond.)* 274:756–761.

164. Summers, J., Smolec, J. M., and Snyder, R. A., 1978, A virus similar to hepatitis B virus associated with hepatitis and hepatoma in woodchucks, *Proc. Natl. Acad. Sci. USA* 75:4533–4537.

165. Marion, P. L., Oshiro, L. S., Regnery, D. C., Scullard, G. H., and Robinson, W. S., 1980, A virus of Beechey ground squirrels that is related to hepatitis B virus of humans, *Proc. Natl. Acad. Sci. USA* 77:2941–2945.

166. Mason, W. S., Seal, G., and Summers, J., 1980, Virus of Pekin duck with structural and biological relatedness to human hepatitis B virus, *J. Virol.* 36:829–836.

167. Gallo, R. C., and Wong-Staal, F., 1984, Current thoughts on the viral etiology of certain human cancers: The Richard and Hinda Rosenthal Foundation Award Lecture, *Cancer Res.* 44:2743–2749.

168. Kurman, R. J., Jenson, A. B., and Lancaster, W. D., 1984, Papilloma virus infection and squamous neoplasia of the cervix, *Pathol. Res. Pract.* 179:24–30.

169. Carswell, E. A., Old, L. J., Kassel, R. L., Green, S., Fiore, N., and Williamson, B., 1975, An endotoxin-induced serum factor that causes necrosis of tumors, *Proc. Natl. Acad. Sci. USA* 72:3666–3670.

170. Beutler, B., Mahoney, J., LeTrang, N., Pekala, P., and Cerami, A., 1985, Purification of cachectin, a lipoprotein lipase-suppressing hormone secreted by endotoxin-induced RAW 264.7 cells, *J. Exp. Med.* 161:984–995.

171. Beutler, B., and Cerami, A., 1986, Cachectin and tumor necrosis factor as two sides of the same biological coin, *Nature (Lond.)* 320:584–588.

172. Hewitt, H. B., 1978, The choice of animal tumors for experimental studies of cancer therapy, *Adv. Cancer Res.* 27:149–200.

173. Fidler, I. J., and Kripke, M. L., 1977, Metastasis results from preexisting variant cells within a malignant tumor, *Science* 197:893–895.

174. Liotta, L. A., Kleinerman, J., Catanzaro, P., and Rynbrandt, D., 1977, Degradation of basement membrane by murine tumor cells, *J. Natl. Cancer Inst.* 58:1427–1431.

175. Brugge, J. S., and Erikson, R. L., 1977, Identification of a transformation-specific antigen induced by an avian sarcoma virus, *Nature (Lond.)* **269**:346–348.
176. Collett, M. S., and Erikson, R. L., 1978, Protein kinase activity associated with the avian sarcoma virus src gene product, *Proc. Natl. Acad. Sci. USA* **75**:2021–2024.
177. Hunter, T., and Sefton, B. M., 1980, Transforming gene product of Rous sarcoma virus phosphorylates tyrosine, *Proc. Natl. Acad. Sci. USA* **77**:1311–1315.
178. Collett, M. S., Purchio, A. F., and Erikson, R. L., 1980, Avian sarcoma virus-transforming protein pp60[src] shows protein kinase activity specific for tyrosine, *Nature (Lond.)* **285**:167–169.
179. Das, M., Miyakawa, T., Fox, C. F., Pruss, R. M., Aharonov, A., and Herschman, H., 1977, Specific radiolabeling of a cell surface receptor for epidermal growth factor, *Proc. Natl. Acad. Sci. USA* **74**:2790–2794.
180. Carpenter, G., and Cohen, S., 1979, Epidermal growth factor, *Annu. Rev. Biochem.* **48**:193–216.
181. Ushiro, H., and Cohen, S., 1980, Identification of phosphotyrosine as a product of epidermal growth factor-activated protein kinase in A-431 cell membranes, *J. Biol. Chem.* **255**:8363–8365.
182. Cohen, S., Carpenter, G., and King, L., Jr., 1980, Epidermal growth factor–receptor–protein kinase interactions. Co-purification of receptor and epidermal growth factor-enhanced phosphorylation activity, *J. Biol. Chem.* **255**:4834–4842.
183. Hunter, T., and Cooper, J. A., 1981, Epidermal growth factor induces rapid tyrosine phosphorylation of proteins in A 431 human tumor cells, *Cell* **24**:741–752.
184. Cohen, S., Ushiro, H., Stoscheck, C., and Chinkers, M., 1982, A native 170,000 epidermal growth factor receptor-kinase complex from shed plasma membrane vesicles, *J. Biol. Chem.* **257**:1523–1531.
185. Cooper, J. A., Bowen-Pope, D. F., Raines, E., Ross, R., and Hunter, T., 1982, Similar effects of platelet-drived growth factor and epidermal growth factor on the phosphorylation of tyrosine in cellular proteins, *Cell* **31**:263–273.
186. Kasuga, M., Zick, Y., Blithe, D. L., Crettaz, M., and Kahn, C. R., 1982, Insulin stimulates tyrosine phosphorylation of the insulin receptor in a cell-free system, *Nature (Lond.)* **298**:667–669.
187. Heldin, C-H., Ek, B., and Rönnstrand, L., 1983, Characterization of the receptor for platelet-derived growth factor on human fibroblasts, *J. Biol. Chem.* **258**:10054–10061.
188. Rubin, J. B., Shia, M. A., and Pilch, P. F., 1983, Stimulation of tyrosine-specific phosphorylation in vitro by insulin-like growth factor 1, *Nature (Lond.)* **305**:438–440.
189. Jacobs, S., Kull, F. C., Jr., Earp, H. S., Svoboda, M. E., Van Wyk, J. J., and Cuatrecasas, P., 1983, Somatomedin-C stimulates the phosphorylation of the β-subunit of its own receptor, *J. Biol. Chem.* **258**:9581–9584.
190. DeLarco, J. E., and Todaro, G. J., 1978, Growth factors from murine sarcoma virus-transformed cells. *Proc. Natl. Acad. Sci. USA* **75**:4001–4005.
191. Todaro, G. J., Fryling, C., and DeLarco, J. G., 1980, Transforming growth factors produced by certain human tumor cells: Polypeptides that interact with epidermal growth factor receptors, *Proc. Natl. Acad. Sci. USA* **77**:5258–5262.
192. Roberts, A. B., Lamb, L. C., Newton, D. L., Sporn, M. B., DeLarco, J. E., and Todaro, G. J., 1980, Transforming growth factors: Isolation of polypeptides from virally and chemically transformed cells by acid/ethanol extraction, *Proc. Natl. Acad. Sci. USA* **77**:3494–3498.
193. Anzano, M. A., Roberts, A. B., Smith, J. M., Sporn, M. B., and DeLarco, J. E., 1983, Sarcoma growth factor from conditioned medium of virally transformed cells is composed of both type α and β transforming growth factors, *Proc. Natl. Acad. Sci. USA* **80**:6264–6268.
194. Poiesz, B. J., Ruscetti, F. W., Gazdar, A. F., Bunn, P. A., Minna, J. D., and Gallo, R. C., 1980, Detection and isolation of type C retrovirus particles from fresh and cultured lymphocytes of a patient with cutaneous T-cell lymphoma, *Proc. Natl. Acad. Sci. USA* **77**:7415–7419.
195. Murray, A. W., and Fitzgerald, D. J., 1979, Tumor promoters inhibit metabolic cooperation in cocultures of epidermal and 3T3 cells, *Biochem. Biophys, Res. Commun.* **91**:395–401.
196. Yotti, L. P., Chang, C. C., and Trosko, J. E., 1979, Elimination of metabolic cooperation in Chinese hamster cells by tumor promoters, *Science* **206**:1089–1091.
197. Shih, C., Shilo, B-Z., Goldfarb, M. P., Dannenberg, A., and Weinberg, R. A., 1979, Passage of phenotypes of chemically transformed cells via transfection of DNA and chromatin, *Proc. Natl. Acad. Sci. USA* **76**:5714–5718.
198. Cooper, G. M., Okenquist, S., and Silverman, L., 1980, Transforming activity of DNA of chemically transformed and normal cells, *Nature (Lond.)* **281**:418–421.
199. Krontiris, T. G., and Cooper, G. M., 1981, Transforming activity of human tumor DNAs, *Proc. Natl. Acad. Sci. USA* **78**:1181–1184.
200. Santos, E., Tronick, S. R., Aaronson, S. A., Pulciani, S., and Barbacid, M., 1982, T24 human bladder

carcinoma oncogene is an activated form of the normal human homologue of BALB—and Harvey—MSV transforming genes, *Nature (Lond.)* **298:**343–347.

201. Shimizu, K., Goldfarb, M., Syard, Y., Perucho, M., Li, Y., Kamata, T., Feramisco, J., Stavnezer, E., Fogh, J., and Wigler, M. H., 1983, Three human transforming genes are related to the viral ras oncogenes, *Proc. Natl. Acad. Sci. USA* **80:**2112–2116.

202. Weinberg, R. A., 1983, A molecular basis of cancer, *Sci. Am.* **249:**126–142.

203. Taparowsky, E., Shimizu, K., Goldfarb, M., and Wigler, M., 1983, Structure and activation of the human N-ras gene, *Cell* **34:**581–586.

204. Shih, T. Y., Weeks, M. O., Young, H. A., and Scolnick, E. M., 1979, Identification of a sarcoma virus-coded phosphoprotein in nonproducer cells transformed by Kirsten or Harvey murine sarcoma virus, *Virology* **96:**64–79.

205. Shih, T. Y., Weeks, M. O., Young, H. A., and Scolnick, E. M., 1979, p21 of Kirsten murine sarcoma virus is thermolabile in a viral mutant temperature sensitive for the maintenance of transformation, *J. Virol.* **31:**546–556.

206. Shih, T. Y., Papageorge, A. G., Stokes, P. E., Weeks, M. O., and Scolnick, E. M., 1980, Guanine nucleotide-binding and autophosphorylating activities associated with p21src protein of Harvey murine sarcoma virus, *Nature (Lond.)* **287:**686–691.

207. McGrath, J. P., Capon, D. J., Goeddel, D. V., and Levinson, A. D., 1984, Comparative biochemical properties of normal and activated human ras p21 protein, *Nature (Lond.)* **301:**644–649.

208. Sweet, R. W., Yokoyama, S., Kamata, T., Feramisco, J. R., Rosenberg, M., and Gross, M., 1984, The product of ras is a GTPase and the T24 oncogenic mutant is deficient in this activity, *Nature (Lond.)* **311:**273–275.

209. Gibbs, J. B., Sigal, I. S., Poe, M., and Scolnick, E. M., 1984, GTPase activity distinguishes normal and oncogenic ras p21 molecules, *Proc. Natl. Acad. Sci. USA* **81:**5704–5708.

210. Driedger, P. E., and Blumberg, P. M., 1980, Specific binding of phorbol ester tumor promoters, *Proc. Natl. Acad. Sci. USA* **77:**567–571.

211. Castagna, M., Takai, Y., Kaibuchi, K., Sano, K., Kikkawa, U., and Nishizuka, Y., 1982, Direct activation of calcium-activated phospholipid-dependent protein kinase by tumor-promoting phobol esters, *J. Biol. Chem.* **257:**7847–7851.

212. Niedel, J. E., Kuhn, L. J., and Vandenbark, G. R., 1983, Phorbol diester receptor copurifies with protein kinase C, *Proc. Natl. Acad. Sci. USA* **80:**36–40.

213. Sporn, M. B., and Todaro, G. J., 1980, Autocrine secretion and malignant transformation of cells, *N. Engl. J. Med.* **303:**878–880.

214. Sporn, M. B., and Roberts, A. B., 1985, Autocrine growth factors and cancer, *Nature (Lond.)* **313:**745–747.

215. Land, H., Parada, L. F., and Weinberg, R. A., 1983, Cellular oncogenes and multistep carcinogenesis, *Science* **222:**771–778.

216. Murphree, A. L., and Benedict, W. F., 1984, Retinoblastoma: clues to human oncogenesis, *Science* **223:**1028–1033.

217. Sager, R., 1986, Genetic suppression of tumor formation: A new frontier in cancer research, *Cancer Res.* **46:**1573–1580.

218. Doolittle, R. F., Hunkapiller, M. W., Hood, L. E., Devare, S. G., Robbins, K. C., Aaronson, S. A., and Antoniades, H. N., 1983, Simian sarcoma virus on gene, v-sis, is derived from the gene (or genes) encoding a platelet-derived growth factor, *Science* **221:**275–277.

219. Waterfield, M. D., Scrace, G. T., Whittle, N., Stroobant, P., Johnsson, A., Wasteson, A., Westermark, B., Heldin, C-H., Huang, J. S., and Deuel, T. F., 1983, Platelet-derived growth factor is structurally related to the putative transforming protein p28sis of simian sarcoma virus, *Nature (Lond.)* **304:**35–39.

220. Downward, J., Yarden, Y., Mayes, E., Scrace, G., Totty, N., Stockwell, P., Ullrich, A., Schlessinger, J., and Waterfield, M. D., 1984, Close similarity of epidermal growth factor receptor and v-erb-B oncogene protein sequences, *Nature (Lond.)* **307:**521–527.

221. Stiles, C. D., 1985, The biological role of oncogenes—Insights from platelet-derived growth factor: Rhoads Memorial Award Lecture, *Cancer Res.* **45:**5215–5218.

222. Weinberg, R. A., 1985, The action of oncogenes in the cytoplasm and nucleus, *Science* **230:**770–776.

223. Eisenman, R. N., Tachibana, C. Y., Abrams, H. D., and Hann, S. R., 1985, v-myc-and c-myc-encoded proteins are associated with the nuclear matrix, *Mol. Cellul. Biol.* **5:**114–126.

224. Goyette, M., Petropoulos, C. J., Shank, P. R., and Fausto, N., 1983, Expression of a cellular oncogene during liver regeneration, *Science* **219:**510–512.

225. Schartl, M., and Barnekow, A., 1984, Differential expression of the cellular src gene during vertebrate development, *Dev. Biol.* **105:**415–422.

226. Pfeifer-Ohlsson, S., Rydnert, J., Goustin, A. S., Larsson, E., Besholtz, C., and Ohlsson, R., 1985, Cell-type-specific pattern of myc proto-oncogene expression in developing human embryos, *Proc. Natl. Acad. Sci. USA* **82:**5050–5054.

227. Corral, M., Tichonicky, L., Gugen-Guillouzo, C., Corcos, D., Raymondjean, M., Paris, B., Kruh, J., and Defer, N., 1985, Expression of c-fos oncogene during hepatocarcinogenesis, liver regeneration, and in synchronized HTC cells, *Exp. Cell Res.* **160:**427–434.

228. Brinster, R. L., Chen, H. Y., Messing, A., van Dyke, T., Levin, A. J., and Palmiter, R. D., 1984, Transgenic mice harboring SV40 T-antigen genes develop characteristic brain tumors, *Cell* **37:**367–379.

229. Stewart, T. A., Pattengale, P. K., and Leder, P., 1984, Spontaneous mammary adenocarcinomas in transgenic mice that carry and express MTV/myc fusion genes, *Cell* **38:**627–637.

230. Hanahan, D., 1985, Heritable formation of pancreatic β-cell tumours in transgenic mice expressing recombinant insulin/simian virus 40 oncogenes, *Nature (Lond.)* **315:**115–122.

231. Fett, J. W., Strydom, D. J., Lobb, R. R., Alderman, E. M., Bethune, J. L., Riordan, J. F., and Vallee, B. L., 1985, Isolation and characterization of angiogenin, an angiogenic protein from human carcinoma cells, *Biochemistry* **24:**5480–5486.

232. Muschel, R. J., Williams, J. E., Lowy, D. R., and Liotta, L. A., 1985, Harvey ras induction of metastatic potential depends upon oncogene activation and the type of recipient cell, *Am. J. Pathol.* **121:**11--8.

233. Friend, S. H., Bernards, R., Rogel, J. S., Weinberg, R. A., Rapaport, J. M., Albert, D. M., and Dryja, T. P., 1986, A human DNA segment with properties of the gene that predisposes to retinoblastoma and osterosarcoma, *Nature (Lond.)* **323:**643–646.

234. Finger, L. R., Harvey, R. C., Moore, R. C. A., Showe, L. C., and Croce, C. M., 1986, A common mechanism of chromosomal translocation in T- and B-cell neoplasia, *Science* **234:**982–985.

235. Thorgeirsson, S. S., Huber, B. E., Sorrell, S., Fojo, A., Pastan, I., and Gottesman, M. M., 1987, Expression of the multidrug-resistant gene in hepatocarcinogenesis and regenerating rat liver, *Science* **236:**1120–1122.

236. Mathew, C. G. P., Chin, K. S., Easton, D. F., Thorpe, K., Carter, C., Liou, G. I., Fong, S.-L., Bridges, C. D. B., Haak, H., Nieuwenhuijzen Kruseman, A. C., Schifter, S., Hansen, H. H., Telenius, H., Telenius-Berg, M., and Ponder, B. A. J., 1987, A linked genetic marker for multiple endocrine neoplasia type 2A on chromosome 10, *Nature (Lond.)* **238:**527–528.

237. Simpson, N. E., Kidd, K. K., Goodfellow, P. J., McDermid, H., Myers, S., Kidd, J. R., Jackson, C. E., Duncan, A. M. V., Farrer, L. A., Brasch, K., Castiglione, C., Genel, M., Gertner, J., Greenberg, C. R., Gusella, J. F., Holden, J. J. A., and White, B. N., 1987, Assignment of multiple endocrine neoplasia type 2A to chromosome 10 by linkage, *Nature (Lond.)* **328:**528–530.

238. Bodmer, W. F., Bailey, C. J., Bodmer, J., Bussey, H. J. R., Ellis, A., Gorman, P., Lucibello, F. C., Murday, V. A., Rider, S. H., Scambler, P., Sheer, D., Solomon, E., and Spurr, N. K., 1987, Localization of the gene for familial adenomatous polyposis on chromosome 5, *Nature (Lond.)* **328:**614–616.

239. Solomon, E., Voss, R., Hall, V., Bodmer, W. F., Jass, J. R., Jeffreys, A. J., Lucibello, F. C., Patel, I., and Rider, S. H., 1987, Chromosome 5 allele loss in human colorectal carcinomas, *Nature (Lond.)* **328:**616–619.

240. Knudson, Jr., A. G., 1971, Mutation and cancer: Statistical study of retinoblastoma, *Proc. Natl. Acad. Sci. USA* **68:**820–823.

241. Reynolds, S. H., Stowers, S. J., Patterson, R. M., Maronpot, R. R., Aaronson, S. A., and Anderson, M. W., 1987, Activated oncogenes in B6C3F1 mouse liver tumors: Implications for risk assessment, *Science* **237:**1309–1316.

242. Nerenberg, M., Hinrichs, S. H., Reynolds, R. K., Khoury, G., and Jay, G., 1987, The tat gene of human T-lymphotropic virus type 1 induces mesenchymal tumors in transgenic mice, *Science* **237:**1324–1329.

243. Hinrichs, S. H., Nerenberg, M., Reynolds, R. K., Khoury, G., and Jay, G., 1987, A transgenic mouse model for human neurofibromatosis, *Science* **237:**1340–1343.

244. Fearon, E. R., Hamilton, S. R., and Vogelstein, B., 1987, Clonal analysis of human colorectal tumors, *Science* **238:**193–197.

245. Egan, S. E., Wright, J. A., Jarolim, L., Yanagihara, K., Bassin, R. H., and Greenberg, A. H., 1987, Transformation by oncogenes encoding protein kinases induces the metastatic phenotype, *Science* **238:**202–205.

246. Liu, E., Hjelle, B., Morgan, R., Hecht, F., and Bishop, J. M., 1987, Mutations of the Kirsten-ras proto-oncogene in human preleukemia, *Nature (Lond.)* **330:**186–188.

247. Jimenez, J. J., and Yunis, A. A., 1987, Tumor cell rejection through terminal cell differentiation, *Science* **238:**1278–1280.

248. Velu, T. J., Beguinot, L., Vass, W. C., Willingham, M. C., Merlino, G. T., Pastan, I., and Lowy, D. R., 1987, Epidermal growth factor-dependent transformation by a human EGF receptor proto-oncogene, *Science* **238:**1408–1410.

249. Leppert, M., Dobbs, M., Scrambler, P., O'Connell, P., Nakamura, Y., Stauffer, D., Woodward, S., Burt, R., Hughes, J., Gardner, E., Lathrop, M., Wasmuth, J., Lalouel, J.-M., and White, R., 1987, The gene for familial polyposis coli maps to the long arm of chromosome 5, *Science* **238:**1411–1413.

250. Collard, J. G., van de Poll, M., Scheffer, A., Roos, E., Hopman, A. H., Geurts van Kessel, Ad H. M., and van Dongen, J. M., 1987, Location of genes involved in invasion and metastasis on human Chromosome 7, *Cancer Res.* **47:**6666–6670.

251. Angel, P., Imagawa, M., Chiu, R., Stein, B., Imbra, R. J., Rahmsdorf, H., Jonat, C., Herrlich, P., and Karin, M., 1987, Phorbol ester-inducible genes contain a common *cis* element recognized by a TPA-modulated trans-acting factor, *Cell* **49:**729 –739.

252. Lee, W., Mitchell, P., and Tjian, R., 1987, Purified transcription factor AP-1 interacts with TPA-inducible enhancer elements, *Cell* **49:**741–752.

253. Lee, W., Haslinger, A., Karin, M., and Tjian, R., 1987, Activation of transcription by two factors that bind promoter and enhancer sequences of the human metallothionein gene and SV 40, *Nature* **325:**369–372.

254. Chiu, R., Imagawa, M., Imbra, R. J., Bockoven, J. R., and Karin, M., 1987, Multiple *cis*- and *trans*-acting elements mediate the transcriptional response to phorbol esters, *Nature* **329:**648–651.

255. Angel, P., Allegretto, E. A., Okino, S. T., Hattori, K., Boyle, W. J., Hunter, T., and Karin, M., 1988, Oncogene *jun* encodes a sequence-specific *trans*- activator similar to AF-1, *Nature* **332:**166–171.

256. Zimmermann, W., Weber, B., Ortlieb, B., Rudert, F., Schempp, W., Fiebig, H. H., Shively, J. E., von Kleist, S., and Thompson, J. A., 1988, Chromosomal localization of the carcinoembryonic antigen gene family and differential expression in various tumors, *Cancer Res.* **48:**2550–2554.

# 1

# *Classification of Neoplasms*

## *Alphonse E. Sirica*

## 1. INTRODUCTION

It is generally agreed by both experimental and clinical pathologists that it is much easier to describe the features that characterize neoplasia* than to try to devise a brief definition that would adequately encompass the total range and complexity of this condition. Nevertheless, two eminent pathologists of this century, Rupert A. Willis and James Ewing, separately provided concise definitions that together come very close to conveying the essence of the neoplastic state. In this regard, Willis[1] stated that a neoplasm "is an abnormal mass of tissue, the growth of which exceeds and is uncoordinated with that of the normal tissues, and persists in the same excessive manner after cessation of the stimuli which evoked the change," while Ewing's definition, with minor modification,[2] declares that "a neoplasm is a *relatively* autonomous growth of tissue." What is implicit here is that (1) the neoplastic change is hereditable, being passed on to succeeding generations of cells; and (2) neoplastic cell proliferation is mostly, but not totally, free of the controls that act to regulate and limit the growth of normal cells and tissues.

It should be evident, when considering the classification of neoplasms, that virtually every cell type of the body can give rise to a neoplasm and that neoplasms can occur just about anywhere in the body. In addition, it is most important to note that neoplasms are subdivided into both benign and malignant forms. A benign neoplasm is one that exhibits a slow, localized growth that usually remains circumscribed. Only rarely does it cause the death of the organism. By contrast, a malignant neoplasm is one that will invade surrounding tissues and vessels and spread to distant body sites; left untreated, it has a high probability of killing the organism. Before giving further details concerning the characteristics that serve to differentiate between benign and malignant neoplasms, it is useful at this point to describe a number of relevant non-neoplastic growth alterations, so that a clearer view of the concept of neoplasia and its classification can be developed.

---

*The term tumor, which denotes a swelling, is commonly used to refer to a neoplasm, while cancer is a generic term for all malignant neoplasms. The use of the term neoplasia is preferred over these others, since it is more focused and connotes a more accurate description than that implied by the word tumor, yet is more encompassing than that indicated by the term cancer.

---

*Alphonse E. Sirica* • Department of Pathology, Medical College of Virginia, Virginia Commonwealth University, Richmond, Virginia 23298.

## 2. NON-NEOPLASTIC ADAPTIVE GROWTH CHANGES

A number of important non-neoplastic adaptive growth changes or disturbances can occur in response either to normal physiologic or to pathologic processes. These are commonly listed as atrophy, hypertrophy, hyperplasia, and metaplasia.

### 2.1. Atrophy

Atrophy refers to a decrease in either the size or number, or both, of constituent cells of an organ or tissue. If enough cells are affected, the normal size of the entire organ or tissue shrinks, and its function is diminished. Mechanistically, atrophy is associated with increased autophagy by the cells and may include cell loss due to apoptosis (controlled cell death) or necrosis.[3,4] In some cases, the lost cells may be replaced by either adipose tissue or fibrous connective tissue, and particular organs (e.g., heart or liver), when undergoing atrophy, may show an intracellular accumulation of lipofuscin pigment (aging pigment). This latter condition is known as brown atrophy, and the lipofuscin pigment, which is an undigested residue of autophagic vacuoles, is believed to be derived from membrane lipid debris rendered indigestible by oxidative changes, caused, for example, by lipid peroxidation.[5] The causes of atrophy include inadequate nutrition, lack of proper blood supply, loss of innervation, decrease in hormonal stimulation, decreased workload and disuse, aging, prolonged tissue compression, and physiologic organ involution.

### 2.2. Hypertrophy

When viewed at the cellular level, hypertrophy is defined as an increase in the size of cells. If sufficient cells are involved, cellular hypertrophy will result in an increase in the total size of the organ or tissue of which they are constituents. Hypertrophy reflects an increase in the synthesis of structural components of the cell and occurs as a result of demand for increased function. This may be (1) a response to increased workload; (2) compensatory due to impaired function of part of an organ system or to a loss of one part of a paired organ, such as kidney; (3) attributable to hormonal stimulation; and (4) in some cases, related to the anabolic effects of specific kinds of chemical inducers, exemplified by the hypertrophic effect of phenobarbital on liver.

### 2.3. Hyperplasia

In comparison with hypertrophy, hyperplasia represents an increase in the actual number of cells of an organ or tissue. It should be noted that increases in the size of most organs and tissues usually occur by a combination of hypertrophy and hyperplasia, although various cell types differ in their ability to exhibit hyperplasia. For example, some adult cells, such as skeletal muscle and cardiac muscle cells and neurons, that have lost their ability to undergo cell division have essentially no capacity for hyperplasia, while others (e.g., those of epidermis, intestinal epithelium, hematopoietic cells, and hepatocytes) can exhibit marked hyperplastic responses. Hyperplasia may be (1) the result of physiologic stimuli or induced by specific mitogenic agents; (2) compensatory after a portion of organ or tissue has been damaged by toxins or disease; or (3) surgically resected, as in the case of liver regeneration after partial hepatectomy or it may be hormonally stimulated. Excessive hormone stimulation can result in pathologic hyperplasia, common examples being endometrial hyperplasia due to an imbalance in estrogen and progesterone production, and bilateral adrenocortical hyperplasia resulting from excessive stimulation by adrenocorticotrophic hormone (ACTH). In many cases, only a single cell type in a given tissue will show a hyperplastic response to a particular physiologic or pathologic stimuli, although in some organs (e.g., prostate or liver), more than one cell type may undergo hyperplasia. In terms of appearance, hyperplasia may present itself in the form of a diffuse cellular pattern or it may be nodular, but the conditions that determine these patterns are not well understood.

## 2.4. Metaplasia

Metaplasia indicates the replacement in an organ or tissue of one adult differentiated cell type by another type of adult differentiated cell. It usually represents a localized adaption to adverse environmental conditions, such as chronic irritation. Thus, metaplasia occurs fundamentally because of a need for another type of cellular function, i.e., one that is ostensibly more protective, although the value of this type of adaptive response is not always evident. Epithelial tissue is the most frequent site of metaplasia. An important example is the change of bronchial epithelium of chronic cigarette smokers from ciliated pseudostratified columnar epithelium to stratified squamous epithelium. This is known as squamous metaplasia. Vitamin A deficiency also results in squamous metaplasia in a variety of epithelia of the body, and the metaplasia of simple cuboidal or columnar epithelium to stratified squamous epithelium can occur as a result of chronic irritation in the excretory ducts of glands and in the gallbladder when irritated by the presence of gallstones. Other examples of epithelial metaplasia include intestinal metaplasia in the biliary tract[6,7] and metaplastic epithelial changes in pancreas[8,9] (see Chapter 24). Furthermore, metaplasia may occur in connective tissue proper, giving rise to bone or cartilage where it normally is not found, such as in tendons. Osseous metaplasia may also be found in some neoplasms. Under these latter conditions, the adaptive aspects underlying osseous or cartilagenous metaplasia are not apparent. Nevertheless, it seems apparent that in a number of instances metaplastic cells may arise from stem cells present in a given adult tissue and are showing an altered pattern of differentiation. There is also evidence to suggest that, under some circumstances, metaplasia may be derived from pre-existing differentiated adult cell types (i.e., see Chapter 24).

## 2.5. Dysplasia

Although technically not an adaptive growth change, dysplasia is considered here because of its relationship to hyperplasia. In fact, a synonymous term for dysplasia is atypical hyperplasia. Dysplasia is defined as an alteration in adult cells characterized by variations in size, shape, and organization. It basically applies to epithelial or mesenchymal cells that have undergone somewhat irregular and atypical proliferative changes in response to chronic irritation or inflammation.[10] Important examples of dysplastic changes include those found in the uterine cervix, in metaplastic squamous epithelium of the bronchi of chronic cigarette smokers, and in the post-hepatitic form of human liver cirrhosis associated with hepatitis B virus (HBV).[11,12]

## 3. PRENEOPLASTIC LESIONS AND MALFORMATIONS

Unlike neoplasia, pathologic forms of non-neoplastic adaptive growth changes are generally not progressive and cease when the specific inciting stimulus has been withdrawn. The tendency is for the resulting cell alterations or lesions to reverse or regress. Dysplastic cells may also disappear with removal of the inciting stimulus, with the possibility of the affected tissues reverting completely to their normal state of structure and function. However, even though certain growth disturbances, such as hyperplasia and metaplasia, and dysplasia are not neoplastic, they can be relevant to the neoplastic process and may precede the development of neoplasia.

Hyperplasia represents a significant change with respect to ensuring the fixation of the initiating event in carcinogenesis, as well as being an important component of tumor promotion.[13] In addition, the presence of dysplasia in the uterine cervix and of atypical metaplasia in the bronchi is closely related to the development of neoplasia in these organs. In this context, these lesions are regarded as preneoplastic. That is, they have a high probability of developing into a neoplasm. Since such lesions as cervical dysplasia or atypical metaplasia of the bronchi may represent intermediate stages in the development of malignant neoplasia, they may also be referred to as precancerous. The term preneoplasia is used in a broader sense to include those non-neoplastic lesions, composed of atypical or phenotypically altered cells, that have been shown to represent actual prestages in the development of both benign and malignant neoplasms.[14] Preneoplasia is discussed in detail in Chapter 9.

A number of developmental aberrations or malformations exist that are tumorlike in appearance. These are represented by the choristomas and the hamartomas, which, despite the ominous sound of their names, are both non-neoplastic lesions. A choristoma is an aberrant mass of tissue cells present in some organ in which such cells are not normally found. Examples include a nodular mass of pancreatic acinar cells in the walls of the stomach or small intestine and a focal mass of disorganized adrenal gland cells located under the kidney capsule or in the wall of the urinary bladder. This is in contrast to ectopia, which designates the presence of a tissue or organ having a normal histologic configuration in an abnormal location of the body. A hamartoma is represented by an irregular focal overgrowth of one or more tissues normally present in a given organ or at a particular body site. A good example is hamartoma of the lung, which may consist of circumscribed growths of well-differentiated cartilage, bronchial epithelium, connective tissue, and mucous glands that are improperly mixed and overgrown in abnormal proportions.

## 4. ANAPLASIA AND DIFFERENTIATION IN NEOPLASMS

Anaplasia, which literally means without form, or to form backward, is typically applied to malignant neoplasms. This term describes two types of disorganization, cytologic and positional, that characterize these lesions. Cytologic anaplasia (Fig. 1) describes the bizarre nuclear and cytoplasmic changes shown by malignant neoplastic cells. These include increased nuclear and nucleolar size, increased nuclear to cytoplasmic ratio, hyperchromatic nuclei, increased cytoplasmic basophilia, increased number of mitoses, atypical and bizarre mitotic figures, cellular pleomorph-

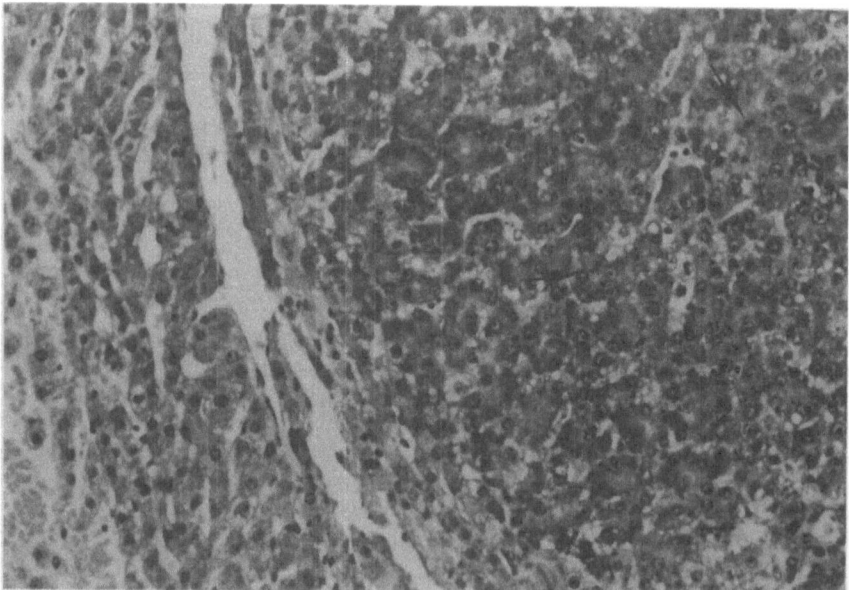

*Figure 1.* Hepatocellular carcinoma of the rat demonstrating the features of cytologic anaplasia. The malignant neoplastic hepatocytes on the right are characterized by such features as increased cytoplasmic basophilia as reflected by their darker staining, enlarged nuclei and nucleoli, increased nuclear to cytoplasmic ratio, hyperchromasia, and pleomorphism. Arrows point to mitotic figures within the hepatocellular carcinoma. By comparison, the normal hepatocytes seen on the left are quite uniform in cytologic appearance and are organized into one-cell or thick cords separated by a paralleling arrangement of sinusoids. (H&E, ×202)

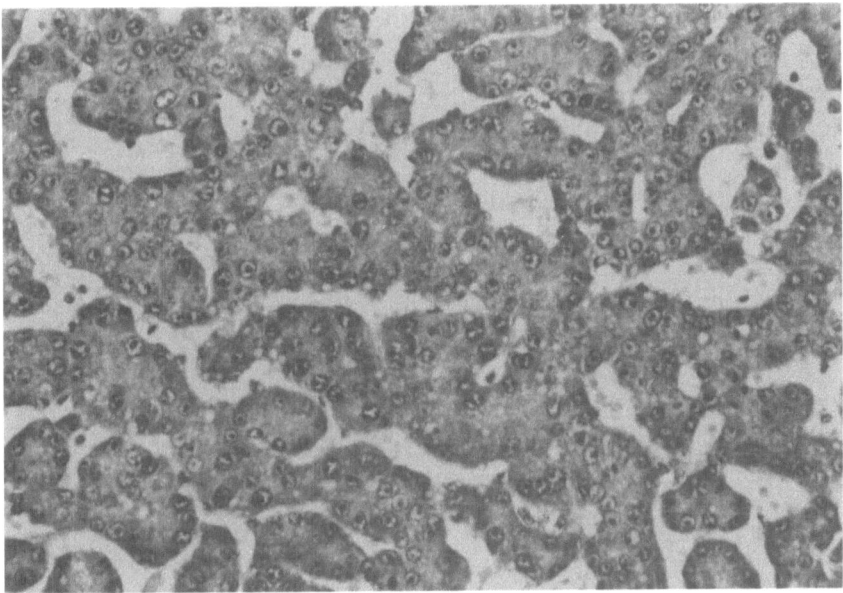

*Figure 2.* The same hepatocellular carcinoma shown in Fig. 1, demonstrating some of the features of positional anaplasia. Instead of being arranged in uniform one-cell thick cords, the malignant neoplastic hepatocytes are organized into multicell thick trabeculae separated by irregular vascular spaces. (H&E, ×320)

ism, and the formation of tumor giant cells. Positional anaplasia (Fig. 2) refers to the disordered relationship of the component cells of the neoplasm to each other. The distinct patterns shown by cells in normal tissues are altered in the form of architectural derangements and abnormal cellular interrelations.

When applied to neoplasms, the term of differentiation designates the degree to which the neoplastic parenchymal cells resemble their normal cell counterparts in both morphology and function. The parenchymal cells of neoplasms show different degrees of differentiation, with benign neoplasms generally well differentiated (Fig. 3) and malignant neoplasms with increasing anaplasia progressively more undifferentiated (Fig. 4).

## 5. PATHOBIOLOGIC CHARACTERISTICS OF BENIGN AND MALIGNANT NEOPLASMS

Benign neoplasms are often, but not always, encapsulated by a fibrous connective tissue capsule (Fig. 5), while malignant neoplasms are invariably nonencapsulated. In addition, benign neoplasms are not invasive, whereas malignant neoplasms characteristically invade adjacent tissues and vasculature (Fig. 6). Benign neoplasms are well differentiated and contain low numbers of mitotic figures, which are normal. Their growth is progressive, but slow. By contrast, malignant neoplasms usually exhibit more rapid growth rates, and mitotic figures are common, with abnormal forms present. These neoplasms are anaplastic and show varying degrees of loss of differentiation. Perhaps the most important distinction between benign and malignant neoplasms is the frequent ability of the latter to spread to other parts of the body to form secondary growths or metastases. Benign neoplasms do not metastasize, while the vast majority of malignant neoplasms can. Exceptions include the gliomas and the basal cell carcinoma of the skin, both of which are quite invasive but rarely spread to distant sites.

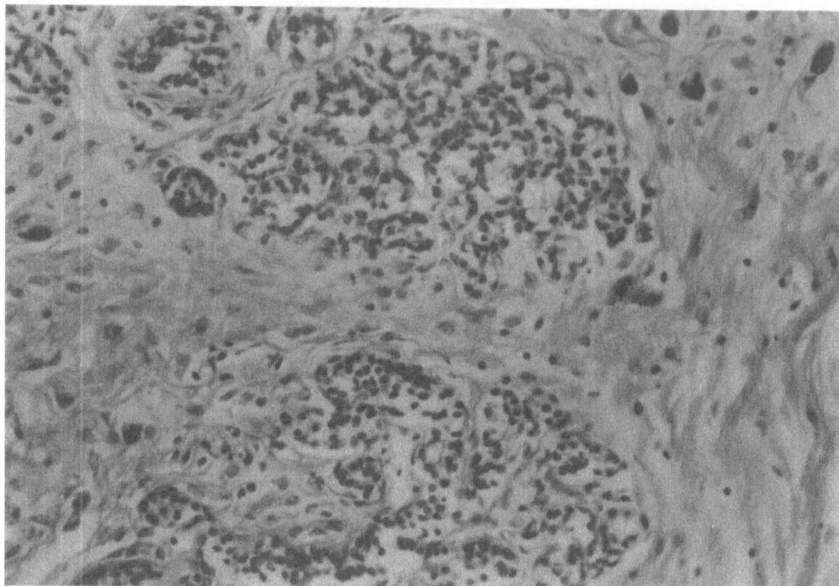

*Figure 3.* Benign well-differentiated fibroadenoma of rat mammary gland. This lesion is composed of nests of slowly proliferating ducts embedded in an expanding periductular fibrous connective tissue. As exemplified here, benign neoplasms are, by nature, well differentiated. (H&E, ×202)

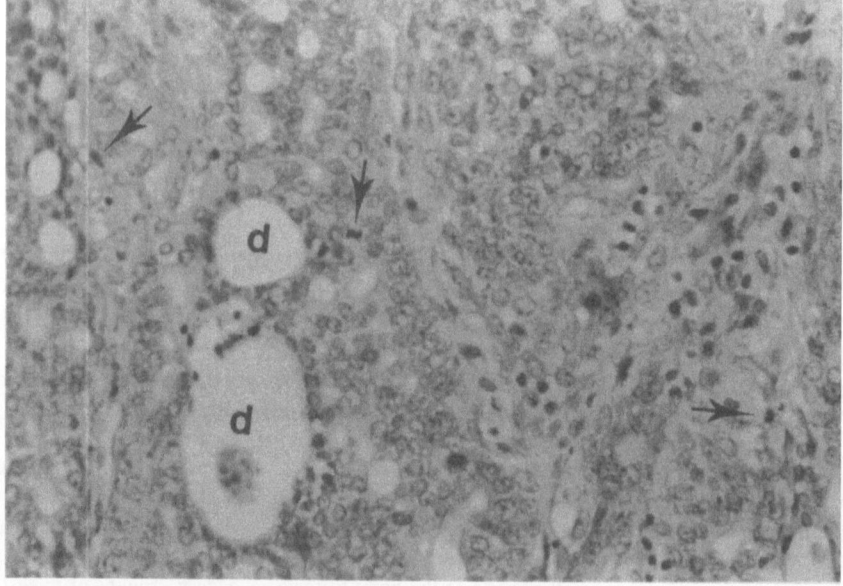

*Figure 4.* Poorly differentiated adenocarcinoma of the mammary gland of the rat. There is very little similarity between the appearance of this malignant neoplasm and normal mammary gland. Note the ductlike structures (d) and the obvious presence of mitotic figures (arrows) within this malignant neoplasm. (H&E, ×256)

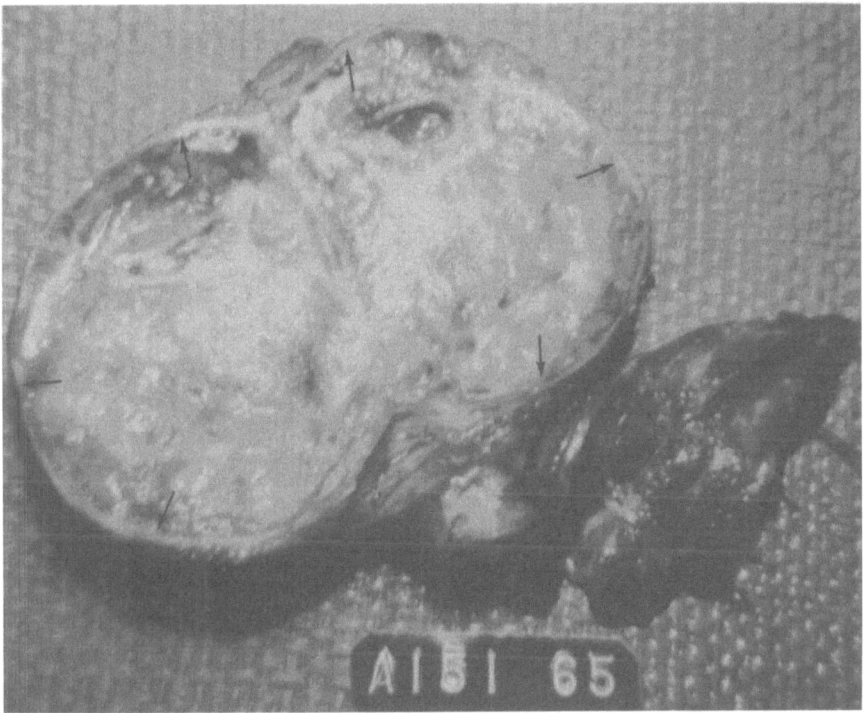

*Figure 5.* Well-circumscribed encapsulated adenoma of a human thyroid gland. Arrows point to the fibrous capsule of this benign neoplasm.

In addition to the proliferating neoplastic cells that make up their parenchyma, both benign and malignant neoplasms have a supportive stroma made up of connective tissue and vascular supply. Desmoplasia is a term used to define the stimulation by neoplastic parenchymal cells of the formation of an excessive collagenous connective tissue stroma. Thus, some neoplasms, such as scirrhous carcinoma of the breast, are quite hard because of extensive dense connective tissue stroma, while others, such as medullary carcinoma of the breast, are soft and fleshy, having a scant fibrous stroma.

The vascularity of a neoplasm can vary greatly, with those that are more slow growing being generally less well vascularized than those that are rapid growing.[15] However, the rapid growth of many malignant neoplasms causes outgrowth or interference with their own blood supply, producing considerable necrosis.[16]

Benign neoplasms commonly produce little tissue damage and usually have minimal effects on the host, while malignant neoplasms are quite destructive to host tissues and have marked effects on the organism as a whole. This is not to imply that benign neoplasms are harmless. In fact, depending on (1) their organ location, (2) their functional activity, such as excessive hormone production, and (3) whether they become infarcted or cause obstructions, benign neoplasms may have adverse consequences for the host, and in some cases may be life threatening and may even cause death. For example, a liver cell adenoma may rupture, causing severe intraperitoneal hemorrhage, and a myxoma of the heart, because of its location, may prove fatal. Nevertheless, because benign neoplasms are both localized and circumscribed in their growth patterns, they are for the most part amenable to surgical removal. By contrast, malignant neoplasms, because of their ability to invade and metastasize, can compromise multiple organ and tissue sites. In addition, malignant neoplasms may be associated with paraneoplastic syndromes[10] and may be the sites of ectopic hormone

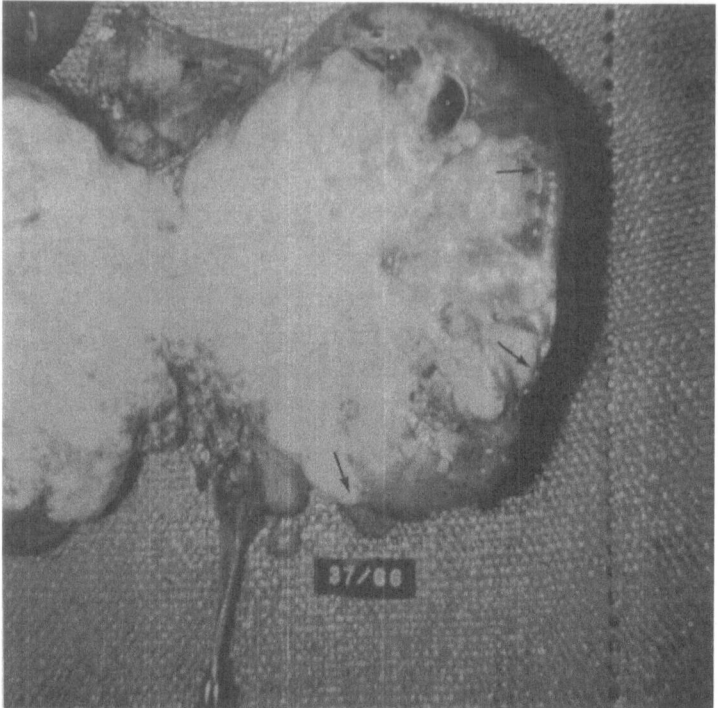

*Figure 6.* Transitional cell carcinoma of the renal pelvis of a human kidney. Arrows point to the irregular margins of the malignant neoplasm as it invades the kidney cortex.

production (see Chapter 23). Furthermore, a common feature of malignant neoplastic disease is cachexia. This is defined as the severe wasting of body tissues, weakness, and ill health that frequently becomes prominent in the end stages of malignant neoplastic disease. The basic mechanism(s) underlying cachexia is still not understood, although recent evidence has implicated the macrophage protein, cachectin, as a central mediator of the wasting that accompanies chronic invasive disease states.[17]

## 6. NOMENCLATURE OF NEOPLASMS

The most practical classification scheme for neoplasms is based on features combining their histogenesis and their pathobiologic behavior. In this regard, some simple rules and definitions related to the naming and classification of neoplasms are presented:

The suffix *-oma* when following the prefix designating a specific tissue generally denotes a benign neoplasms of that particular tissue.
To denote a malignant epithelial neoplasm, the root *carcin-* is combined with the suffix *-oma*, to give carcinoma.
To denote a malignant neoplasm of mesenchymal origin, the root *sarc-* is used with the suffix *-oma* to give sarcoma.
The prefix *adeno-* designates the relationship to a gland. This is used exclusively with neoplasms of epithelial origin.
Descriptive terms, such as papillary, cystic, mucous, medullary (soft), scirrhous (hard), follicular,

exophytic, and polypoid, may be used in naming various histologic types of neoplasms of epithelial origin.

Some common usage exceptions to the above generalities include the terms melanoma, lymphoma, seminoma, hepatoma (the preferred term being hepatocellular carcinoma), multiple myeloma, and diffuse malignant mesothelioma. These are all malignant neoplasms.

Another exception is the term granuloma, which designates a type of non-neoplastic lesion, usually composed of modified macrophages and giant cells, that is associated with a specific type of chronic inflammation.

*Blastoma* is a suffix used to refer to malignant neoplasms that histologically resemble embryonic tissues, e.g., retinoblastoma and hepatoblastoma.

Benign teratoma and its malignant counterpart, teratocarcinoma, are neoplasms that arise from totipotential cells of germinal origin.

Mixed neoplasms, such as a mixed tumor of the salivary gland, refer to those consisting of two or more different kinds of neoplastic tissue, while a carcinosarcoma is a highly malignant neoplasm having the appearance of both carcinoma and sarcoma.

Carcinoma in situ indicates focal lesions that possess all the cytologic features of a malignant epithelial neoplasm, but that remains localized to the epithelium without showing evidence of invasion through the basement membrane.

Leukemias are malignant neoplasms of hematopoietic and lymphoid systems, characterized by progressive infiltration and replacement of hematopoietic organs by proliferating neoplastic cells that circulate freely and may be found in great numbers in the peripheral blood.

Some neoplasms are named after those who first describe them, e.g., Ewing sarcoma, Burkitt lymphoma, and Hodgkin disease.

Table 1 presents a general classification of some neoplasms, exemplifying the rules just mentioned. Figures 7–12 are photomicrographs showing the histopathologic features of some representative benign and malignant neoplasms. This classification is by no means complete and serves as a framework for further understanding the nomenclature used to denote benign and malignant neoplasms. For an extensive classification of neoplasms, the reader is referred to more specialized texts, such as the many excellent fascicles of the *Atlas of Tumor Pathology* published by the Armed Forces Institute of Pathology, Washington, D. C.

*Table I. Examples Demonstrating the Nomenclature of Selected Neoplasms*

| Tissue of origin | Benign | Malignant |
| --- | --- | --- |
| Epidermis | Squamous cell or epidermal papilloma | Squamous cell or epidermal carcinoma |
| Bile duct | Cholangioma | Cholangiocarcinoma |
| Urinary tract epithelium | Transitional cell papilloma | Transitional cell carcinoma |
| Glandular epithelium | Adenoma | Adenocarcinoma |
| Adult fibrous tissue | Fibroma | Fibrosarcoma |
| Cartilage | Chondroma | Chondrosarcoma |
| Bone | Osteoma | Osteosarcoma |
| Adipose tissue | Lipoma | Liposarcoma |
| Smooth muscle | Leiomyoma | Leiomyosarcoma |
| Striated muscle | Rhabdomyoma | Rhabdomyosarcoma |
| Blood vessels | Hemangioma | Hemangiosarcoma |
| Myeloblasts | — | Myeloid leukemia |
| Erythroblasts | — | Erythroid leukemia (e.g., Hodgkin |
| Lymphoid tissue | — | disease) |
| Neurons | Ganglioneuroma | Neuroblastoma |
| Astrocytes | — | Astrocytoma |
| Placenta | Hydatidiform mole | Choriocarcinoma |

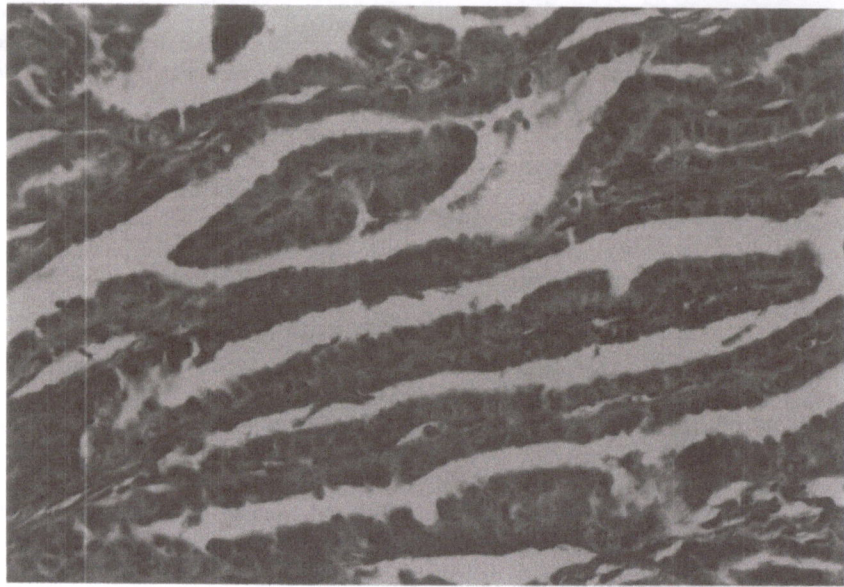

*Figure 7.* Papillary carcinoma of the human thyroid gland. Papillary refers to the fingerlike projections, or papillae, each of which is composed of a fibrovascular core and lined by a single layer of malignant neoplastic cells. (H&E, ×256)

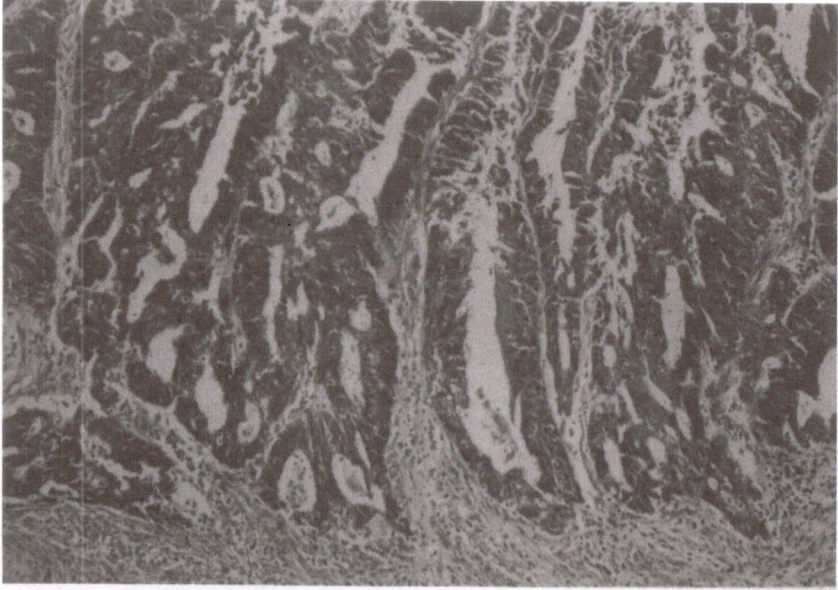

*Figure 8.* Human endometrial adenocarcinoma. Adeno- refers to the glandular character of this malignant neoplasm. (H&E, ×80)

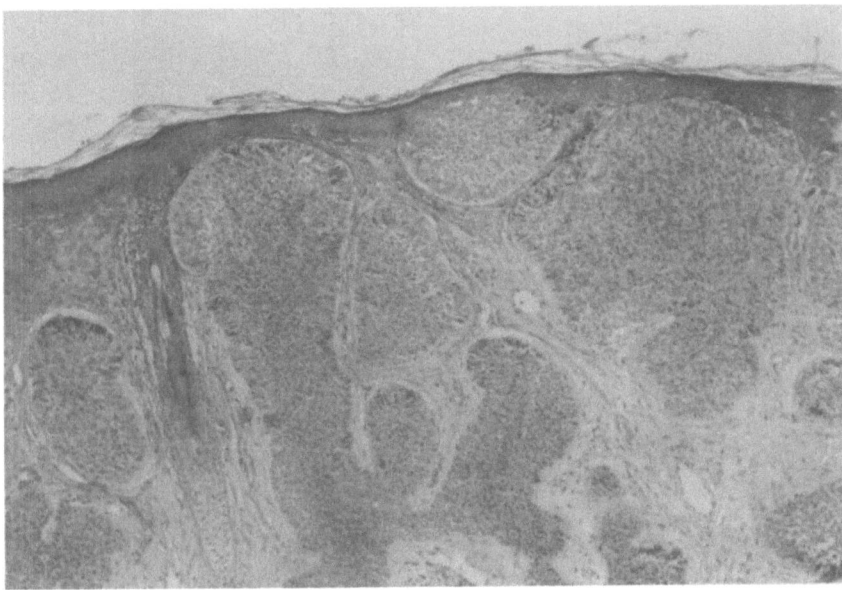

*Figure 9.* Human basal cell carcinoma. This neoplasm is derived from the basal cells of the epidermis. It is highly invasive, but it rarely if ever metastasizes. Note the solid nests of neoplastic basal cells invading the underlying dermis and exhibiting peripheral palisading. (H&E, ×102)

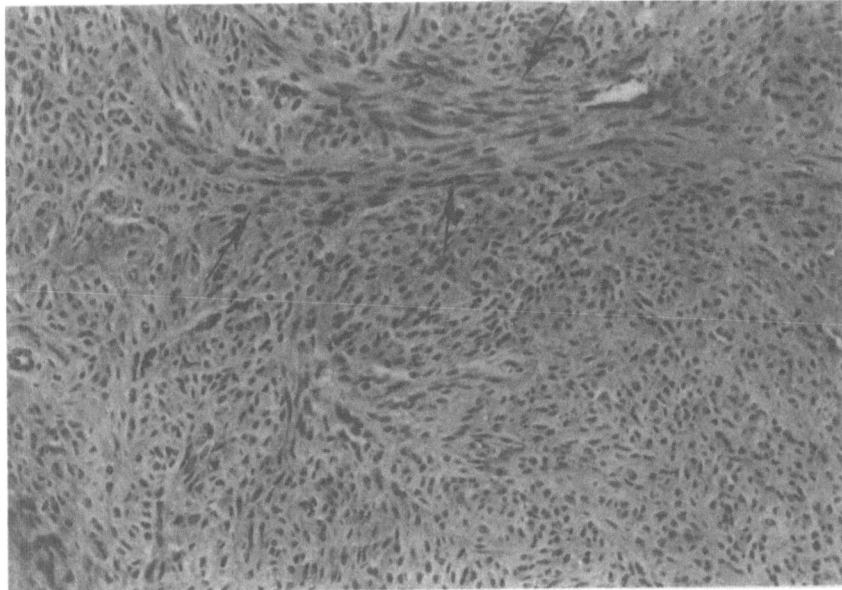

*Figure 10.* Human leiomyoma. This is a benign neoplasm of smooth muscle. Note that the smooth muscle cells of this neoplasm are highly differentiated and that they are organized into intertwining cellular bundles, which are oriented in many directions. Arrows point to one of the regularly arranged bundles of smooth muscle cells characteristic of this neoplasm. (H&E, ×102)

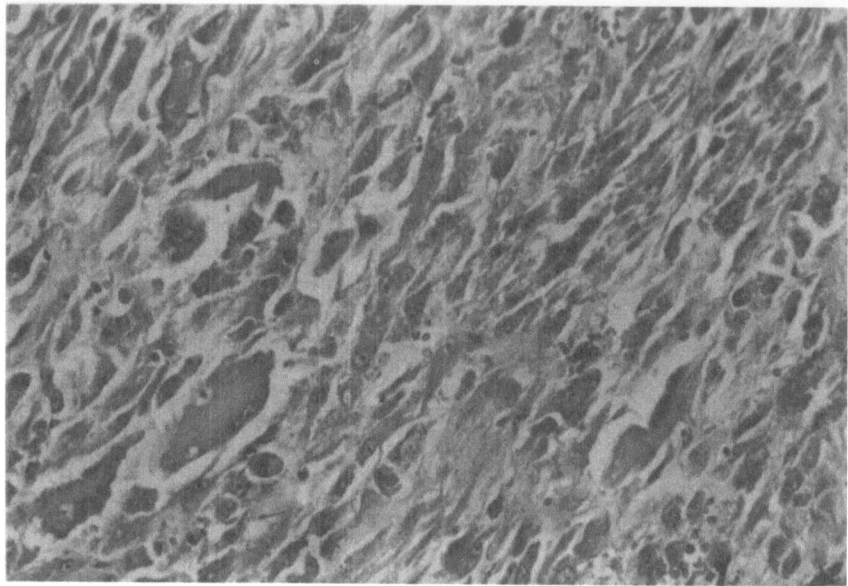

*Figure 11.* Human leiomyosarcoma. This is a malignant neoplasm of smooth muscle. Compare the cytologic features shown here with those shown in Fig. 12. (H&E, ×256)

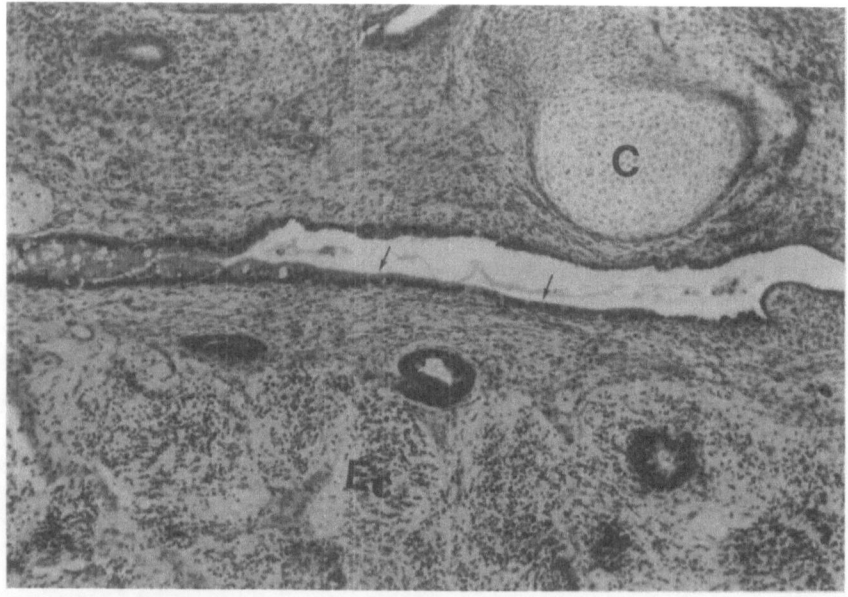

*Figure 12.* Human teratocarcinoma. This malignant neoplasm consists of totipotential embryonal carcinoma cells (Ec), which can differentiate into well-differentiated somatic tissues. Note the obvious presence of cartilage (C) and simple columnar epithelium (arrows) in this section. (H&E, ×80)

## 7. GRADING AND STAGING OF MALIGNANT NEOPLASMS

The grading and staging of malignant neoplasms are primarily for diagnostic reasons and represent efforts to predict their biologic behavior, as well as to serve as a guide for choosing appropriate treatment. The grading of a malignant neoplasm is based on its degree of anaplasia and lack of differentiation. In this regard, it generally follows that the more anaplastic neoplasms show the highest grade of malignancy, while those most closely resembling their normal tissues of origin are lowest in grade. The histopathologic grading of a neoplasm is always done by grading the most anaplastic area of the neoplasm in tissue section. Typically, three or four grades are used, with grade I the least anaplastic and grade IV the most anaplastic. The value of grading is largely dependent on the size of the tissue sample. Unfortunately, the grading of malignant neoplasms has not been a perfect system with respect to making consistent and accurate clinical prognostications. Nevertheless, grading has proved useful in arriving at a prognosis for a number of different types of malignant neoplasms.[18]

The staging of malignant neoplasms is related to their extent of spread and takes into consideration the size and degree of local invasiveness of the primary lesion, its extent of spread to regional lymph nodes, and the presence or absence of distant metastasis. A number of staging classification schemes have been developed. For example, in the colon, the classification established by Duke is most useful.[19] In order to standardize the criteria for the staging of neoplasms, the International Union Against Cancer formulated the TMN System[10] (T = tumor, M = metastasis, N = node). T refers to the malignant primary neoplasm and its size and degree of local invasiveness. It is graded as T 1–4. N refers to lymph nodes and denotes the degree of nodal involvement. No malignant neoplastic involvement is designated by N0, involvement of a few nodes by N1, and of an increasing number of nodes by N2 and N3, respectively. M refers to metastasis, with M0 indicating no metastasis, M1 indicating few metastases, and M2 indicating many metastases. The American Joint Committee on Cancer Staging has also developed a staging scheme employing stages 0–IV to characterize the extent of spread of the malignant neoplasm.[10] The staging of malignant neoplasms has been very useful with respect to selecting and standardizing therapy for specific types of malignant neoplasms.

## REFERENCES

1. Willis, R. A., 1960, *Pathology of Tumors*, 3rd ed., Butterworth, Washington, D.C.
2. Pitot, H. C., 1981, *Fundamentals of Oncology*, 2nd ed., Dekker, New York.
3. Anderson, J. R. (ed.), 1985, *Muir's Textbook of Pathology*, 12th ed., Edward Arnold, Baltimore.
4. Jones, T. C., and Hunt, R. D., 1983, *Veterinary Pathology*, 5th ed., Lea & Febiger, Philadelphia.
5. Scarpelli, D. G., and Chiga, M., 1985, Cell injury and errors of metabolism, in: *Anderson's Pathology*, Vol. 1, 3rd ed. (J. M. Kissane, ed.), pp. 61–112, C. V. Mosby, St. Louis.
6. Terao, K., and Nakano, M., 1974, Cholangiofibrosis induced by short-term feeding of 3'-methyl-4-(dimethylamino)azobenzene: An electron microscopic observation, *Gann* **65**:249–260.
7. Kozuka, S., Kurashina, M., Tsubone, M., Hachisuka, K., and Yasui, A., 1984, Significance of intestinal metaplasia for the evolution of cancer in the biliary tract, *Cancer* **54**:2277–2285.
8. Reddy, J. K., Rao, M. S., Qureshi, S. A., Reddy, M. K., Scarpelli, D. G., and Lalwani, N. D., 1984, Induction and origin of hepatocytes in rat pancreas, *J. Cell Biol.* **98**:2082–2090.
9. Parsa, I., Longnecker, D. S., Scarpelli, D. G., Pour, P., Reddy, J. K., and Lefkowitz, M., 1985, Ductal metaplasia of human exocrine pancreas and its association with carcinoma, *Cancer Res.* **45**:1285–1290.
10. Robbins, S. L., Cotran, R. S., and Kumar, V., 1984, *Pathologic Basis of Disease*, 3rd ed., W. B. Saunders, Philadelphia.
11. Akagi, G., Furuya, K., Kanamura, A., Chihara, T., and Otsuka, H., 1984, Liver cell dysplasia and hepatitis B surface antigen in liver cirrhosis and hepatocellular carcinoma, *Cancer* **54**:315–318.
12. Roncalli, M., Borzio, M., DeBiagi, G., Ferrari, A. R., Macchi, R., Tombesi, V. M., and Servida, E., 1986, Liver cell dysplasia in cirrhosis. A serologic and immunohistochemical study, *Cancer* **57**:1515–1521.

13. Sirica, A. E., 1983, Pathogenesis, in: *Concepts in Cancer Medicine* (S. B. Kahn, R. R. Love, C. Sherman, Jr., and R. Chakravorty, eds.), pp. 157–164, Grune & Stratton, Orlando, Florida.
14. Bannasch, P., 1985, Preneoplastic lesions as endpoints in carcinogenicity testing. 1. Hepatic preneoplasia, *Carcinogenesis,* **7**:689–695.
15. Diamandopoulos, G. T., and Meissner, W. A., 1985, Neoplasia, in: *Anderson's Pathology,* Vol. 1, 8th ed. (J. M. Kissane, ed.), pp. 514–559, C. V. Mosby, St. Louis.
16. Prehn, R. T., 1980, Neoplasia, in: *Principles of Pathobiology,* 3rd ed. (R. B. Hill, Jr., and M. F. LaVia, eds.), pp. 200–254, Oxford University Press, New York.
17. Beutler, B., and Cerami, A., 1986, Cachectin and tumor necrosis factor as two sides of the same biological coin, *Nature (Lond.)* **320**:584–588.
18. Goldfarb, S., 1983, Pathology of neoplasia, in: *Concepts in Cancer Medicine* (S. B. Kahn, R. R. Love, C. Sherman, Jr., and R. Chakravorty, eds.), pp. 127–142, Grune & Stratton, Orlando, Florida.
19. Chakravorty, R. C., 1983, Colorectal cancer, in: *Concepts in Cancer Medicine* (S. B. Kahn, R. R. Love, C. Sherman, Jr., and R. Chakravorty, eds.), pp. 437–461, Grune & Stratton, Orlando, Florida.

# 2

# Chemical Carcinogenesis in Experimental Animals and Humans

## Elizabeth K. Weisburger

## 1. BACKGROUND

The carcinogenic effect of exposure of humans to a mixture of chemical compounds (soot) was reported more than 200 years ago. By 1915, when Japanese research workers demonstrated the carcinogenicity of coal tar in rabbits, many cases of cancer had been noted in workers exposed to oil shales, coal tar, or dyestuff intermediates. In essence, exposed humans were the test organisms that indicated the deleterious effects of long exposure to certain substances. Unfortunately, more recent epidemiologic studies on exposed people have still been the initial indicators of carcinogenicity for some compounds.

By contrast, animal studies prior to use have shown the carcinogenicity of 2-acetylamino-fluorene, thus preventing its widespread use as a pesticide. However, research on this same compound was largely the basis of the concept that for most carcinogens metabolic activation to some reactive intermediate was necessary for the expression of activity,[1] a significant change from some earlier concepts. This chapter discusses the metabolic reactions of the major classes of chemical carcinogens, attempt to provide information on the basis for classification of carcinogens, and the relevance to humans.

## 2. METABOLISM OF CHEMICAL CARCINOGENS

There is no definite trail leading researchers to the mechanism of action of chemical carcinogens. Each must follow the apparent clues in anticipation that they will lead to a solution. Study of the metabolism of chemical carcinogens is one of those faint trails that points to the mechanism of action of chemical carcinogens.

---

*Elizabeth K. Weisburger* • Division of Cancer Etiology, National Cancer Institute, National Institutes of Health, Bethesda, Maryland 20892.

## 2.1. Aromatic Compounds

### 2.1.1. Aromatic Amines and Amino Azo Dyes

Both aromatic amines and amino azo dyes are discussed together because their mode of activation is similar. Furthermore, aromatic amines are generally the starting materials for azo dyes, while certain reductive metabolic pathways, found largely in intestinal bacteria, convert many azo dyes to aromatic amines.

Approximately 30 years after extensive production began of aromatic amines as intermediates in dye manufacture, an increased incidence of bladder cancers in the workers was noted by Rehn. However, actual demonstration of the carcinogenicity of an aromatic amine in animals did not occur until more than 40 years later. During that same decade the hepatocarcinogenicity of an amino azo dye was also discovered.[2,3] Initial studies on the metabolism and mode of action of these two classes of carcinogens indicated apparent differences in their metabolic pathways, but more recent work has shown the convergence in their mode of action.[1,2]

With a few exceptions, the aromatic amines and amino azo dyes were not active at the site of application, leading to the premise that metabolites were responsible for the carcinogenicity of these compounds. However, tests of the initial metabolites identified (i.e., ring-hydroxylated derivatives) were largely negative, leading to the conclusion that these represented detoxification processes rather than activation. Some indication that an oxidative reaction on the nitrogen of aromatic amines was responsible for their deleterious effects came from studies on methemoglobin formation in dogs.[4] However, the discovery that 2-acetylaminofluorene was converted to a nitrogen-hydroxylated metabolite that was more carcinogenic than the parent compound and was active in species resistant to the parent compound led to increased interest in this metabolic pathway. Further research showed it was applicable to other carcinogenic aromatic amines as well. The N-oxidation pathway was not the ultimate activation step, since additional reactions appeared to be necessary.[5]

The enzyme systems involved in the initial metabolic activation and detoxification of aromatic amines and amides are largely the P-450 family of mixed function oxidases, of which there are various forms.[6] The proclivity of certain forms of P-450 to increase detoxification by producing more of the ring hydroxylated derivatives and for other forms to enhance N-hydroxylation of 2-acetylaminofluorene has been reported.[7] As usual, the effects of enzyme inducers are varied, so that some forms are induced readily, while for other forms of P-450 there may be little or no induction. In addition, although the liver is the organ mainly involved in metabolic interactions, the contribution of other organs to the metabolism of xenobiotics should not be overlooked.[8]

Aromatic amines are also oxidized through flavine dependent enzymes[9]; such effects have been best demonstrated *in vitro*. An additional enzyme that activates aromatic amines is a peroxidase, the prostaglandin H (prostaglandin endoperoxide) synthase system. Benzidine is an especially good substrate for this enzyme, but other aromatic amines, such as 2-fluorenamine, are also activated through this pathway.[10,11] Since appreciable levels of prostaglandin synthase occur extrahepatically, local activation of aromatic amines could occur, thus partially explaining the organ-specific effects of some amines.

However, further activation of N-hydroxy-2-acetylaminofluorene is required to show an effect. Some enzymes involved in this process are acetyltransferases and sulfotransferase. Sulfotransferase transports the $SO_3^-$ group from phosphoadenosine phosphosulfate to the N–OH group, to furnish a highly reactive material in which the $SO_3^-$ leaves readily to provide Ar-$\overset{+}{N}$-(arylamidonium ion) and a sulfate residue. The arylamidonium ion, in turn, reacts at the C-8 position of guanosine and to a lesser extent at other locations, to afford DNA adducts (cf. Fig. 1).

Esterification of the N–OH group many also occur via an acyltransferase, to afford a reactive material in which the acetoxy group is a good leaving agent: i.e., Ar-N(COCH$_3$)OH → ArN(COCH$_3$)O(COCH$_3$) → Ar-$\overset{+}{N}$-COCH$_3$ (arylamidonium ion). Another acyltransferase is an N,O-transferase that moves the acetyl group from the nitrogen to the oxygen of the N–OH group to yield ArN(OCOH$_3$)H, a transient material in which the OAc group leaves readily, resulting in the

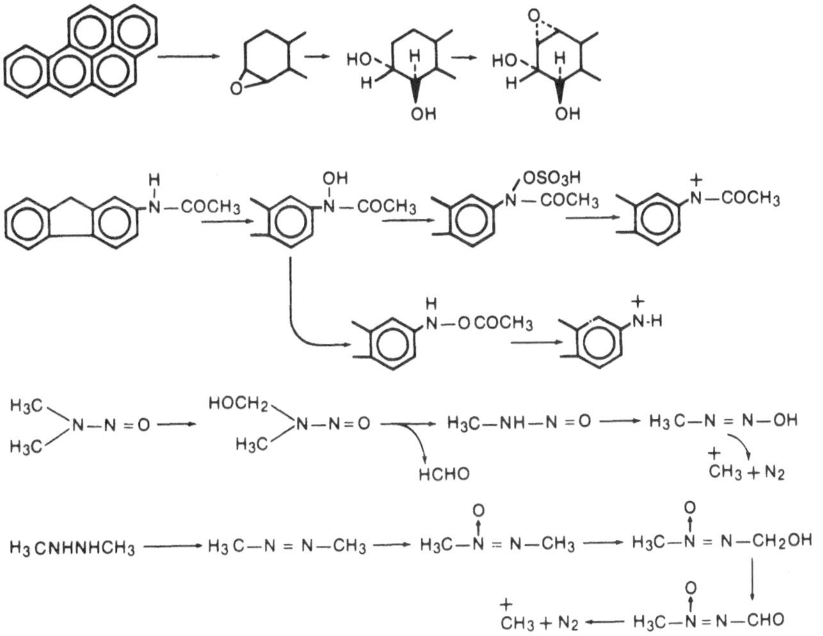

$$H_3C{-}N{=}O \longrightarrow HOCH_2\text{-}N{-}N{=}O \longrightarrow H_3C{-}NH{-}N{=}O \longrightarrow H_3C{-}N{=}N{-}OH$$

$$HCHO \qquad\qquad CH_3 + N_2$$

$$H_3CNHNHCH_3 \longrightarrow H_3C{-}N{=}N{-}CH_3 \longrightarrow H_3C{-}\overset{O}{\overset{\shortparallel}{N}}{=}N{-}CH_3 \longrightarrow H_3C{-}\overset{O}{\overset{\shortparallel}{N}}{=}N{-}CH_2OH$$

$$CH_3 + N_2 \longleftarrow H_3C{-}\overset{O}{\overset{\shortparallel}{N}}{=}N{-}CHO$$

*Figure 1.* Major activation pathway for benzo(a)pyrene, 2-acetylaminofluorene, dimethylnitrosamine, and 1,2-dimethylhydrazine. For more details, see Weisburger and Williams[9] and Dipple *et al.*[15]

arylnitrenium ion (ArN·-H), which may also interact with nucleic acids, proteins and other cellular nucleophiles.[12]

An additional activation possibility for aryl-*N*-hydroxyamides is through a peroxidase which oxides the amide to a nitroxyl radical intermediate.[13,14] In turn, this dismutates to furnish a nitroso compound and the activated *N*-acetoxyarylamide, which then readily forms an arylamidonium ion. The contribution that a glucuronic acid ester of the N-hydroxy compound may make toward activation pathways is probably somewhat less, but it should not be overlooked.[15] Thus, various pathways are available for activation of aromatic amines or amides. At least three enzyme systems are capable of converting them to N-hydroxy derivatives. The latter compounds can be further activated by esterification, trans-esterification, or oxidation. Some amides may also be oxidized to reactive iminoquinones; this pathway has been identified for acetaminophen.[16,17] In order that amino-azo dyes, such as 4-dimethylaminoazobenzene, might follow the activation scheme outlined for aromatic amines, an initial oxidative N-demethylation is required, probably by an amine oxidase or flavine-dependent system. Further steps are N-oxidation and esterification, as for aromatic amines.[2] Detoxification pathways for azo dyes also include ring hydroxylation, glutathione conjugation, and reductive splitting of the azo linkage, also by a flavine-dependent enzyme, azo reductase. However, if the azo dye were originally produced from a relatively potent carcinogenic amine, such as benzidine, the presence of azo reductase may increase the risk by liberating benzidine. Although there is some azo reductase in liver, the intestinal bacteria of mammals are generally very proficient in splitting azo dyes.

## 2.1.2. Aromatic Hydrocarbons

The discovery that tumors could be produced on the ears of rabbits by application of coal tar led to concerted efforts to isolate and identify the responsible substances. For this reason, most of the initial studies on the carcinogenicity of chemical compounds concentrated on polycyclic aromatic hydrocarbons (PAH) and relied on skin painting of any particular material to ascertain its effect. Since the tumors were noted at the site of application, it was long considered that the hydrocarbons were active as such. Thus, intensive investigation on metabolic activation did not occur until after the activated metabolite of 2-acetylaminofluorene was identified.

Although Boyland had proposed an epoxide pathway for polycyclic hydrocarbons to explain the metabolites found in the urine of animals administered such compounds, initial efforts concentrated on K-region (phenanthrene-like double bond) epoxides. The theoretical work of Pullman and Pullman suggested that these regions in a molecule were crucial in reactions with cellular constituents.[18] However, when a K-region epoxide of benzo(a)pyrene became available by synthetic means and was tested, it had less carcinogenic activity than the parent compound. Furthermore, the DNA adducts of K-region epoxides were not the same as those formed from metabolic activation in cultured cell systems. Comparative studies on the microsome-catalyzed binding of benzo(a)pyrene and of its various dihydrodiol metabolites to DNA showed the binding of the *trans*-7,8-dihydrodiol was more than 10-fold that of the parent hydrocarbon. This led to the concept that the dihydrodiols were metabolic intermediates in the activation of benzo(a)pyrene but that further metabolism to an activated agent was probably needed.[15,19] The availability of various diol epoxides, due to improvements in synthetic methods,[20] led to a demonstration that a 7,8-dihydrodiol-9,10-epoxide of benzo(a)pyrene yielded DNA products *in vitro* like those formed in cells exposed to benzo(a)pyrene. This diol epoxide was also a substrate for glutathione transferase, indicating competition between a detoxification reaction and reaction with DNA.

The stereochemical relationships between the diol and epoxide groupings had to be resolved since the diol epoxides have chiral carbons, with the possible existence of four stereoisomers for each diol epoxide. Basically, the benzylic hydroxyl group [7-diol in benzo(a)pyrene] and the epoxide group could be on the same side of the ring (*syn* or *cis*) or on opposite sides (*anti* or *trans*). Hydrolysis of the diol epoxides from benzo(a)pyrene to the corresponding tetrols afforded a reasonable means to delineate their absolute stereochemical configurations and thus that of the parent diol epoxides. Since the *anti* diol epoxide showed the most potent tumor initiating activity, it was concluded this probably is the ultimate activated metabolite of benzo(a)pyrene (cf. Fig. 1). These concepts have been embodied in the bay region hypothesis, introduced by Jerina and associates,[21] which predicts that active dihydrodiol epoxide metabolites would be those in which the epoxide was adjacent to a bay region of a PAH.

The bay region diol epoxide from benzo(a)pyrene has the proper combination of reactivity and stereochemical configuration to be a good initiator and to form a nucleic acid adduct. Not all diol epoxides of PAH have these characteristics. There also are other possible interventions before the entire metabolic pathway of epoxide → diol → diol epoxide can be attained. The initial epoxide may rearrange more or less rapidly to a phenol. If this is rapid, little epoxide remains. Likewise, if the epoxide is a good substrate for glutathione transferase, formation of glutathione conjugates and subsequently mercapturic acids takes place.[22] If these reactions occur to a significant extent, relatively little of the initial epoxide is available for hydration to a *trans*-dihydrodiol by means of the epoxide hydrolase enzyme, followed by a second oxidation to the dihydrodiol epoxide.

Some of the epoxides of polycyclic aromatic hydrocarbons are formed relatively easily, even by ozone in the atmosphere.[23] Likewise, these epoxides are fairly readily converted to phenols, accounting for the numerous phenolic metabolites of benzo(a)pyrene and their sulfuric acid or glucuronic acid conjugates.[24] Thus epoxidation, like other metabolic reactions, may lead to either activation or deactivation of the parent hydrocarbon.

Other pathways for activation of aromatic hydrocarbons have been proposed and have some experimental evidence to support them. Most prominent is one-electron oxidation, probably through peroxidases such as prostaglandin H synthase.[25] It has also been proposed that a peroxyl radical derived from fatty acid hydroperoxides oxidizes benzo(a)pyrene to quinones, or the 7,8-dihydrodiol to a diol epoxide.[26]

Another school holds that biohydroxymethylation, mediated by S-adenosylmethionine, of certain PAH (benzo(a)anthracene, dibenz(a,h)anthracene) leads to L-region methyl derivatives.[27,28] This reaction does occur in rat liver cytosol preparations, but its occurrence *in vivo* has not been demonstrated. The cytosol also oxidized the methyl derivatives to hydroxymethyl compounds with little or no ring oxidation. In turn, the sulfate ester of at least one hydroxymethyl derivative was a highly reactive compound. Activation would thus involve several steps to produce an activated metabolite: biomethylation, oxidation, and sulfate conjugation. Still to be attained is a convincing demonstration that these reactions occur in animals administered PAH.

Although the evidence for a diol-epoxide pathway in the metabolic activation of PAH seems to dominate the scene, the role of other possible modes of activation should not be overlooked. Some of them may explain why the polycyclic aromatics in general are active at the site of application.


## 2.2. Aliphatic Compounds

### 2.2.1. Halogenated Aliphatic Compounds

Halogenated aliphatic compounds that have shown a carcinogenic effect include one-carbon compounds, such as dichloromethane, chloroform, and carbon tetrachloride, as well as many compounds with longer chains, both saturated and unsaturated. Although these substances have many important industrial uses and are produced in large quantities, there is also some natural production of halogenated compounds by marine and terrestial organisms. In addition, trihalomethanes are formed during chlorination of water, probably by reaction with the humic acids in the water. Contamination of water supplies by chlorinated solvents, often trichloroethylene, has increased concern regarding the effects of these compounds.

Dichloromethane (methylene chloride) is metabolized to carbon monoxide and carbon dioxide by animals and humans. *In vitro*, rat liver cytosol converted dichloromethane to formaldehyde. In humans formaldehyde is oxidized to formic acid, which has been detected in the urine of dichloromethane-exposed workers.[29,30] More recent investigations have provided further evidence for both an oxidative cytochrome P-450-mediated pathway and a glutathione-dependent pathway.[31] The first path putatively yields formyl chloride, which decomposes to carbon monoxide, the basis for the elevated carboxyhemoglobin noted following human exposure. Formyl chloride, in turn, may also interact with glutathione to produce formic acid and then carbon dioxide, or it may acylate tissue nucleophiles, specifically microsomal proteins or lipids, as these entities were labeled after administration of [$^{14}$C]dichloromethane.[29,30] As was the case with several other halogenated compounds, minimal or no binding to nucleic acids was observed.[32]

Chloroform is initially metabolized by P-450 enzymes to trichloromethanol, which dehydrochlorinates to yield phosgene, which may interact with water to produce $CO_2$, with protein to yield bound material, with cysteine to afford 2-oxothiazolidine-4-carboxylic acid, and possibly with glutathione, since glutathione levels are depleted in the livers of rats given chloroform.[33] The metabolism of carbon tetrachoride is more complex. Initially, a reductive dechlorination occurs, yielding a P-450–Fe–$CCl_3$ complex that decomposes to give carbon monoxide, carbon dioxide, formic acid, phosgene, dimers (as $C_2Cl_6$), chloroform, and protein or lipid-bound products. However, binding to DNA of metabolites from either chloroform or carbon tetrachloride appears minimal, compared with some other carcinogens.

Halogenated compounds with two-carbon chains are metabolized by various routes. The unsaturated compounds vinyl chloride and trichloroethylene appear to be activated through formation of oxides,[34] although an alternate path involving chlorine migration has also been proposed.[35] These oxides may react with cellular targets or be deactivated, affording halo-alcohols, aldehydes or acids. Similarly, a metabolic study of tetrachloroethylene led to the conclusion that two different pathways were operative. One was P-450-mediated epoxidation leading to reactive metabolites in the liver with eventual excretion in the urine of various chlorinated compounds. The other path involved conjugation with glutathione yielding a mercapturic acid; this path was considered to be implicated in the nephrotoxicity of tetrachloroethylene.[36] In this regard, the toxicity of methyl chloride in mice was prevented by pretreatment of the animals with buthionine sulfoximine, which inhibits glutathione synthesis.[37] Although glutathione conjugation is usually considered a detoxifying mechanism, for several of the aliphatic halogenated compounds, such conjugation leads to toxic intermediates.

For carcinogenic saturated dihalo aliphatic compounds such as 1,2-dibromoethane, two metabolic routes have been identified. One occurs through oxidative dehalogenation, yielding haloalcohol, -aldehyde, and -acetic acid.[38] Another involves coupling with glutathione to yield a sulfur mustard analog which presumably would be an activated type of metabolite.[39,40] Similarly, during the metabolism of hexachlorobutadiene, the formation of a mercapturic acid via glutathione conjugation appeared to be an activating step,[41] but such conjugation led to detoxification of 1,3-dichloropropene.[42] The possible contribution of an epoxide or diepoxide for the dichloropropene, as formed during the metabolism of butadiene,[43] has not been delineated. The carcinogen 1,2-dibromo-3-chloropropane, formerly used as a nematocide, is similarly metabolized to an oxide, alcohols, aliphatic acids, and mercapturic acids.[44]

Although not generally considered as an aliphatic compound, an essential component of the pesticide DDT, or 1,1,1-trichloro-2,2-di(4-chlorophenyl)ethane, is the trichlorinated ethane moiety. DDT is metabolized by reductive dechlorinations or dehydrochlorinations to yield 1,1-dichloro-2,2-bis(4-chlorophenyl)ethane (TDE) and 1,1-dichloro-2,2-bis(4-chlorophenyl)ethylene (DDE). DDE is metabolized slowly through intermediates to 2,2-bis(4-chlorophenyl)ethylene, which is converted by the kidney to the corresponding aldehyde or acid. The acid is excreted readily as free material or as a conjugate with cholanic acid or amino acids. TDE is detoxified more rapidly to the same final products as DDE. However, there is no definitive evidence that DDT or its metabolites cause DNA damage or are mutagenic.[45] Thus, it has been suggested that these compounds may act as inhibitors of intercellular communication *in vivo* and are epigenetic carcinogens rather than genotoxic substances.[46]

The halogenated aliphatics thus represent a class of compounds in which a wide range of carcinogenic effects is noted. Some members, mainly 1,2-dibromoethane and 1,2-dibromo-3-chloropropane, are fairly potent carcinogens and appear to have genotoxic effects. Others, exemplified by DDT, are not so potent, require a long latent period, and may well be epigenetic rather than genotoxic.

## 2.2.2. Hydrazines and Azo and Azoxy Compounds

Hydrazine itself is carcinogenic, but the precise mechanism is unknown. The rapid diacetylation of hydrazine is probably a detoxification process,[47] but monomethylhydrazine is not formed metabolically. Administration of hydrazine leads to an increase in methylation of the guanine of DNA by a circuitous route.[48] The methyl carbon apparently is not derived by capture of the usual biologic methylating agent, S-adenosylmethionine, but through 5-methylcytosine.[49]

It has been proposed that hydrazine may react with endogenous formaldehyde to produce a hydrazone that could be oxidized metabolically to the methylating agent diazomethane.[50] Another possible condensation product of hydrazine and formaldehyde is tetraformyltrisazine; when administered to rats, there was greater methylation of guanine than with hydrazine itself.[51] However, further research on this interesting aspect of the metabolism of hydrazine is needed.

The alkyl derivatives of hydrazine are carcinogenic and 1,2-dimethylhydrazine is a useful model for induction of intestinal cancer in rats and mice.[52] Hydrazine derivatives also occur naturally in mushrooms and may be responsible for their unique effects in laboratory mice.[53]

The prototype, 1,2-dimethylhydrazine, is converted by microsomal oxidases to carcinogenic azomethane, which in turn is also oxidized to azoxymethane, itself an intestinal carcinogen in rats (cf. Fig. 1). Further oxidation affords the relatively unstable methylazoxymethanol, the glycoside of which is cycasin, a carcinogenic neurotoxin produced by the cycad plant.

Methylazoxymethanol might be considered analogous to hydroxymethylmethylnitrosamine, as it decomposes to formaldehyde and methyldiazonium ion, which yields nitrogen and the alkylating agent, methyl carbocation. By means of selective inhibitors of the various oxidation stages for 1,2-dimethylhydrazine, tumor formation can be suppressed.[54] For example, alcohol dehydrogenase is implicated in the metabolism of methylazoxymethanol in the target organ, the colon. Pyrazole, an inhibitor of the dehydrogenase, suppresses the carcinogenic effect of methylazoxymethanol in the colon.[55] The initial N-oxidation of dimethylhydrazine can be reduced by disulfiram, whereas it and a metabolite, carbon disulfide, suppress C oxidation. Thus, both compounds inhibit dimethylhydrazine-induced colon tumors. Alkyl hydrazines with longer or more complex aliphatic chains are handled in a similar fashion by the enzyme systems. Some hydrazine-derived drugs are procarbazine for treatment of cancers and certain amine oxidase inhibitors employed in treatment of depression. The use of the latter drugs should be kept to a minimum, if possible.

## 2.2.3. Nitrosamines

Nitrosamines constitute the most omnipotent carcinogens, for on a comparable basis, they have shown effects in more animal species than any other class of carcinogens.[56] Their metabolic interactions have been investigated thoroughly under varying physiologic conditions and both *in vitro* and *in vivo*. The prototype dialkylnitrosamine, i.e., dimethylnitrosamine, is oxidized by P-450 mono-oxygenase enzymes to an unstable hydroxymethylmethylnitrosamine. This intermediate fragments spontaneously to formaldehyde and nitrosomethylamine, which in turn forms a probable methyldiazonium hydroxide. This dissociates to nitrogen and the activated methyl carbocation which methylates proteins and nucleic acids (cf. Fig. 1). Isotopic studies have demonstrated that diazomethane is not an intermedate and that the initial hydroxylation is a rate-limiting step in tumor initiation.[57]

In part, due to the differing effects of various inducers or inhibitors of dimethylnitrosamine activation, it seems that two forms of dimethylnitrosamine dimethylase are functioning. One operates at low substrate concentrations, while the other is effective at high substrate concentrations. There also are studies that implicate amine oxidases in the metabolism of dimethylnitrosamine, while others point toward a soluble liver enzyme more akin to the enzyme metabolizing dimethylnitrosamine *in vivo*. Furthermore, removal of the nitroso group results in an appreciable amount of amines being produced.

The metabolic process is more complex with respect to dialkylnitrosamines with longer alkyl chains, for oxidation occurs on other carbons besides that in the α-position.[15,57] The prototype, dibutylnitrosamine, is oxidized on the terminal carbon to a hydroxy compound and then to a carboxylic acid. Both these compounds, as well as the parent nitrosamine, are bladder carcinogens in rats. Further oxidation on intermediate carbons may also occur, yielding various hydroxy and keto derivatives as well as shortening of the carbon chain. The significance of all these reactions has not been determined.

In the case of methylalkylnitrosamines, the metabolic pattern depends on the length of the alkyl chain and is analogous to that for fatty acid degradation.[15] Even numbered alkyl chains are degraded by two carbon fragments to a number of substances, including carboxy, hydroxy, and keto compounds. The nitrosamines with odd-numbered carbon chains are also metabolized to ω-carboxylic acids (with and without loss of one carbon) and to keto nitrosamines.

*N*-Nitrosomorpholine, a typical cyclic nitrosamine, is metabolized *in vitro* by rat liver microsomes to *N*-nitroso-2-hydroxymorpholine, in addition to the ring breakdown products acetaldehyde, formaldehyde, and glyoxal.[58] *In vivo*, nitrosomorpholine was metabolized by both α- and β-hydroxylation, but the α-hydroxylation pathway appeared to be the crucial one for activity. Urinary metabolites identified were (2-hydroxyethyl)acetic acid, *N*-nitrosodiethanolamine, and *N*-nitroso(2-hydroxyethyl) glycine. Although not isolated, the diazohydroxide from a ring-opened oxidation product was considered the likely activated intermediate.[59] There has also been extensive study of the metabolism of various cyclic nitrosamines found in tobacco.[60] With *N*-nitrosonornicotine, oxidation on the nitrogen at the 2'-, 5'- and β-carbons was observed, leading to many intermediates and end products.[61] Diazohydroxides, presumably the activated intermediates, were produced both *in vivo* and *in vitro*.[62]

A typical arylalkylnitrosamine, like nitrosomethylaniline, can be denitrosated as well as hydroxylated on the methyl group, yielding formaldehyde and benzenediazonium ion. Aryldiazonium ions are less reactive than the alkyl diazo compounds. Thus, specific reactions involved in the carcinogenic process have not been identified.[15]

## 2.3. Miscellaneous

Numerous other carcinogens which require metabolic activation may occur in the environment, either naturally or as synthetic materials used for specific purposes. Aflatoxin $B_1$, the carcinogenic substance produced by the fungus, *Aspergillus flavus*, presumably is activated metabolically through formation of an epoxide across the 2,3-double bond in the terminal furan ring. Attempts to synthesize or isolate the epoxide have not proved successful, owing to its reactivity. However, investigation of the major DNA and RNA adducts and the hydrolysis product from the RNA adduct, all led to the conclusion that the 2,3-epoxide was involved.[63]

Estragole and safrole are structurally similar natural products that cause liver tumors in mice. Hydroxylation on the 1'-carbon of the propenyl side chain, followed by esterification, by sulfate or by acetate, appeared to be the pathway involved.[64]

Ethyl carbamate or urethan, which causes lung tumors in mice, occurs naturally in products made by fermentation, but it is not used to make polyurethanes. Although N-hydroxylation occurred metabolically, N-hydroxyurethan was not more carcinogenic than the parent compound. Nevertheless, it reacted with nucleic acids and other cellular constituents. It was also more reactive than urethan in systems in which metabolism was suppressed. According to one concept, urethan is activated by metabolic dehydrogenation to vinyl carbamate, with subsequent epoxidation. Isolation of labeled vinyl chloride adducts, from hepatic RNA of mice given labeled urethan seems to support this view.[65]

Dioxane, at high doses, causes liver tumors in rats and guinea pigs. A metabolite has been identified, i.e., 1,4-dioxane-2-one, which is analogous to those resulting from α-oxidation of cyclic nitrosamines.[66] However, further efforts are needed to define more clearly the activated intermediate and its targets.

Pyrrolizidine alkaloids in general contain a long-chain necic acid bound at two points to a pyrrole ring. Only a few (retrosine, petastatine, senkirkine) have been tested, but animal tests of the plant materials from which they are derived, such as coltsfoot, comfrey, and ragworts, have shown these materials to be carcinogenic. These alkaloids are dehydrogenated to pyrrolic compounds that are quite reactive, leading to a redistribution of charges, a leaving group, and the formation of a carbonium ion or similar electrophile derived from the simple pyrrolic nucleus.[67-69] Reaction of one such pyrrole with nucleosides has been investigated. Microsomal metabolism of the pyrrolizidine alkaloid, senecionine, yielded a reactive aldehyde, *trans*-4-hydroxy-2-hexenal, which formed adducts with deoxyguanosine *in vitro*.[70] Not only the pyrrolic nucleus but also aliphatic compounds derived from oxidation of the remainder of the molecule may contribute to the toxic and carcinogenic effects of these alkaloids.

Another carcinogenic natural product is the bracken fern, the fiddleheads of which are eaten as a vegetable in some countries. Although it was suggested that quercetin or shikimic acid might be the substance responsible,[71] more recent investigations point toward ptaquiloside, a relatively unstable norsequiterpene glucoside, as the actual factor.[72] The metabolic interactions of ptaquiloside have not been investigated, but it is conceivable that the cyclopropane ring could open and attach to cellular macromolecules.

## 3. CLASSIFICATION OF CHEMICAL CARCINOGENS

There can be any number of systems to classify chemical carcinogens, based on the viewpoint and requirements of whoever does the classification. However, since this chapter is concerned with the metabolism of chemical carcinogens, a classification based roughly on the reactivity of the parent compound with cellular nucleophiles is employed.

## 3.1. Direct-Acting versus Indirect-Acting Carcinogens

### 3.1.1. Direct-Acting Carcinogens

For direct-acting carcinogens, the required structure to participate in key reactions is innate in the molecule so that generation of an electrophilic reagent by metabolism is not required. Typical examples are β-propiolactone, ethyleneimine, bis(chloromethyl)ether, nitrogen mustard and derivatives, bis(2-chloroethyl)sulfide, diepoxybutane, and propane sultone. However, metabolism may alter the physicochemical characteristics such that the molecule reaches the crucial cellular receptor more readily. An example is cyclophosphamide, which already contains the nitrogen mustard moiety, but it is further converted metabolically to phosphoramide mustard, which appears to be a better carrier to the target area, i.e., bladder in rats and lung in mice.[73,74]

Furthermore, compounds that are too reactive are not potent carcinogens, probably because they combine with water or may be inactivated metabolically before reaching cellular receptors. Compounds of intermediate reactivity appear to be more potent carcinogens *in vivo*. Reactivity constants for a series of alkylating agents and their initial mechanism of action, whether by a unimolecular ($S_N 1$) or a bimolecular ($S_N 2$) step, have been discussed.[75] Because of their inherent reactivity, most direct-acting carcinogens do not survive long enough to present an appreciable hazard to the general population.

### 3.1.2. Indirect-Acting Carcinogens

The indirect-acting compounds, sometimes called pro- or precarcinogens, are stable enough to exist in the environment, but they require metabolic activation before they can interact with cellular macromolecules. However, metabolism of such substances is not an isolated event. There are many factors including, but not limited to species, strain, sex, age, and diet, which influence the rates of metabolic reactions and their course. With respect to species, a study of metabolic pathways showed the guinea pig, which does not develop cancer if fed 2-acetylaminofluorene, lacks the N-hydroxylating enzyme or else destroys very rapidly any *N*-hydroxy-2-acetylaminofluorene formed. As a consequence, the guinea pig is nonresponsive in tests of aromatic amines or their precursors since this species does not N-hydroxylate such compounds. By contrast, rats, mice, and hamsters N-hydroxylate aromatic amines and are good models for such compounds. Some strains of mice do not respond appreciably to the PAH. The presence or absence of an Ah receptor, product of certain Ah (aryl hydrocarbon hydroxylase) regulatory genes, has been implicated.[76]

It is recognized that the responses of males and females to carcinogens and other xenobiotics often differ. Male rats are generally more susceptible to liver cancer from such compounds as 2-acetylaminofluorene. In part, this has been correlated with higher levels of sulfotransferase in the livers of males. However, the correlation is not absolute, for females develop tumors from 2-acetylaminofluorene in tissues having no discernible levels of sulfotransferase, where other activation mechanisms probably hold. In addition to mediating levels of certain enzymes, hormonal status may influence the progression of initiated cells after the original metabolic interactions, but little effort has been expended in this area.

Age is also a factor, as newborn or very young animals generally have low levels of the metabolizing enzymes that detoxify carcinogens or hasten their removal. As a consequence, young animals are often, but not always, more sensitive to carcinogens than are older animals. Diet is a major player in determining response to carcinogens that require metabolism. A diet lacking protein suppressed the metabolism and hepatotoxicity of dimethylnitrosamine in rats, only to have kidney tumors appear many months later. An explanation for the protective action of a riboflavin-containing diet against liver cancer from 4-dimethylaminoazobenzene was that the riboflavin functions as part of an enzyme system (azo reductase), which reduces the azo linkage. The two components thus formed lack carcinogenic activity. Selenium is a constituent of glutathione peroxidase; thus, sufficient selenium might be expected to decrease carcinogenicity if glutathione conjugation represents a detoxication pathway. Conversely, for those carcinogens wherein glutathione conjugation leads to an active intermediate, selenium may increase the effect. There has been an upsurge of interest in diet and carcinogenicity within the past few years,[77] but the metabolic consequences of various recommended dietary regimens have not been exactly delineated.

Overall, the metabolism of indirect-acting or procarcinogens to the activated intermediates can be altered at various points. Systematic study of these reactions may aid eventually in suppressing the effects of carcinogens in persons known to have been exposed.

### 3.1.3. Secondary Effects

Since the testing of compounds for carcinogenicity by intravesical administration is no longer favored, there are fewer situations in which tumors due to secondary effects may arise. The rodent bladder appears especially sensitive with respect to manipulation, the presence of foreign bodies, and other factors. Repeated exposures to water or physiologic saline solution have led to lesions that microscopically resembled bladder papillomas or carcinomas.[78] Metabolism of xenobiotics to oxalates or similar substances that act as a base for bladder calculi has led to labeling of the original compound administered as a carcinogen. Male rats appeared more likely to develop calculi and subsequently bladder tumors. However, when urinary pH was altered by giving ammonium chloride, bladder calculi did not form.[79]

Although feeding rats 2-phenylphenol at levels up to 2% of the diet did not induce tumors, feeding the sodium salt led to bladder tumors, especially in male rats. A metabolic study showed that males excreted seven times more of the glucuronide of 2,5-dihydroxybiphenyl, which was readily converted to a cytotoxic quinone.[80] The combination of cytotoxicity plus the bladder calculi noted in the males may have contributed to the outcome, as well as the effect of the sodium salt on the osmolarity of the bladder membranes. In addition, when one organ affects another through a feedback mechanism, for example, liver and thyroid or thyroid and pituitary, an imbalance in one can lead to a tumor in the other.

Before the advent of barrier-derived laboratory animals, the presence of parasites furthered development of tumors or hyperplastic conditions that resembled tumors, especially of the bladder or liver.[79] The combination of better animals and more attention to sanitation in most bioassays has decreased the possibility of finding such effects.

## 3.2. Genotoxic versus Epigenetic Carcinogens

To the researcher interested in the mechanisms of chemical carcinogenesis, the stages in the process, and the possibility of intervening in these stages, a distinction between genotoxic and epigenetic carcinogens is logical. To the person who has developed a tumor because of exposure to some substance, there is no distinction, as the end result is a carcinogen.

To be genotoxic, a carcinogen either reacts as such or is converted to a reactive substance that interacts covalently with the genetic material of the cell, especially DNA. Epigenetic carcinogens do not form such reactive intermediates and do not react with DNA. However, the difference becomes less distinct for many compounds that form reactive metabolites but that do not bind appreciably to DNA, including some of the carcinogenic halogenated compounds discussed previously. Although 1,2-dibromoethane binds covalently to DNA,[81] several other halogenated compounds do not bind to any appreciable extent. Nonetheless, they caused tumors when administered to animals.

Immunosuppressants, hormones, and solid-state materials (plastic films, fibers) are also generally considered epigenetic carcinogens. Definitely relevant is the discovery that an appreciable number of hypolipidemic drugs and phthalate ester plasticizers are neither mutagenic nor DNA damaging. Nevertheless, they induced liver tumors in rats and mice.[82] As research in these areas continues, the concept may change if details of the interactions of these epigenetic carcinogens can be delineated.

Relationship between Carcinogenicity and Mutagenicity

There is less enthusiasm than previously for relying entirely on mutagenicity tests in classifying a chemical as a carcinogen. Data from many studies have shown that these tests are not totally accurate or specific. One compilation indicates correlations ranging from 6 to 94%, with an average for carcinogenic mutagens of about 90%.[83] Other surveys also showed a relatively wide range in response.[84–86] Since mutagenicity tests can be conducted in bacteria, yeasts, molds, *Drosophila*, and various types of cells in culture as well as in animals, the variation in degree of correlation is plausible. The International Agency for Research on Cancer has evaluated most of the short-term screening assays for carcinogens and has commented on the shortcomings of both the test systems and the lists of compounds in which these systems were applied.[87] Some substances did not respond well, notably some chlorinated hydrocarbons and phthalate esters. Nevertheless, compounds of these types did cause tumors in animals. Thus, the accuracy of mutagenicity tests in predicting carcinogenicity is questionable if applied for all types of structures. For selected groups of compounds, the correlation may be in the order of 90–95%.

## 3.3. Initiators and Promoters

Initiators are compounds with the capability of causing an irreversible alteration in the cell genome. The process is probably rapid but permanent. Since the concept of initiation and promotion was originally developed with experiments from painting of carcinogens on the skins of mice, the first compounds so classified were the PAH such as benzo(a)pyrene. More recent investigations have shown that the concept of initiation can be applied to other organ systems as well, including thyroid, liver, kidney, lungs, colon, and pancreas. The molecular and cellular events involved in initiation have been discussed.[88]

Promoters, by causing clonal expansion of the initiated cells, increase the response when applied after the particular carcinogen. They are noncarcinogenic or have only a weak effect when applied by themselves. Promoters do not bind to DNA, are not mutagenic, and their effects are reversible. The most famous of the promoters is phorbol myristate acetate (PMA), now called 12-O-tetradecanoylphorbol-13-acetate, or TPA, originally isolated from the oil from the seeds of the plant *Croton tiglium*. Other natural materials, i.e., mezerein, teleocidin from *Streptomyces mediocidicus*, and lyngbyatoxin from the alga *Lyngbya majuscula*, also act as promoters.[89] Similarly, dodecane, phenol, and anthralin are promoters. Many theories have been proposed to explain the action of promoters; these range from induction of ornithine decarboxylase to inhibition of intercellular communication.[90]

A mouse model experiment has shown that the promoter could be given as late as 1 year after an initiator and that the incidence of tumors that developed was similar to that in mice treated with a promoter shortly after the initiator. The implications are that a person could be exposed to an initiator of some sort, remain tumor-free for an extended period, and then be exposed to some environmental promoter with subsequent tumor development.

Cocarcinogens are not active alone but enhance the action of a carcinogen when applied along with that substance. Prominent examples are smoking along with asbestos exposure, catechol plus the carcinogens in tobacco smoke, or ethanol along with smoking.

It is obvious that there can be almost unlimited possibilities for interaction between carcinogens, and promoters, or cocarcinogens. Knowledge of these factors may increase the opportunities for intervention in the process of carcinogenesis.

## 4. STRUCTURE–ACTIVITY RELATIONSHIPS

Although the rules of the game of structure–activity relationships are constantly changing as new data become available, they change slowly because of the relatively long time required for completion of animal bioassays. In addition, it must be remembered that the principles outlined are only guidelines and are not entirely accurate in predicting the carcinogenicity of a molecule.

Both physicochemical properties and the chemical structure of a substance should be considered.[91] The physicochemical properties help determine the ability to reach a target cell. High-molecular-weight compounds are usually not absorbed in the mammalian organism and generally do not present a carcinogenic risk unless they are degraded in the gastrointestinal tract by hydrolysis or bacterial action.

The physical state is important, as volatile or dusty compounds can be inhaled and present a risk. Compounds that are soluble due to the presence of hydrophilic groups often are not well absorbed or are conjugated and excreted readily if absorbed, decreasing risk. Furthermore, very reactive substances may hydrolyze, polymerize, or react with noncritical constituents such as body water before reaching a target tissue.

As for structural characteristics, there have been many treatises on the correlations between them and carcinogenicity in one animal system or the other. Therefore, only a summary of some of these principles is presented.

1. *Alkylating agents:* Alkylating agents are suspect because they usually are activated without the need for metabolic interaction. Groups such as epoxy, aziridinyl, strained lactones or sultones, α-haloethers, nitrogen or sulfur mustards, or esters with good leaving groups are usually suspect. Substituents can have fairly substantial effects, probably because they mediate the initial reaction and permit better access to the target tissue.

2. *Aromatic amines or their precursors (nitro compounds) and amino azo dyes:* Such compounds are suspect if the amino or precursor nitro group is in the most reactive position of the molecule or on the terminal carbon atom of the longest conjugated chain of the molecule. Examples are the 2-position of naphthalene, anthracene, and fluorene and the 4- and 4'-positions of biphenyl or stilbene. Additional substituents may increase or decrease the effect relative to the unsubstituted amine. Generally, the addition of OH, COOH, $SO_3H$, or I sometimes decreases carcinogenicity, while $CH_3$, $OCH_3$, F, Cl, or Br (in certain positions) may enhance activity. The heterocyclic analogues (N, O, or S) of many aromatic amines may also be carcinogenic (cf. Fig. 2).

Amino azo dyes follow much the rules for aromatic amines, and addition of substituents may have substantial effects on activity. In addition, if the azo dye is derived from benzidine or analogues, intestinal bacteria can reduce the azo linkage so the carcinogen benzidine, or its analog, is produced. Exceptions can occur if bulky substituents are in the ortho-positions to the azo linkage.

3. *Aromatic hydrocarbons:* An aromatic hydrocarbon generally is not carcinogenic until it contains four to five polycyclic rings, arranged in a nonlinear fashion with an optimal size range (area) of 100 to 135 nm². The effect of substituents such as $CH_3$ groups can be quite dramatic. Heterocyclic (N, S) analogues of carcinogenic aromatic hydrocarbons are often active.

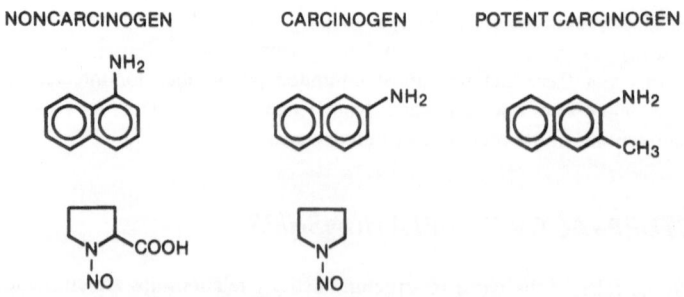

*Figure 2.* Illustration of variations in structure that can alter carcinogenicity. The upper structures represent various naphthylamines, while the lower ones are nitrosoproline and nitrosopyrolidine.

4. *N-Nitroso compounds R(Ar)R'NNO:* Only a few of the more than 200 N-nitroso compounds that have been tested are not carcinogenic. Thus, compounds in which R and R' vary or are the same are suspect. N-Nitroso heterocyclics are often more potent than dialkyl nitroso compounds of comparable molecular weight. Since most dialkylnitroso compounds are activated by oxidation at the α-carbon, if this position is hindered sterically or electronically, or if highly hydrophilic groups are also present in the molecule, the compound may not be a carcinogen. N-Nitrosoureas are under suspicion because metabolic intervention is not required. Some of these compounds affect relatively unusual sites in the animal, such as the nervous system. However, addition of a long aliphatic chain moderates the activity somewhat or alters the site of attack.

5. *Aliphatic hydrazines, azo and azoxy compounds, aryldialkyltriazenes:* Most aliphatic hydrazine derivatives as well as azoalkanes and azoxyalkanes are carcinogenic, especially in mice. Variations in the alkyl groups may alter the site of activity but do not necessarily render the molecule noncarcinogenic. As with other types of carcinogens, substitution by a polar moiety may decrease the activity of a triazene.

Other types of compounds besides those mentioned have exhibited carcinogenic activity. However, the guidelines are less specific for these compounds.

## 5. RELEVANCE TO HUMANS

Most environmental carcinogens are metabolized by mammalian enzymes to activated forms. These enzymes are also present in humans; studies both in exposed persons and in human cells or tissues have shown that the activation pathways observed experimentally occur in humans. In addition, binding of the activated carcinogens to DNA also occurs, and the adducts are the same as found in experimental animals.[92] As a consequence, it appears prudent to treat an animal carcinogen as if it presented a carcinogenic risk to humans, unless proved otherwise. This assumption is strengthened by the fact that all recognized human carcinogens also cause cancer in animals, if tested appropriately. By contrast, some animal carcinogens, such as formaldehyde or saccharin, have not shown evidence of an effect in humans as indicated by several large-scale epidemiologic studies of exposed persons.[93,94] Perhaps the irritating effect of formaldehyde automatically causes people to avoid exposure, which the experimental animals could not do.

However, since it has become impossible to remove all carcinogens from the environment, risk analysis is now used to estimate the risk of cancer from human exposure to very low levels of some animal carcinogens.[95] A risk of $1 \times 10^{-6}$ (1 : 1,000,000) or less is considered societally an acceptable level of risk. These procedures have been applied to estimate the risk from various situations such as chloroform in drinking water and di(ethylhexyl)phthalate in plastics.[96] The risk of developing cancer from the usual low exposure to these compounds is less than that of having an automobile accident. Analyses as those mentioned may aid in bringing a more rational approach to the problem of environmental exposure to various substances and the risk of cancer.

### 5.1. Recognized Human Carcinogens

The International Agency for Research on Cancer (IARC) has evaluated short-term animal and human data on many compounds and has categorized them into recognized human carcinogens, probable human carcinogens, and compounds for which there is insufficient evidence.[97] Several industrial processes associated with a higher risk of cancer have been included as well. However, since manufacturing processes and conditions change, the actual substances responsible have often not been identified.

The compounds recognized as human carcinogens include industrial intermediates, chemotherapeutic agents, metals or their salts, and a mineral fiber. As a result of various regulations,[98] some of the compounds on the IARC list are no longer used in many countries. Others continue to be

### Table I. Recognized Human Carcinogens

4-Aminobiphenyl

Analgesic mixtures containing phenacetin

Arsenic and certain arsenic compounds

Asbestos

Azathioprine

Benzene

Benzidine

N,N-Bis(2-chlorethyl)-2-naphthylamine (chlornaphazine)

Bis(chloromethyl)ether and technical-grade chloromethyl methyl ether

1,4-Butanediol dimethylsulfonate (Myleran)

Certain combined chemotherapy for lymphomas

Chlorambucil

Chromium and certain chromium compounds

Coke oven emissions

Conjugated estrogens

Cyclophosphamide

Diethylstilbestrol

Melphalan

Methoxsalen with ultraviolet A therapy (PUVA)

Mustard gas

2-Naphthylamine

Nickel refining

Thorium dioxide

Vinyl chloride

important intermediates, but the exposure limits have been lowered. Still others are chemotherapeutic agents for which the benefit versus the risk to the patient must be considered (Table I).

Overall, the process of carcinogenesis in humans probably parallels that in animals. Thus, continued high exposure to compounds that are animal carcinogens may well lead to cancer in humans. However, there may not be an absolute correlation, as there are species differences in response to xenobiotics. A balanced approach is needed in extrapolating data from compounds causing cancer in animals to the human situation.

## REFERENCES

1. Miller, E. C. and Miller, J. A., 1981, Mechanisms of chemical carcinogenesis, *Cancer* **47**:1055–1064.
2. Garner, R. C., Martin, C. N., and Clayson, D. B., 1984, Carcinogenic aromatic agents and related compounds, in: *Chemical Carcinogens*, 2nd ed. (C. E. Searle, ed.), pp. 175–276, ACS Monograph 182, American Chemical Society, Washington, D. C.
3. Radomski, J. L., 1979, The primary aromatic amines: Their biological properties and structure–activity relationships, *Annu. Rev. Pharmacol. Toxicol.* **19**:129–157.
4. Kiese, M., 1959, Oxydation von Anilin zu Nitrosobenzol im Hunde, *Naunyn-Schmiedebergs Arch. Pharmakol. Exp. Pathol.* **235**:354–359.
5. Weisburger, J. H., and Weisburger, E. K., 1973, Biochemical formation and pharmacological, toxicological, and pathological properties of hydroxylamines and hydroxamic acids, *Pharmacol. Rev.* **25**:1–66.
6. Nebert, D. W., Eisen, H. J., Negishi, M., Lang, M. A., and Hjelmeland, L. M., 1981, Genetic mechanisms controlling the induction of polysubstrate monooxygenase (P-450) activities, *Annu. Rev. Pharmacol. Toxicol.* **21**:431–462.
7. Thorgeirsson, S. S., Sanderson, N., Park, S. S., and Gelboin, H. V., 1983, Inhibition of 2-acetylaminofluorene oxidations by monoclonal antibodies specific to 3-methylcholanthrene-induced rat liver cytochrome P450, *Carcinogenesis* **4**:639–641.
8. Gram, T. E., Okine, L. K., and Gram, R. A., 1986, The metabolism of xenobiotics by certain extrahepatic organs and its relation to toxicity, *Annu. Rev. Pharmacol. Toxicol.* **26**:259–291.
9. Weisburger, J. H., and Williams, G. M., 1982, Metabolism of chemical carcinogens, in: *Cancer: A Comprehensive Treatise*, 2nd ed. (F. F. Becker, ed.), pp. 241–333, Plenum, New York.
10. Boyd, J. A., Harvan, D. J., and Eling, T. E., 1983, The oxidation of 2-aminofluorene by prostaglandin endoperoxide synthetase, *J. Biol. Chem.* **258**:8246–8254.
11. Wise, R. W., Zenser, T. V., Kadlubar, F. F., and Davis, B. B., 1984, Metabolic activation of carcinogenic aromatic amines by dog bladder and kidney prostaglandin H synthase, *Cancer Res.* **44**:1893–1897.

12. King, C. M., and Weber, W. W., 1981, Formation, metabolic activation by $N,O$-acyltransfer, and hydrolysis of $N$-acyl-$N$-arylamine derivatives, *Natl. Cancer Inst. Monog.* **58**:117–122.
13. Ritter, C. L., Malejka-Giganti, D., and Polnaszek, C. F., 1983, Cytochrome c/$H_2O_2$-mediated one electron oxidation of carcinogenic $N$-fluorenylacetohydroxamic acids to nitroxyl free radicals, *Chem. Biol. Interact.* **46**:317–334.
14. Malejka-Giganti, D., Ritter, C. L., Decker, R. W., and Suilman, J. M., 1986, Peroxidative metabolism of a carcinogen, $N$-hydroxy-$N$-2-fluorenylacetamide, by rat uterus and mammary gland *in vitro, Cancer Res.* **46**:6200–6206.
15. Dipple, A., Michejda, C. J., and Weisburger, E. K., 1985, Metabolism of chemical carcinogens, *Pharmacol. Ther.* **27**:265–296.
16. Corcoran, G. B., Mitchell, J. R., Vaishnav, Y. N., and Horning, E. C., 1980, Evidence that acetaminophen and $N$-hydroxyacetaminophen form a common arylating metabolite, $N$-acetyl-$p$-benzoquinoneimine, *Mol. Pharmacol.* **18**:536–542.
17. Kadlubar, F. F., and Beland, F. A., 1985, Chemical properties of ultimate carcinogenic metabolites of arylamines and arylamides, in: *Polycyclic Hydrocarbons and Carcinogenesis* (R. G. Harvey, ed.), pp. 341–370, *ACS Symposium Series 283*, American Chemical Society, Washington, D. C.
18. Pullman, A., and Pullman, B., 1955, Electronic structure and carcinogenic activity of aromatic molecules. New developments, *Adv. Cancer Res.* **3**:117–169.
19. Dipple, A., Moschel, R. C., and Bigger, C. A. H., 1984, Polynuclear aromatic carcinogens, in: *Chemical Carcinogens*, 2nd ed. (C. E. Searle, ed.), ACS Monograph 182, pp. 41–163, American Chemical Society, Washington, D. C.
20. Harvey, R. G., 1985, Synthesis of the dihydrodiol and diol epoxide metabolites of carcinogenic polycyclic hydrocarbons, in: *Polycyclic Hydrocarbons and Carcinogenesis*, (R. G. Harvey, ed.), pp. 35–62, ACS Symposium Series 283, American Chemical Society, Washington, D. C.
21. Levin, W., Wood, A., Chang, R., Ryan, D., Thomas, P., Yagi, H., Thakker, D., Vyas, K., Boyd, C., Chu, S.-Y., Conney, A., and Jerina, D., 1982, Oxidative metabolism of polycyclic aromatic hydrocarbons to ultimate carcinogens, *Drug Met. Rev.* **13**:555–580.
22. Robertson, I. G. C., and Jernstrom, B., 1986, The enzymatic conjugation of glutathione with bay-region diol-epoxides of benzo[a]pyrene, benz[a]anthracene and chrysene, *Carcinogenesis* **7**:1633–1636.
23. Pitts. J. N., Jr., Lokensgard, D. M., Ripley, P. S., Cauwenberghe, K. A., Van Vaeck, L., Shaffer, S. D., Thill, A. J., and Belser, W. L., Jr., 1980, Atmospheric epoxidation of benzo[a]pyrene by ozone: Formation of the metabolite benzo[a]pyrene-4,5-oxide, *Science* **210**:1347–1349.
24. Gelboin, H. V., 1980, Benzo[a]pyrene metabolism, activation and carcinogenesis: Role and regulation of mixed function oxidases and related enzymes, *Physiol. Rev.* **60**:1107–1166.
25. Cavalieri, E. L., and Rogan, E. G., 1985, One-electron oxidation in aromatic hydrocarbon carcinogenesis, in: *Polycyclic Hydrocarbons and Carcinogenesis* (R. G. Harvey, ed.), ACS Symposium Series 283, pp. 289–305, American Chemical Society, Washington, D. C.
26. Marnett, L. J., 1985, Hydroperoxide-dependent oxygenation of polycyclic aromatic hydrocarbons and their metabolites, in: *Polycyclic Hydrocarbons and Carcinogenesis*, (R. G. Harvey, ed.), ACS Symposium Series 283, pp. 307–326, American Chemical Society, Washington, D. C.
27. Flesher, J. W., Stansbury, K. H., and Sydnor, K. L., 1982, S-Adenosyl-L-methionine is a carbon donor in the conversion of benzo[a]pyrene to 6-hydroxymethylbenzo[a]pyrene by rat liver S-9, *Cancer Lett.* **16**:91–94.
28. Flesher, J. W., Myers, S. R., Bergo, C. H., and Blake, J. W., 1986, Bioalkylation of dibenz[a,h]anthracene in rat liver cytosol, *Chem. Biol. Interact.* **57**:223–233.
29. Anders, M. W., Kubic, V. L., and Ahmed, A. E., 1977, Metabolism of halogenated methanes and macromolecular binding, *J. Environ. Pathol. Toxicol.* **1**:117–124.
30. Ahmed, A. E., and Anders, M. W., 1978, Metabolism of dihalomethanes to formaldehyde and inorganic halide. II. Studies on the mechanism of the reaction, *Biochem. Pharmacol.* **27**:2021–2025.
31. Gargas, M. L., Clewell, H. J. III, and Andersen, M. E., 1986, Metabolism of inhaled dihalomethanes *in vivo:* Differentiation of kinetic constants for two independent pathways, *Toxicol. Appl. Pharmacol.* **82**:211–223.
32. Bolt, H. M., Laib, R. J., Peter, H., and Ottenwalder, H., 1986, DNA adducts of halogenated hydrocarbons, *J. Cancer Res. Clin. Oncol.* **112**:92–96.
33. Davidson, I. W. F., Sumner, D. D., and Parker, J. C., 1982, Chloroform: A review of its metabolism, teratogenic, mutagenic, and carcinogenic potential, *Drug Chem. Toxicol.* **5**:1–87.
34. Bartsch, H., Malavielle, C., Barbin, A., and Planche, G., 1979, Mutagenic and alkylating metabolites of haloethylenes, chlorobutadienes and dichlorobutenes produced by rodent or human liver tissues: Evidence for oxirane formation by P450-linked microsomal mono-oxygenases, *Arch. Toxicol.* **41**:249–277.

35. Miller, R., and Guengerich, F. P., 1982, Oxidation of TCE by liver microsomal cytochrome P-450: Evidence of chlorine migration in a transition state not involving trichloroethylene oxide, *Biochemistry* **21**:1090–1097.
36. Dekant, W., Metzler, M., and Henschler, D., 1986, Identification of S-1,2,2-trichlorovinyl-N-acetylcysteine as a urinary metabolite of tetrachloroethylene: Bioactivation through glutathione conjugation as a possible explanation of its nephrotoxicity, *J. Biochem. Toxicol.* **1**:57–72.
37. Chellman, G. J., White, R. D., Norton, R. M., and Bus, J. S., 1986, Inhibition of the acute toxicity of methyl chloride in male B6C3F$_1$ mice by glutathione depletion, *Toxicol. Appl. Pharmacol.* **86**:93–104.
38. Hill, D. L., Shih, T.-W., Johnston, T. P., and Struck, R. F., 1978, Macromolecular binding and metabolism of the carcinogen 1,2-dibromoethane, *Cancer Res.* **38**:2438–2442.
39. van Bladeren, P. J., Breimer, D. D., Rotteveel-Smigs, G. M. T., de Knijff, P., Mohn, G. R., van Meeteren-Walchli, B., Buijs, W., and van der Gen, A., 1981, The relation between the structure of vicinal dihalogen compounds and their mutagenic activation *via* conjugation of glutathione, *Carcinogenesis* **2**:499–505.
40. Ozawa, N., and Guengerich, F. P., 1983, Evidence for formation of an S-[2-(N$^7$-guanyl)ethyl]glutathione adduct in glutathione-mediated binding of the carcinogen 1,2-dibromoethane to DNA, *Proc. Natl. Acad. Sci. USA* **80**:5266–5270.
41. Reichert, D., and Schutz, S., 1986, Mercapturic acid formation is an activation and intermediary step in the metabolism of hexachlorobutadiene, *Biochem. Pharmacol.* **35**:1271–1275.
42. Climie, I. J. G., Hutson, D. H., Morrison, B. J., and Stoydin, G., 1979, Glutathione conjugation in the detoxification of (Z)-1,3-dichloropropene (a component of the nematocide D-D) in the rat, *Xenobiotica* **9**:149–156.
43. Bond, J. A., Dahl, A. R., Henderson, R. F., Dutcher, J. S., Mauderly, J. L., and Birnbaum, L. S., 1986, Species differences in the disposition of inhaled butadiene, *Toxicol. Appl. Pharmacol.* **84**:617–627.
44. Kluwe, W. M., Gupta, B. N., and Lamb, J. C., IV., 1983, The comparative effects of 1,2-dibromo-3-chloropropane (DBCP) and its metabolites, 3-chloro-1,2-propaneoxide (epichlorohydrin), 3-chloro-1,2-propanediol (alphachlorohydrin), and oxalic acid, upon the urogenital system of male rats, *Toxicol. Appl. Pharmacol.* **70**:67–86.
45. International Agency for Research on Cancer, 1974, *IARC Monographs on the Evaluation of Carcinogenic Risk of Chemicals to Man. Some Organochlorine Pesticides*, Vol. 5, pp. 83–124, IARC, Lyons, France.
46. Williams, G. M., 1981, An epigenetic mechanism of carcinogenicity of organochlorine pesticides, in: *Toxicology of Halogenated Hydrocarbons. Health and Ecological Effects* (M. A. Q. Khan and R. H. Stanton, eds.), pp. 161–170, Pergamon, New York.
47. Colvin, L. B., 1969, Metabolic fate of hydrazines and hydrazides, *J. Pharm. Sci.* **58**:1433–1443.
48. Bosan, W. S., and Shank, R. C., 1983, Methylation of liver DNA guanine in hamsters given hydrazine, *Toxicol. Appl. Pharmacol.* **70**:324–334.
49. Shank, R. C., 1984, Toxicity-induced aberrant methylation of DNA and its repair, *Pharmacol. Rev.* **36**:19S–24S.
50. Bosan, W. S., Lambert, C. E., and Shank, R. C., 1986, The role of formaldehyde in hydrazine-induced methylation of liver DNA guanine, *Carcinogenesis* **7**:413–418.
51. Lambert, C. E., Bosan, W. S., and Shank, R. C., 1986, Tetraformyltrisazine and hydrazine-induced methylation of liver DNA guanine, *Carcinogenesis* **7**:419–422.
52. Zedeck, M. S., 1984, Hydrazine derivatives, azo and azoxy compounds, and methylazoxymethanol and cycasin, in: *Chemical Carcinogens*, 2nd ed. (C. E. Searle, ed.), ACS Monograph 182, pp. 915–944, American Chemical Society, Washington, D. C.
53. Toth, B., and Erickson, J., 1986, Cancer induction in mice by feeding of the uncooked cultivated mushroom of commerce *Agaricus bisporus*, *Cancer Res.* **46**:4007–4011.
54. Wattenberg, L. W., 1978, Inhibitors of chemical carcinogenesis, *Adv. Cancer Res.* **26**:197–226.
55. Fiala, E. S., Kulakis, C., Christiansen, G., and Weisburger, J. H., 1978, Inhibition of the metabolism of the colon carcinogen, azoxymethane, by pyrazole, *Cancer Res.* **38**:4515–4521.
56. Lijinsky, W., 1986, The significance of N-nitroso compounds as environmental carcinogens, *J. Environ. Sci. Health* **C4**:1–45.
57. Preussmann, R., and Stewart, B. W., 1984, N-Nitroso carcinogens, in: *Chemical Carcinogens*, 2nd ed. (C. E. Searle, ed.), ACS Monograph 182, pp. 643–828, American Chemical Society, Washington, D. C.
58. Jarman, M., and Manson, D., 1986, The metabolism of N-nitrosomorpholine by rat liver microsomes and its oxidation by the Fenton system, *Carcinogenesis*, **7**:559–565.
59. Hecht, S. S., and Young, R., 1981, Metabolic α-hydroxylation of N-nitrosomorpholine and 3,3,5,5-tetradeutero-N-nitrosomorpholine in the F344 rat, *Cancer Res.* **41**:5039–5043.

60. Hoffmann, D., and Hecht, S. S., 1985, Nicotine-derived *N*-nitrosamines and tobacco-related cancer: Current status and future directions, *Cancer Res.* **45**:935–944.

61. Hecht, S. S., Castonguay, A., Rivenson, A., Mu, B., and Hoffmann, D., 1983, Tobacco specific nitrosamines: Carcinogenicity, metabolism, and possible role in human cancer, *J. Environ. Sci. Health* **C1**:1–54.

62. Hecht, S. S., Trushin, N., Castonguay, A., and Rivenson, A., 1986, Comparative tumorigenicity and DNA methylation in F344 rats by 4-(methylnitrosamino)-1-(3-pyridyl)-1-butanone and *N*-nitroso-dimethylamine, *Cancer Res.* **46**:498–502.

63. Busby, W. F., Jr., and Wogan, G. N., 1984, Aflatoxins, in: *Chemical Carcinogens*, 2nd ed. (C. E. Searle, ed.), ACS Monograph 182, pp. 945–1136, American Chemical Society, Washington, D. C.

64. Wiseman, R. W., Fennell, T. R., Miller, J. A., and Miller, E. C., 1985, Further characterization of the DNA adducts formed by electrophilic esters of the hepatocarcinogens 1'-hydroxysafrole and 1'-hydroxyestragole *in vitro* and in mouse liver *in vivo*, including new adducts at C-8 and N-7 of guanine residues, *Cancer Res.* **45**:3096–3105.

65. Ribovich, M. L., Miller, J. A., Miller, E. C., and Timmins, L. G., 1982, Labeled 1,$N^6$-ethenoadenosine and 3,$N^4$-ethenocytidine in hepatic RNA of mice given [ethyl-1,2$^3$H or ethyl-1-$^{14}$C]ethyl carbamate (urethan), *Carcinogenesis* **3**:539–546.

66. Woo, Y.-T., Argus, M. F., and Arcos, J. C., 1978, Effect of mixed-function oxidase modifiers on metabolism and toxicity of the oncogen dioxane, *Cancer Res.* **38**:1621–1625.

67. Styles, J., Ashby, J., and Mattocks, A. R., 1980, Evaluation *in vitro* of several pyrrolizidine alkaloid carcinogens: Observations on the essential pyrrolic nucleus, *Carcinogenesis* **1**:161–164.

68. Robertson, K. A., 1982, Alkylation of $N^2$ in deoxyguanosine by dehydroretronecine, a carcinogenic metabolite of the pyrrolizidine alkaloid monocrotaline, *Cancer Res.* **42**:8–14.

69. Wickramanayake, P. P., Arbogast, B. L., Buhler, D. R., Deinzer, M. L., and Burlingame, A. L., 1985, Alkylation of nucleosides and nucleotides by dehydroretronecine; characterization of covalent adducts by liquid secondary ion mass spectrometry, *J. Am. Chem. Soc.* **107**:2485–2488.

70. Winter, C. K., Segall, H. J., and Haddon, W. F., 1986, Formation of cyclic adducts of deoxyguanosine with the aldehydes *trans*-4-hydroxy-2-hexenal and *trans*-4-hydroxy-2-nonenal *in vitro*, *Cancer Res.* **46**:5682–5686.

71. Evans, I. A., 1984, Bracken carcinogenicity, in: *Chemical Carcinogens*, 2nd ed. (C. E. Searle, ed.), ACS Monograph 182, pp. 1171–1204, American Chemical Society, Washington, D. C.

72. Hirono, I., 1985, Recent advances in research on bracken carcinogen and carcinogenicity of betel nut, *J. Environ. Sci. Health* **C3**:145–187.

73. Mehta, J. R., Przybylski, M., and Ludlum, D. B., 1980, Alkylation of guanosine and deoxyguanosine by phosphoramide mustard, *Cancer Res.* **40**:4183–4186.

74. Hemminki, K., 1985, Binding of metabolites of cyclophosphamide to DNA in a rat liver microsomal system and in vivo in mice, *Cancer Res.* **45**:4237–4243.

75. Lawley, P. D., 1984, Carcinogenesis by alkylating agents, in: *Chemical Carcinogens*, 2nd ed. (C. E. Searle, ed.), ACS Monograph 182, pp. 325–484, American Chemical Society, Washington, D. C.

76. Nebert, D. W., and Jensen, N. M., 1979, The Ah locus: Genetic regulation of the metabolism of carcinogens, drugs, and other environmental chemicals by cytochrome P-450-mediated monooxygenases, *CRC Crit. Rev. Biochem.* **8**:401–437.

77. National Research Council, 1982, *Diet, Nutrition and Cancer*, National Academy Press, Washington, D. C.

78. Akaza, H., Murphy, W. M., and Soloway, M. S., 1984, Bladder cancer induced by noncarcinogenic substances, *J. Urol.* **131**:152–155.

79. Clayson, D. B., 1974, Bladder carcinogenesis in rats and mice: Possibility of artifacts, *J. Natl. Cancer Inst.* **52**:1685–1689.

80. Hagiwara, A., Shibata, M., Hirase, M., Fukushima, S., and Ito, N., 1984, Long-term toxicity and carcinogenicity study of sodium *o*-phenylphenate in B6C3F₁ mice, *Fd. Chem. Toxicol.* **22**:809–814.

81. Inskeep, P. B., Koga, N., Cmarik, J. L., and Guengerich, F. P., 1986, Covalent binding of 1,2-dihaloalkanes to DNA and stability of the major DNA adduct, S-[2-($N^7$-guanyl)ethyl]glutathione, *Cancer Res.* **46**:2839–2844.

82. Goel, S. K., Lalwani, N. D., and Reddy, J. K., 1986, Peroxisome proliferation and lipid peroxidation in rat liver, *Cancer Res.* **46**:1324–1330.

83. Brusick, D., 1987, *Principles of Genetic Toxicology*, Plenum, New York.

84. Brown, M. M., Wasson, J. S., Malling, H. V., Shelby, M. D., and Von Halle, E. S., 1979, Literature survey of bacterial, fungal, and *Drosophila* assay systems used in the evaluation of selected chemical compounds for mutagenic activity, *J. Natl. Cancer Inst.* **62**:841–871.

85. Rosenkranz, H. S., and Poirier, L. A., 1979, Evaluation of the mutagenicity and DNA-modifying activity of carcinogens and noncarcinogens in microbial systems, *J. Natl. Cancer Inst.* **62:**873–892.

86. Poirier, L. A., and deSerres, F. J., 1979, Initial National Cancer Institute studies on mutagenesis as a prescreen for chemical carcinogens: An appraisal, *J. Natl. Cancer Inst.* **62:**919–926.

87. International Agency for Research on Cancer, 1980, *Long-term and Short-term Screening Assays for Carcinogens: A Critical Appraisal,* IARC Monograph Supplement 2, IARC, Lyons, France.

88. Weinstein, I. B., Yamasaki, H., Wigler, M., Lee, L.-S., Fisher, P. B., Jeffrey, A., and Grunberger, D., 1979, Molecular and cellular events associated with the action of initiating carcinogens and tumor promoters, in: *Carcinogens: Identification and Mechanisms of Action* (A. C. Griffin and C. R. Shaw, eds.), pp. 399–418, Raven, New York.

89. Fujiki, H., Mori, M., Nakayasu, M., Terada, M., Sugimura, T., and Moore, R. E., 1981, Indole alkaloids: Dihydroteleocodicin B, teleocidin, and lyngbyatoxin A as members of a new class of tumor promoters, *Proc. Natl. Acad. Sci. USA* **78:**3872–3876.

90. Trosko, J. E., and Chang, C. C., 1986, Role of intercellular communications in modifying the consequences of mutations in somatic cells, in: *Antimutagenesis and Anticarcinogenesis Mechanisms* (D. E. Shankel, P. E. Hartman, T. Kada, and A. Hollander, eds.), pp. 439–456, Plenum, New York.

91. Woo, Y.-T., Arcos, J. C., and Lai, D. Y., 1985, Structural and functional criteria for suspecting chemical compounds of carcinogenic activity: State of the art of predictive formalism, in: *Handbook of Carcinogen Testing* (H. A. Milman and E. K. Weisburger, eds.), pp. 2–25, Noyes, Park Ridge, New Jersey.

92. Harris, C. C., 1987, Human tissues and cells in carcinogenesis research, *Cancer Res.* **47:**1–10.

93. Blair, A., Stewart, P., O'Berg, M., Gaffey, W., Walrath, J., Ward, J., Bales, R., Kaplan, S., and Cubit, D., 1986, Mortality among industrial workers exposed to formaldehyde, *J. Natl. Cancer Inst.* **76:**1071–1084.

94. Hoover, R. N., and Strasser, P. H., 1980, Artificial sweeteners and human bladder cancer, *Lancet* **1:**837–840.

95. Silvers, A., and Crump, K. S., 1985, Examination of risk estimation models, in: *Handbook of Carcinogen Testing* (H. A. Milman and E. K. Weisburger, eds.), pp. 502–525, Noyes, Park Ridge, New Jersey.

96. Turnbull, D., and Rodricks, J. V., 1985, Assessment of possible carcinogenic risks to humans resulting from exposure to di(2-ethylhexyl)phthalate(DEHP), *J. Am. Coll. Toxicol.* **4:**111–145.

97. International Agency for Research on Cancer, 1982, *IARC Monographs on the Evaluation of Carcinogenic Risk of Chemicals to Humans,* IARC Monograph Supplement 4, Lyons, France.

98. U.S. Department of Health and Human Services, 1985, *Fourth Annual Report on Carcinogens,* U.S. Department of Health and Human Services, Washington, D. C.

# 3

# DNA Adducts and Carcinogenesis

## Frederick A. Beland and Miriam C. Poirier

## 1. GENERAL CONSIDERATIONS

A central tenet of cancer research is that tumors arise from cells that have undergone a permanent heritable change in their genetic material. This hypothesis originated from the observation that tumor cells have lost normal growth-control mechanisms and transmit this characteristic to their progeny. It is supported by the findings that most chemically induced tumors are monoclonal in origin[1] and that consistent cytogenetic changes are present in certain tumors.[2] Although a number of mechanisms can be envisaged to explain the origin of these heritable genetic changes (e.g., see Chapters 4 and 5), clearly the dominant theme in present-day carcinogenesis is that in most instances they arise from the interaction between chemical carcinogens and DNA. This belief is supported by a number of observations, including the facts that (1) most carcinogens are also mutagens; (2) the mutagenic and carcinogenic properties of many compounds depend on their *in vivo* conversion into electrophilic derivatives that react with nucleophilic sites within DNA to form covalent adducts; (3) the extent of DNA adduct formation can often be correlated with mutagenic and carcinogenic responses; and (4) the activation of specific DNA sequences, termed proto-oncogenes, can be accomplished through the interaction of chemical carcinogens with DNA (see Chapter 14).

There are a number of important reasons for studying the interaction of carcinogens with DNA. As emphasized in Chapter 2, most chemical carcinogens are not directly electrophilic but are converted into electrophilic derivatives through metabolism. These metabolic activation pathways are normally minor pathways, and one or more intermediate steps may be required to form an

*Abbreviations used in this chapter:* 2-AAF, 2-acetylaminofluorene; AcCoA, acetyl coenzyme A; $AFB_1$, aflatoxin $B_1$; $AFB_1$-N7-Gua, *trans*-8,9-dihydro-8-(guan-7-yl)-9-aflatoxin $B_1$; $AFB_1$-N7-dG-DNA, DNA modified with *trans*-8,9-dihydro-8-(deoxyguanosin-7-yl)-9-aflatoxin $B_1$; $AFB_1$-N7-$Pyr_{maj}$, 8,9-dihydro-8-(2,6-diamino-4-oxo-3,4-dihydropyrimid-5-yl formamido)-9-hydroxyaflatoxin $B_1$; $AFB_1$-N7-$Pyr_{min}$, 8,9-dihydro-8-(2-amino-6-formamido-4-oxo-3,4-dihydropyrimid-5-yl amino)-9-hydroxyaflatoxin $B_1$; $AFB_1$-diol, 8,9-dihydro-8,9-dihydroxyaflatoxin $B_1$; BaP, benzo[a]pyrene; dG-C8-AF, *N*-(deoxyguanosin-8-yl)-2-aminofluorene; dG-C8-AAF, *N*-(deoxyguanosin-8-yl)-2-acetylaminofluorene; dG-$N^2$-AAF, 3-(deoxyguanosin-$N^2$-yl)-2-acetylaminofluorene; DMN, *N*-nitrosodimethylamine; ELISA, enzyme-linked immunosorbent assay; HPLC, high-pressure liquid chromatography; MMS, methylmethanesulfonate; MNU, *N*-methyl-*N*-nitrosourea; NNK, 4-(methylnitrosamino)-1-(3-pyridyl)-1-butanone; PAH, polycyclic aromatic hydrocarbons; PAPS, 3'-phosphoadenosine 5'-phosphosulfate; RIA, radioimmunoassay.

*Frederick A. Beland* • National Center for Toxicological Research, Jefferson, Arkansas 72079. *Miriam C. Poirier* • National Cancer Institute, National Institutes of Health, Bethesda, Maryland 20892.

activated species capable of binding to DNA. Elucidation of the structures of adducts in target tissues can provide information concerning these critical metabolic pathways. By determining the identity, quantity, and persistence of DNA adducts, insight may be obtained concerning their effects on DNA structure, transcription, synthesis, and repair. Investigations on the specific types of mutations induced by particular DNA adducts can provide a direct test of the somatic mutation theory of carcinogenesis. Finally, DNA adducts may be considered dosimeters to provide an indication of the relative risk of tumor induction.

## 2. DNA ADDUCT DETERMINATION AND QUANTITATION

The analysis of DNA adducts *in vivo* is complicated by a number of factors, the major one being that they are formed in relatively small quantities. Typical adduct levels in experimental animals administered tumorigenic doses of carcinogens are on the order of 10–100 pmoles/mg DNA, which is equivalent to 3 adducts per $10^5$–$10^6$ nucleotides. As exposure levels decrease, so do adduct concentrations such that adduct levels in humans are estimated to be at least two orders of magnitude lower. A second problem is that in general only limited quantities of DNA are available for analysis. Typically, 1 mg DNA can be isolated from 1 g tissue. Thus, assuming a steady-state adduct concentration of 100 pmoles/mg DNA, only 2 nmoles (~1 μg) adduct will be obtained from 20 g tissue, the size of an adult rat liver. In most situations, both the quantity of tissue and the adduct levels are considerably lower, resulting in the isolation of much smaller amounts of adducts.

A traditional approach to elucidate the structure of DNA adducts has been to conduct *in vitro* reactions between suspected ultimate carcinogens and DNA. The modified DNA is then hydrolyzed, the adducts are isolated by chromatographic techniques, most notably high-pressure liquid chromatography (HPLC), and their structures are elucidated by conventional spectroscopic methods, such as nuclear magnetic resonance and mass spectrometry. These adducts are then compared with the DNA adducts obtained from animals administered radiolabeled carcinogen. The identity of the *in vivo* adducts is typically based on co-chromatography of the radiolabel with the adduct standards prepared from the *in vitro* reactions and is confirmed by comparing their solubility characteristics as a function of either pH or acid–base lability, or both. The sensitivity obtained by using radiolabeled carcinogens can be quite good; however, the expense and general problems associated with the use of radioactive material restrict the types of studies that can be conducted. As a result, alternative approaches have been developed to assay for specific adducts.

The simplest alternative approach for adduct determination has been to change the method of detection associated with HPLC. Certain adducts, such as those derived from benzo[a]pyrene, have high molar extinction coefficients, which has permitted their assay at relatively low quantities by ultraviolet absorbance spectroscopy.[3] Similarly, other adducts fluoresce and this property has been used successfully to analyze specific adducts resulting from alkylating agents.[4] Nevertheless, these methods are generally applicable to only a limited number of adducts and do not possess the sensitivity to be useful at very low adduct concentrations. Thus, in spite of the value of HPLC-based methods, two additional techniques, immunoassays[5] and $^{32}$P-postlabeling,[6] have found increasing use for the identification and quantitation of DNA adducts.

In the immunologic approach, monoclonal or polyclonal antibodies are raised against either carcinogen-modified DNA or carcinogen–nucleoside adducts coupled to a protein carrier.[5] The antibodies are then used to quantify specific adducts by one of two techniques: radioimmunoassay (RIA) or enzyme-linked immunosorbent assay (ELISA). These assays are normally performed competitively with a constant amount of adduct standard (constant competitor) competing with an unknown amount of sample for a limiting quantity of antibody. The unknown sample causes a reduction in the quantity of constant competitor that binds the antibody, and the adduct quantity is determined by comparison with a standard curve prepared with increasing concentrations of known competitor. In RIA, incubations are conducted with adduct-specific antibody, the adduct to be measured, and a specific amount of radiolabeled adduct, which is the constant competitor (Fig. 1). Antibody–antigen complexes form in a concentration-dependent fashion, and these are precipitated

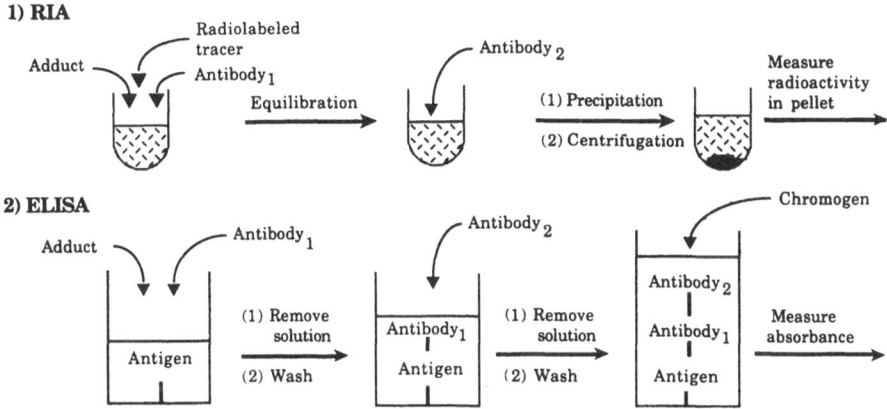

*Figure 1.* DNA adduct determination by immunoassay. Antibody$_1$ is the adduct specific (e.g., rabbit) antibody. Antibody$_2$ is a species-specific (e.g., goat anti-rabbit IgG) antibody. For ELISA, antibody$_2$ is coupled to an enzyme that cleaves the chromogen. RIA, radioimmunoassay; ELISA, enzyme-linked immunosorbent assay.

with a second, anti-IgG antibody. The quantity of radioactivity associated with the precipitated antibody–antigen complex is therefore inversely related to the amount of unknown adduct. In ELISA, the constant competitor is unlabeled immunogen bound to the bottom of a microtiter well (Fig. 1). The adduct-specific antibody competes for the bound immunogen and an unknown concentration of adducts in solution. The antibody–antigen complexes in solution are removed and the bound antibody–antigen complexes are reacted stoichiometrically with a second, enzyme-conjugated antibody that can cleave a chromogen, such as *p*-nitrophenylphosphate. Since each antibody-linked enzyme can cleave many substrate molecules, the magnitude of the initial antibody–antigen complex is amplified significantly. As with RIA, there is an inverse relationship between the quantity of unknown adduct in the competition step and the amount of antibody bound to the microtiter well.

The quantity of adduct detectable by immunoassays depends on the particular method, with ELISA generally giving greater sensitivities ($\sim$1 adduct per $10^7$ nucleotides) than RIA. Both methods are relatively inexpensive, permit simultaneous analysis of many samples, and are sufficiently sensitive for use with human DNA samples. However, they have certain problems. Typically, the sensitivity is limited by the amount of DNA that can be analyzed in a RIA tube or separating specific structurally similar adducts (e.g., by HPLC) before the immunoassay, but this approach is useful only for antibodies elicited against nucleoside adducts and not for those raised against modified DNA. A second problem with immunologic methods is that the antibody may be specific for a broad spectrum of adducts and, thus, may form antibody–antigen complexes with unknown adducts in biologic samples from individuals exposed to environmental carcinogens. Again, a combination of chromatography and immunoassays may permit sufficient characterization of specific adducts.

In the second alternative approach, $^{32}$P-postlabeling,[6] isolated DNA is hydrolyzed with DNase II and micrococcal endonuclease to 3'-nucleotides, which are then converted to $^{32}$P-labeled 3',5'-*bis*-phosphates by incubation with polynucleotide kinase and [$^{32}$P]ATP (Fig. 2). Adducts are then resolved by multidirectional thin-layer chromatography (TLC), located by autoradiography, and quantified by Cerenkov counting. Since specific activities of [$^{32}$P]ATP can range up to 4500 Ci/mmole, this method has the potential to detect vanishing quantities of adducts. However, since both adducted and nonadducted 3'-nucleotides have the possibility of becoming radiolabeled, the sensitivity of the method depends on the ability to discriminate chromatographically between normal and adducted 3',5'-*bis*-phosphates. As might be expected, the greater the difference in physical properties between the adducts and the normal bases, the easier it is to separate the adducts. With alkylated adducts, for example, that differ from normal nucleosides by only a methyl or ethyl

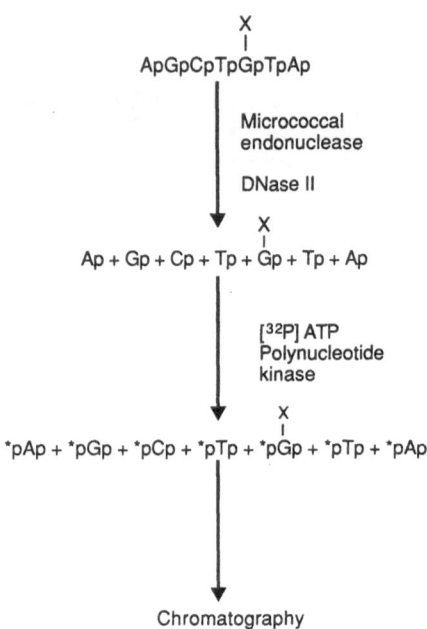

*Figure 2.* DNA adduct determination by [32P]-postlabeling. X, adduct.

group, the limit of detection appears to be in the neighborhood of 1 adduct in $10^6$ nucleotides, whereas with bulky aromatic adducts, which have substantial hydrocarbon moieties, sensitivities approaching 1 adduct in $10^8$ nucleotides have been reported.[6]

Recently, modifications to the original method have increased the sensitivity of this approach. These variations are based on (1) the preferential labeling of adducted 3'-nucleotides in the presence of a limiting quantity of [32P]ATP[7]; (2) the preferential hydrolysis of nonmodified 3'-nucleotides by nuclease $P_1$[8]; and (3) the greater solubility of adducted 3'-nucleotides in organic solvents.[9] Each of these variations permits the preferential [32P]-labeling of adducted 3'-nucleotides and has resulted in sensitivities of adduct detection approaching 1 adduct in $10^{10}$ nucleotides.[8,9]

[32P]-postlabeling is clearly the most powerful method for adduct detection available today, but it is also not without problems. In instances in which the adducts are known, they can be quantified accurately, but in the case of unknown adducts, the quantification is far less certain. Furthermore, this method has the capability of detecting adducts at such low concentrations that in instances in which the carcinogen exposure is unknown, it is virtually impossible to determine the identity of the adducts being measured.

## 3. DNA ADDUCTS FROM SPECIFIC CLASSES OF CARCINOGENS

The remaining sections of this chapter discuss the DNA adducts obtained from four different classes of carcinogens: *N*-nitrosamines, aflatoxins, aromatic amines, and polycyclic aromatic hydrocarbons (PAH). These particular classes were chosen because for each there is substantial evidence of human exposure. Nevertheless, the mechanisms and principles outlined for the study of these compounds are generally applicable to any genotoxic carcinogen. For each class, we consider the metabolic activation pathways and discuss the DNA adducts resulting from this metabolism. We then consider the alterations that result within DNA when these lesions are replicated, and when multiple adducts are present, we attempt to relate the relative importance of each. Finally, we discuss the role played by these adducts in the activation of specific oncogenes by these carcinogens.

## 3.1. N-Nitrosamines

The carcinogenicity of *N*-nitrosamines was first demonstrated by Magee and Barnes in 1956.[10] During the intervening 30 years, more than 300 *N*-nitrosamines and related *N*-nitrosamides have been demonstrated to be tumorigenic in a number of different organs in a wide variety of species. Human exposure to *N*-nitrosamines occurs through a number of sources, including foods, beverages, tobacco, cosmetics, cutting oils, hydraulic fluid, and rubber products. Although conclusive epidemiologic evidence for the carcinogenicity of these compounds in humans is not available (except, perhaps, in the case of the induction of oral cancers in snuff dippers[11]), the fact that *N*-nitrosamines are carcinogenic in such a wide variety of species suggests that they should be carcinogenic in humans. Furthermore, in instances in which there has been known exposure to high levels of *N*-nitrosamines, the DNA adduct profile is similar to that found in the target organs of susceptible species.[12]

The metabolic activation of *N*-nitrosodimethylamine (DMN), a ubiquitously distributed *N*-nitrosamine, and 4-(methylnitrosamino)-1-(3-pyridyl)-1-butanone (NNK), a tobacco-specific *N*-

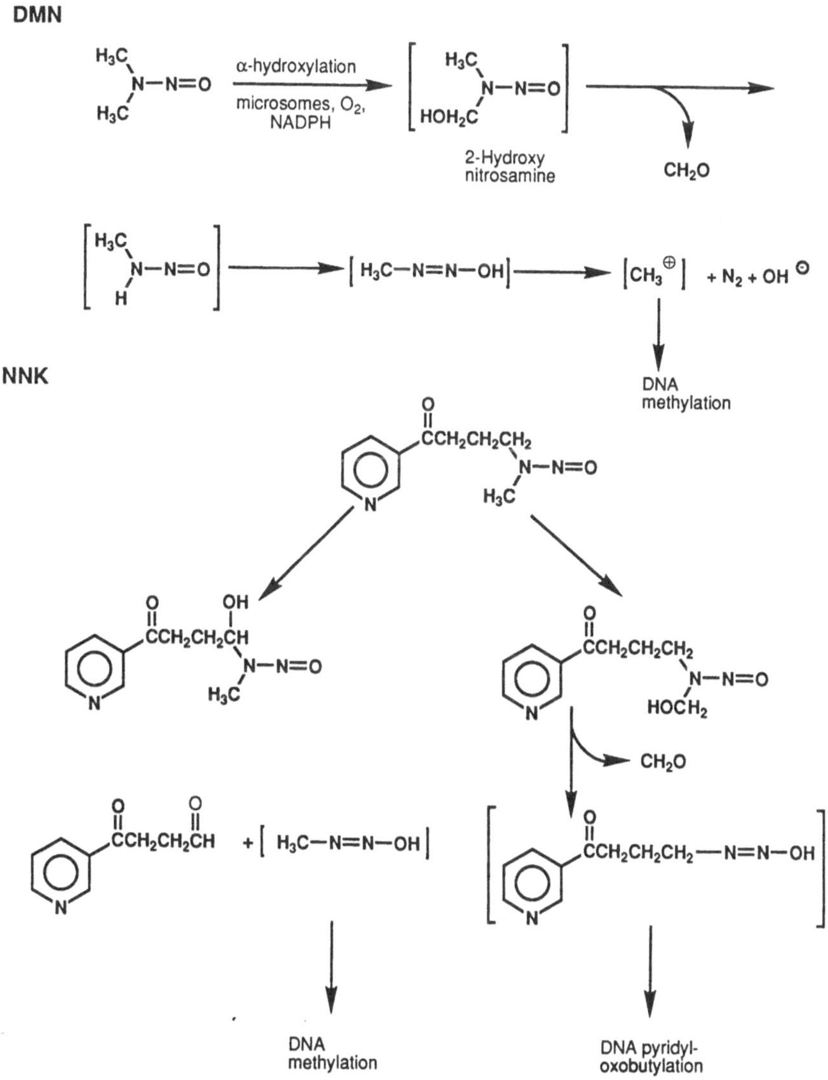

**Figure 3.** Metabolic activation of *N*-nitrosodimethylamine (DMN) and 4-(methylnitrosoamino)-1-(3-pyridyl)-1-butanone (NNK). (Adapted from Hecht *et al.*[13])

nitrosamine, is shown in Fig. 3.[13] The activation sequence for both compounds involves an initial oxidation on the carbon adjacent to the amine nitrogen ($\alpha$-hydroxylation). This oxidation, which gives an unstable $\alpha$-hydroxynitrosamine intermediate, is catalyzed by the microsomal mono-oxygenase, cytochrome P-450. In order for hydroxylation to occur, the $\alpha$-carbon must contain at least one hydrogen; thus, $N$-nitrosamines without $\alpha$-hydrogens are generally regarded as being noncarcinogenic. The importance of $\alpha$-hydrogens is further illustrated by the use of $\alpha$-deuterium analogues, which have decreased carcinogenicity compared with their parent $N$-nitrosamines. Since the strength of a C–D bond is greater than that of a C–H bond, this indicates that the rate-limiting step in the activation sequence is the breaking of the C–H (C–D) bond.

The $\alpha$-hydroxynitrosamine formed from this initial oxidation is an unstable intermediate that rapidly decomposes. In the case of DMN, which is a symmetric $N$-nitrosamine, the products are formaldehyde and methyl diazohydroxide (Fig. 3). This latter intermediate serves as a strong methylating agent. NNK, by comparison, is not symmetric, so two different alkylating species can result. $\alpha$-Hydroxylation of the pyridyloxobutyl moiety will result in the formation of a methylating agent, whereas oxidation of the methyl group yields a pyridyloxobutylating agent (Fig. 3). To date, work concerning the alkylation of DNA by $N$-nitrosamines and other alkylating agents has generally centered around methylation and ethylation. Therefore, these products are emphasized.

A general rule regarding the alkylation of DNA by methylating and ethylating agents is that all primary oxygens and secondary nitrogens have the potential to become substituted. In practice, there are marked differences between the extent of reaction at particular oxygens and nitrogens that depend on both the location of the heteroatom and the specific alkylating agent. Table I gives the extent of reaction of DNA *in vitro* with two direct-acting methylating agents, $N$-methyl-$N$-nitrosourea (MNU) and methyl methanesulfonate (MMS).[14] MNU is a $N$-nitrosamide that, unlike $N$-nitrosamines, will decompose spontaneously to a reactive electrophile. Since MNU and DMN form common reactive intermediates, MNU was selected for illustration to avoid complications associated with metabolism. As shown in Table I, the major site of substitution with both compounds is N7 of guanine. This is followed by N3 of adenine for MMS, and phosphotriesters, and then N3 of adenine for MNU. Under these conditions, the extent of reaction with N7 of guanine by either compound is similar.[14] However, there are marked differences between the two in the extent to which they react with oxygen atoms. MNU has more $S_N1$ character,* and therefore reacts with hard (e.g., oxygen) nucleophilic centers in DNA. By comparison, MMS has more $S_N2$ character, causing it to react with soft nucleophilic sites (e.g., nitrogens). This difference in the extent of oxygen alkylation is important because a single dose of MNU to mice results in a high incidence of thymic lymphoma,[15] whereas an equimolar dose of MMS is not tumorigenic.[16] Since the extent of total alkylation is similar with both compounds, this indicates that specific adducts must be responsible for tumor induction.

The importance of alkylating oxygen atoms in nucleic acid bases for the induction of tumors was first proposed in 1969 by Loveless,[17] who suggested that this could lead to the mis-incorporation of bases during DNA replication. An examination of Table I indicates that three oxygen alkylation products are formed from a carcinogenic alkylating agent such as MNU: $O^6$-methylguanine, $O^4$-methylthymine, and $O^2$-methylthymine. When these adducts are incorporated into synthetic oligonucleotides and their coding properties examined in *in vitro* DNA polymerase assays, two of the adducts, $O^6$-methylguanine and $O^4$-methylthymine, result in the misincorporation of bases.[18–20] The reason for this incorrect incorporation is shown in Fig. 4. Instead of forming a normal base pair with cytosine, $O^6$-methylguanine is held in an abnormal enol as opposed to the normal keto tautomer, hence hydrogen bonds with thymine. Thus, a transition mutation† occurs in which a G–C base pair is converted into an A–T base pair. $O^4$-Methylthymine behaves in a similar

---

*Compounds that have $S_N1$ character are postulated to form carbonium ions; their reactions are unimolecular, typically first order. Compounds with $S_N2$ character do not form carbonium ions; their reactions are bimolecular, typically second order.

†In a transition mutation, a purine is converted into a purine, and a pyrimidine becomes a pyrimidine. In transversion mutations, a pyrimidine is converted into a purine, and vice versa.

Table I. Distribution of Adducts in DNA after in Vitro Reaction with MNU and MMS[a]

| | Adenine | Cytosine | Guanine | Thymine |
|---|---|---|---|---|

| Site of methylation in DNA | Percentage total DNA binding | |
|---|---|---|
| | MNU | MMS |
| **Adenine** | | |
| N1 | 0.9 | 1.9 |
| N3 | 8.4 | 11.3 |
| N7 | 2.0 | 1.8 |
| **Cytosine** | | |
| N3 | 0.5 | nd[b] |
| **Guanine** | | |
| N2 | 0.6 | 0.3 |
| O6 | 5.9 | 0.3 |
| N7 | 66.4 | 81.4 |
| **Thymine** | | |
| O2 | 0.1 | nd[b] |
| N3 | nd[b] | 0.1 |
| O4 | 0.7 | nd[b] |
| Phosphotriester | 12.1 | 0.8 |

[a]Data from Beranek et al.[14]
[b]Not detected; <0.02%.

fashion: It is held in an enol conformation and is misread as a cytosine; therefore, a guanine becomes incorporated during replication, and an A–T base pair is converted into a G–C base pair (again, a transition mutation). Since $O^6$-methylguanine is formed to approximately 10 times the extent of $O^4$-methylthymine, most attention has been focused on the former adduct.

The results of mutagenesis assays in both bacteria and mammalian cells support the data obtained from in vitro DNA polymerase experiments. In bacteria treated with two direct-acting alkylating agents, N-methyl-N'-nitro-N-nitrosoguanidine (a methylating agent) and ethyl methanesulfonate (an ethylating agent), 99% of the resultant base-substitution mutations were attributed to G–C → A–T transitions (i.e., from $O^6$-alkylguanine).[21] Likewise, in Chinese hamster ovary cells treated with methylating and ethylating agents, mutation induction best correlated with the formation of $O^6$-alkylguanine.[22–23] Similar relationships have been found to exist in vivo, hence the high incidence of thymic lymphoma in mice treated with a single dose of MNU versus the inactivity of an equimolar dose of MMS. Analysis of thymic DNA from mice treated with both compounds has indicated a direct relationship between the extent of $O^6$-methylguanine formation and the tumor yield.[15,16] A single dose of MNU will also induce a high incidence of mammary gland tumors in female rats. Sequence analysis of DNA from all these tumors has indicated the presence of G → A transitions in codon 12 of the ras oncogene.[24] Such a mutation is consistent with the formation of $O^6$-methylguanine.

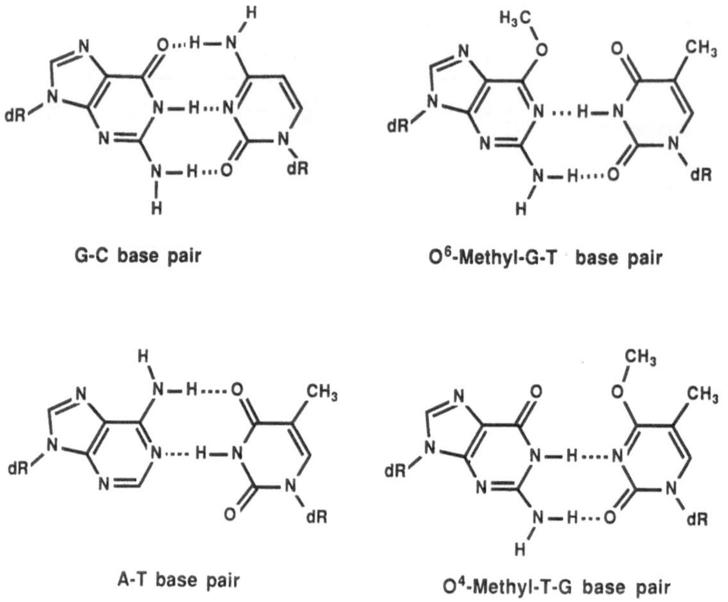

G-C base pair

$O^6$-Methyl-G-T base pair

A-T base pair

$O^4$-Methyl-T-G base pair

*Figure 4.* Normal Watson–Crick base pairing and mispairing caused by formation of $O^6$-methylguanine and $O^4$-methylthymine. Methylation at $O^6$ of guanine and $O^4$ of thymine results in the formation of an "enol" as opposed to the normal "keto" tautomer.

Although $O^6$-alkylguanine is the dominant oxygen-substituted adduct in DNA following a single administration of an alkylating agent, the situation is somewhat more complicated when the carcinogens are administered chronically. A single dose of the liver carcinogen, 1,2-dimethylhydrazine, for example, will result in 100-fold more $O^6$-methylguanine than $O^4$-methylthymine in liver DNA.[25] However, when 1,2-dimethylhydrazine is administered chronically for a period of 30 days, the ratio falls to <2:1. Similarly, after a single dose of the hepatocarcinogen, N-nitrosodiethylamine, $O^6$ of guanine is alkylated three to four times more than $O^4$ of thymine. Under chronic administration of N-nitrosodiethylamine, however, $O^4$-ethylthymine is found in liver DNA at more than 50 times the concentration of $O^6$-ethylguanine.[25] These differences in adduct ratios after single and chronic dosing have been attributed to the preferential repair of $O^6$-alkylguanine by an alkyltransferase, a subject considered in greater detail in Chapter 8.

## 3.2. Aflatoxins

Aflatoxins are another class of carcinogens that humans are exposed to through their diet. These compounds, first implicated as animal hepatocarcinogens during the early 1960s, are produced by molds (primarily *Aspergillus flavus*) that grow on cereals, grains, and nuts. Daily human consumption of these mycotoxins in certain regions of the world, especially Africa and Asia, is estimated to be in the nanogram (ng) to microgram ($\mu$g) range, and there appears to be a positive correlation between the amount of aflatoxin ingested and the incidence of liver cancer in man (summarized by Busby and Wogan[26]).

Four major naturally occurring aflatoxins have been characterized (Fig. 5): aflatoxin $B_1$ ($AFB_1$), aflatoxin $B_2$ ($AFB_2$), aflatoxin $G_1$ ($AFG_1$), and aflatoxin $G_2$ ($AFG_2$). Aflatoxins of the B series contain fused cyclopentanone rings, and G-series derivatives have lactone rings. Compounds designated by the subscript 1 have an ethylenic 8,9-bond (also called the 2,3-position), while this bond is saturated in derivatives with the subscript 2. $AFB_1$ and $AFG_1$ are much more mutagenic and carcinogenic than are $AFB_2$ and $AFG_2$, which implies that the olefinic 8,9-bond is somehow involved in the metabolic activation of these mycotoxins. This interpretation is supported by the

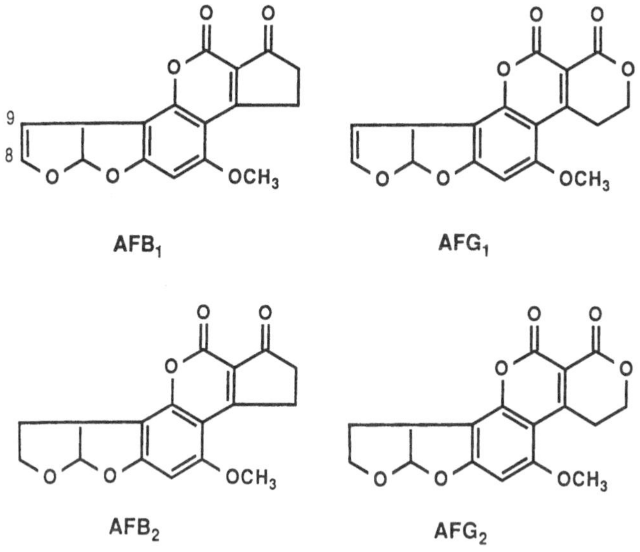

*Figure 5.* Major naturally occurring aflatoxins.

observation that aflatoxin derivatives lacking the furofuran moiety are neither toxic nor tumorigenic. Since $AFB_1$ is the major naturally occurring aflatoxin, as well as the most carcinogenic, most research has centered on this derivative.

As with most chemical carcinogens, $AFB_1$ requires metabolism in order to bind DNA, and the requirement for an 8,9-olefinic bond suggests that a reactive epoxide may be formed. Although this epoxide has so far resisted unambiguous chemical characterization, much indirect evidence supports its existence. Incubation of $AFB_1$ with rat liver microsomes in the presence of DNA results in extensive covalent binding. Upon acid hydrolysis, >90% of this binding can be accounted for by one adduct, *trans*-8,9-dihydro-8-(guan-7-yl)-9-hydroxy $AFB_1$ ($AFB_1$-N7-Gua) (Fig. 6).[27] This structure is consistent with trans opening of an epoxide ring and concomitant attack on N7 of guanine to yield DNA modified with *trans*-8,9-dihydro-8-(deoxyguanosin-7-yl)-9-hydroxy $AFB_1$ ($AFB_1$-N7-dG-DNA). Thus, in contrast to $N$-nitrosamines, which give multiple adducts *in vitro*, $AFB_1$ adduction appears to give only one primary product. Furthermore, while alkylation at $O^6$ of guanine was correlated with mutagenic and tumorigenic responses of $N$-nitrosoamines, this does not appear to be the case with $AFB_1$.

DNA adduct formation by $AFB_1$ at N7 of guanine (Fig. 6) ($AFB_1$-N7-dG-DNA) creates a positive charge that can result in a depurination to give $AFB_1$-N7-Gua. The rate of glycosyl bond breakage increases with decreasing pH, with the adduct having a half-life of approximately 50 hr under neutral conditions.[28] In addition to depurination, $AFB_1$-N7-dG-DNA can also undergo base-catalyzed opening of the imidazole ring to yield two pyrimidine adducts (Fig. 6). The major of these two adducts has been characterized as 8,9-dihydro-8-(2,6-diamino-4-oxo-3,4-dihydropyrimid-5-yl formamido)-9-hydroxy $AFB_1$ ($AFB_1$-N7-$Pyr_{maj}$) (Fig. 6), while the minor adduct has been identified as 8,9-dihydro-8-(2-amino-6-formamido-4-oxo-3,4-dihydropyrimid-5-yl amino)-9-hydroxy $AFB_1$ ($AFB_1$-N7-$Pyr_{min}$) (Fig. 6).[29] A final product that has been reported to occur from the decomposition of $AFB_1$-N7-dG-DNA is 8,9-dihydro-8,9-dihydroxy $AFB_1$ ($AFB_1$-diol) (Fig. 6).[30] This product may result from hydrolysis of the original adduct, in which case the DNA would be restored to its original integrity. Alternatively, the diol has been suggested to arise from hydrolysis of the pyrimidine adducts (Fig. 6),[31] in which case a potentially promutagenic lesion would be introduced into the DNA.

The three $AFB_1$ adducts have markedly different lifetimes *in vivo*. Following a single dose of $AFB_1$ to rats, $AFB_1$-N7-dG-DNA (as assayed by the depurination product, $AFB_1$-N7-Gua) is

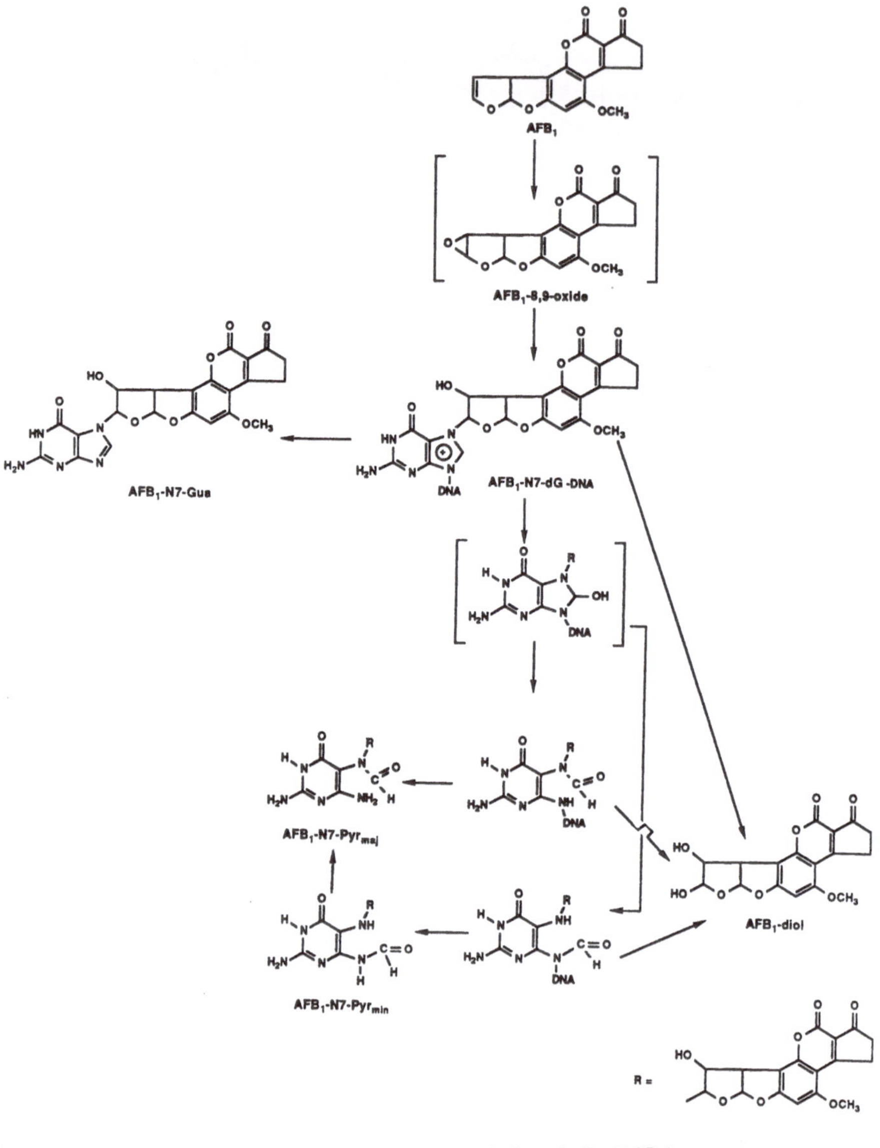

*Figure 6.* Metabolic activation of aflatoxin $B_1$ (AFB$_1$).

initially the major DNA adduct, accounting for >80% of the bound products, but it decreases with a half-life of approximately 7 hr and is only barely detectable after 72 hr.[32] The other two adducts, AFB$_1$-N7-Pyr$_{maj}$ and AFB$_1$-N7-Pyr$_{min}$, do not appear to be repaired; therefore, 72 hr after a single dose, the relative relationship of adducts is AFB$_1$-N7-Pyr$_{maj}$ > AFB$_1$-N7-Pyr$_{min}$ > AFB$_1$-N7-Gua. A similar relationship exists after multiple doses of AFB$_1$. The major adduct is AFB$_1$-N7-Pyr$_{maj}$, which increases in concentration with each dose, AFB$_1$-N7-Pyr$_{min}$ is the next most prevalent, which increases with each dose as well, while $AFB_1$-N7-Gua is present to only a minor extent after repeated intraperitoneal administrations over a 2-week period.[32]

There is uncertainty regarding the biologic significance of each of these $AFB_1$ DNA adducts. When *Salmonella typhimurium* are incubated with $AFB_1$ in the presence of an activating system (e.g., a rat liver postmitochondrial supernatant), both base substitution and frameshift mutations are detected. Analysis of the adducts present in the *Salmonella* genome indicated a single adduct, $AFB_1$-N7-Gua. Thus, this adduct was suggested to give rise to both types of mutations.[31] In similar experiments conducted with *Escherichia coli*, ~90% of the mutations detected were due to G → T transversions, consistent with $AFB_1$ deoxyguanosine adduct formation. However, in this latter study, the mutations were suggested to arise from the apurinic sites that result from glycosyl bond breakage, rather than from the $AFB_1$ adducts themselves.[33] Apurinic sites have also been proposed to be responsible for the mutations induced by $AFB_1$ in cultured diploid human lymphoblasts.[34]

Similar uncertainties exist concerning the adducts involved in tumor induction. When rats are treated with multiple doses of $AFB_1$ over a 2-week period, the pyrimidine adducts are the major products at later time points.[32] If these rats are treated simultaneously with the antioxidant, ethoxyquin, adduct formation is decreased to a greater extent at earlier time points (i.e., day 1) than at later times. Interestingly, ethoxyquin treatment also results in a marked decrease in preoplastic γ-glutamyl transpeptidase-positive hepatocyte foci[35] (see Chapter 9). Since $AFB_1$-N7-Gua is the major adduct at initial time points, this suggests that $AFB_1$-N7-Gua, as opposed to the imidazole ring-opened pyrimidine derivatives, may be more important in tumor initiation. Regardless of which adduct turns out to be the biologically important lesion, the induction of liver tumors in rats by $AFB_1$ is accompanied by a G → A transition in codon 12 that causes activation of the *ras* oncogene,[36] which is consistent with the initial formation of an $AFB_1$ deoxyguanosine adduct.

## 3.3. Aromatic Amines

In contrast to aflatoxins, for which human exposure is primarily through the diet, the induction of tumors by aromatic amines was originally traced to occupational exposure. In 1895, the German physician Rehn noted an increased incidence of bladder cancer in persons involved in the manufacturing of aromatic amine based dyes.[37] Subsequently, Case *et al.*[38] found a similar relationship among British dye and rubber workers, which they attributed to 2-naphthylamine and benzidine (Fig. 7). More recently, exposure to another aromatic amine, 4-aminobiphenyl (Fig. 7), which was used as an antioxidant in the manufacturing of rubber products, was found to lead to an increased incidence of bladder tumors.[39] Although the industrial usage of carcinogenic aromatic amines has been severely curtailed, significant human exposure to this class of carcinogen still occurs. Cigarette smoke, for example, contains nanogram quantities of 2-napthylamine and 4-aminobiphenyl,[40] and these may be responsible for the positive correlation between cigarette smoking and bladder cancer in humans.[41] In addition, carcinogenic heterocyclic aromatic amines formed by the pyrolysis of amino acids during the preparation of certain foods may be important in the etiology of human

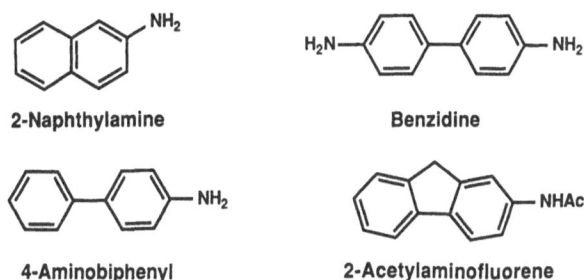

*Figure 7.* Representative carcinogenic aromatic amines and amides.

**2-Naphthylamine**

**Benzidine**

**4-Aminobiphenyl**

**2-Acetylaminofluorene**

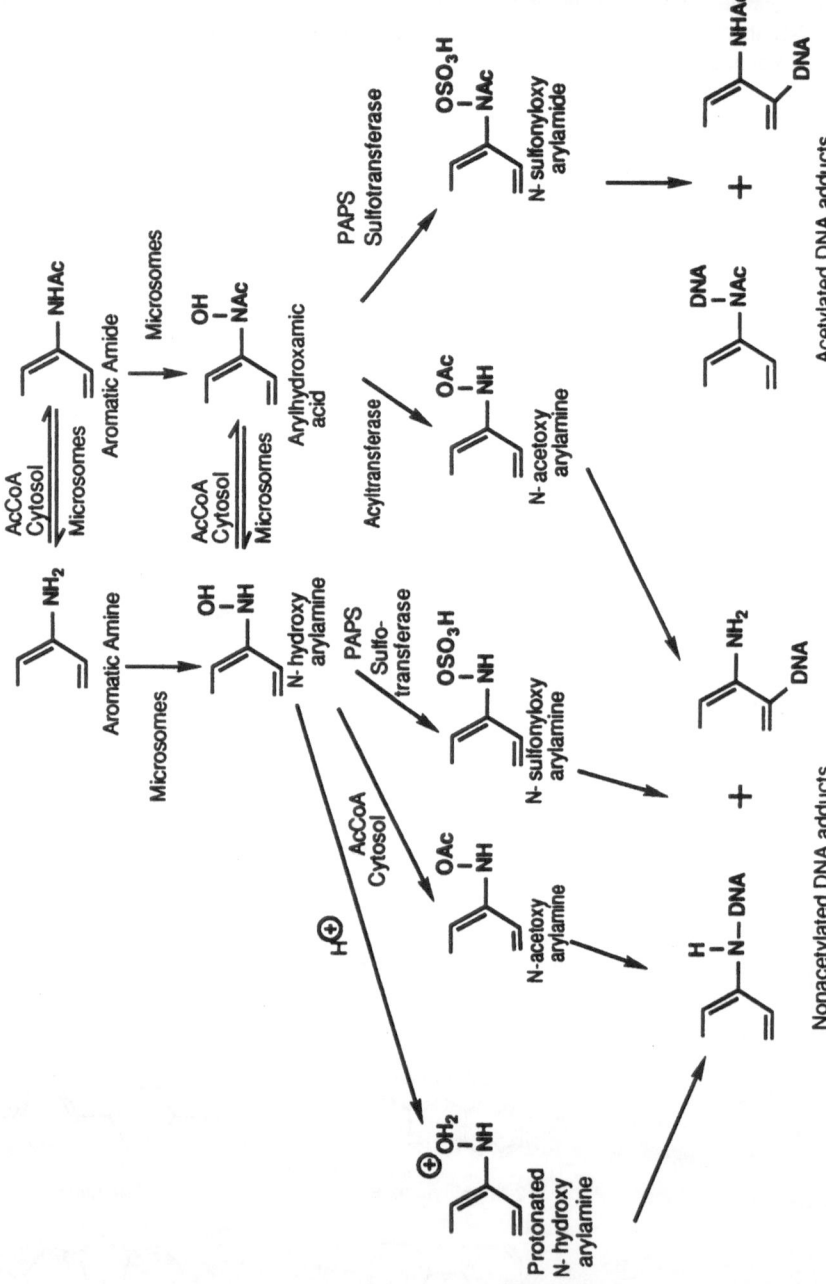

*Figure 8.* Metabolic activation of aromatic amines and amides. AcCoA, acetyl coenzyme A; PAPS, 3'-phosphoadenosine 5'-phosphosulfate.

cancer.[42] There also appears to be widespread exposure to nitro-PAH, which result from the incomplete combustion of organic material such as diesel fuels and are related to aromatic amines by nitroreduction.[43] The incidence of human exposure to aromatic amines seems to be extensive as indicated by the almost universal formation of 4-aminobiphenyl hemoglobin adducts in human blood.[44] The source of this contamination is unknown.

Compared with the two classes of carcinogens discussed previously, the metabolic activation of aromatic amines is considerably more complicated (Fig. 8). Upon absorption, an aromatic amine can undergo a cytosol-catalyzed acetyl coenzyme A (AcCoA)-dependent acetylation to an aromatic amide (Fig. 8). Conversely, aromatic amides can undergo a microsome-catalyzed deacetylation to aromatic amines. These and subsequent acetylation processes may be important for tumorigenesis because there is a positive correlation between persons who have a slow acetylation phenotype (~25% of North Americans of European descent[45]) and the incidence of bladder cancer resulting from aromatic amine exposure.[46] Interestingly, in colon cancer patients with apparently no overt exposure to aromatic amines, persons with a fast acetylator phenotype have a higher tumor incidence than do those with a slow acetylator phenotype.[47,48]

The initial activation of aromatic amines and amides involves a microsome-catalyzed N-oxidation[49] (Fig. 8). In the case of aromatic amines, this yields a N-hydroxy arylamine, while with aromatic amides this gives an arylhydroxamic acid. As with their parent compounds, these N-hydroxy-derivatives are interrelated by acetylation–deacetylation. N-Hydroxyarylamines are electrophilic and will react directly with DNA by an acid-catalyzed reaction. They are also activated by an AcCoA-dependent cytosol-catalyzed O-acetylation, and a 3'-phosphoadenosine-5'-phosphosulfate (PAPS)-dependent sulfotransferase-catalyzed O-sulfonation. Arylhydroxamic acids are not electrophilic and therefore require additional metabolism. The predominant activation pathway appears to be an acyltransferase-catalyzed rearrangement to a reactive N-acetoxy arylamine. An additional pathway is a sulfotransferase-catalyzed formation of a N-sulfonyloxy arylamide.

The metabolic activation of aromatic amines and amides gives rise to acetylated (amide) and nonacetylated (amine) DNA adducts (Fig. 8), and it is a general rule that most adducts will be formed by covalent attachment of the amine or amide nitrogen to C8 of deoxyguanosine[50] (Table II). Minor adducts arise from bond formation between carbons *ortho* to the amine or amide function and exocyclic nitrogens and oxygens of deoxyguanosine and deoxyadenosine (Table II). Depending on the specific carcinogen, the site of substitution on the nucleic acid base, and whether or not the adduct is acetylated, these adducts display markedly different biologic properties and lifetimes *in vivo*. This is illustrated with 2-acetylaminofluorene (2-AAF), undoubtedly the most extensively studied aromatic amine carcinogen.

*Table II. Sites of Modification in DNA in Vivo*
*by Aromatic Amine Carcinogens[a]*

| | Nucleic acid base | | | | |
| | Deoxyguanosine | | | Deoxyadenosine | |
| Carcinogen | C8 | N$^2$ | O$^6$ | C8 | N$^6$ |
|---|---|---|---|---|---|
| 1-Naphthylamine | | | ++ | | |
| 2-Naphthylamine | ++ | + | | | + |
| 4-Aminobiphenyl | ++ | + | | + | |
| 4-Acetylaminobiphenyl | ++[b] | + | | | |
| 4'-Fluoro-4-acetylaminobiphenyl | ++[b] | + | | | |
| 3,2'-Dimethyl-4-aminobiphenyl | ++ | + | | | |
| 2-Acetylaminofluorene | ++[b] | + | | | |
| Benzidine | ++[b] | | | | |

[a]Data from Beland and Kadlubar.[50]
[b]Both nonacetylated and acetylated adducts are found in a ratio ≥ 3 : 1.

Following administration of a single dose of 2-AAF to male rats, three DNA adducts are formed in liver, a target for tumorigenesis by this carcinogen.[50] The major adduct, N-(deoxyguanosin-8-yl)-2-aminofluorene (dG-C8-AF), is nonacetylated, accounts for ~80% of the total binding, and arises primarily from an acyltransferase-catalyzed activation of N-hydroxy-2-AAF (Fig. 9). The other two adducts are acetylated and result from sulfotransferase-catalyzed activation of this arylhydroxamic acid. The major acetylated adduct, N-(deoxyguanosin-8-yl)-2-AAF (dG-C8-AAF), is also substituted through C-8 of deoxyguanosine and accounts for ~15% of the total binding, while an $N^2$-substituted deoxyguanosine adduct, 3-(deoxyguanosin-$N^2$-yl)-2-AAF (dG-$N^2$-AAF) is responsible for the remaining 5%. The N-acetyl moiety of dG-C8-AAF causes significant distortion of the DNA double helix and, as a result, the adduct has a relatively short half-life ($t_{1/2}$ ~7 days) in rat liver DNA. The other two adducts, dG-C8-AF and dG-$N^2$-AAF, do not appear to distort the helix because they reside in the major and minor grooves, respectively. Therefore, these adducts are relatively persistent lesions. The rapid repair of dG-C8-AAF, coupled with a decrease in sulfotransferase activity during chronic 2-AAF feeding, results in the disappearance of this adduct during the first 2 weeks of dietary administration. Thus, dG-C8-AF is essentially the only lesion detected in rat liver DNA after 2–3 weeks of a tumorigenic feeding protocol. Similarly, for nearly all aromatic amines for which DNA adducts have been characterized, the major, if not only, adducts in every species and tissue are nonacetylated C8-substituted deoxyguanosine products[50] (Table II).

The DNA adducts from 2-AAF show marked differences in the types of mutations they induce. As indicated above, the acetylated adduct, dG-C8-AAF, perturbs the DNA double helix. Specifically, instead of being in the normal *anti* conformation, it rotates about the glycosyl bond and adopts a *syn* form. This conformational change is thought to be important for the frameshift mutations that result from this adduct in bacteria.[51] By comparison, the nonacetylated adduct dG-C8-AF maintains a normal *anti* conformation, and this adduct induces primarily base substitution mutations of which the majority are G → T transversions.[51] Similar types of mutations also appear to occur *in vivo*. For example, in mice treated with N-hydroxy-2-AAF, which induces hepatomas, essentially the only adduct detected in hepatic DNA is dG-C8-AF.[52] Tumor induction by this compound has been correlated with a G → T transversion in the c-Ha-*ras* proto-oncogene,[53] a base substitution mutation consistent with dG-C8-AF formation.

## 3.4. Polycyclic Aromatic Hydrocarbons

Of the carcinogens considered in this chapter, the PAH have the longest and perhaps most colorful history. In 1775, the British physician Percival Pott noted an increased incidence of scrotal cancer in chimney sweeps, which he attributed to their exposure to soot and concomitant lack of bathing.[54] Subsequently, industrial exposure to a variety of combustion products was associated with an increased incidence of skin and respiratory tract tumors (reviewed by Kipling and Cooke[55]). These observations led to an intense effort to determine the carcinogenic components of coal tar, culminating in the identification of benzo[a]pyrene (BaP) as the major tumorigenic constituent.[56] Following this initial identification, literally hundreds of PAH and their derivatives were prepared and tested for carcinogenicity. Since many of these have substantial activity, much effort has been expended to elucidate the features that impart carcinogenic activity to this class of compounds. However, it has been primarily through careful metabolism and DNA-binding studies that a clear picture of the pathways involved has evolved.

During the early 1950s, Boyland proposed that each of the known PAH metabolites (i.e., phenols, dihydrodiols, and mercapturic acids) could arise from a common electrophilic intermediate, an epoxide.[57] Theoretical calculations suggested that the K region* of a PAH was essential for carcinogenic activity.[58] Emphasis was therefore placed upon preparing K-region epoxides. However, when BaP-4,5-epoxide (Fig. 10) was synthesized and reacted with DNA, the adduct profile did not correspond to that from BaP *in vivo*.[59] At this same time, an additional experiment

---

*K regions are the areas of a PAH with the greatest double bond character, for example, the 4,5 bond of BaP (Fig. 10).

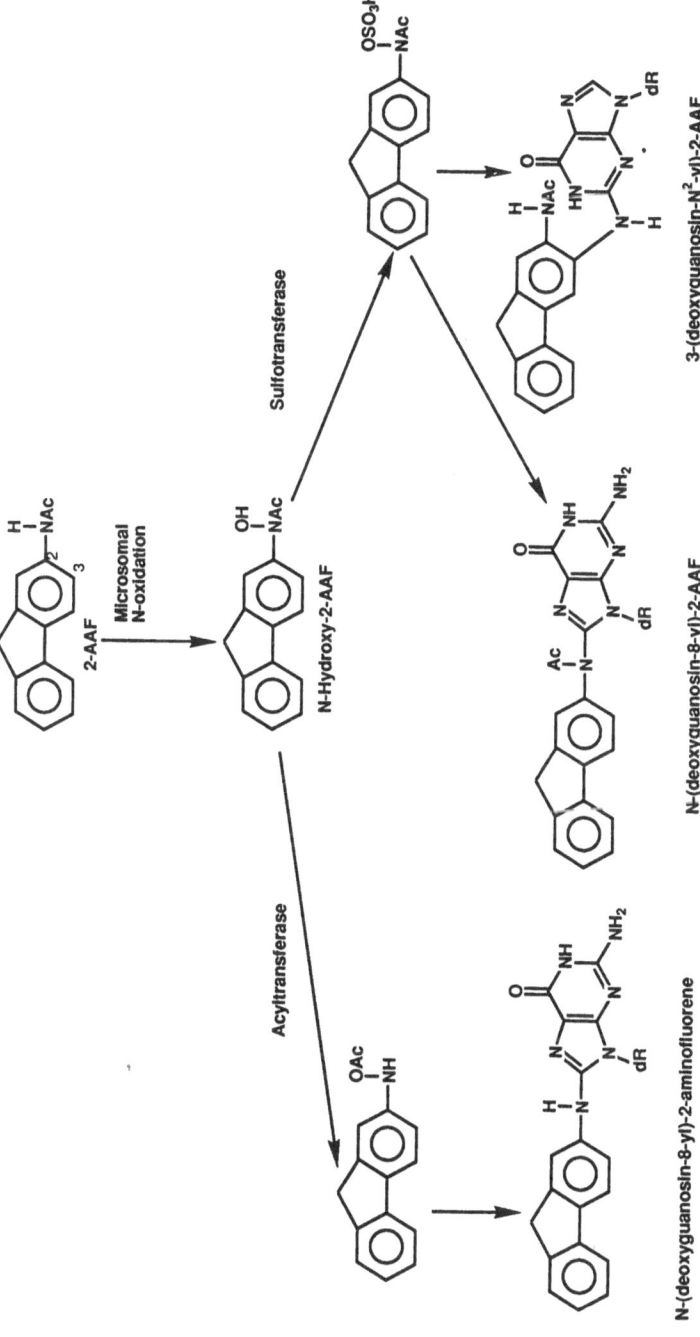

*Figure 9.* Metabolic activation and DNA adducts of 2-acetylaminofluorene (2-AAF).

demonstrated that upon further metabolism, BaP-7,8-dihydrodiol (Fig. 10) bound to DNA to a greater extent than BaP itself.[60] These results led Sims et al.[61] to propose that BaP was activated through a multistep pathway involving an initial epoxidation at the 7,8-position, hydrolysis of this epoxide to a 7,8-dihydrodiol, and then an additional epoxidation on the adjacent 9,10-position to yield a 7,8-diol-9,10-epoxide (Fig. 10).

A factor complicating the metabolism of PAHs is their asymmetry, which leads to the formation of stereoisomers. Thus, the initial epoxidation of BaP can give rise to two enantiomers, (+)- and (−)-BaP-7,8-epoxide, that are converted into (−)- and (+)-BaP-7,8-dihydrodiols, respectively (Fig. 11). Each of these enantiomeric dihydrodiols can then be converted into two diastereomeric diol epoxides. When the epoxide oxygen is on the same side of the aromatic ring system as the 7-hydroxy group, a syn-diol epoxide is formed, whereas epoxidation on the opposite side of the ring results in an anti-diol epoxide. Each of the BaP diol epoxides has different DNA binding and tumorigenic properties. Furthermore, these stereoisomers are not necessarily formed in equal amounts. For example, (+)-BaP-7,8-epoxide, and subsequently (−)-BaP-7,8-dihydrodiol, is formed to a greater extent than (−)-BaP-7,8-epoxide (Fig. 11). Likewise, (−)-BaP-7,8-dihydrodiol is converted primarily into (+)-anti-BaP-7,8-diol-9,10-epoxide, while (+)-BaP-7,8-dihydrodiol is metabolized primarily to (+)-syn-BaP-7,8-diol-9,10-epoxide.[62-64]

With the advent of the diol epoxide activation pathway for BaP, attention turned to other PAH. A critical feature of BaP diol epoxides is that they are located on the terminal benzo ring (i.e., carbons 7–10). Using this as a model, four different diol epoxides (ignoring stereochemistry) can be envisaged for benz[a]anthracene (Fig. 12). Similarly, two diol epoxides can be proposed for chrysene, while BaP, itself, can give rise to two (Fig. 12). After considering data from both tumor studies and theoretical calculations, Jerina and Daly[65] proposed that the particular isomer in which the epoxide moiety was located in the angular bay region should be the biologically significant diol epoxide. Experimental data acquired during the past 10 years with dihydrodiols and diol epoxides from a number of PAH have tended to support this bay region theory (summarized by Dipple et al.[66]).

There are marked differences in the DNA adducts and biologic responses induced by diol epoxide stereoisomers. With BaP diol epoxides, for example, it is quite clear that the racemic

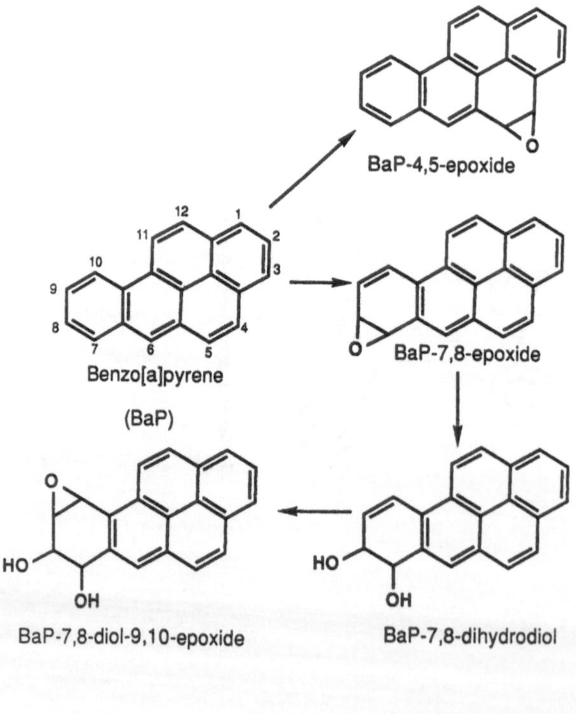

Figure 10. Metabolism of benzo[a]pyrene (BaP) to BaP-4,5-epoxide and BaP-7,8-diol-9,10-epoxide.

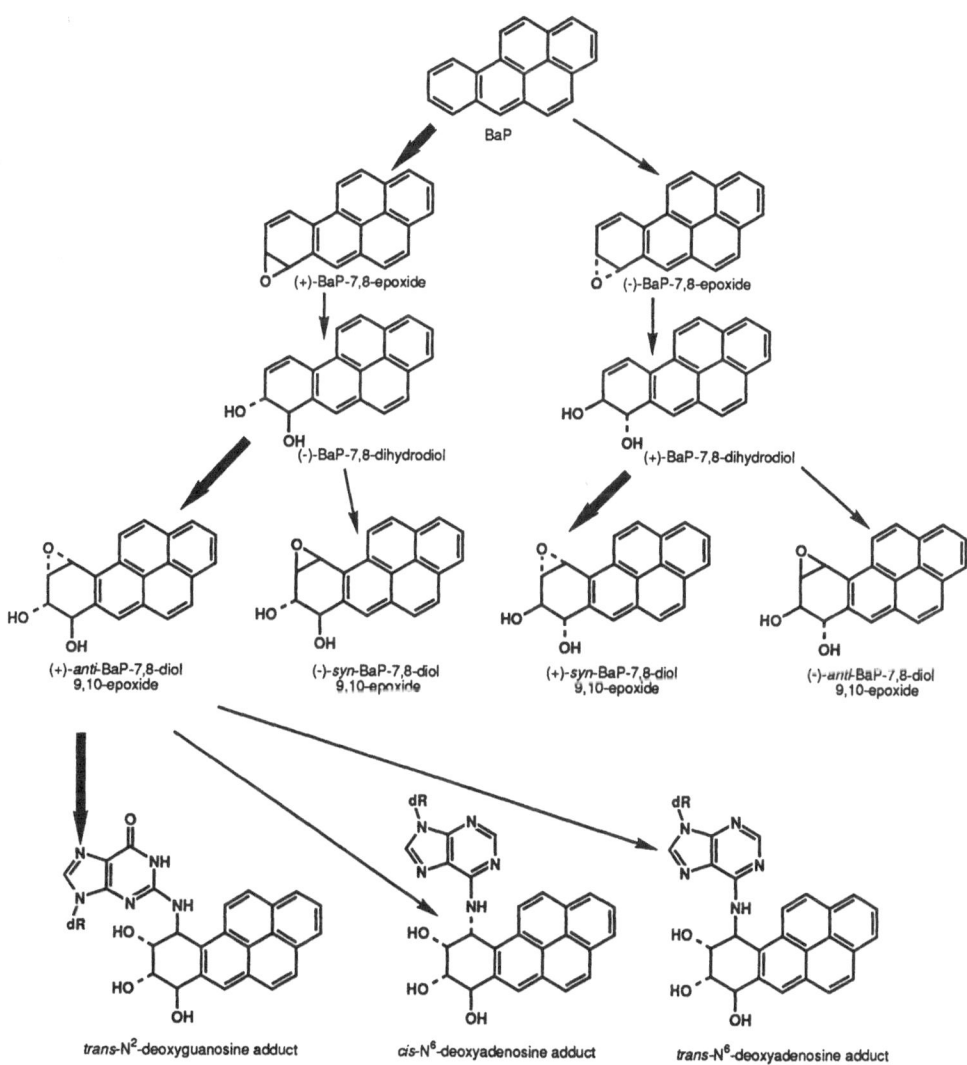

*Figure 11.* Stereospecific metabolism and DNA binding of benzo[a]pyrene (BaP).

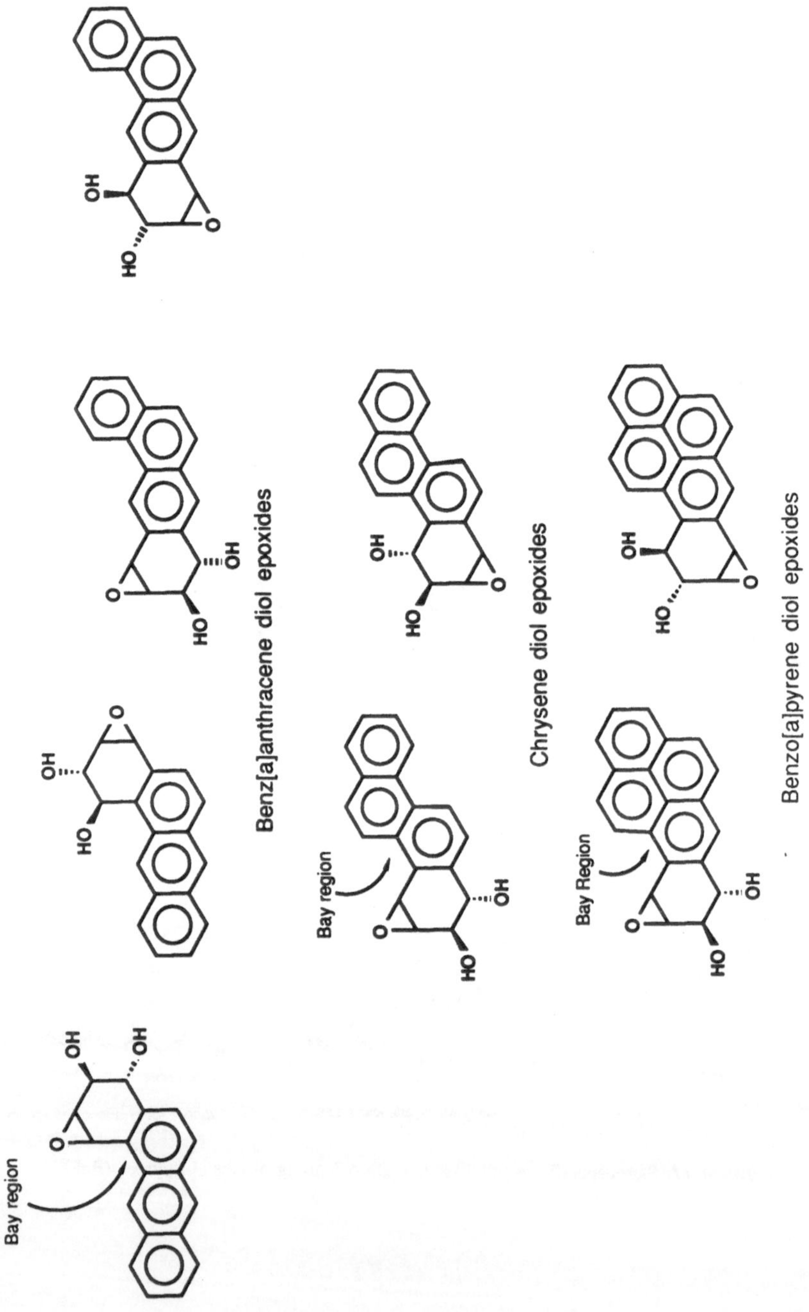

Figure 12. Diol epoxides of benz[a]anthracene, chrysene, and benzo[a]pyrene.

($\pm$)-*anti* isomers are much more tumorigenic than the ($\pm$)-*syn* isomers and that this difference is due primarily to the (+)-*anti* enantiomer.[67,68] Similarly, the ($\pm$)-*anti*-BaP diol epoxide isomers are more mutagenic in mammalian cells than the ($\pm$)-*syn* isomers, and this again appears to be due to the (+)-*anti* enantiomer.[69,70] Interestingly, the opposite relationship is true in bacteria, with ($\pm$)-*syn*-BaP diol epoxide being more mutagenic than the ($\pm$)-*anti* isomers.[71]

The principal DNA adduct obtained *in vitro* from (+)-*anti*-BaP-7,8-diol-9,10-epoxide is an $N^2$-substituted deoxyguanosine adduct formed by trans opening of the epoxide ring at C-10 (Fig. 11).[72,73] This is also the major adduct found in experimental animals and in cells treated with BaP.[72,73] Minor amounts (<10%) of deoxyadenosine adducts have also been reported,[74] and these result from both *cis* and *trans* addition of the $N^6$ position of deoxyadenosine to C-10 of the diol epoxide (Fig. 11).[75] Similar adducts have been found from the (−)-*anti* enantiomer. However, the deoxyguanosine and deoxyadenosine adducts are formed in nearly the same amounts.[74] Because of its lower biologic activity, the adducts obtained from *syn*-BaP diol epoxide have not been characterized as rigorously as those from the *anti*-isomer, although it is known that reactions occur with both deoxyguanosine and deoxyadenosine.[76]

As with the other carcinogens studied, attempts have been made to relate these particular adducts to mutagenic and tumorigenic responses. In mammalian cells treated with ($\pm$)-*anti* BaP diol epoxide, the major mutagenic lesion appears to be the $N^2$-substituted deoxyguanosine adduct obtained from the (+)-*anti*-enantiomer.[77] In bacteria, deoxyguanosine adducts also seem to be the primary mutagenic lesions; however, these adducts seem to arise from the (−)-*anti* and ($\pm$)-*syn* isomers.[76] This segregation in mutagenic response has been attributed to conformational differences between the adducts with the (−)-*anti* and ($\pm$)-*syn* deoxyguanosine adducts having similar conformations that are quite different from that of the (+)-*anti* deoxyguanosine adduct.[78–80] ($\pm$)-*Anti*-BaP diol epoxide will transform NIH 3T3 cells by inducing mutations at both codons 12 and 61 of the c-Ha-*ras* proto-oncogene,[81] and of the codon 61 mutations, approximately 60% are G → T transversions, consistent with the extensive binding (>90%) of ($\pm$)-*anti*-BaP diol epoxide to deoxyguanosine. Although deoxyadenosine adducts represent only a small portion of the binding (~5%), they appear to induce mutations with high efficiency because ~30% of transformants resulting from mutations at codon 61 are due to A → T transversions.[81] The importance of deoxyadenosine adducts in tumorigenic responses is further emphasized from experiments with 7,12-dimethylbenz[a]anthracene[24,82,83] and benzo[c]phenanthrene.[84] With 7,12-dimethylbenz[a]anthracene, mammary gland[24,82] and skin tumor[83] induction has been associated with an A → T transversion in codon 61 of the *ras* oncogene, while with benzo[c]phenanthrene, there is a direct correlation between the binding of its diol epoxide stereoisomers to deoxyadenosine and their oncogenic potential.[84]

## 4. CONCLUSIONS

We have shown that carcinogens are metabolized to electrophilic intermediates that result in the formation of DNA adducts, which makes plausible the notion that DNA damage may produce permanent, heritable neoplastic changes. We have noted that since DNA adduct formation is a relatively rare event *in vivo*, sophisticated methods, including immunoassays and $^{32}$P-postlabeling, have been developed for their detection. We considered the DNA adducts formed by four different classes of genotoxic carcinogens (Table III), and focused on those associated with tumorigenicity, mutagenicity, and proto-oncogene (*ras*) activation. With *N*-nitrosamines, the major DNA adducts are formed through reaction with N7 of deoxyguanosine, the major mutagenic lesion is $O^6$-alkyldeoxyguanosine, and $O^6$-alkyldeoxyguanosine and $O^4$-alkylthymidine are associated with the induction of tumors. Furthermore, the importance of $O^6$-methyldeoxyguanosine is consistent with the G → A transitions of the *ras* proto-oncogene observed during mammary gland tumorigenesis in rats treated with *N*-methyl-*N*-nitrosourea. With aflatoxins, the major site for substitution in DNA is also N7 of deoxyguanosine but, in contrast to the N7-deoxyguanosine adducts formed from *N*-nitrosamines, the N7-deoxyguanosine aflatoxin adduct and/or its ring-opened pyrimidine derivatives are

*Table III. Relationships among Major DNA Adducts, Major Mutagenic Adducts,
and Mutations Observed in ras Oncogene*

| Carcinogen class | Major DNA adduct | Major mutagenic adduct | Adduct associated with tumorigenesis | Predominant mutation in *ras* oncogene |
|---|---|---|---|---|
| *N*-Nitrosamines | N7-dG | $O^6$-dG | $O^6$-dG, $O^4$-dT | G → A transition |
| Aflatoxins | N7-dG | N7-dG | N7-dG | G → A transition |
| Aromatic amines | C8-dG | C8-dG | C8-dG | G → T transversion |
| Polycyclic aromatic hydrocarbons | $N^2$-dG $N^6$-dA | $N^2$-dG $N^6$-dA | $N^2$-dG $N^6$-dA | G → T transversion A → T transversion |

associated with the mutations and tumors induced by this carcinogen. Deoxguanosine adduct formation by aflatoxins is also consonant with the G → A transitions observed in the activation of the *ras* proto-oncogene. Aromatic amines and amides give primarily C8-substituted deoxyguanosine adducts. These lesions appear to be responsible for the mutations induced by these carcinogens and are the major adducts in target tissues. Furthermore, adduct formation at deoxyguanosine is compatible with the G → T transversions observed in the *ras* proto-oncogene of mice treated with *N*-hydroxy-2-acetylaminofluorene. Finally, PAH react primarily with $N^2$ of deoxyguanosine and $N^6$ of deoxyadenosine, and depending on the particular compound both types of adducts have been associated with the mutations and tumors induced by this class of carcinogens as well as with the transformation of the *ras* proto-oncogene.

ACKNOWLEDGMENT. We thank Cindy Hartwick for helping to prepare this manuscript.

## REFERENCES

1. Yuspa, S. H., and Poirier, M. C., 1988, Chemical carcinogenesis: From animal models to molecular models in one decade, *Adv. Cancer Res.* **50**:25–70.
2. Rowley, J. D., 1984, Biological implications of consistent chromosome rearrangements in leukemia and lymphoma, *Cancer Res.* **44**:3159–3168.
3. Weinstein, I. B., 1983, The monitoring of DNA adducts as an approach to carcinogen detection, *Annu. Rev. Public Health* **4**:409–413.
4. Herron, D. C., and Shank, R. C., 1979, Quantitative high-pressure liquid chromatographic analysis of methylated purines in DNA of rats treated with chemical carcinogens, *Anal. Biochem.* **100**:58–63.
5. Poirier, M. C., 1984, The use of carcinogen-DNA adduct antisera for quantitation and localization of genomic damage in animal models and the human population, *Environ. Mutagen.* **6**:879–887.
6. Gupta, R. C., Reddy, M. V., and Randerath, K., 1982, 32P-postlabeling analysis of non-radioactive aromatic carcinogen-DNA adducts, *Carcinogenesis* **3**:1081–1092.
7. Randerath, E., Agrawal, H. P., Weaver, J. A., Bordelon, C. B., and Randerath, K., 1985, 32P-Postlabeling analysis of DNA adducts persisting for up to 42 weeks in the skin, epidermis and dermis of mice treated topically with 7,12-dimethylbenz[a]anthracene, *Carcinogenesis* **6**:1117–1126.
8. Reddy, M. V., and Randerath, K., 1986, Nuclease P1-mediated enhancement of sensitivity of 32P-postlabeling test for structurally diverse DNA adducts, *Carcinogenesis* **7**:1543–1551.
9. Gupta, R. C., 1985, Enhanced sensitivity of 32P-postlabeling analysis of aromatic carcinogen:DNA adducts, *Cancer Res.* **45**:5656–5662.
10. Magee, P. N., and Barnes, J. M., 1956, The production of malignant primary hepatic tumours in the rat by feeding dimethylnitrosamine, *Br. J. Cancer* **10**:114–122.
11. Winn, D. M., 1986, Smokeless tobacco and oral/pharynx cancer: The role of cofactors, in: *Banbury Report 23: Mechanisms in Tobacco Carcinogenesis* (D. Hoffmann and C. C. Harris, eds.), pp. 361–375, Cold Spring Harbor Laboratory, New York.

12. Herron, D. C., and Shank, R. C., 1980, Methylated purines in human liver DNA after probable di-methylnitrosamine poisoning, *Cancer Res.* **40**:3116–3117.

13. Hecht, S. S., Foiles, P. G., Carmella, S. G., Trushin, N., Rivenson, A., and Hoffmann, D., 1986, Recent studies on the metabolic activation of tobacco-specific nitrosamines: Prospects for dosimetry in humans, in: *Banbury Report 23: Mechanisms in Tobacco Carcinogenesis* (D. Hoffmann and C. C. Harris, eds.), pp. 245–257, Cold Spring Harbor Laboratory, New York.

14. Beranek, D. T., Weis, C. C., and Swenson, D. H., 1980, A comprehensive quantitative analysis of methylated and ethylated DNA using high pressure liquid chromatography, *Carcinogenesis* **1**:595–606.

15. Frei, J. V., Swenson, D. H., Warren, W., and Lawley, P. D., 1978, Alkylation of deoxyribonucleic acid *in vivo* in various organs of C57BL mice by the carcionogens *N*-methyl-*N*-nitrosourea, *N*-ethyl-*N*-nitrosourea and ethyl methanesulphonate in relation to induction of thymic lymphoma. Some applications of high-pressure liquid chromatography, *Biochem. J.* **174**:1031–1044.

16. Frei, J. V., and Lawley, P. D., 1976, Tissue distribution and mode of DNA methylation in mice by methyl methanesulphonate and *N*-methyl-*N'*-nitro-*N*-nitrosoguanidine: Lack of thymic lymphoma induction and low extent of methylation of target tissue DNA at O-6 of guanine, *Chem. Biol. Interact.* **13**:215–222.

17. Loveless, A., 1969, Possible relevance of O-6 alkylation of deoxyguanosine to the mutagenicity and carcinogenicity of nitrosamines and nitrosamides, *Nature (Lond.)* **223**:206–207.

18. Abbott, P. J., and Saffhill, R., 1977, DNA synthesis with methylated poly(dA-dT) templates: Possible role of $O^4$-methylthymine as a pro-mutagenic base, *Nucleic Acids Res.* **4**:761–769.

19. Saffhill, R., and Abbott, P. J., 1978, Formation of $O^2$-methylthymine in poly(dA-dT) on methylation with N-methyl-N-nitrosourea and dimethyl sulphate. Evidence that $O^2$-methylthymidine does not miscode during DNA synthesis, *Nucleic Acids Res.* **5**:1971–1978.

20. Abbott, P. J., and Saffhill, R., 1979, DNA synthesis with methylated poly(dC-dG) templates. Evidence for a competitive nature to miscoding by $O^6$-methylguanine, *Biochim. Biophys. Acta* **562**:51–61.

21. Coulondre, C., and Miller, J. H., 1977, Genetic studies of the *lac* repressor. IV. Mutagenic specificity in the *lacI* gene of *Escherichia coli*, *J. Mol. Biol.* **117**:577–606.

22. Heflich, R. H., Beranek, D. T., Kodell, R. L., and Morris, S. M., 1982, Induction of mutations and sister–chromatid exchanges in Chinese hamster ovary cells by ethylating agents. Relationship to specific DNA adducts. *Mutat. Res.* **106**:147–161.

23. Beranek, D. T., Heflich, R. H., Kodell, R. L., Morris, S. M., and Casciano, D. A., 1983, Correlation between specific DNA-methylation products and mutation induction at the HGPRT locus in Chinese hamster ovary cells, *Mutat. Res.* **110**:171–180.

24. Zarbl, H., Sukumar, S., Arthur, A. V., Martin-Zanca, D., and Barbacid, M., 1985, Direct mutagenesis of Ha-*ras*-1 oncogenes by *N*-nitroso-*N*-methylurea during initiation of mammary carcinogenesis in rats, *Nature (Lond.)* **315**:382–386.

25. Richardson, F. C., Dyroff, M. C., Boucheron, J. A., and Swenberg, J. A., 1985, Differential repair of $O^4$-alkylthymidine following exposure to methylating and ethylating hepatocarcinogens, *Carcinogenesis* **6**:625–629.

26. Busby, W. F., Jr., and Wogan, G. N., 1984, Aflatoxins, in: *Chemical Carcinogens*, Vol. 2 (C. E. Searle, ed.), pp. 945–1136, American Chemical Society, Washington, D.C.

27. Essigmann, J. M., Croy, R. G., Nadzan, A. M., Busby, W. F., Jr., Reinhold, V. N., Büchi, G., and Wogan, G. N., 1977, Structural identification of the major DNA adduct formed by aflatoxin $B_1$ *in vitro*, *Proc. Natl. Acad. Sci. USA* **74**:1870–1874.

28. Groopman, J. D., Croy, R. G., and Wogan, G. N., 1981, *In vitro* reactions of aflatoxin $B_1$-adducted DNA, *Proc. Natl. Acad. Sci. USA* **78**:5445–5449.

29. Hertzog, P. J., Smith, J. R. L., and Garner, R. C., 1982, Characterisation of the imidazole ring-opened forms of *trans*-8,9-dihydro-8-(7-guanyl)9-hydroxy aflatoxin $B_1$, *Carcinogenesis* **3**:723–725.

30. Lin, J.-K., Miller, J. A., and Miller, E. C., 1977, 2,3-Dihydro-2-(guan-7-yl)-3-hydroxy-aflatoxin $B_1$, a major acid hydrolysis product of aflatoxin $B_1$-DNA or -ribosomal RNA adducts formed in hepatic microsome-mediated reactions and in rat liver *in vivo*, *Cancer Res.* **37**:4430–4438.

31. Stark, A. A., Essigmann, J. M., Demain, A. L., Skopek, T. R., and Wogan, G. N., 1979, Aflatoxin $B_1$ mutagenesis, DNA binding, and adduct formation in *Salmonella typhimurium*, *Proc. Natl. Acad. Sci. USA* **76**:1343–1347.

32. Croy, R. G., and Wogan, G. N., 1981, Temporal patterns of covalent DNA adducts in rat liver after single and multiple doses of aflatoxin $B_1$, *Cancer Res.* **41**:197–203.

33. Foster, P. L., Eisenstadt, E., and Miller, J. H., 1983, Base substitution mutations induced by metabolically activated aflatoxin $B_1$, *Proc. Natl. Acad. Sci. USA* **80**:2695–2698.

34. Kaden, D. A., Call, K. M., Leong, P.-M., Komives, E. A., and Thilly, W. G., 1987, Killing and mutation

of human lymphoblast cells by aflatoxin B₁: Evidence for an inducible repair response, *Cancer Res.* **47:**1993–2001.

35. Kensler, T. W., Egner, P. A., Davidson, N. E., Roebuck, B. D., Pikul, A., and Groopman, J. D., 1986, Modulation of aflatoxin metabolism, aflatoxin-$N^7$-guanine formation, and hepatic tumorigenesis in rats fed ethoxyquin: Role of induction of glutathione *S*-transferases, *Cancer Res.* **46:**3924–3931.

36. McMahon, G., Davis, E., and Wogan, G. N., 1987, Characterization of c-Ki-*ras* oncogene alleles in rat liver tumors induced by aflatoxin B₁, *Proc. Am. Assoc. Cancer Res.* **28:**150.

37. Rehn, C., 1895, Blasengeschwülste bei Fuchsinarbeitern, *Arch. Klin. Chir.* **50:**588–600.

38. Case, R. A. M., Hosker, M. E., McDonald, D. B., and Pearson, J. T., 1954, Tumours of the urinary bladder in workmen engaged in the manufacture and use of certain dyestuff intermediates in the British chemical industry. I. The role of aniline, benzidine, alpha-naphthylamine and beta-naphthylamine, *Br. J. Indust. Med.* **11:**75–104.

39. Melick, W. F., Escue, H. M., Naryka, J. J., Mezera, R. A., and Wheeler, E. P., 1955, The first reported cases of human bladder tumors due to a new carcinogen—xenylamine, *J. Urol.* **74:**760–766.

40. Patrianakos, C., and D. Hoffmann, 1979, Chemical studies on tobacco smoke. LXIV. On the analysis of aromatic amines in cigarette smoke, *J. Anal. Toxicol.* **3:**150–154.

41. Mommsen, S., and Aagaard, J., 1983, Tobacco as a risk factor in bladder cancer, *Carcinogenesis* **4:**335–338.

42. Sugimura, T., 1986, Past, present, and future of mutagens in cooked foods, *Environ. Health Persp.* **67:**5–10.

43. Tokiwa, H., and Ohnishi, Y., 1986, Mutagenicity and carcinogenicity of nitroarenes and their sources in the environment, *CRC Crit. Rev. Toxicol.* **17:**23–60.

44. Bryant, M. S., Skipper, P. L., Tannebaum, S. R., and Maclure, M., 1987, Hemoglobin adducts of 4-aminobiphenyl in smokers and nonsmokers, *Cancer Res.* **47:**602–608.

45. Weber, W. W., and Hein, D. W., 1985, N-Acetylation pharmacogenetics, *Pharmacol. Rev.* **37:**25–79.

46. Cartwright, R. A., Rogers, H. J., Barham-Hall, D., Glashan, R. W., Ahmad, R. A., Higgins, E., and Kahn, M. A., 1982, Role of N-acetyltransferase phenotypes in bladder carcinogenesis: A pharmacogenetic epidemiological approach to bladder cancer, *Lancet* **ii:**842–846.

47. Lang, N. P., Chu, D. Z. J., Hunter, C. F., Kendall, D. C., Flammang, T. J., and Kadlubar, F. F., 1986, Role of aromatic amine acetyltransferase in human colorectal cancer, *Arch. Surg.* **121:**1259–1261.

48. Ilett, K. F., David, B. M., Detchon, P., Castleden, W. M., and Kwa, R., 1987, Acetylation phenotype in colorectal carcinoma, *Cancer Res.* **47:**1466–1469.

49. Kadlubar, F. F., and Beland, F. A., 1985, Chemical properties of ultimate carcinogenic metabolites of arylamines and arylamides, in: *Polycyclic Hydrocarbons and Carcinogenesis* (R. G. Harvey, ed.), pp. 341–370, American Chemical Society, Washington, D.C.

50. Beland, F. A., and Kadlubar, F. F., 1985, Formation and persistence of arylamine DNA adduct *in vivo*, *Environ. Health Persp.* **62:**19–30.

51. Bichara, M., and Fuchs, R. P. P., 1985, DNA binding and mutation spectra of the carcinogen N-2-aminofluorene in *Escherichia coli*. A correlation between the conformation of the premutagenic lesion and the mutation specificity, *J. Mol. Biol.* **183:**341–351.

52. Lai, C.-C., Miller, E. C., Miller, J. A., and Liem, A., 1987, Initiation of hepatocarcinogenesis in infant male B6C3F₁ mice by N-hydroxy-2-aminofluorene or N-hydroxy-2-acetylaminofluorene depends primarily on metabolism to N-sulfooxy-2-aminofluorene and formation of DNA-(deoxyguanosin-8-yl)-2-aminofluorene adducts, *Carcinogenesis* **8:**471–478.

53. Wiseman, R. W., Stowers, S. J., Miller, E. C., Anderson, M. W., and Miller, J. A., 1986, Activating mutations of the c-Ha-*ras* protooncogene in chemically induced hepatomas of the male B6C3 F₁ mouse, *Proc. Natl. Acad. Sci. USA* **83:**5825–5829.

54. Pott, P., 1775, *Chirurgical Observations Relative to the Cataract, the Polypus of the Nose, the Cancer of the Scrotum, the Different Kinds of Ruptures, and the Mortification of the Toes and Feet*, Hawes, Clarke and Collins, London. (Reprinted in: *Natl. Cancer Inst. Monogr.* **10:**7–13, 1963.)

55. Kipling, M. D., and Cooke, M. A., 1984, Soots, tars, and oils as causes of occupational cancer, in: *Chemical Carcinogens*, Vol. 1 (C. E. Searle, ed.), pp. 165–174, American Chemical Society, Washington, D.C.

56. Cook, J. W., Hewett, C., and Hieger, I., 1932, Coal-tar constituents and cancer, *Nature (Lond.)* **130:**926.

57. Boyland, E., 1950, The biological significance of metabolism of polycyclic compounds, *Biochem. Soc. Symp.* **5:**40–54.

58. Pullman, A., and Pullman, B., 1955, Electronic structure and carcinogenic activity of aromatic molecules. New developments, *Adv. Cancer Res.* **3:**117–169.

59. Baird, W. M., Harvey, R. G., and Brookes, P., 1975, Comparison of the cellular DNA-bound products of benzo(a)pyrene with the products formed by the reaction of benzo(a)pyrene-4,5-oxide with DNA, *Cancer Res.* **35**:54–57.

60. Borgen, A., Darvey, H., Castagnoli, N., Crocker, T. T., Rasmussen, R. E., and Wang, I. Y., 1973, Metabolic conversion of benzo[a]pyrene by Syrian hamster liver microsomes and binding of metabolites to deoxyribonucleic acid, *J. Med. Chem.* **16**:502–506.

61. Sims, P., Grover, P. L., Swaisland, A., Pal, K., and Hewer, A., 1974, Metabolic activation of benzo(a)pyrene proceeds by a diol-epoxide, *Nature (Lond.)* **252**:326–328.

62. Yang, S. K., McCourt, D. W., Leutz, J. C., and Gelboin, H. V., 1977, Benzo[a]pyrene diol epoxides: Mechanism of enzymatic formation and optically active intermediates, *Science* **196**:1199–1201.

63. Thakker, D. R., Yagi, H., Akagi, H., Koreeda, M., Lu, A. Y. H., Levin, W., Wood, A. W., Conney, A. H., and Jerina, D. M., 1977, Metabolism of benzo[a]pyrene. VI. Stereoselective metabolism of benzo[a]pyrene and benzo[a]pyrene 7,8-dihydrodiol to diol epoxides, *Chem. Biol. Interact.* **16**:281–300.

64. Levin, W., Buening, M. K., Wood, A. W., Chang, R. L., Kedzierski, B., Thakker, D. R., Boyd, D. R., Gadaginamath, G. S., Armstrong, R. N., Yagi, H., Karle, J. M., Slaga, T. J., Jerina, D. M., and Conney, A. H., 1980, An enantiomeric interaction in the metabolism and tumorigenicity of (+)- and (−)-benzo[a]pyrene 7,8-oxide, *J. Biol. Chem.* **255**:9067–9074.

65. Jerina, D. M., and Daly, J. W., 1976, Oxidation at carbon, in: *Drug Metabolism* (D. V. Parke and R. L. Smith, eds.), pp. 13–32, Taylor and Francis, London.

66. Dipple, A., Moschel, R. C., and Bigger, C. A. H., 1984, Polynuclear aromatic carcinogens, in: *Chemical Carcinogens*, Vol. 1 (C. E. Searle, ed.), pp. 41–163, American Chemical Society, Washington, D.C.

67. Slaga, T. J., Bracken, W. J., Gleason, G., Levin, W., Yagi, H., Jerina, D. M., and Conney, A. H., 1979, Marked differences in the skin tumor-initiating activities of the optical enantiomers of the diastereomeric benzo(a)pyrene 7,8-diol-9,10-epoxides, *Cancer Res.* **39**:67–71.

68. Buening, M. K., Wislocki, P. G., Levin, W., Yagi, H., Thakker, D. R., Akagi, H., Koreeda, M., Jerina, D. M., and Conney, A. H., 1978, Tumorigenicity of the optical enantiomers of the diastereomeric benzo[a]pyrene 7,8-diol-9,10-epoxides in newborn mice: Exceptional activity of (+)-7β,8α-dihydroxy-9α,10α-epoxy-7,8,9,10-tetrahydrobenzo[a]pyrene, *Proc. Natl. Acad. Sci. USA* **75**:5358–5361.

69. Newbold, R. F., and Brookes, P., 1976, Exceptional mutagenicity of a benzo[a]pyrene diol epoxide in cultured mammalian cells, *Nature (Lond.)* **261**:52–54.

70. Brookes, P., and Osborne, M. R., 1982, Mutation in mammalian cells by stereoisomers of *anti*-benzo[a]pyrene-diolepoxide in relation to the extent and nature of the DNA reaction products, *Carcinogenesis* **3**:1223–1226.

71. Wood, A. W., Wislocki, P. G., Chang, R. L., Levin, W., Lu, A. Y. H., Yagi, H., Hernandez, O., Jerina, D. M., and Conney, A. H., 1976, Mutagenicity and cytotoxicity of benzo(a)pyrene benzo-ring epoxides, *Cancer Res.* **36**:3358–3366.

72. Jeffrey, A. M., Weinstein, I. B., Jennette, K. W., Grzeskowiak, K., Nakanishi, K., Harvey, R. G., Autrup, H., and Harris, C., 1977, Structures of benzo(a)pyrene-nucleic acid adducts formed in human and bovine bronchial explants, *Nature (Lond.)* **269**:348–350.

73. Koreeda, M., Moore, P. D., Wislocki, P. G., Levin, W., Conney, A. H., Yagi, H., and Jerina, D. M., 1978, Binding of benzo[a]pyrene 7,8-diol-9,10-epoxides to DNA, RNA, and protein of mouse skin occurs with high stereoselectivity, *Science* **199**:778–781.

74. Meehan, T., and Straub, K., 1979, Double-stranded DNA stereoselectively binds benzo(a)pyrene diol epoxides, *Nature (Lond.)* **277**:410–412.

75. Jeffrey, A. M., Grzeskowiak, K., Weinstein, I. B., Nakanishi, K., Roller, P., and Harvey, R. G., 1979, Benzo(a)pyrene-7,8-dihydrodiol 9,10-oxide adenosine and deoxyadenosine adducts: Structure and stereochemistry, *Science* **206**:1309–1311.

76. Burgess, J. A., Stevens, C. W., and Fahl, W. E., 1985, Mutation at separate gene loci in *Salmonella typhimurium* TA100 related to DNA nucleotide modification by stereoisomeric benzo(a)pyrene 7,8-diol-9,10-epoxides, *Cancer Res.* **45**:4257–4262.

77. Stevens, C. W., Bouck, N., Burgess, J. A., and Fahl, W. E., 1985, Benzo[a]pyrene diol-epoxides: Different mutagenic efficiency in human and bacterial cells, *Mutat. Res.* **152**:5–14.

78. Jernström, B., Lycksell, P.-O., Gräslund, A., and Nordén, B., 1984, Spectroscopic studies of DNA complexes formed after reaction with *anti*-benzo[a]pyrene-7,8-dihydrodiol-9,10-oxide enantiomers of different carcinogenic potency, *Carcinogenesis* **5**:1129–1135.

79. Geacintov, N. E., Ibanez, V., Gagliano, A. G., Jacobs, S. A., and Harvey, R. G., 1984, Stereoselective covalent binding of anti-benzo(a)pyrene diol epoxide to DNA. Conformation of enantiomer adducts, *J. Biomol. Struct. Dynam.* **1**:1473–1484.

80. Geacintov, N. E., Zinger, D., Ibanez, V., Santella, R., Grunberger, D., and Harvey, R. G., 1987, Properties of covalent benzo[a]pyrene diol epoxide—DNA adducts investigated by fluorescence techniques, *Carcinogenesis* **8:**925–935.

81. Vousden, K. H., Bos, J. L., Marshall, C. J., and Phillips, D. H., 1986, Mutations activating human c-Ha-*ras*1 protooncogene (*HRAS1*) induced by chemical carcinogens and depurination, *Proc. Natl. Acad. Sci. USA* **83:**1222–1226.

82. Dandekar, S., Sukumar, S., Zarbl, H., Young, L. J. T., and Cardiff, R. D., 1986, Specific activation of the cellular Harvey-*ras* oncogene in dimethylbenzanthracene-induced mouse mammary tumors, *Mol. Cell. Biol.* **6:**4104–4108.

83. Quintanilla, M., Brown, K., Ramsden, M., and Balmain, A., 1986, Carcinogen-specific mutation and amplification of Ha-*ras* during mouse skin carcinogenesis, *Nature (Lond.)* **322:**78–80.

84. Dipple, A., Pigott, M. A., Agarwal, S. K., Yagi, H., Sayer, J. M., and Jerina, D. M., 1987, Optically active benzo[c]phenanthrene diol epoxides bind extensively to adenine in DNA, *Nature (Lond.)* **327:**535–536.

# 4

# *Oncogenic Viruses*

## *Mario R. Escobar*

## *1. INTRODUCTION*

### *1.1. Purpose*

This chapter begins with a brief account of the important events that have occurred during the history of viral oncology. After this is a description of the major subgroups of DNA and RNA oncogenic viruses followed by a discussion of the pathobiology and unifying features of viral oncogenesis and cell transformation. Next, there is a review of established animal models of human cancer and an examination of the most widely investigated oncogenic human viruses. Finally, the immunologic aspects of neoplasia are considered in some detail, concluding with remarks on the future perspectives in the field of viral oncology.

### *1.2. Overview and Historic Events*

From the turn of this century until about 1970, many advances have been made in the field of experimental viral oncology. It was during the latter part of this period that Temin proposed his provirus theory for Rous sarcoma,[1] which reflected his foresight and led in 1970 to the independent discovery by two research groups, including that of Temin's, of reverse transcriptase.[2,3] The significance of this discovery was not realized immediately so that the impetus in tumor virus research actually declined during the early seventies. The seminal observation made by these two groups that genetic information could be processed from RNA to DNA—rather than only from DNA to RNA, as had been previously thought—greatly affected oncoviral research, and after a brief lag phase of several years, triggered the recent explosion of research on the molecular biology of retroviruses. It was really not until the present decade that research on oncogenic viruses has been brought to the cutting edge of biomedical sciences. This switch may best be explained by (1) the stronger conviction of a direct relevance of viruses to human neoplasia, due mostly to the advent of recombinant DNA biotechnology and the recent discovery of cellular oncogenes and human oncogenic retroviruses, and (2) the use of defined oncogenes and oncogenic retroviruses to develop powerful model systems in which to probe the molecular biology of eukaryotic cells and, in particular, the subcellular mechanisms of animal cell transformation. Oncogenic viruses can be distinguished from other viruses by their unique ability to transform cells, using the information encoded in only one or a few transforming genes.[4]

---

*Mario R. Escobar* • Department of Pathology, Medical College of Virginia, Virginia Commonwealth University, Richmond, Virginia, 23298-0106.

The great promise of viral oncology is that the ongoing investigations, which are being focused on the functions of the transforming proteins that are encoded by the viral oncogenes, will lead to the elucidation of the mechanisms of transformation at the cellular and molecular levels. Furthermore, such studies will inevitably provide new insights into growth regulation in normal cells as well.

Some of the milestones in viral oncology that have made a major impact on the field are outlined below in chronologic order.

| Year | Event | References |
|------|-------|-----------|
| DNA viruses | | |
| 1814–1931 | Bateman (1814) was the first to describe the disease of molluscum contagiosum and Goodpasture and Woodruff (1931) were the first to conclude that this disease was caused by a virus. | 5,6 |
| 1960 | Vogt and Dulbecco demonstrated that polyoma virus was the first DNA virus capable of transforming cells in culture. | 7 |
| 1961 | Yaba monkey tumor virus was first recovered by Niven and associates from subcutaneous tumors that occurred in a colony of Rhesus monkeys in Nigeria; the viral etiology of progressive multifocal leukoencephalopathy was suspected by Richardson. | 8, 9 |
| 1962 | Trentin et al. reported the first virus of human origin known to be oncogenic in animals. | 10 |
| 1964 | Epstein et al. simultaneously with Pulvertaft, reported in the same issue of the *Lancet* the presence of virus particles in cultured lymphoblasts from Burkitt lymphoma. | 11,12 |
| 1969 | Rawls and co-workers associated herpes virus type 2 and carcinoma of the uterine cervix. | 13 |
| 1973 | Albrecht and Rapp showed that both human and nonhuman cells can undergo oncogenic transformation when inoculated with infectious or UV-irradiated cytomegalovirus. These cells can produce malignant tumors when inoculated into appropriate animal models. | 14 |
| 1976 | zur Hausen associated papillomaviruses with human genital cancer. | 15 |
| 1977 | Gardner provided evidence that progressive multifocal leukoencephalitis was the first human disease associated with polyoma virus (JC virus). | 16 |
| 1978 | Szmuness provided evidence for a causal association between hepatocellular carcinoma and the hepatitis B virus. | 17 |
| 1986 | A novel human herpeslike virus (human B lymphotropic virus or HBLV) was isolated from patients with associated lymphoproliferative disorders by Salahuddin et al. | 18 |

| Year | Event | References |
|------|-------|-----------|
| RNA Viruses | | |
| 1908 | Ellerman and Bang observed an ultrafiltrable agent in avian leukosis. | 19 |
| 1911 | Rous induced sarcomas in chickens with cell-free filtrates from sarcomas. | 20 |
| 1914 | Fujinami and Inamoto produced sarcomas in chickens and ducks using tumor ultrafiltrates. | 21 |
| 1936 | Bittner demonstrated mammary tumors through a milk factor. | 22 |
| 1951 | Gross provided the first conclusive evidence for an etiologic role of viruses in murine leukemia. | 23 |
| 1955 | Graffi *et al.* discovered another virus in sarcoma filtrates, which causes myeloid leukemia in mice. | 24 |
| 1957 | Friend obtained a filtrable agent from the spleen of a leukemic Swiss mouse, which consistently produced erythroleukemia. | 25 |
| 1959 | Lieberman and Kaplan found leukemogenic activity in cell-free filtrates from radiation-induced leukemias of mice. | 26 |
| 1960,1962 | Moloney and Rauscher described viral agents, murine leukemia virus (MuLV), which efficiently produced lymphoid leukemia in adult animals of most inbred strains of mice. | 27,28 |
| 1964–1967 | Harvey, Moloney, Finkel *et al.,* and Kirsten and Mayer linked induction of murine sarcomas to RNA tumor viruses. Except for Finkel, Biskis and Jinkins virus, none of these murine sarcoma viruses was isolated from naturally occurring sarcomas. | 29–31 |
| 1964–1969 | Jarrett *et al.,* Kawakami *et al.,* and Rickart *et al.* associated cat leukemias and sarcomas with RNA tumor viruses. | 33–35 |
| 1969–1971 | Snyder and Theilen, Gardner and Arnstein, and McDonough and Sarma described the first isolates of feline sarcoma virus. | 32,36 |
| 1970 | Chopra and Mason discovered the first primate retrovirus in a mammary carcinoma of a Rhesus monkey. | 37 |
| | Temin and Mizutani and Baltimore identified reverse transcriptase in RNA tumor viruses. | 2,3,38,39 |
| 1971 | Wolfe *et al.* isolated a primate retrovirus from a fibrosarcoma of a woolly monkey that transformed cells in culture and induced fibrosarcomas in infected marmoset monkeys. | 40 |
| 1972 | Theilen and Wolfe isolated a primate retrovirus from spontaneous lymphosarcomas and leukemias of Gibbon apes that induces granulocytic and lymphocytic leukemias in Gibbons. | 32 |

| Year | Event | References |
|------|-------|-----------|
| 1973–1980 | Duesberg and Vogt detected the first oncogene in Rous sarcoma virus (RSV) on the basis of biochemical and genetic analysis. The subsequent isolation of this oncogene (*src*) in 1976 was by Stehelin *et al.*, and the determination of its complete nucleotide sequence in 1980 by Bishop defined this oncogene and led to the detection of other oncogenes in retroviruses and also in transformed and normal vertebrate cells. | 41–43 |
| | Poiesz *et al.* detected the first human leukemia/lymphoma virus (HTLV-1) in cultured T cells of two adult black American patients with aggressive forms of T-cell malignancy. | 44,45 |

## 1.3. Classification

Viruses are unique because, unlike all other microorganisms, they contain either DNA or RNA in their genome, but not both. Therefore, like other viruses, tumor viruses are also classified among different families into DNA and RNA tumor viruses, depending on their type of nucleic acid. They may be further subdivided according to the biophysical characteristics of their virions. Poxviruses are larger (i.e., 230–400 µm in diameter) than any other DNA or RNA tumor virus. In fact, their size overlaps with that of the smallest bacteria (e.g., *Chlamydia*, *Rickettsia*, *Mycoplasma*), with which they share certain biologic features (e.g., susceptibility to rifamycin). The smallest of all tumor viruses are the members of the hepadnavirus group (e.g., 42 µm). All the retroviruses (oncoviruses) are intermediate in size (100–120 µm). It is remarkable, however, that notwithstanding the deep taxonomic dichotomy between the DNA and RNA tumor viruses, there are also many points of convergence which make the distinction between the two groups regarding their role in neoplasia much more difficult to interpret than was previously believed.

### 1.3.1. DNA Tumor Viruses

All DNA tumor viruses known to date consist of double-stranded DNA (dsDNA). DNA viruses are further subdivided into those whose nucleocapsid is surrounded by an outer lipid-containing envelope or membrane and those which lack this important outer structure.

As shown in Table I, the dsDNA enveloped tumor viruses include the pox-, herpes-, and hepadnaviruses. The members of each of these three groups are tabulated therein according to the host, species of origin, and the general morphologic characteristics of the virion (e.g., size and type of symmetry) and the genome (e.g., molecular weight and nucleic acid configuration). The newest member of the herpes virus group, human B lymphotropic virus (HBLV), was discovered recently.[18] Although morphologically similar to the members of this group, it is readily distinguishable from the known human and primate herpesviruses by host range, *in vitro* biologic effects, and antigenic features.

As shown in Table II, the dsDNA tumor viruses where the viral nucleocapsid is deprived of an outer lipid-containing envelope include the adeno-, papilloma-, and polyomaviruses. The members of each of these three groups are also tabulated according to the same criteria used as in Table I.

### 1.3.2. RNA Tumor Viruses (Oncoviruses)

RNA tumor viruses were once called oncornaviruses (i.e., oncogenic RNA) but are now classified as retroviruses because they contain RNA-dependent DNA polymerase (reverse transcriptase). Retroviruses characteristically induce a variety of neoplastic diseases and are very widely distributed among vertebrate species. They are recognized by their morphology, the structure of their

*Table I. dsDNA Tumor Virus Groups in which the Virus Is Surrounded by an Outer Lipid-Containing Envelope*

| Virus group and subgroup | Host species of origin | General morphologic characteristics | | | |
| | | Virion | | Genome | |
| | | Size (nm) | Structure | Molecular weight ($\times 10^6$) | Configuration |
| --- | --- | --- | --- | --- | --- |
| Pox | | | | | |
| Molluscum contagiosum | Human | | | | |
| Yaba | Monkey | 230–300 | Complex | 130–240 | Linear |
| Fibroma–myxoma | Rabbit, squirrel deer | | symmetry | | |
| Herpes | | | | | |
| Simplex, types 1 and 2 | Human | | | | |
| Epstein-Barr | Human | | | | |
| Cytomegalo | Human | | | | |
| Human B-lymphotropic[a] | Human | | | | |
| Saimiri | Monkey (squirrel) | 100–200 | Icosahedral | 100 | Linear |
| Ateles | Monkey (spider) | | symmetry | | |
| Melendez | Monkey | | | | |
| Equine, type 1 | Horse | | | | |
| Marek | Avian | | | | |
| Lucké | Frog | | | | |
| Hinze | Rabbit | | | | |
| Hepadna | | | | | |
| Hepatitis B | Human | | | | |
| Woodchuck hepatitis | Woodchuck | 42 | Complex | 1.6 | Circular[b] |
| Ground squirrel hepatitis | Squirrel | | symmetry | | |
| Duck hepatitis | Peking duck | | | | |

[a]Human B-lymphotropic virus is herpeslike but has unique antigenic features.
[b]One DNA strand of hepatitis B is incomplete and variable in length; a viral DNA polymerase can complete it.

RNA viral genomes, and their reverse transcriptase. Retroviruses are divided into three subfamilies of unequal size: oncoviruses, lentiviruses (*lente:* slow), and spumaviruses (*spuma:* foam). The oncoviruses form by far the largest subfamily of retroviruses and have been isolated from virtually all vertebrate species in which they have been diligently sought, including humans. They are categorized in Table III according to their host species of origin, their morphologic particle type, and the neoplasia with which each subgroup is associated. The other two subfamilies of retroviruses are not oncogenic and will not be addressed in this chapter. Suffice it to say that although the spumaviruses may induce persistent infection *in vivo* or in culture, they have not yet been associated with a distinct pathologic entity. The lentiviruses, on the other hand, are known to be pathogenic. The two lentiviruses which have been best characterized thus far are the visna and maedi viruses. The human T-cell lymphotropic virus (HTLV-III), the etiologic agent of the acquired immune deficiency syndrome (AIDS), and recently redesignated as the human immunodeficiency virus (HIV), is the newest member of this group of retroviruses.

## 2. HOST CELLS, TUMOR VIRUSES, AND THEIR INTERACTIONS

### 2.1. Host Cells

Host cells are either permissive or nonpermissive for replication of a given virus. Permissive cells support virus growth, whereas nonpermissive cells do not. As a general rule, permissive cells

*Table II. dsDNA Tumor Virus Groups in which the Virus Is Deprived of an Outer Lipid-Containing Envelope*

| | | General morphologic characteristics | | | |
| | | Virion | | Genome | |
| Virus group and subgroup | Host species of origin | Size (nm) | Structure | Molecular weight ($\times 10^6$) | Configuration |
|---|---|---|---|---|---|
| Adeno | | | | | |
| Human types 3, 7, 9, 11, 12, 14, 16, 18, 21, and 31 | Human | | | | |
| Simian types (some) | Monkey | 70–90 | Icosahedral symmetry | 20–25 | Linear |
| Bovine, type 3 | Cow | | | | |
| Avian (CELO) | Chicken | | | | |
| Papova | | | | | |
| Papilloma | | | | | |
| Human | Human | | | | |
| Shope | Rabbit | | | | |
| Bovine, type 1[a] | Cow | | | | |
| Canine | Dog | 45–55 | Icosahedral symmetry | 3–5 | Circular |
| Polyoma[b] | Mouse | | | | |
| SV40[c] | Monkey | | | | |
| BK/JC | Human | | | | |

[a]DNA genome size is 7.9 kb.
[b]DNA genome size is 5.3 kb.
[c]DNA genome size is 5.2 kb.

are not transformed by the virus, but nonpermissive cells may be transformed. It is noteworthy that not all cells from the natural host species are susceptible to either virus infection or transformation, or both. Most tumor viruses are remarkably tissue specific, a feature that most likely has to do with the variable presence of surface cell receptors for the virus or intracellular factors required for viral gene expression.[46]

## 2.2. Tumor Viruses

### 2.2.1. DNA Tumor Viruses

These viruses usually replicate in certain cells of their natural host (i.e., homologous cells) but are rarely, if ever, oncogenic in those hosts. Conversely, DNA tumor viruses cannot replicate in heterologous host cells but do occasionally transform them. SV40, a prototype DNA tumor virus that naturally infects Rhesus monkeys, replicates in monkey kidney cell monolayers but does not transform them. This virus is unable to replicate in cells of rodent origin (i.e., heterologous cells), but it induces their transformation, albeit at low efficiency. The role played by the DNA tumor viruses in the oncogenic process has been critically evaluated by Monier and Salzman,[47] who attempted to define those viral functions that could control the various steps in cell transformation.

### 2.2.2. RNA Tumor Viruses

In contrast to the scenario presented above, RNA tumor viruses may cause neoplasia in their natural hosts. They can both replicate in and transform homologous cells. Certain RNA tumor viruses can also transform heterologous cells, usually without virus replication. In short, the main

## Table III. ssRNA Tumor Virus Groups (Oncoviruses)

| Virus group and subgroup | Abbreviations used | Host species of origin | Particle type[c] | Type of malignancy |
|---|---|---|---|---|
| Primate | | | | |
| Human T-cell lympho-tropic | HTLV-1[a] | Human | C | Lymphoma/leukemia |
| Simian sarcoma | SiSV-1[a] | Woolly monkey | C | Sarcoma |
| Gibbon | GALV[a] | Ape | C | Leukemia |
| Mason–Pfizer | MPMV[a] | Rhesus monkey | D | Mammary carcinoma |
| Murine complex | | | | |
| Murine leukemia | MuLV[b] | Mouse | C | Leukemia |
| Murine sarcoma | MuSV[a] | Mouse | C | Sarcoma |
| Bittner | MMTV[b] | Mouse | B | Mammary tumor |
| Feline complex | | | | |
| Feline leukemia | FeLV[b] | Cat | C | Leukemia |
| Feline sarcoma | FeSV[a] | Cat | C | Sarcoma |
| Avian complex | | | | |
| Avian erythroblastosis | AEV[a] | Chicken | C | Sarcoma, erythroblastosis |
| Avian leukosis | ALV[b] | Chicken | C | Leukemia |
| Rous sarcoma | ASV[a] | Chicken | C | Sarcoma |
| Reticuloendotheliosis | REV[a] | Birds | C | Lymphoma |
| Other | | | | |
| Bovine leukemia | BLV[a] | Cow | C | Leukemia |
| Hamster leukemia | HaLV[b] | Hamster | C | Leukemia |
| Rat leukemia | RaLV[b] | Rat | C | Leukemia |

[a]These viruses are exogenous.
[b]Some of these viruses are endogenous and some are exogenous.
[c]B, C, and D particles are found extracellularly; diameters: B = 100–130 nm, C = 90–110 nm, and D = 100–120 nm.

difference between RNA and DNA tumor viruses is that the former can transform both permissive and nonpermissive host cells.

Retroviruses possess a number of unusual properties. In marked contrast to most other viruses, which kill the cells they infect, retroviruses typically establish a chronic infection in susceptible host cells. The continual expression of the viral genes is not usually cytotoxic, since most retroviruses are not cytocidal. On the contrary, often retroviral infection either enhances the rate of cell proliferation or has no detectable effect on cell growth. For example, cells infected with sarcoma viruses exhibit morphologic changes and proliferate like tumor cells, while cells infected with leukemia viruses show no morphologic or cytopathic changes and continue to grow normally. In order to induce chronic infection, the viral genome of retroviruses has developed a unique strategy for its replication. Although the viral genome inside retrovirus virions consists of single-stranded RNA, the virus replicates in the host cell through a double-stranded viral DNA intermediate that is integrated efficiently into the host cell DNA. This conversion of the virion RNA to a DNA genome is catalyzed by the virally encoded RNA-dependent DNA polymerase or reverse transcriptase.[48]

Another unusual feature that is also related to their mode of replication is that certain retroviruses behave as cellular genes insofar as they are carried in the germ line as endogenous proviruses (i.e., integrated viral genomes linked to host-cell DNA) that are transmitted vertically as Mendelian elements from parent to offspring.[49] Other retroviruses are spread horizontally, as are most infectious agents (e.g., HTLV-I).

## 2.3. Interactions: Proto-Oncogenes and Retro-Oncogenes

The concept emerging is that recognized oncogenes probably represent individual components of complicated pathways responsible for regulating cell growth. Incorrect expression of any component might interrupt that regulation, hence leading to uncontrolled proliferation and the onset of neoplastic growth. Representative cellular proto-oncogenes (c-*onc*) and retro-oncogenes (v-*onc*), of primates, cats, and rodents are shown in Table IV. Those of avian species appear in Table V. They are characterized according to the host species of origin (c-*onc*), prototype virus (v-*onc*), type of tumor with which they are associated, and their protein products, including functional activity, subcellular location, and molecular weight. Listed in these tables are 20 pairs of homologous c-*onc* (where a human proto-oncogene has been found, its human chromosome location is indicated) and v-*onc* genes, 13 v-*onc* genes only, and 3 c-*onc* genes which have no counterpart in a retrovirus genome. Although at least 30 different cellular oncogenes have been identified by virtue of their presence in retrovirus isolates, there are probably other potential cellular oncogenes that have not been segregated into retrovirus vectors. Gene-transfer techniques have been successful in recovering a few novel oncogenes from tumors of nonviral origin. Oncogenes are covered in greater depth in Chapters 13 and 14 of this book.

## 2.3.1. Proto-Oncogenes

Oncogenes were first identified in neoplastic tissues and were thought to be disseminated by retroviruses. They were shown to cause neoplastic transformation of cells *in vitro* and were, therefore, regarded as "the genes that cause cancer." They occur in all eukaryotes, including humans, and are not normally tumorigenic; indeed, they appear to be critically involved in a number of cellular processes. Of more than 30 cellular oncogenes that have been discovered, at least 28 have been mapped to the human karyotype. When the protein products of these oncogenes were investigated, they were found to be very similar to known substances that are normally involved in the control of cell division—growth factors, plasma membrane receptors, modulators of the transduction of exogenous signals through the plasma membrane, and nuclear DNA-binding substances. These findings changed the original concept of oncogenes. They are now regarded as playing vital roles in the normal control of mitosis, and they should be properly called *mitogenes* rather than *oncogenes*. Like all other genes, if a mitogene is mutated, rearranged, translocated, or otherwise deranged, its effects will change; it may then become an oncogene that will promote disorderly cell division and thus contribute to the pathogenesis of cancer.[50]

## 2.3.2. Retro-Oncogenes

Retroviral oncogenes (designated v-*onc*) are derived from progenitor DNA sequences of normal cells (designated c-*onc*).[51] These sequences are thought to have been acquired by retroviruses upon passage through rodents, cats, chickens, or primates. The source of these new sequences has been traced in most cases to the genomes of the host animal through which the original virus was passed. It seems that a larger number of transforming retroviruses exist than there are oncogenes. The same or similar oncogenes have been observed in different viral isolates, e.g., *fps* and *fms* in feline sarcoma virus (FeSV) are closely related, or *src* and *mos* in RSV and Moloney-murine sarcoma virus (Mo-MuSV). The cellular progenitors of retroviral oncogenes seem to have been highly conserved during evolution.[52] This assertion is supported by the finding that sequences homologous to *src* are not only found in the DNAs of vertebrate species such as chicken, calf, mouse, man and salmon, but also in the DNA of *Drosophila melanogaster*.[53] The identification of *Drosophila* genes that are structurally similar to vertebrate oncogenes provides a mechanism to identify the function of these genes. Through sophisticated genetic manipulations available in *Drosophila*, it should be possible to determine whether cellular oncogene products are essential during development and in which tissues they are required.[52] Similar observations have been made with sequences homologous to other oncogenes. Evidence is accumulating that human DNA as well as the DNAs of all other vertebrate species contain progenitors for most of the oncogenes analyzed. As shown in Tables IV and V, sequences related to the following viral oncogenes have been detected in human DNA: v-*myc* of avian myelocytomatosis virus MC29 in human chromosome 8; v-*myb* of avian myeloblastosis virus in human chromosome 6; v-*mos* of Moloney murine sarcoma

Table IV. Representative Cellular Proto-Oncogenes (c-Onc) and Retroviral Oncogenes (v-Onc) of Primates, Cats, and Rodents

| Designation | | Host species | Prototype virus | Type of tumor | Protein product[a] | | |
|---|---|---|---|---|---|---|---|
| c-Onc | v-Onc | | | | Activity | Subcellular location | $M_r$ ($\times 10^3$) |
| N-ras | | Human | None | Neuroblastoma | | | |
| sis(22)[b] | sis | Woolly monkey | SiSV | Sarcoma | PDGF-like | Cyt, secreted | p28 |
| fes(15)[b] | fes | Cat | STFeLV | Sarcoma | Tyrosine kinase | PM, Cyt | p85 |
| fes(15)[b] | fes | Cat | GAFeLV | Sarcoma | Tyrosine kinase | Cyt | p110 |
| | fgr | Cat | GRFeLV | Sarcoma | Tyrosine kinase | | |
| fms(5)[b] | fms | Cat | MSFeLV | Sarcoma | CSF-1 receptor, glycoprotein | PM, ER | p170 |
| abl(9)[b] | abl | Mouse | A-MuLV | Leukemia | Tyrosine kinase | PM, Cyt | p120 |
| | bas | Mouse | BALB MuSV | Sarcoma | | | p21 |
| fos(14)[c] | fos | Mouse | FBJ-MuSV | Osteosarcoma | | Nucleus | P39, p55 |
| mos(8)[b] | mos | Mouse | Mo-MuSV | Sarcoma | | Cyt | p37 |
| mos(8)[b] | mos | Mouse | Gz-MuSV | Sarcoma | | Cyt | p37, p62 |
| | raf | Mouse | 3611-MuSV | Fibrosarcoma | | | p90, p75 |
| neu | | Rat | None | Neuroglioblastoma | | | |
| Ha-ras(11,X)[b,d] | Ha-ras | Rat | Ha-MuSV | Sarcoma | GDP/GTP binding | PM | p21 |
| Ki-ras(6,12)[b,e] | Ki-ras | Rat | Ki-MuSV | Sarcoma | GDP/GTP binding | PM | P21 |
| | ras | Rat | Ra-RaSV | Sarcoma | | | p29 |

[a] Abbreviations used: PM, plasma membrane; Cyt, cytoplasm; ER, endoplasmic reticulum; PDGF, platelet-derived growth factor; GDP/GTP, guanosine di- and triphosphate; CSF-1, colony stimulating factor-1.

[b] A human proto-oncogene for this c-onc exists.

[c] Chromosome localization data taken from Garrett (see also Chapter 13).

[d] Human proto-oncogene for Ha-ras-1 and Ha-ras-2, respectively.

[e] Human proto-oncogene for Ki-ras-1 and Ki-ras-2, respectively.

## Table V. Representative Cellular Proto-Oncogenes (c-Onc) and Retroviral Oncogenes (v-Onc) of Avian Species

| Designation | | Host species | Prototype virus | Type of tumor | Protein product[a] | | |
| --- | --- | --- | --- | --- | --- | --- | --- |
| c-Onc | v-Onc | | | | Activity | Subcellular location | $M_r$ ($\times 10^3$) |
| erb A(17)[b] | erb A | Chicken | AEV | Leukemia | | | p75, p135 |
| erb B | erb B | Chicken | AEV | Sarcoma | EGF receptor | PM, ER | p61 |
| ets | ets | Chicken | E26V | | | Nucleus | |
| fps(15)[b] | fps | Chicken | FSV | Sarcoma | Tyrosine kinase | PM, ER | p140 |
| | fps | Chicken | PRCII | Sarcoma | Tyrosine kinase | | p105 |
| | fps | Chicken | UR1 | Sarcoma | Tyrosine kinase | | p150 |
| | fps | Chicken | 16L | Sarcoma | Tyrosine kinase | | p142 |
| | mil | Chicken | MH2 | | | | |
| myb(6)[b] | myb | Chicken | AMV | Leukemia | | Nucleus | |
| myc(8)[b] | myb | Chicken | E26 | Leukemia | | | |
| | myc | Chicken | MC29 | Carcinoma, leukemia | DNA binding | Nucleus | p110 |
| | myc | Chicken | CMII | Sarcoma | | | p90 |
| | myc | Chicken | MH2 | Leukemia, sarcoma, carcinoma | | | p100 |
| | ros | Chicken | UR2 | Sarcoma | Tyrosine kinase | | p68 |
| | ski | Chicken | SKV | | | | |
| src(2p)[b] | src | Chicken | RSV | Sarcoma | Tyrosine kinase | PM | p60 |
| yes | yes | Chicken | Y73 | Sarcoma | Tyrosine kinase | | p90 |
| yes | yes | Chicken | ESV | Sarcoma | Tyrosine kinase | | p80 |
| B-lym | | Chicken | | Lymphoma | | | |
| rel | rel | Turkey | REV-T | Lymphoma | | | |

[a] Abbreviations used: PM, plasma membrane; ER, endoplasmic reticulum; EGF, epidermal growth factor. Numbers in parentheses indicate the human chromosome location.
[b] A human proto-oncogene for this c-onc exists.

virus in human chromosome 8; v-Ha-*ras* (i.e., c-Ha-*ras*-1 and c-Ha-*ras*-2) of Harvey murine sarcoma virus in human chromosomes 11 and X, respectively; v-Ki-*ras* (i.e., c-Ki-*ras*-1 and c-Ki-*ras*-2) of Kirsten murine sarcoma virus in human chromosomes 6 and 12, respectively; v-*abl* of Abelson murine leukemia virus in human chromosome 9; v-*fes* of feline sarcoma virus in human chromosome 15; and, v-*sis* of simian sarcoma virus in human chromosome 22. It is also of great interest that a recent study[54] has revealed that hepatitis B virus (HBV) integration places the viral DNA sequence next to a liver cell DNA sequence which bears a striking resemblance to both an oncogene, v-*erb* A, and the supposed DNA-binding domain of the human glucocorticoid receptor and human estrogen receptor genes. The authors of this finding suggested that this gene, usually silent or transcribed at a very low level in normal hepatocytes, becomes inappropriately expressed as a consequence of HBV integration, and thus may contribute to cell transformation of these cells. In another study,[55] integrated HBV DNAs from two single-integration hepatocellular carcinomas have been cloned, and the cellular integration sites have been analyzed. The integrated hepatitis B DNA in one of these two carcinomas contained a large inverted repeat of viral DNA, in which each repeat consisted of a linear DNA segment similar to the other carcinoma, but in addition, it was accompanied by a cellular DNA translocation at the viral integration site. The translocation occurred between chromosomes 17 and 18, along with a deletion of at least 1.3 kilobases of chromosome 18 DNA at the translocation site. On the basis of these findings, it was suggested that postintegration rearrangement of integrated hepatitis B virus and hepatocyte DNA results in the generation of chromosomal aberrations.[55] These chromosomal aberrations may function in a multistage mechanism leading to the development and progression of hepatocellular carcinoma.

## 3. COMMON PATHWAYS OF CELL TRANSFORMATION AND NEOPLASIA: UNIFYING FEATURES OF VIRAL ONCOGENESIS

### 3.1. Virus-Induced Transformation

In theory, transformation is defined as a stable, heritable alteration in the growth control of cells in culture. In practice, transformation can be recognized by the cells' permanent acquisition of some growth property not exhibited by the parental cell type.[49] However, it must be emphasized that no set of characteristics invariably distinguishes transformed cells from their normal counterparts. For example, the properties of the transformed cell often depend on the selection procedure and the host species and type of cell used in the transformation assay.[4] Although there are many phenotypic changes that occur as a result of transformation, the most notable ones are (1) certain alterations in cell-growth patterns consisting of growth to a higher cell density, increased rate of growth, decreased requirement for serum growth factors, decreased cell adhesion to a substrate, enhanced ability to grow in semisolid medium (anchorage independence), and loss of contact inhibition (the latter is determined by the number of foci induced and, therefore, can serve as the basis for a quantitative assay for certain tumor viruses); (2) alterations in cell surface demonstrated by the increased rate of transport of cell nutrients, increased secretion of proteases or protease activators, increased agglutinability by plant lectins, and changes in composition of glycoproteins and glycolipids, sometimes including the presence of virus-coded proteins; (3) detection of viral DNA, mRNA, and viral-coded proteins associated with changes in cell cytoskeleton, often resulting in more rounded cell shape; as well as the alteration of certain biochemical processes,[56] including increased metabolic rate, increased glycolysis, abnormal levels of cyclic nucleotides, and the activation or repression of particular cellular genes; and, finally (4) the property of tumorigenicity expressed by the production of tumors when transformed cells are inoculated into appropriate experimental animals, particularly animals immunodeficient as a result of experimentally induced or natural (e.g., newborn) immunosuppression. Sometimes, many transformed cells exhibit changes in growth behavior in culture, but may not be transplantable *in vivo*. This indicates that no *in vitro* growth characteristic can successfully predict tumorigenicity.

### 3.1.1. Transforming Genes and DNA Tumor Viruses

Cells in culture have been used for nearly 30 years as a study model of transformation by DNA tumor viruses. Historically, polyoma was the first DNA virus shown to transform cultured cells. Cells were immortalized, grew at an increased rate, and produced tumors.[57] These studies initiated the investigation of virus-induced cell transformation at the molecular level. The purpose of these studies was to elucidate the mechanism(s) by which the expression of a small amount of defined viral genetic information could alter the regulation of growth of normal cells through the transformation process. The model assumed that transformation in culture by DNA tumor viruses is germane to naturally occurring tumorigenesis. In general, comparison of the properties of cells transformed in culture by DNA tumor viruses with those derived from experimentally induced or spontaneous tumors supports this assumption. On the other hand, similar studies on the molecular biology and pathobiology of oncogenesis with RNA tumor viruses were slow to develop until the discovery of reverse transcriptase.[38,39] The molecular mechanisms underlying transformation by DNA tumor viruses can be exemplified by the SV40 model. In this model, the genome contains "early" and "late" regions. The late region consists of genes that code for the synthesis of coat proteins; they are not expressed in transformed cells. The early region is expressed soon after infection of cells; it contains genes that code for early proteins, e.g., the SV40 tumor (T) antigens, which are necessary for the replication of viral DNA in permissive cells and for transformation of nonpermissive cells. The transforming protein must be continuously synthesized for the cells to stay transformed. Even with the larger DNA viruses (e.g., adenoviruses) only one or two genes are involved in cell transformation.[46]

It must be emphasized that with very few exceptions, DNA tumor viruses are not oncogenic under natural circumstances in their native host species. One such exception is the papillomaviruses, which are different from conventional DNA tumor viruses. They are natural causes of benign neoplasms in their native host species.[58] They are also causes of highly invasive and metastatic tumors in several animal species and quite possibly in humans, as will be discussed later. Another possible exception is herpes simplex virus, type 2 (HSV-2), which since the late 1960s has been suspected of having a link with human cancer of the uterine cervix.[59] More recently, however, HSV-2, has taken second place as the cause of cervical cancer in humans. The weight of evidence falls rather on the papillomaviruses based on molecular cloning, DNA sequencing, and transcription analysis using cloned viral DNA as probes. Accordingly, papillomaviruses are the prime candidates for an etiologic role not only in cervical cancer but in other types of human urogenital cancers as well.[15,60,61] It has been suggested as another possibility that HSV-2 may induce cervical tumors by a hit-and-run mechanism; i.e., the virus is necessary to initiate but not to maintain the tumor cell.[62] zur Hausen[63] proposed the hypothesis that both HSV-2 and papillomaviruses play a synergistic role in the genesis of cervical cancer. A third exception may be the Epstein–Barr virus. Although a great deal has been learned about this virus, and it seems almost certain that it is the etiologic agent of both the African type of Burkitt lymphoma and nasopharyngeal carcinoma, conclusive proof for this is still lacking. In this regard, it has been suggested that Burkitt lymphoma may actually be the end result of a complex multistep carcinogenic process involving several factors. Lastly, three of the four hepatitis B-like viruses (i.e., hepatitis B, woodchuck hepatitis, and duck hepatitis B) appear to cause primary hepatocellular carcinoma in their native host species.[64,65]

### 3.1.2. Oncogenes by RNA Tumor Viruses: Retroviral and Cellular Oncogenes

Carcinogenesis by RNA tumor viruses is believed to follow several pathways. Experimental support exists for several distinct theories of viral carcinogenesis. It appears that the rapid induction of sarcomas or carcinomas by the acute transforming viruses, whose oncogenes form recombinants with the cellular oncogenes, is different from the slower induction of leukemia by the chronic leukemia viruses. The latter have no viral oncogenes, although they may utilize cellular oncogenes. With respect to the acute transforming RNA tumor viruses, a cellular gene becomes inserted by recombination into the viral genome to be expressed as a viral gene under the control of the viral promoter. With respect to the chronic leukemia viruses, the viral promoter or enhancer element is inserted adjacent to or near the cellular gene in the cell chromosome.

The avian sarcoma virus (RSV), which is one of the most intensively studied agents, represents a useful model to illustrate summarily some aspects of the transformation process. The product of the v-*onc* gene of this virus (i.e., *src* gene) is a phosphoprotein that localizes primarily in plasma membranes of transformed cells, functions as a protein kinase, and phosphorylates proteins at tyrosine residues.

Leukemogenesis by certain recombinant retroviruses, or via chronic mitogenic stimulation as a result of viral infection, may not be associated with oncogenes of either viral or cellular origin. A hypothetical second step, which could be DNA or chromosomal rearrangement, would be required for irreversible transformation or carcinogenesis.[32]

Viral genetic information that is a constant part of the genetic constitution of an organism is designated as endogenous.[46] Important features of an integrated retroviral provirus or endogenous virus are: (1) DNA copies of RNA viral genome are covalently linked to cellular DNA and are present in all somatic and germ cells in the host; (2) endogenous viral genomes are transmitted genetically from parent to offspring; (3) the integrated state subjects the endogenous viral genomes to host genetic control; and (4) the endogenous virus may be induced to replicate either spontaneously or by treatment with extrinsic (e.g., chemical or physical) agents.

Endogenous v-*onc* proviruses are ubiquitous in nature.[66–69] Many of these viral genomes are replication-defective, usually because of minor structural defects that are similar to those found among proviruses acquired via exogenous infection with a replication-competent virus.[70] The defective proviruses may, however, express one or more viral replication genes, and nondefective endogenous proviruses may give rise to an infectious virus. It has been suggested that endogenous viral genomes may serve an essential normal growth function for the host.[60,71] Although this possibility has been attractive, it has not been verified experimentally. In fact, certain studies[67,72] have directly indicated that at least certain endogenous viral genomes are not absolutely required for normal growth. Although chickens that are negative for endogenous viruses grow normally, exogenous infection with an avian leukosis virus induces disease after a much shorter latent period than that induced in chickens containing endogenous viral loci.[73] This latter finding is consistent with the view that the presence of endogenous viral genes in host cell DNA may confer at least a partial protection of the host against disease induced by exogenous infection with a related retrovirus. Endogenous proviruses generally are less oncogenic for the animal in which they are found than are exogenous viruses. In addition to their bearing mutations, even the replication-competent endogenous proviruses usually exhibit low oncogenicity. This reduced oncogenicity can be explained by the several differences between most endogenous and exogenous viruses. The former characteristically have a xenotropic host range. This prevents them from infecting the majority of cells in the natural host. There are also significant differences between them with regard to certain regions of their genome. It is likely that such differences result in less viral progeny being produced per endogenous provirus than is the case with exogenous viruses.[74,75]

## 3.2. Unifying Features of Viral Carcinogenesis

Very recent studies[4] suggested that the same cellular genes may be activated by DNA tumor viruses, by retroviruses, and by chemical carcinogens. Thus, there may be a limited number of pathways to oncogenesis, and aberrant regulation of a small group of cellular genes may serve as the basis of malignancy.

Cells transformed by oncogenic viruses display complex new biological biochemical properties as described earlier in this section. These new properties probably reflect the activation and possibly the repression of specific cellular genes as a consequence of the pleiotropic action of virus-coded transforming proteins.[4] The origin of the transforming genes of DNA tumor viruses is still at best a point of conjecture. If they have evolved from cellular genes, they must have diverged considerably, because the transforming genes of DNA tumor viruses have not thus far been found to hybridize to cellular DNA. On the other hand, the retroviral oncogenes (i.e., v-*onc* genes) appear to have evolved from cellular genes, since cellular homologues of retroviral oncogenes are present in a large number of vertebrate species. A recent observation having important biological significance is that segments of the DNA adenovirus E1A transforming gene are structurally related to the two retroviral v-*onc* genes, *myc* and *myb*, as shown by computer analysis of recently determined DNA sequences.[76] This finding is quite intriguing because the *myc* and the E1A gene products are both nuclear proteins associated with immortalization of primary cells. Furthermore, nucleotide sequences related to the v-*myc* oncogene of the avian and myelocytomatosis virus and to the human c-*myc* proto-oncogene have been shown to be homologous to several regions of the human cytomegalovirus genome.[74,77,78] A comparison of the nucleotide sequences of 11 cloned mammalian hepadnavirus isolates with sequences of retrovirus genomes has revealed regions of homology between specific regions of the genomes of viruses in the two families.[79,80] These investigations further demonstrated that hepadnavirus and retroviruses share both genome homology and similar features of replication.

DNA tumor virus transforming genes and retroviral oncogenes encode interchangeable and complementary functions. Also, the oncogenic activity of human cancer oncogenes, i.e., cellular homologues of retroviral oncogenes, can be complemented by DNA tumor virus transforming genes. These findings indicate that the latter encode functions that mimic those of cellular genes. Incidentally, studies are underway in an attempt to identify the target cellular genes that become activated in oncogenesis. These studies have led to investigation of the regulation of eukaryotic gene expression and cell growth. Some of these recent studies have been reviewed in the literature.[4,81] Future studies related to the functional characterization of cellular genes whose expression is modified in transformed cells are necessary in order to elucidate molecular mechanisms involved both in embryonic development and in neoplasia.

## 4. PATHOBIOLOGY OF ONCOGENIC VIRUSES AND EXPERIMENTAL ANIMAL MODELS OF VIRUS-INDUCED HUMAN NEOPLASIA

### 4.1. DNA Tumor Viruses

#### 4.1.1. Polyomaviruses

The BK and JC viruses usually infect children and are ubiquitous in the human population. BK virus has been isolated from the urine of immunodeficient individuals but it does not cause clinical infections. BK virus can, however, induce tumors experimentally in newborn hamsters and mice. BK virus can transform cells from a variety of animal species, including hamster, rat, mouse, rabbit, and African green monkey. BK virus DNA can also transform rat and hamster cells.

In contrast, JC virus causes progressive multifocal leukoencephalitis (PML), a relatively rare and fatal demyelinating disease often associated with immunodeficiency. JC virus is highly oncogenic in newborn hamsters, induces a wide variety of tumors, and shows a predilection for neuroectodermal cells. Furthermore, JC virus can induce brain tumors in adult owl monkeys. JC virus and its DNA can transform primary cultures of newborn hamster glial cells, and transformed hamster cells produce tumors in weanling hamsters.

Although both BK and JC viruses are ubiquitous and oncogenic, they do not seem to play a significant role in the etiology of human neoplasia. Extensive molecular hybridization analysis has excluded the presence of DNA sequences incriminating these two viruses in those human cancer types that represent about 90% of the total cancer incidence in the United States.[82]

#### 4.1.2. Papillomaviruses

These viruses are unique among the DNA viruses in that they are the natural causes of benign tumors in their animal species of origin (i.e., warts in humans), which may be spread horizontally.

They are also the causes of malignant neoplasia in a number of animal species, quite possibly including humans. These viruses can induce three types of benign neoplastic lesions: (1) papillomas, which are tumors derived from the epithelium; (2) fibropapillomas, which contain a considerable amount of fibrous connective tissue in addition to neoplastic epithelium; and (3) fibromas, which consist mainly of fibrous connective tissue containing proliferating fibroblasts. Three animal papillomaviruses are oncogenic in their native host species: bovine papillomaviruses-type 4, which results in a high incidence of alimentary tract and urinary bladder cancer in cattle feeding on bracken fern;[83] cottontail rabbit papillomavirus (CRPV), which causes carcinomas under natural conditions;[84] and the *Mastomys natalensis* papillomavirus (MnPV), a papillomavirus endemic in the multimammate mouse *Mastomys natalensis*.[85] Five papillomaviruses have been shown to induce tumors following inoculation into hamsters: bovine papillomaviruses, types 1 and 2; the sheep papillomavirus, the European elk papillomavirus, and the deer fibroma virus.

CRPV provides an interesting model to study viral carcinogenesis and the progression of a nonmalignant papilloma to a carcinoma. It produces an enzootic disease of wild cottontail rabbits in the high plains of the midwestern United States. Although papillomas often regress, about 25% of them progress to carcinomas. Experimentally, CRPV induces cutaneous papillomas in domestic rabbits, and as many as 75% of the papillomas progress to carcinomas. CRPV DNA can induce papillomas in domestic rabbits.[86]

There are about 25 human papillomavirus (HPV) types that have been reported in the literature, most of which have been described in the past few years. A new HPV type has been defined as a virus isolate exhibiting less than 50% DNA homology with other known HPV types, as determined under stringent conditions.[87] Of eight different HPV types infecting patients with epidermodysplasia veruciformis, three (HPV-5, HPV-8, and HPV-10 in that order of frequency) have been associated with squamous cell carcinomas (Bowen disease). HPV-5 was isolated from the tumor tissues of these patients. Of great significance to human clinical medicine is that HPV types 6, 10, 11, and 16 have been detected with high frequency in human urogenital cancers. A number of studies involving molecular hybridization[60,88–90] have provided very strong support for the etiologic role of several HPVs in urogenital cancer. In addition, this role is also consistent with the results of clinical, histologic, immunologic, and epidemiologic studies. HPVs have also been associated by Kreider *et al.* with carcinoma of the human uterine cervix.[91] These investigators have described a unique nude mouse model that may be useful in the analysis of transformation mechanisms by HPVs.

A new type of condylomatous lesion, a microscopically invisible flat wart often referred to as subclinical papillomavirus infection (SPI), has been recognized during the past few years. SPI has been associated frequently with cervical epithelial dysplasia and neoplasia.[92–94] In addition to playing a possible role in urogenital and anorectal malignancies, HPVs may also be involved in the etiology of other types of human cancer. Squamous cell carcinomas of the larynx, esophagus, and lung have been reported to exhibit a striking histological similarity to HPV-associated lesions that are characteristic of dysplasia of the uterine cervix.[92,95–97] Finally, two new HPVs have been isolated recently from potential target tissues: HPV-11 from laryngeal papillomas[98] and HPV-13 from oral focal hyperplasia.[99] It has also been suggested that subclinical lesions induced by latent infection with an unidentified HPV in the respiratory tract may convert to carcinomas because of heavy exposure to carcinogens present in tobacco smoke.[4]

## 4.1.3. Adenoviruses

All human adenoviruses thus far examined can transform rodent fibroblasts in culture. However, they differ in their ability to induce tumors in newborn hamsters. Accordingly, group A adenoviruses (i.e., types 12, 18, and 31) induce tumors in most animals within 4 months.[4] Those in group B (i.e., types 3, 7, 14, 16, and 21) induce tumors in a small fraction of animals within 4–18 months.[100] Those in groups C, D, and E do not induce tumors in newborn hamsters. It is interesting, however, that adenovirus type 9 (i.e., group D), which does not induce tumors in hamsters, will specifically induce mammary fibroadenomas with a high frequency in female rats.[101] Recent studies at the molecular level[102,103] have revealed that the adenovirus E1A T antigen specifically represses the expression of class I transplantation antigens involved in the host immune response. Although the human adenoviruses are ubiquitous, oncogenic, and frequently cause latent infections, there is no evidence of adenovirus DNA sequences in the common types of human cancers found in the United States.[4] Hence, these viruses probably do not play a significant role in the etiology of human cancers.

## 4.1.4. Herpesviruses

Although all the members of the herpesvirus family have the same morphology, they differ widely in their biologic properties.[104] Herpesviruses typically cause acute infections followed by latency and eventual recurrence in each host, including humans. Herpesviruses replicate in cells of their natural hosts. Some herpesviruses are associated with tumors in lower animals. Marek's disease is a highly contagious lymphoproliferative disease of chickens that can be prevented by vaccination with an attenuated strain of the Marek disease virus. The prevention of cancer by vaccination in this instance establishes the etiologic role of this virus and provides a model for the control of human neoplasia by a similar approach. Other examples of herpesvirus-induced neoplasia in animals include lymphomas of certain species of monkeys and adenocarcinoma of frogs.[46] Four members have oncogenic properties with potential relevance to human neoplasias: herpes simplex virus (HSV), cytomegalovirus (CMV), Epstein–Barr virus (EBV), and, the new addition to the family, human B-lymphotropic virus (HBLV). Each of these four herpesviruses will be discussed briefly below.

*4.1.4a. Herpes Simplex Viruses.* Morphologic transformation of hamster embryo cells in culture by herpes simplex virus type 1 (HSV-1)[105] and herpes simplex virus type 2 (HSV-2)[106] was first accomplished during the early 1970s. Since these viruses have a high lytic activity, it was necessary to inactivate their infectivity by UV irradiation. Later experiments demonstrated that photodynamic inactivation, elevated temperatures, or the use of temperature-sensitive viral mutants at the nonpermissive temperature were equally successful. Under these conditions, it was observed that virus-specific RNA was actually transcribed in those cells. However, the role of persisting viral genetic information in maintaining the transformed state of the cell is unclear, since viral DNA sequences were reported to be lost from the transformed cell lines after serial passages. *In vitro* transformation of embryonic rat cells and the NIH 3T3 cell line have also been demonstrated,[4] but the process is rather inefficient and the mechanism of transformation is obscure. Despite the ability of HSV-2 to induce the transformation of human cells *in vitro*, DNA sequences have been found only rarely in cervical tumors. On the other hand, *in situ* DNA–RNA hybridization studies[107,108] have revealed that virus-specific RNA is detectable in 35–67% of the cervical tumor cells that were examined. In order to reconcile these differences, it has been suggested[62] that the virus may be necessary to initiate but not to maintain oncogenicity, or that HSV-2 and the human papillomaviruses play a synergistic role in the induction of carcinoma of the uterine cervix in humans.[63]

The involvement of HSV-2 in human cervical neoplasia has been seriously questioned in recent years. The reason is that there is a glaring discrepancy between the findings from the retrospective seroepidemiologic study[59] of the late 1960s (i.e., which demonstrated that women with cervical cancer had a higher rate of seropositivity and a higher titer of HSV-2 specific antibodies than did matched controls) and a prospective study reported in 1984.[109] The latter study failed to show any difference between the two study population groups, thus leading the authors to conclude that women previously infected with HSV-2 are not at a significant risk for developing cervical neoplasia.

*4.1.4b. Human Cytomegalovirus.* This virus is similar to HSV-2, inasmuch as both viruses have two distinct transforming regions. However, the transforming fragments of these two viruses are unlikely to code for transforming proteins because they do not contain appropriate open reading frames.[110] By contrast, transforming DNA fragments of cytomegalovirus (CMV) and HSV-2 may insert into the cellular genome, thereby activating cellular genes that may regulate cell growth.[110] These two transforming regions of the human CMV have been identified by transfection with cloned restriction fragments.[111] Nonetheless, viral DNA sequences were not detected in the transformed cell. In contrast, human CMV DNA sequences (0.2–6 copies of viral DNA per cell) have been detected in cancers of the prostate, colon, and cervix and in Kaposi sarcoma, as well as in normal prostate, colon, and cervical tissues according to DNA reassociation kinetics.[112] This again has raised a serious question regarding the role of this virus in human neoplasia, since both normal and malignant tissues are commonly infected with this virus.

Several factors have suggested that CMV may be involved in the development of Kaposi sarcoma in AIDS patients. Since not all HIV-seropositive individuals develop AIDS, there is a possibility that a viral cofactor might either activate T cells, allowing for HIV infection, or may enhance HIV replication in persistently infected cells, thus allowing for a cytopathic infection.[113] Evidence also indicates that HSV-1 can reactivate the transcription of latent HIV, resulting in high-level expression of HIV-specific RNA.[114]

*4.1.4c. Epstein–Barr Virus.* EBV is the most common etiologic agent of acute infectious mononucleosis (the other two etiologic agents being CMV and *Toxoplasma gondii*, but with a much lower incidence). EBV is B lymphotropic in susceptible humans. In a few immunodeficient children, infections with this virus have progressed to a B-cell lymphoma. One tragic case of severe combined immunodeficiency recently demonstrated that this virus can cause B-cell lymphoma. A 12-year-old child kept in a gnotobiotic chamber since birth received a bone marrow transplant and died 124 days later of multiple B-cell proliferations proven to be due to EBV.[46] This virus has also been linked to Burkitt lymphoma, a tumor most frequently found in children in central Africa, and to nasopharyngeal carcinoma, the incidence of which is higher in Chinese male populations in Southeast Asia than elsewhere. Normal human lymphocytes have a limited life span *in vitro*, but EBV can transform such lymphocytes into lymphoblastoid cell lines that grow indefinitely in culture. With the exception of the case of severe combined immunodeficiency mentioned above, no definitive proof exists to date that any herpesvirus is directly responsible for any human tumor. It has been suggested that, because of their low efficiencies of transformation *in vitro* and the difficulties in defining a transforming gene, herpesvirus effects represent only one step in a complex sequence leading to neoplasia. For example, EBV appears to be one cofactor in the pathogenesis of Burkitt lymphoma. A chromosomal translocation that activates the c-*myc* proto-oncogene also may play a role in this transformation[46] (see Chapter 15). A summary of studies on the interaction between EBV and tumor promoters, with special reference to potential mechanisms of virus induction and transformation of normal human lymphocytes, was recently published.[115]

Epstein–Barr virus has oncogenic properties *in vitro* and *in vivo*. The virus efficiently transforms B lymphocytes of human and subhuman primates *in vitro* to produce permanent cell lines that are capable of indefinite growth in culture and are tumorigenic in monkeys. It can induce lymphoproliferative disease when injected into marmosets and owl monkeys. Viral DNA and viral nuclear antigens are readily detected in lymphoid cells derived by *in vitro* transformation and in cell lines established from biopsies of Burkitt lymphoma and nasopharyngeal carcinoma tissues.[4]

A small Colombian monkey, the cottontop tamarin, is the susceptible experimental animal of choice for biological experiments with EBV. This animal was used for the development of an effective experimental vaccine against EBV. This vaccine was derived from a viral membrane antigen, the high molecular weight glycoprotein gp340.[116]

*4.1.4d. Human B Lymphotropic Virus.* This virus is the newest member of the family of human herpesviruses. Although it is morphologically indistinguishable from the other herpesviruses, it is different from them with regard to biological properties, host range, and antigenic features. For example, although probes obtained from each of the known human herpesvirus readily detected the homologous viral DNA, they did not hybridize to genomic human B lymphotropic virus (HBLV) DNA, and vice versa.[117] With regard to the host range, the HBLV only infects freshly isolated B cells. Attempts to transmit the virus to a number of T and B lymphoblastoid cell lines, and to a variety of other commonly used cell types, were unsuccessful. By contrast, EBV infects most B cells and some epithelial cells. Cytomegalovirus, HSV, and varicella–zoster virus infect a variety of cell types. Furthermore, unlike Epstein–Barr infected cells, B cells infected with the HBLV are not immortalized.[18] It is likely that this virus might be associated with at least some of the lymphoproliferative disorders observed in HIV-infected individuals, but the final proof is still lacking.

### 4.1.5. Hepatitis B-Like Viruses

Within the past decade, significant evidence has evolved to show an association between persistent infection with hepatitis B virus (HBV) and the development of primary hepatocellular carcinoma. Hepatitis B virus surface antigen (HBsAg) is frequently found in the nontransformed hepatocytes of patients with hepatocellular carcinoma (Fig. 1), but is usually not defined within the malignant hepatocytes.[118] These lines of evidence are based on epidemiologic studies of populations in areas endemic for persistent HBV infection, on molecular studies of hepatocellular carcinoma cell lines obtained from carriers of the virus who have developed liver cancer, and on animal models infected with viruses closely related to the human HBV. Despite substantial evidence for such an association, the mechanism(s) by which HBV infection and hepatocellular carcinoma are related remains largely unknown.[119,120] During the past several years, three additional hepatitis B-like viruses, the duck hepatitis B virus (DHBV), the woodchuck hepatitis virus (WHV), and the ground squirrel hepatitis virus (GSHV), have been discovered. These viruses and their DNA genomes are very similar in size and organization to that of the human HBV. These nonhuman viruses also cause liver disease and appear to cause hepatocellular carcinoma in their native species. The genomes of the human HBV and the WHV have been shown to be integrated into the host-cell genome. On the other hand, direct experimental proof that these viruses are oncogenic is currently unavailable; i.e., they have not been shown to transform cells in culture or to induce tumors in experimental animals. Nevertheless, the epidemiologic evidence is strong, and it is possible that these viruses induce neoplasia by a previously unidentified mechanism. Integrated viral DNA has been detected in human and woodchuck hepatocellular carcinomas by DNA blot hybridization. The tumor tissue of most patients with this type of malignancy contains HBV DNA sequences.[121,122] Tumor cells appear to be clonal, since identical integration patterns were seen in different portions of the same tumor, but tumors from individual patients showed different banding patterns, thus suggesting that viral DNA is not integrated at a unique cellular DNA site.

The WHV provides a working model to investigate the molecular biology of cell transformation by hepatitis B-like viruses. However, results obtained with this model have not indicated a common cellular locus for viral DNA integration. Furthermore, they have also not been consistent with the promoter-insertion model of cell transformation in which viral DNA integrates near a cellular oncogene and activates its expression, as is the case with the avian leukosis viruses.[123–125] By contrast, the pattern of HBV DNA integration in a human cell line derived from hepatocellular carcinoma tissue[126] demonstrated that the site of integration of viral DNA was localized to the single-stranded gap region in HBV DNA, indicating that a specific sequence on the viral genome is used for integration.

## 4.2. RNA Tumor Viruses

The similarities between certain human malignancies (e.g., leukemias, lymphomas, sarcomas, breast cancer) and a number of virus-induced tumors in animals have been the major reason for the rigorous search for a viral etiology in human cancer. The leukemias are undoubtedly the human neoplasias most widely investigated for their possible association with retroviruses.[127,128] These efforts have included the detection of complete viral particles by electron microscopy and tissue culture, as well as the search for viral RNA, reverse transcriptase, viral structural proteins, and antiviral antibodies. The presence of reverse transcriptase analogous to that of mammalian C-type

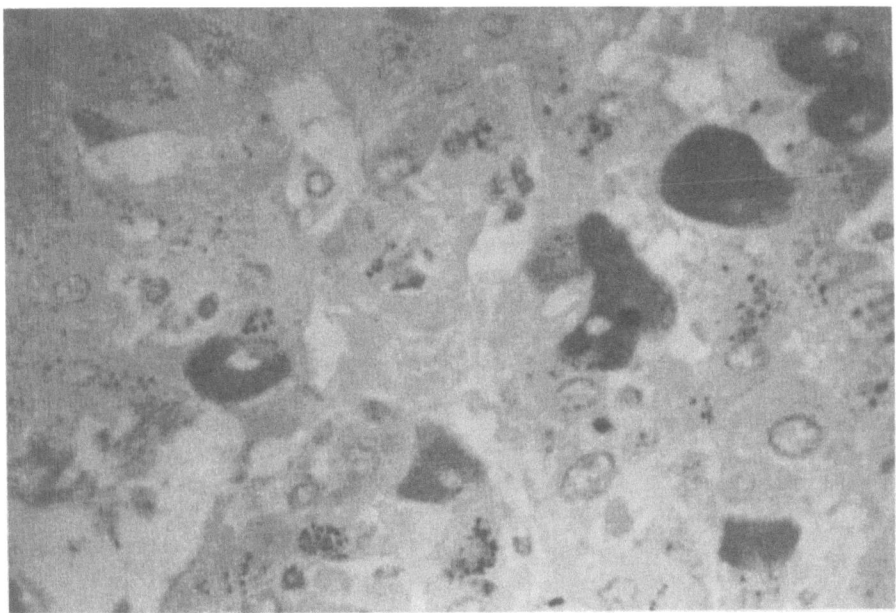

*Figure 1.* Positively stained HBsAg (dark areas) in the cytoplasm of nontumorous hepatocytes of a patient with a hepatocellular carcinoma (not shown). (Aldehyde fuschsin, ×250)

retroviruses in at least some of the human leukemias has been documented by several independent investigators,[127–129] and the detection of retrovirus-specific RNA in certain human leukemias[128] has been confirmed. The RNA detected exhibits partial homology with the RNAs of murine leukemia virus (MuLV), murine simian virus (MuSV), and simian sarcoma virus (SiSV). In addition, it has a high molecular weight with poly-A sequences similar to those of retroviral RNA.[128] Some human leukemias have antigens related to the core structural proteins p30 of the primate retroviruses SiSV and baboon erythroleukemia virus (BaEV) and p70 of SiSV.[130] Antibodies against the core proteins (p30) of SiSV, BaEV, and MuLV were detected in human sera and exudate fluids,[131] whereas antibodies against the reverse transcriptase of feline leukemia virus (FeLV) and of SiSV have been identified on the surface of leukocytes from patients with acute myelogenous leukemia and chronic myelogenous leukemia in blast crisis.[132] Several successful isolations of retroviruses from cultured human leukemic and embryonic cells were reported that showed an RNA and antigenic relationship of the presumable human isolates with SiSV and BaEV.[133–136] Finally, retrovirus-related sequences have been found in human nuclear DNA.[137–140]

The successful propagation of human T lymphocytes with the help of the T-cell growth factor or interleukin-2 led to the discovery of the human T-cell leukemia/lymphoma viruses. These exogenous viruses exhibited C-type morphology and were different from all the other retroviruses known at that time.[44,45,141] These viruses represent the only bona fide human retroviruses with disease association known to date. Retroviruses have also been associated with human breast cancer,[142–145] osteosarcomas,[143,146,147] and melanomas.[148–150] but research efforts in these areas have been less intensive than in leukemia.[128]

The presence of endogenous viruses in many vertebrate species connotes that endogenous retroviruses also exist in humans. Retrovirus-like structures have been detected in human embryonal tissues as well as in human placentas.[151–153] Some of the viral components were related serologically to SiSV and BaEV.[154] Other particles, detected in human amnion cells, resemble the D-type virus Mason Pfizer mammary tumor virus (MPMV). Support for the existence of human endogenous retroviruses comes from the demonstration of gene sequences in normal human tissue that are related to the genomes of known RNA tumor viruses (MuLV, BaEV, mouse mammary tumor virus [MMTV]).[137–140,155]

## 5. IMMUNOLOGIC ASPECTS OF VIRUS-INDUCED NEOPLASIA

The immunology and immunopathology of neoplasia should include the antigenic properties of transformed cells, the host immune responses to these neoplastic cells, the immunologic conse- quences to the host as a result of the proliferation of the tumor cells and, finally, the mechanisms by which the immune system can be modulated to control and eradicate transformed cells. Tumor cells are significantly more complex than bacteria, which can be more easily distinguished as being foreign to the host. This is so because tumor cells have many similarities with normal cells even though they exhibit abnormal tendencies to proliferate, spread throughout the host, and interfere with the vital physiological functions of organ systems. Elucidation of the mechanisms that make a cancerous cell different from normal cells should lead to the understanding of how these malignant cells might be controlled or destroyed by the immune system. To provide a comprehensive review of this important area in immunology is indeed a formidable task beyond the scope of this chapter. Instead, a brief overview of the immunologic aspects of viral oncology will be discussed briefly in this section.

### 5.1. Virus-Associated Antigens

Virus-induced tumors are of particular interest in tumor immunology owing to the great likelihood that cells transformed by the integration of viral genes or oncogenes will lead to the expression of new virus-associated antigens that can be recognized by the immune system. The central theme of tumor immunology is the process of transformation of a normal cell into a malignant one. Such a process can result from a variety of events, the specific nature of which may help determine whether the competence of the immune system is adequate to control the outgrowth of the neoplasm. These transforming events may occur spontaneously by random mutations or gene rearrangements, or they may be induced by viral, chemical, or physical carcinogenic agents.

### 5.1.1. DNA Viruses

Most cells infected by potentially oncogenic DNA viruses do not become transformed. In contrast to the infection of permissive cells, infection of nonpermissive cells can result in the integration of viral DNA into the host genome and expression of only some of the viral genes, so that lytic viral particles are not produced. Transformation may then result either from direct trigger- ing of cellular genes by the integrated viral DNA or from the host aberrantly splicing viral DNA sequences to synthesize new proteins that promote transformation.

DNA viruses induce unique nuclear and cell-surface antigens. Each virus induces the ex- pression of the same antigens regardless of the tissue or animal species of origin. It must be noted that these virus-induced antigens are distinct from the virion antigens, even though they are encoded by the virus; they are designated tumor-associated antigens. In addition to these antigens, virus- induced tumors may also express other antigens that are instead encoded by the host genome as a result of host gene deregulation by the transforming event. These newly expressed antigens can be manifested either as tumor-specific transplantation antigens (TSTA) or oncodevelopmental antigens (ODA).[156]

### 5.1.2. RNA Viruses

Following infection of the host cell by RNA tumor viruses, a double-stranded copy of the viral RNA genome is synthesized (i.e., by means of the retroviral reverse transcriptase). Integration of this complementary DNA (cDNA) into the host cell genome results in the production of new infectious viruses that bud from the cell membrane (so-called C-type particles), expression of structural and other virus-associated antigens on the cell membrane, and potentially, transformation. Retroviruses can be separated into rapidly transforming and slow transforming types. The former contain oncogenic genes that can directly transform cells, whereas slowly transforming viruses lack such oncogenes and must aberrantly activate host genes that in turn induce transformation. Regardless of the mechanism by which retroviruses induce neoplasia, the resulting tumors are likely to express new surface antigens than can be recognized by the immune system.[157] These antigens coded for by both the viral and host genomes include viral envelope antigens consisting for the most part of the envelope glycoprotein gp70 (all gp70 determinants of murine oncornaviruses crossreact extensively), intrinsic viral proteins, and cell-surface antigens. Whereas antibodies to gp70 will block infectivity, immunity against the tumor cell surface antigens are distinct from the viral antigens as well as from the H-2 histocompatibility antigens. The complexity of neoantigens expressed in virus-induced tumors can be illustrated by the experimental hamster model of Rous sarcoma virus. In this system, the antigens comprise (1) the virus envelope antigen (VEA), (2) virus group-specific antigens (gs antigens), (3) virus-coded nonviral proteins, (4) cell-coded determinants activated by the virus, and (5) oncodevelopmental antigens encoded for by cellular genes that are activated by virus-induced transformation.[156]

## 5.2. Effector Mechanisms of Virus-Induced Tumor Immunity

If tumors express antigens that are recognizable by the authochthonous host, then such antigens may stimulate an immune response that will eradicate the proliferating neoplastic cells. Virus-induced experimental tumors share common antigens; whereas those that are induced by specific chemical carcinogens or which occur spontaneously, usually do not. The shared virus-induced antigens may be products encoded by the viral genome or cellular products not expressed in the virus itself. In contrast to the poorly antigenic or nonantigenic antigens of spontaneous tumors, the antigens of virus-induced tumors are highly immunogenic. Hence, it is disappointing that most human tumors appear to exhibit a low degree of antigenicity. A further complication of this problem is that the features that apply to one tumor may not apply to the next. In fact, even tumors of similar histologic type and growth patterns may provoke entirely different immune responses.[156] All the above have enormous implications in terms of immunodiagnostic, immunoprophylactic, and immunotherapeutic approaches to the management of human cancer (see Chapter 28).

A tumor cell, either transplanted or induced, represents a foreign configuration to the host in which it arises. The immune mechanisms operable against tumor cells are basically the same as those marshalled in response to any other foreign configuration.[158] Essentially, five general mechanisms for immune-mediated destruction of tumor cells have been described[156]: (1) complement-mediated lysis, (2) antibody-dependent cell-mediated cytotoxicity, (3) T-cell-mediated cytolysis by T cytotoxic or T killer cells, (4) activated macrophage killing, and (5) killing by natural cytotoxic or natural killer (NK) cells, or lymphokine-activated killer (LAK) cells. Studies of these *in vitro* mechanisms have resulted in new insights into how immune mechanisms might restrict the growth or kill tumor cells. Nonetheless, the major *in vivo* mechanism for tumor cell killing is delayed hypersensitivity. The *in vivo* contribution of T killer cells, natural killer cells, and antibody-dependent cell-mediated cytotoxicity as defined by *in vitro* assays is uncertain.[156]

An aberration or imbalance in the immunosurveillance mechanisms of the host is thought to contribute in part to the frank expression of cancer. Although this concept has emerged from studies in animals for decades, its relevance to humans is less clear. One of the lines of evidence in support of this concept originates from investigations showing that the widespread use of immunosuppressive agents in graft recipients is associated with an increased incidence of malignancy following organ transplantation. Also, other studies have shown that children with immunodeficiency disorders have a greater risk of neoplasia.[159] A more recent finding which supports the likely role of the immune system in tumor resistance is the high incidence of Kaposi's sarcoma in male homosexuals or other individuals infected with HIV. There are a number of possible explanations for the role of immunosuppression in the development of neoplasia. At first, most of the attention was placed on the role of specific T-cell-mediated immunity in reacting against new or altered antigens on the surface of transformed cells. More recently, however, it has been found that a natural surveillance system also appears to play an important role in resistance against the development and progressive growth of tumors.[158]

Whereas there is considerable evidence in support of immune surveillance, there are also enough conflicting data to indicate that this system operates either ineffectively or not at all. During the past two decades, there have been many studies that have challenged the concept of immunologic surveillance. Some have suggested that immunodeficiency is mainly associated with lymphoreticular malignancy and not with solid tumors of other organ systems. Others have provided evidence in mice and rats that congenital absence, or neonatal removal, of the thymus is not associated with increased susceptibility to the development of spontaneous or chemically induced tumors. In this regard, it is worth mentioning that in contrast to the host-immune response to DNA tumor viruses, adults previously thymectomized in neonatal life show a decreased tumor incidence when infected with RNA tumor viruses during adult life.[158]

## 6. CONCLUDING REMARKS

Although the potential for viruses to induce neoplasia has been demonstrated by investigations in animals since the beginning of this century, the implications of this finding to human cancer were not realized until human oncogenic viruses were finally identified. Oncogenic viruses are important experimental tools that can assist us in the elucidation of the molecular mechanisms of carcinogenesis. Studies of the role that viruses play in the pathobiology of human neoplasia have been greatly facilitated by recent progress in recombinant DNA biotechnology and, particularly, by the timely discovery of cellular oncogenes and human oncogenic retroviruses. As enumerated in this review, important advances have been made over the past twenty years concerning the molecular biology of viral carcinogenesis. It can confidently be expected that research efforts in this area will continue and are likely to open broader avenues for the advancement of novel methods in cancer diagnosis, prophylaxis, and treatment. Results of recent work indicating that the same cellular genes may be activated by DNA tumor viruses, by retroviruses, and by chemical carcinogens have suggested that there may be a limited number of pathways to oncogenesis, and aberrant replication of a small group of cellular genes may set the stage for the neoplastic process.

Convincing evidence shows that an immune response against certain human tumors is actually elicited and that such a reaction may, in rare cases, be responsible for the regression of inoperable primary cancers. Nevertheless, clear-cut proof of an effective tumor resistance in humans as a result of an immune response to the tumor itself is an exception to the general rule. It is for that reason that early attempts at using immunologic approaches in the treatment of human cancer proved unsuccessful.

By contrast, there are many mechanisms by which tumor cells can nonspecifically interfere with the development of immunity in the host. Certain tumors can be shown to release soluble factors that directly inhibit the immune response. In addition, protein-calorie malnutrition, which is usually associated with progressive tumor growth, can evoke a generalized depression of humoral and/or cellular immunity. For example, prostaglandins secreted by macrophages from tumor-bearing hosts are known to suppress the immune response. The specificity of this effect was confirmed when it was demonstrated that indomethacin, a cyclooxygenase inhibitor, was able to overcome the inhibitory effect attributed to the macrophage prostaglandins. However, further research needs to be done before indomethacin can be considered viable in the treatment of cancer patients. Vaccination is another promising alternative approach to the prophylactic control of virus-induced human neoplasia. Accordingly, immunization against hepatitis B virus infection should eventually lower the incidence of primary hepatocellular carcinoma in certain parts of the world.

# REFERENCES

1. Temin, H. M., 1981, Nature of the provirus of Rous sarcoma. *Natl. Cancer Inst. Monog.* **17:**557–570.
2. Temin, H. M., and Mizutani, S., 1970, RNA-dependent DNA polymerase in virions of Rous sarcoma virus. *Nature (Lond.)* **226:**1211–1213.
3. Baltimore, D., 1970, RNA-dependent DNA polymerase in virions of RNA tumor viruses. *Nature (Lond.)* **226:**1209–1211.
4. Green, M., 1985, Transformation and oncogenesis: DNA viruses, in: *Virology* (B. N. Fields, ed.), pp. 183–234, Raven, New York.
5. Bateman, T., 1814, *A Practical Synopsis of Cutaneous Diseases,* 3rd ed., Longman, Hurst, Rees, Orme and Brown, London.
6. Goodpasture, E. W., and Woodruff, C. E., 1931, A comparison of the inclusion bodies of the fowlpox and molluscum contagiosum, *Am. J. Pathol.* **7:**1–7.
7. Vogt, M., and Dulbecco, R., 1960, Virus-cell interaction with a tumor producing virus, *Proc. Natl. Acad. Sci. USA* **46:**365–370.
8. Niven, J. S. F., Armstrong, J. A., Andrews, C. H., Pereira, H. G., and Valentine, R. C., 1961, Subcutaneous "growths" in monkeys produced by a poxvirus, *J. Pathol.* **81:**1–14.
9. Richardson, E. 1961, Progressive multifocal leukoencephalopathy, *N. Engl. J. Med.* **265:**815–823.
10. Trentin, J. J., Yabe, Y., and Taylor, G., 1962, The quest for human cancer viruses, *Science* **137:**835–841.
11. Epstein, M. A., Anchong, B. G., and Barr, Y. M., 1964, Virus particles in cultured lymphoblasts from Burkitt's lymphoma, *Lancet* **1:**702–703.
12. Pulvertaft, R. J. V., 1964, Cytology of Burkitt's tumor (African lymphoma), *Lancet* **1:**238–240.
13. Rawls, W. E., Tompkins, W. A. F., and Melnick, J. L., 1969, The association of herpes virus type 2 and carcinoma of the uterine cervix, *Am. J. Epidemiol.* **89:**547–554.
14. Albrecht, T., and Rapp, F., 1973, Malignant transformation of cancer embryo fibroblasts following exposure to ultraviolet-irradiated human cytomegalovirus, *Virology* **55:**53–61.
15. zur Hausen, H., 1976, Condyloma acuminata and human genital cancer, *Cancer Res.* **36:**794.
16. Gardner, S., 1977, The new human papovaviruses: Their nature and significance, in: *Recent Advances in Clinical Virology* (A. P. Waterson, ed.), pp. 93–115, Livingston, New York.
17. Szmuness, W., 1978, Hepatocellular carcinoma and the hepatitis B virus: Evidence for a causal association, *Prog. Med. Virol.* **24:**40–69.
18. Salahuddin, S. Z., Ablashi, D. V., Markham, P. D., Josephs, S. F., Sturzenegger, S., Kaplan, M., Halligan, G., Biberfield, P., Wong-Staal, F., Kramarsky, B., and Gallo, R. C., 1986, Isolation of a new virus, HBLV, in patients with lymphoproliferative disorders, *Science* **234:**596–601.
19. Ellermann, V., and Bang, O., 1908, Experimentelle Leukamie bei Huhnern, *Zentralbl. Bakteriol.* **46:**595.
20. Rous, P. A., 1911, Sarcoma of the fowl transmissible by an agent separable from the tumor cells, *J. Exp. Med.* **13:**397.
21. Fujinami, A., and Inamoto, K., 1914, Uber Geschwulste bei japanischen Haushuhnern insbesondere uber einen Transplantablen Tumor, *Zeitschr. Krebsforsch.* **14:**94–119.
22. Bittner, J. J., 1936, Some possible effects of nursing on the mammary gland tumor incidence of mice, *Science* **84:**162–163.
23. Gross, L., 1951, "Spontaneous" leukemia developing in C3H mice following inoculation in infancy, with AK leukemic extracts, or AK embryos, *Proc. Soc. Exp. Biol. Med.* **76:**27.
24. Graffi, A., Bielka, H., Fey, F., and Marchiani, P., 1955, Gehauftes Aufreten von Leukamien nach Injection von Sarkomfiltraten, *Wien. Klin. Wochenschr.* **105:**61.
25. Friend, C., 1957, Cell-free transmission in adult Swiss mice of a disease having the character of a leukemia, *J. Exp. Med.* **105:**307–318.
26. Lieberman, M., and Kaplan, H. S., 1959, Leukemogenic activity of filtrates from radiation-induced lymphoid tumors of mice, *Science* **130:**387–388.
27. Moloney, J. B., 1960, Biological studies on a lymphoid leukemia virus extracted from sarcoma S37. I. Origin and introductory investigations, *J. Natl. Cancer Inst.* **24:**933–951.
28. Rauscher, F. J., 1962, A virus-induced disease of mice characterized by erythrocytopoiesis and lymphoid leukemia, *J. Natl. Cancer Inst.* **29:**515–543.
29. Harvey, J. J., 1964, An unidentified virus which causes the rapid production of tumours in mice, *Nature (Lond.)* **204:**1104–1105.
30. Moloney, J. B., 1966, A virus-induced rhabdomyosarcoma of mice, *Natl. Cancer Inst. Monog.* **22:**139–142.

31. Finkel, M. P., Biskis, B. O., and Jinkins, P. B., 1966, Virus induction of osteosarcomas in mice, *Science* **151:**698–701.
32. Hehlmann, R., Schetters, H., and Erfle, V., 1984, RNA tumor viruses. in: *Human Virology* (R. B. Belshe, ed.), PSG, pp. 139–178, Littleton, Massachusetts.
33. Jarrett, W. F. H., Martin, W. B., Crighton, G. W., Dalton, R. G., and Stewart, M. F., 1964, Leukemia in the cat: Transmission experiments with leukemia (lymphosarcoma), *Nature (Lond.)* **202:**566–568.
34. Kawakami, T. G., Theilen, G. H., Dungworth, D. L., Munn, R. J., and Beall, S. G., 1967, "C"-type viral particles in plasma of cats with feline leukemia, *Science* **158:**1049–1050.
35. Rickard, C. G., Post, J. E., Noronha, F., and Barr, L. M., 1969, A transmissable virus-induced lymphocytic leukemia of the cat, *J. Natl. Cancer Inst.* **42:**987–1014.
36. Snyder, S. P., and Theilen, G. H., 1969, Transmissible feline fibrosarcoma, *Nature (Lond.)* **221:**1074–1075.
37. Chopra, H. S., and Mason, M. M., 1970, A new virus in a spontaneous mammary tumor of a Rhesus monkey, *Cancer Res.* **30:**2081–2086.
38. Verma, I. M., 1977, The reverse transcriptase, *Biochim. Biophys. Acta* **473:**1–38.
39. Alberts, B., Bray, D., Lewis, J., Raff, M., Roberts, K., and Watson, J. D., 1983, *Molecular Biology of the Cell,* Garland, New York.
40. Wolfe, L. G., Deinhardt, F., Theilen, G. H., Rabin, H., Kawakami, T., and Bustad, L. K., 1971, Induction of tumors in marmoset monkeys by simian sarcoma virus, type 1 (lagothrix): A preliminary report, *J. Natl. Cancer Inst.* **47:**1115–1120.
41. Duesberg, P. H., and Vogt, P. K., 1973, Differences between the ribonucleic acids of transforming and nontransforming avian tumor viruses, *Proc. Natl. Acad. Sci. USA* **67:**1673–1680.
42. Stehelin, D., Varmus, H. E., Bishop, J. M., and Vogt, P. K., 1976, DNA related to the transforming gene(s) of avian sarcoma viruses is present in normal DNA, *Nature (Lond.)* **260:**170–173.
43. Bishop, J. M., 1980, The molecular biology of RNA tumor viruses: A physician's guide, *N. Engl. J. Med.* **303:**675–682.
44. Poiesz, B. J., Ruscetti, F. W., Gazdar, A. F., Bunn, P. A., Minna, J. D., and Gallo, R. C., 1980, Detection and isolation of type C retrovirus particles from fresh and cultured lymphocytes of a patient with cutaneous T-cell lymphoma, *Proc. Natl. Acad. Sci. USA* **77:**7415–7419.
45. Poiesz, B. J., Ruscetti, F. W., Reitz, M. S., Kalyanaraman, V. S., and Gallo, R. C., 1981, Isolation of a new type C retrovirus (HTLV) in primary uncultured cells of a patient with Sezary T-cell leukemia, *Nature (Lond.)* **294:**268–271.
46. Jawetz, E., Melnick, J. L., and Adelberg, E. A., 1987, Tumor viruses and oncogenes, in: *Review of Medical Microbiology* (E. Jawetz, J. L. Melnick, and E. A. Adelberg, eds.), pp. 519–532, Appleton & Lange, E. Norwalk, Connecticut.
47. Monier, R., and Salzman, N. P., 1983, History and overview of oncogenic DNA viruses, in: *Viruses Associated with Human Cancer* (L. A. Phillips, ed.), pp. 3–35, Marcel, New York.
48. Lowy, D. R., 1985, Transformation and oncogenesis: Retroviruses, in: *Virology* (B. N. Fields, ed.), pp. 235–263, Raven, New York.
49. Coffin, J. M., 1982, Structure of the retroviral genomes, in: *Molecular Biology of Tumor Viruses: RNA Tumor Viruses* (R. A. Weiss, N. Teich, H. E. Varmus, and J. M. Coffin, eds.) pp. 261–368, Cold Spring Harbor Laboratory, Cold Spring Harbor, New York.
50. Gordon, H., 1985, Oncogenes, *Mayo Clin. Proc.* **60:**697–713.
51. Graf, T., and Stehelin, D., 1982, Avian leukemia viruses. Oncogenes and genome structure, *Biochim. Biophys. Acta* **651:**245–271.
52. Shilo, B. Z., 1984, Evolution of cellular oncogenes, *Adv. Virol. Oncol.* **4:**29–44.
53. Shilo, B. Z., and Weinberg, R. A., 1981, DNA sequences homologous to vertebrate oncogenes are conserved in *Drosophila melanogaster, Proc. Natl. Acad. Sci. USA* **78:**6789–6792.
54. Dejean, A., Bougueleret, L., Grzeschik, K. H., and Tiollais, P., 1986, Hepatitis B virus DNA integration in a sequence homologous to v-erb-A and steroid receptor genes in a hepatocellular carcinoma, *Nature (Lond.)* **322:**70–72.
55. Hino, O., Shows, T. B., and Rogler, C. E., 1986, Hepatitis B virus integration site in hepatocellular carcinoma at chromosome 17;18 translocation, *Proc. Natl. Acad. Sci. USA* **83:**8338–8342.
56. Macara, I. G., 1985, Oncogenes, ions and phospholipids, *Am. J. Physiol.* **248**(pt. 1):C3–C11.
57. Vogt, M., and Dulbecco, R., 1960, Virus-cell interaction with a tumor-producing virus, *Proc. Natl. Acad. Sci. USA* **46:**365–370.
58. Lancaster, W. D., and Olson, C., 1982, Animal papillomaviruses, *Microbiol. Rev.* **46:**191–207.

59. Rawls, W. E., Clarke, A., Smith, K. O., Docherty, J. J., Gilman, S. C., and Graham, S., 1980, Specific antibodies to herpes simplex virus type 2 among women with cervical cancer, in: *Viruses in Naturally Occurring Cancers*, Vol. 7 (M. Essex, G. Todaro, and H. zur Hausen, eds.), pp. 117–133, Cold Spring Harbor Laboratory, Cold Spring Harbor, New York.

60. Green, M., Brackmann, K. H., Sanders, P. R., Loewenstein, P. M., Freel, J. H., Eisinger, M., and Switlyk, S. A., 1982, Isolation of a human papillomavirus from a patient with epidermodysplasia verruciformis: Presence of related viral DNA genomes in human urogenital tumors, *Proc. Natl. Acad. Sci. USA* **79**:4437–4441.

61. Orth, G., Favre, M., Breitburd, F., Croissant, O., Jablonska, S., Obalek, S., Jarzabet-Chorzelska, M., and Rzesa, G., 1980, Epidermodysplasia verruciformis: A model for the role of papilloma viruses in human cancer, in: *Viruses in Naturally Occurring Cancers*, Vol. 7 (M. Essex, G. Todaro, and H. zur Hausen, eds.), pp. 259–282, Cold Spring Harbor Laboratory, Cold Spring Harbor, New York.

62. Galloway, D. A., and McDougall, J. K., 1983, The oncogenic potential of herpes simplex viruses: Evidence of a "hit-and-run" mechanism, *Nature (Lond.)* **302**:21–24.

63. zur Hausen, H., 1982, Human genital cancer: Synergism between two virus infections or synergism between a virus infection and initiating events?, *Lancet* **2**:1370–1372.

64. London, W. T., 1983, Hepatitis B virus and primary hepatocellular carcinoma, in: *Advances in Viral Oncology*, Vol. 3 (G. Klein, ed.), pp. 325–341, Raven, New York.

65. Summers, J., and Mason, W. S., 1982, Properties of the hepatitis B-like viruses related to their taxonomic classification, *Hepatology* **2**:61S–66S.

66. Coffin, J. M., 1982, Endogenous proviruses, in: *Molecular Biology of Tumor Viruses: RNA Tumor Viruses* (R. A. Weiss, N. Teich, H. E. Varmus, and J. M. Coffin, eds.), pp. 1109–1204, Cold Spring Harbor Laboratory, Cold Spring Harbor, New York.

67. Crittenden, L. B., 1981, Exogenous and endogenous leukosis virus genes, *Avian Pathol.* **10**:101–112.

68. Jaenisch, R., 1983, Endogenous retroviruses, *Cell* **32**:5–6.

69. Pincus, T., 1980, The endogenous murine type C virus, in: *Molecular Biology of RNA Tumor Viruses* (J. Stephenson, ed.), pp. 77–130, Academic, New York.

70. O'Rear, J. J., and Temin, H. M., 1982, Spontaneous changes in nucleotide sequences in provirus of spleen necrosis virus, an avian retrovirus, *Proc. Natl. Acad. Sci. USA* **79**:1230–1234.

71. Todaro, G. J., 1980, Interspecies transmission mammalian retroviruses, in: *Molecular Biology of RNA Tumor Viruses* (J. R. Stephenson, ed.), pp. 47–76, Academic, New York.

72. Cohen, J. C., and Varmus, H. E., 1979, Endogenous mammary tumour virus DNA varies among wild mice and segregates during inbreeding, *Nature (Lond.)* **278**:418–423.

73. Robinson, H. L., Astrin, S. M., Senior, A. M., and Salzar, F. H., 1981, Host susceptibility to endogenous viruses: Defective, glycoprotein-expressing proviruses interfere with infections, *J. Virol.* **40**:745–751.

74. Robinson, H. L., Blais, B. M., Tsichlis, P. N., and Coffin, J. M., 1982, At least two regions of the viral genome determine the oncogenic potential of avian leukosis viruses, *Proc. Natl. Acad. Sci. USA* **79**:1225–1229.

75. Cullen, B. R., Skalka, A. M., and Ju, G., 1983, Endogenous avian retroviruses contain deficient promoter and leader sequences, *Proc. Natl. Acad. Sci. USA* **80**:2946–2950.

76. Ralston, R., and Bishop, J. M., 1983, The protein products of the *myc* and *myb* oncogenes and adenovirus E1a are structurally related, *Nature (Lond.)* **306**:803–806.

77. Gelmann, H. P., Clanton, D. J., Jariwalla, R. J., and Rosenthal, L. J., 1983, Characterization and location of *myc* homologous sequences in human cytomegalovirus DNA, *Proc. Natl. Acad. Sci. USA* **80**:5107–5111.

78. Spector, D. H., and Vacquier, J. P., 1983, Human cytomegalovirus (strain AD169) contains sequences related to the avian retrovirus oncogene v-*myc*, *Proc. Natl. Acad. Sci. USA* **80**:3889–3893.

79. Robinson, W. S., Miller, R. H., and Marion, P. L., 1987, Hepadnaviruses and retroviruses share genome homology and features of replication, *Hepatology* **7**:64S–73S.

80. Miller, R. H., and Robinson, W. S., 1986, Common evolutionary origin of hepatitis B virus and retroviruses, *Proc. Natl. Acad. Sci. USA* **83**:2531–2535.

81. Bishop, J. M., 1983, Cellular oncogenes and retroviruses, *Annu. Rev. Biochem.* **52**:301–354.

82. Wold, W. S. M., Mackey, J. K., Brackmann, K. H., Takemori, N., Rigden, P., and Green, M. 1978. Analysis of human tumors and human malignant cell lines for BK virus specific DNA sequences, *Proc. Natl. Acad. Sci. USA* **75**:454–458.

83. Jarrett, W. F. H., McNeil, P. E. Grimshaw, W. T. R., Selman, I. E., and McIntyre, W. I. M., 1978,

High incidence area of cattle cancer with a possible interaction between an environmental carcinogen and a papilloma virus, *Nature (Lond.)* **274:**215–217.

84. Kidd, J. G., and Rous, P., 1940, Cancers deriving from the virus papillomas of wild rabbits under natural conditions, *J. Exp. Med.* **71:**469–494.

85. Mueller, H., and Grissmann, L., 1978, *Mastomys natalensis* papilloma virus (MnPV), the causative agent of epithelial proliferations: Characterization of the virus particle, *J. Gen. Virol.* **41:**315–323.

86. Ito, Y., 1960, A tumor-producing factor extracted by phenol from papillomatous tissue (Shope) of cottontail rabbits, *Virology* **12:**596–601.

87. Coggin, J. R., Jr., and zur Hausen, H., 1979, Workshop on papillomaviruses and cancer, *Cancer Res.* **39:**545–546.

88. Zachow, K. R., Ostrow, R. S., Bender, M., Watts, S., Okagaki, T., Pass, F., and Faras, A. J., 1982, Detection of human papillomavirus DNA in anogenital neoplasias, *Nature (Lond.)* **300:**771–773.

89. Durst, M., Grissmann, L., Ikenberg, H., and zur Hausen, H., 1983, A papillomavirus DNA from a cervical carcinoma and its prevalence in cancer biopsy samples from different geographic regions, *Proc. Natl. Acad. Sci. USA* **80:**3812–3815.

90. Grissman, L., Wolnik, L., Ikenberg, H., Koldovsky, U., Schurch, H. G., and zur Hausen, H., 1983, Human papillomavirus types 6 and 11 DNA sequences in genital and laryngeal papillomas and in some cervical cancer, *Proc. Natl. Acad. Sci. USA* **80:**560–563.

91. Kreider, J. W., Howett, M. K., Wolfe, S. A., Bartlett, G. L., Zaino, R. J., Sedlacek, T. V., and Mortel, R., 1985, Morphological transformation *in vivo* of human uterine cervix with papillomavirus from condylomata acuminata, *Nature (Lond.)* **317:**639–641.

92. Syrjanen, K. J., 1980, Epithelial lesions suggestive of a condylomatous origin found closely associated with invasive bronchial squamous cell carcinomas, *Respiration* **40:**150–160.

93. Kurman, R. J., Shah, K. H., Lancaster, W. D., and Jenson, A. B., 1981, Immunoperoxidase localization of papillomavirus antigens in cervical dysplasia and vulvar condylomas, *Am. J. Obstet. Gynecol.* **140:**931–935.

94. Woodruff, J. D., Braun, L., Cavalieri, R., Gupta, P., Pass, F., and Shah, K., 1981, Immunological identification of papillomavirus antigen in paraffin-processed condyloma tissues from the female genital tract, *Obstet. Gynecol.* **56:**727–732.

95. Syrjanen, K. J., 1984, Current concepts of human papillomavirus infections in the genital tract and their relationship to intraepithelial neoplasia and squamous cell carcinoma, *Obstet. Gynecol.* **39:**252–265.

96. Syrjanen, K. J., 1982, Histological changes identical to those of condylomatous lesions found in esophageal squamous cell carcinomas, *Arch. Geschwulstforsch.* **52:**S283–S292.

97. Syrjanen, K. J., and Syrjanen, S. M., 1981, Histological evidence for the presence of condylomatous epithelial lesions in association with laryngeal squamous cell carcinoma, *ORLJ Otorhinolaryngol. Relat. Spec.* **43:**181–194.

98. Grissmann, L., Diehl, V., Schultz-Coulon, H.-J., and zur Hausen, H., 1982, Molecular cloning and characterization of human papilloma virus DNA derived from a laryngeal papilloma, *J. Virol.* **44:**393–400.

99. Pfister, H., Hettich, I., Runne, U., Grissmann, L., and Chilf, G. N., 1983, Characterization of human papillomavirus type 13 from focal epithelial hyperplasia neck lesions, *J. Virol.* **47:**363–366.

100. Green, M., 1971, Search for adenovirus messenger RNA in cancers of man, in: *Oncology* (L. Clark, R. W. Gumley, J. E. McCay, and M. M. Copeland, eds.), pp. 156–165, Year Book Medical Publishers, Chicago.

101. Jonsson, N., and Ankerst, J., 1977, Studies on adenovirus type 9-induced mammary fibroadenomas in rats and their malignant transformation, *Cancer* **39:**2513–2519.

102. Bernards, R., Schrier, P. I., Houweling, A., Box, J. L., and van der Eb, A. J., 1983, Tumorigenicity of cells transformed by adenovirus type 12 by evasion of T-cell immunity, *Nature (Lond.)* **305:**776–779.

103. Schrier, P. I., Bernards, R., Vaessen, R. T. M. J., Houweling, A., and van der Eb, A. J., 1983, Expression of class I major histocompatibility antigens switched off by highly oncogenic adenovirus 12 in transformed rat cells, *Nature (Lond.)* **305:**771–775.

104. Roizman, B., 1982, The family herpesviridae: General description, taxonomy, and classification, in: *The Viruses. The Herpesviruses,* Vol. 1 (B. Roizman, ed.), pp. 1–23, Plenum, New York.

105. Duff, R., and Rapp, F., 1973, Oncogenic transformation of hamster embryo cells after exposure to inactivated herpes simplex virus type 1, *J. Virol.* **12:**209–217.

106. Duff, R., and Rapp, F., 1971, Oncogenic transformation of hamster cells after exposure to herpes simplex virus type 2, *Nature (Lond.)* **233:**48–50.

107. Maitland, N. J., Kinross, J. H., Busuttil, A., Ludgate, S. M., Smart, G. E., and Jones, K. W., 1981, The detection of DNA tumour virus-specific RNA sequences in abnormal human cervical biopsies by *in situ* hybridization, *J. Gen. Virol.* **55:**123–127.

108. McDougall, J. K., Crum, C. P., Fenoglio, C. M., Goldstein, L. C., and Galloway, D. A., 1982, Herpesvirus-specific RNA and protein in carcinoma of the uterine cervix, *Proc. Natl. Acad. Sci. USA* **79:**3853–3857.

109. Vonka, V., Kanka, J., Jelinek, J., Subrt, I., Suchanek, A., Havrankova, A., Vachal, M., Hirsch, I., Domorazkova, E., Zavadova, H., Richterova, V., Naprstkova, J., Dvorakova, V., and Svoboda, B., 1984, Prospective study on the relationship between cervical neoplasia and herpes simplex type-2 virus I. Epidemiological characteristics, *Int. J. Cancer* **33:**49–60.

110. Galloway, D. A., Nelson, J. A., and McDougall, J. K., 1984, Small fragments of herpesvirus DNA with transforming activity contain insertion sequence-like structures, *Proc. Natl. Acad. Sci. USA* **81:**4736–4740.

111. Nelson, J. A., Fleckenstein, B., Galloway, D. A., and McDougall, J. K., 1982, Transformation of NIH 3T3 cells with cloned fragments of human cytomegalovirus strain AD169, *J. Virol.* **43:**83–91.

112. Huang, E.-S., Boldogh, I., and Mar, E.-C., 1983, Human cytomegaloviruses: Evidence for possible association with human cancer, in: *Viruses Associated with Human Cancer* (L. A. Phillips, ed.), pp. 161–194, Dekker, New York.

113. Zagury, D., Bernard, J., Leonard, R., Cheynier, R., Feldman, M., Sarin, P. S., and Gallo, R. C., 1986, Long-term cultures of HTLV-III-infected T cells: A model of cytopathology of T-cell depletion in AIDS, *Science* **231:**850–853.

114. Mosca, J. D., Bednarik, D. P., Raj, N. B. K., Rosen, C. A., Sodroski, J. G., Haseltine, W. A., and Pitha, P. M., 1987, HSV-1 can reactivate transcription of latent HIV, *Nature (Lond.)* **325:**67–70.

115. Yamamoto, N., 1984, Interaction of viruses with tumor promotors, *Rev. Physiol. Biochem. Pharmacol.* **101:**111–159.

116. Epstein, M. A., 1986, Vaccination against Epstein-Barr virus: Current progress and future strategies, *Lancet* **2:**1425–1427.

117. Josephs, S. F., Salahuddin, S. Z., Ablashi, D. V., Schachter, F., Wong-Staal, F., and Gallo, R. C., 1986, Genomic analysis of the human B-lymphotropic virus (HBLV), *Science* **234:**601–603.

118. Swenson, P. D., Escobar, M. R., and Silverman, J. F., 1980, Hepatitis B virus and core antigens in the liver of primary hepatocellular carcinoma cases in Virginia, *Acta Biol. Acad. Sci. Hung.* **31:**321–328.

119. Lieberman, H. M., and Shafritz, D., 1986, Persistent hepatitis B virus infection and hepatocellular carcinoma, in: *Progress in Liver Diseases VIII* (H. Popper and F. Schaffner, eds.), pp. 395–415, Grune & Stratton, New York.

120. Wu, T. C., Tong, M. J., Hwang, B., Lee, S. D., and Hu, M. M., 1987, Primary hepatocellular carcinoma and hepatitis B infection during childhood, *Hepatology* **7:**46–48.

121. Brechot, C., Pourcel, C., Louise, A., Rain, B., and Tiollais, P., 1980, Presence of integrated hepatitis B virus DNA sequences in cellular DNA of human hepatocellular carcinoma, *Nature (Lond.)* **286:**533–535.

122. Shafritz, D. A., and Kew, M. C., 1981, Identification of integrated hepatitis B virus DNA sequences in human hepatocellular carcinomas, *Hepatology* **1:**1–8.

123. Hayward, W. S., Neel, B. G., and Astrin, S. M., 1981, Activation of a cellular *onc* gene by promoter insertion in ALV-induced lymphoid leukosis, *Nature (Lond.)* **290:**475–480.

124. Neel, B. G., Hayward, W. S., Robinson, H. L., Fang, J., and Astrin, S. M., 1981, Avian leukosis virus-induced tumors have common proviral integration sites and synthesize discrete new RNA's: Oncogenesis by promoter insertion, *Cell* **23:**323–334.

125. Payne, G. S., Courtneidge, S. A., Crittenden, L. B., Fadly, A. M., Bishop, J. M., and Varmus, H. E., 1981, Analysis of avian leukosis virus DNA and RNA in bursal tumors: Viral gene expression is not required for maintenance of the tumor state, *Cell* **23:**311–322.

126. Koshy, R., Koch, S., von Loringhoven, A. F., Kahmann, R., Murray, R., and Hofschneider, P. H., 1983, Integration of hepatitis B virus DNA: Evidence for integration in the single-stranded gap, *Cell* **34:**215–223.

127. Gallo, R. C., Wong-Staal, F., and Ruscetti, F., 1982, Viruses and adult leukemia–lymphoma of man and relevant animal models, in: *Adult Leukemias* (C. D. Bloomfield, ed.), pp. 141–215, Martinus Nijhoff, The Hague.

128. Hehlmann, R., Schetters, H., and Erfle, V., 1984, Current understanding of viral etiology in leukemia, in: *Leukemia, Recent Results in Cancer Research* (E. Thiel and S. Thierfelder, eds.), pp. 1–28, Springer-Verlag, Berlin.

129. Chandra, P., and Steel, L. K., 1977, Purification, biochemical characterization and serological analysis of cellular deoxyribonucleic acid polymerases and a reverse transcriptase from spleen of a patient with myelofibrotic syndrome, *Biochem. J.* **167**:315–523.

130. Hehlmann, R., Schetters, H., Erfle, V., and Leib-Mosch, C., 1983, Detection and biochemical characterization of antigens in human leukemic sera that crossreact with primate C-type viral p30 proteins, *Cancer Res.* **43**:392–399.

131. Herbrink, P., Moen, J. E. T., Brouwer, J., and Warnaar, S. O., 1980, Detection of antibodies cross-reactive with type-C RNA tumor viral p30 protein in human sera and exudate fluids, *Cancer Res.* **40**:166–173.

132. Jacquemin, P. C., Saxinger, C., and Gallo, R. C., 1978, Surface antibodies of human myelogenous leukemia leukocytes reactive with specific type-C viral reverse transcriptases, *Nature (Lond.)* **276**:230–236.

133. Gallagher, R. E., and Gallo, R. C., 1975, Type-C RNA tumor virus isolated from cultured human acute myelogenous leukemia cells, *Science* **187**:350–353.

134. Nooter, K., Aarson, A. M., Bentvelze, P., deGroot, F. G., and Van Pelt, F. G., 1975, Isolation of infectious C-type oncornavirus from human leukemic bone marrow cells, *Nature (Lond.)* **256**:595–597.

135. Panem, S., Prochownik, E. V., Reale, F. R., and Kirsten, W. H., 1975, Isolation of type C virions from a normal human fibroblast strain, *Science* **189**:297–299.

136. Kaplan, H. S., Goodenow, R. S., Epstein, A. L., Gartner, S., Decleve, A., and Rosenthal, P. N., 1977, Isolation of a type C RNA virus from an established human histiocytic lymphoma cell line, *Proc. Natl. Acad. Sci. USA* **74**:2564–2568.

137. Bonner, T. I., Connell, C. O., and Cohen, M., 1982, Cloned endogenous retroviral sequences from human DNA, *Proc. Natl. Acad. Sci. USA* **79**:4709–4713.

138. Martin, M. A., Bryan, T., Rasheed, S., and Kahn, A. S., 1981, Identification and cloning of endogenous retroviral sequences present in human DNA, *Proc. Natl. Acad. Sci. USA* **78**:4892–4896.

139. O'Brien, S. J., Bonner, T. I., Cohen, M., O'Connell, C., and Nash, W. G., 1983, Mapping of an endogenous retroviral sequence to human chromosome 18, *Nature (Lond.)* **303**:74–77.

140. Repaske, R., O'Neill, R. R., Steele, P. E., and Martin, M. A., 1983, Characterization and partial nucleotide sequence of endogenous type C retrovirus segments in human chromosomal DNA, *Proc. Natl. Acad. Sci. USA* **80**:678–682.

141. Poiesz, B. J., Ruscetti, F. W., Mier, J. W., Woods, A. M., and Gallo, R. C., 1980, T-cell lines established from human T-lymphocytic neoplasias by direct response to T-cell growth factor, *Proc. Natl. Acad. Sci. USA* **77**:6815–6819.

142. Hehlmann, R., 1976, RNA tumor viruses and human cancer, in: *Current Topics in Microbiology and Immunology*, Vol. 73, pp. 141–215, Springer-Verlag, Berlin.

143. Pimentel, E., 1979, Human oncovirology, *Biochim. Biophys. Acta* **560**:169–216.

144. Ohno, T., and Spiegelman, S., 1977, Antigenic relatedness of the DNA polymerase of human breast cancer particles to the enzyme of the Mason–Pfizer monkey virus. *Proc. Natl. Acad. Sci. USA* **74**:2144–2148.

145. Dion, A. S., Farwell, D. C., Pomenti, A. A., and Girardi, A. J., 1980, A human protein related to the major envelope protein of murine mammary tumor virus: Identification and characterization, *Proc. Natl. Acad. Sci. USA* **77**:1301–1305.

146. Welte, K., Ebener, U., and Chandra, P., 1979, Serological characterization of a purified reverse transcriptase from osteosarcoma of a child, *Cancer Lett.* **7**:189–195.

147. Zurcher, C., Brinkhof, J., Bentvelzen, P., and deMan, J. C. H., 1975, C-type virus antigens detected by immunofluorescence in human bone tumor cultures, *Nature (Lond.)* **254**:457–459.

148. Chandra, P., Balikcioglu, S., and Mildner, B., 1978, Biochemical and immunological characterization of a reverse transcriptase from human melanoma tissue, *Cancer Lett.* **5**:299–310.

149. Balda, B. R., Hehlmann, R., Cho, J. R., and Spiegelman, S., 1975, Oncornavirus-like particles in human skin cancers, *Proc. Natl. Acad. Sci. USA* **72**:3697–3700.

150. Parsons, P. G., Klucis, E., Gross, P. D., Pope, J. H., Little, J. H., and Davis, N. C., 1976, Oncornavirus-like particles in malignant melanoma and control biopsies, *Int. J. Cancer* **18**:757–763.

151. Kalter, S. S., Helmke, R., Heberling, R. L., Panigel, M., Fowler, A.K., Strickland, J. E., and Hellman, A., 1973, C-type particles in normal human placentas, *J. Natl. Cancer Inst.* **50**:1081–1084.

152. Dirksen, E. R., and Levy, J. A., 1977, Virus-like particles in placentas from normal individuals and patients with systemic lupus erythematosus, *J. Natl. Cancer Inst.* **59**:1187–1192.

153. Sawyer, M. H., Nachlas, Jr., N. E., and Panem, S., 1978, C-type viral antigen expression in human placenta, *Nature (Lond.)* **275**:62–64.

154. Thiry, L., Sprecher-Goldberger, S., Bossens, M., and Neurax, F., 1978, Cell-mediated immune response to simian oncornavirus antigens in pregnant women, *J. Natl. Cancer Inst.* **60:**527–532.

155. Callahan, R., Drohan, W., Tronick, S., and Schlom, J., 1982, Detection and cloning of human DNA sequences related to the mouse mammary tumor virus genome, *Proc. Natl. Acad. Sci. USA* **79:**5503–5507.

156. Sell, S., 1987, *Immunology, Immunopathology and Immunity*, Elsevier, New York.

157. Stites, D. P., Stobo, J. D., and Wells, J. V., 1987, Tumor immunology. in: *Basic and Clinical Immunology* (D. P. Stites, J. D. Stobo, and J. V. Wells, eds.), pp. 186–196, Appleton & Lange, E. Norwalk, Connecticut.

158. Herberman, R. B., and Bellanti, J. A., 1985, Immune defense mechanisms in tumor immunity, in: *Immunology*, Vol. III (J. A. Bellanti, ed.), pp. 330–345, W. B. Saunders, Philadelphia.

159. Church, J. A., and Schlegel, R. J., 1985, Immune deficiency disorders, in: *Immunology*, Vol. III (J. A. Bellanti, ed.), pp. 471–507. W. B. Saunders, Philadelphia.

# 5

# Radiation Carcinogenesis

## R. Timothy Mulcahy

## 1. INTRODUCTION

### 1.1. Historic Perspective

Ionizing radiation is perhaps the most universally recognized and most intensely studied carcinogen known to man. Certainly no other single environmental carcinogen has attracted as much public attention, elicited such strong emotional responses, or been the subject of more regulatory legislation than radiation. Public awareness of the cancer-inducing property of radiation is relatively recent and is certainly linked to the experience of the survivors of the atomic bomb detonations at Hiroshima and Nagasaki and of persons exposed to fall-out secondary to nuclear weapons testing. Public concern over radiation safety has become even more acute with the proliferation of nuclear arms, the growth of the nuclear power industry and recent accidents at nuclear power plants, such as Chernobyl. However, the oncogenic potential of radiation exposure was recognized early in its history, with the first published report of radiation-induced cancer appearing in the scientific literature shortly after the turn of the twentieth century.[1] Indeed, it is believed that Madam Curie and her daughter Irene both succumbed to leukemia attributable to intense radiation exposure associated with their pioneering work with radioactivity. Since these early days in radiation research, the carcinogenic properties of ionizing radiation have been repeatedly substantiated in human populations, experimental animals, and, more recently, tissue-culture systems. More importantly, this accumulating evidence for the cancer-inducing ability of radiation has been accompanied by a growing understanding of potential mechanisms of radiation carcinogenesis, factors influencing the expression of radiation-induced neoplasia, and the risks associated with low-level exposures. It is the intent of this chapter to review the human and experimental experience in the area of radiation carcinogenesis, summarizing cellular and tissue responses, and discussing potential mechanisms involved in the pathogenesis of radiation-induced neoplasms.

### 1.2. Ionizing Radiation and Its Interaction with Matter

A brief introduction to the properties of ionizing radiations and the manner in which they interact with biologic matter to produce damage is helpful for issues discussed in subsequent sections. Many of the data discussed involve the use of photon irradiation, exposure to $\gamma$- or X-rays. Both are very energetic forms of electromagnetic radiation, with identical properties but different origins. $\gamma$-Rays are produced by the decay of unstable atomic nuclei, while X-rays typically result

R. Timothy Mulcahy • Department of Human Oncology, University of Wisconsin–Madison, Madison, Wisconsin 53792.

from the bombardment of a target (i.e., tungsten) with accelerated electrons. These photons interact with electrons of atoms in an absorbing material, ejecting them from their orbits (ionization). The resulting energetic electrons then interact with other molecules to produce ion pairs and highly reactive free radicals. In this way, the energy of the incident photon is transferred, via electrons, to biologically important molecules, producing chemical alterations that, under appropriate conditions, may themselves be expressed as some form of biologic damage, such as cell death or neoplastic transformation.

Another form of ionizing radiation important in radiation carcinogenesis are neutrons. These uncharged particles produce ionizations in an absorbing material by primarily interacting with atomic nuclei, particularly hydrogen nuclei, setting in motion protons or other charged particles capable of producing ionizations in the molecules of the absorbing material. In contrast to photon-induced ionizations, which are distributed widely and randomly, ionizations associated with the absorption of neutrons are more concentrated spatially. As a consequence of this dense ionization pattern, neutrons are frequently more effective at causing various types of biologic damage than are γ- or X-rays at comparable absorbed doses.

Certain wavelengths of electromagnetic radiation in the ultraviolet (UV) range are also known to be either mutagenic or carcinogenic, or both. Unlike ionizing radiation, damage resulting from UV exposure is the consequence of molecular excitation as opposed to ionization. While a relatively extensive literature pertaining to the carcinogenic effects of UV radiation exists, the remainder of this chapter is restricted to a consideration of the carcinogenic effects of ionizing radiations.

## 2. RADIATION CARCINOGENESIS IN VIVO

### 2.1. The Human Experience

While much of what is known about radiation carcinogenesis and factors influencing its expression has been derived from experimental systems, a rather extensive compilation of data based on tumorigenesis in exposed human populations has accumulated over the past 85 years. This vast human experience makes radiation unique among carcinogenic agents in providing a data base from which risk estimates for humans can be calculated. As will become evident, these estimates of risk are fraught with problems and characterized by considerable uncertainties—they are indeed estimates. However, they do provide some valuable information concerning radiation carcinogenesis in the species of ultimate concern, man.

A large proportion of the data relating radiation exposure and tumor induction in man, and perhaps the best known to the general populace, is based on the thorough follow-up of the Japanese survivors of the atomic bomb blasts in Hiroshima and Nagasaki. The estimated increased risk of dying from cancers of various sites for persons exposed to 200 or more rad,* as compared with unexposed persons, is shown in Fig. 1. The risk of dying of leukemia was increased approximately 10-fold in this cohort, whereas the mortality associated with certain other malignancies, such as those arising in pancreas, uterus, or rectum had at the time of the report not shown a significant increase as compared to the control population. For most other tissues, as well as for the collective risk of dying from any malignancy excluding leukemia, there was approximately a twofold increase in the irradiated population. With the exception of the leukemia risk estimate, most other estimates are still subject to change, as peak tumor incidence for many of the solid neoplasms had not occurred during the 28-year interval (1950–1978) over which these data were collected. Consequently, many of these risk calculations may represent conservative estimates, although, given the large confidence intervals associated with many of the relative risk factors presented in Fig. 1, the final risk estimates may not prove to be significantly different.

One generally required criterion for establishing a causal relationship between radiation exposure and tumor induction is a dose–response relationship, i.e., correlation between tumor inci-

*rad = unit of absorbed dose, equal to 100 erg/g.

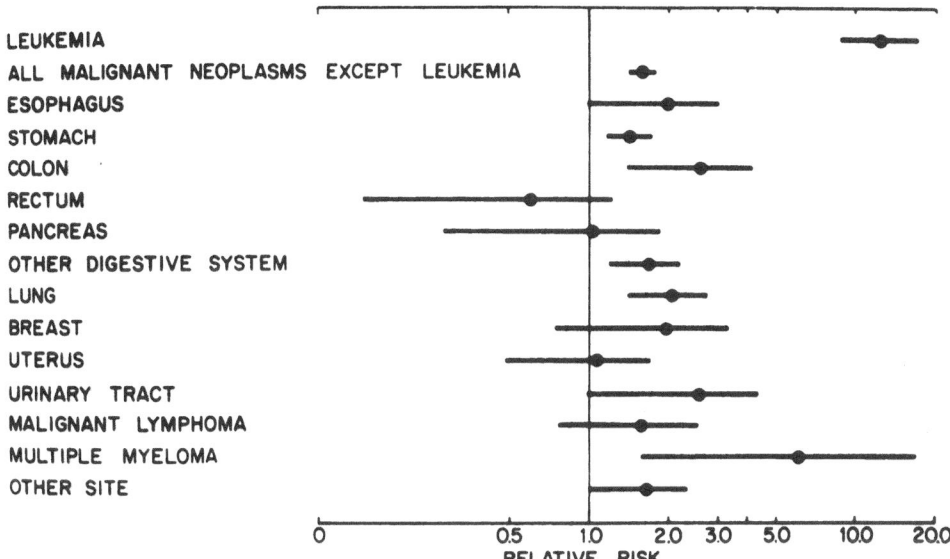

*Figure 1.* Site-specific cancer mortality for persons exposed to doses of 200 rad and over following the bombings at Hiroshima and Nagasaki. The period of observation was 1950–1978. Error bars are 90% confidence intervals. (From Kato and Schull.[2])

dence within the irradiated field and exposure dose. Such a relationship between dose and incidence has been established from the Japanese data for age-adjusted cancer incidence in general (excluding leukemia), as well as for leukemia incidence and breast cancer incidence,[3] thus unambiguously linking radiation exposure and tumor induction in this irradiated population.

Similarly, causal relationships have been identified in studies of cohorts exposed to ionizing radiation in medical settings for the treatment or diagnosis of various relatively benign conditions. The exposure in these cases often differs significantly from the A-bomb situation in two important ways: (1) smaller tissue volumes were irradiated, thereby limiting the risk of cancer-induction specifically to those tissues in the field; (2) and total exposure was frequently fractionated over a protracted period of time. Nevertheless, the data conclusively confirm the association between radiation exposure and the induction of neoplasia. Table I summarizes the data from medically exposed populations, indicating the disease or disorder treated and the major types of neoplasms observed to be increased in the treated groups.

Certain occupations have involved, and others continue to involve exposure to ionizing radiation or radioactive isotopes in the work environment. The collective experience from various occupationally exposed populations, some of which are also summarized in Table I, is consistent with the rest of the human exposure data in defining a significant correlation between radiation exposure and an increased cancer risk in many exposed tissues. It should also be noted that a relationship between increased risk of cancer induction and radiation exposure for several other tissues is strongly suggested on the basis of observations of the human populations described in Table I, as well as in other studies. Collectively, the epidemiologic data either establish or strongly suggest that virtually every tissue in the body is susceptible to the carcinogenic effects of ionizing radiation.

While risk estimates useful in the establishment of exposure limits for the general population can be derived from analyses of the dose–response relationships for several of these groups of exposed persons, such values are associated with considerable uncertainties and must be interpreted with caution. The uncertainties reflect several factors, not the least of which include difficulties in accurately assessing dose, an inability to normalize adequately for host and environmental factors

Table I. Tumor Induction in Humans following Medical
or Occupational Exposure

Cancer induction associated with medical radiation exposure
with therapeutic intent

| Conditions treated | Type of neoplasm(s) induced |
| --- | --- |
| Ankylosing spondylitis | Leukemia (predominantly granulocytic)[3-5] |
| | Bronchogenic carcinoma[3] |
| Postpartum mastitis | Breast carcinoma[3,6,7] (all histologies) |
| Benign head and neck conditions (tinea capitis, thymic enlargement, acne) | Thyroid carcinoma[3,8,9] (predominantly papillary) |
| Ankylosing spondylitis, bone tuberculosis treated with injections of $^{224}Ra^a$ | CNS tumors[9] Bone sarcomas[3,10] |

Cancer induction associated with medical radiation exposure
for diagnostic purposes

| Diagnostic procedures | Types of neoplasms induced |
| --- | --- |
| Multiple fluoroscopies in female tuberculosis patients | Breast carcinomas[3,7,11,12] (all histologies) |
| Use of Thorotrast[b] contrast medium | Liver neoplasms[3,13,14] (most commonly angiosarcomas and cholangiocarcinomas) |

Cancer induction associated with occupational exposure

| Occupation | Source of exposure | Types of neoplasms induced |
| --- | --- | --- |
| Watch-dial painters | $^{224}Ra^a$ | Bone sarcomas and carcinomas of the paranasal sinuses[3,15] |
| Underground miners | Radon daughters[c] | Bronchogenic carcinomas[3,16] |

[a]A bone-seeking radioactive isotope which emits alpha particles (densely ionizing).
[b]Contains thorium-232, an α-emitter.
[c]α-emitting isotopes.

that could conceivably modulate neoplastic expression (described in more detail in Section 5), and an inability to define accurately the shape of the dose–response relationship at low doses. Ideally, radiation protection standards would be based on risk estimates derived from data for groups of persons exposed to very low protracted doses reflective of the exposure history of the general population. However, in the absence of human data in this dose range, it has been necessary to establish radiation protection standards based on extrapolation from high dose data. The problem with this approach can be appreciated by examining Fig. 2, which represents dose–response data for the induction of thyroid cancer in persons exposed during childhood.[17] While a correlation between exposure dose and incidence is obvious, the data can be fit by any one of three different mathematical models, each yielding unique risk estimates for low-dose exposures. For cancers at other sites, the problem may be even more exaggerated because the thyroid data are somewhat unusual in having incidence data for doses below 20 rad. A discussion regarding selection of appropriate curve-

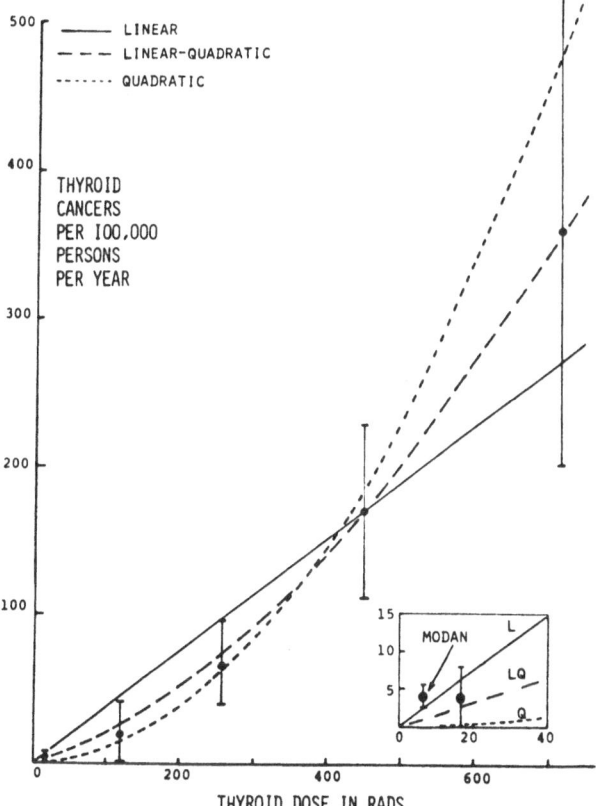

*Figure 2.* Dose–response curves for thyroid tumor induction in individuals exposed to X-rays during child-hood. The three different curves represent three different mathematical models that can be used to describe the data; each yields unique risk estimates for low doses as indicated in the insert. (From Webster.[18])

fitting models is beyond the scope of this chapter; interested readers should consult the BEIR III report[3] and reports by Land,[17] Webster,[18] and Upton[19] for further details. It should be obvious that use of risk estimates based on any of the different models could potentially have significantly different health and economic impact.

## 2.2. Radiation Carcinogenesis in Animal Models

The carcinogenic properties of ionizing radiation have been extensively studied using animal models. Numerous species and strains of animals have been employed in radiation carcinogenesis experiments over the past several decades and, while tumors have been induced in each, the type of tumors induced, the time to peak tumor incidence, and the relative sensitivity of various tissues can vary widely from species to species or from strain to strain within a given species.[20,21] As a consequence of the intraspecies variation in radiation response, estimation of human cancer risk from quantitative extrapolation from animal data is considered inappropriate. Rather, the true value of animal studies lies in their use to probe mechanisms of radiation oncogenesis and factors influencing its expression. As pointed out by Fry,[21] while a number of factors will act collectively to influence the ultimate expression of neoplasia and contribute to cross-species differences, the initial events involved in carcinogenesis are likely to be relatively species independent. Similarly, controlled examination of factors capable of modulating tumor induction in animals will likely have implications and applicability to the human situation as well. The versatility and power of animal investigations have been augmented by the recent introduction of quantitative transplantation models in which epithelial cells are removed from irradiated or unirradiated donor animals and transplanted into ectopic sites (i.e., interscapular fat pad of the rat) in syngeneic recipients.[22] The recipients can then be observed for tumor growth at the graft sites, or the sites can be removed to determine the percentage of irradiated cells surviving the radiation exposure. Consequently, carcinogenic risk and factors influencing risk can be assessed on a per-surviving-cell basis.

Animals studies have also established that radiation exposure can result in tumor induction in tissue outside the irradiated field by disrupting normal homeostatic relationships among various cells and tissues. This particular effect of radiation has been encountered most commonly in hormonally responsive tissue and is exemplified by the induction of thyrotrophic pituitary tumors in mice subsequent to radiation ablation of the thyroid gland.[23]

# 3. PATHOLOGY OF RADIATION CARCINOGENESIS IN VIVO

## 3.1. Incidence and Morphology

Unfortunately for cancer biologists and epidemiologists alike, tumors induced in irradiated populations of animals or humans are morphologically indistinguishable from those occurring spontaneously. Consequently, radiation-induced neoplasms must be detected against a background of spontaneous incidence and radiation causation inferred from significantly increased observed–expected ratios in the exposed groups. With rare exceptions, all neoplastic morphologic variants for a given tissue type have been observed to be induced by radiation.[3] The most notable exception to this generalization is chronic lymphocytic leukemia, the incidence of which, in contrast to all other types of leukemia, has not been observed to be increased following radiation exposure.[24] While virtually all histologic variants for a given tissue can be observed with increased frequency following irradiation of that tissue, re-examination of Table I will show that the induction frequency for individual histologies is not uniform, with certain tumor types being observed with relatively high frequency in irradiated groups. In the case of radiation leukemogenesis, the predominant histologic type observed is the granulocytic variant. Similarly, papillary carcinomas are induced with high frequency following exposure of the thyroid gland.

## 3.2. Relative Tissue Sensitivity

In addition to identifying marked interspecies variation in susceptibility to the carcinogenic effect of ionizing radiation, animal studies have shown that the various tissues of any given individual species or strain display differential sensitivity to the oncogenic effects of radiation. Tissue-dependent sensitivity has also been observed in epidemiologic studies of irradiated human populations. The variation in sensitivity among different organs and tissues is considerable and can be summarized as in Table II, derived from the BEIR III report.[3] According to this analysis, tissue can be divided into four different categories with respect to susceptibility to radiation carcinogenesis. The most sensitive tissues include mammary and thyroid glands and bone marrow. For these tissues there is incontrovertible evidence for a causal relationship between radiation exposure and tumor induction. The opposite end of the sensitivity spectrum includes prostatic and uterine tissue, for which an association between exposure and tumor induction is uncertain at best.

Spontaneous tumor incidence also displays a marked tissue dependency.[3] However, tissue sensitivity to the oncogenic effects of radiation and spontaneous tumor incidence are not correlated (refer to Table II). Although the underlying mechanisms responsible for the variation in tissue sensitivity remain unclear, several factors, including differences in inherent cellular sensitivity to radiation, repair differences, tissue-dependent variations in cellular kinetics, and the number of clonogenic cells present at the time of irradiation, are all believed to play prominent roles. Other

*Table II. Sensitivity of Various Tissues to Oncogenic Influence of Ionizing Radiation*

| Site or type of cancer | Spontaneous incidence of cancer | Relative sensitivity to radiation induction of cancer |
|---|---|---|
| Major radiation-induced cancers | | |
| Female breast | Very high | High |
| Thyroid | Low | Very high, especially in females |
| Lung (bronchus) | Very high | Moderate |
| Leukemia | Moderate | Very high |
| Alimentary tract (especially colon) | High | Moderate to low |
| Minor radiation-induced cancers | | |
| Pharynx | Low | Moderate |
| Liver and biliary tract | Low | Moderate |
| Pancreas | Moderate | Moderate |
| Lymphomas | Moderate | Moderate |
| Kidney and bladder | Moderate | Low |
| Brain and nervous system | Low | Low |
| Salivary glands | Very low | Low |
| Bone | Very low | Low |
| Skin | High | Low |
| Sites or tissues in which magnitude of radiation-induced cancer is uncertain | | |
| Larynx | Moderate | Low |
| Nasal sinuses | Very low | Low |
| Parathyroid | Very low | Low |
| Ovary | Moderate | Low |
| Connective tissues | Very low | Low |
| Sites or tissues in which radiation-induced cancer has not been observed | | |
| Prostate | Very high | Absent? |
| Uterus and cervix | Very high | Absent? |
| Testis | Low | Absent? |
| Mesentery and mesothelium | Very low | Absent? |
| Chronic lymphatic leukemia | Low | Absent? |

extrinsic or environmental variables, such as hormonal responsiveness and interaction among cells, may also contribute by functioning to promote or inhibit neoplastic expression.

## 3.3. Latency

Cancer induction by radiation is characterized by a prolonged interval between the time of irradiation and the appearance of detectable tumors. The length of the induction period, commonly referred to as latency, is generally such that tumors induced in any given irradiated tissue occur at approximately the same time as spontaneous tumors in that particular tissue.[25] In the case of leukemias, the relationship between incidence and time after irradiation can be described as a wave function, with peak tumor incidence occurring somewhere between 5 and 15 years postexposure.[26] Also, the length of the latent period associated with the development of leukemia is highly dependent on the age of the person at the time of irradiation and differs considerably depending on the histologic variant examined.

The latencies for most solid tumors are commonly much longer than those characteristic of the leukemias and average in excess of 15 years. This difference may be related to the rapid cellular turnover characteristic of hematopoietic tissues. In further contrast to the leukemias, the relationship between cancer risk and time after irradiation for solid neoplasms is not wavelike.[25] Rather, epidemiologic and experimental data suggest that risk continues to increase as a constant proportion of the baseline incidence throughout the lifetime of exposed persons.

## 4. RADIATION TRANSFORMATION IN VITRO

### 4.1. Experimental Techniques

Efforts to understand the mechanisms by which cells are transformed to the neoplastic phenotype by ionizing radiation have been greatly advanced by the development of quantitative *in vitro* techniques for assaying neoplastic transformation. Most radiation transformation studies have made use of either of two different assay systems. The first is based on the use of fresh explants of cells derived from hamster embryos, while the second involves the use of immortalized fibroblastic lines originally derived from mouse embryos, most commonly the BALB/c 3T3 line derived by Kakunaga[27] from lines originally developed by Todaro and Green[28] or the C3H 10T1/2 line developed by Reznikoff *et al.*[29] In addition to permitting the quantitative assessment of effects at the cellular level, both assays are relatively inexpensive and quick. Each system offers unique strengths and weaknesses, but enumeration of the relative advantages and disadvantages is beyond the scope of this discussion and have recently been summarized by Hall and Hei.[30] Substantial methodologic differences between the two systems also exist. In the interest of simplicity, a description of only one, the C3H 10T1/2 system, is provided. It is noteworthy that the results obtained with either system are comparable in spite of their inherent differences. Interested readers should refer to reports by Borek[31] and Terzaghi and Little[32] for more detailed information on the application of the hamster embryo and C3H 10T1/2 systems, respectively, to the study of radiation transformation.

A typical protocol for assaying radiation transformation in C3H 10T1/2 cells is as follows[33]: exponentially growing cells are plated onto plastic dishes approximately 24–72 hr before radiation exposure and then replated in fresh culture dishes at a concentration of ~150–400 viable cells per dish. These cells grow to confluence in approximately 2–3 weeks and are then incubated for an additional 3–4 weeks, at which time the plates are fixed and stained. Transformants are identified as foci of cells with markedly different morphologic characteristics and growth patterns overgrowing a background of nontransformed cells (Fig. 3). It is also possible to determine the fraction of cells that survive the initial radiation exposure by plating aliquots of the original cell suspension at low concentrations for colony formation. Thus, transformation frequency can be expressed as a function of the number of cells surviving the treatment.

### 4.2. Properties of Transformed Cells

Three varieties (types I–III) of morphologically distinct transformed foci have been identified, each associated with different oncogenic potential.[34] Type I foci are composed of densely packed cells that, when isolated and inoculated into nude mice, fail to give rise to tumors. For this reason, type I foci are not quantitated in transformation assays. Type II and III foci are characterized by a pronounced piling up of cells against a monolayer background of nontransformed C3H 10T1/2 cells. Type III foci are differentiated morphologically from type II by a characteristic criss-cross pattern of densely staining cells not observed in the type II foci. Cells cloned from type II and III foci are capable of anchorage-independent growth in soft agar, a property frequently expressed by neoplastic cells but not by their nontransformed counterparts and can give rise to progressively growing tumors when inoculated into nude mice. Cells cloned from type III foci induced by

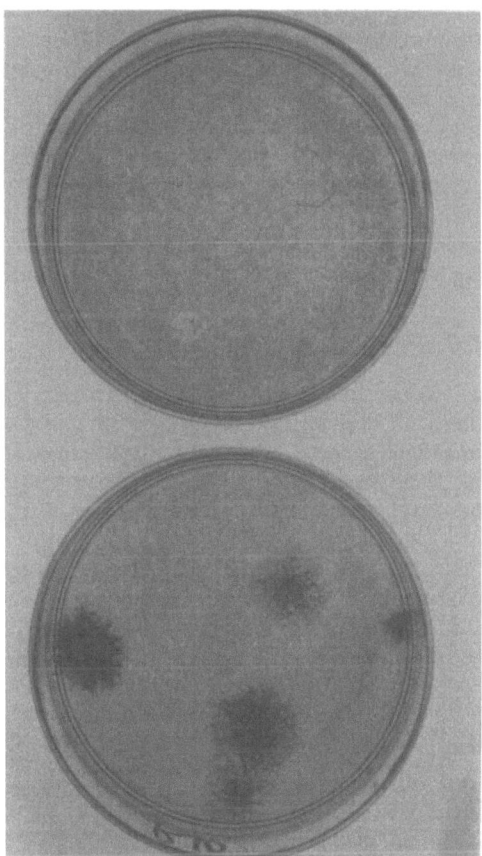

*Figure 3.* Plate of nontransformed C3H 10T1/2 cells (a) and a plate showing multiple foci of transformed cells (b).

exposure to chemical carcinogens, as well as by photon and neutron radiation, are highly tumorigenic, giving rise to fibrosarcomas with very high frequency. Tumor yield following injection of cells from type II foci is lower, but the tumors are also typically fibrosarcomas.

The fibroblastic origin of these cells and the tumors arising from them is an often-cited criticism of the use of these systems for the study of radiation carcinogenesis, since most radiation-induced tumors are epithelial in origin. Bertram[35] addressed this particular issue, concluding that the validity of the *in vitro* assays was confirmed by the "close correspondence between *in vivo* and *in vitro* phenomenon," despite differences in the embryonic origin of the cells involved. The close agreement between the *in vitro* and *in vivo* observations will become evident in the next section, which describes factors that have been shown to modulate the oncogenic effects of ionizing radiation. The commonality of response underscores the applicability of the *in vitro* systems for the study of radiation carcinogenesis.

## 5. FACTORS INFLUENCING RADIATION CARCINOGENESIS OR TRANSFORMATION

Epidemiologic studies and investigations employing animals or *in vitro* transformation systems have identified several factors that can modify the response of cells or tissue to the transforming properties of radiation. As discussed in more detail in the following sections, the carcinogenicity or transforming efficiency of radiation can be influenced by the physical properties of the radiation itself, such as radiation quality (i.e., γ-rays versus neutrons), as well as by a number of host and environmental factors. It is interesting to note that, with rare exceptions, whenever a modifier has been examined in terms of its effect on tumor induction *in vivo* and transformation frequency *in vitro*, qualitatively similar effects (i.e., enhancement or inhibition) have been detected. This close agreement would seem to support the conclusion of Bertram[35] and others regarding the value of *in vitro* transformation systems in the study of carcinogenesis. In addition to providing valuable information regarding the mechanism of radiation carcinogenesis, recognition of the role of modifying factors could result in improved risk assessment and the identification of intervention strategies.

## 5.1. Physical Factors

*Dose:* Transformation frequency typically increases in a dose-dependent manner, reaching a maximum at some intermediate dose and then decreasing as the dose is escalated. This downward trend at higher doses is attributable to the killing of transformed cells, which are equally sensitive to the lethal effects of radiation, as are their nontransformed counterparts.[36] A similar relationship between dose and tumor incidence has been observed for a number of neoplasms, including murine myeloid leukemia and for thyroid tumors in rats treated with radioactive iodine.[37] In some situations, *in vivo* cell killing resulting from exposure to high radiation doses may actually serve to promote tumor induction by stimulating proliferation of surviving cells. Such an effect has been shown to play an important role in the induction of thymic lymphomas in irradiated mice[38] and has been implicated in the pathogenesis of osteogenic sarcomas in dogs treated with $^{226}$Ra.[39]

*Radiation quality, dose rate, and fractionation:* The type of radiation used (radiation quality) and the rate or manner in which it is delivered can have a profound effect on tumorigenicity or transformation frequency.[40] The relationship between radiation quality and transformation frequency is illustrated in Fig. 4a for C3H 10T1/2 cells exposed to single doses of neutrons (□) and γ-rays (○) at high dose rates. Neutrons are more efficient transforming agents than are equivalent doses of γ-rays, presumably because of their higher ionization density. It is also important to note that the relative biologic effectiveness (RBE)* of neutrons is greatest at low doses. The effect of protracting dose delivery in the C3H 10T1/2 system is shown in Fig. 4b. The transformation frequency of γ-rays is significantly reduced when the dose rate is decreased. By contrast, a reduction in the neutron dose rate results in a markedly enhanced transforming efficiency, that is particularly prominent at low doses (Fig. 4b, inset). A sparing effect can also be produced by delivering the total γ-ray dose as a number of small fractions as opposed to a single large dose (Fig. 4c). Miller *et al.*[47] demonstrated that this sparing effect may be dose dependent and that at low doses (<100 rad) split-dose treatment can actually enhance the transforming ability of X-rays. In the case of neutrons, however, the transformation frequency associated with fractionation is again increased relative to that observed following single doses, and in the case illustrated in Fig. 4c, is comparable to the effect of dose protraction at low doses. As indicated by the observed divergence of the dose–response curves, the RBE for low-dose fractionated neutron irradiation is particularly large, approaching a value of 70–75.[45] The decreased transforming efficiency of low dose rate or fractionated γ-rays has been attributed to error-free repair of subeffective transformation damage during an extended exposure interval, whereas the enhancement of transformation by lowering dose rate or fractionating neutrons may be associated with an error-prone repair process.[41]

These same physical factors have been shown to modify radiation carcinogenesis in much the same manner in numerous *in vivo* studies, as exemplified in Fig. 5, which represents a composite of data reported by Ullrich[48,49] and Ullrich and Storer[50] for mammary carcinoma induction in BALB/c mice. It must be emphasized, however, that in addition to reflecting changes in the physical

---

*RBE = Relative biological effectiveness, the ratio of X-ray and neutron doses required to produce the same end point, i.e., transformation.

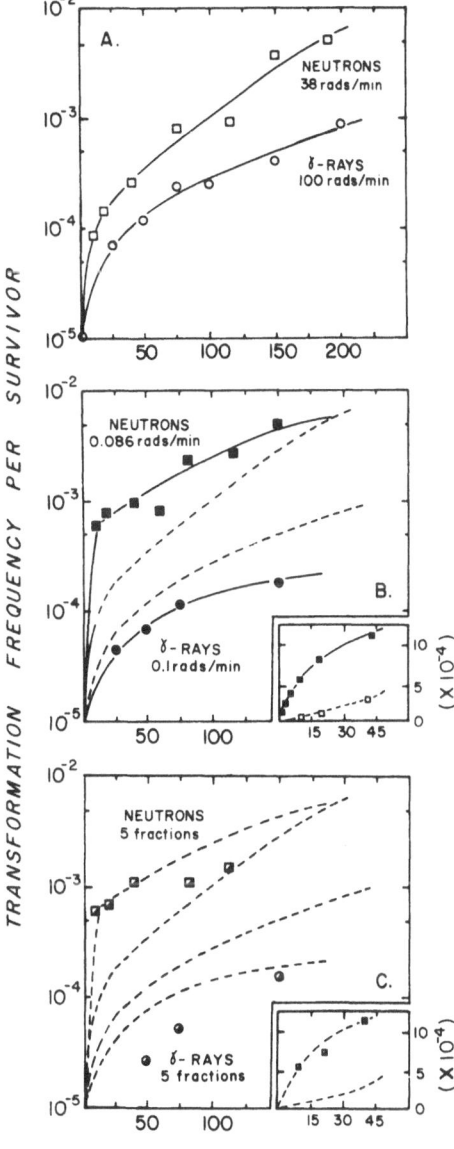

*Figure 4.* Comparison of the transforming efficiencies of single doses of neutrons (□) and γ-rays (○) at high dose rates in C3H 10T1/2 cells. (Redrawn from Elkind *et al.*,[41] using data from Han *et al.*[42] and Hill *et al.*[43]) The effect of reduced dose rates on transformation of C3H 10T1/2 cells by γ-rays (●) and neutrons (■). (---) Redrawn from A. The insert compares the effect of low dose rate (■) and high dose rate (□) neutrons at low doses. Note that the transformation frequency axis for the insert is linear. (Redrawn from Elkind *et al.*[41] using data from Han *et al.*[42] and Hill *et al.*[44]) The effect of dose fractionation on neutron and γ-ray-induced transformation in C3H 10T1/2 cells. The insert is again for low doses of neutrons and makes use of a linear transformation axis. (Redrawn from Hill *et al.*[45] using data from Hill *et al.*[46]) The error bars included in all the original graphs were omitted for clarity.

parameters of radiation delivery, the shapes of *in vivo* tumor-induction curves, such as those shown in Fig. 5, also reflect the net outcome of a complex interplay of other factors including, but not limited to, cell killing, dose-distribution characteristics, and host influences. It is not surprising that all tissues do not respond to changes in radiation characteristics in an entirely predictable manner.

## 5.2. Host/Environmental Factors

*Age:* The age of a person at the time of irradiation is currently recognized as one of the most important response determinants for assessing cancer risk associated with radiation exposure. An age dependence has been clearly demonstrated for leukemia, thyroid cancer, and breast cancer induction and is strongly suggested for other sites.[3] Breast cancer risk among survivors of the A

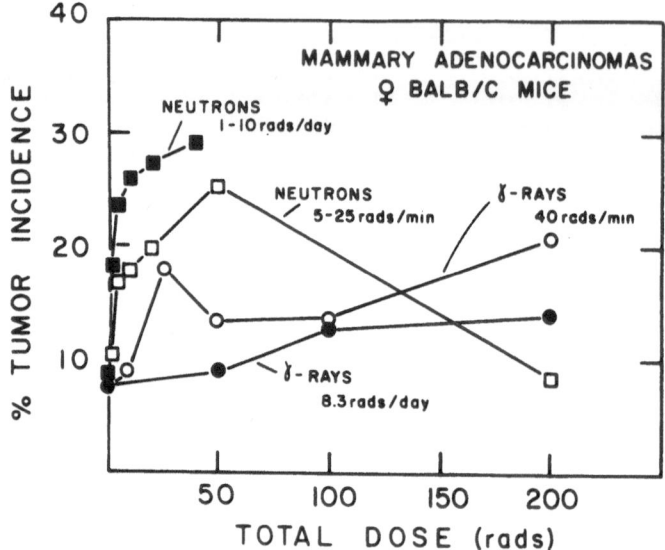

*Figure 5.* Comparison of the effectiveness of neutrons and γ-rays at high and low dose rates for the induction of mammary adenocarcinomas in female BALB/c mice. (Drawn from data of Ullrich[48,49] and Ullrich and Storer.[50]) The data for high-dose-rate γ-radiation (○) were pooled from Ullrich[48] and Ullrich and Storer.[50]

bombs, previously thought to be greatest for those women who were 10–19 years of age in 1945, has been shown to be even greater in those under age 10 at the time of the bombings.[51] Beyond this age, risk decreases progressively with age at the time of the bombings. Similarly, those irradiated during childhood for a number of head and neck conditions are at higher risk of thyroid tumor induction than are those irradiated at older ages.[8,9] The incidence of radiation-induced leukemias is particularly interesting in having a bimodal susceptibility pattern, one peak associated with irradiation during childhood and the second with irradiation beyond the age of 50.[52] Not only does age influence the probability of tumor induction but, in the case of leukemias, it is a prominent determinant of the histologic type induced. The greatest relative risk for chronic granulocytic leukemia was observed in those who were under 9 years of age at the time of the bombings at Hiroshima and Nagasaki, whereas for older persons the risk of developing acute leukemia was increased.

Evidence from a few studies dating back to the mid-1950s had suggested that exposure to very low doses of radiation during intrauterine life was associated with a higher risk of cancer-related mortality in childhood.[53,54] This relationship could not be confirmed in several other studies, nor has it been supported by data from Hiroshima and Nagasaki.[55] A positive association between prenatal exposure and childhood cancer was detected in a large study based in the northeastern United States but, in a recent update, the investigators state that the relationship is probably not causal, although a confounding variable could not be identified.[56] Owing to the conflicting data, the relative sensitivity of the embryo to the oncogenic properties of ionizing radiation cannot be clearly defined. Nevertheless, it has been recommended that the elective use of X-rays in females of reproductive age be limited to early in the menstrual cycle when the probability of pregnancy is very low.

*Sex:* Cancer induction rates for different tissues frequently demonstrate sex-dependent differential sensitivity. This is particularly true for tumors induced in endocrine organs and can frequently be attributed to male–female hormonal differences. Epidemiologic studies have shown that the risk of tumor induction in certain tissues, such as the thyroid gland, can be three to four times greater in irradiated females than in age-matched males.[8,9] Interestingly, the spontaneous rate is also higher in females.

*Hormones:* Hormones have long been known to play a significant role in tumor induction following exposure to radiation and chemical carcinogens, particularly in endocrine tissues or their peripheral targets, or both.[57] Enhancement or inhibition of tumorigenesis through hormonal manipulations in experimental animals depends on the particular experimental conditions employed but, in general, hormonal stimulation results in augmented tumor expression, while suppression reduces tumor incidence. Under appropriate conditions, tumors can also be induced in endocrine tissues outside the radiation field secondary in radiation-induced disruption of normal homeostatic mechanisms.

Hormonal factors have also been shown to influence radiation transformation *in vitro.* Cortisone and dexamethasone, both glucocorticoids, and β-estradiol enhance transformation in C3H 10T1/2 cells[58] and diploid human cells,[59] respectively. Guernsey *et al.*[60,61] reported that physiologic concentrations of the thyroid hormone, triiodothyronine (T3), play an integral role in the transformation of hamster cells or C3H 10T1/2 cells by radiation. In their studies, no transformants were detected in cultures irradiated in the absence of T3, while in the presence of T3 a typical dose-dependent increase in transformation frequency was observed. The potentiating effect of T3 was most pronounced when added 12 hr prior to irradiation, suggesting that the hormone was involved in the initiation phase of radiation transformation.

*Tumor promoters and anti-carcinogens:* The phorbol ester, 12-*O*-tetradecanoyl-phorbol 13-acetate (TPA), is a potent promoter of carcinogenesis *in vivo* when administered subsequent to treatment with carcinogens. TPA has also been shown to enhance radiation-induced transformation of cells in culture significantly.[40] Experiments described by Kennedy *et al.*[62,63] demonstrate that promotion by TPA requires chronic TPA administration after radiation exposure, suggesting that TPA expresses its promoting effect during the postirradiation proliferative phase, analogous to its effect *in vivo.*

In contrast to the effects of TPA, a number of compounds have been identified that effectively suppress or inhibit the carcinogenic effects of chemical and physical agents, including radiation.[40] These agents are frequently referred to as anti-carcinogens, examples of which are protease inhibitors, retinoids, vitamin E, and selenium. They represent a broad spectrum of compounds that affect the yield of radiation-induced transformants by quite diverse mechanisms. Selenium reduces transformation presumably by augmenting the cell's ability to handle oxidative challenges and detoxify peroxides.[64] Anti-oxidants, such as vitamin E, effectively scavenge radiation-induced reactive oxygen species and damaging free radicals. The mechanism of action of vitamin A analogues[65] (retinoids) is complex and may involve scavenging of radicals but also may reversibly inhibit the progression of initiated cells to the transformed phenotype.[66] The retinoids have also been reported to inhibit the promoting effects of TPA. The protease inhibitors represent an interesting class of compounds that, like TPA, exert their effect during postirradiation proliferation of initiated cells to reverse the initiated state, thereby inhibiting transformation in the presence or absence of TPA.[67]

The modulating effects of these various compounds is not limited to transformation *in vitro,* as similar effects have been observed *in vivo* with chemical carcinogens as well as with radiation.

# 6. PATHOGENESIS OF RADIATION CARCINOGENESIS

## 6.1. Multistep Process: Initiation and Promotion

Like cancer induction by chemical agents, radiation carcinogenesis can be conceptualized as a complex multistep process (see Chapter 6). The nature and actual number of steps involved in the process is unknown, but in the simplest case can be thought of as involving at least two distinct phases: initiation and promotion. In the first step of the transformation process (initiation) exposure to ionizing radiation results in some heritable change in a proportion of the exposed cells. During the promotion phase of carcinogenesis, there is a selective expansion of cells derived from initiated cells under the influence of environmental or growth factors, ultimately leading to the emergence of cell populations with the potential for autonomous growth. Tumor-promoting agents, such as TPA, exert their effects during this second phase of carcinogenesis to increase the yield of transformants *in vitro* or tumors *in vivo*. Realistically, it is likely that many more steps are involved in the conversion of a normal cell to a neoplastic one following exposure to chemical or physical carcinogens (see Chapter 6). Nevertheless, initiation has traditionally been thought to involve some type of damage (e.g., mutation) occurring in a very small number of exposed cells, whereas promotion has been considered common. However, recent evidence from *in vitro* (reviewed by Little[68]) and *in vivo*[69-71] studies with chemical carcinogens and radiation have been interpreted as indicating that the first step in transformation occurs in a large fraction of the exposed cell population and that the final step resulting in conversion to the transformed phenotype is the rare event. If confirmed, this interpretation will have profound ramifications for the current understanding of the mechanism of radiation transformation. For example, these data suggest that the first step in transformation is unlikely to involve a specific mutation, as the probability of inducing a common mutation in a large fraction of the irradiated population is exceedingly small. Furthermore, according to this hypothesis, some later change is the actual transforming event, and this occurs with a frequency of $\sim 10^{-6}$/cell/generation in the progeny of initiated cells.[72,73] Therefore, such a later-occurring change may itself be mutational. Work testing these possibilities is continuing and should provide interesting information concerning the nature of initiation and promotion.

## 6.2. DNA as a Critical Target

DNA, as carrier of the genetic code, has long been considered the critical target for radiation damage ultimately responsible for neoplastic transformation. This conclusion was primarily supported by inference based on the observation that many carcinogens, including radiation, are also mutagens capable of inducing DNA damage. Evidence that selective direct damage to DNA was sufficient for transformation of cells *in vitro* was provided by Barrett *et al.*[74] Using hamster embryo cells that had incorporated 5-bromodeoxyuridine in place of thymidine in their DNA, these investigators induced transformation by exposing the cells to near-UV radiation. Under the conditions of their experiments, the interaction between light and 5-bromodeoxyuridine produced damage restricted to DNA, indicating that such damage could indeed result in transformation. A similar approach was applied by Little,[75] who demonstrated that the transforming efficiency of X-rays in C3H 10T1/2 cells was enhanced by 5-bromodeoxyuridine incorporation. Again, the effect was attributed to enhanced DNA damage in these cells, since incorporation of 5-bromodeoxyuridine into cellular DNA had previously been shown to enhance radiation-induced DNA damage.

More direct evidence implicating DNA damage in radiation transformation has recently been provided by *in vitro* transformation experiments. LeMotte *et al.*[76] reported that radioactive $^{125}I$ incorporated in DNA as iododeoxyuridine had a higher transforming efficiency in the BALB/c 3T3 system than did the incorporation of radioactive [$^3H$]thymidine. The differences in transforming efficiencies were attributed to differences in the decay properties of these two isotopes. Specifically, the radiation from the [$^{125}I$]iododeoxyuridine was confined to the DNA itself, whereas that associated with tritium decay was widely distributed throughout the nucleus. Further putative evidence has been provided by DNA-mediated gene transfer experiments in which cellular DNA is isolated and then transferred to another cell type, typically NIH-3T3 cells. Borek[77] reported that the DNA from X-ray transformed hamster embryo cells or X-ray transformed C3H 10T1/2 cells encoded information capable of inducing the transformed phenotype in normal NIH-3T3 cells, but DNA from nontransformed hamster or C3H 10T1/2 cells did not. While these results indicate that the DNA from transformed cells may have been altered, there is no evidence that DNA was an important target for radiation. Nevertheless, considering the available data *in toto*, it seems safe to conclude that DNA is an important target in radiation transformation and carcinogenesis. The actual nature of DNA involvement requires further elucidation.

## 6.3. *Oncogenes in Radiation Carcinogenesis*

No chapter on carcinogenesis would be complete without a consideration of the role of oncogenes in tumor induction (see also Chapter 13). In light of the spectrum of damage detected in DNA and chromosomes following radiation exposure, it is not unreasonable to postulate that radiation exerts its oncogeneic effect through the activation of one or more oncogenes. The data available on the role of oncogenes in radiation carcinogenesis and transformation are scant compared with those reported with chemical carcinogens. Numerous investigators[77-80] have detected the expression of various oncogenes (e.g., *myc*, K-*ras*, N-*ras*, II-*ras*, *abl*) in radiation-induced tumors or transformed cells and have successfully transfected NIH-3T3 cells with DNA derived from these sources. In general, the mechanisms by which radiation activates specific oncogenes are unknown. A notable exception is the activation of N- or K-*ras* genes in radiation-induced thymic lymphomas. Guerrero *et al.*[81] reported that a significant proportion (50%) of the thymic lymphomas induced in multiple strains of mice express either an activated N- or K-*ras* oncogene. In all cases, the activation was the result of a single base mutation either in the 12th or 61st codon of the gene and resulted in single amino acid substitutions in the *ras*-encoded p21 protein. The same alterations in the coding regions of the ras genes were detected in DNA from thymic lymphomas induced by the direct-acting chemical carcinogen, nitrosomethylurea, indicating that radiation-induced activation of the ras genes is not unique to this agent. These elegant studies clearly indicate that activated oncogenes can be detected in cells from radiation-induced tumors and transformed foci, but what still remains to be determined is whether the changes in oncogene expression occur as a late secondary event in neoplastic transformation or are causally involved.

## 7. CONCLUSION

A great deal has been learned since 1902, when Freiben[1] first suggested that radiation is carcinogenic. The oncogenic potential of ionizing radiation has since been well documented in human populations, animal models, and *in vitro* transformation systems. The conversion of normal cells to malignant ones following irradiation is now known to be a very complex multiphase process, sensitive to the stimulatory and inhibitory influences of various modulating factors operative between the time of exposure and the detection of the neoplastic phenotype, be it a tumor *in vivo* or a transformed foci *in vitro*. However, in spite of impressive strides, much remains to be resolved before achieving the goal of understanding the process of radiation carcinogenesis. Extrapolating from the rate of progress over the past two decades, it does not seem overly optimistic to hope for realization of this ambitious goal by the centennial of Freiben's report.

ACKNOWLEDGMENTS. I am grateful to my colleagues Dr. Kelly H. Clifton and Dr. Michael N. Gould for helpful discussions and critiques of this chapter. I am especially grateful to Dr. Catherine A. Reznikoff and Dr. Brian J. Christian for kindly providing Fig. 3 of the C3H 10T1/2 cells. Finally, I would like to thank Peggy Shager for assistance in the preparation of the manuscript.

## REFERENCES

1. Freiben, A., 1902, Demonstration eines Cancroides des rechten Handrueckens, das sich nach langdauernder Einwirkung von Roentgenstrahlen entwickelt hat, *Fortschr. Roentgenstr.* **6**:106–111.
2. Kato, H., and Schull, W. J., 1982, Studies of the mortality of A-bomb survivors. 7. Mortality, 1950–1978. Part I. Cancer mortality, *Radiat. Res.* **90**:395–432.
3. National Academy of Sciences, 1980, *The Effects on Population of Exposure to Low Levels of Ionizing Radiation: 1980*, National Academy Press, Washington, D. C.

4. Court-Brown, W. M., and Doll, R., 1965, Mortality from cancer and other causes after radiotherapy for ankylosing spondylitis, *Br. Med. J.* **2**:1327–1332.
5. Smith, P. G., 1984, Late effects of x-ray treatment in ankylosing spondylitis, in: *Progress in Cancer Research and Therapy,* Vol. 26: *Radiation Carcinogenesis: Epidemiology and Biological Significance* (J. D. Boice and J. F. Fraumeni, eds.), pp. 107–118, Raven, New York.
6. Shore, R. E., Hempelmann, L. H., Kowaluk, E., Mansur, P. S., Pasternak, B. S., Albert, R. E., and Haughie, G. E., 1977, Breast neoplasms in women treated with x-rays for acute post-partum mastitis, *J. Natl. Cancer Inst.* **59**:813–822.
7. Howe, G. R., 1984, Epidemiology of radiogenic breast cancer, in: *Progress in Cancer Research and Therapy,* Vol. 26: *Radiation Carcinogenesis: Epidemiology and Biological Significance* (J. D. Boice and J. F. Fraumeni, eds.), pp. 119–129, Raven, New York.
8. Shore, R. E., Woodward, E. D., and Hempelmann, L. H., 1984, Radiation-induced thyroid cancer, in: *Progress in Cancer Research and Therapy,* Vol. 26: *Radiation Carcinogenesis: Epidemiology and Biological Significance* (J. D. Boice and J. F. Fraumeni, eds.), pp. 131–138, Raven, New York.
9. Ron, E., and Modan, B., 1984, Thyroid and other neoplasms following childhood scalp irradiation, in: *Progress in Cancer Research and Therapy,* Vol. 26: *Radiation Carcinogenesis: Epidemiology and Biological Significance* (J. D. Boice and J. F. Fraumeni, eds.), pp. 139–151, Raven, New York.
10. Mays, C. W., and Spiess, H., 1984, Bone sarcomas in patients given Radium-224, in: *Progress in Cancer Research and Therapy,* Vol. 26: *Radiation Carcinogenesis: Epidemiology and Biological Significance* (J. D. Boice and J. F. Fraumeni, eds.), pp. 241–252, Raven, New York.
11. Boice, J. R., and Monson, R. R., 1977, Breast cancer in women after repeated fluoroscopic examination of the chest. *J. Natl. Cancer Inst.* **59**:823–832.
12. Howe, G. R., Miller, A. B., and Sherman, G. J., 1982, Breast cancer mortality following fluoroscopic irradiation in a cohort of tuberculosis patients, *Cancer Detect. Prev.* **5**:175–178.
13. Mole, R. H., 1978, The radiobiological significance of the studies with $^{224}$Ra and thorotrast (surveys in Denmark, Portugal and Germany), *Health Phys.* **35**:167–174.
14. van Kaick, G., Muth, H., Kaul, A., Immick, H., Liebermann, D., Lorenz, D., Lorenz, W. J., Luhrs, H., Scheer, K. E., Wagner, G., Wegener, K., and Wesch, H., 1984, Results of the German thorotrast study, in: *Progress in Cancer Research and Therapy,* Vol. 26: *Radiation Carcinogenesis: Epidemiology and Biological Significance* (J. D. Boice and J. F. Fraumeni, eds.), pp. 253–262, Raven, New York.
15. Rowland, R. E., and Lucas, H. F., 1984, Radium-dial workers, in: *Progress in Cancer Research and Therapy,* Vol. 26: *Radiation Carcinogenesis: Epidemiology and Biological Significance* (J. D. Boice and J. F. Fraumeni, eds.), pp. 231–240, Raven, New York.
16. Radford, E. P., 1984, Radiogenic cancer in underground miners, in: *Progress in Cancer Research and Therapy,* Vol. 26: *Radiation Carcinogenesis: Epidemiology and Biological Significance* (J. D. Boice and J. F. Fraumeni, eds.), pp. 225–230, Raven, New York.
17. Land, C. E., 1980, Estimating cancer risks from low doses of ionizing radiation, *Science* **209**:1197–1203.
18. Webster, E. W., 1981, On the question of cancer induction by small x-ray doses, *AJR* **137**:647–666.
19. Upton, A. C., 1985, Biological basis for assessing carcinogenic risk of low-level radiation, in: *Carcinogenesis—A Comprehensive Survey,* Vol. 10: *The Role of Chemicals and Radiation in the Etiology of Cancer* (E. Huberman and S. H. Barr, eds.), pp. 381–401, Raven, New York.
20. Upton, A. C., 1984, Biological aspects of radiation carcinogenesis, in: *Progress in Cancer Research and Therapy,* Vol. 26: *Radiation Carcinogenesis: Epidemiology and Biological Significance* (J. D. Boice and J. F. Fraumeni, eds.), pp. 9–19, Raven, New York.
21. Fry, R. J. M., 1984, Relevance of animal studies to the human experience, in: *Progress in Cancer Research and Therapy,* Vol. 26: *Radiation Carcinogenesis: Epidemiology and Biological Significance* (J. D. Boice and J. F. Fraumeni, eds.), pp. 337–346, Raven, New York.
22. Clifton, K. H., 1980, Quantitative studies of the radiobiology of hormone responsive normal cell populations, in: *Radiation Biology in Cancer Research* (R. E. Meyn and H. R. Withers, eds.), pp. 501–513, Raven, New York.
23. Furth, J., Haran-Ghera, N., Curtis, H. J., and Buffett, R. F., 1959, Studies on the pathogenesis of neoplasms by ionizing radiation. I. Pituitary tumors, *Cancer Res.* **19**:550–556.
24. Miller, R. W., and Beebe, G. W., 1986, Leukemia, lymphoma and multiple myeloma, in: *Radiation Carcinogenesis* (A. C. Upton, R. E. Albert, F. J. Burns, and R. E. Shore, eds.), pp. 245–260, Elsevier, New York.
25. Land, C. E., and Tokunaga, M., 1984, Induction period, in: *Progress in Cancer Research and Therapy,* Vol. 26: *Radiation Carcinogenesis. Epidemiology and Biological Significance* (J. D. Boice and J. F. Fraumeni, eds.), pp. 421–436, Raven, New York.

26. Ichimaru, M., Ishimaru, T., and Belsky, J. L., 1975, Incidence of leukemia in atomic bomb survivors belonging to a fixed cohort in Hiroshima and Nagasaki, 1950–1971. Radiation dose, years after exposure, age at exposure, and type of leukemia, *J. Radiat. Res.* **19**:262–282.

27. Kakunaga, T., 1973, A quantitative system for assay of malignant transformation by chemical carcinogens using a clone derived from Balb/3T3, *Int. J. Cancer* **12**:463–472.

28. Todaro, G. J., and Green, H., 1963, Quantitative studies of the growth of mouse embryo cells in culture and their development into established lines, *J. Cell Biol.* **17**:299–313.

29. Reznikoff, C. A., Brankow, D. W., and Heidelberger, C., 1973, Establishment and characterization of a cloned line of C3H mouse embryo cells sensitive to post-confluence inhibition of division, *Cancer Res.* **33**:3231–3238.

30. Hall, E. J., and Hei, T. K., 1986, Oncogenic transformation of cells in culture: Pragmatic comparisons of oncogenicity, cellular and molecular mechanisms, *Int. J. Radiat. Oncol. Biol. Phys.* **12**:1909–1921.

31. Borek, C., 1982, Radiation oncogenesis in culture, *Adv. Cancer Res.* **37**:159–232.

32. Terzaghi, M., and Little, J. B., 1976, X-radiation induced transformation in a C3H mouse embryo-derived cell line, *Cancer Res.* **36**:1367–1374.

33. Elkind, M. M., Han, A., Hill, C. K., and Buonaguro, F., 1983, Repair mechanisms in radiation-induced cell transformation, in: *Radiation Research, Proceedings of the Seventh International Congress of Radiation Research* (J. J. Broerse, G. W. Barendsen, H. B. Kal, and A. J. van der Kogel, eds.), pp. 33–42, Martinus Nijhoff, Amsterdam.

34. Reznikoff, C. A., Bertram, J. S., Brankow, D. W., and Heidelberger, C., 1973, Quantitative and qualitative studies on chemical transformation of cloned C3H mouse embryo cells sensitive to post-confluence inhibition of cell division, *Cancer Res.* **33**:3239–3249.

35. Bertram, J. S., 1985, Neoplastic transformation in cell cultures: *In vitro/in vivo* correlations, in: *Transformation Assay of Established Cell Lines: Mechanisms and Application*, IARC Scientific publications No. 67 (T. Kakunaga and H. Yamasaki, eds.), pp. 77–91, International Agency for Research on Cancer, Lyons, France.

36. Han, A., Hill, C. K., and Elkind, M. M., 1979, Repair of cell killing and neoplastic transformation at reduced dose rates of $^{60}$Co-x-rays, *Cancer Res.* **40**:123–130.

37. Upton, A. C., 1961, The dose–response relationship in gamma-radiation-induced cancer, *Cancer Res.* **21**:717–729.

38. Kaplan, H. S., 1967, On the natural history of the murine leukemias: Presidential address, *Cancer Res.* **27**:1325–1340.

39. Marshall, J. H., and Groer, P. G., 1977, A theory on the induction of bone cancer by alpha radiation, *Radiat. Res.* **71**:149–192.

40. Chan, G. L., and Little, J. B., 1986, Neoplastic transformation *in vitro*, in: *Radiation Carcinogenesis* (A. C. Upton, R. E. Albert, F. J. Burns, and R. E. Shore, eds.), pp. 107–136, Elsevier, New York.

41. Elkind, M. M., Han, A., and Hill, C. K., 1984, Error-free and error-prone repair in radiation-induced neoplastic cell transformation, in: *Progress in Cancer Research and Therapy*, Vol. 26: *Radiation Carcinogenesis: Epidemiology and Biological Significance* (J. D. Boice and J. F. Fraumeni, eds.), pp. 303–318, Raven, New York.

42. Han, A., Hill, C. K., and Elkind, M. M., 1979, Repair of cell killing and neoplastic transformation at reduced dose rates of $^{60}$Co gamma-rays, *Cancer Res.* **40**:3328–3332.

43. Hill, C. K., Buonaguro, F. M., Myers, C. P., Han, A., and Elkind, M. M., 1982, Fission-spectrum neutrons at reduced dose rates enhance neoplastic transformation, *Nature (Lond.)* **298**:67–69.

44. Hill, C. K., Han, A., and Elkind, M. M., 1984, Fission spectrum at a low dose rate enhance neoplastic transformation in the linear, low dose region (0–10 cGy), *Int. J. Radiat. Biol.* **46**:11–15.

45. Hill, C. K., Carnes, B. A., Han, A., and Elkind, M. M., 1985, Neoplastic transformation is enhanced by multiple low doses of fission-spectrum neutrons, *Radiat. Res.* **102**:404–410.

46. Hill, C. K., Han, A., Buonaguro, F., and Elkind, M. M., 1984, Multifractionation of $^{60}$Co gamma-rays reduces neoplastic transformation *in vitro*, *Carcinogenesis* **5**:193–197.

47. Miller, R. C., Hall, E. J., and Rossi, H. H., 1979, Oncogenic transformation of mammalian cells *in vitro* with split doses of x-rays, *Proc. Natl. Acad. Sci. USA* **76**:5755–5758.

48. Ullrich, R. L., 1983, Tumor induction in Balb/c female mice after fission neutron or gamma irradiation, *Radiat. Res.* **93**:506–515.

49. Ullrich, R. L., 1984, Tumor induction in Balb/c mice after fractionated or protracted exposures to fission spectrum neutrons, *Radiat. Res.* **97**:587–597.

50. Ullrich, R. L., and Storer, J. B., 1979, Influence of gamma-irradiation on the development of neoplastic disease in mice. III. Dose-rate effects, *Radiat. Res.* **80**:325–342.

51. Tokunaga, M., Land, C. E., Yamamoto, T., Asano, M., Tokuoka, S., Ezaki, H., Nishimori, I., and Fukikara, T., 1984, Breast cancer among atomic bomb survivors, in: *Progress in Cancer Research and Therapy*, Vol. 26: *Radiation Carcinogenesis: Epidemiology and Biological Significance* (J. D. Boice and J. F. Fraumeni, eds.), pp. 45–56, Raven, New York.

52. Finch, S. C., 1984, Leukemia and lymphoma in atomic bomb survivors, in: *Progress in Cancer Research and Therapy*, Vol. 26: *Radiation Carcinogenesis: Epidemiology and Biological Significance* (J. D. Boice and J. F. Fraumeni, eds.), pp. 37–44, Raven, New York.

53. Stewart, A., Webb, J., Giles, D., and Hewitt, D., 1956, Malignant disease in childhood and diagnostic irradiation in utero, *Lancet* 2:447.

54. MacMahon, B., 1962, Prenatal x-ray exposure and childhood cancer, *J. Natl. Cancer Inst.* 28:1173–1191.

55. Jablon, S., and Kato, H., 1970, Childhood cancer in relation to prenatal exposure to atomic bomb radiation, *Lancet* 2:1000–1003.

56. Monson, R. R., and MacMahon, B., Prenatal x-ray exposure and cancer in children, in: *Progress in Cancer Research and Therapy*, Vol. 26: *Radiation Carcinogenesis: Epidemiology and Biological Significance* (J. D. Boice and J. F. Fraumeni, eds.), pp. 97–105, Raven, New York.

57. Furth, J., 1982, Hormones as etiological agents in neoplasia, in: *Cancer. A Comprehensive Treatise*, Vol. 1, 2nd ed. (F. F. Becker, ed.), pp. 89–134, Plenum, New York.

58. Kennedy, A. R., and Weichselbaum, R. R., 1981, Effects of dexamethasone and cortisone with x-ray irradiation on the transformation of C3H 10T1/2 cells, *Nature (Lond.)* 294:97–98.

59. Borek, C., 1980, X-ray-induced *in vitro* neoplastic transformation of human diploid cells, *Nature (Lond.)* 283:776–778.

60. Guernsey, D. L., Ong, A., and Borek, C., 1980, Thyroid hormone modulation of x-ray-induced *in vitro* neoplastic transformation, *Nature (Lond.)* 288:591–592.

61. Guernsey, D. L., Borek, C., and Edelman, I. S., 1981, Crucial role of thyroid hormone in x-ray-induced neoplastic transformation in cell culture, *Proc. Natl. Acad. Sci. USA* 78:5709–5711.

62. Kennedy, A. R., Murphy, G., and Little, J. B., 1980, The effect of time and duration of exposure to 12-*O*-tetradecanoylphorbol-13-acetate (TPA) on x-ray transformation in C3H10T1/2 cells, *Cancer Res.* 40:1915–1920.

63. Kennedy, A. R., and Little, J. B., 1980, An investigation of the mechanism for the enhancement of radiation transformation *in vitro* by TPA, *Carcinogenesis* 1:1039–1047.

64. Borek, C., Ong, A., Mason, H., Donahue, L., and Biaglow, J. E., 1986, Selenium and Vitamin E inhibit radiogenic and chemically induced transformation *in vitro* via different mechanisms, *Proc. Natl. Acad. Sci. USA* 83:1490–1494.

65. Harisiadis, L., Miller, R. C., Hall, E. J., and Borek, C., 1978, Vitamin A analogue inhibits radiation induced oncogenic transformation, *Nature (Lond.)* 274:486–487.

66. Merriman, R. L., and Bertram, J. S., 1979, Reversible inhibition by retinoids of 3-methylcholanthrene-induced neoplastic transformation in C3H/10T1/2 clone 8 cells, *Cancer Res.* 39:1661–1666.

67. Kennedy, A. R., 1985, The conditions for the modification of radiation transformation *in vitro* by a tumor promoter and protease inhibitors, *Carcinogenesis* 6:1441–1445.

68. Little, J. B., 1985, Cellular mechanisms of oncogenic transformation *in vitro*, in: *Transformation Assay of Established Cell Lines: Mechanisms and Application*, IARC Scientific publications No. 67, (T. Kakunaga and H. Yamasaki, eds.), pp. 9–29, International Agency for Research on Cancer, Lyons, France.

69. Terzaghi, M., and Nettesheim, P., 1979, Dynamics of neoplastic development in carcinogen-exposed tracheal mucosa, *Cancer Res.* 39:4003–4010.

70. Mulcahy, R. T., Gould, M. N., and Clifton, K. H., 1984, Radiogenic initiation of thyroid cancer: A common cellular event, *Int. J. Radiat. Biol.* 45:419–426.

71. Clifton, K. H., Kamiya, K., Mulcahy, R. T., and Gould, M. N., 1985, Radiogenic neoplasia in the thyroid and mammary clonogens: Progress, problems and possibilities, in: *Assessment of Risk from Low Level Exposure to Radiation and Chemicals* (A. D. Woodhead, C. J. Shellabarger, V. Pond, and A. Hollaender, eds.), pp. 329–344, Plenum, New York.

72. Kennedy, A. R., Cairns, J., and Little, J. B., 1984, Timing of the steps in transformation of C3H10T1/2 cells by x-irradiation, *Nature (Lond.)* 307:85–86.

73. Kennedy, A. R., and Little, J. B., 1984, Evidence that a second step in x-ray induced oncogenic transformation *in vitro* occurs during cellular proliferation, *Radiat. Res.* 99:228–248.

74. Barrett, J. C., Tsutsui, T., and Ts'o, P. O. P., 1978, Neoplastic transformation induced by a direct perturbation of DNA, *Nature (Lond.)* 274:229–232.

75. Little, J. B., 1977, Radiation carcinogenesis *in vitro*: Implications for mechanisms, in: *Origins of Human*

*Cancer,* Vol. IV (H. Hiatt, J. D. Watson, and J. A. Winston, eds.), pp. 923–939, Cold Spring Harbor Laboratory, Cold Spring Harbor, New York.

76. LeMotte, P. K., Adelstein, S. J., and Little, J. B., 1982, Malignant transformation induced by incorporated radionuclides in Balb/3T3 mouse embryo fibroblasts, *Proc. Natl. Acad. Sci. USA* **79:**7763–7767.

77. Borek, C., 1985, Oncogenes and cellular controls in radiogenic transformation of rodent and human cells, in: *Carcinogenesis—A Comprehensive Survey,* Vol. 10: *The Role of Chemicals and Radiation in the Etiology of Cancer* (E. Huberman and S. H. Barr, eds.), pp. 303–316, Raven, New York.

78. Kaminsky, S., Mulcahy, R. T., and Zain, S., 1985, Oncogene expression in a radiation induced rat thyroid carcinoma, *Proc. Am. Assoc. Cancer Res.* **26:**256.

79. Sarvey, M. J., and Garte, S. J., 1986, Activation of myc and ras oncogenes in radiation-induced rat skin tumors, *Proc. Am. Assoc. Cancer Res.* **27:**21.

80. Mizuki, K., Nose, K., Okamoto, H., Tsuchida, N., and Hayashi, K., 1985, Amplification of c-Ki-ras gene and aberrant expression of c-myc in WI-38 cells transformed *in vitro* by gamma-irradiation, *Biochem. Biophys. Res. Commun.* **128:**1037–1043.

81. Guerrero, I., Villasante, L., Diamond, L., Berman, J. W., Newcomb, E. W., Steinberg, J. J., Lake, R., and Pellier, A., 1986, Oncogene activation and surface markers in mouse lymphomas induced by radiation and nitrosomethylurea, *Leukemia Res.* **10:**851–858.

# 6

# The Multistage Concept of Carcinogenesis

## Carl Peraino and Carol A. Jones

## 1. TYPES OF TUMORIGENIC ENHANCEMENT

The recognition of carcinogenesis as a complex multievent process has developed from evidence gained over the past 50 years of research in experimental oncology demonstrating that tumors can be induced in high yield by the combined administration of agents that may have little or no carcinogenic activity when given singly. Three major types of tumorigenic enhancement may be defined on the basis of the types of inducing agents used and of the temporal relationships of their administration:

1.  *Syncarcinogenesis:* Synergistic enhancement of tumor formation by simultaneous[1] or sequential treatment[2] with two carcinogens that separately may have relatively little carcinogenic activity
2.  *Cocarcinogenesis:* Enhancement of tumor formation by simultaneous administration of a carcinogen and an additional agent (cocarcinogen) that has no intrinsic carcinogenic activity but facilitates carcinogen action[3-8]
3.  *Two-stage, or initiation-promotion carcinogenesis:* Enhancement of tumor formation by the sequential administration of a carcinogen (initiator) and an additional agent (promoter) that has no intrinsic carcinogenic activity but facilitates expression of prior carcinogen-induced cryptic cellular changes.[3] In this context, an initiating agent is exemplified by a subcarcinogenic dose of carcinogen, i.e., one that will not elicit neoplasms within the life span of an animal but that will produce an irreversible fundamental change (i.e., mutation) in the cells of a target organ or tissue so as to predispose them to neoplastic transformation

*Abbreviations used in this chapter:* AAF, 2-acetylaminofluorene; BHT, butylated hydroxytoluene; DAG, diacylglycerol; DDT, dichlorodiphenyltrichloroethane; DMN, dimethylnitrosamine; HGPRT, hypoxanthine-guanine phosphoribosyltransferase; MNNG, $N$-methyl-$N'$-nitro-$N$-nitrosoguanidine; PCB, polychlorinated biphenyls; PKC, protein kinase C; TCDD, 2,3,7,8-tetrachlorodibenzo-$p$-dioxin; TPA, 12-$O$-tetradecanoylphorbol 13-acetate.

*Carl Peraino and Carol A. Jones* • Biological, Environmental, and Medical Research Division, Argonne National Laboratory, Argonne, Illinois 60439. The submitted manuscript has been authored by a contractor of the U. S. Government under contract No. W-31-109-ENG-38. Accordingly, the U. S. Government retains a nonexclusive, royalty-free license to publish or reproduce the published form of this contribution, or allow others to do so, for U. S. Government purposes.

when they are further subjected to an appropriate tumor promoting stimulus. A tumor promoter, exemplified by certain plant products, hormones, and xenobiotics acts to affect gene expression and to stimulate a hyperplastic expansion of the initiated cell population. This process ultimately results in the development of persistent precancerous nodules, papillomas, or polyps within the target tissue or organ. Some of these lesions can then undergo progression to malignant neoplasms (see Chapter 10).

Of the foregoing three categories of combined treatments, the initiation–promotion system has been the predominant experimental approach used in oncologic research and has provided the greatest insight into the elements of the carcinogenic process. This chapter is concerned with the sequential multistage nature of carcinogenesis as revealed through the application of the initiation–promotion strategy.

## 2. MULTISTAGE SKIN TUMORIGENESIS

The first documented evidence for a causal relationship between carcinogenesis and exposure to specific agents was described in 1775 by the British surgeon, Percival Pott, who traced the high incidence of scrotal cancer in chimney sweeps to their chronic exposure to soot.[9] Over a subsequent interval of approximately 140 years, considerable epidemiologic evidence accumulated showing increased carcinogenic risk associated with exposure to a variety of agents such as paraffin oil, tobacco, and aniline dyes.[10] Despite numerous attempts,[10] however, clear-cut experimental induction of cancer was not attained until 1915, when Yamigawa and Ichikawa[11] demonstrated that repeated applications of coal tar to the ears of rabbits produced metastasizing carcinomas. These observations were exhaustively confirmed in many subsequent studies by these and other investigators, using mice as experimental animals.[10]

In view of the marked inflammatory changes noted in skin treated with coal tar in these early experiments, attention turned during the 1920s to the influence of induced rapid cell division on the carcinogenic process. The first such investigations showed that mouse skin tumorigenesis was enhanced by physical wounding, following repeated applications of coal tar to the point of first tumor appearance.[12] This approach represents the earliest known application of the initiation–promotion protocol. A subsequent modification of this approach replaced physical trauma with oleic acid,[13] an agent known to produce epidermal hyperplasia.[14] A systematic application of this experimental strategy by Rous and colleagues[15,16] led to the formalization of the multistage concept of carcinogenesis by Rous,[16] who coined the now classic terms initiation and promotion to denote, respectively, (1) the production of potentially tumorigenic cells by limited exposure to carcinogen, and (2) the completion of the neoplastic transformation by subsequent treatment with agents that are not intrinsically carcinogenic.

Major additional advances in the characterization of the *in vivo* skin tumor initiation–promotion system occurred over the next three decades. These advances include (1) the discovery of croton oil as the quintessential skin tumor promotor[17,18]; (2) the demonstration that only a single application of carcinogen is required for initiation[19]; (3) the demonstration that the cellular changes produced by initiator action are irreversible and persist indefinitely[20] (whereas promotor action is reversible and requires frequent promoter treatments over a prolonged interval[3]); (4) the observation that the reversal of the initiation–promotion treatment sequence is ineffective, demonstrating the existence of a unidirectional multistage process[21,22]; and (5) the isolation and identification of phorbol esters, the most active of which is 12-*O*-tetradecanoylphorbol 13-acetate (TPA), as the tumor-promoting principles from croton oil[23,24] (Fig. 1).

The subdivision of skin tumor promotion into different stages was first proposed on the basis of evidence that limited exposure of initiated skin (generated by a prior single treatment with carcinogen) to croton oil produced few tumors, whereas many tumors quickly emerged if the brief croton oil treatment was followed by inflammatory stimuli (e g , chemical irritation or wounding) that had little promoting activity in the absence of the croton oil pretreatment.[3] The limited croton

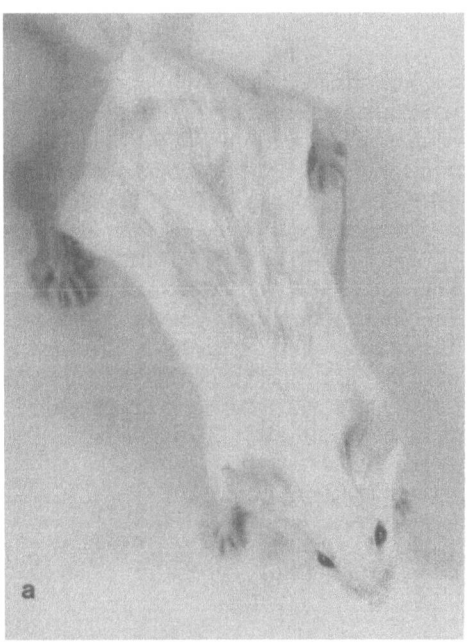

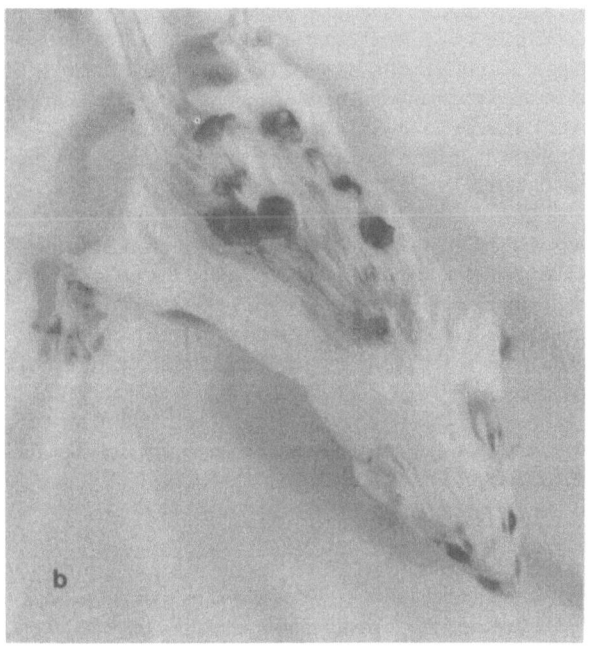

*Figure 1.* Multistage tumorigenesis in mouse skin. (a) Control female SENCAR mouse previously given a noninitiating treatment with acetone (0.2 ml) followed 2 weeks later by biweekly applications to skin of the tumor-promoting agent TPA (3.4 nmoles) for a period of 18 weeks. (b) Tumor-bearing mouse previously initiated with a low dose of the carcinogen, 7,12-dimethylbenz(a)anthracene (10 nmoles), followed 2 weeks later by promotion with TPA (3.4 nmoles) applied to skin 2×/week for 18 weeks. (Courtesy of Dr. John DiGiovanni, University of Texas System Cancer Center.)

oil treatment was postulated to change the initiated cells into dormant tumor cells (the conversion stage), which were then induced to form visible tumors by proliferative stimulation (the propagation stage).

The two-stage promotion concept has since been refined and extended in several investigations involving comparisons of skin tumor yields in initiated mice exposed to various sequential combinations of pure compounds that differ substantially in their promoting activities but are similar in other epidermal effects such as proliferative stimulation and inflammation[25-30] (see Chapter 12). It has been learned that the conversion stage (which involves DNA synthesis, but not DNA mutation, and is obligatory for tumor formation under conditions of initiation by a subtumorigenic dose of carcinogen) can be elicited by a single topical application of TPA, administered either postinitiation or up to several weeks before initiation.[26,28,29] The propagation stage (elicited by repeated treatments with weak or nonpromoting epidermal hyperplasiogens such as mezerein or 12-deoxyphorbol-13-2,4,6-decatrienoate) occurs only after the initiation and conversion stages and is also essential for tumor formation under subtumorigenic initiation conditions.[25-29]

On the basis of evidence that the TPA-induced conversion step is persistent and does not require prior initiation, it has been suggested[26,28,29] that true promotion, as classically defined, involves only the propagation step. TPA-induced conversion may constitute a mechanistically distinct process that renders the cell sensitive to promotion if initiation occurs within the interval when the cell remains converted. The delineation of skin tumorigenesis as a multistage process has helped to explain the existence of the phenomenon of tumor latency, which refers to the prolonged period between the first exposure to a carcinogen and the actual appearance of a malignant neoplasm.

# 3. MULTISTAGE TUMORIGENESIS IN NONEPIDERMAL SYSTEMS

## 3.1. Bladder

In a historical sequence analogous to that described for the skin tumorigenesis model, evidence for a multistage mechanism of bladder carcinogenesis was first obtained in studies showing that the combination of a longlasting bladder-implanted cholesterol pellet and a separately administered single dose of a rapidly metabolized tryptophan metabolite (the 8-methyl ether of xanthurenic acid) induced bladder tumors more effectively than either agent alone.[31] Because the cholesterol pellet was considered a physical (rather than chemical) irritant,[32] this observation in effect recapitulated Deelman's findings on the enhancement of chemically initiated skin tumorigenesis by physical wounding.[12]

In further analogy with the evolution of the skin model, subsequent bladder studies showed that replacement of the physical irritant by a chemical stimulus (i.e., the feeding of saccharin or cyclamate) also enhanced bladder tumorigenesis in rats previously treated with a single dose of methylnitrosourea infused into the bladder.[33] Additional refinement and mechanistic analysis of the multistage bladder carcinogenesis model has centered on the use of brief (2-week) exposure to dietary FANFT (N-[4-(5-nitro-2-furyl)-2-thiazolyl]formamide) as the initiating agent followed by physical stimuli (e.g., freezing of bladder epithelium) or chemical enhancers (e.g., dietary saccharin, constituents of normal urine). These studies are designed to examine the role of increased cellularity and mitotic rate in the enhancement of tumor formation and to determine the identities and modes of action of enhancing factors.[32]

## 3.2. Liver

The first unequivocal evidence that liver tumorigenesis occurs in qualitatively distinct sequential stages emerged from an investigation of the effect of phenobarbital on 2-acetylaminofluorene-(AAF) induced hepatocarcinogenesis in rats.[34] This study showed that the chronic feeding of the noncarcinogenic xenobiotic phenobarbital together with AAF in the diet (simultaneous treatment protocol) reduced hepatic tumor incidence in comparison with that in rats receiving only dietary AAF, whereas prolonged administration of dietary phenobarbital after a brief interval of dietary AAF exposure (sequential treatment protocol) markedly enhanced hepatic tumorigenesis over that seen after the brief AAF treatment alone. Additional studies of the sequential treatment protocol revealed the persistence of the latent tumorigenic changes induced by the brief initiation stimulus (2-week AAF feeding) and the requirement for prolonged promoter administration (phenobarbital feeding) to produce enhancement.[35,36]

The demonstration of hepatic tumor initiation and promotion by the AAF-phenobarbital sequential treatment protocol stimulated the development of several alternative multistage hepatocarcinogenesis systems, representative examples of which are summarized in Table I. Application of
these protocols has identified a variety of agents as promoters of rat hepatocarcinogenesis. In
addition to phenobarbital, these agents include DDT, PCB, BHT, TCDD, contraceptive steroids,
choline deficiency, α-hexachlorocyclohexane, and hepatic peroxisome proliferators.[37]

The similarities between the liver tumorigenesis model and the skin model constituted strong
empirical support for the general applicability of the multistage concept of carcinogenesis. Further
evolution of the liver multistage system has involved efforts in many laboratories to characterize the
developmental relationships of the various types of putative preneoplastic hepatocellular changes
occurring (see Chapter 9) between the initiation event and the appearance of grossly observable
tumors, with the expectation that such information will provide insight into the sequential events of
the neoplastic process.[37]

## 3.3. Respiratory Tract

Numerous epidemiologic studies of human respiratory tract carcinogenesis have demonstrated
synergistic interactions among disparate factors, such as asbestos and cigarette smoke or radiation
and cigarette smoke, in the induction of respiratory tract tumors.[38] Although these observations
suggest a multievent mechanism for tumorigenesis, they do not provide appropriate information for
distinguishing whether these multiple events occur simultaneously as in syncarcinogenesis and
cocarcinogenesis or sequentially as in the initiation–promotion model.

Experimental evidence for a sequential, multistage model of respiratory tract tumorigenesis
was first obtained by Armuth and Berenblum,[39] who observed that repeated injections of mice with
phorbol over a prolonged interval, after a single injection of dimethylnitrosamine (DMN) at birth,
produced a high incidence of lung tumors among the survivors. Treatment with DMN alone
produced few tumors, and phorbol alone showed no tumorigenic activity. Subsequently, Witschi et
al.[40] demonstrated that weekly injections of Swiss–Webster mice with the antioxidant butylated
hydroxytoluene (BHT) for 2–3 months after a single injection of urethan significantly enhanced
lung tumor frequency over that in mice receiving only urethan, whereas coadministration of BHT
with urethan in several injections did not alter the frequency of urethan-induced lung tumorigenesis.
The enhancing effect of BHT was attributed to its simulation of proliferative activity in type II

### Table I. Representative Multistage Rat Hepatocarcinogenesis Protocols[a]

| Experimental model | Year | Basic protocol |
|---|---|---|
| Peraino sequential feeding model | 1971 | Feeding of carcinogen for 2 weeks, beginning at weaning, followed by prolonged promoter feeding |
| Solt–Farber selection model | 1976 | Single treatment with a necrogenic dose of carcinogen followed by the application of a proliferative stimulus (partial hepatectomy or carbon tetrachloride administration) midway through the 2-week feeding of AAF as a cytotoxic growth suppressant |
| Pitot partial hepatectomy model | 1978 | Single treatment with subtoxic dose of carcinogen during surgically induced proliferative stimulation, followed by prolonged promoter feeding |
| Shinozuka–Lombardi lipotrope deficiency model | 1979 | Production of lipotrope deficiency by feeding a choline-devoid diet following exposure to a hepatocarcinogen |
| Kitagawa in vivo initiation–in vitro promotion model | 1980 | Administration of carcinogen in vivo followed by culturing of initiated hepatocytes and exposure to promoter in vitro |
| Peraino neonatal rat model | 1981 | Single administration of subtoxic dose of carcinogen at birth followed by prolonged promoter feeding after weaning |

[a]From Peraino et al.[37] and references cited therein.

alveolar cells, which serve as stem cells for the alveolar epithelium.[40] Recent studies showed that the chronic administration of glycerol, another proliferative stimulant for this stem cell population, also promoted lung tumorigenesis in mice initiated by a single treatment with 4-nitroquinoline 1-oxide.[41]

Topping and Nettesheim[42,43] studied multistage respiratory tract tumorigenesis by means of a heterotopic tracheal transplant system. Rat tracheas transplanted to the backs of isogenic hosts were given a limited intraluminal exposure to 1,2-dimethylbenz(a)anthracene at a borderline tumorigenic level, followed by prolonged exposure to a subtumorigenic dose of asbestos fibers or to phorbol ester. In both cases, this sequential treatment protocol produced a synergistic induction of carcinomas in the transplants. With these *in vivo* studies providing a definitive indication of the multistage nature of respiratory tract carcinogenesis, subsequent investigations have focused primarily on the use of cultured tracheal explants and cultured respiratory epithelial cells for examining the multistage mechanism in this system.[38]

In the development of the tracheal explant system, freshly cultured pieces of rat trachea were exposed to carcinogen and subsequently maintained so as to permit the establishment of epithelial outgrowths.[44] These outgrowths were then compared with those from cultured, untreated tracheas to identify carcinogen-induced cellular changes indicative of neoplastic transformation. Evidence for such changes included aberrant behavior of carcinogen-treated cells in culture (as characterized by anchorage-independent growth, escape from senescence, and atypical morphology and tumorigenicity upon reimplantation *in vivo*).[38]

The successful demonstration of transformation in tracheal explant outgrowths led to the use of this system for *in vitro* initiation–promotion studies.[45] Tracheal organ cultures were briefly exposed to low levels of the initiator N-methyl-N'-nitro-N-nitrosoguanidine (MNNG), then given multiple treatments with the promoter TPA. This combined treatment protocol accelerated and enhanced the occurrence of neoplastically transformed colonies over that seen with MNNG treatment alone.[45] The TPA treatment alone produced no transformed colonies but did engender escape from senescence and the establishment of immortal tracheal epithelial cell lines.[46,47] The subsequent improvement of this experimental system has involved the replacement of explant cultures with primary tracheal epithelial cell cultures as a means of increasing control over exposure conditions and enabling clonal analysis of cellular changes occurring during the transformation process.[38]

## 3.4. Intestine

As noted for respiratory tract carcinogenesis, considerable epidemiologic evidence suggests that intestinal carcinogenesis in humans is a multievent process involving interactions of different classes of tumorigenic stimuli including fecal carcinogens and co-carcinogens derived from high meat consumption, as well as fecal promoting agents associated with the ingestion of high levels of dietary fat.[48] Mechanistic studies of intestinal carcinogenesis by experimental oncologists have verified the sequential stepwise nature of this process,[48–51] by analogy with tumorigenesis in the various systems described above, and have focused principally on the mechanism by which high dietary fat promotes colon tumor formation.

Such studies began during the mid-1970s with the observation that yields of experimentally induced rat intestinal tumors were increased by high levels of dietary fat, which was itself not intrinsically tumorigenic.[52,53] The finding that administered bile acids (which normally show elevated gut levels following high fat intake) also enhanced intestinal tumor formation[54–57] implicated these compounds in the fat-mediated promotion process.[48] The possibility of additional, more direct involvement of dietary fat in intestinal tumor promotion was raised by studies showing a correlation between the polyunsaturated fatty acid content of the fat and its promoting activity.[58,59] This effect was attributed in part to the enhanced secretion of bile acids stimulated by the polyunsaturated fat[58] but suggested additional contributory factors include highly active fatty acid metabolites such as prostaglandins[58,59] and fatty acid hydroperoxides.[60]

Investigation of intestinal tumor promotion mechanisms demonstrated an enhanced proliferation of colonic tissue as a consequence of exposure to bile acids, fats, or fatty acids.[60,61] This enhancement was associated with increased tissue levels of ornithine decarboxylase, an enzyme linked to proliferative stimulation in a variety of tissues.[60,62] Extension of mechanistic studies to *in vitro* systems showed that bile acids can exert co-mutagenic activity with intestinal carcinogens in a bacterial mutagenesis assay[7] and can also promote the transformation of previously initiated mouse fibroblasts.[63]

### 3.5. Mammary Gland

The multistage nature of mammary carcinogenesis was inferred from epidemiologic studies pointing to a variety of nongenotoxic risk factors (such as dietary fat and hormonal imbalances) in the development of human breast cancer[64,65] and was demonstrated directly in many investigations of the murine mammary tumor model.[66–73] On the basis of these investigations, mammotropic hormones and dietary fat were identified as two major types of rodent mammary tumor promoters.

Important endocrine factors involved in mammary tumor promotion were identified as the pituitary hormone prolactin and the ovarian hormones estrogen and progesterone.[73] The pituitary and ovarian factors appeared to act in a complementary fashion in the promotion process, since both endocrine sources were required for the optimum tumorigenic response.[73] In addition, the facilitative participation of insulin in mammary tumor promotion was suggested by studies demonstrating modulatory effects of insulin on tumor cell estrogen receptor levels. The direct stimulation of tumor cell DNA synthesis by insulin was also observed.[73]

With regard to promotion by dietary fat, polyunsaturated fat exhibited greater promoting activity than did saturated fat in both rats and mice.[66–73] The constituent fatty acids that imparted this enhanced activity were linoleic acid[71,73] and oleic acid.[73] The promoting effects of dietary fat were manifested as increases both in tumor yields when the high-fat diet was fed after an initiating dose of carcinogen[68,70,72–74] and in the growth rates of implanted mammary carcinoma cells.[66,67,69,71,72] Numerous candidate mechanisms for mammary tumor promotion by dietary fat have been investigated, including enhancement of mammotropic hormone secretion, alteration of target cell hormone responsiveness, immune suppression, direct stimulation of tumor cell proliferation, modulation of tumor cell membrane fluidity, inhibition of cell–cell communication, stimulation of prostaglandin production, free radical generation, and modulation of protein kinase C (PKC) activity,[67,70,72,73] but as yet no mechanistic frontrunner has clearly emerged from this list.

### 3.6. Other Nonepidermal Systems

Additional tissues in which multistage carcinogenesis has been demonstrated experimentally include thyroid,[75–77] pancreas,[78] and stomach. There is also evidence in the human that alcohol in combination with heavy cigarette smoking significantly increases the risk of malignant neoplasms of the oral cavity, esophagus, and larynx, although it is not clear whether alcohol is acting as a promoting agent for these types of tumors. Some of these systems are discussed further in other chapters.

## 4. MULTISTAGE MODELS OF NEOPLASIA IN CELL-CULTURE SYSTEMS

Investigations of multistage transformation at the cellular and molecular levels have centered on the simplification of experimental systems as a means of achieving better control over experimental conditions and of reducing the range of unknown factors that might influence results. These simplification efforts have involved the development of *in vitro* cultures of cells that manifest phenotypic changes analogous to those exhibited by tissues undergoing multistage carcinogenesis *in vivo*. It is important to remember, however, that most cells in culture undergo adaptive changes and thus deviate from their status in the living animal. Immortalized cell lines are often aneuploid or genetically unstable and may have already accumulated preneoplastic events.[79] Furthermore, most tumor-promoting agents induce a plethora of phenotypic changes in cultured cells, of which probably very few are related to tumor promotion. Thus, it is difficult to identify *in vitro* the relevant events that underlie the promotion process. Nevertheless, *in vitro* studies have yielded valuable information not only about the process of neoplastic development but also about the basic processes of growth and differentiation that are disrupted during carcinogenesis. The following major approaches to the study of promotion have been pursued in cellular systems.

## 4.1. Measurement of Multistage Development of Cell Transformation

Transformation of normal cells to malignant cells *in vitro* by chemical agents has been achieved in a number of fibroblast and epithelial cell systems.[80–84] Early neoplastic changes in the cells are indicated by altered patterns of morphology or growth. Such changes have formed the basis for quantitative assays to predict carcinogenic risk.[83] The development of a fully neoplastic (i.e., tumorigenic) phenotype is a progressive multistage process in these cell systems, analogous to neoplastic development *in vivo*. Thus, these systems are also important in studying the cellular events underlying each stage in the process of carcinogenesis. Lasne *et al.*[85] first reported that the addition of TPA to carcinogen-treated rat embryo fibroblasts could increase the yield of transformed cells. The first quantitative demonstration of a two-stage phenomenon in cell culture was achieved by Heidelberger and co-workers in mouse C3H 10T1/2 cells[86] and by Sivak and Van Duuren in mouse 3T3 cells.[87] To date there have been many studies of promotion in cultured cells, but most have used either the C3H 10T1/2 cell system or the Syrian hamster embryo cell transformation assay. The *in vitro* protocol parallels that developed for mouse skin *in vivo*. Cells are exposed initially to a single low (nontransforming) dose of carcinogen. This treatment is followed by prolonged or repetitive exposure to the promoter, which is also nontoxic and nontransforming when added to cells without the carcinogen pretreatment.

Although C3H 10T1/2 cells are nontumorigenic, they are aneuploid and appear to be preneoplastic.[79,88] In the transformation assay, the cultured fibroblasts are treated with carcinogens and then reseeded at low density. During a period of 4–6 weeks, the cells form contact-inhibited monolayers. Transformed cells within the monolayer overcome the constraint of contact-inhibited growth and continue to proliferate, forming foci of piled-up cells.[89] The addition of promoters throughout the assay period results in an elevated yield of transformed foci.[86,90] A similar assay protocol is used for mouse 3T3 cells.[87]

Syrian hamster cells are normal diploid fibroblasts that have a limited life span in culture. The cells are nontumorigenic and in culture form colonies with flat ordered morphologies. Upon carcinogen treatment, a fraction of the colonies that develop during a 7- to 10-day culture period display disoriented criss-crossed patterns. These colonies are presumed to have developed from initiated cells.[80,91] The addition of promoters during the clonal development of carcinogen-treated cells results in a markedly elevated frequency of morphologically transformed colonies.[92–94]

Ionizing and nonionizing radiations, as well as chemical carcinogens, have been used as initiators in these systems. Promoting agents that can effectively increase the yield of transformed foci after the threshold initiation dose is given include phorbol esters, phenobarbital, saccharin, bile salts, fatty acids, cigarette smoke extracts, and epidermal growth factor.[90]

The mechanisms underlying the action of promoters in transformation assays have yet to be defined. Promoters of morphologic transformation in the Syrian hamster embryo cell transformation assay may act either at the DNA or at the cellular level. Promoters that alter gene expression could turn on genes coding for expression of the transformed phenotype that were activated during the carcinogen exposure. Selection of initiated cell types is not a likely mechanism in this clonal assay, because the colony-forming efficiency of the cell population is not affected by the promoter. Promoters could also act on the plasma membrane and alter cell–cell communication (as discussed in Section 4.2). This factor could influence expression of the transformed phenotype within the colony. The action of promoters has been shown to be highly reversible in this system.[95]

The action of TPA has been studied in detail in the C3H 10T1/2 cells by Kennedy and Little and co-workers.[96,97] Promotion in this system seems to involve a change in the population dynamics rather than changes in the genome.[90] Mordan *et al.*[98] observed that TPA reduces the minimum size of the colony necessary to produce a transformed focus. Kennedy showed that initiation in this cell line is potentially a very common event, affecting most of the cells in a carcinogen-treated population. By contrast, promoters increase the probability of the second, more rare event required for expression of the transformed phenotype.[97] This action requires that the cells be in a proliferative state, although proliferation itself is not the mechanism of promotion, nor is the induction of an error-prone repair system.[90]

There are few epithelial cell models for promotion studies. In addition to the previously described tracheal system devised by Nettesheim *et al.*,[45,46] Kaufman and colleagues developed a human endometrial stromal cell system.[99] Phenotypic alterations resembling those found in endometrial sarcomas are acquired in these cells in a stepwise manner following long-term carcinogen treatment. These phenotypic changes include altered morphology and growth requirements and increased γ-glutamyltranspeptidase activity.[99] Following an initiating dose of MNNG, prolonged exposure to TPA or diethylstilbestrol (DES) produces a promotionlike enhancement of transformed phenotypes in the cell population.[100,101]

Promotion of hepatocarcinogenesis in cultured cells isolated from rats exposed *in vivo* to AAF was achieved by using phenobarbital but not TPA, consistent with the organ/tissue specificity of these agents *in vivo*.[102,103] Proliferative foci of enzymatically altered cells could be identified in the carcinogen-initiated hepatocyte cultures. Growth of foci was greatly enhanced by the addition of phenobarbital but was inhibited by TPA.[103]

In a skin cell culture model developed by Yuspa and Hennings, and co-workers,[104] basal epidermal cells could be propagated in medium containing reduced calcium levels (0.5 mM). High-calcium (1.2 mM) medium, however, acted as a terminal differentiation signal to the cells, causing keratinization and the cessation of cell division. A quantitative assay of epidermal cell differentiation was subsequently developed.[105] Addition of TPA to cultures of these normal basal cells resulted in a dual response. Most cells responded with high rates of proliferation and DNA synthesis and with increased ornithine decarboxylase activity but decreased transglutaminase activity. This pattern was characteristic of the TPA response of undifferentiated basal cells *in vivo*.[106,107] In subpopulations of the cultured cells, however, terminal differentiation was induced or accelerated by TPA as it is by growth in high-calcium medium.[107–109] Epidermal cells isolated either from mouse skin treated with carcinogens or carcinogen plus promoter,[108] or from carcinogen-induced papillomas,[110] were predominantly resistant to TPA and calcium differentiation signals and continued to proliferate under conditions favoring terminal differentiation. A series of terminally differentiation-resistant cell lines have been characterized for their keratinocyte patterns, morphology, and malignant potential.[111] Although there was marked biochemical heterogeneity among the lines, those exhibiting a highly malignant potential were, in general, poorly differentiated, as characterized by their loss of keratinizing capacity.[111]

The action of TPA in carcinogen-treated epidermal cells is therefore contrary to its action in fibroblast cells, where increased frequency and rate of transformation are observed. Mouse skin carcinogens seem to alter the regulation of epidermal cell differentiation, causing induction of cell types that are resistant to undergoing terminal differentiation.[108] Promoters such as TPA that modulate cell differentiation can also induce terminal differentiation in some basal cell populations and thereby, it is argued, provide a growth advantage for initiated cells resistant to the TPA differentiation signal.[106,108,110]

Somewhat different observations have been reported by Colburn and co-workers for a series of cell lines derived from the long-term culture or carcinogen treatment of epidermal cells from newborn mouse skin. These cells (JB6 lines) will grow in soft agar and will induce tumors in animals after exposure to TPA.[112] The cells have been subcloned into promotion-sensitive or -resistant lines.[113] TPA promotion in the sensitive cells was found to be genetically determined; two promotion-sensitive genes, termed pro-1 and pro-2, have been characterized.[114]

In human epidermal cells, TPA produces an accelerated rate of terminal differentiation[115] that is accompanied by inhibition of DNA synthesis and ornithine decarboxylase activity.[116] Similarly, epithelial cells derived from the human bronchus, colon, or esophagus, upon exposure to TPA or related promoters, show inhibited growth and the onset of terminal differentiation.[117–119] Thus, as was observed by Yuspa for mouse epidermal cells,[108] TPA appears to induce differentiation in normal human epithelial cells, which in turn facilitates the proliferation of initiated cells that have lost the ability to respond to the signals of terminal differentiation.

### 4.2. Measurement of Promoter-Induced Changes in Intercellular Relationships

The maintenance of specialized cellular and tissue functions associated with the normal differentiated state presumably requires, in part, the existence of intercellular communication mechanisms. One such mechanism is the direct transfer of intercellular signals via specialized membrane junctions (gap junctions) between cells in contact (see Chapter 16). The disruption or modification of this communication pathway by promoter-induced membrane changes is thought to represent a principal mechanism by which initiated cells escape from normal proliferative constraints and consequently undergo clonal expansion to form tumors.[120,121]

The first evidence for a possible relationship between tumor promotion and the disruption of cell–cell communication was obtained in studies measuring the effects of tumor promoters on metabolic cooperation between cells *in vitro*.[122,123] These studies used two different types of metabolic cooperation systems. Murray and Fitzgerald[122] prelabeled mouse epidermal cells (HEL/37) with [$^3$H]uridine, co-cultured the labeled cells with unlabeled mouse fibroblasts (3T3), and visually scored by autoradiography the proportion of HEL/37-3T3 contact pairs in which label had been transferred to the 3T3 cells. The addition of tumor promoters such as TPA to this system inhibited label transfer.

The metabolic cooperation system developed by Yotti *et al.*[123] involved the addition of 6-thioguanine to cocultures of 6-thioguanine-sensitive, wild-type Chinese hamster lung fibroblasts (V79) and mutant V79 cells that were 6-thioguanine resistant. The resistance of the mutants derived from their deficiency in the enzyme hypoxanthine-guanine phosphoribosyl transferase (HGPRT), which converts 6-thioguanine to the lethal metabolite 6-thioguanosine monophosphate. Metabolic cooperation, involving the gap-junctional transfer of this metabolite between wild-type and mutant cells in direct contact, resulted in the death of both cell types. The addition of tumor promoters to this system inhibited the transfer of the 6-thioguanosine monophosphate to the HGPRT($-$) mutants, thereby permitting their survival and growth in the presence of 6-thioguanine, although the cocultured nonmutant V79 cells did not survive under these conditions.

The evidence that metabolic cooperation is inhibited by a wide variety of agents with tumor-promoting activity[120,124] has stimulated speculation that the mechanism of tumor promotion involves the interruption of the flow of intercellular growth-regulatory signals (e.g., chalones) and the consequent facilitation of the clonal expansion of carcinogen-altered cells to a size that permits autonomous growth.[120] Recently, however, the putative relationship between cell–cell communication and promotion has been clouded by several observations: (1) exposure of gap-junctionally associated rat liver epithelial cells in culture to tumor-promoting agents had relatively little effect on cell–cell communication,[125] although liver tumorigenesis clearly proceeds via an initiation-promotion mechanism (see Section 3.2); (2) incomplete (second stage) promoters and complete promoters inhibited metabolic cooperation[30]; and (3) metabolic cooperation was inhibited by agents that antagonize tumor promotion.[126–128] These studies indicate that gap-junctional disruption can be mechanistically dissociated from tumor promotion. Therefore, although tumor promoters may be useful for studying mechanisms regulating intercellular communication, the relevance of this information to mechanisms of tumor promotion remains problematic.

### 4.3. Measurement of Promoter–Induced Changes in Membrane Function

While initiators interact primarily with DNA, the primary site of some tumor promoters, most notably the phorbol esters, is the cell membrane, with consequential pleiotropic effects on cell growth, function, and differentiation. Extensive research into the biochemical action of phorbol esters has led to the following proposed mechanism of action. The promoters interact with highly specific cellular cytosolic receptors found in most mammalian cell types including human cells.[129] Following promoter binding, these receptors are translocated to the plasma membrane.[130] The receptors constitute a family of calcium- and phospholipid-dependent PKC enzymes with specificity for serine and threonine (see Chapter 18). Several PKC genes have been recently cloned.[131,132] The endogenous substrate for the PKC enzymes is diacylglycerol (DAG).[131] TPA and related promoters can act in place of DAG to activate PKC.[133,134] PKC activation plays a central role in the process of signal transduction[129] and leads to a cascade of biochemical events, including a burst of intracellular calcium; activation of many enzymes such as phosphatases, kinases, and phosphodiesterases; and alterations in the cytoskeleton.[129] Signals conveyed to the nucleus result in altered expression, activation, or suppression of many genes, some of which have been identified as oncogenes.[135–137]

The interaction of TPA with the cell membrane is analogous to that of other agents important in the regulation of cell growth and differentiation, i.e., epidermal growth factor and platelet-derived growth factor, both of which bind to another protein kinase, tyrosine kinase.[137] The mechanism(s) underlying TPA-induced signal transduction are unknown. In particular, it is unclear whether this process involves translocation of the promoter-PKC complex to the nucleus.[130,138] The persistent effects of TPA after it is no longer present in the cell are believed to result from the PKC-mediated phosphorylation of a DNA methylase enzyme, which produces altered patterns of DNA methylation.[139] Prolonged activation of PKC also results in altered levels of poly ADP ribose, which is a post-translational modification of nuclear protein that plays a role in the regulation of chromatin structure and function. This might therefore constitute another mechanism whereby TPA can induce stable changes in DNA function.[140] Such persistent alterations may be responsible for the enhancement of tumorigenesis by TPA administered prior to initiation.[26,28,29] It should be noted, however, that the liver tumor promoter phenobarbital (1) does not exert persistent tumorigenic enhancing effects when it is no longer present in the liver,[141] and (2) exerts an inactivating effect on PKC,[142] as opposed to the previously noted activation of this enzyme by TPA. These discrepancies between the cellular effects of the promoters TPA and phenobarbital suggest that (1) promotion may occur via more than one mechanism, or (2) promotion involves a single mechanism that is obscured by a plethora of agent-specific cellular responses.

### 4.4. Measurement of Changes in Cellular Differentiation

Established myeloid, lymphoid, and leukemic cell lines, in which the stages of cellular differentiation are characterized by specific enzymic or antigenic markers, have been used to study the action of promoters on the regulation of gene expression and cell differentiation[30,143–145] (see Chapter 22). TPA and related promoting agents have been shown to inhibit cell replication and induce cell differentiation in these hematopoietic cells. For example, TPA will induce human promyelocytic HL-60 leukemia cells to differentiate into macrophage-like cells[146] and human T-cell leukemic cells to differentiate into mature suppressor T-lymphocytes.[145] In myeloid leukemic cells, these TPA-mediated phenotypic alterations are characterized by specific modifications in the patterns of cell surface or nuclear antigens and by alterations in the glycosphingolipid pattern of the cell membranes.[146,147] The study of cell variants that are sensitive or resistant to TPA-induced differentiation should yield valuable insights into the processes controlling normal cell growth and differentiation in these systems.[148] However, because these studies have been restricted to cell-culture systems, the relevance of the observations to a mechanism of tumor promotion in hematopoietic cells *in vivo* remains to be proven.

### 5. CONCLUSIONS

Since the first demonstration of a two-stage mechanism for the development of skin tumors, growing evidence has suggested that tumorigenesis in general proceeds by means of a multistage process involving the initiation of tumorigenic genomic changes and the promotion of their phenotypic expression. It is also becoming increasingly apparent from *in vitro* studies that promotion mechanisms are closely intertwined with the normal processes of cell growth and differentiation, which are themselves only poorly understood. Moreover, the actions of promoting agents are so manifold and diverse, especially in cultured cell models, that it is difficult to distinguish those effects that are relevant to the tumor promotion mechanism. Therefore, the identification of the specific cellular mechanisms involved in promotion and the development of systems for the identification of promoting agents represent major continuing challenges in experimental oncology. Successfully meeting these challenges will substantially increase our understanding of the elements of neoplasia and will provide a means for the assessment and mitigation of human tumorigenic risk from environmental promoters.

ACKNOWLEDGMENTS. This work was supported by the United States Department of Energy, Office of Health and Environmental Research, under contract W-31-109-ENG-38, and by the National Toxicology Program under Interagency Agreement Y01-ES-20091.

# REFERENCES

1. Mori, H., Kunyasu, T., Sugie, S., Shima, H., and Takahashi, T., 1985, Syncarcinogenic effects of methyl methanesulfonate with methylazoxymethanol acetate in rat small intestine and liver, *Carcinogenesis* **6**:1529–1531.
2. Michejda, C. J., Kroeger-Koepke, M. B., and Kovatch, R. M., 1986, Carcinogenic effects of sequential administration of two nitrosamines in Fischer 344 rats, *Cancer Res.* **46**:2252–2256.
3. Boutwell, R. K., 1964, Some biological aspects of skin carcinogenesis, in: *Progress in Experimental Tumor Research*, Vol. 4 (F. Homburger, ed.), pp. 207–250, S. Karger, New York.
4. Berenblum, I., 1969, A re-evaluation of the concept of cocarcinogenesis, in: *Progress in Experimental Tumor Research*, Vol. 11 (F. Homburger, ed.), pp. 21–30, S. Karger, New York.
5. Van Duuren, B. L., and Goldschmidt, B. M., 1976, Cocarcinogenic and tumor-promoting agents in tobacco carcinogenesis, *J. Natl. Cancer Inst.* **56**:1237–1242.
6. Sivak, A., 1979, Cocarcinogenesis, *Biochim. Biophys. Acta* **560**:67–89.
7. Wilpart, M., and Robertfroid, M., 1986, Effects of secondary biliary acids on the mutagenicity of *N*-methyl-*N'*-nitro-*N*-nitrosoguanidine, 2-acetylaminofluorene and 2-nitrofluorene towards *Salmonella typhimurium* strains, *Carcinogenesis* **7**:703–706.
8. Deml, E., and Oesterle, D., 1986, Enhancing effect of co-administration of polychlorinated biphenyls and diethylnitrosamine on enzyme-altered islands induced by diethylnitrosamine in rat liver, *Carcinogenesis* **7**:1697–1700.
9. Potter, M., 1963, Percival Pott's contributions to cancer research, in: *Conference on Biology of Cutaneous Cancer*, NCI Monograph No. 10 (F. Urbach, ed.), pp. 1–13, National Cancer Institute, Washington, D.C.
10. Shimkin, M. B., and Triolo, V. A., 1969, History of chemical carcinogenesis: Some prospective remarks, in: *Progress in Experimental Tumor Research*, Vol. 11 (F. Homburger, ed.), pp. 1–20, S. Karger, New York.
11. Yamigawa, K., and Ichikawa, K., 1918, Experimental study of the pathogenesis of carcinoma, *J. Cancer Res.* **3**:1–21.
12. Deelman, H. T., 1927, The part played by injury and repair in the development of cancer; with remarks on the growth of experimental cancers, *Br. Med. J.* **1**:872.
13. Twort, J. M., and Twort, C. C., 1939, Comparative activity of some carcinogenic hydrocarbons, *Am. J. Cancer* **35**:80–85.
14. Twort, C. C., and Ing, H. R., 1928, Untersuchungen uber Krebserzeugende agenzien, *Z. Krebsforsch.* **27**:309–351.
15. Rous, P., and Kidd, J. G., 1941, Conditional neoplasms and subthreshold neoplastic states: a study of the tar tumors of rabbits, *J. Exp. Med.* **73**:365–390.
16. Friedewald, W. F., and Rous, P., 1944, The initiating and promoting elements in tumor production: An analysis of the effects of tar, benzpyrene, and methylcholanthrene on rabbit skin, *J. Exp. Med.* **80**:101–125.
17. Berenblum, I., 1941, The cocarcinogenic action of croton resin, *Cancer Res* **1**:44–48.

18. Berenblum, I., and Shubik, P., 1947, A new quantitative approach to the study of stages of chemical carcinogenesis in the mouse's skin, *Br. J. Cancer* **1**:383–391.

19. Mottram, J. C., 1944, A developing factor in experimental blastogenesis, *J. Pathol.* **56**:181–187.

20. Berenblum, I., and Shubik, P., 1949, The persistence of latent tumor cells induced in the mouse's skin by a single application of 9,10-dimethyl-1,2-benzanthracene, *Br. J. Cancer* **3**:384–386.

21. Berenblum, I., and Haran, N., 1955, The significance of the sequence of initiating and promoting actions in the process of skin carcinogenesis in the mouse, *Br. J. Cancer* **9**:268–271.

22. Roe, F. J. C., 1959, The effect of applying croton oil before a single application of 9,10-dimethyl-1,2-benzanthracene, *Br. J. Cancer* **13**:87–91.

23. Van Duuren, B. L., 1965, The tumor enhancing principles of *Croton tiglium* L., *Cancer Res.* **25**:1871–1875.

24. Hecker, E., 1971, Isolation and characterization of the cocarcinogenic principles from croton oil, in: *Methods in Cancer Research*, Vol. 6 (H. Busch, ed.), pp. 439–484, Academic, New York.

25. Furstenberger, G., Berry, D. L., Sorg, B., and Marks, F., 1981, Skin tumor promotion by phorbol esters is a two-stage process, *Proc. Natl. Acad. Sci. USA* **78**:7722–7726.

26. Furstenberger, G., Sorg, B., and Marks, F., 1983, Tumor promotion by phorbol esters in mouse skin: Evidence for a memory effect, *Science* **220**:89–91.

27. Slaga, T. J., 1984, Multistage skin tumor promotion and specificity of inhibition, in: *Mechanisms of Tumor Promotion*, Vol. II: *Tumor Promotion and Skin Carcinogenesis* (T. J. Slaga, ed.), pp. 189–196, CRC Press, Boca Raton, Florida.

28. Furstenberger, G., Kinzel, V., Schwarz, M., and Marks, F., 1985, Partial inversion of the initiation-promotion sequence of multistage tumorigenesis in the skin of NMRI mice, *Science* **230**:76–78.

29. Kinzel, V., Furstenberger, G., Loehrke, H., and Marks, F., 1986, Three-stage tumorigenesis in mouse skin: DNA synthesis as a prerequisite for the conversion stage induced by TPA prior to initiation, *Carcinogenesis* **7**:779–782.

30. Yamasaki, H., Aguelon-Pegouries, A.-M., Enomoto, T., Martel, N., Furstenberger, G., and Marks, F., 1985, Comparative effects of a complete tumor promoter, TPA, and a second-stage tumor promoter, RPA, on intercellular communication, cell differentiation and cell transformation, *Carcinogenesis* **6**:1173–1179.

31. Bryan, G. T., and Springberg, P. D., 1966, Role of the vehicle in the genesis of bladder carcinomas in mice by the pellet implantation technic, *Cancer Res.* **26**:105–109.

32. Cohen, S. M., Murasaki, G., Ellwein, L. B., and Greenfield, R. E., 1983, Tumor promotion in bladder carcinogenesis, in: *Mechanisms of Tumor Promotion*, Vol. 1: *Tumor Promotion in Internal Organs* (T. J. Slaga, ed.), pp. 131–149, CRC Press, Boca Raton, Florida.

33. Hicks, R. M., Wakefield, J., and Chowaniec, J., 1975, Evaluation of a new model to detect bladder carcinogens or cocarcinogens: Results obtained with saccharine, cyclamate, and cyclophosphamide, *Chem. Biol. Interact.* **11**:225–233.

34. Peraino, C., Fry, R. J. M., and Staffeldt, E., 1971, Reduction and enhancement by phenobarbital of hepatocarcinogenesis induced in the rat by 2-acetylaminofluorene, *Cancer Res.* **31**:1506–1512.

35. Peraino, C., Fry, R. J. M., Staffeldt, E., and Kisieleski, W. E., 1973, Effects of varying the exposure to phenobarbital on its enhancement of 2-acetylaminofluorene-induced hepatic tumorigenesis in the rat, *Cancer Res.* **33**:2701–2705.

36. Peraino, C., Fry, R. J. M., and Staffeldt, E., 1977, Effects of varying the onset and duration of exposure to phenobarbital on its enhancement of 2-acetylaminofluorene-induced hepatic tumorigenesis, *Cancer Res.* **37**:3623–3627.

37. Peraino, C., Richards, W. L., and Stevens, F. J., 1983, Multistage hepatocarcinogenesis, in: *Mechanisms of Tumor Promotion*, Vol. 1: *Tumor Promotion in Internal Organs* (T. J. Slaga, ed.), pp. 1–53, CRC Press, Boca Raton, Florida.

38. Steele, V. E., and Nettesheim, P., 1983, Tumor promotion in respiratory tract carcinogenesis, in: *Mechanisms of Tumor Promotion*, Vol. 1: *Tumor Promotion in Internal Organs* (T. J. Slaga, ed.), pp. 91–105, CRC Press, Boca Raton, Florida.

39. Armuth, V., and Berenblum, I., 1972, Systemic promoting action of phorbol in liver and lung carcinogenesis in AKR mice, *Cancer Res.* **32**:2259–2262.

40. Witschi, H. P., Williamson, D., and Lock, S., 1977, Enhancement of urethan tumorigenesis in mouse lung by butylated hydroxytoluene, *J. Natl. Cancer Inst.* **58**:301–305.

41. Inayama, Y., 1986, Promoting action of glycerol in pulmonary tumorigenesis model using a single administration of 4-nitroquinoline 1-oxide in mice, *Jpn. J. Cancer Res.* **77**:345–350.

42. Topping, D. C., and Nettesheim, P., 1980, Two stage carcinogenesis studies with asbestos fibers in Fischer 344 rats, *J. Natl. Cancer Inst.* **65**:627–630.

43. Topping, D. C., and Nettesheim, P., 1980, Promotion-like enhancement of tracheal carcinogenesis in rats by 12-O-tetradecanoyl-phorbol-13-acetate, *Cancer Res.* **40**:4352–4355.

44. Marchok, A. C., Cone, V., and Nettesheim, P., 1975, Induction of squamous metaplasia in tracheal organ cultures, *Lab. Invest.* **33**:451–460.

45. Steele, V. E., Marchok, A. C., and Nettesheim, P., 1980, Enhancement of carcinogenesis in cultured respiratory tract epithelium by 12-O-tetradecanoylphorbol-13-acetate, *Int. J. Cancer* **26**:343–348.

46. Steele, V. E., Marchok, A. C., and Nettesheim, P., 1978, Establishment of epithelial cell lines following exposure of cultured tracheal epithelium to 12-O-tetradecanoylphorbol-13-acetate, *Cancer Res.* **38**:3563–3565.

47. Steele, V. E., and Beeman, D. K., 1981, Relationships of increased growth capacity and tumor promotion in cultured rat tracheal cells, *In Vitro* **17**:202–203.

48. Reddy, B. S., 1983, Tumor promotion in colon carcinogenesis, in: *Mechanisms of Tumor Promotion*, Vol. I: *Tumor Promotion in Internal Organs* (T. J. Slaga, ed.), pp. 107–129, CRC Press, Boca Raton, Florida.

49. Watanabe, K., Reddy, B. S., Wong, C. Q., and Weisburger, J. H., 1978, Effect of dietary undegraded carageenin on colon carcinogenesis in F344 rats treated with azoxymethane or methylnitrosourea, *Cancer Res.* **38**:4427–4430.

50. Pollard, M. S., and Luckert, P. H., 1979, Promotional effect of sodium barbiturate on intestinal tumors induced in rats by dimethyl hydrazine, *J. Natl. Cancer Inst.* **63**:1089–1092.

51. Lindenschmidt, R. C., Tryka, A. F., Goad, M. E., and Witschi, H. P., 1986, The effects of dietary butylated hydroxytoluene on liver and colon tumor development in mice, *Toxicology* **38**:151–160.

52. Nigro, N. D., Singh, D. V., Campbell, R. L., and Pak, M. S., 1975, Effect of dietary beef fat on intestinal tumor formation by azoxymethane in rats, *J. Natl. Cancer Inst.* **54**:439–442.

53. Reddy, B. S., Watanabe, K., and Weisburger, J. H., 1977, Effect of high fat diet on colon carcinogenesis in F344 rats treated with 1,2-dimethylhydrazine, methylazoxymethanol acetate, or methylnitrosourea, *Cancer Res.* **37**:4156–4159.

54. Chomchai, C., Bhadarachari, N., and Nigro, N. D., 1974, The effect of bile on the induction of experimental intestinal tumors in rats, *Dis. Colon Rectum* **17**:310–312.

55. Narisawa, T., Magadia, N. E., Weisburger, J. H., and Wynder, E. L., 1974, Promoting effect of bile acids on colon carcinogenesis after intrarectal instillation of N-methyl-N'-nitro-N-nitrosoguanidine in rats, *J. Natl. Cancer Inst.* **53**:1093–1097.

56. Reddy, B. S., and Watanabe, K., 1979, Effect of cholesterol metabolites and promoting effect of lithocholic acid in colon carcinogenesis in germ-free and conventional F344 rats, *Cancer Res.* **39**:1521–1524.

57. Cohen, B. I., Raicht, R. F., Deschner, E. E., Takahashi, M., Sarwal, A. N., and Fazzini, E., 1980, Effect of cholic acid feeding on N-methyl-N-nitrosourea-induced colon tumors and cell kinetics in rats, *J. Natl. Cancer Inst.* **61**:573–578.

58. Reddy, B. S., and Maeura, Y., 1984, Tumor promotion by dietary fat in azoxymethane-induced colon carcinogenesis in female F344 rats: Influence of amount and source of dietary fat, *J. Natl. Cancer Inst.* **72**:745–750.

59. Reddy, B. S., Tanaka, T., and Simi, B., 1985, Effect of different levels of dietary trans fat or corn oil on azoxymethane-induced colon carcinogenesis in F344 rats, *J. Natl. Cancer Inst.* **75**:791–798.

60. Bull, A. W., Nigro, N. D., Golembieski, W. A., Crissman, J. D., and Marnett, L. J., 1984, In vivo stimulation of DNA synthesis and induction of ornithine decarboxylase in rat colon by fatty acid hydroperoxides, autoxidation products of unsaturated fatty acids, *Cancer Res.* **44**:4924–4928.

61. Bull, A. D., Marnett, L. J., Dawe, E. J., and Nigro, N. D., 1983, Stimulation of deoxythymidine incorporation in the colon of rats treated intrarectally with bile acids and fats, *Carcinogenesis* **4**:207–210.

62. Rozhin, J., Wilson, P. S., Bull, A. W., and Nigro, N. D., Ornithine decarboxylase activity in the rat and human colon, *Cancer Res.* **44**:3226–3230.

63. Kaibara, N., Yurugi, E., and Koga, S., 1984, Promoting effect of bile acids on the chemical transformation of C3H/10T1/2 fibroblasts in vitro, *Cancer Res.* **44**:5482–5485.

64. Wynder, E. L., 1984, Nutrition, diet, and cancer, an evaluation, *Curr. Concepts Nutr.* **13**:171–193.

65. Moore, D. H., Moore, D. H. II, and Moore, C. T., 1983, Breast carcinoma etiological factors, *Adv. Cancer Res.* **40**:189–253.

66. Abraham, S., Faulkin, L. J., Hillyard, L. A., and Mitchell, D. J., 1981, Effect of dietary fat on tumorigenesis in the mouse mammary gland, *J. Natl. Cancer Inst.* **72**:1421–1429.

67. Gabor, H., Hillyard, L. A., and Abraham, S., 1985, Effect of dietary fat on growth kinetics of transplantable mammary adenocarcinoma in BALB/c mice, *J. Natl. Cancer Inst.* **74**:1299–1305.

68. Hopkins, G. J., Hard, G. C., and West, C. E., 1978, Carcinogenesis induced by 7,12-dimethyl-

benz(a)anthracene in C3H-A(vy)fB mice: Influence of different dietary fats, *J. Natl. Cancer Inst.* **60**:849–853.

69. Hopkins, G. J., and West, C. E., 1977, Effect of dietary polyunsaturated fat on the growth of a transplantable adenocarcinoma in C3HA(vy)fB mice, *J. Natl. Cancer Inst.* **58**:753–756.

70. Lane, H. W., Butel, J. S., Howard, C., Shepherd, F., Halligan, R., and Medina, D., 1985, The role of high levels of dietary fat in 7,12-dimethylbenzanthracene-induced mouse mammary tumorigenesis: Lack of an effect on lipid peroxidation, *Carcinogenesis* **6**:403–407.

71. Rao, G. A., and Abraham, S., 1976, Enhanced growth rate of transplanted mammary adenocarcinoma induced in C3H mice by dietary linoleate, *J. Natl. Cancer Inst.* **56**:431–432.

72. Welsch, C. W., and Aylsworth, C. F., 1983, Enhancement of murine mammary tumorigenesis by feeding high levels of dietary fat: A hormonal mechanism, *J. Natl. Cancer Inst.* **70**:215–221.

73. Welsch, C. W., 1985, Host factors affecting the growth of carcinogen-induced rat mammary carcinomas: A review and tribute to Charles Brenton Huggins, *Cancer Res.* **45**:3415–3443.

74. Hopkins, G. J., and Carroll, K. K., 1979, Relationship between amount and type of dietary fat in promotion of mammary carcinogenesis induced by 7,12-dimethylbenz(a)anthracene, *J. Natl. Cancer Inst.* **62**:1009–1012.

75. Hiasa, Y., Kitahori, Y., Oshima, M., Fujita, T., Yuasa, T., Konishi, N., and Miyashiro, A., 1982, Promoting effects of phenobarbital and barbital on development of thyroid tumors in rats treated with N-bis(2-hydroxypropyl)nitrosamine, *Carcinogenesis* **3**:1187–1190.

76. Tsuda, H., Fukushima, S., Imaida, K., Kurata, Y., and Ito, N., 1983, Organ-specific promoting effects of phenobarbital and saccharin in induction of thyroid, liver, and urinary bladder tumors in rats after initiation with *N*-nitrosomethylurea, *Cancer Res.* **43**:3292–3296.

77. Diwan, B. A., Palmer, A. E., Oshima, M., and Rice, J. M., 1985, *N*-nitroso-*N*-methylurea initiation in multiple tissues for organ-specific tumor promotion in rats by phenobarbital, *J. Natl. Cancer Inst.* **75**:1099–1105.

78. Roebuck, B. D., Longnecker, D. S., and Yager, J. D., Jr., 1983, Initiation and promotion in pancreatic carcinogenesis, in: *Mechanisms of Tumor Promotion*, Vol. 1: *Tumor Promotion in Internal Organs* (T. J. Slaga, ed.), pp. 151–171, CRC Press, Boca Raton, Florida.

79. Barrett, J. C., and Elmore, E., 1985, Comparison of carcinogenesis and mutagenesis of mammalian cells in culture, in: *Mechanisms and Toxicity of Chemical Carcinogens and Mutagens* (W. G. Flamm and R. J. Lorentzen, eds.), pp. 171–206, Princeton Publishing Co., Princeton, New Jersey.

80. Berwald, Y., and Sachs, L., 1965, *In vitro* transformation of normal cells to tumor cells by carcinogenic hydrocarbons, *J. Natl. Cancer Inst.* **35**:641–661.

81. Kakunaga, T., 1973, A quantitative system for assay of malignant transformation by chemical carcinogens using a clone derived from Balb/3T3, *Int. J. Cancer* **12**:463–473.

82. Marchok, A. C., Rhoton, J. C., and Nettersheim, P., 1978, *In vitro* development of oncogenicity in cell lines established from tracheal epithelium pre-exposed *in vivo* to 7,12-dimethylbenz(a)anthracene, *Cancer Res.* **38**:2030–2037.

83. Heidelberger, C., Freeman, A. E., Pienta, R. J., Sivak, A., Bertram, J. S., Casto, B. C., Dunkel, V. C., Francis, M. C., Kakunaga, T., Little, J. B., and Schechtman, L. M., 1983, Cell transformation by chemical agents: A review and analysis of the literature, *Mutat. Res.* **114**:283–385.

84. Barrett, J. C., and Thomassen, D. G., 1985, Use of quantitative cell transformation assays in risk estimation, in: *Methods for Estimating Risk of Chemical Injury: Human and Nonhuman Biota and Ecosystems* (V. B. Vouk, G. C. Butler, D. G. Hoel, and D. B. Peakall, eds.), pp. 201–234, Wiley, New York.

85. Lasne, C., Gentil, A., and Chouroulinkov, I., 1974, Two-stage malignant transformation of rat fibroblasts in tissue culture, *Nature (Lond.)* **274**:490–491.

86. Mondal, S., Brankow, D. W., and Heidelberger, C., 1976, Two-stage chemical oncogenesis in cultures of C3H 10T1/2 cells, *Cancer Res.* **36**:2254–2260.

87. Sivak, A., and Van Duuren, B. L., 1970, A cell culture system for the assessment of tumor-promoting activity, *J. Natl. Cancer Inst.* **44**:1091–1097.

88. Boone, C. S., and Jacobs, J. B., 1976, Sarcomas routinely produced from putatively nontumorigenic Balb/3T3 and C3H 10T1/2 cells by subcutaneous inoculation attached to plastic platelets, *J. Supramol. Struct.* **5**:131–137.

89. Reznikoff, C. A., Bertram, J. S., Brankow, D. W., and Heidelberger, C., 1973, Quantitative and qualitative studies of chemical transformation of cloned C3H mouse embryo cells sensitive to postconfluence inhibition of cell division, *Cancer Res.* **33**:3239–3249.

90. Kennedy, A. R., 1984, Promotion and other interactions between agents in the induction of transformation

*in vitro* in fibroblast-like cell culture systems, in: *Mechanisms of Tumor Promotion*, Vol. 3: *Tumor Promotion and Carcinogenesis In Vitro* (T. J. Slaga, ed.), pp. 13–55, CRC Press, Boca Raton, Florida.

91. DiPaolo, J. A., Nelson, R. L., and Donovan, P. J., 1969, Sarcoma-producing cell lines derived from clones transformed *in vitro* by benzo(a)pyrene, *Science* **165**:917–918.

92. Popescu, N. C., Amsbaugh, S. C., and DiPaolo, J. A., 1980, Enhancement of N-methyl-N'-nitro-N-nitrosoguanidine transformation of Syrian hamster cells by a phorbol diester is independent of sister chromatid exchanges and chromosome aberrations, *Proc. Natl. Acad. Sci. USA* **77**:7282–7286.

93. Rivedal, E., and Sanner, T., 1982, Promotional effect of different phorbol esters on morphological transformation of hamster embryo cells, *Cancer Lett.* **17**:1–8.

94. Jones, C. A., Callaham, M. C., and Huberman, E., 1984, Enhancement of chemical-carcinogen-induced cell transformation in hamster embryo cells by $1\alpha,25$-dihydroxycholecalciferol, the biologically active metabolite of vitamin $D_3$, *Carcinogenesis* **5**:1155–1159.

95. DiPaolo, J. A., Demarinis, A. J., Evans, C. H., and Doniger, J., 1981, Expression of initiated and promoted stages of irradiation carcinogenesis *in vitro*, *Cancer Lett.* **14**:243–249.

96. Kennedy, A. R., Mondal, S., Heidelberger, C., and Little, J. B., 1978, Enhancement of x-ray transformation by phorbol 12-myristate 13-acetate in a cloned line of C3H mouse embryo cells, *Cancer Res.* **38**:439–443.

97. Kennedy, A. R., and Little, J. B., 1980, Investigations of the mechanisms for enhancement of radiation transformation *in vitro* by 12-O-tetradecanoylphorbol-13-acetate, *Carcinogenesis* **1**:1039–1047.

98. Mordan, L. J., Markner, J. E., and Bertram, J. S., 1983, Quantitative neoplastic transformation of C3H/10T1/2 cells: Dependence on colony size of initiated cells at confluence, *Cancer Res.* **43**:4062–4067.

99. Dorman, B. H., Siegfried, J. M., and Kaufman, D. G., 1983, Alterations of human endometrial stromal cells produced by N-methyl-N'-nitro-nitrosoguanidine, *Cancer Res.* **43**:3348–3357.

100. Siegfried, J. M., Nelson, K. G., Martin, J. L., and Kaufman, D. G., 1984, Promotional effect of diethylstilbestrol on human endometrial stromal cells pretreated with a direct acting carcinogen, *Carcinogenesis* **5**:641–646.

101. Siegfried, J. M., Nelson, K. G., and Kaufman, D. G., 1985, Promotion-like enhancement of transformed phenotypes in human endometrial stromal cells, in: *Carcinogenesis: A Comprehensive Survey*, Vol. 8 (M. J. Mass, J. G. Kaufman, J. M. Siegfried, V. E. Steele, and S. Nesnow, eds.), pp. 279–292, Raven, New York.

102. Kitagawa, T., Watanabe, R., Kayano, T., and Sugano, H., 1980, *In vitro* carcinogenesis of hepatocytes obtained from acetylaminofluorene-treated rat liver and promotion of their growth by phenobarbital, *Gann* **71**:747–754.

103. Kayano, T., Nomura, K., Mino, O., and Kitagawa, T., 1982, Failure of phorbol ester TPA to promote growth of *in vivo*-initiated rat hepatocytes transferred into a culture system, *Gann* **73**:354–357.

104. Hennings, H., Michael, D., Cheng, C., Steinert, P., Holbrook, K., and Yuspa, S. H., 1980, Calcium regulation of growth and differentiation of mouse epidermal cells in culture, *Cell* **19**:245–254.

105. Kulesz-Martin, M. F., Koehler, B., Hennings, H., and Yuspa, S. H., 1980, Quantitative assay for carcinogen altered differentiation in mouse epidermal cells, *Carcinogenesis* **1**:995–1006.

106. Yuspa, S. H., 1984, Tumor promotion in epidermal cells in culture, in: *Mechanisms of Tumor Promotion*, Vol. 3: *Tumor Promotion and Carcinogenesis In Vitro* (T. J. Slaga, ed.), pp. 1–11, CRC Press, Boca Raton, Florida.

107. Yuspa, S. H., Ben, T., Hennings, H., and Lichti, U., 1982, Divergent responses in epidermal basal cells exposed to the tumor promoter 12-O-tetradecanoylphorbol-13-acetate, *Cancer Res.* **42**:2344–2349.

108. Yuspa, S. H., and Morgan, D. L., 1981, Mouse skin cells resistant to terminal differentiation associated with initiation of carcinogenesis, *Nature (Lond.)* **293**:72–74.

109. Reiners, J. J., and Slaga, T. J., 1983, Effects of tumor promoters on the rate and commitment to terminal differentiation of subpopulations of murine keratinocytes, *Cell* **32**:247–255.

110. Yuspa, S. H., Morgan, D., Lichti, U., Spangler, E. F., Michael, D., Kilkenny, A., and Hennings, H., 1986, Cultivation and characterization of cells derived from mouse skin papillomas induced by an initiation–promotion protocol, *Carcinogenesis* **7**:949–958.

111. Kulesz-Martin, M., Kilkenny, A. E., Holbrook, K. A., Digernes, V., and Yuspa, S. H., 1983, Properties of carcinogen altered mouse epidermal cells resistant to calcium-induced terminal differentiation, *Carcinogenesis* **4**:1367–1377.

112. Colburn, N. H., Vorder Bruegge, W. F., Bates, J. R., Gray, R. H., Rossen, J. D., Kelsey, W. H., and Shimada, T., 1978, Correlation of anchorage-independent growth with tumorigenicity of chemically transformed mouse epidermal cells, *Cancer Res.* **38**:624–634.

113. Colburn, N. H., 1980, Tumor promoter produces anchorage independence in mouse epidermal cells by an induction mechanism, *Carcinogenesis* **1**:951–954.

114. Lerman, M. I., Hegamyer, G. A., and Colburn, N. H., 1986, Cloning and characterization of putative genes that specify sensitivity to neoplastic transformation by tumor promoters, *Int. J. Cancer* **37**:293–302.

115. Mawley Nelson, P., Stanley, J., Schmidt, J., Gullino, M., and Yuspa, S. H., 1982, The tumor promoter 12-*O*-tetradecanoylphorbol-13-acetate accelerates keratinocyte differentiation and stimulates growth of an identified cell type in cultured human epidermis, *Exp. Cell Res.* **137**:117–155.

116. Chida, K., and Kuroki, T., 1984, Inhibition of DNA synthesis and sugar uptake and lack of induction of ornithine decarboxylase in human epidermal cells treated with mouse skin tumor promoters, *Cancer Res.* **44**:875–879.

117. Willey, J. C., Moser, C. E., Jr., Lechner, J. F., and Harris, C. C., 1984, Differential effects of 12-*O*-tetradecanoylphorbol-13-acetate on cultured normal and neoplastic human bronchial epithelial cells, *Cancer Res.* **44**:5124–5126.

118. Friedman, E. A., 1981, Differential response of premalignant epithelial cell classes to phorbol ester tumor promoters and to deoxycholic acid, *Cancer Res.* **41**:4588–4599.

119. Sasajima, K., Willey, J. C., Banks-Schlegel, S. P., and Harris, C. C., 1987, Effects of tumor promoters and cocarcinogens on growth and differentiation of cultured human esophageal epithelial cells, *J. Natl. Cancer Inst.* **78**:419–423.

120. Trosko, J. E., and Chang, C. C., 1984, Role of intercellular communication in tumor promotion, in: *Mechanisms of Tumor Promotion*, Vol. IV: *Cellular Responses to Tumor Promoters* (T. J. Slage, ed.), pp. 119–145, CRC Press, Boca Raton, Florida.

121. Trosko, J. E., 1987, Mechanisms of tumor promotion. Possible role of inhibited intercellular communication, *Eur. J. Cancer Clin. Oncol.* **23**:599–601.

122. Murray, A. W., and Fitzgerald, D. J., 1979, Tumor promoters inhibit metabolic cooperation in co-cultures of epidermal and 3T3 cells, *Biochem. Biophys. Res. Commun.* **91**:395–401.

123. Yotti, L. P., Chang, C. C., and Trosko, J. E., 1979, Elimination of metabolic cooperation in Chinese hamster cells by a tumor promoter, *Science* **206**:1089–1091.

124. Trosko, J. E., Yotti, L. P., Warren, S. T., Tsushimoto, G., and Chang, C. C., 1982, Inhibition of cell-cell communication by tumor promoters, in: *Carcinogenesis: A Comprehensive Survey*, Vol. 7: *Cocarcinogenesis and Biological Effects of Tumor Promoters* (E. Hecker, N. E. Fusenig, W. Kunz, F. Marks, and H. W. Thielmann, eds.), pp. 565–585, Raven, New York.

125. Walder, L., and Lutzelschwab, R., 1984, Effects of 12-*O*-tetradecanoylphorbol-13-acetate (TPA), retinoic acid and diazepam on intercellular communication in a monolayer of rat liver epithelial cells, *Exp. Cell Res.* **152**:66–76.

126. Radner, B. S., and Kennedy, A. R., 1984, Effects of agents known to antagonize the enhancement of *in vitro* transformation by 12-tetradecanoylphorbol-13-acetate (TPA) on the TPA suppression of metabolic cooperation, *Cancer Lett.* **25**:139–144.

127. Davidson, J. S., Baumgarten, I. M., and Harley, E. H., 1985, Effects of 12-*O*-tetradecanoylphorbol-13-acetate and retinoids on intercellular junctional communication measured with a citrulline incorporation assay, *Carcinogenesis* **6**:645–650.

128. Tsuda, H., and Okamoto, H., 1986, Elimination of metabolic cooperation by glycyrrhetinic acid, an anti-tumor promoter, in cultured Chinese hamster cells, *Carcinogenesis* **7**:1805–1807.

129. Blumberg, P. M., 1981, *In vitro* studies on the mode of action of the phorbol esters, potent tumor promoters: Parts 1 and 2, *CRC Critical Rev. Toxicol.* **8**:153–234.

130. Kraft, A. S., and Andess, W. B., 1983, Phorbol esters increase the amount of $CA^{2+}$, phospholipid-dependent protein kinase associated with plasma membrane, *Nature (Lond.)* **301**:621–623.

131. Nishizuka, Y., 1986, Perspectives on the role of protein kinase C in stimulus-response coupling, *J. Natl. Cancer Inst.* **76**:363–370.

132. Housey, G. M., O'Brian, C. A., Johnson, M. D., Kirschmeier, P., and Weinstein, I. B., 1987, Isolation of cDNA clones encoding protein kinase C: Evidence for a protein kinase C-related gene family, *Proc. Natl. Acad. Sci. USA* **84**:1065–1069.

133. Dreidger, P. E., and Blumberg, P. M., 1980, Specific binding of phorbol ester tumor promoters, *Proc. Natl. Acad. Sci. USA* **77**:571–567.

134. Horowitz, A., Greenebaum, E., and Weinstein, I. B., 1981, Identification of receptors for phorbol ester tumor promoters in intact mammalian cells and of an inhibitor of receptor binding in biologic fluids, *Proc. Natl. Acad. Sci. USA* **78**:2315–2319.

135. Bishop, J. M., 1985, Viral oncogenes, *Cell* **42**:23–38.

136. Vande Woude, G. F., Levine, A. J., Topp, W. C., and Watson, J. D. (eds.), 1984, *The Cancer Cell,* Vol. II: *Oncogenes and Viral Genes,* Cold Spring Harbor Laboratory, Cold Spring Harbor, New York.

137. Weinstein, I. B., 1987, Growth factors, oncogenes, and multistage carcinogenesis, *J. Cell Biochem.* **33:**213–224.

138. Cambier, J. C., Newell, M. K., Justeman, L. B., McGuire, J. C., Leach, K. L., and Chen, Z. Z., 1987, Ia binding ligands and cAMP stimulate nuclear translocation of PKC in β lymphocytes, *Nature (Lond.)* **327:**629–632.

139. DePaoli-Roach, A., Roach, P. J., Zucker, K. E., and Smith, S. S., 1986, Selective phosphorylation of human DNA methyltransferase by protein kinase C, *FEBS Lett.* **197:**149–153.

140. Singh, N., Leduc, Y., Poirier, G., and Cerutti, P., 1985, Non-histone chromosomal protein acceptors for poly(ADP)-ribose in phorbol-12-myristate-13-acetate treated mouse embryo fibroblasts (C3H10T1/2), *Carcinogenesis* **6:**1489–1494.

141. Williams, G. M., and Furuya, K., 1984, Distinction between liver neoplasm promoting and syncarcinogenic effects demonstrated by exposure to phenobarbital or diethylnitrosamine either before or after N-2-fluorenylacetamide, *Carcinogenesis* **5:**171–174.

142. Chauhan, V. P. S., and Brockerhoff, H., 1987, Phenobarbital competes with diacylglycerol for protein kinase C, *Life Sci.* **40:**89–93.

143. Rovera, G., O'Brien, T. A., and Diamond, L., 1977, Tumor promoters inhibit spontaneous differentiation of Friend erythroleukemia cells in cultures, *Proc. Natl. Acad. Sci. USA* **74:**2894–2898.

144. Huberman, E., and Callaham, M. F., 1979, Induction of terminal differentiation in human promyelocytic leukemia cells by tumor-promoting agents, *Proc. Natl. Acad. Sci. USA* **76:**1293–1297.

145. Ryffel, B., Henning, C. B., and Huberman, E., 1982, Differentiation of human T-lymphoid leukemia cells into cells that have a suppressor phenotype is induced by phorbol 12-myristate 13-acetate, *Proc. Natl. Acad. Sci. USA* **79:**7336–7340.

146. Murao, S., Epstein, A. L., Clevenger, O. V., and Huberman, E., 1985, Expression of maturation-specific nuclear antigens in differentiating human myeloid leukemia cells, *Cancer Res.* **45:**791–795.

147. Kiguchi, K., Henning-Chubb, C., and Huberman, E., Alteration in glycosphingolipid pattern during phorbol-12-myristate-13-acetate-induced cell differentiation in human T-lymphoid leukemia cells, *Cancer Res.* **46:**3027–3033.

148. Homma, Y., Henning-Chubb, C. B., and Huberman, E., 1986, Translocation of protein kinase C in human leukemia cells susceptible or resistant to differentiation induced by phorbol 12-myristate 13-acetate, *Proc. Natl. Acad. Sci. USA* **83:**7316–7319.

# 7

# Organ and Species Specificity in Chemical Carcinogenesis and Tumor Promotion

## Bhalchandra A. Diwan and Jerry M. Rice

### 1. INTRODUCTION

Chemical carcinogens include substances as diverse as mineral fibers (e.g., asbestos), plastic films, certain metals and their salts, and organic compounds of low molecular weight. All these categories include specific compounds or preparations that are carcinogenic both for humans and for experimental animals. Far more substances have been tested and found positive for carcinogenicity in rodents than have been shown to cause cancer in humans, especially among the organic compounds that constitute by far the largest group of known carcinogens.

In both humans and animals, it is commonly observed that exposure to almost any carcinogen causes tumors selectively at a limited number of sites. The spectrum of sites varies from one carcinogen to another and, for a given carcinogen, may or may not be the same in humans as in any other species. Some specific sites and kinds of tumors are so characteristically associated with one specific causative agent that diagnosis of a case of the disease automatically suggests the likelihood of previous exposure to the agent, for example, pleural mesothelioma and certain forms of asbestos.[1,2] Another example is carcinoma of the urinary bladder in humans who were occupationally exposed to 2-aminonaphthalene in the manufacture of dyes, usually a result of combined inhalation, ingestion, and percutaneous exposure. Similar neoplasms developed in hamsters, dogs, and monkeys during prolonged feeding of the same compound.[3-5] More recently, occupational exposure to vinyl chloride by inhalation was found to cause hemangiosarcomas, especially of the liver. Experimental inhalation of this compound caused histologically and anatomically comparable neoplasms in many other species including mice, rats, and hamsters.[6,7]

It has often been found, however, that the tumors caused by a substance in experimental rodents include, or in fact are limited to, neoplasms that are different from those that occur in humans exposed to that substance, with regard to both cell of origin and anatomic site. In mice, tumors of the peripheral lung (originating from type II pneumocytes) and the liver (originating from hepatocytes) are commonly seen in bioassays, irrespective of apparent selectivity for other tissues in humans and other species. There thus exist both tissue and organ specificity and differences between

*Bhalchandra A. Diwan and Jerry M. Rice* • Biological Carcinogenesis Development Program, Program Resources, Inc.; and Laboratory of Comparative Carcinogenesis, National Cancer Institute, National Institutes of Health, Frederick Cancer Research Facility, Frederick, Maryland 21701.

species in response to chemical carcinogens. These limit the extent to which one can extrapolate from rodent bioassays to humans in predicting the nature of carcinogenic risk. A species may be extremely susceptible or totally resistant to a given carcinogenic agent. For example, 2-aminonaphthalene, a bladder carcinogen in humans, causes only liver tumors in mice and is inactive in rats.[2,3] Similarly, 2-acetylaminofluorene (2-AAF), which has been tested in at least 15 species, shows remarkable interspecies differences. Guinea pig, cotton rat, monkey, and some other mammals are resistant, while laboratory rats, several strains of mice, and hamsters are susceptible to its hepatocarcinogenic effects.[8] Such all-or-none effects are rare, however, and more commonly a given carcinogen affects a different spectrum of organs, or different cell types within the organ, in different species.

This chapter discusses examples of some of the most important kinds of tissue specificities and interspecies differences in carcinogenesis by organic compounds of low molecular weight. When the underlying mechanisms are known, they are described, but it must be emphasized that in many, perhaps most cases, such mechanisms are not yet understood. A number of factors can be identified that contribute to interspecies differences and to organ and tissue specificity. Some of the most important of these are the following:

1. *Toxicodynamics*, the temporal and spatial patterns of distribution of the carcinogen within the organism: These vary with the solubility of the parent compound and its metabolites, and their chemical reactivity under biological conditions. Toxicodynamics change with the magnitude of an individual dose, the rate and duration of dosing, and the route of exposure.
2. *Metabolism*, the enzyme-mediated biotransformation of a compound to a derivative that is either less toxic or nontoxic (detoxification) or to a derivative that is chemically reactive and genotoxic (activation): Metabolism is highly variable from one tissue to another and from species to species. Multiple molecular pathways may exist for the metabolism of a compound; these often vary with age, and some may be inducible (i.e., may increase in activity) in response to the carcinogen or to other foreign substances.
3. *Target affinity*, reactivity with critical cellular constituents (e.g., the purine and pyrimidine bases in DNA) that constitute potentially mutagenic or clastogenic molecular lesions: There are hot spots in DNA where reactivity is greater than expected by chance alone, and some where mutation occurs more frequently; these two types of hot spot may or may not coincide.
4. *DNA repair*, which occurs by a number of different mechanisms, depending on the nature of the lesion: Repair capacity is limited, varies from one type of cell to another and from one species to another, and can be poisoned or overwhelmed by very large doses of carcinogens.
5. *Cell cycle*, the early part of the S phase (DNA synthesis phase) of which is especially susceptible to damage by carcinogens: This is a major factor in the high susceptibility of rapidly proliferating tissues to carcinogenesis, including intestinal mucosa and most fetal tissues.
6. *Homeostatic control of proliferation*, which can suppress expression of the transformed phenotype: This control appears to be mediated in part by intercellular communication via gap junctions between cells and can be interrupted by tumor promoters.

A simplified classification of organic carcinogens is given in Table I, based on whether they form reactive intermediates that combine irreversibly with intracellular target molecules including DNA, with mutation or clastogenic damage as a demonstrable result (genotoxicity). Compounds that do this are subclassified according to whether they are dependent on metabolism and on the degree of complexity of metabolic path(s) involved. It must be emphasized that characteristic and striking examples of tissue specificity occur within each of these categories of substances. Direct-acting carcinogens—those that do not require metabolism to act and that do so through a genotoxic mechanism—include many of the most potent carcinogens known. They provide an excellent example of toxicodynamic control of tissue specificity, determined by the absorption and distribu-

*Table I. Categories of Carcinogenic*
*Organic Compounds*[a]

---

Genotoxic
 Direct acting (independent of metabolism)
  Example: *N*-nitrosomethylurea
 Metabolism dependent
  Single pathway, phase I
   Example: *N*-nitrosodimethylamine
    Activating: α-C-hydroxylation
  Successive phase I and II reactions
   Example: 2-acetylaminofluorene
    Activating: *N*-hydroxylation, sulfate esterification
    Detoxifying: Arene oxide formation, hydrolysis, glucuronidation
Nongenotoxic
 Example: phenobarbital

---

[a]For a more complete classification, see Chapter 2.

tion of the agent within the organism. The spectrum of tumors that may result from exposure to any of these agents is highly dependent on the route of administration and the intrinsic chemical reactivity of the agent, as well as on the dose administered and the duration and frequency of exposure. Results also vary with characteristics of the organism at risk, including age, sex, and genetic background.

Although also direct acting in the sense that neoplasms develop in proximity to the carcinogen and that no biotransformation appears to be required, carcinogens such as asbestos, plastic films, and metal prostheses are by convention not included in this category.

## 2. ORGAN AND SPECIES SPECIFICITY ATTRIBUTABLE TO METABOLISM

The overwhelming majority of genotoxic organic carcinogens are metabolism dependent, and differences in metabolic capacity for either phase I or phase II reactions, or both, from one tissue to another must clearly contribute to the observed patterns of selective tumor induction in certain tissues. It has proved extremely difficult, however, to quantify the rates of competing metabolic paths in many if not most cases and to explain tissue or even species specificity on the basis of metabolism. Polynuclear aromatic hydrocarbons (PAH), such as benzo[a]pyrene, are metabolized by a remarkable diversity of pathways, the most potently activating of which involve a succession of three steps: oxidation to an arene oxide, hydrolysis of the oxide to a diol, and introduction of a second arene oxide function. These compounds are adequately metabolized, however, by so many different types of cells that the PAH are effective carcinogens for nearly any tissue into which they are introduced (at least in rats and mice), and for a long time it was considered possible that they were in fact direct acting. By contrast, the polynuclear aromatic amines provide a clear and classic example of metabolism as an absolute determinant of both species and tissue specificity in carcinogenesis.

### 2.1. Polycyclic Aromatic Amines

Several polycyclic aromatic amines have been shown to cause cancer in humans and in experimental animals. For many aromatic amines, the major target organ is the urinary bladder (Table II). Thus, 2-aminonaphthalene, benzidine, and 4-aminobiphenyl characteristically and selectively induce bladder carcinomas in humans. In hamsters, dogs, and monkeys, 2-aminonaphthalene is also carcinogenic for the urinary bladder, but in the mouse, it does not affect urinary bladder but is carcinogenic for the liver.[2–4] Likewise, 2'3-dimethyl-4-biphenylamine produces tumors of the intestine and of Zymbal's gland in rats but induces mainly bladder tumors in hamsters.[9]

*Table II. Carcinogenic Activity of Polynuclear Aromatic Amines in Different Species[a]*

| Species | Bladder | Kidney | Liver | Intestine | Zymbal's gland | Breast | Other |
|---|---|---|---|---|---|---|---|
| | | | 2-Acetylaminofluorene | | | | |
| Rat | + | − | + | − | + | + | |
| Mouse | + | + | + | + | − | + | |
| Hamster | − | − | + | − | − | − | Cholangioma |
| Rabbit | + | − | − | − | − | − | Ureter |
| Guinea pig | − | − | − | − | − | − | |
| | | | 2-Aminonaphthalene | | | | |
| Mouse | − | − | + | − | − | − | |
| Hamster | + | − | − | − | − | − | |
| Dog | + | − | − | − | − | − | |
| Monkey | + | − | − | − | − | − | |
| Man | + | − | − | − | − | − | |
| Rat | − | − | − | − | − | − | |
| Rabbit | − | − | − | − | − | − | |
| | | | 4-(o-Tolylazo)-o-toluidine | | | | |
| Hamster | + | − | + | − | − | + | |
| Mouse | + | − | + | − | − | − | Lung |
| Rat | + | − | + | − | − | − | |
| Dog | + | − | ? | − | − | − | Gallbladder |
| Rabbit | ? | − | − | − | − | − | |
| | | | 4-Aminobiphenyl | | | | |
| Mouse | + | − | + | − | − | − | |
| Rat | − | − | − | + | − | − | Mammary gland |
| Rabbit | + | − | − | − | − | − | |
| Dog | + | − | − | − | − | − | |

[a]Modified from Clayson and Garner.[4]

In rats, 2-AAF induces tumors predominantly of liver but also of the urinary bladder, mammary gland, Zymbal's gland, and other organs. 2-AAF is carcinogenic for the urinary bladder and the ureter in the rabbit but exerts no such effects in the hamster.[10] These interspecies differences appear to be related to differences in the metabolism of these compounds. It had long been known that phenols were major metabolites of the polycyclic amines, and these were postulated during the 1950s to play a significant role in the carcinogenic process. It was not then recognized that the phenols were formed via arene oxide intermediates or that in fact this phase I reaction was detoxifying and competed with another more important activating reaction, N-hydroxylation. In 1960, it was shown for the first time that 2-AAF is converted to N-hydroxy-AAF (N-OH-AAF), which is a more potent carcinogen than AAF itself when fed to rats.[11] Guinea pigs, which are resistant to the carcinogenic action of 2-AAF, are unable to N-hydroxylate the amine to any appreciable extent. 2-AAF remains one of the best examples of a critical phase I metabolic step absolutely determining susceptibility or resistance of a species to the carcinogenic effects of a potent compound and in fact to the entire class of compounds of which it is a member. N-Hydroxylation itself is, however, only the first of two steps in the metabolic activation and is insufficient by itself; subsequent phase II formation of an ester is required. Available data suggest that the sulfate ester of N-hydroxy-AAF is an important metabolite in the induction of liver tumors by these compounds.

The proposed mechanism for the initiation of bladder cancer focuses on metabolic activation

(N-oxidation) of the arylamine followed by N-glucuronidation in the liver. The *N*-hydroxy-*N*-glucuronide product is subsequently transported through the kidney to the bladder urothelium, where it is hydrolyzed under mildly acidic conditions within the bladder to yield free *N*-hydroxyarylamines that covalently bind to urothelial DNA.[12] Recent investigations have suggested, however, that bladder urothelium from humans and other species has the metabolic capacity necessary to activate arylamine carcinogens. Arylamines readily undergo N-acetylation catalyzed by acetyl coenzyme A-dependent *N*-acetyltransferase enzyme(s). Hepatic N-acetylation capacity in humans and other mammalian species is controlled by inheritance of two codominant alleles at a single genetic locus (reviewed by Cartwright[13]). Recent epidemiologic studies in humans suggested that persons can be identified as rapid, intermediate, or slow acetylator phenotypes and that slow acetylators may show a genetic predisposition to arylamine-induced bladder cancer.

## 3. BIOLOGIC EFFECTS OF ALKYLATING AGENTS

Alkylating agents react with DNA to form relatively simple, easily identified products, and a substantial literature exists relating the chemistry of alkylating agents to their biologic effects, especially their mutagenic action. A remarkable range of carcinogenic effects is seen following exposure to these substances; they provide useful tools for identifying and studying the many factors that determine susceptibility to chemical carcinogenesis.

### 3.1. Direct-Acting Compounds

A wide variety of chemical classes that are considered reactive alkylating agents include carcinogenic compounds of varying potency. Among these are epoxides, lactones, alkyl sulfates, and sulfonates, 2-chloroalkylamines and sulfides (mustards), α-haloethers, *N*-nitrosoamides, and others. Not all direct-acting alkylating agents are carcinogenic; extremely unstable and highly reactive compounds, and conversely those that are very stable, tend to be weakly carcinogenic or inactive. The most reactive of the alkylating agents produce tumors only locally, in tissues directly exposed to the agent, and not in distant organs, access to which would require systemic distribution. For example, bis(chloromethyl)ether (BCE) produces skin tumors in the mouse after percutaneous administration,[14] lung and nasal cavity tumors in the rat after inhalation,[15] and skin and soft tissue tumors in the mouse and only soft tissue tumors in the rat following subcutaneous administration.[16] The only tumors induced at remote sites are lung tumors in mice after subcutaneous administration. Other less reactive alkylating agents, such as β-propiolactone and methyl methanesulfonate, produce a variety of both local and systemic tumors in rodents, depending on the route of administration.[17,18]

As might be predicted *a priori*, certain alkylating agents have a level of stability/reactivity under physiologic conditions such that, if administered appropriately, these compounds can induce neoplasms in practically all tissues. Such universal carcinogens are to be found among the lower homologues in the series of *N*-nitroso-*n*-alkylureas.[19]

### 3.1.1. N-Nitrosoalkylureas

The simplest compounds in this series, *N*-nitrosomethylurea (NMU) and *N*-nitrosoethylurea (ENU), can induce tumors in rodents literally from the teeth (compound odontomas, NMU, rat[20]) to the tips of the toes (melanoma, ENU, Mongolian gerbil[21]), when given intravenously. NMU has been studied in a wide variety of species, including mice, rats, hamsters, guinea pigs, dogs, and monkeys.[22] Each species has been found to yield a distinctive spectrum of tumors following systemic exposure to these agents. Intraperitoneal and intravenous injections of NMU produce numerous malignant gliomas of the brain and spinal cord and schwannomas of the peripheral nervous system in the rat.[23,24] Similar treatment in the mouse produces high yields of thymic lymphomas and pulmonary adenomas; tumors of the brain and other parts of the nervous system are rare.[25] Hamsters develop an entirely different spectrum of tumors that include adenocarcinomas of large and small intestine, odontogenic tumors, and epidermoid carcinomas.[26,27] Intravenous injections of NMU in adult gerbils produce only tumors of the oral cavity and carcinomas and adenomas of the mid-ventral sebaceous gland[28] (contrast this with the melanomas induced by ENU). Both rabbits and dogs develop mostly brain tumors (sarcomas, gliomas, or multiform glioblastomas), although vascular tumors of different organs have also been found in these species.[29,30] A single intraveous injection of NMU induces a high incidence of mammary carcinomas in rats,[31] while only leukemias occur in mice.[32] Similar interspecies differences in target organ susceptibilities have been observed following other routes of administration.

### 3.1.2. Azaserine

Azaserine (O-diazoacetyl-L-serine) is an antibiotic produced by *Streptomyces fragilis*. It is a strong mutagen in several *in vitro* and *in vivo* test systems and has been shown to induce pancreatic atypical acinar cell nodules (AACN), adenoma, and carcinomas in rats.[33] Wistar and W/LEW rats are highly susceptible to nodule induction; F344 are less susceptible and develop about 10% as many AACN as Wistar rats. Female rats are less susceptible than males. The mouse shows a response intermediate between that of F344 and Wistar rats.[34] Syrian hamsters and guinea pigs are relatively resistant to azaserine-induced pancreatic carcinogenesis. *Mastomys natalensis* is susceptible to the development of azaserine-induced AACN and adenomas of the pancreas, while *Mystromys albicaudatus* is nonresponsive.[35]

In addition to pancreatic tumors, azaserine induces a low but significant incidence of kidney (renal cell epithelium) and liver (hepatocellular) tumors in rats.[34] By contrast, neither kidney nor liver tumors occur in mice or hamsters; however, intraperitoneal administration of azaserine induces lung tumors in strain A/J mice.[36] In dogs, intravenous perfusion of azaserine produces toxic effects in kidney, salivary glands and prostate but not in pancreas.[33] Male rats, like humans, develop a higher incidence of pancreatic tumors than do females. Sex steroids play a major role in the higher incidence of pancreatic cancer in male rats. Orchiectomy decreases the number and size of atypical acinar cell foci and AACN of pancreas in azaserine-treated male rats. Testosterone treatment partially reverses the effect of orchiectomy. This effect of testosterone is not mediated through the high-affinity receptors characteristic of gonadal tissue.[37]

Several dietary factors modulate the incidence and pathogenesis of pancreatic cancer in rats. Diets high in unsaturated fat and raw soybean products greatly enhance pancreatic carcinogenesis initiated by azaserine. The enhancement of pancreatic carcinogenesis by raw soy protein appears to be mediated by cholecystokinin, since plasma cholecystokinin values increase significantly in rats fed this protein diet.[38] Diet containing raw soybean products causes pancreatic enlargement and increases the incidence of pancreatic nodules in rats. Mice fed a similar diet have pancreatic hypertrophy but a relatively low incidence of AACN. By contrast, hamsters do not exhibit pancreatic enlargement in response to this diet and have a very low incidence of pancreatic tumors. Two pancreatic peptides, bombesin and caerulein, promote the growth (size and number) of pre-neoplastic acinar cell nodules initiated by azaserine.[39] DL-Ethionine-induced pancreatitis potentiates pancreatic carcinogenesis in azaserine-treated rats.[33]

## 3.2. Metabolism-Dependent Compounds

1,2-Dialkylhydrazines, aliphatic azo compounds, and aliphatic N-nitrosamines are the most intensively studied of the metabolism-dependent aklylating agents. While a few hydrazines and N-nitrosamines have been isolated as natural products, the great majority are of synthetic origin. Unlike the methylating agents of intermediary metabolism, such as S-adenosylmethionine, which participate in methyl group transfer reactions that are enzyme catalyzed and metabolically controlled, the carcinogenic metabolism-dependent alkylating agents are activated by P-450-dependent mixed-function oxidases that generate highly reactive alkylating intermediates that react indiscriminately. The *N*-nitrosamines are remarkable both for their carcinogenic potency and for the extreme variations in organ specificity among homologous members of a selected series, such as *N*-nitrosodialkylamines of increasing chain length.

## Nitrosamines

The symmetric *N*-nitrosodialkylamines, *N*-nitrosodiethylamine (DEN) and *N*-nitrosodimethylamine (DMN), induce liver tumors in all laboratory animal species,[40,41] including nonhuman primates.[42] Nasal cavity tumors (adenocarcinomas, undifferentiated carcinomas) and esophageal neoplasms (squamous papillomas and carcinomas) also occur in rats following single or chronic administration of DEN.[40] Neither nasal cavity nor esophageal tumors appear in mice, but in this species squamous papillomas of the forestomach are commonly observed after single or multiple exposures to this agent. Tumors of the upper respiratory tract, particularly the trachea, occur in hamsters following DEN administration.[40] Like DEN, multiple injections of DMN produce liver tumors in rats (hepatocellular carcinomas and cholangiocellular tumors), mice (hepatocellular adenomas and carcinomas, hemangiomas, and hemangioendotheliomas) and hamsters (cholangiomas, cholangiocarcinomas, and hemangiomas).[41] Adenomas and adenocarcinomas of the peripheral lung are most common in mice; a few such tumors are found in rats, but none in hamsters. A single intraperitoneal injection of DMN also induces a high incidence of kidney tumors in young and adult rats. Tumors induced in young rats are mostly renal mesenchymal tumors, while those in adult rats are almost all epithelial tumors of the renal cortex, with a few transitional cell tumors of the renal pelvis.[43] *N*-Nitrosodi-*n*-butylamine (DBN) induces predominantly liver and bladder tumors in rats while only bladder tumors occur in both mice and hamsters.[44] *N*-Nitrosodi-*n*-propylamine produces mainly esophageal tumors in rats. Its β-oxidized derivative *N*-nitrosobis(2-oxypropyl)amine is a potent carcinogen for the hamster pancreas and liver, while in rats this compound induces tumors in a wide spectrum of organs, but the pancreas remains resistant.[44,45]

Species differences in organotropism are also observed after exposure to cyclic nitrosamines. Thus, while nitrosopyrrolidine induces liver tumors in rats, lung tumors occur in mice and Syrian hamsters. *N*-Nitrosopiperidine induces esophageal tumors in both mice and rats but only lung tumors in hamsters.[44] The liver is a main target organ for *N*-nitrosomorpholine in rats and mice. However, its structural analogue, *N*-nitroso-2,6-dimethylmorpholine, induces esophageal tumors in rats, both pancreatic and liver tumors in hamsters, and hemangiosarcomas in the liver of guinea pigs.[44,45]

The rat esophagus is very sensitive to the carcinogenic effect of asymmetrical nitrosamines. *N*-Nitrosomethyl-*n*-dodecylamine, however, is found to have a different pattern of organotropism. This compound produces bladder tumors in both rats and hamsters, but only liver tumors in guinea pigs.[46] *N*-Nitrosomethyl-*n*-butylamine, a strong esophageal carcinogen in rats, fails to induce such tumors in mice or hamsters.[44]

While α-hydroxylation is postulated to be the principal activation pathway for nitrosamines,[40,41] other pathways have also been suggested. Figure 1 shows three proposed pathways for the metabolism of DMN.[47] In path a, DMN is activated by rapid metabolism to formaldehyde, nitrogen gas, and a methylating agent, considered an ultimate carcinogenic metabolite. However, one recent study[48] reported less than theoretical yields of labeled nitrogen after administration of $^{15}$N-labeled DMN to rats, while another study[49] found labeled methylamine as a major urinary metabolite in rats dosed with $^{14}$C-labeled DMN. Thus, although the α-hydroxylation pathway is an important pathway, it is not an exclusive route for nitrosamine metabolism. According to path b, N–N bond cleavage initially produces nitric oxide (NO), which can be converted to nitrite by an ambient oxidizing agent. Dimethylamine would be a biproduct of nitrite generation in this scheme. In path c, denitrosation is accomplished by an initial oxidative pathway closely related to the α-oxidation of DMN. This pathway should result in fragmentation of DMN to the imine ($CH_3 - N = CH_2$), which in turn should hydrolyze to produce formaldehyde and methylamine. In a recent study,[47] when DMN was incubated with liver microsomes from ethanol-treated rats, no net increase in dimethylamine concentration was observed, but the yield of monomethylamine was equimolar with that of nitrite. Accordingly, DMN

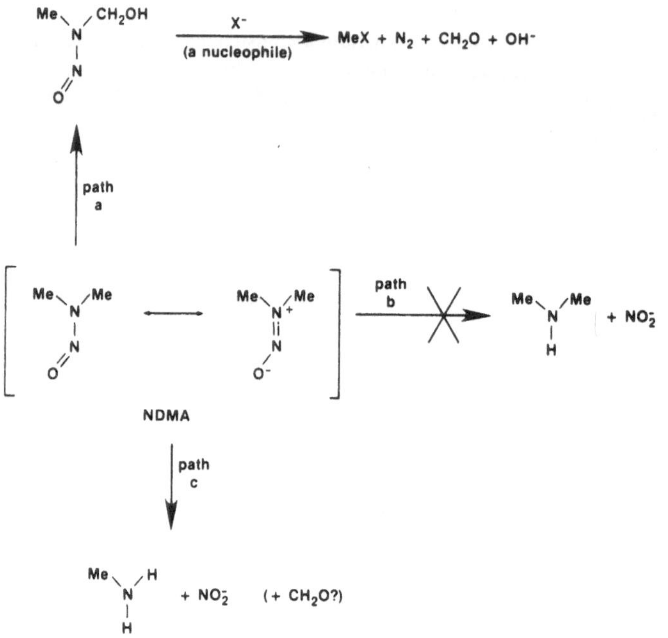

Figure 1. Alternate metabolic pathways for the metabolism of N-nitrosodimethylamine. (From Keefer et al.[47])

metabolism would involve a competition between at least two important pathways, i.e., demethylation (activating) and denitrosation (deactivating).

In the case of DBN and more complex nitrosamines, the oxidation occurs not only at the α-position but also at all the other carbons. Preussmann and Stewart[50] suggested that ω-oxidation of DBN is important in bladder carcinogenesis. N-Nitrosobis(2-hydroxypropyl)(2-oxopropyl)amine (HPOP), a pancreatic carcinogen in hamsters, has no effect on the pancreas of the adult rat.[51] This is because of differences in the metabolism and activation of this carcinogen by rats and hamsters. Hamsters sulfate HPOP several times more rapidly and reduce it to N-nitrosobis(2-oxopropyl)amine (BOP) more efficiently than rats. By contrast, rats excrete more unchanged HPOP and its glucuronic acid conjugate than do hamsters. Furthermore, glucuronidation of HPOP is catalyzed by an enzyme, the activity of which is three times greater in rats than in hamsters. In contrast to glucuronidation, sulfation of HPOP in liver cytosol from hamsters is catalyzed at least 10 times faster than in comparable preparations from rats.

Little is known about the metabolism of cyclic nitrosamines. However, in hamsters, α-hydroxylation appears to be the important pathway for N-nitroso-2,6-dimethylmorpholine, a pancreatic carcinogen in this species.[44]

## 3.3. Molecular Targets of Alkylating Agents

All carcinogenic alkylating agents combine irreversibly with the same nucleophilic reaction centers in DNA. These include the phosphate esters and specific heteroatoms (N,O) either within the purine ring systems or that are extranuclear. Some, but not all, of such reaction products have been shown to be mutagenic, causing misreading of the DNA message, and therefore appear to be logical candidates for molecular lesions that could be initial stages in the carcinogenic process. Alkylating agents differ in the relative amounts of different adducts that they form and in the rate and extent of reaction. Adducts differ in the ease with which they can be repaired, which may also vary among species and from one tissue to another, and in the molecular mechanisms by which they are removed.

## 3.3.1. Pyrimidines and Purines in DNA

As a direct alkylating agent, NMU alkylates nucleic acid both *in vivo* and *in vitro*.[17] Thus, following *in vivo* NMU treatment, alkylation of nucleic acids has been detected in various organs. Although several methylated products were formed, removal of $O^6$-methylguanine from DNA of the brain and, to a lesser extent, from that of kidney (organs that are relatively susceptible to the carcinogenic action of NMU), was slower than from the liver, which is relatively resistant to carcinogenesis by this agent. These data provided support for the hypothesis that $O^6$-alkylguanine is the DNA adduct responsible for brain tumor induction.[52,53] More recent investigations have shown that gerbil, hamster, and mouse brains develop concentrations of $O^6$-alkylguanine similar to rats, yet are resistant to brain tumor induction by NMU.[54] Several studies have emphasized the importance of cellular proliferation in carcinogenesis. Thus, although the DNA of neuronal cells of the brains of young rats treated with NMU was alkylated to the same extent as the DNA from the glial cells, brain tumors produced by this agent originate from glial cells, which proliferate, and not from neurons, which do not.[55]

A high correlation was also found between $O^6$-alkylguanine formation following exposure to *N*-nitrosamines and tumor incidence in many tissues but not in liver. In liver, $O^6$-methylguanine accumulates in the nonparenchymal cells but not in hepatocytes. Therefore, $O^6$-methylguanine may be an important mutagenic lesion responsible for the induction of angiosarcomas after exposure to methylating agents, but it probably does not play a major role in the induction of hepatocellular carcinomas.[56,57] The main promutagenic DNA adduct that accumulates in the liver of rats continuously exposed to DEN is $O^4$-ethyldeoxythymidine. Thus, the major promutagenic product responsible for induction of hepatocellular carcinomas by ethylating agents may be $O^4$-ethyldeoxythymidine.[57]

Azaserine causes DNA damage in the rat pancreas, as detected by alkaline sucrose gradient and alkaline elution techniques. However, in pyridoxal-deficient rats, it fails to induce such pancreatic DNA damage. Furthermore, the pyridoxal antagonist 4'-deoxypyridoxine inhibits the initiation of pancreatic carcinogenesis in azaserine-treated rats.[58] These studies confirm the relationship of the induction of DNA damage by azaserine to its ability to induce pancreatic tumors and support earlier findings that azaserine metabolism *in vivo* is pyridoxal dependent. A comparison of biochemical effect of azaserine in different species (rats, mice, hamster, and guinea pigs), however, indicates that neither the degree nor the persistence of DNA damage shows any correlation with the differing responses of these species to induction of preneoplastic and neoplastic pancreatic lesions by azaserine.[59]

## 3.3.2. Oncogene Activation

The origin, nature, and mechanisms of activation of the cellular oncogenes that have sequence homology to the transforming genes of known retroviruses have been the subject of extensive recent reviews.[60,61] These genes exist in all mammalian cells and apparently function in various regulatory mechanisms that normally control cellular proliferation, by encoding proteins that function as (1) growth factors; (2) transmembrane receptors for growth factors and other protein kinases that are either tyrosine-specific or serine-threonine specific; (3) intracytoplasmic regulatory proteins that bind GTP or GDP; or (4) intranuclear regulatory proteins. (These genes are treated in more detail in Chapters 13, 14, and 20.) Some are found as activated (transforming) variants in a proportion of human tumors, but *not* in normal tissues of the same individual. Homologous genes are similarly present in some carcinogen-induced tumors of experimental animals, but not in non-neoplastic tissues of carcinogen-treated tumor-bearing individuals. They must have appeared in the course of development of the tumors in which they are found and may reasonably be considered to have played a role in the growth of those neoplasms.

Oncogenes in their activated forms are usually detected by their ability to induce multilayered transformed foci after transfection of tumor-derived DNA into subconfluent monolayers of NIH 3T3 mouse fibroblasts. Activation of cellular oncogenes (proto-oncogenes) to transforming genes is known to occur by a variety of mechanisms. These mechanisms can be grouped into two functional categories: (1) increased expression of an otherwise normal gene product, and (2) expression of an altered gene product. Most oncogenes detected in chemically transformed rodent cells and chemically induced animal tumors by DNA transfection belong to members of the *ras* gene family; H-, K-, and N-*ras,* all of which encode closely related GDP/GTP-binding proteins of 21,000 $M_r$ designated p21. Several recent studies demonstrated that the *ras* oncogenes are commonly activated by a single point mutation in coding regions in either the 12th or the 61st codons. These codons appear to be hot spots for the activation of *ras* genes in primary rodent and human tumors. Altered protein products are produced that vary from the normal p21 by a single amino acid and have distinctly different electrophoretic mobilities. Because genotoxic carcinogens are mutagens, and because the known chemistry of some of these agents is consistent with the nature of the activating mutations found in *ras* genes in tumors, it may be that these specific genomic sequences are among the targets of chemical carcinogens that are significant in initiating or otherwise contributing to tumor development in certain tissues.

The expression and/or activation of certain oncogenes in tumor cells induced by chemical carcinogens varies with target organ and species, as well as the nature of the chemical carcinogen used to produce the tumors (Table III). Barbacid and co-workers[62,63] demonstrated that activated

### Table III. Activated Proto-Oncogenes in Different Tumors Induced by Chemical Carcinogens

| Chemical carcinogens[a] | Neoplasm | Activated oncogenes (incidence) | Activating mutation | References |
|---|---|---|---|---|
| | | Rats | | |
| NMU | Mammary carcinoma | H-*ras* (86%) | G → A, codon 12 | 62, 63 |
| DMBA | Mammary carcinoma | H-*ras* (23%) | codon 61 | 63 |
| 1,8-Dinitropyrene | Fibrosarcoma | K-*ras* (14%) | | 73 |
| Aflatoxin B₁ | Hepatocellular adenoma, carcinoma | K-*ras* (20%) | | 70, 87 |
| DMN-OMe | Kidney mesenchymal tumor | N-*ras* (4%), K-*ras* (40%) | [codon 12] | 71 |
| TNM | Lung carcinoma | K-*ras* (74%) | G → A | 74 |
| ENU | Schwannoma | *neu* (47%) | A → T | 78 |
| MMS | Nasal carcinoma | Unidentified | | 18 |
| | | Mice | | |
| DMBA | Skin carcinoma | H-*ras* (75%) | A → T, codon 61 | 67 |
| DMBA, TPA[b] | Skin papilloma | H-*ras* (90%) | A → T, codon 61 | 67, 82 |
| β-Propiolactone | Skin carcinoma | H-*ras* (40%) | | 18 |
| MCA | Fibrosarcoma | K-*ras* (50%) | | 72 |
| MCA | Thymic lymphoma | K-*ras* (83%) | | 83 |
| NMU | Lymphoma | N-*ras* (100%) | | 84 |
| DMBA | Mammary carcinoma | H-*ras* (75%) | A → T, codon 61 | 85 |
| N-OH-AAF | Hepatocellular carcinoma | H-*ras* (100%) | C → A, codon 61 | 69 |
| VC | Hepatocellular carcinoma | H-*ras* (100%) | A → T, codon 61 | 69 |
| HO-DHE | Hepatocellular carcinoma | H-*ras* (100%) | A → G, codon 61 | 69 |
| Furfural | Hepatocellular adenoma, carcinoma | H-*ras* (70%), K-*ras* (8%) | | 86 |
| TNM | Lung adenoma, carcinoma | K-*ras* (100%) | G → A | 74 |
| Furan | Hepatocellular adenoma, carcinoma | H-*ras* (78%), K-*ras* (15%) | | 86 |

[a] Abbreviations used: DMBA, 7,12-dimethylbenz[a]anthracene; TPA, 12-*O*-tetradecanoylphorbol-13-acetate; MCA, 3-methylcholanthrene; NMU, *N*-nitrosomethylurea; N-OH-AAF, *N*-hydroxy-2-acetylaminofluorene; VC, vinyl carbamate; HO-DHE, 1'-hydroxy-2'3'-dehydroestragole; TNM, tetranitromethane; DMN-OMe, *N*-nitrosomethylaminomethyl methyl ether; ENU, *N*-nitrosoethylurea; MMS, methyl methanesulfonate.
[b] DMBA initiation followed by TPA promotion.

H-*ras* oncogenes were present in virtually all mammary carcinomas induced by a direct-acting carcinogen, NMU, in young female rats. The mechanism of activation of this oncogene was shown to involve a single point mutation in codon 12. This is the same genetic alteration previously identified in the H-*ras* oncogene isolated from human tumors. Their studies, moreover, suggested that the single point mutation induced by NMU resulted from methylating the O-6 position of guanine, resulting in a G→A transition, and that this was probably responsible for activation of the rat H-*ras* oncogene to a transforming variant. In contrast to this finding with NMU, H-*ras* oncogenes present in mammary tumors induced in female rats by 7,12-dimethylbenz[a]anthracene (DMBA) did not possess mutations in the 12th codon but had undergone a mutation in the 61st codon, another hot spot in the *ras* genes.[63] This shift in location of the mutation with the inducing agent, within the same gene in the same variety of tumor in a single species, is one of the strongest arguments both for a mechanistic role of the oncogene involved and for direct chemical interaction of the carcinogen with cellular DNA encoding that oncogene.

Cellular homologues of the H-*ras* oncogene have been shown to be activated in papillomas and squamous cell carcinomas induced in mouse skin.[64,65] Pelling and co-workers[66] extend these studies further and showed that H-*ras* activation can occur in benign tumors or papillomas and that the enhanced expression of H-*ras* RNA was apparently not due to amplification of the murine H-*ras* proto-oncogene, since tumors possessed the same gene copy number present in untreated epidermis or in epidermis immediately following initiation and brief periods of promotion. Bizub and associates[67] induced skin carcinomas by repetitive applications of DMBA or by an initiation–promotion model using a single application of dibenz[c,h]acridine or benzo[a]pyrene (BP) followed by chronic treatment with 12-*O*-tetradecanoylphorbol-13-acetate (TPA). DNAs isolated from carcinomas induced by DMBA or dibenz[c,h]acridine, but not BP, transformed NIH 3T3 cells, and a high percentage of transformed foci (but not all) had an amplified H-*ras* gene. Furthermore, the amplified H-*ras* of the NIH 3T3 transformants and the primary carcinomas were found to have an A→T transversion in the second position of the 61st codon. These results show two additional classes of hydrocarbon-induced squamous carcinomas: tumors whose DNA efficiently transform 3T3 cells but lack mutated *ras* genes, and tumors whose DNA fail to transform 3T3 cells.

In the spontaneous hepatomas of B6C3F$_1$ mice, H-*ras* oncogenes are activated by random mutations in the first two nucleotides of codon 61.[68] Activation of H-*ras* oncogenes has also been demonstrated in the hepatomas induced by three different carcinogens: *N*-hydroxy-2-acetylaminofluorene (*N*-OH-AAF), vinyl carbamate, or 1'-hydroxy-2',3'-dehydroestragole. One such tumor also contained an activated K-*ras* gene. The activating mutations in most tumors were localized in the 61st codon of the cellular H-*ras* oncogene. Moreover, an AT→TA transversion at the second position of codon 61 was detected in DNA from many of the vinyl carbamate-induced hepatomas, a CG→AT transversion at the first position of the 61st codon was observed in *N*-OH-AAF-induced hepatomas, while AT→GC transitions at the second position of codon 61 were the activating mutations in 1'-hydroxy-2',3'-dehydroestragole-induced tumors.[69] By contrast, spontaneous liver tumors in Fischer rats show no evidence of activated oncogenes. However, when such tumors were induced by the carcinogen aflatoxin B$_1$, activated K-*ras* oncogenes could be detected in some DNAs from these tumors.[70]

Recently, activated cellular K-*ras* and N-*ras* oncogenes were detected in *N*-methyl-*N*-methoxymethylnitrosamine-induced mesenchymal kidney tumors in rats.[71] Activated oncogenes (unidentified) have also been found in nasal carcinomas induced by methyl methanesulfonate in rats.[18] In some fibrosarcomas induced by either 3-methylcholanthrene (MCA) in mice or by 1,8-dinitropyrene in rats, activated K-*ras* oncogenes were detected.[72,73] Activation of K-*ras* oncogenes was recently demonstrated in lung tumors from rats and mice chemically exposed to tetranitromethane.[74] Thus, long-term chronic exposure to a carcinogen is capable of reproducibly activating oncogenes similar to those observed in both single-dose and initiation–promotion models. A K-*ras* oncogene was also detected in human lung tumors in an earlier study.[75] These human and rodent data on the activation of the K-*ras* oncogene in the lung suggest a tissue-specific activation of a particular proto-oncogene.

The *neu* oncogene was originally isolated from cultured rat cell lines derived from ENU-induced intracranial tumors believed to be of central nervous system (CNS) origin.[76] Activation of *neu* was shown to result from a consistent specific T→A transversion in the sequence that encodes the transmembrane region of the *neu* gene product.[77] By contrast, activated *neu* oncogene sequences were recently detected in ENU-induced rat tumors of the peripheral nervous system (schwannomas), but not in tumors of the CNS.[78]

The respective roles played by carcinogenic initiators and noncarcinogenic promoters in influencing the activation of H-*ras* proto-oncogenes at various stages of tumorigenesis have recently been investigated in mouse skin and to some extent in mouse and rat liver.[60,61] Balmain and co-workers were first to show that cellular H-*ras* oncogene activation occurs in DMBA-TPA-induced skin tumors (papillomas).[64,65] This observation implies that *ras* activation is an early event in mouse skin carcinogenesis. Similar observations were made by Pelling and associates,[66] who demonstrated enhanced expression of H-*ras* proto-oncogenes in TPA-promoted papillomas as early as 7 weeks after initiation. As papillomas progressed under the influence of continued promotion with TPA, the incidence of H-*ras* expression decreased. The concept that an activated *ras* gene is the initiating event, necessary but not sufficient for the causation of squamous papillomas in mice, finds further support from recent *in vitro* studies in which infection of epidermal skin cells with Harvey–MSV (murine sarcoma virus) was found to generate initiated cells that did not express neoplastic properties unless they were subsequently treated with the promoter TPA.[79]

Activated *ras* genes have been identified in spontaneous as well as in chemically induced hepatocellular adenomas in mice; the presence of an activated H-*ras* oncogene in benign liver tumors indicates that *ras* gene activation can occur at a premalignant stage of liver tumor development.[68,69] The detection of activated K-*ras* genes in benign mouse lung tumors also suggests that activation of this gene may be an early event in tetranitromethane-induced lung tumors.[74]

The accumulating evidence tends to support the argument that the activated *ras* genes can participate in the initiation of chemical carcinogenesis, at least in certain tissues. The evidence is based mainly on the observations that mouse skin papillomas contain mutated H-*ras* genes at early stages. Moreover, other studies have suggested that activation of *ras* proto-oncogenes may also play a part in the progression of some tumors toward a more malignant phenotype (see Chapter 10). Introduction of *myc* or the Ela oncogene of adenovirus 5 makes it possible for primary embryo fibroblast cells to grow indefinitely in culture, while the *ras* oncogene appears to be responsible for the final neoplastic transformation of the cultured cells.[80] Newbold and Overell[81] showed that mutationally activated human H-*ras* can transform primary diploid hamster fibroblasts only if those cells have been immortalized previously by treatment with chemical carcinogens. These observations suggest that, under certain circumstances, *ras* genes may also participate in the promotion of neoplastic development.

## 4. ORGAN AND SPECIES SPECIFICITY IN TUMOR PROMOTION

Extensive research in experimental animals during the past four decades has shown that chemical carcinogenesis frequently involves separate steps of initiation and promotion. This phenomenon was first demonstrated during the early 1940s in rabbit skin by Rous and associates and in mouse skin by Berenblum and Motram.[88] Subsequent studies by Berenblum and Shubik and by Boutwell provided strong support for the multistage mechanism of skin carcinogenesis in mice.[88]

Tumor promoters, in the strict sense, are specific substances, for the most part organic compounds of low molecular weight, that by nongenotoxic mechanism(s) magnify the effect of a genotoxic carcinogen if given after exposure to the genotoxic substance, or initiator. The sequence of exposures is essential to the definition. Many potent promoters may have a very different effect if given concurrently with a genotoxic compound. Phenobarbital (PB), for example, a promoter of hepatocellular carcinogenesis, may so modify metabolism of many carcinogens that it effectively induces detoxification enzymes and reduces, rather than increases, the carcinogenicity of some carcinogenic compounds with which it has been given concurrently.[89] The nongenotoxic mechanism(s) also appear essential to the definition, although this point is currently a subject of debate. Genotoxic carcinogens, given in combination or sequentially, commonly have an additive or even synergistic effect on target tissues that are vulnerable to all agents in the combination; to include them as promoters or to speak of such agents as being both initiating and promoting for a given target tissue is to confuse the issue and to dilute the values of an important concept to such an extent that it loses all meaning.[90]

A useful unifying hypothesis, demonstrable by a number of methods that can be applied to cells in monolayer culture, is that tumor promoters as a group inhibit or block intercellular communication mediated via exchange of substances through gap junctions between cells.[91] Nearly all kinds of cells have gap junctions, but tumor promotion as defined by quantitative *in vivo* experiments is limited to epithelia. Isolated published studies indicate an enhancement by known promoters of carcinogenesis in cells of mesenchymal origin, but this data base is too limited to analyze. Tumor promoters are generally also very selective, affecting a single kind of epithelium or, exceptionally, several. Most promoters that are effective on mouse skin are effective in other squamous epithelia (vagina, forestomach, esophagus), but to a limited or negligible extent in nonsquamous epithelia; this division serves as a convenient framework for discussing organ and species specificity.

Susceptibility to tumor promoters is genetically controlled, varying widely both among species and among inbred strains or outbred individuals within a species.

## 4.1. Promotion in Squamous Epithelia

The prototypes of all tumor promoters, and the active ingredient of the natural product, croton oil, is 12-*O*-tetradecanolyphorbol-13-acetate (TPA), which elicits squamous papillomas when applied repeatedly to the skin of mice previously exposed to a genotoxic initiator at that site (or, less efficiently, exposed systemically—even transplacentally during fetal life). In the model of initiation and promotion proposed by Boutwell,[88,92] promotion in mouse skin was divided into two phases: conversion (of a latent, nonproliferating initiated cell to an autonomous neoplastic cell) and propagation (of the neoplastic cell to form first a clone and then a tumor). Accordingly, croton oil could act as a converting agent, and turpentine, an inducer of cell proliferation in the mouse skin, would bring about propagation. This model of two-stage promotion (so far applicable only to mouse skin) was later refined by Slaga, who used SENCAR mice, TPA as a converting agent (stage I), and mezerein as a propagating agent (stage II).[93] Recently, Japanese workers isolated many new classes of compounds from plants, microorganisms, marine blue algae, and coelenterates that possess strong tumor-promoting activity (with both converting and propagating capacity) in mouse skin[93–97] (Table IV).

Phorbol esters were initially believed to be promoters only for mouse skin, but several reports now suggest that these compounds are active promoters for other squamous epithelia in the mouse, including forestomach and vagina, and possibly certain nonsquamous epithelia such as colon as well. Phorbol esters are now thought to act by activating protein kinase C in target tissues (see Chapter 18).

Shubik in 1950[98] reported that the skins of rats, guinea pigs, and rabbits are resistant to two-stage skin carcinogenesis. However, using higher doses of DMBA and TPA, Goerttler and colleagues were able to induce skin tumors in rats that included epithelial (fibroepitheliomas, squamous cell carcinomas) as well as nonepithelial tumors (sarcomas).[99] Exposure to DMBA alone resulted in development of similar skin tumors in some rats in this system. Experiments with hamsters, using intragastric initiation with DMBA followed by repeated topical applications of either TPA or benzoyl peroxide, reportedly led to the appearance of melanotic melanomas,[100] but this observation has not yet been independently confirmed.

Rats and hamsters, unlike mice, are relatively resistant to two-stage skin carcinogenesis. TPA induces many morphologic and biochemical effects in the mouse skin, including hyperplasia, induction of ornithine decarboxylase, and stimulation of protein kinase C. Siskin and Barret[101] showed that a single treatment with TPA induces hyperplasia in hamster skin, but this responsiveness is lost after multiple treatments. Shoyab and associates[102] reported that the resistance of rat and hamster skin to TPA promotion may be related to the high levels of phorbol diester-inactivating enzyme in the skin tissue in these species. No other factors have been carefully studied that would account for the resistance of these species to two-stage skin carcinogenesis.

*Table IV. Tumor-Promoting Activity of Different Chemicals for Squamous Epithelia in Rodents[a]*

| Compound | Tissues and organs affected | | | References |
|---|---|---|---|---|
| | Mouse | Rat | Syrian hamster | |
| TPA | Skin | Skin | Skin–dermal melanocytes | 93, 99, 100 |
| | Forestomach, vagina, colon | Neg/skin | Neg/skin | 88 |
| Teleocidin | Skin, forestomach | NT[b] | NT | 94, 95 |
| Lyngbyatoxin A | Skin | NT | NT | 94 |
| Des-*O*-methylolivoretin C | Skin | NT | NT | 96 |
| Aplysiatoxin | Skin | NT | NT | 94 |
| Thapsigargin | Skin | NT | NT | 97 |
| Benzoyl peroxide | Skin | NT | Skin–dermal melanocytes | 93, 100 |
| Anthralin | Skin | NT | NT | 93 |
| 1-Fluoro-2,4-dinitrobenzene | Skin | NT | NT | 93 |
| Palytoxin | Skin | NT | NT | 96 |
| Polyhalogenated hydrocarbons (PCB, PBB, TCDD, α-HCH) | Liver, skin (TCDD) | Liver | NT | 103 |
| Di(2-ethylhexyl)phthalate | Liver, skin[c] | Neg | NT | 104 |
| BHA | Neg | Forestomach | Forestomach | 105 |

[a]Abbreviations used: TPA, 12-*O*-tetradecanoylphorbol-13-acetate; PCB, polychlorinated biphenyls; PBB, polybrominated biphenyls; TCDD, 2,3,7,8-tetrachlorodibenzo-*p*-dioxin; α-HCH, α-hexachlorocyclohexane; BHA, butylated hydroxyanisole.
[b]NT, not tested.
[c]Second stage only.

In the course of studies on promotion in tissues other than skin, a number of compounds with structures quite unlike that of TPA have been found to have promoting activity for mouse skin[74,103,104] or for other squamous epithelia in other species[105] (Table IV). It remains to be seen whether the capacity of such agents to promote in both squamous and selected nonsquamous epithelia reflects the capacity to act via more than one mechanism.

## 4.2. Promotion in Nonsquamous Epithelia

The concept of two-stage carcinogenesis is valid not only in mouse skin but in several other organs and tissues of both rats and mice. In 1971, Peraino and associates first discovered that an anticonvulsant drug, phenobarbital (PB), is an effective promoter of hepatocarcinogenesis initiated by 2-AAF in rats.[89] Since then, many other agents have been shown to enhance carcinogenesis in hepatocytes and in other tissues and organ systems (Tables V and VI). For example, two dietary sweeteners, saccharin and cyclamate, and certain metabolites of tryptophan promote bladder carcinogenesis in rats.[106] Similarly, high-fat diet and a number of bile acids have been shown to promote colon carcinogenesis in rats and mice.[107] This list is getting longer each year as several laboratories all over the world are routinely testing newer and hitherto untested chemical agents for tumor-promoting activity in different organs.

Phenobarbital, a long-acting barbiturate sedative and anticonvulsant, has been widely used as a promoter of hepatocarcinogenesis in rats and mice (Table V). Unlike the rat and the mouse, in the Syrian hamster, liver parenchymal cells were totally resistant to the tumor-promoting effects of PB.[108] DDT, another strong liver tumor promoter in rats and mice, also failed to promote liver carcinogenesis in hamsters.[109] On the other hand, in *Patas* monkeys, PB is also found to promote hepatocarcinogenesis initiated by DEN.[110] In rats and mice, PB is known to increase liver weight (and size) and to induce NADPH cytochrome P-450 reductase and one or more species of cytochrome P-450 together with associated monooxygenase activity toward a wide variety of substances. Nims et al.[111] recently showed that a good correlation exists between tumor-promoting activity of various barbiturate derivatives[112,113] and their abilities to induce PB-specific cytochrome P-450II B1. In hamsters, although PB enhanced total cytochrome P-450 activity. no significant increase was observed in liver weight, PB-specific cytochrome P-450, or aminopyrine N-demethylase activities.[108] The correlation of hepatic cytochrome P-450II B1 inducibility with promotion of hepatocarcinogenesis and its possibility as a marker for susceptibility to tumor promotion require further study.

The promoting ability of PB is not restricted to liver alone, as it has also proved to be a strong promoter of thyroid follicular epithelium in the rat. Sodium PB, but not PB itself, has been shown to promote bladder carcinogenesis in rats.[114] Barbital (5,5-diethylbarbituric acid), which is struc-

### Table V. Tumor-Promoting Activity of Different Chemicals for Nonsquamous Epithelia[a] in Rodents

| Compound | Tissues and organs affected[b] | | | |
| | Mouse | Rat | Syrian hamster | References |
| --- | --- | --- | --- | --- |
| Drugs | | | | |
| Phenobarbital | Liver, thyroid | Liver, thyroid | Neg/liver | 89, 108 |
| Sodium phenobarbital | Liver | Liver, thyroid, bladder | NT | 114 |
| Sodium barbital | Liver, kidney | Liver, thyroid, bladder, kidney[c] | NT | 115 |
| Aprobarbital | NT | Liver | NT | 112 |
| Allobarbital | NT | Liver | NT | 112 |
| Pentobarbital | NT | Liver, thyroid | NT | 113 |
| Nirvanol | NT | Liver, thyroid | NT | 117 |
| Hypolipidemic drugs (clofibrate, nafenopin, WY-14,643) | Liver | Liver | NT | 112 |
| Diazepam | Liver | Neg/liver | NT | 118, 120 |
| Oxazepam | Liver | Liver | NT | 119 |
| Suxibuzone | NT | Liver | NT | 123 |
| Miscellaneous compounds | | | | |
| 5-Azacytidine | NT | Liver | NT | 124 |
| DDT | Liver | Liver | Neg/liver | 103 |
| TCPOBOP | Liver | Neg/liver | NT | 125 |
| Estrogens (estradiol, mestranol) | Liver | Liver | NT | 103 |
| Progestins (progesterone, cyproterone acetate) | Liver | Liver | NT | 103 |
| BHT | Lung | Liver | NT | 103 |
| Ethoxyquin | NT | Kidney, bladder | NT | 105 |
| N-(3,5-dichlorophenyl) succinimide | NT | Kidney | NT | 126 |
| β-Cyclodextrin | NT | Kidney | NT | 127 |
| Potassium bromate | NT | Kidney | NT | 128 |
| Lead acetate | NT | Kidney | NT | 126 |

[a]Abbreviations used: DDT. dichlorodiphenyltrichloroethane; TCPOBOP, 1,4-bis[2-(3,5-dichloropyridyloxy)]benzene; BHT, butylated hydroxytoluene; NT, not tested.
[b]Liver = hepatocytes; thyroid = follicular epithelium; kidney = cortical proximal tubular epithelium (except where otherwise noted); bladder = urothelium (transitional epithelium).
[c]Cortical proximal tubular epithelium and pelvic transitional urothelium.

*Table VI. Dietary Factors and Additives That Enhance Carcinogenesis in Rodents*

| Compound or diets | Species | | | References |
| | Mouse | Rat | Syrian hamster | |
|---|---|---|---|---|
| Bile acids (deoxy-cholic acid, cheno-deoxycholate) | NT | Colon, liver | NT | 107 |
| Choline-deficient diet | Liver | Liver | NT | 129 |
| L-Isoleucine, L-leucine | NT | Bladder | NT | 130 |
| Sodium ascorbate | NT | Bladder | NT | 105 |
| Sodium erythrobate | NT | Bladder | NT | 105 |
| Folic acid | NT | Kidney | NT | 126 |
| DL-Serine | NT | Kidney | NT | 131 |
| Orotic acid | NT | Liver, intestine | NT | 132 |
| High-fat diet | Liver, colon, mammary gland | Liver, colon, mammary gland, pancreas | Pancreas | 107 |
| Raw soybean protein | Neg/pancreas | Pancreas | Neg/pancreas | 38 |
| Pancreaticotropic peptides (bombesin, caerulein) | NT | Pancreas | NT | 39 |
| Nicotinamide | Kidney | Kidney | NT | 133 |
| Iodine-deficient diet | NT | Thyroid | NT | 134 |
| Saccharin, cyclamate, tryptophan derivatives | Bladder | Bladder | NT | 106 |

*a*NT: Not tested.

turally similar to PB (5-ethyl-5-phenylbarbituric acid), is found to be a broad-spectrum tumor promoter in rats, as it promotes tumor development in liver, thyroid, kidney, and urinary bladder.[115,116] Pentobarbital also promotes carcinogenesis in both the liver and thyroid of rats, while most other barbiturate derivatives were active only in liver. Nirvanol (5-ethyl-5-phenylhydantoin), a structural analogue of PB, was likewise effective in promoting both liver and thyroid carcinogenesis in rats.[117] Some bile acids have been shown to promote tumor development in both the colon and liver. However, most promoters are active at only one site. For example, tumor-promoting activity of saccharin and other sweeteners appears to be restricted to bladder urothelium.[106]

The most widely used benzodiazepine tranquilizers, diazepam and oxazepam, promote liver carcinogenesis in mice.[118] Oxazepam,[119] but not diazepam,[120] is also a liver tumor promoter in rats. In mice, diazepam, an effective liver tumor promoter, is metabolized by two successive P-450-mediated oxidative steps, $N$-demethylation and $N$-$\alpha$-C-hydroxylation, to produce oxazepam which in turn is further metabolized only by conjugation reactions.[115] Diazepam, which does not promote hepatocarcinogenesis in rats, is metabolized differently in the rat than in the mouse.[121,122] In the rat, the N-demethylation step is replaced by hydroxylation of the phenyl substituent, resulting in the formation of polar phenolic derivatives of diazepam. Very little desmethyldiazepam and no oxazepam is detectable in the urine or feces of rats after intraperitoneal or oral administration of this drug. This difference in the metabolism (detoxification and elimination) of diazepam could account for the observed differences in tumor-promoting activity of this drug between these two species. It is of interest that the predominant metabolic path for diazepam in humans is the same as that seen in mice.

During the course of our studies on the promotion of hepatocarcinogenesis in mice,[104,118] we found some significant differences in the promotion process between this species and the rat. Promotion of hepatocellular carcinogenesis in mice by both PB and the benzodiazepine derivatives strongly suggests an acceleration of the overall neoplastic process. In mice, foci tend to progress to adenomas and adenomas to carcinomas more inexorably than do comparable lesions in rats. The neoplastic process was qualitatively more advanced and quantitatively more extensive in promoted mice than in mice that had been given DEN alone. This contrasts with the promoting effects of PB in rats initiated with 2-AAF,[89,114] in which increasing the dose of the promoter increased the final tumor yield but did not affect the time of onset or attainment of the plateau phase of tumor promotion. Thus, in rats PB does not appear to influence the character of the neoplastic phenotype or the kinetics of its expression. The kinetics of expression of the DEN-initiated neoplastic phenotype in mice clearly are affected by PB and the benzodiazepines, and the promotion phenomenon in this species is at least in this respect different from that in rats.

A substantial number of other drugs and miscellaneous chemicals have also been shown to promote carcinogenesis in nonsquamous epithelia in rodents (Table V). Many of these, such as suxibuzone,[123] 5-azacytidine,[124] and 1,4 bis[2-(3,5-dichloropyridyloxy)]benzene,[125] are specific for hepatocellular tumor promotion in rats or mice or both. Others, including ethoxyquin,[105] $N$-(3,5-dichlorophenyl)succinimide,[126] $\beta$-cyclodextrin,[127] and certain inorganic salts, such as potassium bromate[128] and lead acetate,[126] appear to be specific for the kidney or the bladder, at least in rats. It is to be expected that more such substances will be identified. Evaluating their potential risk to humans will most likely require clarification of the mechanisms of action by which these diverse substances promote carcinogenesis in rodents.

It is generally found that tumor promoters are weakly active in long-term bioassays and thus appear to be carcinogens by the purely phenomenologic meaning of the term. This may occur because a significant number of cells become initiated naturally in the course of a lifetime in the rodents used for bioassays, and exposure to a promoter increases the probability that such cells will proliferate to generate tumors.

## 4.3. Dietary Factors That Promote Carcinogenesis

Not only foreign substances (xenobiotics), but also diets that are seriously deficient or excessive in certain nutrients may enhance carcinogenesis in certain organs (Table VI). Diets deficient in choline[129] or that contain large excesses of the amino acids leucine,[130] isoleucine,[130] or serine,[131] or of other substances including orotic acid[132] or nicotinamide,[133] have definite enhancing effects that are methodologically indistinguishable from those of promotion by drugs or miscellaneous chemicals. These effects may well be mediated by a variety of metabolic derangements and are likely to differ mechanistically from promotion by xenobiotics. Dietary iodine deficiency is both goitrogenic and promoting for thyroid follicular epithelium in rats[134] and provides possibly the closest linkage between experimental tumor promotion studies in rodents and actual human experience.

ACKNOWLEDGMENT. This project was funded in part with federal funds from the Department of Health and Human Services under contract NO1-CO-74102. The content of this publication does not necessarily reflect the views or policies of the Department of Health and Human Services, nor does mention of trade names, commercial products, or organizations imply endorsement by the U.S. government.

## REFERENCES

1. Peto, J., Seidman, H., and Selikoff, I. J., 1982, Mesothelioma mortality in asbestos workers: Implications for models of carcinogenesis and risk assessments, *Br. J. Cancer* **45:**124–129.
2. IARC, 1973, Some inorganic and organometallic compounds. *IARC Monographs on the Evaluation of Carcinogenic Risk of Chemicals to Man,* Vol. 2, pp. 17–47, International Agency for Research on Cancer, Lyons, France.

3. Wilbourn, J., Haroun, L., Haseltine, E., Kaldor, J., Partensky, C., and Vainio, H., 1986, Responses of experimental animals to human carcinogens: An analysis based upon the IARC monographs program, *Carcinogenesis* **7**:1853–1863.

4. Clayson, D. B., and Garner, R. C., 1976, Carcinogenic aromatic amines and related compounds, in: *Chemical Carcinogens* (C. E. Searle, ed.), pp. 366–461, American Chemical Society, Washington, D.C.

5. IARC, 1974, Some aromatic amines, hydrazine and related substances, N-nitroso compounds, and miscellaneous alkylating agents. *IARC Monographs on the Evaluation of Carcinogenic Risk of Chemicals to Man*, Vol. 4, pp. 97–111, International Agency for Research on Cancer, Lyons, France.

6. Maltoni, C., 1977, Vinyl chloride carcinogenicity: An experimental model for carcinogenesis studies, in: *Origins of Human Cancer* (H. H. Hiatt, J. D. Watson, and J. A. Winsten, eds.), pp. 119–146, Cold Spring Harbor Laboratory, Cold Spring Harbor, New York.

7. Creech, J. L., and Johnson, M. N., 1974, Angiosarcomas of the liver in the manufacture of polyvinyl chloride, *J. Occup. Med.* **16**:150–153.

8. Weisburger, E. K., 1981, N-Substituted aryl compounds in carcinogenesis and mutagenesis, *Natl. Cancer Inst. Monog.* **58**:1–7.

9. So, B. H., and Wynder, E. L., 1972, Introduction of hamster tumors of the urinary bladder by 3,2′-dimethyl-4-aminobiphenyl, *J. Natl. Cancer Inst.* **48**:1733–1738.

10. Irving, C. C., Wieseman, J. R., and Young, J. M., 1967, Carcinogenicity of 2-acetylaminofluorene in the rabbit, *Cancer Res.* **27**:838–848.

11. Miller, E. C., Miller, J. A., and Enomoto, M., 1964, The comparative carcinogenicities of 2-acetylaminofluorene and its N-hydroxy metabolite in mice, hamsters, and guinea pigs, *Cancer Res.* **24**:2018–2031.

12. Thorgeirsson, S. S., 1984, Metabolic determinants in the carcinogenicity of aromatic amines, in: *Biochemical Basis of Chemical Carcinogenesis* (H. Geim, ed.), pp. 47–54, Raven, New York.

13. Cartwright, R. A., 1984, Epidemiological studies on N-acetylation and C-center oxidation in neoplasia, in: *Genetic Variability in Responses to Chemical Exposure, Banbury Reports*, Volume 16 (G. S. Omenn and H. V. Gelboin, eds.), pp. 359–365, Cold Spring Harbor Laboratory, Cold Spring Harbor, New York.

14. Van Duuren, B. L., Katz, C., Goldschmidt, M., Frenkel, K., and Sivak, A., 1972, Carcinogenicity of halo-ethers. II. Structure–activity relationships of analogs of bis(chloromethyl)ether, *J. Natl. Cancer Inst.* **48**:1431–1439.

15. Laskin, S., Kuschner, M., Drew, R. T., Cappiello, V. P., and Nelson, N., 1971, Tumors of the respiratory tract induced by inhalation of bis(chloromethyl)ether, *Arch. Environ. Health* **23**:135–136.

16. Leong, B. K. J., MacFarland, H. N., and Reese, W. H., Jr., 1971, Induction of lung adenomas by chronic inhalation of bis(chloromethyl)ether, *Arch. Environ. Health* **22**:663–666.

17. Bartsch, H., Terracokini, B., Malaveille, C., Tomatis, L., Wahrendorf, J., Burn, G., and Dodet, B., 1983, Quantitative comparison of carcinogenicity, mutagenicity, and electrophilicity of 10 direct-acting alkylating agents and the initial $O^6$ : 7 alkylguanine ratio in DNA with carcinogenic potency in rodents, *Mutat. Res.* **110**:181–219.

18. Garte, S. J., Hood, A. T., Hochwalt, A. E., D'Eustachio, P., Snyder, C. A., Segal, A., and Albert, R. E., 1985, Carcinogen specificity in the activation of transforming genes by direct-acting alkylating agents, *Carcinogenesis* **6**:1709–1712.

19. IARC, 1978, Some nitroso compounds, *IARC Monographs on the Evaluation of the Carcinogenic Risk of Chemicals to Humans*, Vol. 17, pp. 191–215, International Agency for Research on Cancer, Lyons, France.

20. Berman, J. J., and Rice, J. M., 1980, Odontogenic tumours produced in Fischer rats by a single intraportal injection of methylnitrosourea, *Arch. Oral Biol.* **25**:213–220.

21. Kleihues, P., Bucheler, J., and Riede, U. N., 1978, Selective induction of melanomas in gerbils (*Meriones unguiculatus*) following postnatal administration of N-ethyl-N-nitrosourea, *J. Natl. Cancer Inst.* **61**:859–863.

22. IARC, 1978, Some nitroso compounds, *IARC Monographs on the Evaluation of Carcinogenic Risk of Chemicals to Humans*, Vol. 17, pp. 227–255, International Agency for Research on Cancer, Lyons, France.

23. Thomas, C., Sierra, J. L., and Kersting, G., 1968, Neurogene Tumoren bei Ratten nach intraperitonealer Applikation von N-Nitroso-N-methyl-harnstoff, *Naturwissenschaften* **55**:183.

24. Swenberg, J. A., Koestner, A., and Wechsler, W., 1972, The induction of tumors of the nervous system with intravenous methylnitrosourea, *Lab. Invest.* **26**:75–85.

25. Joshi, V. V., and Frei, J. V., 1970, Effects of dose and schedule of methylnitrosourea on incidence of malignant lymphoma in adult female mice, *J. Natl. Cancer Inst.* **45**:335–339.

26. Reznik, G., Mohr, U., and Kmock, N., 1976, Carcinogenic effect of different nitroso-compounds in Chinese hamsters: *N*-dibutylnitrosamine and *N*-nitrosomethylurea, *Cancer Lett.* **1**:183–188.

27. Mohr, U., Haas, H., and Hilfrich, J., 1974, The carcinogenic effects of dimethylnitrosamine and nitrosomethylurea in European hamsters (*Cricetus cricetus* L.), *Br. J. Cancer* **29**:359–364.

28. Haas, H., Hilfrich, J., Kmoch, N., and Mohr, U., 1975, Specific carcinogenic effect of *N*-methyl-*N*-nitrosourea on the midventral sebaceous gland of the gerbil (*Meriones unguiculatus*), *J. Natl. Cancer Inst.* **55**:637–640.

29. Stavrou, D., Haglid, K. G., and Weidenbach, W., 1975, Experimentelle Induktion neurogener Tumoren beim Hund durch chronische parenterale Applikation von Methylnitrosoharnstoff, in: *Proceedings of the Eighth International Congress of Neuropathology, Budapest, 1974*, pp. 425–431, Excerpta Medica, Amsterdam.

30. Denlinger, R. J., Koestner, A., and Swenberg, J. A., 1978, Neoplasms in purebred boxer dogs following long-term administration of *N*-methyl-*N*-nitrosourea, *Cancer Res.* **38**:1711–1717.

31. Bots, G. T. A. M., and Willinghagen, R. G. T., 1975, Tumors in the mammary gland induced in Lewis rats by intravenous methylnitrosourea, *Br. J. Cancer* **31**:372–374.

32. Terracini, B., and Testa, M. C., 1970, Carcinogenicity of a single administration of *N*-nitrosomethylurea: A comparison between newborn and 5-week-old mice and rats, *Br. J. Cancer* **24**:588–598.

33. IARC, 1976, Some naturally occurring substances, *IARC Monographs on the Evaluation of Carcinogenic Risk of Chemicals to Man*, Vol. 10, pp. 73–77, International Agency for Research on Cancer, Lyons, France.

34. Roebuck, B. D., and Longnecker, D. S., 1977, Species and rat strain variation in pancreatic nodule induction by azaserine, *J. Natl. Cancer Inst.* **59**:1273–1278.

35. Roebuck, B. D., and Longnecker, D. S., 1979, Response of two rodents, *Mastomys natalensis* and *Mystromys albicaudatus*, to the pancreatic carcinogen, azaserine, *J. Natl. Cancer Inst.* **62**:1264–1272.

36. Stoner, G. D., Lonram, P. B., Greisiger, E. A., Stober, J., Morgan, M., and Pereira, M. A., 1986, Comparison of two routes of chemical administration on the lung adenoma response in strain A/J mice, *Toxicol. Appl. Pharmacol.* **82**:19–31.

37. Lhoste, E. F., Roebuck, B. D., Brinck-Johnsen, T., and Longnecker, D. S., 1987, Effect of castration and hormone replacement on azaserine-induced pancreatic carcinogenesis in male and female F344 rats, *Carcinogenesis* **8**:699–703.

38. Liener, I. E., and Hasdai, A., 1986, The effect of the long-term feeding of raw soy flour on the pancreas of the mouse and hamster, *Adv. Exp. Med. Biol.* **199**:189–197.

39. Lhoste, E. F., and Longnecker, D. S., 1987, Effect of bombesin and caerulein on the early stages of carcinogenesis induced by azaserine in the rat pancreas, *Cancer Res.* **47**:3273–3277.

40. IARC, 1978, Some N-nitroso compounds, *IARC Monographs on the Evaluation of the Carcinogenic Risk of Chemicals to Humans*, Vol. 17, pp. 83–124, International Agency for Research on Cancer, Lyons, France.

41. IARC, 1978, Some N-nitroso compounds, *IARC Monograph on the Evaluation of the Carcinogenic Risk of Chemicals to Humans*, Vol. 17, pp. 125–175, International Agency for Research on Cancer, Lyons, France.

42. Adamson, R. H., and Sieber, S. M., 1983, Chemical carcinogenesis studies in nonhuman primates, in: *Organ and Species Specificity in Chemical Carcinogenesis* (R. Langenbach, S. Nesnow, and J. M. Rice, eds.), pp. 129–156, Plenum, New York.

43. Hard, G. C., 1979, Effect of age at treatment on incidence and type of renal neoplasm induced in the rat by a single dose of dimethylnitrosamine, *Cancer Res.* **39**:4965–4970.

44. Lijinsky, W., 1983, Species specificity in nitrosamine carcinogenesis, in: *Organ and Species Specificity in Chemical Carcinogenesis* (R. Langenbach, S. Nesnow, and J. M. Rice, eds.), pp. 63–75, Plenum, New York.

45. Lijinsky, W., Saavedra, J. E., Nutsen, G. L., and Kovach, R. M., 1984, Comparison of the carcinogenic effectiveness of *N*-nitroso-bis(2-hydroxypropyl)amine, *N*-nitroso-bis(2-oxypropyl)amine, *N*-nitroso(2-hydroxypropyl(2-oxypropyl)amine and *N*-nitroso-2,6-dimethylmorpholine in Syrian hamsters, *J. Natl. Cancer Inst.* **72**:685–688.

46. Cardy, R. H., and Lijinsky, W., 1980, Comparison of the carcinogenic effects of five nitrosamines in guinea pigs, *Cancer Res.* **40**: 1879–1884.

47. Keefer, L. K., Anjo, T., Wade, D., Wang, T., and Yang, C. S., 1987, Concurrent generation of methylamine and nitrite during denitrosation of *N*-nitrosodimethylamine by rat liver microsomes, *Cancer Res.* **47**:447–452.

48. Michejda, C. J., Kroeger-Koepke, M. B., Koepke, S. R., Magee, P. N., and Chu, C., 1982, Nitrogen formation during *in vivo* and *in vitro* metabolism of *N*-nitrosamines, *Banbury Rep.* **12**:69–85.

49. Heath, D. F., and Dutton, A., 1958, The detection of metabolic products from dimethylnitrosamine in rats and mice, *Biochem. J.* **70:**619–626.

50. Preussmann, R., and Stewart, B. W., 1984, *N*-nitroso carcinogens, in: *Chemical Carcinogens*, 2nd ed. (C. E. Searle, ed.), pp. 643–828, American Chemical Society Monograph 182, American Chemical Society, Washington, D.C.

51. Kokkinakis, D. M., Scarpelli, D. G., Subbarao, V., and Hollenberg, P. F., 1987, Species differences in the metabolism of *N*-nitroso(2-hydroxypropyl)(2-oxypropyl)amine, *Carcinogenesis* **8:**295–303.

52. Kleihues, P., and Margison, G. P., 1974, Carcinogenicity of *N*-methyl-*N*-nitrosourea. Possible role of excision repair of $O^6$-methylguanine from DNA, *J. Natl. Cancer Inst.* **53:**1839–1842.

53. Margison, G. P., and Kleihues, P., 1975, Chemical carcinogenesis in the nervous system. Preferential accumulation of $O^6$-methylguanine in rat brain deoxyribonucleic acid during repetitive administration of *N*-methyl-*N*-nitrosourea, *Biochem. J.* **148:**521–525.

54. Kleihues, P., Hodgson, R. M., Veit, C., Schweinsberg, F., and Wiessler, M., 1983, DNA modification and repair *in vivo:* Towards a biochemical basis of organo-specific carcinogenesis by methylating agents, in: *Organ and Species Specificity in Chemical Carcinogenesis* (R. Langenbach, S. Nesnow, and J. M. Rice, eds.), pp. 509–528, Plenum, New York.

55. Kleihues, P., Magee, P. N., Austoker, J., Cox, D., and Mathias, A. P., 1973, Reaction of *N*-methyl-*N*-nitrosourea with DNA of neuronal and glial cells *in vivo*, *FEBS Lett.* **32:**105–108.

56. Pegg, A. E., 1984, Methylation of $O^6$ positions of guanine in DNA is the most likely initiating event in carcinogenesis by methylating agents, *Cancer Invest.* **2:**223–231.

57. Swenberg, J. A., Dyroff, M. C., Bedell, M. A., Popp, J. A., Huh, N., Kirstein, A., and Rajewsky, M. F., 1984, $O^4$-Ethyldeoxythymidine, but not $O^6$-ethyldeoxyguanosine, accumulates in DNA of hepatocytes of rats exposed continuously to diethylnitrosamine, *Proc. Natl. Acad. Sci. USA* **81:**1692–1695.

58. Zurlo, J., Roebuck, B. D., Rutkowski, J. V., Curphey, T. J., and Longnecker, D. S., 1984, Effect of pyridoxal deficiency on pancreatic DNA damage and nodule induction by azaserine, *Carcinogenesis* **5:**555–558.

59. Roebuck, B. D., Lilja, H. S., Curphey, T. J., and Longnecker, D. S., 1980, Pathological and biochemical effects of azaserine in inbred Wistar/Lewis rats and noninbred CD1 mice, *J. Natl. Cancer Inst.* **65:**383–389.

60. Bishop, J. M., 1983, Cellular oncogenes and retroviruses, *Annu. Rev. Biochem.* **52:**301–354.

61. Barbacid, M., 1987, *ras* Genes, *Annu. Rev. Biochem.* **56:**779–827.

62. Sukumar, S., Notario, V., Martin-Zanca, D., and Barbacid, M., 1983, Induction of mammary carcinomas in rats by nitrosomethylurea involves malignant activation of H-*ras*-1 locus by single point mutations, *Nature (Lond.)* **306:**658–661.

63. Zarbl, H., Sukumar, S., Arthur, A. V., Martin-Zanca, D., and Barbacid, M., 1985, Direct mutagenesis of H-*ras*-1 oncogenes by *N*-nitroso-*N*-methylurea during initiation of mammary carcinogenesis in rats, *Nature (Lond.)* **315:**382–385.

64. Balmain, A., and Pragneil, I. B., 1983, Mouse skin carcinomas induced *in vivo* by chemical carcinogens have a transforming Harvey-*ras* oncogene, *Nature (Lond.)* **303:**72–74.

65. Balmain, A., Ramsden, M., Bowden, G. T., and Smith, J., 1984, Activation of the mouse cellular Harvey-*ras* gene in chemically induced benign skin papillomas, *Nature (Lond.)* **307:**658–660.

66. Pelling, J. C., Ernst, S. M., Strawhecker, J. M., Johnson, J. A., Nairn, R. S., and Slaga, T. J., 1986, Elevated expression of Ha-*ras* is an early event in two stage skin carcinogenesis in SENCAR mice, *Carcinogenesis* **7:**1599–1602.

67. Bizub, D., Wood, A. W., and Skulka, A. M., 1986, Mutagenesis of the H-*ras* oncogene in mouse skin tumors induced by polycyclic aromatic hydrocarbons, *Proc. Natl. Acad. Sci. USA* **83:**6048–6052.

68. Reynolds, S. H., Stowers, S. J., Maronpot, R. R., Anderson, M. W., and Aaronson, S. A., 1986, Detection and identification of activated oncogenes in spontaneously occurring benign and malignant hepatocellular tumors of the B6C3F1 mouse, *Proc. Natl. Acad. Sci. USA* **83:**33–37.

69. Wiseman, R. W., Stowers, S. J., Miller, E. C., Anderson, M. W., and Miller, J. A., 1986, Activating mutations of the c-Ha-*ras* proto-oncogene in chemically induced hepatomas of the male B6C3F1 mouse, *Proc. Natl. Acad. Sci. USA* **83:**5825–5829.

70. McMahon, G., Hanson, L., Lee, J. J., and Wogan, G. N., 1986, Identification of an activated c-Ki-*ras* oncogene in rat liver tumors induced by aflatoxin $B_1$, *Proc. Natl. Acad. Sci. USA* **83:**9418–9422.

71. Sukumar, S., Perantoni, A., Reed, C., Rice, J. M., and Wenk, M., 1986, Activated K-*ras* and N-*ras* oncogenes in primary renal mesenchymal tumors induced in F344 rats by methyl(methoxymethyl)nitrosamine, *Mol. Cell. Biol.* **6:**2716–2720.

72. Eva, A., and Aaronson, S. A., 1983, Frequent activation of c-Ki-*ras* as a transforming gene in fibrosarcomas induced by methylcholanthrene, *Science* **220:**955–956.

73. Tahira, T., Hayashi, K., Ochiai, M., Tsuchidu, N., Nagao, M., and Sugimura, T., 1986, Structure of the c-K-*ras* gene in a rat fibrosarcoma induced by 1,8-dinitropyrene, *Mol. Cell. Biol.* **6:**1349–1351.

74. Stowers, S. J., Glover, P. L., Reynolds, S. H., Boone, L. R., Maronpot, R. R., and Anderson, M. W., 1987, Activation of the K-*ras* proto-oncogene in lung tumors from rats and mice chronically exposed to tetranitromethane, *Cancer Res.* **47:**3212–3219.

75. Santos, E., Martin-Zanca, D., Reddy, P., Pierotti, M., Della Porta, G., and Barbacid, M., 1984, Malignant activation of a K-*ras* oncogene in lung carcinoma but not in normal tissue of the same patient, *Science* **223:**661–664.

76. Schechter, A. L., Stern, D. F., Vaidyanathan, L., Decker, S. J., Drebin, J. A., Greene, M. I., and Weinberg, R. A., 1984, The *neu* oncogene: An erb-B-related gene encoding a 185,000-$M_r$ tumor antigen, *Nature (Lond.)* **312:**513–516.

77. Bargmann, C., Hung, M., and Weinberg, R., 1986, Multiple independent activations of the *neu* oncogene by a point mutation altering the transmembrane domain of p185, *Cell* **45:**644–657.

78. Perantoni, A. O., Rice, J. M., Reed, C. D., Watatani, M., and Wenk, M. L., 1987, Activated *neu* oncogene sequence in primary tumors of the peripheral nervous system induced in rats by transplacental exposure to ethylnitrosourea, *Proc. Natl. Acad. Sci. USA* **84:**6317–6321.

79. Brown, K., Quintanilla, M., Ramsden, M., Kerr, I. B., Young, S., and Balmain, A., 1986, V-*ras* genes from Harvey and BALB murine sarcoma viruses can act as initiators of two-stage mouse skin carcinogenesis, *Cell* **46:**447–456.

80. Kinsella, A. R. and Radman, M., 1978, Tumor promoter induces sister chromatid exchanges: Relevance to mechanisms of carcinogenesis, *Proc. Natl. Acad. Sci. USA* **75:**6149–6153.

81. Newbold, R. F., and Overell, R. W., 1983, Fibroblast immortality is a prerequisite to transformation by EJ c-Ha-*ras* oncogene, *Nature (Lond.)* **304:**468–651.

82. Quintanilla, M., Brown, K., Ramsden, M., and Balmain, A., 1986, Carcinogen-specific mutation and amplification of Ha-*ras* during mouse skin carcinogenesis, *Nature (Lond.)* **322:**78–80.

83. Eva, A., and Trimmer, R. W., 1986, High frequency of c-K-*ras* activation in 3-methylcholanthrene-induced mouse thymomas, *Carcinogenesis* **7:**1931–1933.

84. Guerrero, I., Calzada, P., Mayer, A., and Pellicer, A., 1984, A molecular approach to leukemogenesis: mouse lymphomas contain an activated c-*ras* oncogene, *Proc. Natl. Acad. Sci. USA* **81:**202–205.

85. Dandekar, S., Sukumar, S., Zarbl, H., Young, L. J., and Cardiff, R. D., 1986, Specific activation of the cellular Harvey-*ras* oncogene in dimethylbenzanthracene-induced mouse mammary tumors, *Mol. Cell. Biol.* **6:**4104–4108.

86. Reynolds, S. H., Stowers, S. J., Patterson, R. M., Maronpot, R. R., Arronson, S. A., and Anderson, M. W., 1987, Activated oncogenes in B6C3F1 mouse liver tumors: Implications for risk assessment, *Science* **237:**1309–1316.

87. McMahon, G., Davis, E., and Wogan, G. N., 1987, Characterization of c-K-*ras* oncogene alleles by direct sequencing of enzymatically amplified DNA from carcinogen-induced tumors, *Proc. Natl. Acad. Sci. USA* **84:**4974–4978.

88. Montesano, R., and Slaga, T. J., 1983, Initiation and promotion in carcinogenesis: An appraisal, *Cancer Surv.* **2:**613–621.

89. Peraino, C., Fry, R. J., and Staffeldt, E., 1971, Reduction and enhancement by phenobarbital of hepatocarcinogenesis induced in the rat by 2-acetylaminofluorene, *Cancer Res.* **31:**1506–1512.

90. Williams, G. M., and Furuya, K., 1984, Distinction between liver neoplasm promoting and syncarcinogenic effects demonstrated by exposure to phenobarbital or diethylnitrosamine either before or after *N*-2-fluorenylacetamide, *Carcinogenesis* **5:**171–174.

91. Chen, T.-H., Kavanagh, T. J., Chang, C. C., and Trosko, J. E., 1984, Inhibition of metabolic cooperation in Chinese hamster V79 cells by various organic solvents and simple compounds, *Cell Biol. Toxicol.* **1:**155–171.

92. Boutwell, R. K., 1964, Some biological aspects of skin carcinogenesis, *Progr. Exp. Tumor Res.* **4:**207–250.

93. Slaga, T. J., 1983, Cellular and molecular mechanisms of tumor promotion, *Cancer Surv.* **2:**595–612.

94. Fujiki, H., and Sugimura, T., 1983, New potent tumor promoters: Teleocidin, lyngbyatoxin A and aplysiatoxin, *Cancer Surv.* **2:**539–556.

95. Suganuma, M., Fujiki, H., Morino, K., Takayama, S., and Sugimura, T., 1987, Tumor producing activity of teleocidin in skin and forestomach of mice initiated transplacentally with 7,12-dimethylbenz(a)-anthracene, *J. Cancer Res. Clin. Oncol.* **113:**123–125.

96. Nimomiya, M., Fujiki, H., Paik, N. S., Hakii, H., Suganuma, M., Hitotsuyanagi, Y., Aimi, N., Sakai, S., Endo, Y., Shudo, K., and Sugimura, T., 1986, Des-*O*-methylolivoretin C is a new member of the teleocidin class of tumor promoters, *Jpn. J. Cancer Res.* **77:**222–225.

97. Fujiki, H., Suganuma, M., Nakayasu, M., Hakii, H., Horiuchi, T., Takayama, S., and Sugimura, T., 1986, Palytoxin is a non-12-O-tetradecanoylphorbol-13-acetate type tumor promoter in two-stage mouse skin carcinogenesis, *Carcinogenesis* **7**:707–710.

98. Shubik, P., 1950, Studies on the promoting phase in the stages of carcinogenesis in mice, rabbits and guinea pigs, *Cancer Res.* **10**:13–17.

99. Goerttler, K., Loehrke, H., Schweizer, J., and Hesse, B., 1980, Positive two stage carcinogenesis in female Sprague-Dawley rats using DMBA as initiator and TPA as promoter, *Virchows Arch.* **385**:181–186.

100. Schweizer, J., Loehrke, H., Edler, L., and Goerttler, K., 1987, Benzoyl peroxide promotes the formation of melanotic tumors in the skin of 7,12-dimethylbenz[a]anthracene-initiated Syrian golden hamsters, *Carcinogenesis* **8**:479–482.

101. Siskin, E. E., and Barret, J. C., 1987, Hyperplasia of Syrian hamster epidermis induced by single but not multiple treatments with 12-O-tetradecanoylphorbol-13-acetate, *Cancer Res.* **41**:346–350.

102. Shoyab, M., Warren, T. C., and Todaro, C. J., 1982, Phorbol 12,13-diester, 12-ester hydrolase may prevent tumor promotion by phorbol diesters in skin, *Nature (Lond.)* **295**:152–154.

103. Schulte-Hermann, R., 1985, Tumor promotion in liver, *Arch. Toxicol.* **57**:147–158.

104. Ward, J. M., Rice, J. M., Creasia, D., Lynch, P., and Riggs, C., 1983, Dissimilar patterns of promotion by di(2-ethylhexyl)phthalate and phenobarbital of hepatocellular neoplasia initiated by diethylnitrosamine in B6C3F1 mice, *Carcinogenesis* **4**:1021–1029.

105. Ito, N., Fukushima, S., and Tsuda, H., 1986, Carcinogenicity and modification of the carcinogenic response by BHA, BHT, and other antioxidants, in: *CRC Critical Reviews in Toxicology*, Vol. 15 (D. B. Clayson, D. Krewski, and I. Munro, eds.), pp. 109–149, CRC Press, Boca Raton, Florida.

106. Hicks, M. R., 1982, Promotion in bladder cancer, in: *Carcinogenesis and Biological Effects of Tumor Promoters*, Vol. 7 (E. Hecker, N. E. Fusenig, W. Kunz, F. Marks, and H. W. Thielman, eds.), pp. 139–154, Raven, New York.

107. Narisawa, T., Magadia, N. E., Weisburger, J. H., and Wynder, E. L., 1974, Promoting effect of bile acids on colon carcinogenesis after intrarectal instillation of N-methyl-N-nitro-N-nitrosoguanidine in rats, *J. Natl. Cancer Inst.* **53**:1093–1097.

108. Diwan, B. A., Ward, J. M., Anderson, L. M., Hagiwara, A., and Rice, J. M., 1986, Lack of effect of phenobarbital on hepatocellular carcinogenesis initiated by N-nitrosodiethylamine or methylazoxymethanol acetate in male Syrian golden hamsters, *Toxicol. Appl. Pharmacol.* **86**:298–307.

109. Tanaka, T., Mori, H., and Williams, G. M., 1987, Enhancement of dimethylnitrosamine-initiated hepatocarcinogenesis in hamster by subsequent administration of carbon tetrachloride but not phenobarbital or p,p'-dichlorodiphenyltrichloroethane, *Carcinogenesis* **8**:1171–1178.

110. Palmer, A. E., Rice, J. M., Ward, J. M., Ohshima, M., Cicmanec, J. L., Dove, L. F., and Lynch, P. H., 1984, Promotion by sodium phenobarbital of liver tumors initiated by diethylnitrosamine in the patas monkey, *Proc. Am. Assoc. Cancer Res.* **25**:141.

111. Nims, R. W., Devor, D. E., Henneman, J. R., and Lubet, R. A., 1987, Induction of alkoxyresorufin O-dealkylases, epoxide hydrolase, and liver weight gain, correlation with liver tumor-promoting potential in a series of barbiturates, *Carcinogenesis* **8**:67–71.

112. Diwan, B. A., Rice, J. M., Hu, H., and Ward, J. M., 1986, Barbiturate structure/tumor promotion relationships: Tumor promoting effects of two long-acting hypnotic barbiturates, 5,5-diallylbarbituric acid and 5-allyl-5-isopropylbarbituric acid, and two monosubstituted analogs of phenobarbital, 5-ethyl- and 5-phenyl-barbituric acid in rat liver, *Proc. Am. Assoc. Cancer Res.* **27**:141.

113. Shinozuka, H., Lombardi, B., and Abanobi, S. E., 1982, A comparative study of the efficacy of four barbiturates as promoters of the development of γ-glutamyltranspeptidase-positive foci in the liver of carcinogen treated rats, *Carcinogenesis* **3**:1017–1020.

114. Peraino, C., 1981, Initiation and promotion of liver tumorigenesis, *Natl. Cancer Inst. Monog.* **58**:55–61.

115. Diwan, B. A., Rice, J. M., Ohshima, M., Ward, J. M., and Dove, L. F., 1985, Comparative tumor promoting activities of phenobarbital, amobarbital, barbital sodium, and barbituric acid on livers and other organs of male F344/NCr rats following initiation with N-nitrosodiethylamine, *J. Natl. Cancer Inst.* **74**:325–336.

116. Hagiwara, A., Diwan, B. A., Rice, J. M., and Ward, J. M., 1987, Toxic and tumor promoting effects of sodium salts of phenobarbital and barbital on bladder tumors initiated by FANFT in F344 rats, *Toxicologist* **7**:103.

117. Diwan, B. A., Rice, J. M., Nims, R. A., and Ward, J. M., 1987, Tumor promoting effects of two hydantoin derivatives, 5-ethyl-5-phenyl hydantoin and 5,5-diethylhydantoin in rat liver, *Proc. Am. Assoc. Cancer Res.* **28**:169.

118. Diwan, B. A., Rice, J. M., and Ward, J. M., 1986, Tumor-promoting activity of benzodiazepine tranquilizers, diazepam and oxazepam, in mouse liver, *Carcinogenesis* **7**:789–794.

119. Preat, V., de Gerlache, J., Lans, M., and Roberfroid, M., 1987, Promoting effect of oxazepam in rat hepatocarcinogenesis, *Carcinogenesis* **8**:97–100.

120. Hino, O., and Kitagawa, T., 1982, Effect of diazepam on hepatocarcinogenesis in the rat, *Toxicol. Lett.* **11**:155–157.

121. Schwartz, M. A., Bommer, P., and Vane, F. M., 1983, Diazepam metabolites in the rat: Characterization by high resolution mass spectrometry and nuclear magnetic resonance, *Arch. Biochem. Biophys.* **121**:508–516.

122. Marcucci, F., Fanelli, R., Mussini, E., and Garattini, S., 1970, Further studies on species differences in diazepam metabolism, *Eur. J. Pharmacol.* **9**:253–256.

123. Yanagi, S., Sakamoto, M., Takahashi, S., Tsutsumi, M., Konishi, Y., Shibata, K., and Kamiya, T., 1987, Promotion of hepatocarcinogenesis by suxibuzone in rats initiated with 3′-methyl-4-dimethylamino-azobenzene, *Cancer Lett.* **36**:11–18.

124. Carr, B. J., Reilly, J. G., and Riggs, A. D., 1984, 5-Azacytidine: Promotion activity for rat hepatocellular carcinoma, in: *Models, Mechanisms and Etiology of Tumor Promotion* (M. Borszonyi, N. E. Day, K. Lapis, and H. Yamasaki, eds.), pp. 409–412. IARC Scientific Publication No. 56, International Agency for Research on Cancer, Lyons, France.

125. Dragani, T. A., Manenti, G., Galliani, G., and Della Porta, G., 1985, Promoting effects of 1,4-bis[2-(3,5-dichloropyridyloxy)]benzene in mouse hepatocarcinogenesis, *Carcinogenesis* **6**:225–228.

126. Shirai, T., Ohshima, M., Masuda, A., Tamano, S., and Ito, N., 1984, Promotion of 2-(ethylnitrosamino)-ethanol-induced renal carcinogenesis in rats by nephrotoxic commpounds: Positive responses with folic acid, basic lead acetate, and N-(3,5-dichlorophenyl)succinimide but not with 2,3-dibromo-1-propanol phosphate, *J. Natl. Cancer Inst.* **72**:477–482.

127. Hiasa, Y., Ohshima, M., Kitahori, Y., Konishi, N., Fujita, T., and Yuasa, T., 1983, β-cyclodextrin: Promoting effect on the development of renal tubular cell tumors in rats treated with N-ethyl-N-hydroxy-ethylnitrosamine, *J. Natl. Cancer Inst.* **69**:963–967.

128. Kurokawa. Y., Takashi, M., Kokubo, T., Ohno, Y., and Hayashi, Y., 1983, Enhancement by potassium bromate of renal tumorigenesis initiated by N-ethyl-N-hydroxyethylnitrosamine in F344 rats, *Gann* **74**:607–610.

129. Shinozuka, H., Abanobi, S. E., and Lombardi, B., 1983, Modulation of tumor promotion in liver carcinogenesis, *Environ. Health Perspect.* **50**:163–168.

130. Nishio, Y., Kakizoe, T., Ohtani, M., Sato, S., Sugimura, T., and Fukushima, S., 1985, L-Isoleucine and L-leucine: Tumor promoters of bladder cancer in rats, *Science* **231**:843–845.

131. Hiasa, Y., Enoki, N., Kitahori, Y., Konishi, N., and Shimoyama, T., 1984, DL-Serine: Promoting activity on renal tumorigenesis by N-ethyl-N-hydroxyethylnitrosamine in rats, *J. Natl. Cancer Inst.* **73**:297–299.

132. Rao, P. M., Laconi, E., Rajalakshmi, S., and Sarma, D. S. R., 1986, Orotic acid (OA), a liver tumor promoter, also promotes carcinogenesis of the intestine in the rat, *Proc. Am. Assoc. Cancer Res.* **27**:142.

133. Rosenberg, M. R., Novicki, D. L., Jirtle, R. L., Novotny, A., and Michalopoulos, G., 1985, Promoting effect of nicotinamide on the development of renal tubular cell tumors in rats initiated with diethylnitros-amine, *Cancer Res.* **45**:809–814.

134. Ohshima, M., and Ward, J. M., 1984, Promotion of N-methyl-N-nitrosourea-induced thyroid tumors by iodine deficiency in F344/NCr rats, *J. Natl. Cancer Inst.* **73**:289–296.

# 8

# DNA Repair Mechanisms and Carcinogenesis

## Steven L. Dresler

## 1. INTRODUCTION

The study of cellular mechanisms for repairing damaged DNA remains as an important element of modern carcinogenesis research. The impetus for investigating DNA repair mechanisms arises from several fundamental observations. First, many carcinogens, both natural and experimental, are known to be DNA-damaging agents,[1,2] and cellular removal of DNA damage has been shown to correlate with a diminished incidence of neoplastic transformation in experimental systems.[3] Second, human patients genetically deficient in DNA repair have a greatly increased incidence of malignant neoplasms.[4] Third, the great majority of known carcinogens have been found to be mutagens as well[5,6]; it has been inferred from this that the carcinogenic potential of these agents is mediated by interactions with and damage to DNA. These observations have led to the conclusion that DNA repair mechanisms form one of the major anticarcinogenic defenses of the mammalian cell. A key goal of much current research in carcinogenesis is to understand why carcinogens are able to produce cancer in spite of the extensive cellular capacity to repair DNA damage. This review concludes with a consideration of this question.

## 2. DAMAGE TO DNA

Before discussing the mechanisms of DNA repair, it is appropriate to present a brief review of the types of damage to DNA and their consequences. Representatives of the major classes of DNA damage are shown in Fig. 1. Two types of pyrimidine dimers[7] are induced by exposure to ultraviolet (UV) radiation. The bulk of UV damage consists of cyclobutyl pyrimidine dimers (Fig. 1a), produced by a symmetric reaction between the $C^5$, $C^6$ bonds of adjacent pyrimidines in the DNA strand. Cyclobutyl pyrimidine dimers most often involve adjacent thymines (as depicted in Fig. 1a), but cytosine–thymine and cytosine–cytosine dimers occur as well. Cyclobutyl pyrimidine dimers appear to produce substantial kinking and unwinding of the DNA at the site of damage.[8] A second type of pyrimidine dimer, the so-called 6–4-photoproduct (Fig. 1b), has a stable bond linking the C-6 position of the pyrimidine ring 5' in the DNA strand to the C-4 position of the 3'-pyrimidine.[9] The exocyclic amino or keto group attached to the participating C-4 is also lost during the reaction.

*Steven L. Dresler* • Department of Pathology, Washington University School of Medicine, St. Louis, Missouri 63110.

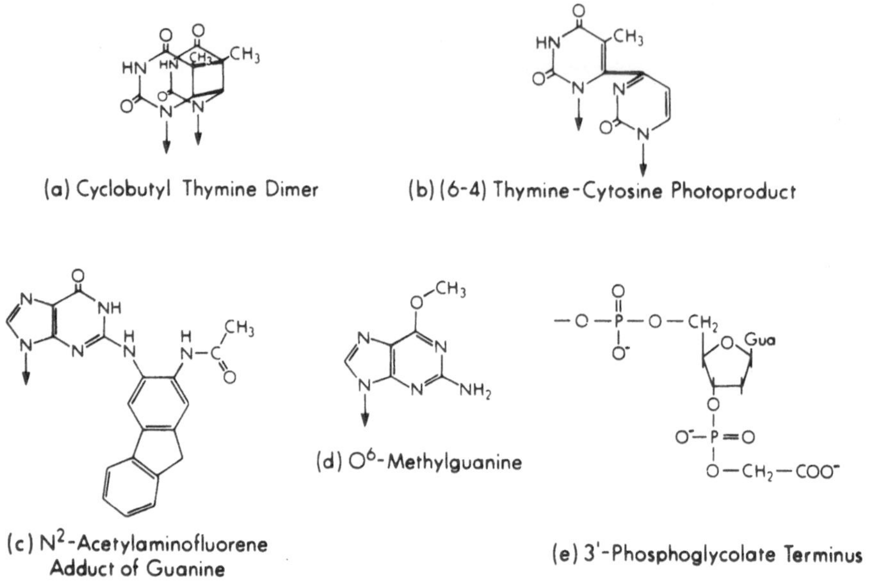

(a) Cyclobutyl Thymine Dimer     (b) (6-4) Thymine-Cytosine Photoproduct

(d) O⁶-Methylguanine

(c) N²-Acetylaminofluorene
Adduct of Guanine

(e) 3'-Phosphoglycolate Terminus

*Figure 1.* Examples of several types of DNA damage. The arrows in (a), (b), (c), and (d) represent bonds to C¹ of a deoxyribose residue in the DNA sugar-phosphate backbone. Darker lines in (a) and (b) represent bonds formed during the dimerization reaction. See text for details.

The 3'-pyrimidine in (6-4) lesions is typically cytosine, as depicted in Fig. 1b. These 6–4 lesions are much less frequent than cyclobutyl pyrimidine dimers but are significant because they are apparently much more mutagenic.[9] Pyrimidine dimers are of great biologic significance because they act as blocks to the progression of DNA replication forks.[10]

A second important class of DNA damage includes bulky chemical adducts of the purine and pyrimidine bases (see Chapter 3). Agents producing this type of damage, represented by such compounds as benzo(a)pyrene, aflatoxin, 7,12-dimethylbenz(a)anthracene, and 2-acetylamino-fluorene, include many of the classic chemical carcinogens.[1,2] A representative bulky chemical lesion, the N²-acetylaminofluorene adduct of guanine, is shown in Fig. 1c. Bulky base adducts, like pyrimidine dimers, distort the DNA helix[11] and can act as blocks to DNA replication.[12,13] In addition, bulky chemical adducts may be mutagenic,[14] producing either point mutations or, by intercalating between bases in the DNA strand, frameshift mutations.[15]

Simple base modifications, the third class of DNA damage, differ from bulky adducts in that they do not distort the DNA helix. Examples of such lesions are the thymine and cytosine hydrates induced by UV,[7] the numerous altered pyrimidine and purine bases induced by ionizing radiation,[16] and the alkylated bases observed after damage by agents such as N-methyl-N-nitrosourea (MNU), methylmethanesulfonate (MMS), and N-methyl-N'-nitro-N-nitrosoguanidine (MNNG).[14] A typical lesion, O⁶-methylguanine, is seen in Fig. 1d. Simple base modifications do not generally lead to arrested DNA replication, but they can be highly mutagenic.[14,15] A special form of base modification is the DNA–DNA crosslink. These lesions are formed by difunctional agents such as nitrogen mustard[17] and cis-diaminedichloroplatinum (II),[18] which can react with bases on opposite DNA strands, linking the strands together. Because DNA crosslinks prevent strand separation, they form complete blocks to DNA replication and transcription.

The final class of damage is DNA strand breaks. Such lesions are generated by ionizing radiation,[16] by drugs such as bleomycin,[19] and by endogenously generated active oxygen species.[20] Most DNA strand breaks generated by these agents cannot be simply religated. The breaks are generated by oxidative fragmentation of a deoxyribose sugar residue in the DNA backbone, and most of them have a phosphate or phosphoglycolate group blocking the 3'-terminal[21] (Fig. 1e).

Such lesions must be repaired by the excision repair process. Breaks in the DNA may involve one or both strands. Single-strand breaks act as blocks to replication and transcription; double strand breaks may form substrates for illegitimate recombinational events.[22]

## 3. DNA REPAIR SYSTEMS

The various forms of DNA damage can lead to cell death, mutation, and DNA recombination and rearrangement. To ameliorate the consequences of DNA damage, mammalian cells have well-developed DNA repair systems. This section reviews the mechanisms of DNA repair known to operate in mammalian cells with emphasis on the excision repair process and the $O^6$-methyltransferases, the systems that are understood in greatest detail. Further information about DNA repair mechanisms is available in an excellent book by Friedberg.[23]

### 3.1. Direct Repair of Damage

#### 3.1.1. Enzymatic Photoreactivation

The simplest DNA repair systems directly transform damaged bases back to their native structure without removing them from the DNA strand. One such system is the enzymatic photoreactivation of cyclobutyl pyrimidine dimers.[24] Photoreactivating enzymes directly monomerize dimers in DNA using energy obtained by absorption of visible light. Enzymatic photoreactivation has been clearly shown to have biologic significance in prokaryotes and lower eukaryotes. Photoreactivating activities have been identified in extracts from a variety of mammalian tissues, and a 40,000-$M_r$ protein with photoreactivating activity has been purified from human leukocytes.[25] However, the actual involvement of such an enzyme in repairing pyrimidine dimers in intact mammalian cells has not been demonstrated.

#### 3.1.2. $O^6$-Methyltransferases

The modified purine base $O^6$-methylguanine, induced by alkylating agents such as MNU and MNNG, is a lesion of particular biologic significance. It appears to be highly mutagenic when induced in cultured mammalian cells.[26] Furthermore, the carcinogenic potency of alkylating agents appears to correlate with their ability to modify the $O^6$ of guanine, and the production of tumors by alkylating agents in several experimental systems is related to the accumulation of $O^6$-alkylguanine in the involved tissues.[27–29] Because of the high mutagenic and carcinogenic potential of $O^6$-methylguanine, the discovery that mammalian cells possess $O^6$-methyltransferases, enzymes that directly remove $O^6$-methyl adducts from guanine in DNA, has generated much interest.

$O^6$-Methyltransferases from mammalian sources are proteins of about 20,000 $M_r$.[29] These proteins catalyze the transfer of $O^6$-methyl, $O^6$-ethyl, and substituted $O^6$-alkyl groups from guanine residues in DNA to specific cysteine residues on the methyltransferase molecules themselves. The methyltransferase thus acts as both catalyst and acceptor for the group transfer and is consumed in stoichiometric amounts during the reaction. There appears to be no cellular mechanism for recycling $O^6$-methyltransferase and, following an episode of damage and repair, methyltransferase activity can be restored only by protein synthesis.

Levels of $O^6$-methyltransferase activity vary dramatically among mammalian species and among various organs in a given species. Rodent cells generally show lower methyltransferase levels than do human cells.[30,31] The pattern of variation between organs, however, is similar in rat and humans, with methyltransferase activities highest in liver; intermediate in kidney, spleen, and gut; and lowest in brain.[30,32–34] Levels of $O^6$-methyltransferase also vary with the level of cellular differentiation in human T lymphocytes; mature T cells in the blood show activities per cell four to five times greater than those found in immature T cells in the thymus.[35] In some cases, biologic responses to alkylation damage have been compared for organs and cell types having different levels of methyltransferase activity. In rat organs, the *in vivo* rates of removal of $O^6$-alkyl adducts from guanine were found to correlate well with $O^6$-methyltransferase levels; removal was most rapid in liver; intermediate in spleen, kidney, and gut; and very slow in brain.[36,37] Also, sensitivity to killing by MNNG in human T lymphocytes at different stages of differentiation correlates inversely with $O^6$-methyltransferase levels.[35] Thus, in normal mammalian cells, $O^6$-methyltransferases appear to be significant in ameliorating the biologic effects of alkylation damage to DNA.

Marked variations in $O^6$-methyltransferase activities have also been seen in human tumor and virus-transformed cell lines. An analysis of a number of human tumor cell lines for ability to repair methylation damage using reactivation of MNNG-treated adenovirus 5 as an assay yielded a sizable group that failed to reactivate the virus[38]; these were designated Mer⁻. Subsequent study revealed that Mer⁻ cells uniformly have little or no $O^6$-methyltransferase activity while Mer⁺ cells (those able to reactivate MNNG-treated adenovirus 5) all display significant methyltransferase activity.[39] A study of Epstein-Barr virus-transformed lymphoblastoid cell lines revealed a group that was unable to remove $O^6$-methylguanine from their DNA[40]; these cells were designated Mex⁻. These cells also lacked $O^6$-methyltransferase activity.[41] Virtually all Mer⁻ and Mex⁻ cells are substantially more sensitive to killing by MNNG than are their Mer⁺ and Mex⁺ counterparts,[39,40,42] indicating again that $O^6$-methyltransferase activity forms a significant defense against alkylation damage to DNA in mammalian cells. A contrary note is provided by a study in which a Mex⁺ human lymphoma cell line was specifically depleted of $O^6$-methyltransferase activity by growth in medium containing free $O^6$-methylguanine.[43] The methyltransferase-depleted cells showed no increase in sensitivity to killing by MNNG, leading Karran and Williams[43] to suggest that the increased killing by MNNG seen in Mer⁻ and Mex⁻ cells may be attributable to factors other than methyltransferase deficiency. It is also possible, however, that the growth of cells in $O^6$-methylguanine induces other repair systems that compensate for the methyltransferase deficiency. This issue has yet to be resolved.

A major feature of the repair of alkylation damage in *Escherichia coli* is the adaptive response, a mechanism by which cells exposed to a low dose of an alkylating agent become resistant to the cytotoxic and mutagenic effects of subsequent exposure to alkylating agents by producing high levels of several DNA repair enzymes, among them $O^6$-methyltransferase.[44] Considerable effort has been expended to determine whether such a response also occurs in mammalian cells. Although early efforts produced equivocal results, it has now been clearly demonstrated that treatment with alkylating agents induces $O^6$-methyltransferase activity in rat hepatoma cells.[45] The response differs in several ways, however, from that seen in *E. coli*. First, a wide range of insults other than alkylating agents, including UV, γ-irradiation, heat, and bleomycin, can induce the phenomenon.[46] Second, the magnitude of the induced increase in methyltransferase activity is much less in the mammalian cells (two- to fivefold) than in *E. coli* (several hundredfold).[45,46] Finally, the stimulation of methyltransferase activity does not appear to occur in cells that have low constitutive levels of methyltransferase.[46] The wide range of inducers active in mammalian cells suggests that the observed induction of $O^6$-methyltransferase may be related to the so-called heat-shock response.[47] It is of interest, however, that the induction of $O^6$-methyltransferase in rat hepatoma cells is associated with a decrease in mutagenic response to MNNG,[45] providing further support for the concept that $O^6$-methyltransferase activity is an important determinant of the biologic effect of alkylation damage to DNA in mammalian cells.

## 3.2. Excision Repair

### 3.2.1. Overview

The overall scheme of DNA excision repair in mammalian cells, which has been developed partly by analogy with prokaryotic systems, is presented in Fig. 2. The process involves incision of the damaged DNA strand adjacent to the site of damage, excision of the damaged nucleotide(s) along with a variable number of undamaged nucleotides, synthesis of a DNA repair patch to fill the gap thus created, and ligation of the free 3′ end of the repair patch to the 5′ end of the pre-existing DNA strand. In mammalian cells, excision repair acts on DNA in chromatin and, as expected,

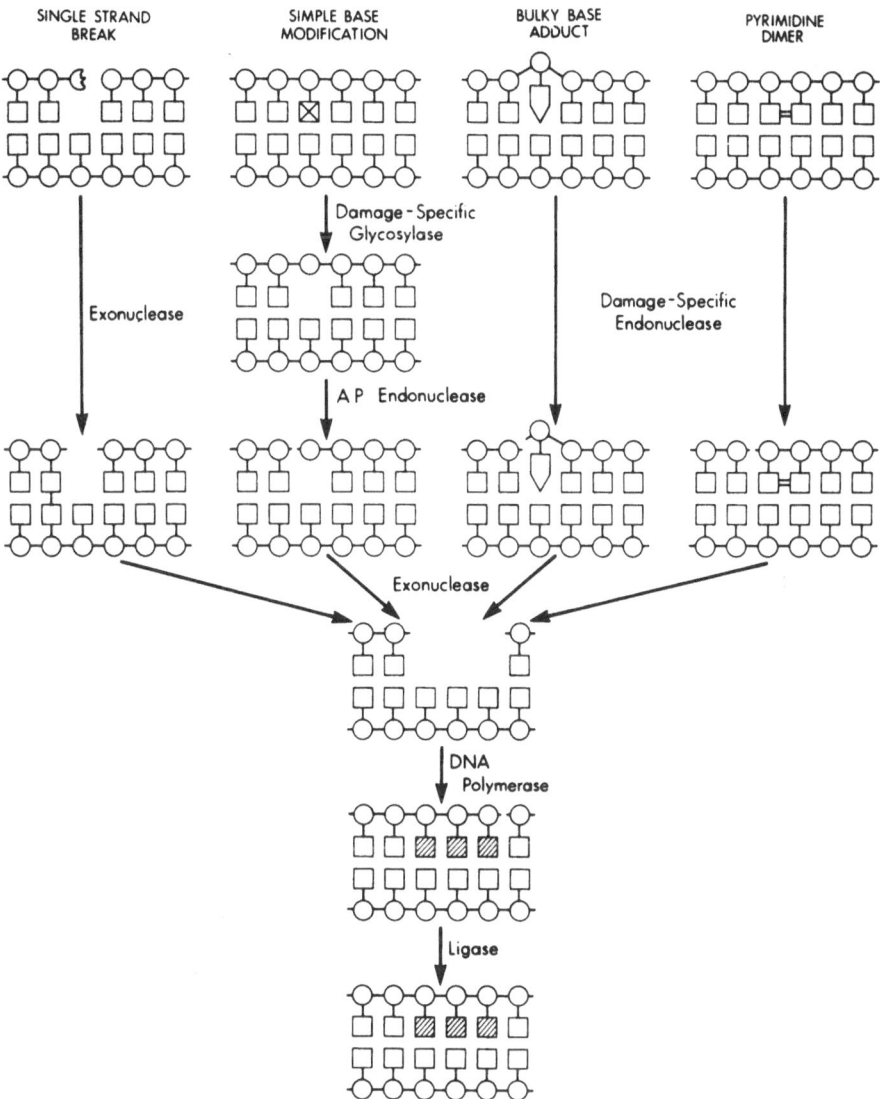

*Figure 2.* An outline of pathways for excision repair of various types of DNA damage. Squares represent purine or pyrimidine bases and circles represent deoxyribose residues in the sugar-phosphate backbone of DNA. Shaded squares represent bases newly incorporated by DNA repair synthesis. Lengths of actual repair patches may vary from the number shown (see text for details). In each example, the 5' end of the damaged DNA strand lies to the left.

chromatin changes that increase the accessibility of the damaged DNA to repair enzymes accompany the excision repair process. Each of the individual elements of DNA excision repair is discussed.

### 3.2.2. Incision

Studies in prokaryotes have revealed two general mechanisms for incision of DNA at sites of damage.[48] One mechanism involves initial breakage of the bond between a damaged base and its associated deoxyribose residue by a damage-specific N-glycosylase, followed by actual scission of the phosphodiester backbone of the DNA by an apurinic/apyrimidinic (AP) endonuclease. A number of damage specific N-glycosylases have been isolated from mammalian cells. These include enzymes that recognize and remove uracil,[49] hypoxanthine,[50] 3-methyladenine,[51–53] and 7-methylguanine.[51,53,54] Two major AP endonucleases have also been found in mammalian cells.[55–57] These N-glycosylases and AP endonucleases, acting in concert, are conceivably capable of incising DNA at sites of damage. Owing to the paucity of repair mutants in eukaryotic cells, however, *in vivo* roles for these enzymes have not been established.

The second mechanism for incision at sites of DNA damage is direct scission of the phosphodiester backbone in a single step, without base release.[48] The prime example of an enzyme using this mechanism is the uvr endonuclease of *E coli*, an ATP-dependent enzyme that directly incises UV-damaged DNA both 3' and 5' to the damaged bases, releasing an oligonucleotide about 12 bases long.[58–60] Several attempts have been made to isolate enzymes from mammalian cells that might be analogous to the uvr endonuclease. Such enzymes have proven to be extremely labile,[61,62] and characterizations of them have been limited. Damage-specific DNA binding proteins without known enzymatic activity have been reported.[63,64] Presumably such proteins could associate with nonspecific endonucleases to form damage-specific enzyme complexes.

Recent studies of pyrimidine dimer-containing DNA fragments excised by UV-damaged normal human fibroblasts[65] led Paterson *et al.*[66] to suggest an entirely new model for incision of UV-damaged DNA. These workers propose that the DNA backbone is initially cleaved between the dimerized pyrimidine residues by a damage-specific phosphodiesterase (Fig. 3) followed by a second cleavage 5' to the dimer by a damage-specific endonuclease. It is suggested that the initial incision within the dimer is required to induce a conformational change at the dimer-containing site, which enables it to be recognized by a generalized bulky lesion repair endonuclease, similar to the uvr endonuclease of *E. coli*.[66] Convincing data indicate that incisions such as those depicted in Fig. 3 do occur in human cells; the nature of the enzymes involved is still a matter for speculation.

Human cells derived from patients with the genetic disease xeroderma pigmentosum (XP) have contributed greatly to our functional understanding of the incision process in mammalian cells.[67] XP patients show extreme photosensitivity of the skin and have a high incidence of skin neoplasms.[68] Cells from these patients show varying degrees of increased sensitivity to UV,[67] and biochemical analyses indicate that these cells are deficient in excision repair of UV damage at or before the incision step.[69–71] (XP cells are also deficient in repair of some bulky chemical DNA adducts, but repair of alkylation and strand break damage is normal.[67]) The localization of the XP defect to the incision step is strengthened by the finding that the excision repair defect in XP cell lines can be complemented *in vivo*[72,73] and *in vitro*[74–76] using pyrimidine dimer-specific endonucleases isolated from *E. coli* infected with bacteriophage T4 and from *Micrococcus luteus*.

One of the most striking features of the XP excision repair defects is the finding that they may be divided into multiple (currently nine) complementation groups using cell-fusion techniques.[77–81]

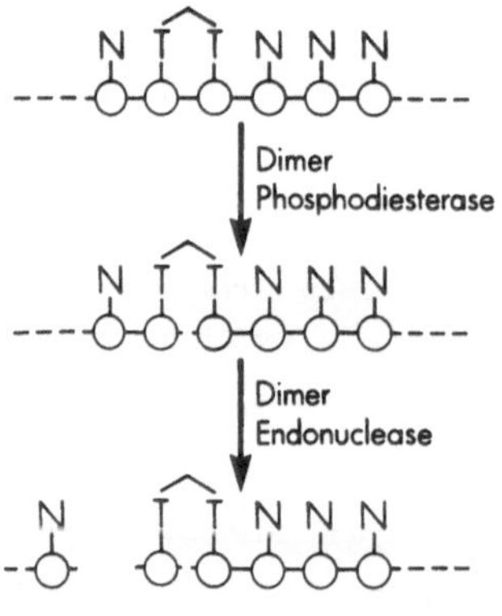

*Figure 3.* A two-step model for incision at pyrimidine dimer sites in DNA in human cells, proposed by Paterson *et al.*[66] The letter N represents any purine or pyrimidine base. The letter T represents thymine. In the first step, the sugar-phosphate backbone is incised between the dimerized thymines. A incision is then made 5' to the dimer.

The groups vary in their degrees of UV sensitivity[82] and in the magnitude of their excision repair defects,[83] with a fairly good correlation between these two factors.[67] The large number of complementation groups, all leading to a defect in incision at sites of DNA damage, has produced much speculation about the nature of the proteins defective in XP. Some have suggested that mammalian cells require as many as nine proteins for incision of UV-damaged DNA, while bacteria require only three (i.e., *uvrA, uvrB, uvrC*), because of additional complications introduced by the packaging of eukaryotic DNA into chromatin.[67] In fact, two research groups have reported that extracts of normal human cells can excise thymine dimers from both purified DNA and from chromatin but that extracts of XP cells (complementation group A) can excise dimers only from DNA and not from chromatin.[61,84] Similar results have been obtained using extracts from cells of two other XP complementation groups, C and G.[84] These findings suggest that the proteins deficient in XP cells of groups A, C, and G may be involved in preparing DNA in chromatin for dimer removal.

It has been suggested that the factors absent in some XP cell lines might be regulatory proteins not directly involved in excision repair.[85,86] Studies of the kinetics and response to protein synthesis inhibitors of complementation between normal cells and cells from XP groups, A, C, and D suggest that in these three groups the factors deficient in XP are directly involved in the excision repair process.[85,86] It has also been found that XP group D cells lack one of the two AP endonucleases found in normal human cells[56,87] and that XP group A cells contain an AP endonuclease with an altered $K_m$ for AP sites.[87] In addition, Paterson *et al.*[66] found evidence that XP group A and group D cells are deficient in the second step of their two-step scheme for incision at pyrimidine dimer sites (see Fig. 3). The relationship of this defect to the altered AP endonucleases also found in these cells is not known. Using permeable human fibroblasts,[76] it has been shown that ATP is required for a step at or before the incision of UV-damaged DNA.[88] ATP could be involved directly in the incision process, as is the case in *E. coli,* or it could be required for a pre-incision chromatin alteration, perhaps mediated by a type II topoisomerase[89] or a protein kinase.

## 3.2.3. Excision

Several exonucleases capable of removing damaged nucleotides from DNA have been isolated from mammalian cells. These include DNase IV from rabbit tissue,[90] several enzymes isolated from human KB cells,[91] an exonuclease isolated from placenta,[92] and an exonuclease that copurifies with an AP endonuclease from human lymphoblasts.[93] None of these enzymes has been specifically implicated in excision repair *in vivo*. In *E. coli,* the 5'-exonucleases of DNA polymerases I and III are capable of excising damaged nucleotides from DNA,[94,95] suggesting that excision may be coupled to repair patch synthesis. Although none of the mammalian DNA polymerases that have been isolated has such an exonuclease,[96] there is some evidence that excision of damage and repair patch synthesis may be coupled in mammalian cells. A dimer-excising activity in human cell extracts is stimulated by addition of deoxyribonucleoside triphosphates (dNTPs),[97] consistent with a linkage between excision and repair patch synthesis. *In vivo* evidence for such coupling is provided by the inhibition of both dimer excision and repair patch synthesis, but not of damage-specific incision of the DNA, which is seen when UV-irradiated human fibroblasts are treated with aphidicolin,[98] a specific inhibitor of DNA polymerases $\alpha$ and $\delta$. During excision repair in mammalian cells, an exonuclease may associate with a DNA polymerase to form a complex functionally similar to bacterial polymerases I and III.

It is generally thought that damaged DNA strands in mammalian cells are incised 5' to sites of pyrimidine dimers and chemical adducts leaving free 3'-hydroxyls to act as primers for repair patch synthesis (see Fig. 2); only the 5'-end of damaged DNA incised in this fashion must be subjected to nucleolytic processing before repair patch synthesis and ligation. Combined action of a damage-specific glycosylase and a 3' AP endonuclease, analogous to the mechanism of incision at pyrimidine dimer sites in *M. luteus,*[48] would leave, however, a 3'-apurinic deoxyribose that would not act as a primer for DNA repair patch synthesis.[99] Action of a 5'-AP endonuclease or a 3'-exonuclease would be required to generate a 3'-primer terminal.[99,100] A similar situation exists for strand breaks generated by $\gamma$-irradiation or drugs, such as bleomycin. These strand breaks do not require incision, but the 3'-phosphate and 3'-phosphoglycolate terminals generated by these agents[19,21] must be excised by a 3'-exonuclease before they can serve as primers for repair patch synthesis[101] (see Figs. 1 and 2). The identity of the exonuclease that performs this excision function in mammalian cells is unknown.

### 3.2.4. Repair Patch Synthesis

Four DNA polymerases have been isolated from mammalian cells: $\alpha$, $\beta$, $\gamma$, and $\delta$.[96] Three of these, $\alpha$, $\beta$, and $\delta$, are located primarily in the nucleus. The nuclear DNA polymerases can be differentiated functionally by their responses to inhibitors. Polymerases $\alpha$ and $\delta$ are both inhibited strongly by aphidicolin and by sulfhydryl-blocking reagents such as $N$-ethylmaleimide.[102] Polymerase $\beta$ is insensitive to aphidicolin and sulfhydryl blockers but is inhibited very strongly by dideoxythymidine triphosphate (ddTTP).[96] Polymerase $\delta$ is also inhibited by ddTTP, although less strongly than polymerase $\beta$, providing one means of differentiating $\delta$ from polymerase $\alpha$, which is quite resistant to ddTTP.[103] Polymerases $\alpha$ and $\delta$ can also be distinguished using butylphenyl-deoxyguanosine triphosphate (BuPh-dGTP), which inhibits $\alpha$ very strongly and $\delta$ weakly.[104,105] None of the mammalian polymerases has a 5'-exonuclease of the sort found in association with $E.$ $coli$ polymerases I and III,[94,95] but polymerase $\delta$ has a 3'-exonuclease that apparently performs a proofreading function on newly incorporated nucleotides[106] and thereby increases the fidelity of DNA synthesis by about 10-fold.[107] Whether the 3'-exonuclease of polymerase $\delta$ is capable of excising 3'-AP deoxyribose, 3'-phosphate, or 3'-phosphoglycolate terminals is unknown.

The availability of specific DNA polymerase inhibitors has facilitated determination of which polymerases are involved in excision repair. Synthesis of DNA repair patches following damage by UV, the bulky heterocyclic carcinogen $N$-acetoxy-2-acetylaminofluorene (AAAF), and alkylating agents such as MNU and MNNG is sensitive to aphidicolin, indicating involvement of DNA polymerase $\alpha$ and/or $\delta$.[108,109] Aphidicolin also inhibits the removal of pyrimidine dimers from the DNA of UV-damaged cells[98] and potentiates killing of human cells by UV,[110] indicating that the aphidicolin-sensitive component of repair synthesis is biologically important. Further investigations using BuPh-dGTP[111] and ddTTP[112] suggest that the enzyme that mediates UV-induced DNA repair synthesis is DNA polymerase $\delta$. Studies using aphidicolin,[113] BuPh-dGTP,[111] and ddTTP[112] also indicate that the polymerase that mediates UV-induced DNA repair synthesis is the same as that which mediates semiconservative DNA replication. This is a striking result, given the great differences between the products of replication and repair synthesis. Careful kinetic studies in permeable human fibroblasts have shown that the $K_m$ for dNTPs of UV-induced repair synthesis is about 10-fold lower than that of replication.[113] Thus, although UV-induced repair synthesis and semiconservative replication involve the same DNA polymerase, that polymerase is altered in specific and distinct ways, presumably by association with specific accessory proteins, for each task. It seems appropriate that repair synthesis, which must function efficiently even in nongrowing cells that have low dNTP levels,[114] has a very low $K_m$ for dNTP.

DNA polymerase $\beta$ is also involved in DNA repair synthesis, primarily in the repair of damage induced by strand-breaking agents such as bleomycin and neocarzinostatin. At concentrations specific for DNA polymerase $\beta$, ddTTP inhibits 50–80% of bleomycin-induced repair synthesis in permeable human cells.[108,109] (The remainder of the bleomycin-induced repair synthesis is mediated by an aphidicolin-sensitive polymerase, which has not been further identified.) Polymerase $\beta$ also mediates repair synthesis following UV damage in rat brain neurons, which lack the aphidicolin-sensitive DNA polymerases, $\alpha$ and $\delta$.[115]

DNA repair patches synthesized in mammalian cells have a striking length heterogeneity. Regan and Setlow[116] separated DNA damaging agents into two classes: "long patch agents," which induce repair patches approximately 100 nucleotides in length, and "short patch agents," which induce patches three to four nucleotides long. Initially, the long patch agents were thought to comprise UV and bulky chemical damaging agents, and the short patch agents were thought to include ionizing radiation and alkylating agents. Subsequent studies indicate that alkylating agents actually induce long repair patches.[117–119] In addition, recent more direct measurement techniques indicate that "long patch" length is in the range of 20–40 nucleotides.[118–121] The molecular mechanism by which repair patch size is determined is not known; apparently, it is not dictated by which DNA polymerase synthesizes the patch.[122]

## 3.2.5. Ligation

Mammalian cells contain two DNA ligases, known as ligase I and ligase II, both of which are ATP dependent.[123] Ligase I levels are elevated in rapidly dividing cells, while ligase II levels are not.[124] From this, it has been hypothesized that ligase I functions in DNA replication, while ligase II participates in DNA repair. The ADP-ribosylation-dependent stimulation of ligase II activity seen following alkylation damage to mouse leukemia cells[125] supports the involvement of ligase II in repair. A cell line with delayed strand break rejoining following both UV[126] and alkylation[127] damage also shows a delayed joining of DNA fragments produced in the DNA replication process.[128] This finding has led to the suggestion that ligase I may participate in DNA repair as well.

## 3.2.6. Chromatin Alterations

Numerous studies have demonstrated that chromatin structure is altered during DNA excision repair. One widely used chromatin structural probe is digestion with staphylococcal nuclease (SN), a procedure that divides nuclear DNA into two classes: nuclease sensitive and nuclease resistant. In unperturbed cells, the nuclease-sensitive fraction represents nucleosome linker DNA and the nuclease-resistant component represents DNA of the nucleosome core.[129] SN studies of cells following DNA damage indicate that newly synthesized repair patches are initially highly nuclease sensitive[130,131] but, with time, acquire the same nuclease sensitivity as bulk DNA in chromatin.[132–135] Studies of damage removal indicate that the nuclease sensitivity of newly synthesized repair patches does not result from preferential repair of damage sites in pre-existing nuclease-sensitive regions but is due instead to a transient structural change in regions of chromatin undergoing excision repair.[133,135,136] This change in chromatin structure, which has been called rearrangement,[132] accompanies repair of damage produced by a wide variety of agents, including UV,[130–135] the bulky chemicals AAAF,[137] 7-bromomethylbenz(a)anthracene,[136] and angelicin,[135] and the alkylating agents MNU and MMS.[138] Chromatin rearrangement thus appears to be a general feature of DNA excision repair. The loss of nuclease sensitivity of nascent repair patches does not occur until the patches are completed and ligated,[139–141] and a careful analysis of SN digestion kinetics indicates that there are at least two intermediate steps in the rearrangement process.[140] The point in the excision repair pathway at which repaired regions acquire a high degree of nuclease sensitivity is unknown, although it has been suggested that it accompanies a structural change occurring early in the repair process that is required to give repair enzymes access to the damaged DNA[142] (Fig. 4).

We have only a vague understanding of the chromatin alterations responsible for the accentuated nuclease sensitivity of new repair patches. Nucleotides newly incorporated by excision repair are not found in the 160 base-pair nucleosomal DNA repeat seen on gel electrophoresis of SN digestion products[132,143] nor in the 10-base repeat produced by DNase I digestion.[143] These results indicate that the DNA–protein interactions normally present in the nucleosome core are extensively disrupted during excision repair. It has been shown that following the completion of rearrangement, DNA repair patches are overrepresented in the 3'- and 5'-ends of nucleosome core DNA and underrepresented in the central regions of core DNA.[144] This nonuniformity suggests that nucleosomal DNA–protein interactions are not totally abolished during the excision repair process. Neither removal of histone H1 from chromatin[145] nor histone hyperacetylation induced by sodium butyrate[146] affects the rearrangement process. A clear understanding of the chromatin changes that accompany excision repair may necessitate the physical isolation and direct analysis of chromatin regions undergoing repair.

Certain biochemical alterations of chromatin proteins, the functions of which are poorly understood, are also known to accompany DNA damage and repair. The best studied of these is the attachment of single ADP-ribose residues (mono-ADP-ribosylation) or polymeric chains of ADP-

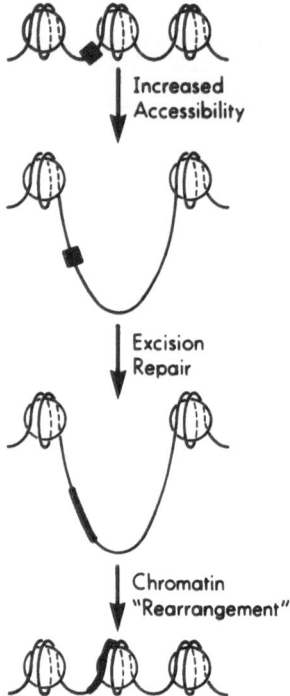

Increased
Accessibility

Excision
Repair

Chromatin
"Rearrangement"

*Figure 4.* A schematic model of chromatin changes occurring during DNA excision repair. Nucleosome structure may be lost in the region of damage permitting repair enzymes access to the damage site. Following repair patch synthesis and ligation, normal chromatin structure is restored. The square represents a site of DNA damage. The thickened line represents a DNA repair patch.

ribose residues (poly-ADP-ribosylation) to various chromatin proteins. Increased incorporation of labeled NAD into protein-bound ADP-ribose is seen following DNA damage by many chemical and physical agents.[147–150] Damage-induced ADP-ribosylation follows DNA strand breakage produced either directly by the damaging agent or by enzymatic incision.[151–153] Increased ADP-ribosylation is not seen following UV irradiation of incision-deficient XP cells unless they are complemented with prokaryotic UV endonuclease.[152] Functions suggested for damage-induced ADP-ribosylation include stimulation of the DNA ligase required for ligating completed repair patches,[125] inhibition of a repair-associated topoisomerase,[154] partial disruption of chromatin structure to permit access of repair enzymes,[153] and provision of a scaffold to prevent excessive disruption of chromatin structure during the repair process.[155] It has also been suggested that damage-induced ADP-ribosylation may mediate the supression of semiconservative replication[156] and transcription[157] that follow DNA damage.

An increase in nuclear histone acetylation for 2–6 hr following UV irradiation of human fibroblasts has also been observed.[158] This period of hyperacetylation is prolonged if the rate of repair synthesis is slowed by the addition of hydroxyurea, suggesting that it is linked to the repair process. Histone acetylation is known to alter DNA–protein interactions in chromatin; it has previously been shown that histone hyperacetylation induced by sodium butyrate increases the rate of repair of UV damage in human cells.[121,159] The acetylation induced by UV radiation may also serve to stimulate DNA repair.

## 3.2.7. Distribution of Excision Repair in the Mammalian Genome

It is now clear that the chromatin structure of the mammalian genome is quite heterogeneous. As might be expected, this heterogeneity exerts a potent modulating influence on the excision repair process. An early intimation of this fact was the finding that repair patches induced by UV irradiation of human fibroblasts are introduced into the genome in a distinctly nonrandom fashion.[160] Up to 36 hr after irradiation, the patches are highly clustered. At 72 hr, a time when essentially all damage sites have been repaired, the distribution of repair patches becomes random, indicating that the underlying distribution of repairable damage is random. The nonrandomness seen at early times of repair could be due to preferential repair of certain regions of chromatin. Such a pattern could also be produced by DNA repair enzymes that act in a processive manner, that is, enzymes that move linearly along the DNA strand and repair damage sites as they are encountered. It is interesting that a prokaryotic DNA repair enzyme, the UV endonuclease of bacteriophage T4, has been found to act processively.[161,162]

Other examples of nonrandomness of excision repair have been discovered by comparing repair in specific DNA sequences with repair in the genome as a whole.[163] The first sequence used in this way was the highly repetitive α-satellite DNA of the African green monkey. This sequence comprises 15–20% of the genome in this species and is present in the nucleus as compact heterochromatin. Repair of UV damage in α-satellite DNA is indistinguishable from that in the genome as a whole.[164] Repair of bulky chemical adducts produced by monofunctional and difunctional furocoumarins[164,165] and by aflatoxin $B_1$,[166] however, is decreased by about 70% in α-DNA. Repair of damage produced by another bulky chemical, AAAF, is also reduced, but only by about 40%.[164] These data suggest that the structure of α-DNA sequences in nuclear chromatin impedes the repair of some kinds of lesions in the DNA. Interestingly, removal of aflatoxin adducts from α-DNA is increased when cells are exposed to low doses of UV.[167] This suggests that UV damage directly or indirectly alters the structure of α chromatin in such a way that DNA damage becomes more accessible to repair enzymes. Apparently furocoumarin and aflatoxin adducts are not capable of inducing this chromatin change.

Using molecular probes, it has also been possible to examine excision repair in specific nonrepetitive sequences.[163] The first target of such analysis was the amplified dihydrofolate reductase (DHFR) gene in methotrexate-resistant Chinese hamster ovary (CHO) cells. Repair of UV damage in this transcribed gene was severalfold more efficient than repair in the CHO genome as a whole.[168] Subsequently, preferential repair of UV damage was found to occur in other transcriptionally active genes, including the amplified DHFR gene in a methotrexate-resistant human cell line,[169] single-copy DHFR genes in the parental CHO line and in normal human fibroblasts,[170] and the c-*abl* gene in mouse cells.[171] Its wide occurrence suggests that preferential repair of active genes may be a general feature of DNA excision repair in mammalian cells. This phenomenon may explain the rapid recovery of RNA synthesis (i.e., transcription) following UV damage seen in repair-proficient cells.[172]

Studies to define the mechanism responsible for preferential repair of active genes are beginning. Using molecular probes, it has been possible to measure rates of repair of UV damage in small regions within and adjacent to the CHO DHFR gene.[173] Maximal repair occurs at the 5′-end of the transcribed region of the gene and repair efficiency decreases as one moves either 3′ or 5′ from this point. This pattern of repair efficiency is similar to the general pattern of nuclease sensitivity observed within transcribed genes,[129] raising the possibility that preferential repair may be a passive phenomenon resulting from the open configuration of active genes. The finding that partially repair-deficient XP group C cells lack the capacity to preferentially repair active genes[170] suggests, however, that the preferential repair may result from the action of specific repair factors that are lacking in group C cells.

## 4. RELATIONSHIP OF DNA REPAIR TO CARCINOGENESIS

With existing knowledge of the mechanisms of DNA repair as a background, one can consider ways in which DNA repair processes relate to carcinogenesis. Data from experimental systems and human genetic deficiency states support the concept that DNA repair forms a major defense against carcinogenic agents. As a corollary to this concept, it is believed that initiation of carcinogenesis, in at least some cases, results from failures of DNA repair. It is also possible that DNA repair intermediates may serve occasionally as precursors for genetic or epigenetic alterations that initiate the carcinogenic process. Both possibilities are discussed in detail below.

## 4.1. Causes of Incomplete DNA Repair

### 4.1.1. Genetic Deficiency

The study of patients with XP, who have gross deficiencies in the repair of UV and bulky chemical damage, has contributed greatly to modern concepts of the relationship between DNA repair and carcinogenesis. Patients with this autosomal-recessive genetic trait have incidences of epidermoid carcinoma and malignant melanoma of the skin several thousandfold higher than those seen in the general population.[174] Epidemiologic evidence indicates that these cancers are induced by the carcinogenic action of UV radiation in sunlight, even in normal individuals.[175] The increased incidence of a UV-induced cancer in patients with a UV repair defect strongly supports the concept that incomplete repair of DNA damage has a carcinogenic effect *in vivo*. Patients with XP also have increased incidence of tumors of the brain and of areas of the oral cavity that are unlikely to be exposed to UV.[174] This suggests that repair of bulky chemical lesions, which is also deficient in XP, may have a significant anticarcinogenic effect at these sites. Carcinogens in the diet may be important factors in the increased incidence of oral carcinoma in XP patients. It has been found, for example, that cultured XP cells are hypersensitive to killing by two bulky chemical carcinogens, 3-amino-1,4-dimethyl-5*H*-pyrido[4,3-*b*]indole and 3-amino-1-methyl-5*H*-pyrido[4,3-*b*]indole, both of which are tryptophan pyrolysis products known to occur in broiled meat and fish.[176] Interestingly, there is apparently no increase in the incidence of other common cancers, such as those of the gastrointestinal (GI) tract, lung, and female genitalia, in XP patients.[174] This finding may indicate that DNA damage by bulky chemicals is not important in carcinogenesis at these sites.[177] The fact that XP patients commonly succumb to metastatic skin neoplasms at an early age[4,67] suggests an alternate possibility—that, in general, XP patients do not survive long enough to develop malignancies at most internal sites.[174]

Ataxia telangiectasia (AT) is a second autosomal-recessive syndrome with an apparent defect in DNA repair. The clinical features of AT include immunodeficiency, central nervous system (CNS) dysfunction, a high frequency of chromosomal aberrations, and a markedly increased incidence of malignancy.[178,179] AT homozygotes who do not die of infections brought on by their immune defect typically develop neoplasms, the great majority of which are lymphomas. AT heterozygotes have a two- to threefold increased risk of developing cancer of any type, and women who are AT heterozygotes have a sevenfold increased risk of developing breast cancer.[180] Original concepts of the molecular lesion in AT were quite simple. AT cells are hypersensitive to killing by X- and γ-irradiation[181] and by radiomimetic drugs such as bleomycin.[182] Thus, AT was regarded as an X-ray analogue of XP. Biologic evidence supporting this concept is provided by confluent holding experiments. Normal human cells that are X-irradiated during density-dependent inhibition of growth and held in that state for a period of time before re-entering the cell cycle showed a marked reduction in X-ray-induced cytotoxicity and chromosomal aberrations. This reduction is evidence that repair of X-ray-induced damage has taken place during the confluent holding period.[183] AT fibroblasts held in the growth-inhibited state fail to show a reduction in X-ray-induced cytotoxicity and chromosome aberrations, suggesting that they lack the ability to repair some important fraction of the X-ray-induced lesions. Biochemical studies have failed to clearly define the nature of this putative AT-repair defect. AT cells are hypersensitive to killing by a number of agents, all of which produce DNA strand breaks by free radical destruction of deoxyribose residues in the sugar–phosphate backbone producing 3'-phosphate and 3'-phosphoglycolate termini[184] (see Fig. 1). Closure of single-strand breaks by AT cells appears to proceed normally,[185] however, and deficient repair of double-strand breaks has been found in only a single AT cell line.[186,187] An early report indicated that AT cells are defective in excision of a form of base damage produced by ionizing radiation under anoxic conditions.[185] However, other studies have failed to confirm this finding.[188] Recent experiments using gene-transfer techniques suggest the existence of a qualitative rather than quantitative defect in double-strand break repair in AT cells.[189] Cloned genes, when cut with a restriction endonuclease prior to transfer into AT cells, develop deletions and/or rearrangements around the cleavage site that are not seen following transfer into normal cells. It is suggested that excessive cellular exonuclease activity may be responsible for these deletions. An intriguing feature of ataxia telangiectasia is that the cells exhibit replicative DNA synthesis that is not inhibited by damage produced by X- or γ-irradiation or by radiomimetic drugs.[190,191] In normal cells, such damage inhibits both replicon initiation[190,191] and elongation.[192] Although the mechanism that mediates this inhibition of replication is unknown, its absence in AT cells suggests that the molecular lesion in AT may involve more than a simple DNA repair defect.

Several other heritable syndromes with increased incidence of malignant neoplasms have been proposed to involve DNA repair defects. Of this group, Bloom syndrome (BS) is the most thoroughly studied. BS patients exhibit sunlight hypersensitivity, growth retardation, and an increased incidence of malignancies, particularly of acute leukemias.[193] Cells from BS patients have a high frequency of spontaneous sister chromatid exchange and spontaneous chromosome aberrations and, in some instances, have been observed to secrete substances in culture which will induce sister chromatid exchange in normal cells.[194] However, no DNA repair defect has been documented. Recently, several Bloom syndrome cell lines have been found to have deficiencies in DNA ligase I that produce delayed Okazaki fragment joining during DNA replication.[195,196] Such a defect could certainly be responsible for the high level of chromosomal abnormalities seen in BS, without the need to invoke a DNA repair defect as well. Analysis of cells from additional patients will determine whether the DNA ligase defect is universal in BS.

Fanconi anemia (FA) is another genetic disorder in which a DNA repair defect has been proposed.[197] Clinical features of FA are anemia, growth retardation, various congenital anomalies, an increased incidence of acute leukemia, and a high frequency of spontaneous chromosome aberrations. Cultured cells from FA patients are hypersensitive to killing by DNA crosslinking agents such as mitomycin C and trimethylpsoralen,[197,198] leading to the suggestion that FA might result from a DNA repair defect. Attempts to identify such a defect biochemically have proved unsuccessful.[199] The molecular basis of FA remains to be elucidated.

Another hereditary disorder that may be related to a DNA repair defect is Cockayne syndrome (CS). The major clinical features of CS are dwarfism, mental retardation, premature aging, and sunlight hypersensitivity. Although CS patients do not show any great increase in cancer incidence, their cells have markedly increased sensitivity to killing by UV and chemical carcinogens.[200] CS cells appear to have no gross defect in the repair of DNA damage but do have pronounced delay in recovery from damage-induced depressions of replication[201] and transcription.[172] These findings suggest that CS cells may have a subtle defect in repair of DNA damage in a small but significant genomic domain.[202] If the molecular defect in CS can be clearly defined, it will be of particular interest because it apparently leads to increased cytotoxicity of DNA damage without an increase in carcinogenicity.

## 4.1.2. Less Severe Repair Deficiencies

Patients with severe repair defects such as XP have obvious clinical symptoms that make them easily identifiable. As a result, the link between these repair deficiencies and an increased incidence of cancer has been easy to demonstrate. Persons with less severe DNA repair deficiencies that do not produce recognizable symptom complexes cannot be identified unless their repair competence is specifically tested. Thus, the relationship of minor repair deficiencies to carcinogenesis is less well understood. It has been shown, however, that the capacity for excision repair of DNA damage induced by the bulky chemical AAAF varies among individuals and that this variability appears to correlate with the propensity to develop colorectal cancer. Following a dose of 10 µM AAAF, mononuclear leukocytes isolated from the blood of patients with pathologically proven colorectal malignancies showed a similar level of DNA damage but 20% less repair synthesis than cells from normal controls.[203] A similar reduction in AAAF-induced repair synthesis was seen in cells from disease-free members of pedigrees showing hereditary predisposition to develop colorectal cancer. Longitudinal studies indicate that these variations in the excision repair response are consistent at least over periods of months,[204] and twin studies suggest that at least a portion of such variability may be heritable.[205] In another study, a four- to fivefold range of $O^6$-methyltransferase and uracil-$N$-glycosylase activities was seen in extracts prepared from fresh epidermal biopsies taken from a group of patients with nonmalignant dermatologic conditions.[206] These results suggest that variations in DNA repair capacity may be widespread in human populations. Further screening studies should demonstrate the extent to which such variations contribute to carcinogenesis.

### 4.1.3. Regional Inaccessibility of DNA Damage

Mammalian genomes appear to be divided into domains with widely varying rates of DNA excision repair.[163] For example, actively transcribed genes seem to be repaired much more rapidly than do quiescent genes. This phenomenon is well demonstrated by comparing repair of UV damage in the active c-*abl* and inactive c-*mos* oncogenes in mouse fibroblasts. In 24 hr, 85% of the pyrimidine dimers are removed from c-*abl*, while only 22% are removed from c-*mos*.[171] Delayed removal of dimers in XP cells leads to hypermutability following UV[207]; one would expect that inactive genes such as c-*mos*, being repaired more slowly, would also be subject to increased rates of mutation. Subsequent expression of such a mutated oncogene might contribute to the development of malignancy (see Chapter 13).

Intrinsic structural features of DNA also influence the efficiency of DNA repair. It is now known that under certain conditions, the secondary structure of DNA may change from the normal right-handed helix (B-DNA) to a left-handed helical form known as Z-DNA.[208] Conversion from B- to Z-DNA may be an important element in the regulation of gene expression. For this reason, it is of great interest that some DNA repair enzymes function very poorly on damage contained in Z-form DNA. For example, the $O^6$-methyltransferase of *E. coli* does not repair $O^6$-methylguanine in Z-DNA.[209] Similarly, *E. coli* formamidopyrimidine–DNA glycosylase does not remove its substrate, 2,6-diamino-4-oxo-methylformamidopyrimidine (a ring-opened product of the alkylated base 7-methylguanine), from Z-DNA.[210] Although analogous studies using enzymes from mammalian sources have not been performed, it is reasonable to assume that the results would be similar. The inability of certain repair enzymes to act on lesions in Z-DNA could increase the mutagenic potency of some DNA damaging agents and could contribute to carcinogenesis by promoting mutation in potential gene-regulatory sequences.

### 4.1.4. Inactivation and Depletion of Repair Enzymes

Except perhaps in occupational settings, persons are rarely exposed to toxic agents one at a time. Natural sources such as smoke are complex mixtures of harmful chemicals. It is therefore important to understand how one noxious agent may alter the repair of DNA damage produced by another. Several studies have addressed this issue. One group has shown that repair of UV damage to DNA is potently inhibited by prior exposure of cells to the alkylating agents MNNG and MMS.[211,212] Because XP cells repair alkylation damage normally but are deficient in UV repair,[67] it is unlikely that UV and alkylation damage compete for a single-repair pathway. The inhibition of UV repair by MMS and MNNG probably results from a direct effect of these chemicals on UV repair enzymes. Alkylating agents such as these do react with proteins as well as DNA,[1] and alkylation is a well-known mechanism of enzyme inactivation.[96] Thus, this explanation is quite plausible. In another study, it was shown that exposure of cultured human bronchial fibroblasts either to 4-hydroxy-$\alpha$,$\beta$-unsaturated aldehydes generated by lipid peroxidation or to acrolein, an $\alpha$,$\beta$-unsaturated aldehyde found in tobacco smoke, markedly inhibited cellular $O^6$-methyltransferase activity.[213] These agents also markedly diminished cellular thiol content, and it was proposed that this led to methyltransferase inactivation as a result of oxidation of the essential cysteine residue in the enzyme's active site. In a third study, it was found that pretreatment of human colon carcinoma cells and normal human fibroblasts with the alkylating agent MNU inhibited subsequent $O^6$-methyltransferase repair of damage produced by the difunctional alkylating agent chloroethylnitrosourea.[214] Because the inhibition was seen following pretreatment with MNU, which methylates the $O^6$ of guanine, but not following pretreatment with MMS, an alkylating agent that does not generate $O^6$-methylguanine in significant amounts, the effect was considered to result from saturation of the $O^6$-methyltransferase system. (It will be remembered that $O^6$-methyltransferase molecules are consumed stoichiometrically during repair of $O^6$-methylguanine and that there is no cellular system for regenerating spent enzyme molecules.) Clearly, there are multiple paths by which exogenous and endogenous chemicals can inhibit repair of DNA damage. An understanding of the relationship between DNA damage and repair and carcinogenesis must take these into account.

## 4.2. Mechanisms for Tolerating Unrepaired DNA Damage

There are many reasons why unrepaired DNA damage might persist in the genome of a mammalian cell. The potential effects of such lesions on propagation of genetic information are twofold (see Section 2). Damaged bases that lead to mispairing at the time of DNA synthesis will produce mutations. Other base adducts, notably bulky chemical lesions and pyrimidine dimers, will arrest progression of the replication fork. Replication arrest is particularly deleterious and must be overcome if cell growth and division are to continue. Cells have developed tolerance mechanisms that permit replication past sites of unrepaired DNA damage. *E. coli,* which has been best studied in this regard, has multiple systems for tolerance of damage. In one of these, DNA synthesis arrests at a damage site but reinitiates at a point downstream from the damage. This arrest and reinitiation creates a daughter–strand gap that is filled by recombination with the sister–DNA duplex on the other limb of the replication fork.[215] This process, known as postreplication repair or daughter–strand gap repair, is the predominant form of damage tolerance operative in *E. coli* at early times after damage. At later times, a second mechanism is induced (as part of the general SOS response to DNA damage) that permits DNA synthesis to continue past sites of damage without arrest.[216] This translesion DNA synthesis apparently results from an alteration in the replication apparatus, the biochemical nature of which has not been clearly defined. The onset of translesion DNA synthesis is accompanied by an increase in mutation rate; thus, the process has been called error prone. Some studies indicate that mutations resulting from translesion synthesis are entirely due to base misinsertion that occurs opposite sites of damage (known as targeted mutations).[217] Other work suggests, however, that the altered replication apparatus that performs translesion DNA synthesis has decreased replicative fidelity, resulting in misinsertion opposite normal template sites (untargeted mutations).[218] The relative contributions of targeted and untargeted mutation to the total spectrum of induced mutagenesis in *E. coli* is unknown.

Mechanisms for tolerance of DNA damage in mammalian cells are less well understood.[219] DNA synthesized during a short pulse-labeling period following UV irradiation of human or mouse cells is of lower molecular weight than that synthesized in undamaged cells.[220,221] With time, this low-molecular-weight DNA is joined to create higher-molecular-weight forms in a process that superficially resembles the daughter–strand gap-repair mechanism of *E. coli.* The existence of multiple replicons in the mammalian genome (compared with a single replicon per genome in *E. coli*) introduces interpretive difficulties, however. It is possible that the slow joining of lower-molecular-weight DNA observed in irradiated cells merely represents a delay in the joining of newly synthesized DNA from adjacent replicons, which is a feature of normal mammalian replication. Similarly, evidence consistent with recombinational repair of daughter–strand gaps has been obtained for human cells,[222] but alternate explanations are equally plausible.

The possible existence of inducible mechanisms for damage tolerance in mammalian cells has been explored as well. Suggestive evidence for such processes is provided by split-dose experiments, in which replicative DNA synthesis in human cells exposed to a single dose of 10 J/m² UV was compared with that seen in cells given a dose of 1 J/m² UV followed 2 hr later by a dose of 9 J/m² UV. Cells exposed to split-dose UV returned to the preirradiation level of replication much more rapidly than do those given the single large UV dose.[223] This result suggests that the initial low-dose UV exposure induced a mechanism that permitted replication to resume prior to repair of all the UV damage produced by the second larger UV dose.

Virus reactivation systems have provided the best evidence for inducible damage tolerance mechanisms in mammalian cells. For example, prior irradiation of monkey cells with 10 J/m² UV increased their ability to reactive UV-irradiated simian virus 40 (SV40) by almost 10-fold compared with reactivation of the virus by unirradiated cells.[224] Prior UV irradiation of the host cells also increased the rate of mutation of the UV-damaged virus. These results suggest that (1) UV irradiation of host cells induces a system that facilitates either repair or replication of UV-damaged virus, and (2) the inducible system is mutagenic. DNA sequence analysis of virus reactivated by the UV-irradiated cells showed that the mutagenic process in this case is a targeted one; all mutations were observed to be opposite to potential pyrimidine dimer sites.[225] These data are most consistent with induction of a translesion DNA replication system in UV-irradiated mammalian cells. Further study will be required to determine whether this mutagenic system plays a significant role in tolerance to DNA damage in the host genome.

Because systems for tolerating DNA damage can lead to both recombination and mutation, they clearly could have significance in the carcinogenic process. Further study will be required to determine the degree to which tolerance mechanisms operate in mammalian cells.

## 5. SUMMARY

DNA-damaging agents are clearly linked to the development of cancer in both experimental animals and humans. The multiple pathways for cellular repair of DNA damage form a major defense against carcinogenesis. In various circumstances, DNA repair may be slow or incomplete allowing persistence of DNA lesions which can cause mutation or arrest of replication. Mammalian cells may have tolerance mechanisms for replication in the presence of DNA damage; however, these mechanisms may in themselves lead to mutation or genetic recombination, or both. Because mutation and recombination have been implicated in carcinogenesis, the long-term consequences of unrepaired DNA damage are serious.

## REFERENCES

1. Miller, E. C., 1978, Some current perspectives on chemical carcinogenesis in humans and experimental animals: Presidential address, *Cancer Res.* **38**:1479–1496.
2. Farber, E., 1981, Chemical carcinogenesis, *N. Engl. J. Med.* **305**:1379–1389.
3. McCormick, J. J., Fry, D. G., and Maher, V. M., 1986, Transformation of human fibroblasts by carcinogens or transfections of oncogenes, *Prog. Clin. Biol. Res.* **209A**:295–303.
4. Cleaver, J. E., 1983, Xeroderma pigmentosum, in: *The Metabolic Basis of Inherited Disease* (J. B. Stanbury, J. B. Wyngaarden, D. S. Fredrickson, J. L. Goldstein, and M. S. Brown, eds.), pp. 1227–1248, McGraw-Hill, New York.
5. McCann, J., Choi, E., Yamasaki, E., and Ames, B. N., 1975, Detection of carcinogens as mutagens in the *Salmonella*/microsome test: Assay of 300 chemicals, *Proc. Natl. Acad. Sci. USA* **72**:5135–5139.
6. McCann, J., and Ames, B. N., 1976, Detection of carcinogens as mutagens in the *Salmonella*/microsome test: Assay of 300 chemicals: Discussion, *Proc. Natl. Acad. Sci. USA* **73**:950–954.
7. Wang, S. U., 1976, *Photochemistry and Photobiology of Nucleic Acids*, Academic, New York.
8. Pearlman, D. A., Holbrook, S. R., Pirkle, D. H., and Kim, S.-H., 1985, Molecular models for DNA damaged by photoreaction, *Science* **227**:1304–1308.
9. Haseltine, W. A., 1983, Ultraviolet light repair and mutagenesis revisited, *Cell* **33**:13–77.
10. Berger, C. A., and Edenberg, H. J., 1986, Pyrimidine dimers block simian virus 40 replication forks, *Mol. Cell Biol.* **6**:3443–3450.
11. Santella, R. M., Grunberger, D., and Weinstein, I. B., 1983, Carcinogens can induce alternate conformations in nucleic acid structures, *Cold Spring Harbor Symp. Quant. Biol.* **48**:339–346.
12. Moore, P. D., Rabkin, S. D., Osborn, A. L., King, C. M., and Strauss, B. S., 1982, Effect of acetylated and deacetylated 2-aminofluorene adducts on *in vitro* DNA synthesis, *Proc. Natl. Acad. Sci. USA* **79**:7166–7170.
13. Yoshida, S., Koiwai, O., Suzuki, R., and Tada, M., 1984, Arrest of DNA elongation by DNA poly-

merases at guanine adducts on 4-hydroxyaminoquinoline 1-oxide-modified DNA template, *Cancer Res.* **44:**1867–1870.

14. Singer, B., and Kusmierek, J. T., 1982, Chemical mutagenesis, *Annu. Rev. Biochem.* **52:**655–693.
15. Miller, J. H., 1983, Mutational specificity in bacteria, *Annu. Rev. Genet.* **17:**215–238.
16. Ward, J. F., 1975, Molecular mechanisms of radiation-induced damage to nucleic acids, *Adv. Radiat. Biol.* **5:**181–239.
17. Kohn, K. W., Spears, C. L., and Doty, P., 1966, Interstrand crosslinking of DNA by nitrogen mustard, *J. Mol. Biol.* **19:**266–288.
18. Roberts, J. J., and Thomson, A. J., 1979, The mechanism of action of antitumor platinum compounds, *Prog. Nucleic Acids Res. Mol. Biol.* **22:**71–133.
19. Hecht, S. M., 1986, DNA strand scission by activated bleomycin group antibiotics, *Fed. Proc.* **45:**2784–2791.
20. Birnboim, H. C., 1982, DNA strand breakage in human leukocytes exposed to a tumor promoter, phorbol myristate acetate, *Science* **215:**1247–1249.
21. Henner, W. D., Rodriguez, L. O., Hecht, S. M., and Haseltine, W. A., 1983, γ ray induced deoxyribonucleic acid strand breaks. 3′ glycolate termini, *J. Biol. Chem.* **258:**711–713.
22. Szostak, J. W., Orr-Weaver, T. L., Rothstein, R. J., and Stahl, F. W., 1983, The double-strand break repair model for recombination, *Cell* **33:**25–35.
23. Friedberg, E. C., 1984, *DNA Repair,* W. H. Freeman, San Francisco.
24. Sutherland, B. M., 1978, Enzymatic photoreactivation of DNA, in: *DNA Repair Mechanisms* (P. C. Hanawalt, E. C. Friedberg, and C. F. Fox, eds.), pp. 113–122, Academic, New York.
25. Sutherland, B. M., 1974, Photoreactivating enzyme from human leukocytes, *Nature (Lond.)* **48:**109–112.
26. Newbold, R. F., Warren, W., Medcalf, A. S. C., and Amos, J., 1980, Mutagenicity of carcinogenic methylating agents is associated with a specific DNA modification, *Nature (Lond.)* **283:**596–599.
27. Singer, B., 1979, *N*-nitrosoalkylating agents: Formation and persistence of alkyl derivatives in mammalian nucleic acids as contributing factors in carcinogenesis, *J. Natl. Cancer Inst.* **62:**1329–1339.
28. Doniger, J., Day, R. S., and Dipaulo, J. A. 1985, Quantitative assessment of the role of $O^6$-methylguanine in the initiation of carcinogenesis by methylating agents, *Proc. Natl. Acad. Sci. USA* **82:**421–425.
29. Yarosh, D. B., 1985, The role of $O^6$-methylguanine-DNA methyltransferase in cell survival, mutagenesis, and carcinogenesis, *Mutat. Res.* **145:**1–16.
30. Grafstrom, R., Pegg, A. E., Trump, B. F., and Harris, C. C., 1984, $O^6$-alkylguanine-DNA alkyltransferase activity in normal human tissues and cells, *Cancer Res.* **44:**2855–2857.
31. Yagi, T., Yarosh, D. B., and Day, R. S., 1984, Comparison of repair of $O^6$-methylguanine produced by *N*-methyl-*N*′-nitro-*N*-nitrosoguanidine in mouse and human cells, *Carcinogenesis* **5:**593–600.
32. Singer, B., Spengler, S., and Bodell, W. J., 1981, Tissue dependent enzyme-mediated repair or removal of *O*-ethyl pyrimidines and ethyl purines in carcinogen-treated rats, *Carcinogenesis* **2:**1069–1073.
33. Myrnes, B., Giercksky, K. E., and Krokan, H., 1983, Interindividual variation in the activity of $O^6$-methylguanine-DNA methyltransferase and uracil-DNA glycosylase in human organs, *Carcinogenesis* **4:**1565–1568.
34. Krokan, H., Haugen, A., Myrnes, B., and Guddal, P. H., 1983, Repair of premutagenic DNA lesions in human fetal tissues: Evidence for low levels of $O^6$-methylguanine-DNA methyltransferase and uracil-DNA glycosylase activity in some tissues, *Carcinogenesis* **4:**1559–1564.
35. Cohen, A., and Leung, C., 1986, $O^6$-methylguanine-DNA methyltransferase activity and sensitivity to *N*-methyl-*N*′-nitro-*N*-nitrosoguanidine during human T-lymphocyte differentiation, *Carcinogenesis* **7:**1877–1879.
36. O'Connor, P. J., Saffhill, R., and Margison, G. P., 1979, *N*-nitroso compounds: Biochemical mechanisms of action, in: *Environmental Carcinogenesis* (P. Emmelot and E. Kriek, eds.), pp. 73–96, Elsevier/North-Holland, Amsterdam.
37. Den Engelse, L., DeGraaf, A., DeBrij, R.-J., and Menkveld, G. J., 1987, $O^2$- and $O^4$-ethylthymine and the ethylphosphotriester dTp(Et)dT are highly persistent DNA modifications in slowly dividing tissues of the ethylnitrosourea-treated rat, *Carcinogenesis* **8:**751–757.
38. Day, R. S., Ziolkowski, C. H. J., Scudiero, D. A., Meyer, S. A., and Mattern, M. R., 1980, Human tumor cell strains defective in the repair of alkylation damage, *Carcinogenesis* **1:**21–32.
39. Yarosh, D. B., Rice, M., Ziolkowski, C. H. J., Day, R. S., Scudiero, D. A., Foote, R. S., and Mitra, S., 1983, $O^6$-methylguanine-DNA methyltransferase in human tumor cells in: *Cellular Responses to DNA Damage* (E. C. Friedberg and B. A. Bridges, eds.), pp. 261–270, Alan R. Liss, New York.

40. Sklar, R., and Strauss, B., 1981, Removal of $O^6$-methylguanine from DNA of normal and xeroderma pigmentosum-derived lymphoblastoid cell lines, *Nature (Lond.)* **289:**417–420.

41. Harris, A. L., Karran, P., and Lindahl, T., 1983, $O^6$-methylguanine-DNA methyltransferase of human lymphoid cells: Structural and kinetic properties and absence in repair-deficient cells, *Cancer Res.* **43:**3247–3252.

42. Scudiero, D. A., Meyer, S. A., Clutterbuck, B. E., Mattern, M. R., Ziolkowski, C. H. J., and Day, R. S., 1984, Relationship of DNA repair phenotypes of human fibroblast and tumor strains to killing by *N*-methyl-*N'*-nitro-*N*-nitrosoguanidine, *Cancer Res.* **44:**961–969.

43. Karran, P., and Williams, S. A., 1985, The cytotoxic and mutagenic effects of alkylating agents on human lymphoid cells are caused by different DNA lesions, *Carcinogenesis* **6:**789–792.

44. Walker, G. C., 1984, Mutagenesis and inducible responses to deoxyribonucleic acid damage in *E. coli*, *Microbiol. Rev.* **48:**60–93.

45. Frosina, G., and Laval, F., 1987, The $O^6$-methylguanine-DNA-methyltransferase activity of rat hepatoma cells is increased after a single exposure to alkylating agents, *Carcinogenesis* **8:**91–95.

46. Lefebvre, P., and Laval, F., 1986, Enhancement of $O^6$-methylguanine-DNA-methyltransferase activity induced by various treatments in mammalian cells, *Cancer Res.* **46:**5701–5705.

47. Schlesinger, M. J., Ashburner, M., and Tessieres, A. (eds.), 1982, *Heat Shock: From Bacteria to Man*, Cold Spring Harbor Laboratory, Cold Spring Harbor, New York.

48. Lindahl, T., 1982, DNA repair enzymes, *Annu. Rev. Biochem.* **51:**61–87.

49. Krokan, H., and Wittwer, C. U., 1981, Uracil DNA glycosylase from HeLa cells: General properties, substrate specificity and effect of uracil analogs, *Nucleic Acids Res.* **9:**2599–2613.

50. Karran, P., and Lindahl, T., 1980, Hypoxanthine in deoxyribonucleic acid: Generation by heat-induced hydrolysis of adenine residues and release in free form by a deoxyribonucleic acid glycosylase from calf thymus, *Biochemistry* **19:**6005–6011.

51. Cathcart, R., and Goldthwait, D. A., 1981, Enzymatic excision of 3-methyladenine and 7-methylguanine by a rat liver nucleic fraction, *Biochemistry* **20:**273–280.

52. Brnt, T. P., 1979, Partial purification and characterization of a human 3-methyladenine DNA glycosylase, *Biochemistry* **18:**911–916.

53. Singer, B., and Brent, T. P., 1981, Human lymphoblasts contain DNA glycosylase activity excising N-3 and N-7 methyl and ethyl purines but not $O^6$-alkylguanines or 1-alkyladenines, *Proc. Natl. Acad. Sci. USA* **78:**856–860.

54. Margison, G. P., and Pegg, A. E., 1981, Enzymatic release of 7-methylguanine from methylated DNA by rodent liver extracts, *Proc. Natl. Acad. Sci. USA* **78:**861–865.

55. Verly, W. G., Colson, P., Zocchi, G., Goffin, C., Liuzzi, M., Buschenschmidt, G., and Muller, M., 1981, Localization of the phosphodiester bond hydrolyzed by the major apurinic/apyrimidinic endodeoxyribonuclease from rat-liver chromatin, *Eur. J. Biochem.* **118:**195–201.

56. Mosbaugh, D. W., and Linn, S., 1980, Further characterization of human fibroblast apurinic/apyrimidinic DNA endonucleases, *J. Biol. Chem.* **255:**11743–11752.

57. Kane, C. M., and Linn, S., 1981, Purification and characterization of an apurinic/apyrimidinic endonuclease from HeLa cells, *J. Biol. Chem.* **256:**3405–3414.

58. Sancar, A., and Rupp, W. D., 1983, A novel repair enzyme: UVRABC excision nuclease of *Escherichia coli* cuts a DNA strand on both sides of the damaged region, *Cell* **33:**249–260.

59. Seeberg, E., and Steinum, A. L., 1983, Properties of the uvrABC endonuclease from *E. coli*, in: *Cellular Responses to DNA Damage* (E. C. Friedberg and B. A. Bridges, eds.) pp. 39–49, Alan R. Liss, New York.

60. Yeung, A. T., Mattes, W. B., Oh, E. Y., and Grossman, L., 1983, Enzymatic properties of purified *Escherichia coli* uvrABC proteins, *Proc. Natl. Acad. Sci. USA* **80:**6157–6161.

61. Mortelmans, K., Friedberg, E. C., Slor, H., Thomas, G., and Cleaver, J. E., 1976, Evidence for a defect in thymine dimer excision in extracts of xeroderma pigmentosum cells, *Proc. Natl. Acad. Sci. USA* **73:**2757–2761.

62. Waldstein, E. A., Peller, S., and Setlow, R. B., 1979, UV-endonuclease from calf thymus with specificity toward pyrimidine dimers in DNA, *Proc. Natl. Acad. Sci. USA* **76:**3746–3750.

63. Feldberg, R. S., and Grossman, L., 1976, A DNA binding protein from human placenta specific for ultraviolet damaged DNA, *Biochemistry* **15:**2402–2408.

64. Feldberg, R. S., Lucas, J. L., and Dannenberg, A., 1982, A damage-specific DNA binding protein. Large scale purification from human placenta and purification, *J. Biol. Chem.* **257:**6394–6401.

65. Weinfield, M., Gentner, N. E., Johnson, L. D., and Paterson, M. C., 1986, Photoreversal-dependent release of thymidine and thymidine monophosphate from pyrimidine dimer-containing DNA excision fragments isolated from ultraviolet-damaged human fibroblasts, *Biochemistry* **25:**2656–2664.

66. Paterson, M. C., Middlestadt, M. V., MacFarlane, S. J., Gentner, N. E., and Weinfield, M., 1987, Molecular evidence for cleavage of intradimer phosphodiester linkage as a novel step in excision repair of cyclobutyl pyrimidine photodimers in cultured human cells, *J. Cell. Sci. (Suppl.)* **6:**161–176.

67. Friedberg, E. C., Ehmann, U. K., and Williams, J. I., 1979, Human diseases associated with defective DNA repair, *Adv. Radiat. Biol.* **8:**85–174.

68. Kramer, K. H., 1977, Progressive degenerative diseases associated with defective DNA repair: Xeroderma pigmentosum and ataxia teleangectasia, in: *DNA Repair Processes* (W. W. Nichols and D. G. Murphy, eds.), pp. 37–71, Symposium Specialists, Miami.

69. Fornace, A. J., Kohn, K. W., and Kann, H. E., 1976, DNA single-strand breaks during repair of UV damage in human fibroblasts and abnormalities of repair in xeroderma pigmentosum, *Proc. Natl. Acad. Sci. USA* **73:**39–43.

70. Erixon, K., and Ahnstrom, G., 1979, Single-strand breaks in DNA during repair of UV-induced damage in normal human and xeroderma pigmentosum cells as determined by alkaline DNA unwinding and hydroxylapatite chromatography, *Mutat. Res.* **59:**257–271.

71. Cook, P. R., Brazell, I. A., Pawsey, S. A., and Gianelli, F., 1978, Changes induced by ultraviolet light in the superhelical DNA of lymphocytes from subjects with xeroderma pigmentosum and normal controls, *J. Cell Sci.* **29:**117–127.

72. Tanaka, K., Sekiguchi, M., and Okada, Y., 1975, Restoration of ultraviolet-induced unscheduled DNA synthesis of xeroderma pigmentosum cells by the concomitant treatment with bacteriophage T4 endonuclease V and HVJ (Sendai virus), *Proc. Natl. Acad. Sci. USA* **72:**4071–4075.

73. Tanaka, H., Hagakawa, H., Sekiguchi, M., and Okada, Y., 1977, Specific action of T4 endonuclease V on damaged DNA in xeroderma pigmentosum cells *in vivo*, *Proc. Natl. Acad. Sci. USA* **74:**2958–2962.

74. Smith, C. A., and Hanawalt, P. C., 1978, Phage T4 endonuclease V stimulates DNA repair replication in isolated nuclei from ultraviolet-irradiated human cells, including xeroderma pigmentosum fibroblasts, *Proc. Natl. Acad. Sci. USA* **75:**2598–2602.

75. Ciarrocchi, G., and Linn, S., 1978, A cell-free assay measuring repair DNA synthesis in human fibroblasts, *Proc. Natl. Acad. Sci. USA* **75:**1887–1891.

76. Dresler, S. L., Roberts, J. D., and Lieberman, M. W., 1982, Characterization of deoxyribonucleic acid repair synthesis in permeable human fibroblasts, *Biochemistry* **21:**2557–2564.

77. Kraemer, K. H., de Weerd-Kastelein, E. A., Robbins, J. H., Keijzer, W., Barrett, S. F., Petinga, R. A., and Bootsma, D., 1975, Five complementation groups in xeroderma pigmentosum, *Mutat. Res.* **33:**327–340.

78. Arase, S., Kozuka, T., Tanaka, K., Ikenaga, M., and Takebe, H., 1979, A sixth complementation group in xeroderma pigmentosum, *Mutat. Res.* **59:**143–146.

79. Keijzer, W., Jaspers, N. G. J., Abrahams, P. J., Taylor, A. M. R., Arlett, C. F., Zelle, B., Takebe, H., Kinmont, P. D. S., and Bootsma, D., 1979, A seventh complementation group in excision-deficient xeroderma pigmentosum, *Mutat. Res.* **62:**183–190.

80. Robbins, J. H., Moshell, A. N., Lutzner, M. A., Ganges, M. D., and Dupuy, J.-M., 1983, A new patient with both xeroderma pigmentosum and Cockayne syndrome is in a new xeroderma pigmentosum complementation group, *J. Invest. Dermatol.* **80:**331.

81. Fischer, E., Keijzer, W., Thielman, H. W., Popanda, O., Bohnert, E., Edler, L., Jung, E. G., and Bootsma, D., 1985, A ninth complementation group in xeroderma pigmentosum, XP I, *Mutat. Res.* **145:**217–225.

82. Andrews, A. D., Barrett, S. F., and Robbins, J. H., 1978, Xeroderma pigmentosum neurological abnormalities correlate with colony-forming ability after ultraviolet radiation, *Proc. Natl. Acad. Sci. USA* **75:**1984–1988.

83. Kraemer, K. H., Coon, H. B., Petinga, R. A., Barrett, S. F., Rahe, A. E., and Robbins, J. H., 1975, Genetic heterogeneity in xeroderma pigmentosum: Complementation groups and their relation to DNA repair rates, *Proc. Natl. Acad. Sci. USA* **72:**59–63.

84. Kano, Y., and Fujiwara, Y., 1983, Defective thymine dimer excision from xeroderma pigmentosum chromatin and its characteristic catalysis by cell-free extracts, *Carcinogenesis* **4:**1419–1424.

85. Matsukama, S., Zelle, B., Keijzer, W., Berends, F., and Bootsma, D., 1981, Different rates of restoration of repair capacity in complementing xeroderma pigmentosum cells after fusion, *Exp. Cell Res.* **134:**103–112.

86. Gianelli, F., Pawsey, S. A., and Avery, J. A., 1982, Differences in patterns of complementation of the more common groups of xeroderma pigmentosum: Possible implications, *Cell* **29:**451–458.

87. Kuhnlein, U., Penhoet, E. E., and Linn, S., 1976, An altered apurinic DNA endonuclease activity in group A and group D xeroderma pigmentosum fibroblasts, *Proc. Natl. Acad. Sci. USA* **73:**1169–1173.

88. Dresler, S. L., and Lieberman, M. W., 1983, Requirement of ATP for specific incision of ultraviolet-damaged DNA during excision repair in permeable human fibroblasts, *J. Biol. Chem.* **258**:12269–12273.

89. Dresler, S. L., and Robinson-Hill, R. M., 1987, Direct inhibition of u.v.-induced DNA excision repair in human cells by novobiocin, coumermycin and nalidixic acid, *Carcinogenesis* **8**:813–817.

90. Lindahl, T., Galley, J. A., and Edelman, G. M., 1969, Deoxyribunuclease IV: A new exonuclease from mammalian tissues, *Proc. Natl. Acad. Sci. USA* **62**:597–603.

91. Cook, K. H., and Friedberg, E. C., 1978, Multiple thymine dimer excising nuclease activities in extracts of human KB cells, *Biochemistry* **17**:850–857.

92. Doniger, J., and Grossman, L., 1976, Human correxonuclease. Purification and properties of a DNA repair exonuclease from placenta, *J. Biol. Chem.* **251**:4579–4587.

93. Bose, K., Karran, P., and Strauss, B., 1978, Repair of depurinated DNA *in vitro* by enzymes purified from human lymphoblasts, *Proc. Natl. Acad. Sci. USA* **75**:794–798.

94. Kelly, R. B., Atkinson, M. R., Huberman, J. A., and Kornberg, A., 1969, Excision of thymine dimers and other mismatched sequences by DNA polymerase of *Escherichia coli, Nature (Lond.)* **224**:495–501.

95. Livingston, D. M., and Richardson, C. C., 1975, Deoxyribonucleic acid polymerase III of *Escherichia coli*. Characterization of associated exonuclease activities, *J. Biol. Chem.* **250**:470–478.

96. Kornberg, A., 1980, *DNA Replication*, W. H. Freeman, San Francisco.

97. Friedberg, E. C., Rude, J. M., Cook, K. H., Ehmann, U. K., Mortelmans, K., Cleaver, J. E., and Slor, H., 1977, Excision repair in mammalian cells and the current status of xeroderma pigmentosum, in *DNA Repair Processes* (W. W. Nichols and D. G. Murphy, eds.), pp. 21–36, Symposium Specialists, Miami.

98. Snyder, R. D., and Regan, J. D., 1982, Differential responses of log and stationary phase human fibroblasts to inhibition of DNA repair by aphidicolin, *Biochim. Biophys. Acta* **697**:229–234.

99. Mosbaugh, D. W., and Linn, S., 1982, Characterization of the action of *Escherichia coli* DNA polymerase I at incisions produced by repair endodeoxyribunucleases, *J. Biol. Chem.* **257**:575–583.

100. Warner, H. R., Demple, B. F., Deutsch, W. A., Kane, C. M., and Linn, S., 1980, Apurinic/apyrimidinic endonucleases in repair of pyrimidine dimers and other lesions in DNA, *Proc. Natl. Acad. Sci. USA* **77**:4602–4606.

101. Henner, W. D., Grunberg, S. M., and Haseltine, W. A., 1983, Enzyme action at 3′ termini of ionizing radiation-induced DNA strand breaks, *J. Biol. Chem.* **258**:15198–15205.

102. Lee, M. Y. W. T., Tan, C.-K., Downey, K. M., and So, A. G., 1981, Structural and functional properties of calf thymus DNA polymerase δ, *Prog. Nucleic Acids Res. Mol. Biol.* **26**:83–96.

103. Wahl, A. F., Crute, J. J., Sabatino, R. D., Bodner, J. B., Marraccino, R. L., Harwell, L. W., Lord, E. M., and Bambara, R. A., 1986, Properties of two forms of DNA polymerase delta from calf thymus, *Biochemistry* **25**:7821–7827.

104. Byrnes, J. J., 1985, Differential inhibitors of DNA polymerases α and δ, *Biochem. Biophys. Res. Commun.* **132**:628–634.

105. Lee, M. Y. W. T., Toomey, N. L., and Wright, G. E., 1985, Differential inhibition of human placental DNA polymerases δ and α by BuPdGTP and BuAdATP, *Nucleic Acids Res.* **13**:8623–8630.

106. Loeb, L. A., and Kunkel, T. A., 1982, Fidelity of DNA synthesis, *Annu. Rev. Biochem.* **51**:429–457.

107. Kunkel, T. A., Sabatino, R. D., and Bambara, R. A., 1987, Exonucleolytic proofreading by calf thymus DNA polymerase δ, *Proc. Natl. Acad. Sci. USA* **84**:4865–4869.

108. Miller, M. R., and Chinault, D. N., 1982, The roles of DNA polymerases α, β, and γ in DNA repair synthesis induced in hamster and human cells by different DNA damaging agents, *J. Biol. Chem.* **257**:10204–10209.

109. Dresler, S. L., and Lieberman, M. W., 1983, Identification of DNA polymerases involved in DNA excision repair in diploid human fibroblasts, *J. Biol. Chem.* **258**:9990–9994.

110. Tyrrell, R. M., 1983, Specific toxicity of aphidicolin to ultraviolet-irradiated excision proficient human skin fibroblasts, *Carcinogenesis* **4**:327–329.

111. Dresler, S. L., and Frattini, M. G., 1986, DNA replication and UV-induced DNA repair synthesis in human fibroblasts are much less sensitive than DNA polymerase α to inhibition by butylphenyl-deoxyguanosine triphosphate, *Nucleic Acids Res.* **14**:7093–7102.

112. Dresler, S. L., and Kimbro, K. S., 1987, 2′,3′-dideoxythymidine 5′-triphosphate inhibition of DNA replication and ultraviolet-induced DNA repair synthesis in human cells: Evidence for involvement of DNA polymerase δ, *Biochemistry* **26**:2664–2668.

113. Dresler, S. L., 1984, Comparative enzymology of ultraviolet-induced DNA repair synthesis and semiconservative DNA replication in permeable diploid human fibroblasts, *J. Biol. Chem.* **259**:13947–13952.

114. Hauschka, P. V., 1973, Analysis of nucleotide pools in animal cells, *Methods Cell Biol.* **7**:361–462.

115. Hubscher, U., Kuenzle, C. C., and Spadari, S., 1979, Functional roles of DNA polymerases β and γ, *Proc. Natl. Acad. Sci. USA* **76**:2316–2320.

116. Regan, J. D., and Setlow, R. D., 1974, Two forms of repair in the DNA of human cells damaged by chemical carcinogens and mutagens, *Cancer Res.* **34**:3318–3325.

117. Snyder, R. D., and Regan, J. D., 1982, DNA repair in normal human and xeroderma pigmentosum group A fibroblasts following treatment with various methane sulfonates and the demonstration of a long-patch (u.v.-like) repair component, *Carcinogenesis* **3**:7–14.

118. Walker, I. G., and Th'ng, J. P. H., 1982, Excision repair patch size in DNA from human KB cells treated with UV-light, or methyl methanesulfonate, *Mutat. Res.* **105**:277–285.

119. Th'ng, J. P. H., and Walker, I. G., 1983, DNA repair patch measurements with nucleosomal DNA, *Carcinogenesis* **4**:975–978.

120. Hanawalt, P. C., Cooper, P. K., and Smith, C. A., 1981, Repair replication schemes in bacteria and human cells, *Prog. Nucleic Acids Res. Mol. Biol.* **26**:181–196.

121. Dresler, S. L., 1985, Stimulation of deoxyribonucleic acid excision repair in human fibroblast pretreated with sodium butyrate, *Biochemistry* **24**:6861–6869.

122. Miller, M. R., and Liu, L. H., 1982, Participation of different DNA polymerases in mammalian DNA repair synthesis is not related to "patch size," *Biochem. Biophys. Res. Commun.* **108**:1676–1682.

123. Soderhall, S., and Lindahl, T., 1976, DNA ligases of eukaryotes, *FEBS Lett.* **67**:1–8.

124. Soderhall, S., and Lindahl, T., 1975, Mammalian DNA ligases: Serological evidence for two separate enzymes, *J. Biol. Chem.* **250**:8438–8444.

125. Creissen, D., and Shall, S., Regulation of DNA ligase activity by poly(ADP-ribose), *Nature (Lond.)* **296**:271–272.

126. Squires, S., and Johnson, R. T., 1983, U.V. induces long-lived DNA breaks in Cockayne's Syndrome and cells from an immunodeficient individual (46BR): Defects and disturbance in post incision steps of excision repair, *Carcinogenesis* **4**:565–572.

127. Teo, I. A., Broughton, B. C., Day, R. S., James, M. R., Karran, P., Mayne, L. V., and Lehmann, A. R., 1983, A biochemical defect in the repair of alkylated DNA in cells from an immunodeficient patient (46BR), *Carcinogenesis* **4**:559–564.

128. Henderson, L. M., Arlett, C. F., Harcourt, S. A., Lehmann, A. R., and Broughton, B. C., 1985, Cells from an immunodeficient patient (46BR) with a defect in DNA ligation are hypomutable but hypersensitive to the induction of sister chromatid exchange, *Proc. Natl. Acad. Sci. USA* **82**:2044–2048.

129. Igo-Kemenes, T., Horz, W., and Zachau, H. G., 1982, Chromatin, *Annu. Rev. Biochem.* **51**:89–121.

130. Cleaver, J. E., 1977, Nucleosome structure controls the rate of excision repair in the DNA of human cells, *Nature (Lond.)* **270**:451–453.

131. Smerdon, M. J., Tlsty, T. D., and Lieberman, M. W., 1978, Distribution of ultraviolet-induced DNA repair synthesis in nuclease sensitive and resistant regions of human chromatin, *Biochemistry* **17**:2377–2386.

132. Smerdon, M. J., and Lieberman, M. W., 1978, Nucleosome rearrangement in human chromatin during UV-induced DNA repair synthesis, *Proc. Natl. Acad. Sci. USA* **75**:4238–4241.

133. Williams, J. I., and Friedberg, E. C., 1979, Deoxyribonucleic acid excision repair in chromatin after ultraviolet irradiation of human fibroblasts in culture, *Biochemistry* **18**:3965–3972.

134. Bodell, W. J., and Cleaver, J. E., 1981, Transient conformational changes in chromatin during excision repair of ultraviolet damage to DNA, *Nucleic Acids Res.* **9**:359–370.

135. Zolan, M. E., Smith, C. A., Calvin, N. M., and Hanawalt, P. C., 1982, Rearrangement of mammalian chromatin structure following excision repair, *Nature (Lond.)* **299**:461–464.

136. Oleson, F. B., Mitchell, B. L., Dipple, A., and Lieberman, M. W., 1979, Distribution of DNA damage in chromatin and its relation to repair in human cells treated with 7-bromomethyl-benz(a)anthracene, *Nucleic Acids Res.* **7**:1343–1361.

137. Tlsty, T. D., and Lieberman, M. W., 1978, The distribution of DNA repair synthesis in chromatin and its rearrangement following damage with *N*-acetoxy-2-acetylaminofluorene, *Nucleic Acids Res.* **5**:3261–3273.

138. Sidik, K., and Smerdon, M. J., 1984, Nuclease sensitivity of repair-incorporated nucleotides in chromatin and nucleosome rearrangement in human cells damaged by methylmethanesulfonate and methylnitrosourea, *Carcinogenesis* **5**:245–253.

139. Bodell, W. J., Kaufmann, W. K., and Cleaver, J. E., 1982, Enzyme digestion of intermediates of excision repair in human cells irradiated with ultraviolet light, *Biochemistry* **21**:6767–6772.

140. Hunting, D. J., Dresler, S. L., and Lieberman, M. W., 1985, Multiple conformation states of repair patches in chromatin during DNA excision repair, *Biochemistry* **24**:3219–3226.

141. Smerdon, M. J., 1986, Completion of excision repair in human cells. Relationship between ligation and nucleosome formation, *J. Biol. Chem.* **261**:244–252.

142. Lieberman, M. W., Smerdon, M. J., Tlsty, T. D., and Oleson, F. B., 1979, The role of chromatin

structure in DNA repair in human cells damaged with chemical carcinogens and ultraviolet radiation, in: *Environmental Carcinogenesis* (P. Emmelot and E. Kriek, eds.), pp. 345–363, Elsevier/North-Holland, Amsterdam.

143. Smerdon, M. J., and Lieberman, M. W., 1980, Distribution within chromatin of deoxyribonucleic acid repair synthesis occurring at different times after ultraviolet irradiation, *Biochemistry* **19**:2992–3000.

144. Lan, S. Y., and Smerdon, M. J., 1985, A nonuniform distribution of excision repair synthesis in nucleosome core DNA, *Biochemistry* **24**:7771–7783.

145. Smerdon, M. J., Watkins, J. F., and Lieberman, M. W., 1982, Effect of histone H1 removal on the distribution of ultraviolet-induced deoxyribonucleic acid repair synthesis within chromatin, *Biochemistry* **21**:3879–3885.

146. Smerdon, M. J., 1983, Rearrangements of chromatin structure in newly repaired regions of deoxyribonucleic acid in human cells treated with sodium butyrate or hydroxyurea, *Biochemistry* **22**:3516–3525.

147. Thi Man, M., and Shall, S., 1982, The alkylating agent, dimethyl sulfate, stimulates ADP-ribosylation of histone H1 and other proteins in permeabilized mouse lymphoma (L1210) cells, *Eur. J. Biochem.* **126**:83–88.

148. Jacobson, E. L., Antol, K. M., Juarez-Salinas, H., and Jacobson, M. K., 1983, Poly(ADP-ribose) metabolism in ultraviolet irradiated human fibroblasts, *J. Biol. Chem.* **258**:103–107.

149. Adamietz, P., and Rudolph, A., 1984, ADP-ribosylation of nuclear proteins *in vivo*. Identification of histone H2B as a major acceptor for mono- and poly(ADP-ribose) in dimethyl sulfate-treated hepatoma AH 7974 cells, *J. Biol. Chem.* **259**:6841–6846.

150. Kreimeyer, A., Wielckens, K., Adamietz, P., and Hilz, H., 1984, DNA repair-associated ADP-ribosylation *in vivo*. Modification of histone H1 differs from that of the principal acceptor proteins, *J. Biol. Chem.* **259**:890–896.

151. Benjamin, R. C., and Gill, D. M., 1980, ADP-ribosylation in mammalian cell ghosts. Dependence of poly(ADP-ribose) synthesis on strand breakage in DNA. *J. Biol. Chem.* **255**:10502–10508.

152. Berger, N. A., and Sikorski, G. W., 1981, Poly(adenosine diphosphoribose) synthesis in ultraviolet-irradiation xeroderma pigmentosum cells reconstituted with *Micrococcus luteus* UV endonuclease, *Biochemistry* **20**:3610–3614.

153. Cohen, J. J., Catino, D. M., Petzold, S. J., and Berger, N. A., 1982, Activation of poly(adenosine diphosphate ribose) polymerase by SV40 minichromosomes: Effects of deoxyribonucleic acid damage and histone H1, *Biochemistry* **21**:4931–4940.

154. Ferro, A. M., Higgins, N. P., and Olivera, B. M., 1983, Poly(ADP-ribosylation) of a DNA topoisomerase, *J. Biol. Chem.* **258**:6000–6003.

155. Thraves, P. J., and Smulson, M. E., 1982, Acceptors for the poly ADP-ribosylation modification of chromatin structure are altered by carcinogen-induced DNA damage, *Carcinogenesis* **3**:1143–1148.

156. Edwards, M. J., and Taylor, A. M. R., 1980, Unusual levels of (ADP-ribose)$_n$ and DNA synthesis in ataxia teleangiectasia cells following γ-ray irradiation, *Nature (Lond.)* **287**:745–747.

157. Taniguchi, T., Agemori, M., Kameshita, I., Nishikimi, M., and Shizuta, Y., 1982, Participation of poly (ADP-ribosyl)ation in the depression of RNA synthesis caused by treatment of mouse lymphoma cells with methylnitrosourea, *J. Biol. Chem.* **257**:4027–4030.

158. Ramanathan, B., and Smerdon, M. J., 1986, Changes in nuclear protein acetylation in u.v.-damaged human cells, *Carcinogenesis* **7**:1087–1094.

159. Smerdon, M. J., Lan, S. Y., Calza, R. E., and Reeves, R., 1982, Sodium butyrate stimulates DNA repair in UV-irradiated normal and xeroderma pigmentosum human fibroblasts, *J. Biol. Chem.* **257**:13441–13447.

160. Cohn, S. M., and Lieberman, M. W., 1984, The distribution of DNA excision-repair sites in human diploid fibroblasts following ultraviolet irradiation, *J. Biol. Chem.* **259**:12463–12469.

161. Ganesan, A. K., Seawell, P. C., Lewis, R. J., and Hanawalt, P. C., 1986, Processivity of T4 endonuclease V is sensitive to NaCl concentration, *Biochemistry* **25**:5751–5755.

162. Gruskin, E. A., and Lloyd, R. S., 1986, The DNA scanning mechanism of T4 endonuclease V. Effect of NaCl concentration on processive nicking activity, *J. Biol. Chem.* **261**:9607–9613.

163. Smith, C. A., 1987, DNA repair in specific sequences in mammalian cells, *J. Cell. Sci. (Suppl.)* **6**:225–241.

164. Zolan, M. E., Cortopassi, G. A., Smith, C. A., and Hanawalt, P. C., 1982, Deficient repair of chemical adducts in α DNA of monkey cells, *Cell* **28**:613–619.

165. Zolan, M. E., Smith, C. A., and Hanawalt, P. C., 1984, Formation and repair of furocoumarin adducts in α deoxyribonucleic acid and bulk deoxyribonucleic acid of monkey cells, *Biochemistry* **23**:63–69.

166. Leadon, S. A., Zolan, M. E., and Hanawalt, P. C., 1983, Restricted repair of aflatoxin B1 induced damage in alpha DNA of monkey cells, *Nucleic Acids Res.* **11:**5675–5689.

167. Leadon, S. A., and Hanawalt, P. C., 1984, Ultraviolet irradiation of monkey cells enhances the repair of DNA adducts in alpha DNA, *Carcinogenesis* **5:**1505–1510.

168. Bohr, V. B., Smith, C. A., Okumoto, D. S., and Hanawalt, P. C., 1985, DNA repair in an active gene: Removal of pyrimidine dimers from the DHFR gene of CHO cells is much more efficient than in the genome overall, *Cell* **40:**359–369.

169. Mellon, I., Bohr, V. A., Smith, C. A., and Hanawalt, P. C., 1986, Preferential repair of an active gene in human cells, *Proc. Natl. Acad. Sci. USA* **83:**8878–8882.

170. Bohr, V. A., Okumoto, D. S., and Hanawalt, P. C., 1986, Survival of UV-irradiated mammalian cells correlates with efficient DNA repair in an essential gene, *Proc. Natl. Acad. Sci. USA* **83:**3830–3833.

171. Madhani, H. D., Leadon, S. A., Smith, C. A., and Hanawalt, P. C., 1986, Differential DNA repair in transcriptionally active and inactive proto-oncogenes: c-*abl* and c-*mos*, *Cell* **45:**417–422.

172. Mayne, L. V., and Lehmann, A. R., 1982, Failure of RNA synthesis to recover after UV irradiation: An early defect in cells from individuals with Cockayne's syndrome and xeroderma pigmentosum, *Cancer Res.* **42:**1473–1478.

173. Bohr, V. A., Okumoto, D. S., Ho, L., and Hanawalt, P. C., 1986, Characterization of a DNA repair domain containing the dihydrofolate reductase gene in Chinese hamster ovary cells, *J. Biol. Chem.* **261:**16666–16672.

174. Kraemer, K. H., Lee, M. M., and Scotto, J., 1984, DNA repair protects against cutaneous and internal neoplasia: Evidence from xeroderma pigmentosum, *Carcinogenesis* **5:**511–514.

175. Granstein, R. D., and Sober, A. J., 1982, Current concepts in ultraviolet carcinogenesis, *Proc. Soc. Exp. Biol. Med.* **170:**115–125.

176. Protic-Sabljic, M., Whyte, D. B., and Kraemer, K. H., 1985, Hypersensitivity of xeroderma pigmentosum cells to dietary carcinogens, *Mutat. Res.* **145:**89–94.

177. Cairns, J., 1981, The origin of human cancers, *Nature (Lond.)* **289:**353–357.

178. Paterson, M. C., and Smith, P. J., 1979, Ataxia telangiectasis: An inherited human disorder involving hypersensitivity to ionizing radiation and related DNA damaging chemicals, *Annu. Rev. Genet.* **13:**291–318.

179. Boder, E., 1984, Ataxia telangiectasia: An overview, in: *Ataxia Telangiectasia: Genetics, Neuropathology, and Immunology of a Degenerative Disease of Childhood*, Kroc Foundation Series, Vol. 19 (R. A. Gatti and M. Swift, eds.), pp. 1–61, Alan R. Liss, New York.

180. Swift, M., Reitnauer, P. J., Morrell, D., and Chase, C. L., 1987, Breast and other cancers in families with ataxia-telangectasia, *N. Engl. J. Med.* **316:**1289–1294.

181. Taylor, R. M., Harnden, D. G., Arlett, C. F., Harcourt, S. A., Lehmann, A. R., Stevens, S., and Bridges, B. A., 1985, Ataxia telangiectasia: A human mutation with abnormal radiation sensitivity, *Nature (Lond.)* **258:**427–429.

182. Taylor, R. M., Rosney, C. M., and Campbell, J. B., 1979, Unusual sensitivity of ataxia telangiectasia cells to bleomycin, *Cancer Res.* **39:**1046–1050.

183. Little, J. B., and Nagasawa, H., 1985, Effect of confluent holding on potentially lethal damage repair, cell cycle progression, and chromosomal aberrations in human normal and ataxia-telangiectasia fibroblasts, *Radiat. Res.* **101:**81–93.

184. Shiloh, Y., Tabor, E., and Becker, Y., 1983, Abnormal response of ataxia telangiectasia cells to agents that break the deoxyribose moiety of DNA via a targeted free radical mechanism, *Carcinogenesis* **4:**1317–1322.

185. Paterson, M. C., Smith, B. P., Lohman, P. M. H., Anderson, A. K., and Fishman, L., 1976, Defective excision repair of gamma-ray damaged DNA in human (ataxia telangiectasia) fibroblasts, *Nature (Lond.)* **260:**444–447.

186. Lehman, A. R., and Stevens, S., 1977, The production and repair of double-strand breaks in cells from normal humans and from patients with ataxia-telangiectasia, *Biochim, Biophys. Acta* **474:**49–60.

187. Coquerelle, T. M., Weibezahn, K. F., and Lucke-Huhle, C., 1987, Rejoining of double strand breaks in normal human and ataxia-telangiectasia fibroblasts after exposure to $^{60}$Co γ-rays, $^{241}$Am α-particles or bleomycin, *Int. J. Rad. Biol.* **51:**209–218.

188. Fornace, A. J., Kinsella, T. J., Dobson, P. P., and Mitchell, J. B., 1986, Repair of ionizing radiation DNA base damage in ataxia telangiectasia cells, *Cancer Res.* **46:**1703–1706.

189. Cox, R., Debenham, P. G., Masson, W. K., and Webb, M. B., 1986, Ataxia-telangiectasia: A human mutation giving high frequency misrepair of DNA double-stranded scissions, *Mol. Biol. Med.* **3:**229–244.

190. Painter, R. B., and Young, B. R., 1980, Radiosensitivity in ataxia-telangiectasia: A new explanation, *Proc. Natl. Acad. Sci. USA* **77:**7315–7317.

191. Painter, R. B., 1981, Radioresistant DNA synthesis: An intrinsic feature of ataxia-telangiectasia, *Mutat. Res.* **84:**183–190.

192. Mohamed, R., Ford, M., and Lavin, M. F., 1986, Ionizing radiation and DNA-chain elongation in ataxia telangiectasia lymphoblastoid cells, *Mutat. Res.* **165:**117–122.

193. German, J., Bloom, D., and Passarge, E., 1979, Bloom's syndrome. VII. Progress report for 1978, *Clin. Genet.* **15:**361–367.

194. Emerit, I., and Cerutti, P., 1981, Clastongenic activity from Bloom syndrome fibroblast cultures, *Proc. Natl. Acad. Sci. USA* **78:**1868–1872.

195. Willis, A. E., and Lindahl, T., 1987, DNA ligase I deficiency in Bloom's syndrome, *Nature (Lond.)* **325:**355–357.

196. Chan, J. Y. H., Becker, F. F., German, J., and Ray, J. H., 1987, Altered DNA ligase I activity in Bloom's syndrome cells, *Nature (London)* **325:**357–359.

197. Sasaki, M. S., 1978, Fanconi's anemia: A condition possibly associated with defective DNA repair, in: *DNA Repair Mechanisms* (P. C. Hanawalt, E. C. Friedberg, and C. F. Fox, eds.), pp. 675–684, Academic, New York.

198. Fujiwara, Y., Tatsumi, M., and Sasaki, M. S., 1977, Crosslink repair in human cells and its possible defect in Fanconi's anemia cells, *J. Mol. Biol.* **113:**635–649.

199. Poll, E. H. A., Arwert, F., Kortbeek, H. T., and Eriksson, A. W., 1984, Fanconi anemia cells are not uniformly deficient in unhooking of DNA interstrand crosslinks, induced by mitomycin C or 8-methoxy-psoralen plus UVA, *Hum. Genet.* **68:**228–234.

200. Wade, M. H., and Chu, E. H. Y., 1979, Effects of DNA damaging agents on cultured fibroblasts derived from patients with Cockayne syndrome, *Mutat. Res.* **59:**49–60.

201. Lehmann, A. R., Kirk-Bell, S., and Mayne, L., 1979, Abnormal kinetics of DNA synthesis in UV light irradiated cells from patients with Cockayne's syndrome, *Cancer Res.* **39:**4237–4241.

202. Hanawalt, P. C., and Sarasin, A., 1986, Cancer-prone hereditary diseases with DNA processing abnormalities, *Trends Genet.* **2:**124–129.

203. Pero, R. W., Miller, D. G., Lipkin, M., Markowitz, M., Gupta, S., Winawer, S. J., Enker, W., and Good, R., 1983, Reduced capacity for DNA repair synthesis in patients with or genetically predisposed to colorectal cancer, *J. Natl. Cancer Inst.* **70:**867–875.

204. Pero, R. W., and Lund-Pero, M., 1983, The reproducibility of individual estimations in the covalent binding of N-acetoxy-2-acetylaminofluorene to DNA and the induction of unscheduled DNA synthesis, *Mutat. Res.* **120:**219–224.

205. Pero, R. W., Bryngelsson, C., Bryngelsson, T., and Norden, A., 1983, A genetic component of the variance of N-acetoxy-2-acetylaminofluorene-induced DNA damage in mononuclear leukocytes determined by a twin study, *Hum. Genet.* **65:**181–184.

206. Myrnes, B., Eggset, G., Volden, G., and Krokan, H., 1984, Enzymatic repair of premutagenic DNA lesions in human epidermis. Quantitation of $O^6$-methylguanine-DNA methyltransferase and uracil-DNA glycosylase activities, *Mutat. Res.* **131:**183–186.

207. Maher, V. M., Dorney, D. J., Konze-Thomas, B., and McCormick, J. J., 1979, DNA excision-repair processes in human cells can eliminate cytotoxic and mutagenic consequences of ultraviolet radiation, *Mutat. Res.* **62:**311–339.

208. Rich, A., Nordheim, A., and Wang, A. H.-J., 1984, The chemistry and biology of Z-DNA, *Annu. Rev. Biochem.* **53:**791–846.

209. Boiteux, S., Costa de Oliviera, R., and Laval, J., 1985, The *Escherichia coli* $O^6$-methylguanine-DNA methyltransferase does not repair promutagenic $O^6$-methylguanine residues when present in Z-DNA, *J. Biol. Chem.* **260:**8711–8715.

210. Lagravere, C., Malfoy, B., Leng, M., and Laval, J., 1984, Ring-opened alkylated guanine is not repaired in Z-DNA, *Nature (Lond.)* **310:**798–800.

211. Park, S. D., Choi, K. H., Hong, S. W., and Cleaver, J. E., 1981, Inhibition of excision-repair of ultraviolet damage in human cells by exposure to methylmethanesulfonate, *Mutat. Res.* **82:**365–371.

212. Park, S. D., and Cleaver, J. E., 1982, Inactivation of nucleotide excision repair in Chinese hamster ovary cells by exposure to an alkylating agent, *Photochem. Photobiol.* **35:**419–421.

213. Krokan, H., Grafstrom, R. C., Sundqvist, K., Esterbauer, H., and Harris, C. C., 1985, Cytotoxicity, thiol depletion and inhibition of $O^6$-methylguanine-DNA methyltransferase by various aldehydes in cultured human bronchial fibroblasts, *Carcinogenesis* **12:**1755–1759.

214. Zlotogorski, C., and Erickson, L. C., 1984, Pretreatment of human colon tumor cells with DNA methylating agents inhibits their ability to repair chloroethyl monoadducts, *Carcinogenesis* **5**:83–87.
215. Howard-Flanders, P., 1983, Workshop summary: Recombination repair, in: *Cellular Responses to DNA Damage* (E. C. Friedberg and B. A. Bridges, eds.), pp. 577–583, Alan R. Liss, New York.
216. Witkin, E. M., 1976, Ultraviolet mutagenesis and inducible DNA repair in *E. coli, Bacteriol. Rev.* **40**:869–907.
217. Miller, J. H., 1982, Carcinogens induce targeted mutations in *Escherichia coli, Cell* **31**:5–7.
218. Brandenburger, A., Godson, G. N., Radman, M., Glickman, B. W., Van Sluis, C. A., and Doubleday, O. P., 1981, Radiation-induced base substitution mutagenesis in single-stranded DNA phage M13, *Nature (Lond.)* **294**:180–182.
219. Meneghini, R., Menck, C. F. M., and Schumacher, R. I., 1981, Mechanisms of tolerance to DNA lesions in mammalian cells, *Quant. Rev. Biophys.* **14**:381–432.
220. Lehmann, A. R., 1972, Postreplication repair of DNA in ultraviolet-irradiated mammalian cells, *J. Mol. Biol.* **66**:319–337.
221. Buhl, S. N., Stillman, R. M., Setlow, R. B., and Regan, J. D., 1972, DNA chain elongation and joining in normal human and xeroderma pigmentosum cells after ultraviolet irradiation, *Biophys. J.* **12**:1183–1191.
222. Lehmann, A. R., and Kirk-Bell, S., 1978, Pyrimidine dimer sites associated with the daughter DNA strands in UV-irradiated human fibroblasts, *Photochem. Photobiol.* **27**:297–307.
223. Moustacchi, E., Ehmann, U. K., and Friedberg, E. C., 1979, Defective recovery of semiconservative DNA synthesis in xeroderma pigmentosum cells following split dose ultraviolet-irradiation, *Mutat. Res.* **62**:159–171.
224. Sarasin, A., and Benoit, A., 1980, Induction of an error-prone mode of DNA repair in UV-irradiated monkey kidney cells, *Mutat. Res.* **70**:71–81.
225. Bourre, F., and Sarasin, A., 1983, Targeted mutagenesis of SV40 DNA induced by UV light, *Nature (Lond.)* **305**:68–70.

# 9

# *Preneoplasia and Precancerous Lesions*

## *Alphonse E. Sirica*

## 1. INTRODUCTION

Many forms of experimental animal and human neoplasms have been observed to be preceded in their development by characteristic precursor lesions. As defined in Chapter 1, those lesions that serve as precursors for neoplasms in general, either benign or malignant, are commonly referred to as *preneoplastic,* while the precursors of malignant neoplasms are regarded as *precancerous* or *premalignant.*

Both preneoplastic and precancerous stages have been associated more often with the development of epithelial neoplasms. However, a number of leukemic conditions, particularly myelogenous leukemias, are also known to be preceded by specific preleukemic states.[1] On the other hand, many sarcomas usually demonstrate malignant characteristics to be present at very early stages in their development.[2]

Dysplasia is most commonly associated with epithelial preneoplasia, whereas the presence of carcinoma in situ usually heralds the development of overt malignant change. In addition, some benign neoplasms, such as villous adenomas of the colon, are at relatively high risk of giving rise to malignant neoplasms, while other types, such as mammary fibroadenomas, rarely if ever become cancerous. It is also important to emphasize here that although specific preneoplastic and/or precancerous lesions have been detected in most organ systems, most of these do not exhibit transition to malignant neoplasia. In fact, the actual percentage of preneoplastic lesions or benign neoplasms that give rise to malignant ones is usually quite low.[2] Nevertheless, under the appropriate circumstances, the cell populations comprising such precursor lesions show an apparently greater probability of undergoing malignant transformation than do their normal cell counterparts. As might be expected, the risk of developing malignant neoplasia associated with the appearance of specific precursor lesions becomes amplified when multiple lesions are present. This phenomenon is seen in human familial polyposis coli, in the initiation–promotion models of hepatocarcinogenesis in the rat, and in epidermal carcinogenesis in the mouse (see Chapter 6).

A most important limitation in being able to define clearly those precursor cell stages that are directly involved in the multistep development of malignant neoplasia is the lack of specific markers capable of distinguishing between such lesions that are likely to undergo the transition to malignancy and those that may develop in parallel, but that either remain as end-point lesions or those that

*Alphonse E. Sirica* • Department of Pathology, Medical College of Virginia, Virginia Commonwealth University, Richmond, Virginia 23298.

regress or become remodeled (see Chapter 19). However, it is also evident that to begin the search for such markers first requires a full understanding of the pathobiology of the precursor stages, with identification of those lesions that persist and those that reverse upon removal of a carcinogenic or tumor-promoting stimulus.

The aim of this chapter is to provide an overview of preneoplastic and precancerous lesions, whether putative or actual, in experimental animals and in humans, as well as to illustrate with select examples the pathobiologic features that characterize some well-defined precursor lesions for specific experimental and naturally occurring malignancies.

## 2. PRENEOPLASTIC AND PRECANCEROUS LESIONS IN EXPERIMENTAL ANIMALS

Carcinogenesis research in experimental animals, and in particular rodents, has provided the strongest support for the existence of discrete preneoplastic and/or precancerous stages in cancer development. Table I lists examples of precursor lesions that have been observed to be associated with the development of specific types of malignant neoplasms in rodents treated with chemical carcinogenesis. While all these examples may be considered precancerous, some are also preneoplastic, such as the atypical hyperplastic and metaplastic lesions, while others, such as the persistent papillomas and adenomatous polyps, may be considered benign neoplasms.

It is not possible to describe in detail the pathologic features characterizing each of these precursor lesions here. For this, the reader is referred to the references listed in Table I. However, because there is now convincing evidence to support the role of squamous cell papillomas as precursors for squamous cell carcinoma in mouse skin and of hyperplastic hepatocellular foci and nodules as precursors of hepatocellular carcinomas in rat, some further discussion of their pathology is in order.

### 2.1. Squamous Cell Papilloma as a Precancerous Lesion in Mouse Skin Carcinogenesis

Cutaneous papillomas are irregular-shaped cauliflowerlike lesions that are elevated above the skin surface and attached by either a narrow stalk (pedunculated) or a broad base (sessile). Each is composed of a series of epidermal folds exhibiting a thickened stratified squamous cell epithelium with basal cell hyperplasia, acanthosis, and hyperkeratinization.[3] Areas of epithelial atypia are also frequently observed.

Each epidermal fold of the papilloma is supported by a central connective tissue dermal core that may either be less predominant (acanthopapilloma) or more prominent (fibropapilloma) than the epithelial component. In addition, two distinct behavioral types of papillomas have been shown to be produced in the initiation–promotion model of mouse skin carcinogenesis.[3] The first of these types, which is in the majority, was found to regress upon discontinuation of the tumor-promoter treatment, while the second type was observed to be more autonomous, having a decreased tendency to regress when the promoter treatment was stopped. It is this persistent or autonomous papilloma that has been described as being a known site of origin of squamous cell carcinoma,[3,39] with the overall rate of transition from papillomas to squamous cell carcinomas estimated at 10–30% in this model.[3]

Although the papilloma to carcinoma sequence has been most commonly seen in mouse skin carcinogenesis with initiation–promotion protocols, this is not the only pathway that has been described for the development of this type of malignant neoplasm. In this regard, Klein-Szanto[3] reported that in complete carcinogenesis protocols, i.e., repetitive applications to skin of carcinogenic polycyclic aromatic hydrocarbons (PAH) such as 7,12-dimethylbenz(a)anthracene, a large percentage of the resulting squamous cell carcinomas arose from nonpapillomatous skin.

*Table I. Examples of Preneoplastic and/or Precancerous Lesions Expressed during Experimental Carcinogenesis in Rodents*

| Animal | Tissue or organ | Putative or actual precursor lesion(s) | Associated malignant neoplasm(s) | References |
|---|---|---|---|---|
| Mouse | Skin | Squamous cell papilloma | Squamous cell carcinoma | 3 |
| Mouse | Skin | Pigmented nevi (cellular blue nevi) | Malignant spindle cell melanoma | 4 |
| Rat | Liver | Hyperplastic foci and nodules of phenotypically altered hepatocytes | Hepatocellular carcinoma | 5–8 |
| Rat, hamster | Liver | Cholangiofibrosis | Intrahepatic cholangiocarcinoma, anaplastic mixed cholangiohepatocellular carcinomas | 9–12 |
| Rat | Pancreatic acinus | Hyperplastic foci and nodules of atypical acinar cells | Acinar cell adenocarcinoma | 13–16 |
| Rat | Pancreatic duct and/or acinus? | Dysplastic ductal epithelium | Ductal adenocarcinoma | 17–20 |
| Rat | Forestomach | Downward basal cell hyperplasia, squamous cell papilloma | Squamous cell carcinoma | 21–24 |
| Rat | Glandular stomach | Dysplastic gland tubules, adenomatous anastomotic polyp with glandular dysplasia | Adenocarcinoma | 25 |
| Rat | Small intestine | Mainly adenomatous villous polyps (tubulovillous adenomas) | Adenocarcinoma | 26 |
| Rat | Colon | Mucosal dysplasia, adenomatous polyps | Adenocarcinoma | 27, 28 |
| Rat | Lung | Adenomatous hyperplasia | Alveolar-bronchial carcinoma | 29 |
| Hamster, rat | Tracheobronchial epithelium | Marked atypical squamous cell metaplasia | Squamous cell carcinoma or combined squamous cell and adenocarcinoma | 30–32 |
| Rat | Kidney | Proliferative clear cell, basophilic, and oncocytic tubules | Clear and granular cell adenocarcinomas, basophilic renal epithelioma, renal oncocytoma | 11, 33, 34 |
| Rat | Urinary bladder | Papillary hyperplasias, urothelial papilloma | Transitional cell carcinoma | 35 |
| Aging male ACI/Seg rat | Ventral prostate | Dysplasia | Prostatic carcinoma | 36 |
| Mouse | Mammary gland | Alveolar hyperplasia (hyperplastic alveolar nodule) | Adenocarcinoma | 37, 38 |

However, no definitive lesions representing the early progeny of the initiated cell in mouse skin carcinogenesis have been identified.

## 2.2. Precursor Lesions Associated with Hepatocarcinogenesis in the Rat

One of the best experimental systems for investigating the precursor cell stages in the development of malignant neoplasia is the rat liver. During hepatocarcinogenesis in the rat, whether based on complete carcinogen or initiation–promotion regimens, there is almost invariably a sequential development of focal and nodular hyperplastic lesions of atypical hepatocytes that precede the actual appearance of hepatocellular carcinomas. The demonstration of hepatocellular carcinoma arising within some of the persistent forms of the nodular lesions has been further cited as very strong evidence that they are precancerous.[39]

The earliest apparent precursor lesions to be seen in rat liver during hepatocarcinogenesis are the microscopic hyperplastic foci or islands of atypical hepatocytes. Since these early lesions have been shown to be readily distinguished from normal liver parenchyma by their histochemically demonstrable patterns of altered marker enzyme activities, they have also been frequently called enzyme-altered foci.[5,40] In addition, because data supporting their precursor role in rat hepatocarcinogenesis is more indirect than that obtained from studies on the more advanced hepatic nodular lesions, they, as well as earlier-appearing hyperplastic nodules, have been described as being putative preneoplastic lesions.[41] By contrast, it is generally believed that a number of these hepatocellular foci progress to give rise to hepatocellular nodules.[8,12,43] Furthermore, those foci that remain stable have been postulated to represent the clonal progeny of the initiated liver cell.[40]

In histologic liver sections stained with hematoxylin and eosin (H&E), at least three types of early hyperplastic foci of atypical hepatocytes have been described.[6,43] Depending on their cytoplasmic staining characteristics, these have been classified as the clear cell focus, the acidophilic cells focus, and the mixed cell focus. The most distinguishing feature of clear cell hepatocytes is the washed-out appearance or emptiness of their cytoplasm. This clear portion of cytoplasm has been shown to exhibit an abundant glycogen storage. By contrast, in liver tissue sections stained with H&E, the cytoplasm of the altered hepatocytes comprising an acidophilic focus is characterized by an intense acidophilic staining and ground glass appearance. This staining feature is related in large part to hypertrophy of their agranular endoplasmic reticulum. In addition, these cells contain increased amounts of cytoplasm, possess an enlarged nucleus (or nuclei) with a prominent centrally located nucleolus, and are also enriched in glycogen.

Mixed-cell hepatocellular foci (Fig. 1a) appear some weeks to several months after the more uniformly stained clear cell and acidophilic cell foci.[6] As implied by this classification, they are composed of a mixture of altered hepatocytes that may include in addition to clear cells and acidophilic cells, vacuolated neutral fat-storing cells, basophilic cells that are rich in ribosomes but deficient in glycogen content, and various intermediate cell types.

The lipid storage exhibited by some of these cells has been viewed by Bannasch[44] as representing a transitory stage associated with the conversion of the glycogenotic clear and acidophilic cells to the basophilic cell type. When and if this conversion takes place within a focus, it has been further reported to coincide with an increase in nuclear DNA synthesis and cell proliferation.[44] In this regard, collections or foci of basophilic cells are more frequently observed in the nodular hepatocellular lesions and are seldom found in those that are focal.[6] These cells further appear to be more closely related to the development of frank hepatocellular carcinoma than are the clear and acidophilic cells.[6,7,44] Bannasch and associates[7] also described foci composed of basophilic cells that contained some measurable glycogen. They in turn, classified this type as the tigroid cell focus.

While the various types of altered hepatocellular foci are observed microscopically in H&E-stained liver sections, they are far more clearly delineated from the surrounding normal liver tissue by the use of specific histochemical and immunohistochemical markers, including staining for increased glycogen, altered iron storage, some novel antigens, and a variety of altered enzymatic activities[5–7,40] (see also Chapter 19). In rat liver, many but not all of the hyperplastic hepatocellular foci induced by direct carcinogenic treatments, as well as by most liver tumor initiation: promotion

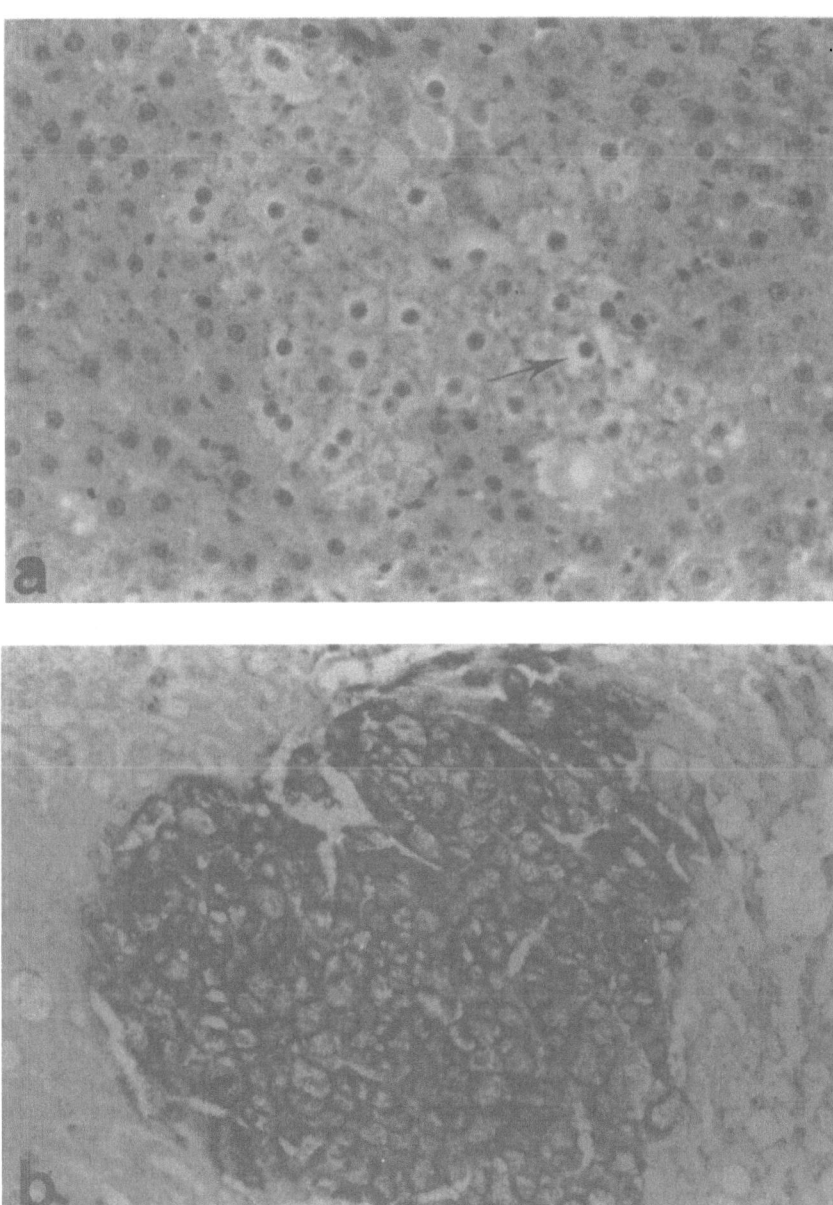

*Figure 1.* Examples of hyperplastic foci of atypical hepatocytes induced in rat liver during chemical hepatocarcinogenesis. (a) Very early mixed-cell focus composed essentially of acidophilic cells, but also containing at least one clear cell (arrow) (H&E ×128). (b) Histochemical demonstration of γ-glutamyl transpeptidase activity in a preneoplastic hepatocellular focus induced in rat liver by a hepatocarcinogenic regimen involving initiation with diethylnitrosamine and tumor promotion with phenobarbital (×160).

regimens can be distinguished from normal liver parenchyma by their histochemically demonstrated γ-glutamyl transpeptidase activity (Fig. 1b).

Grossly visible nodular proliferative lesions composed of phenotypically altered hepatocytes typically develop within weeks to months after the first appearance of the foci. Several terms have been used to describe these lesions, including hyperplastic nodule,[43] neoplastic nodule,[43] hepatic cell adenoma,[43] and, more recently, hepatocyte nodule[8,39] and proliferating hepatic nodule.[7] However, such terms as neoplastic nodule or hepatic cell adenoma should be avoided when making general statements about these lesions, since many of the nodules have been demonstrated to be reversible. In addition, it would appear to be of further value to use adjectives, such as altered or atypical, to complement more accurate descriptive terms like hepatocyte nodule.

In the rat, there is considerable evidence to support the view that the nodular liver lesions have evolved during hepatocarcinogenesis from at least some of the microscopic foci. Like the mixed-cell foci, the nodules have also been found in H&E-stained tissue preparation to be composed of varying mixtures of cell types, including not only acidophilic and clear cells, but also fat-storing cells, basophilic cells, and diverse intermediate cell types.[6] They also have been shown to exhibit similar but not identical phenotypic marker alterations to those shown by the focal lesions,[5,42] with nodules produced by a number of different hepatocarcinogenic regimens showing remarkable uniformity in architecture, cytology, blood supply, and altered metabolic patterns.[8,39] These atypical hepatocyte nodules are roughly spherical in shape and are frequently observed to be elevated above the liver surface. Unlike the hepatocytes of normal liver, which are organized in a regular manner into single-cell thick plates, those of the nodule are arranged in irregular plates that are two to three cells thick.[39] Farber[39,45] further pointed out that the nodules are anatomically distinct from embryonic, fetal, neonatal, and regenerating liver and show a unique phenotype.

Portal triads (branches of the hepatic artery, portal vein, and intrahepatic bile duct) are not formed within the nodules, although an occasional one may be observed that had enveloped such portal structures during its expansion. In addition, as a result of their expansive growth, the nodules produce a compression of the surrounding normal liver parenchyma so that in histologic section they appear as being sharply demarcated from the normal liver. They are, however, not encapsulated by a regular connective tissue sheath, although regions of oval cell proliferation may be found at the periphery and within some nodules. The blood supply of the nodules has also been shown to be different from that of normal liver, as well as of the microscopic foci. In this regard, nodules are supplied by blood derived mainly from the hepatic artery and not the portal vein.[39]

Many, but not all, of the nodules produced in different rat models of hepatocarcinogenesis have been found to disappear or to exhibit reversibility upon discontinuation of hepatocarcinogenic or tumor-promoting treatments. Terms used to describe this phenomenon have included regression, phenotypic reversion, phenotypic instability, maturation, and remodeling.[6–8,39,40,46] Farber and associates[8,45] have provided convincing evidence to indicate that this reversion of the nodule back to normal-appearing liver is accomplished in large part by a complex process of redifferentiation. However, the nodules have been shown to exhibit an increase in single-cell death, or apoptosis, which may also be partially related in part to their regression.[42,47] Apoptosis has also been observed in hyperplastic foci;[42] in some models of hepatocarcinogenesis, some foci have also been shown to undergo reversion after the inciting treatment is stopped.[40,48] By contrast, Pitot and associates[49,50] obtained results indicating that the hyperplastic hepatocellular foci induced in the livers of rats that received a single subcarcinogenic dose of diethylnitrosamine at 24 hr after partial hepatectomy, followed by chronic administration of the hepatic tumor promoter, phenobarbital, are phenotypically stable and not reversible upon removal of the promoting stimulus.* Evidence has also been

---

*In a recent study from Pitot's laboratory, it was found that withdrawal of the hepatic tumor promoting agent phenobarbital for relatively short periods of time from rats previously fed the promoting agent for 6 months following initiation with diethylnitrosamine did result in a marked decrease in the number of hyperplastic hepatocyte foci. However, subsequent readministration of the promoting agent following the period of its withdrawal resulted in the reappearance of at least the same number of foci as was originally present. This has been interpreted to mean that in this model of hepatocarcinogenesis the potential number of altered hepatocyte foci remains constant within the liver, even though they may actually disappear upon removal of the tumor-promoting treatment.[100]

presented which suggests that treatments with hepatic tumor-promoting agents like phenobarbital may be acting to prevent remodeling or reversion of the hyperplastic liver lesions,[51] as well as to inhibit apoptosis.[42]

The persistent atypical hepatocyte nodules, that is, those remaining after discontinuation of the hepatocarcinogenic or hepatic tumor-promoting treatment, are considered the most likely precursors of hepatocellular carcinoma in the rat.[6,8,12,39] However, as yet there is no clear-cut way to distinguish these persistent nodular lesions from those that can revert,[8,40] except by the use of stop experiments[7] wherein the carcinogenic or tumor-promoting stimulus is withdrawn. By contrast, Farber and associates[8,47] recently presented data to indicate that the hepatocytes of the persistent nodules exhibit different cell kinetics than do those of normal liver or of early nodules. They also exhibit alterations in their growth control that are reflected by seemingly autonomous cell proliferation. That the persistent hepatic nodules are precancerous lesions is strongly supported by studies that have demonstrated the development of actual microhepatocellular carcinomas within them, without evidence of hepatic tumor formation elsewhere in the liver.[6,8,12,39] Whether the persistent hepatic nodule is an obligatory lesion in the development of hepatocellular carcinoma remains controversial,[8] although evidence has been presented for microhepatocellular carcinomas arising within hepatic foci without passing through a nodular intermediate stage.[6,7] Microscopic hyperbasophilic foci of altered hepatocytes have also been described in the livers of mice previously given a single carcinogenic dose of diethylnitrosamine by intraperitoneal injection when they were infants.[12,52,53] Goldfarb and associates[12] proposed that these focal lesions may actually be microhepatocellular carcinomas, since they were observed to contain a high incidence of $\alpha$-fetoprotein-(AFP) producing cells and, more to the point, showed venous invasion. In addition, oval cells, which are believed to be derived from the bile ductular cell, have been postulated to be precursor cells for at least some of the preneoplastic and neoplastic hepatocellular lesions in the rat.[54-58] In this regard, Tsao and Grisham[58] recently showed the development of hepatocellular carcinomas, as well as cholangiocarcinomas and hepatoblastomas when chemically transformed cultured rat liver epithelial cells with oval cell properties were transplanted into 1-day-old isogeneic rats.

It should be reiterated that the development of hepatocellular carcinoma within carcinogen-induced hepatic nodules and foci is a relatively rare event, so that even after many months of a specific hepatocarcinogenic treatment, the actual number of such malignant neoplasms that become apparent is greatly outnumbered by the foci, and to a lesser extent, by the nodules that develop.[7,42] Bannasch[7] interpreted this discrepancy between the number of foci (and nodules) and the final tumor yield as possibly being related only to temporal factors, or that it may actually indicate that only a small number of foci and nodules have the potential for undergoing the transition to malignancy.

## 3. PRENEOPLASTIC AND PRECANCEROUS LESIONS IN HUMANS

As is the case with experimental animals, the human also has been shown to exhibit a variety of specific conditions and atypical proliferative lesions which predispose for the development of malignant neoplasia. Some examples are listed in Table II, but this listing is not meant to be comprehensive. Further attention is paid to describing a number of the better studied tumor precursor relationships that have been identified in humans.

### 3.1. Cervical Dysplasia and Carcinoma in Situ of the Uterine Cervix

One of the better known examples in humans that illustrates the role of precursor lesions in tumor development relates to the pathogenesis of invasive squamous cell carcinoma of the uterine cervix. This malignant neoplasm originates from the stratified squamous epithelial layer (Fig. 2a) at or close to the squamo-columnar junction of the exocervical os, and it is generally believed to represent the final stage in a continuum of increasingly atypical epithelial changes.[59,60] This atypia is first manifested by mild dysplasia, followed by moderate and then severe dysplasia, and subsequently by carcinoma in situ, before evolving into frank malignancy. Unlike dysplastic cervical

*Table II. Examples of Conditions and Lesions That Predispose for the Development of Malignant Neoplasms in Humans*

| Classification | Example | Associated malignant neoplasm(s) |
|---|---|---|
| Inherited disorders | Familial polyposis coli | Colon and rectal adenocarcinoma |
| | Fanconi anemia | Myelogenous leukemia |
| | Xeroderma pigmentosum | Basal and squamous cell carcinomas of skin |
| | Basal cell nevus syndrome | Basal cell carcinoma of skin |
| | Familial dysplastic nevus syndrome | Malignant melanoma |
| | Hereditary neurofibromatosis (von Recklinghausen disease) | Neurofibrosarcoma |
| Preneoplastic/precancerous | Epithelial dysplasias, including those of uterine cervix, endometrium, gastrointestinal and respiratory tract mucosa | Various carcinomas and adenocarcinomas |
| | Leukoplakia of the oral cavity and external genitalia | Squamous cell carcinoma |
| | Chronic ulcerative colitis | Colon adenocarcinoma |
| | Atypical squamous metaplasia of bronchial epithelium | Bronchogenic carcinoma |
| | Actinic (solar) keratosis of skin | Squamous cell carcinoma |
| | Fibrocystic breast disease | Mammary carcinomas |
| | Dysplastic nevi | Malignant melanoma |
| Neoplastic/precancerous | Adenomatous polyps of the colon and rectum | Colon and rectal adenocarcinoma |
| | Diffuse adenomatous polyposis of stomach | Gastric adenocarcinoma |
| | Villous papilloma of urothelium | Transitional cell carcinoma of the urinary bladder |
| | Carcinoma in situ | Various invasive carcinomas and adenocarcinomas |
| Preleukemia | Polycythemia vera | Myelogenous leukemia |
| | Idiopathic myelofibrosis | Myelogenous leukemia |
| | Idiopathic acquired sideroblastic anemia | Myelogenous leukemia |
| | Pancytopenia with hyperplastic marrow | Myelogenous leukemia |

epithelium, the atypical cells of carcinoma in situ extend the entire thickness of the epithelial cell layer, from the basement membrane to its uppermost surface (Fig. 2b). These cells are characterized by a marked degree of anaplasia, showing a high nuclear to cytoplasmic ratio, increased basophilia, hyperchromatic nuclei, poor maturation, and scattered mitoses, which are not just confined to the basal cell layer. However, even though they exhibit the cytologic features of cervical carcinoma cells, they have not as yet acquired the malignant cell property of invasiveness.

That carcinoma in situ of the cervix should be considered precancerous is supported by observations that indicate that it may be more than 8–20 years before women with this lesion develop invasive carcinoma.[59–61] However, if left untreated, a highly significant number of women with carcinoma in situ of the cervix will develop malignancy. In comparison, it was found that populations of women whose cervical carcinoma in situ was treated by conization showed almost no subsequent development of invasive carcinoma.[2,60] By contrast, it is quite common to find areas of carcinoma in situ occurring within a cervix that also contains invasive carcinoma,[59] and focal invasion of cells through the basement membrane (microinvasion) has been observed to be originating from cervical carcinoma in situ.[2]

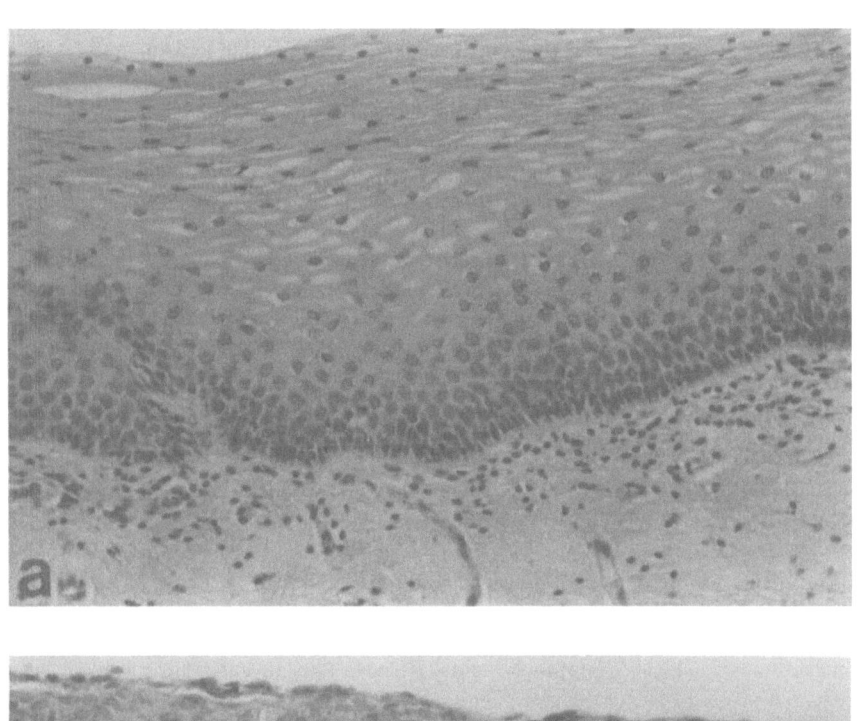

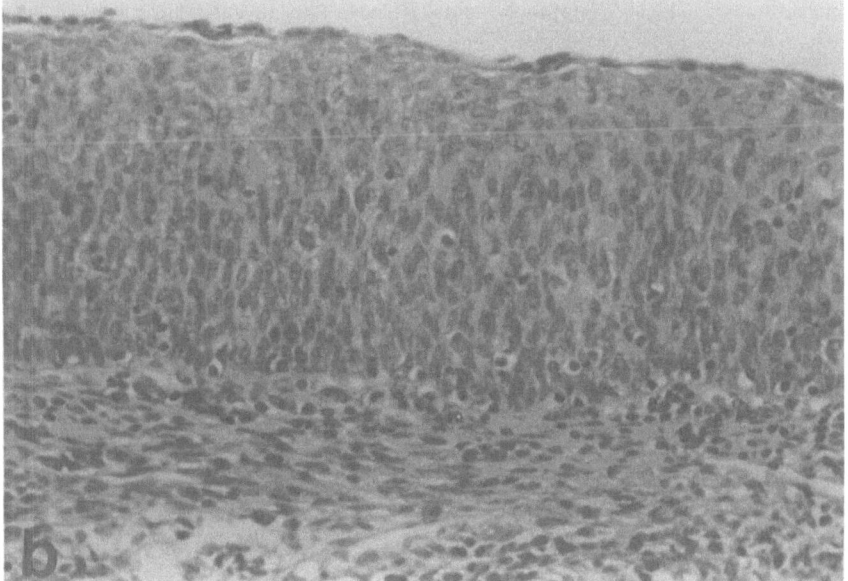

*Figure 2.* Carcinoma in situ of the human uterine cervix. (a) Normal stratified squamous epithelium of cervix (H&E, ×250). (b) Carcinoma in situ (H&E, ×250).

## 3.2. Adenomatous Polyps of the Colon and Rectum

Two kinds of polyps may develop within the colon and rectum, the hyperplastic polyp and the adenomatous polyp. Of the two kinds, the hyperplastic polyps are by far the more common, and for the most part are small innocuous lesions. By contrast, the rarer adenomatous polyps are true neoplasms (adenomas) that have the potential to undergo the transition to malignancy.

Approximately 70–80% of adenomatous polyps occur in the sigmoid colon and rectum. These may be pedunculated or sessile and are classified into three histologic types: tubular adenoma, villous adenoma, and tubulovillous adenoma.[62] Pure tubular adenomas rarely give rise to colorectal adenocarcinoma, whereas the more ominous villous adenomas have been found to contain malignant cells in more than one third of cases. The risk of malignancy is also increased with larger polyps, as well as with multiple polyps.

Evidence supporting the precancerous nature of the adenomatous colorectal polyps has been derived from pathologic, clinical, and epidemiologic data.[27,62–64] This can be enumerated as follows: (1) microscopic adenocarcinoma has commonly been found in adenomatous polyps, but only rarely has it been observed to arise *de novo* within normal colonic or rectal mucosa; (2) the distribution within colon and rectum of the large adenomatous polyps that are most apt to give rise to malignancy is quite similar to that of colorectal adenocarcinomas; (3) persons with polyposis syndromes, such as familial polyposis coli, an autosomal-dominant condition characterized by the multiple development of mainly sessile adenomatous polyps within the colon and rectum, also show a very high incidence of colorectal adenocarcinoma; (4) populations that develop adenomatous polyps of the colon and rectum were further observed to develop colorectal adenocarcinomas; and (5) a 25-year follow-up study of 18,158 patients that was performed at the University of Minnesota Cancer Detection Center demonstrated an 85% reduction in statistically anticipated colorectal adenocarcinomas as a result of the removal of benign polyps and adenomatous lesions upon their detection by sigmoidoscopic examination.[65] Thus, in the human, there is strong support for the adenomatous polyp as being the precursor lesion for most sporadic colon and rectal adenocarcinomas.[64]

## 3.3. Dysplastic Nevi

Extensive studies done on families exhibiting familial dysplastic nevus syndrome, an autosomal-dominant condition associated with a very high incidence of cutaneous malignant melanoma, have focused attention on the dysplastic nevus as being the precursor lesion for this malignant neoplasm.[66] The dysplastic nevus has also been observed to be present in a nonfamilial sporadic form; it has further been postulated by Reed[67] that many malignant melanomas may evolve from precancerous dysplasias. In this regard, invasive melanomas have frequently been found to be in direct association with an adjacent dysplastic nevus, and remnants of dysplastic nevi have been noted in up to 35% of primary melanomas.[66] Clark *et al.*[68] also pointed out that while the vast majority of nevi showing dysplasia do not undergo the transition to melanoma, when melanoma does develop from a precursor lesion, the dysplastic nevus is that precursor. This relationship between the dysplastic nevus and superficial spreading and nodular melanoma has, in turn, served as the basis for an interesting model of tumor progression in humans.[68]

## 3.4. Liver Cell Dysplasia and Adenomatous Hyperplastic Liver Nodules

Anthony[69] was the first to suggest that liver cell dysplasia may be a precursor for hepatocellular carcinoma in humans. Subsequently, there have been a number of studies indicating a frequent association between this lesion and chronic hepatitis B virus (HBV) infection, certain types of liver cirrhosis, particularly the posthepatitic HBV-associated form, and hepatocellular carcinoma.[70,71]

Histologically, liver cell dysplasia is characterized by cellular enlargement, nuclear hyperchromasia, pleomorphism, and multinucleation of the altered hepatocytes, which may occur focally in cell groups, or may occupy whole cirrhotic liver nodules.[69] In cases of HBV infection, a significant correlation has been reported between liver cell dysplasia and the presence of hepatitis B surface antigen (HBsAg) in noncancerous hepatic tissue.[72] Roncalli *et al.*[70,71] further observed that, despite the close relationship between liver cell dysplasia and HBV infection,* the dysplastic hepatocytes only rarely displayed HBsAg as compared with the surrounding liver parenchyma, and they were essentially negative for tissue hepatitis B core antigen (HBcAg). However, when HBsAg was seen in dysplastic hepatocytes, it frequently showed a peculiar perinuclear pattern. Hepatocellular carcinomas have also been shown to contain a low incidence of HBsAg-positive cells, and infected neoplastic cells did not contain detectable core antigen in their nucleus.[70,71] Kew *et al.*[73] also reported a similar perinuclear staining pattern for HBsAg in a moderately differentiated hepatocellular carcinoma containing cells that were positive for this antigen.

While these findings suggest that liver cell dysplasia may be a preneoplastic lesion for hepatocellular carcinoma, direct evidence for this relationship is still lacking.[74] Furthermore, a number of Japanese pathologists recently questioned the view that liver cell dysplasia may be a preneoplastic lesion. In this regard, Akagi *et al.*[72] indicated that the incidence of liver cell dysplasia in cirrhotic liver with hepatocellular carcinoma is quite variable. Henmi *et al.*[75] further reported that liver cell dysplasia did not resemble hepatocellular carcinomas with respect to their degree of nuclear atypism and their intracytoplasmic iron content. In addition, histochemical and immunohistochemical marker studies have revealed dysplastic hepatocytes to be phenotypically more similar to normal hepatocytes than to neoplastic hepatocytes.[70,74,75] Finally, to this author's knowledge, there have been no studies to date that have demonstrated the selective integration of HBV–DNA into the genome of dysplastic hepatocytes, as has been shown for hepatocellular carcinoma cells.[76,77] Nevertheless, it is generally believed that when liver cell dysplasia is observed in biopsied liver, it should not be treated lightly, but rather, it may indicate that the patient with this lesion may develop or may already have hepatocellular carcinoma.[74]

Arakawa *et al.*[78] recently described the emergence of microhepatocellular carcinomas within adenomatous hyperplastic nodules that were resected from the livers of patients with nonalcoholic cirrhosis. The emerging malignant hepatic neoplasms within these hyperplastic liver lesions were seen as small nodules within nodules, reminiscent of hepatocellular carcinoma developing within persistent carcinogen-induced hyperplastic nodules of rat liver. On the basis of these findings, it was postulated that in nonalcoholic cirrhotic patients from Japan and Southeast Asia, in whom hepatocellular carcinoma is endemic, an adenomatous hyperplastic liver nodule or similar hyperplastic liver lesions are likely representative of preneoplastic or precancerous lesions that may already be committed to malignant transformation.

## 3.5. Other Examples of Putative Epithelial Cell Preneoplasia

Some other specific examples of putative preneoplastic and/or precancerous epithelial cell lesions reported for the human include intraductal dysplasia of the prostate,[79] gastric epithelial dysplasia,[80] atypical lobules and intraductal papillomas of the female breast,[81] squamous cell metaplasia with marked atypia in the bronchus,[82] and dysplastic ductal lesions of the pancreas.[83] In the case of pancreatic ductal carcinoma, controversy still exists as to the cellular origin of this malignant neoplasm in both experimental animals and humans. Some investigators believe it to be derived from pre-existing duct cells and proliferating intralobular ductular cells, while others consider it to originate from pancreatic acinar cells that have undergone ductal metaplasia.[83] Recent studies of human cholecystectomy specimens have also suggested a precursor relationship between dysplasia and carcinoma in situ and the subsequent development of invasive carcinoma of the gall bladder.[84,85] In this regard, Albores-Saavedra *et al.*[84] reported the mean age of persons with epithelial dysplasia of the gall bladder to be 5 years less than the mean age of those with carcinoma in situ. Furthermore, there was a 10-year difference between the mean age of those with carcinoma in situ and

---

*In addition to being associated with HBV infection, liver cell dysplasia was recently identified in the livers of patients with non-A, non-B hepatitis. Three of 17 of those with liver cell dysplasia and non-A, non-B hepatitis were also found to have hepatocellular carcinoma with a predominant giant cell pattern.[101]

patients with invasive carcinoma, suggesting a sequential or stepwise pattern of development of this malignant neoplasm.

## 4. CONCLUSIONS

The identification and characterization of preneoplastic, and particularly precancerous, lesions is important not only from the standpoint of being able to better understand the natural histories of malignant neoplasms but also because such information may offer possibilities for either prevention or an appropriate early therapeutic intervention. In addition, several investigators have proposed the use of defined preneoplastic lesions in rat liver[7,40,86,87] and in other organ systems[11] of experimental animals as being suitable endpoints for the *in vivo* evaluation of carcinogenic and tumor-promoting substances. For a more complete analysis of the use of preneoplastic lesions as end points in carcinogenicity testing, the reader is referred to the recent Commentaries by Bannasch.[7,11]

Farber[39] recently hypothesized that precancerous stages actually represent a new form of physiologic adaptation to a cytotoxic environment brought about by carcinogenic exposures. Schulte-Hermann *et al.*[88] recently demonstrated that the hyperplastic foci of atypical hepatocytes induced in rat liver during hepatocarcinogenesis also exhibit adaptive responses to the hepatic tumor promoter, phenobarbital. In Farber's view, the pathway to the development of malignant neoplasia is considered to be related to an aberration of such an adaptation, so that a small subset of the affected cells lose their ability to redifferentiate even when the inciting stimulus is removed.[39] These cells can then continue to expand to form those types of persistent lesions that are believed to be more relevant to cancer development.

The relationship between oncogene expression and preneoplasia or precancer is not clear. Balmain *et al.*[89] reported the presence of an activated Harvey-ras gene (c-$ras^H$) in many carcinogen-induced skin papillomas, as well as epidermal carcinomas of the mouse. However, more recent studies by Slaga and associates[90] and by Toftgard *et al.*[91] have been unable to demonstrate a specific correlation between increased expression or rearrangement of known oncogenes (or proto-oncogenes) and each of the different stages of skin tumor development in the mouse, including epidermal hyperplasia, papillomas, and carcinomas. Beer *et al.*[92] have further found that γ-glutamyl transpeptidase-positive hepatocytes isolated from the liver of rats at 6 months after a regimen involving initiation with diethylnitrosamine and hepatic tumor promotion with phenobarbital showed no major differences from other hepatocyte populations (i.e., those from the same liver, but without histochemical γ-glutamyl transpeptidase activity) in either the size or amount of messenger RNA (mRNA) transcripts for the proto-oncogenes c-*myc* and H-*ras*. These investigators did find an apparent elevation of c-*myc* RNA, however, in at least some persistent atypical hepatocyte nodules with associated regions of hepatocellular carcinoma. Furthermore, DNA from normal human fibroblasts of persons with high cancer-risk syndromes, including familial polyposis coli, Gardner syndrome, site-specific familial tumor aggregations, and xeroderma pigmentosum, was observed to lack transforming activity in the NIH 3T3 transfection assay.[93] It is therefore possible that increased proto-oncogene or oncogene expression may in some cases be more related to tumor progression, which includes the stage at which a precancerous lesion undergoes the transition to malignancy (see Chapter 10). The reader is referred to Chapters 7, 14, and 20 for alternative views.

A number of studies have demonstrated an increasing chromosomal instability or altered karyotypes within cells of precancerous skin and liver lesions that were experimentally induced in rodents. Aneuploid cells were observed by Conti *et al.*[90] in at least one half of skin papillomas that developed in mice after initiation with dimethylbenz(a)anthracene followed by 10 weeks of tumor promotion with 12-*O*-tetradecanoyl-phorbol-13-acetate. By the 20th week of tumor promotion, almost every papilloma were found to contain several aneuploid cells, and the squamous cell carcinomas that subsequently developed in these animals were all highly aneuploid.* Mori *et al.*[94]

---

*More recently, Aldaz *et al.* reported that dysplasia and aneuploidy are both characteristic features of most skin papillomas induced in SENCAR mice by a two-stage carcinogenesis regimen involving 20 weeks of tumor promotion with phorbol 12-myristate 13-acetate (PMA).[102]

also observed that hyperbasophilic foci of atypical hepatocytes induced in rat liver by a chronic dietary administration of 0.02% 2-acetylaminofluorene exhibited an aneuploid pattern resembling those of cells in hepatocellular carcinomas. More recently, Sarafoff *et al.*[95] reported that while most ATPase-deficient hepatocyte foci induced in rat liver by a single dose of *N*-methyl-*N*-nitrosourea followed by a chronic administration of phenobarbital consisted of an almost exclusive diploid cell population, others showed a tetraploid pattern, and a few of the larger foci contained a mixture of di-, tetra-, and octoploid hepatocytes. While these experimental findings are limited, they do suggest that chromosomal variations, and in particular aneuploidy, may be related to an increased risk of conversion of precancerous stages to malignancy. The relationship between aneuploidy and tumor progression is discussed in further detail in Chapter 10.

Lastly, a number of studies have been reported that were directed toward the isolation and, in some cases, the culturing of cells from presumptive precursor lesions for some types of malignant neoplasms in experimental animals and humans. For example, the laboratories of Thorgeirsson[96] and Pitot[92] have both described procedures for the isolation of cell populations highly enriched in γ-glutamyl transpeptidase-positive hepatocytes from the whole livers of rats containing enzyme-altered hepatocellular foci and/or nodules. Atypical cells were also isolated directly from hyper-plastic hepatocellular nodules induced in rat liver by the feeding of 2-acetylaminofluorene;[97,98] Kitagawa *et al.*[97] further demonstrated the maintenance of such cells in primary culture. Willson *et al.*[99] recently described culture methods that were used to derive cell lines from human colon adenomas and adenocarcinomas. In this study, the cell lines were developed from tubular and villous polyps, primary adenocarcinomas, and hepatic metastases that occurred in patients with colon adenocarcinomas. Interestingly, culture cells from the tubular polyps were found to have a normal human karyotype, while those from villous polyps and all the adenocarcinomas were aneuploid with stable marker chromosomes. In this regard, the culturing of cells isolated from precursor lesions may provide useful models for investigating the sequential steps underlying the development of malignant neoplastic disease.

# REFERENCES

1. Lichtman, M. A., and Brennan, J. K., 1983, Dyshemopoietic (preleukemic) disorders, in: *Hematology*, 3rd ed. (A. J. Williams, E. Beutler, A. J. Erslev, and M. A. Lichtman, eds.), pp. 175–184, McGraw-Hill, New York.
2. Goldfarb, S., 1983. Pathology of neoplasia, in: *Concepts in Cancer Medicine* (S. B. Kahn, R. R. Love, C. Sherman, Jr., and R. Chakravorty, eds.), pp. 127–142, Grune & Stratton, Orlando, Florida.
3. Klein-Szanto, A. J. P., 1984, Morphological evaluation of tumor promoter effects on mammalian skin, in: *Mechanisms of Tumor Promotion: Tumor Promotion and Skin Carcinogenesis*, Vol. 2 (T. J. Slaga, ed.), pp. 41–72. CRC Press, Boca Raton, Florida.
4. Berkelhammer, J., and Oxenhandler, R. W., 1987, Evaluation of premalignant and malignant lesions during the induction of mouse melanomas, *Cancer Res.* **47:**1251–1254.
5. Sirica, A. E., and Pitot, H. C., 1982, Phenotypic markers of hepatic ''pre-neoplasia'' and neoplasia in the rat, in: *Cancer-Cell Organelles*, Vol. 11 (E. Reid, G. M. W. Cook, and D. J. Morre, eds.), pp. 131–143, Ellis Horwood, Chichester.
6. Bannasch, P., Moore, M. A., Klimek, and Zerban, H., 1982, Biological markers of preneoplastic foci and neoplastic nodules in rodent liver, *Toxicol. Pathol.* **10:**19–36.
7. Bannasch, P., 1986, Preneoplastic lesions as end points in carcinogenicity testing. I. Hepatic preneoplasia, *Carcinogenesis* **7:**689–695.
8. Farber, E., and Sarma, D. S. R., 1987, Hepatocarcinogenesis: A dynamic cellular perspective, *Lab. Invest.* **56:**4–22.
9. McD. Herrold, K., 1967, Histogenesis of malignant liver tumors induced by dimethylnitrosamine. An experimental study in Syrian hamsters, *J. Natl. Cancer Inst.* **39:**1099–1111.
10. Reddy, K. P., Buschmann, R. J., and Chomet, B., 1977, Cholangiocarcinomas induced by feeding 3′-methyl-4-dimethylaminoazobenzene to rats, *Am. J. Pathol.* **87:**189–204.
11. Bannasch, P., 1986, Preneoplastic lesions as end points in carcinogenicity testing. II. Preneoplasia in various non-hepatic tissues, *Carcinogenesis* **7:**849–852.

12. Goldfarb, S., and Pugh, T. D., 1986, Multistage rodent hepatocarcinogenesis, *Prog. Liver Dis.* **8:**597–620.

13. Longnecker, D. S., and Crawford, B. G., 1974, Hyperplastic nodules and adenomas of exocrine pancreas in azaserine-treated rats, *J. Natl. Cancer Inst.* **53:**573–577.

14. Mori, H., Tanaka, T., Takahashi, M., and Williams, G. M., 1983, Exclusion of cellular iron and reduced γ-glutamyl transpeptidase activity in rat pancreas acinar cell hyperplastic nodules and adenomas induced by azaserine, *Gann* **74:**497–501.

15. Roebuck, B. D., Baumgartner, K. J., Thron, C. D., and Longnecker, D. S., 1984, Inhibition by retinoids of the growth of azaserine-induced foci in the rat pancreas, *J. Natl. Cancer Inst.* **73:**233–236.

16. Longnecker, D. S., Roebuck, B. D., and Kuhlmann, E. T., 1985, Enhancement of pancreatic carcinogenesis by a dietary unsaturated fat in rats treated with saline or N-nitroso(2-hydroxypropyl) (2-oxopropyl) amine, *J. Natl. Cancer Inst.* **74:**219–222.

17. Sindelar, W. F., and Kurman, C. C., 1982, Nitrosamine-induced pancreatic carcinogenesis in outbred and inbred Syrian hamsters, *Carcinogenesis* **3:**1021–1026.

18. Scarpelli, D. G., Rao, M. S., and Subbarao, V., 1983, Augmentation of carcinogenesis by N-nitrosobis(2-oxopropyl)amine administered during S phase of the cell cycle in regenerating hamster pancreas, *Cancer Res.* **43:**611–616.

19. Ishikawa, O., Wade, A., Oohigashi, H., Imaoka, S., and Iwanaga, T., 1984, Relationship between goblet cells and carcinoma of the pancreas during N-nitrosobis(2-hydroxypropyl)amine-induced carcinogenesis in Syrian golden hamsters, *Cancer Res.* **44:**1630–1634.

20. Pour, P. M., 1984, Histogenesis of exocrine pancreatic cancer in the hamster model, *Environ. Health Perspect.* **56:**229–243.

21. Wattenberg, L. W., Jerina, D. M., Lam, L. K. T., and Yagi, H., 1979, Neoplastic effects of oral administration of (±)-trans-7,8-dihydroxy-7,8-dihydrobenzo(a)pyrene and their inhibition by butylated hydroxyanisole, *J. Natl. Cancer Inst.* **62:**1103–1106.

22. Ito, N., Fukushima, S., Hagiwara, A., Shibata, M., and Ogiso, T., 1983, Carcinogenicity of butylated hydroxyanisole in F344 rats, *J. Natl. Cancer Inst.* **70:**343–352.

23. Masui, T., Asamoto, M., Hirsoe, M., Fukushima, S., and Ito, N., 1986, Disappearance of upward proliferation and persistence of downward basal cell proliferation in rat forestomach papillomas induced by butylated hydroxyanisole, *Jpn. J. Cancer Res. (Gann)* **77:**854–857.

24. Chan, P. C., Haseman, J. K., Boorman, G. A., Huff, J., Manus, A. G., and Cardy, R. H., 1986, Forestomach lesions in rats and mice administered 3-chloro-2-methylpropene by gavage for two years, *Cancer Res.* **46:**6349–6352.

25. Schlake, W., and Nomura, K., 1979, Histogenesis of carcinoma in the glandular stomach of the rat after BI resection, in: *Current Topics in Pathology: Carcinogenesis,* Vol. 67 (E. Grundmann, ed.), pp. 1–67, Springer-Verlag, Berlin.

26. Höhn, P., 1979, Morphology and morphogenesis of experimentally induced small intestinal tumors, in: *Current Topics in Pathology: Carcinogenesis,* Vol. 67 (E. Grundmann, ed.), pp. 69–144, Springer-Verlag, Berlin.

27. Reddy, B. S., 1983, Tumor promotion in colon carcinogenesis, in: *Mechanism of Tumor Promotion: Tumor Promotion in Internal Organs,* Vol. 1 (T. J. Slaga, ed.), pp. 107–129, CRC Press, Boca Raton, Florida.

28. Shioda, Y., Brown, W. R., and Ahnen, D. J., 1987, Serial observations of colonic carcinogenesis in the rat: Premalignant mucosa binds *Ulex europeus* agglutinin, *Gastroenterology* **92:**1–12.

29. Dunnick, J. K., Boorman, G. A., Haseman, J. K., Langloss, J., Cardy, R. H., and Manus, A. G., 1986, Lung neoplasms in rodents after chronic administration of dimethyl hydrogen phosphite, *Cancer Res.* **46:**264–270.

30. Nettesheim, P., Griesemer, R. A., Martin, D. H., and Caton, Jr., J. E., 1977, Induction of preneoplastic and neoplastic lesions in grafted rat tracheas continuously exposed to benzo(a)pyrene, *Cancer Res.* **37:**1272–1278.

31. Becci, P. J., McDowell, E. M., and Trump, B. F., 1978, The respiratory epithelium. IV. Histogenesis of epidermoid metaplasia and carcinoma *in situ* in the hamster, *J. Natl. Cancer Inst.* **61:**577–586.

32. Becci, P. J., McDowell, E. M., and Trump, B. F., 1978, The respiratory epithelium. VI. Histogenesis of lung tumors induced by benzo(a)pyrene-ferric oxide in the hamster, *J. Natl. Cancer Inst.* **61:**607–618.

33. Hard, G. C., and Butler, W. H., 1971, Morphogenesis of epithelial neoplasms induced in the rat kidney by dimethylnitrosamine, *Cancer Res.* **31:**1496–1505.

34. Tsuda, H., Hacker, H. J., Katayama, H., Masui, T., Ito, N., and Bannasch, P., 1986, Correlative histochemical studies on preneoplastic and neoplastic lesions in the kidney of rats treated with nitrosamines, *Virchows Arch.* **51:**385–404.

35. Kunze, E., 1979, Development of urinary bladder cancer in the rat, in: *Current Topics in Pathology: Carcinogenesis*, Vol. 67 (Grundmann, E., ed.), pp. 145–232, Springer-Verlag, Berlin.

36. Isaacs, J. T., 1984, The aging ACI/Seg. versus Copenhagen male rat as a model system for the study of prostatic carcinogenesis, *Cancer Res.* **44:**5785–5791.

37. Asch, H. L., and Asch, B. B., 1985, Heterogeneity of keratin expression in mouse mammary hyperplastic alveolar nodules and adenocarcinomas, *Cancer Res.* **45:**2760–2768.

38. Gray, D. A., McGrath, C. M., Jones, R. F., and Morris, V. L., 1986, A common mouse mammary tumor virus integration site in chemically induced precancerous mammary hyperplasias, *Virology* **148:**360–368.

39. Farber, E., 1984, Pre-cancerous steps in carcinogenesis: Their physiological adaptive nature, *Biochim. Biophys. Acta* **738:**171–180.

40. Pitot, H. C., and Sirica, A. E., 1980, The stages of initiation and promotion in hepatocarcinogenesis, *Biochim. Biophys. Acta* **605:**191–215.

41. Ogawa, K., Solt, D. B., and Farber, E., 1980, Phenotypic diversity as an early property of putative preneoplastic hepatocyte populations in liver carcinogenesis, *Cancer Res.* **40:**725–733.

42. Schulte-Hermann, R., 1985, Tumor promotion in the liver, *Arch. Toxicol.* **57:**147–158.

43. Institute of Laboratory Animal Resources, NRC, 1980, Introduction to histologic typing of liver tumors of the rat, *J. Natl. Cancer Inst.* **64:**181–191.

44. Bannasch, P., 1984, Sequential cellular changes during chemical carcinogenesis, *J. Cancer Res. Clin. Oncol.* **108:**11–22.

45. Farber, E., 1984, The multistep nature of cancer development, *Cancer Res.* **44:**4217–4223.

46. Teebor, G. W., and Becker, F. F., 1971, Regression and persistence of hyperplastic hepatic nodules induced by *N*-2-fluorenylacetamide and their relationship to hepatocarcinogenesis, *Cancer Res.* **31:**1–3.

47. Rotstein, J. Sarma, D. S. R., and Farber, E., 1986, Sequential alterations in growth control and cell dynamics of rat hepatocytes in early precancerous steps in hepatocarcinogenesis, *Cancer Res.* **46:**2377–2385.

48. Moore, M. A., Hacker, H.-J., and Bannasch, P., 1983, Phenotypic instability in focal and nodular lesions induced in a short term system in the rat liver, *Carcinogenesis* **4:**595–603.

49. Goldsworthy, T., Campbell, H. A., and Pitot, H. C., 1984, The natural history and dose-response characteristics of enzyme-altered foci in rat liver following phenobarbital and diethylnitrosamine administration, *Carcinogenesis* **5:**67–71.

50. Goldsworthy, T. L., and Pitot, H. C., 1985, The quantitative analysis and stability of histochemical markers of altered hepatic foci in rat liver following initiation by diethylnitrosamine administration and promotion with phenobarbital, *Carcinogenesis* **6:**1261–1269.

51. Sirica, A. E., Jicinsky, J. K., and Heyer, E. K., 1984, Effect of chronic phenobarbital administration on the gamma-glutamyl transpeptidase activity of hyperplastic liver lesions induced in rats by the Solt/Farber initiation: Selection process of hepatocarcinogenesis, *Carcinogenesis* **5:**1737–1740.

52. Goldfarb, S., Pugh, T. D., Koen, H., and He, Y.-Z., 1983, Preneoplastic and neoplastic progression during hepatocarcinogenesis in mice injected with diethylnitrosamine in infancy, *Environ. Health Perspect.* **50:**149–161.

53. Vesselinovitch, S. D., Hacker, H. J., and Bannasch, P., 1985, Histochemical characterization of focal hepatic lesions induced by single diethylnitrosamine treatment in infant mice, *Cancer Res.* **45:**2774–2780.

54. Lombardi, B., 1982, On the nature, properties and significance of oval cells, in: *Recent Trends in Chemical Carcinogenesis*, Vol. 1 (P. Pani, F. Feo, and A. Columbano, eds.), pp. 37–56, ESA, Cagliari.

55. Sell, S., and Leffert, H. L., 1982, An evaluation of cellular lineages in the pathogenesis of experimental hepatocellular carcinoma, *Hepatology* **2:**77–86.

56. Hayner, N. T., Braun, L., Yaswen, P., Brooks, M., and Fausto, N., 1984, Isozyme profiles of oval cells, parenchymal cells, and biliary cells isolated by centrifugal elutriation from normal and preneoplastic livers, *Cancer Res.* **44:**332–338.

57. Sirica, A. E., and Cihla, H. P., 1984, Isolation and partial characterizations of oval and hyperplastic bile ductular cell-enriched populations from the livers of carcinogen and noncarcinogen-treated rats, *Cancer Res.* **44:**3454–3466.

58. Tsao, M.-S., and Grisham, J. W., 1987, Hepatocarcinomas, cholangiocarcinomas, and hepatoblastomas produced by chemically transformed cultured rat liver epithelial cells, *Am. J. Pathol.* **127:**168–181.

59. Robbins, S. L., Cotran, R. S., and Kumar, V., 1984, *Pathologic Basis of Disease*, 3rd ed., W. B. Saunders, Philadelphia.

60. Kraus, F. T., 1985, Female genitalia, in: *Anderson's Pathology*, 8th ed., Vol. 2 (J. M. Kissane, ed.), pp. 1451–1545, C. V. Mosby, St. Louis.

61. Buchler, D. A., 1983, Cervical cancer, in *Concepts in Cancer Medicine* (S. B. Kahn, R. R. Love, C. Sherman, Jr., and R. Chakravorty, eds.), pp. 463–471, Grune & Stratton, Orlando, Florida.

62. Robbins, S. L., Cotran, R. S., and Kumar, V., 1984, *Pathologic Basis of Disease*, 3rd ed., W. B. Saunders, Philadelphia.

63. Fine, G., and Ma, C. K., 1985, Alimentary tract, in: *Anderson's Pathology*, 8th ed. Vol. 2 (J. M. Kissane, ed.), pp. 1055–1095, C. V. Mosby, St. Louis.

64. Chakravorty, R. C., 1983, Colorectal cancer, in: *Concepts in Cancer Medicine* (S. B. Kahn, R. R. Love, C. Sherman, Jr., and M. D. Chakravorty, eds.), pp. 437–461, Grune & Stratton, Orlando, Florida.

65. Gilbertsen, V. A., 1974, Proctosigmoidoscopy and polypectomy in reducing the incidence of rectal cancer, *Cancer* **34**:936–939.

66. Greene, M. H., Clark, W. H., Jr., Tucker, M. A., Elder, D. E., Kraemer, K. H., Guerry IV, D., Witmer, W. K., Thompson, J., Matozzo, I., and Fraser, M. C., 1985, Acquired precursors of cutaneous malignant melanoma: The familial dysplastic nevus syndrome, *N. Engl. J. Med.* **312**:91–97.

67. Reed, R. J., 1984, A classification of melanocytic dysplasias and malignant melanomas, *Am. J. Dermatopathol.* **6**:195–206.

68. Clark Jr., W. H., Elder, D. E., Guerry IV, D., Epstein, M. N., Greene, M. H., and Van Horn, M., 1984, A study of tumor progression: The precursor lesions of superficial spreading and nodular melanoma, *Hum. Pathol.* **15**:1147–1165.

69. Anthony, P. P., 1976, Precursor lesions for liver cancer in humans, *Cancer Res.* **36**:2579–2583.

70. Roncalli, M., Borzio, M., DeBiagi, G., Servida, E., Cantaboni, A., Sironi, M., and Taccagni, G. L., 1985, *Histopathology* **9**:209–221.

71. Roncalli, M., Borzio, M., DeBiagi, G., Ferrari, A. R., Macchi, R., Tombesi, V. M., and Servida, E., 1986, Liver cell dysplasia in cirrhosis: A serologic and immunohistochemical study, *Cancer* **57**:1515–1521.

72. Akagi, G., Furuya, K., Kanamura, A., Chihara, T., and Otsuka, H., 1984, Liver cell dysplasia and hepatitis B surface antigen in liver cirrhosis and hepatocellular carcinoma, *Cancer* **54**:315–318.

73. Kew, M. C., Ray, M. B., Desmet, J. V., and Desmeiter, J., 1980, Hepatitis B surface antigen in tumour tissue and non-tumorous liver in black patients with hepatocellular carcinoma, *Br. J. Cancer* **41**:399–406.

74. Okuda, K., 1986, Early recognition of hepatocellular carcinoma, *Hepatology* **6**:729–738.

75. Henmi, A., Uchida, T., and Shikata, T., 1985, Karyometric analysis of liver cell dysplasia and hepatocellular carcinoma: Evidence against precancerous nature of liver cell dysplasia, *Cancer* **55**:2594–2599.

76. Yaginuma, K., Kobayashi, M., Yoshida, E., and Koike, K., 1985, Hepatitis B virus integration in hepatocellular carcinoma DNA: Duplication of cellular flanking sequences at the integration site, *Proc. Natl. Acad. Sci. USA* **82**:4458–4462.

77. Hino, O., Shows, T. B., and Rogler, C. E., 1986, Hepatitis B virus integration site in hepatocellular carcinoma at chromosome 17,18 translocation, *Proc. Natl. Acad. Sci. USA* **83**:8338–8342.

78. Arakawa, M., Kage, M., Sugihara, S., Nakashima, T., Suenaga, M., and Okuda, K., 1986, Emergence of malignant lesions within an adenomatous hyperplastic nodule in a cirrhotic liver: Observations in five cases, *Gastroenterology* **91**:198–208.

79. McNeal, J. E., and Bostwick, D. G., 1986, Intraductal dysplasia: A premalignant lesion of the prostate, *Hum. Pathol.* **17**:64–71.

80. Jarvis, L. R., and Whitehead, R., 1985, Morphometric analysis of gastric dysplasia, *J. Pathol.* **147**:133–138.

81. Squartini, F., Bistocchi, M., Sarnelli, R., and Basolo, F., 1986, Early pathologic changes in experimental and human breast cancer: facts and comments, *Ann. NY Acad. Sci.* **464**:231–261.

82. Auerbach, O., Stout, A. P., Hammond, E. C., and Garfinkel, L., 1961, Changes in bronchial epithelium in relation to cigarette smoking and in relation to lung cancer, *N. Engl. J. Med.* **265**:253–267.

83. Parsa, I., Longnecker, D. S., Scarpelli, D. G., Pour, P., Reddy, J. K., and Lefkowitz, M., 1985, Ductal metaplasia of human exocrine pancreas and its association with carcinoma, *Cancer Res.* **45**:1285–1290.

84. Albores-Saavedra, J., Alcántra-Vazquez, A., Cruz-Ortiz, H., and Herrera-Goepfert, R., 1980, The precursor lesions of invasive gallbladder carcinoma: Hyperplasia, atypical hyperplasia and carcinoma *in situ*, *Cancer* **45**:919–927.

85. Ojeda, V. J., Shilkin, K. B., and Walters, M.N-I., 1985, Premalignant epithelial lesions of the gallbladder: A prospective study of 120 cholecystectomy specimens, *Pathology* **17**:451–454.

86. Tatematsu, M., Shirai, T., Tsuda, H., Miyata, Y., Shinohara, Y., and Ito, N., 1977, Rapid production of hyperplastic liver nodules in rats treated with carcinogenic chemicals: A new approach for an *in vivo* short-term screening test for hepatocarcinogens, *Gann* **68**:499–507.

87. Sirica, A. E., Barsness, L., Goldsworthy, T., and Pitot, H. C., 1978, Definition of stages during hepatocarcinogenesis in the rat: Potential application of the evaluation of initiating and promoting agents in the environment, *J. Environ. Pathol. Toxicol.* **2**:21–28.

88. Schulte-Hermann, R., Timmermann-Trosiener, I., and Schuppler, J., 1986, Facilitated expression of adaptive responses to phenobarbital in putative pre-stages of liver cancer, *Carcinogenesis* **7**:1651–1655.

89. Balmain, A., Ramsden, M., Bowden, G. T., and Smith, J., 1984, Activation of the mouse cellular Harvey-ras gene in chemically induced benign skin papillomas, *Nature (Lond.)* **307**:658–660.

90. Conti, C. J., Aldaz, C. M., O'Connell, J., Klein-Szanto, A. J. P., and Slaga, T. J., 1986, Aneuploidy, an early event in mouse skin tumor development, *Carcinogenesis* **7**:1845–1848.

91. Toftgard, R., Roop, D. R., and Yuspa, S. H., 1985, Proto-oncogene expression during two-stage carcinogenesis in mouse skin, *Carcinogenesis* **6**:655–657.

92. Beer, D. G., Schwarz, M., Sawada, N., and Pitot, H. C., 1986, Expression of H-ras and c-myc protooncogenes in isolated γ-glutamyl transpeptidase-positive rat hepatocytes and in hepatocellular carcinomas induced by diethylnitrosamine, *Cancer Res.* **46**:2435–2441.

93. Needleman, S. W., Yuasa, Y., Shivastava, S., and Aaronson, S. A., 1983, Normal cells of patients with high cancer risk syndromes lack transforming activity in the NIH/3T3 transfection assay, *Science* **222**:173–175.

94. Mori, H., Tanaka, T., Sugie, S., Takahashi, M., and Williams, G. M., 1982, DNA content of liver cell nuclei of *N*-2-fluorenylacetamide-induced altered foci and neoplasms in rats and human hyperplastic foci, *J. Natl. Cancer Inst.* **69**:1277–1282.

95. Sarafoff, M., Rabes, H. M. and Dörmer, P., 1986, Correlations between ploidy and initiation probability determined by DNA cytophotometry in individual altered hepatic foci, *Carcinogenesis* **7**:1191–1196.

96. Evarts, R. P., Marsden, E., Hanna, P., Wirth, P. J., and Thorgeirsson, S. S., 1984, Isolation of preneoplastic rat liver cells by centrifugal elutriation and binding to asialofetuin, *Cancer Res.* **44**:5718–5724.

97. Kitagawa, T., Michalopoulos, G., and Pitot, H. C., 1975, Unscheduled DNA synthesis in cells from *N*-2-fluorenylacetamide-induced hyperplastic nodules of rat liver maintained in a primary culture system, *Cancer Res.* **35**:3682–3692.

98. DeGerlache, J., Lans, M., Taper, H., and Roberfroid, M., 1980, Separate isolation of cells from nodules and surrounding parenchyma of the same precancerous rat liver: Biochemical and cytochemical characterization, *Toxicology* **18**:225–232.

99. Willson, J. K. V., Bittner, G. N., Oberley, T. D., Meisner, L. F., and Weese, J. L., Cell culture of human colon adenomas and carcinomas, *Cancer Res.* **47**:2704–2713.

100. Hendrich, S., Glauert, H. P., and Pitot, H. C., 1986, The phenotypic stability of altered hepatic foci: Effects of withdrawal and subsequent readministration of phenobarbital, *Carcinogenesis* **7**:2041–2045.

101. Lefkowitch, J. H., and Apfelbaum, T. F., 1987, Liver cell dysplasia and hepatocellular carcinoma in non-A, non-B hepatitis, *Arch. Pathol. Lab. Med.* **111**:170–173.

102. Aldaz, C. M., Conti, C. J., Klein-Szanto, A. J. P., and Slaga, T. J., 1987, Progressive dysplasia and aneuploidy are hallmarks of mouse skin papillomas: Relevance to malignancy, *Proc. Natl. Acad. Sci. USA* **84**:2029–2032.

# 10

# Tumor Progression and the Clonal Evolution of Neoplasia

## Alphonse E. Sirica

## 1. INTRODUCTION

Tumor progression has for many years been recognized as an important stage in the development of malignant neoplasia. In 1935, Peyton Rous[1] first used the term progression to describe the development in rabbits of carcinoma from viral-induced cutaneous papillomas. However, it was Leslie Foulds in the late 1940s who first generalized the concept of tumor progression.[2-4] According to Foulds, "the concept of progression is one of stepwise neoplastic development through qualitatively different stages."[5] In particular, he has stated that tumors gain or lose characters such as growth rate, invasiveness, powers of metastasis, hormone responsiveness, and morphologic characteristics independently. Furthermore, these changes were considered by Foulds to be essentially irreversible and to result in an increased autonomy.[4] That such changes may in fact undergo apparent reversibility is discussed at the end of this chapter.

A number of other related definitions of tumor progression have also been presented (i.e., see Chapter 19). In this regard, Farber[5] recently defined progression as being "the stepwise process whereby the occasional expanded initiated cell, the [precancerous] nodule, the polyp, or the papilloma, evolves into a cancer and further steps the cancer undergoes as it becomes progressively more malignant." He has further indicated that the sequence characterizing the transition from a precancerous lesion to a malignant neoplasm is the least understood of any segment of the carcinogenic process.[5]

Closely linked to tumor progression is the phenomenon of tumor heterogeneity.[6] Pleomorphism or cellular variability within tumors has been known since the nineteenth century to be a characteristic of malignant neoplasms. During the 1960s, Van Potter and colleagues[7,8] eloquently demonstrated a marked degree of heterogeneity in the enzyme patterns of a variety of transplantable diploid and some aneuploid hepatocellular carcinomas of the rat. Further, malignant neoplasms have now been demonstrated to exhibit heterogeneity with respect to such diverse phenotypic properties as growth rate, metastatic capability, susceptibility to the cytotoxic actions of chemotherapeutic agents, antigenicity and immunogenicity, cell membrane glycoprotein composition, hormone receptors, cellular products, enzymes, and karyotype.[6,9-12] However, phenotypic heterogeneity is not just limited to malignant neoplasms but has also been found in preneoplastic lesions such as the hyperplastic foci of atypical hepatocytes manifested in rat liver during chemical

---

*Alphonse E. Sirica* • Department of Pathology, Medical College of Virginia, Virginia Commonwealth University, Richmond, Virginia 23298.

hepatocarcinogenesis.[12–14] Likewise, cells of normal tissues have been shown to exhibit hetero-geneity in a number of characteristics, but this has usually not been as pronounced as that seen in malignant neoplasms.[6,11]

There is now considerable evidence to indicate that most animal and human neoplasms are derived from a single altered cell.[15,16] On the other hand, that many primary malignant neoplasms appear to have a monoclonal origin seems at first glance to be in conflict with their observed phenotypic heterogeneity. In an effort to relate the single-cell origin of malignant neoplasms with tumor progression and heterogeneity, Peter Nowell[16,17] proposed the concept of clonal evolution in neoplastic populations. In brief, this concept implies that tumor progression represents the result of sequential selection over time of increasingly variant subpopulations within the original clone. It has been further suggested that such a clonal evolution might be the result of an enhanced genetic instability within the neoplastic cell population.[16,17]

The aim of this chapter is to review tumor progression within the context of Foulds' general principles, clonality, and possible underlying mechanisms. For further treatment of this complex phenomenon, the reader is referred to recent reviews by Heppner,[6] Nicolson,[11] Nowell,[16] and Rubin.[18]

## 2. STRUCTURAL VARIATION IN TUMORS

Structural variation is a common feature of malignant neoplasms. Considerable variability, including difference in stromal content and composition, inflammatory cell response, vascular supply, tumor architecture, and degrees of anaplasia and tumor cell differentiation, can be encoun-tered not only within different tumors of a particular type, but also within different regions of an individual tumor. The histologic appearance of tumors can also change over time, generally in the direction of increasing malignancy, and metastatic tumors often correspond in their appearance to the less well-differentiated components of the original primary tumor.[19]

Invasive breast cancer represents a good example of a malignant neoplasm illustrating such structural variation. These tumors can vary in amount of connective tissue (i.e., scirrhous versus medullary carcinomas), secretory activity (i.e., colloid carcinoma), and growth patterns (i.e., papillary versus tubular carcinomas).[20,21] In the dog, for example, one may observe within a single tissue section of a given malignant breast tumor, areas of papillary, tubular, and medullary car-cinoma.[22] Similarly, combined histologic types are found in human breast cancers, with a reported incidence of around 22%.[20] Furthermore, as exemplified by the rat mammary gland adenocar-cinoma shown in Fig. 1a,b, different areas of malignant breast tumors can usually be found to show higher degrees of anaplasia and loss of differentiation than others, even within the same tissue section.

## 3. FOULDS' GENERAL PRINCIPLES OF TUMOR PROGRESSION

As a result of his pioneering studies on mammary neoplasms in the mouse, Foulds originally proposed six general principles or rules of tumor progression.[4] Perhaps the most important of these are his rules of (1) "independent progression of multiple tumors," which maintains that progression occurs independently in different neoplasms in the same animal[3,4]; and (2) "independent progres-sion of characters," which states that different characters (e.g., growth rate, metastatic capability, loss of differentiated functions) generally undergo progression independent of one another in the same tumor.[3,4] Foulds[4] further pointed out that "the concept of independently variable characters is crucially important in the study of neoplastic development." In addition, he was among the first to clearly recognize the importance of taking into account the independent variability and consequent individuality of tumors, and he correctly noted that many of the reported biochemical, enzymatic, and antigenic changes seen in particular classes of malignant neoplasms are likely not in themselves "essential components of the neoplastic process, but are only incidental consequences of it."[3,4]

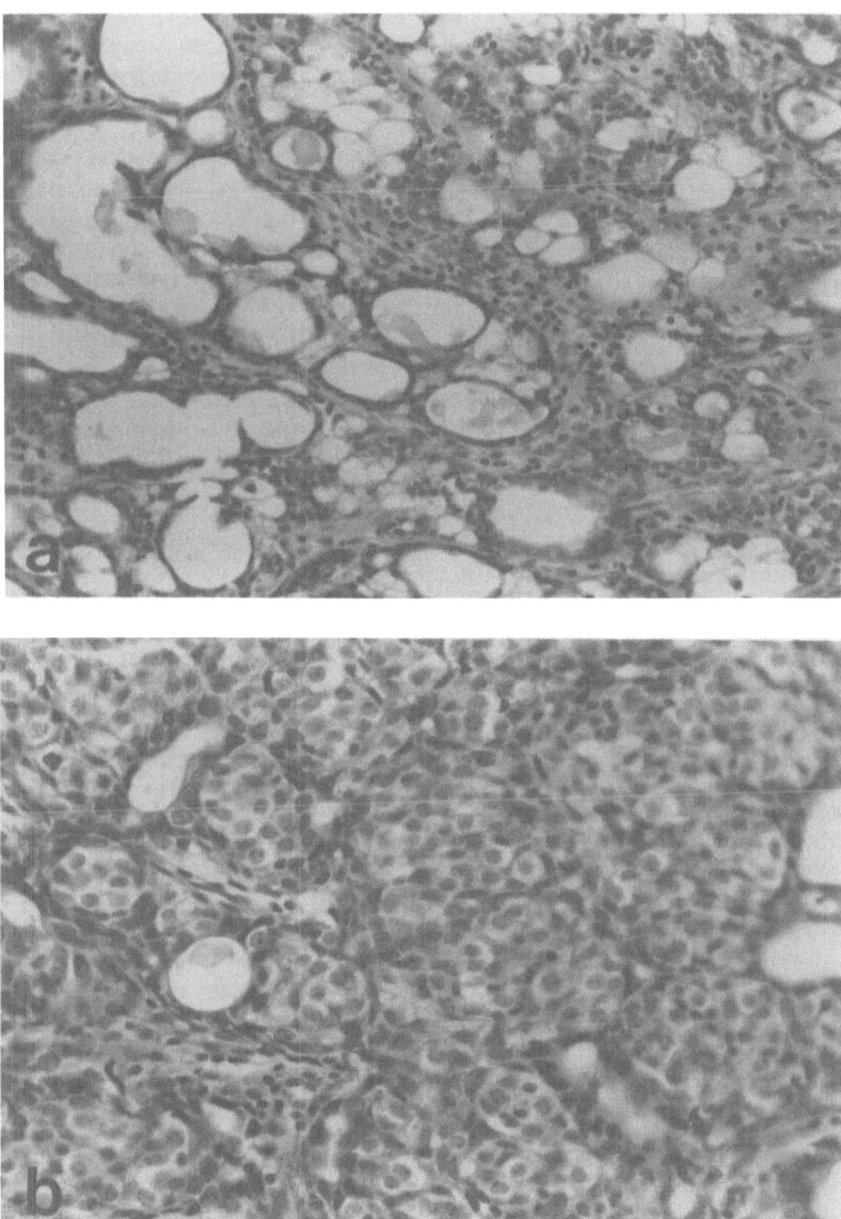

*Figure 1.* Photomicrographs of two separate regions of an individual mammary gland adenocarcinoma induced by the administration of 7,12-dimethylbenz(a)anthracene to a female rat. (a) The region shown demonstrates mainly a well-differentiated cystic glandular appearance of the tumor (H&E, ×128). (b) This region is composed of a highly anaplastic nest of poorly differentiated mammary carcinoma cells (H&E, ×250).

## 4. CLONAL ORIGINS OF NEOPLASMS IN HUMANS AND EXPERIMENTAL ANIMALS

Obviously, heterogeneity in neoplasms would be more easily explained if they were shown to have multiple cell origins, and indeed, data are available to support this form of development for at least some types of neoplasms (i.e., human neurofibromas).[15] However, there is now a substantial amount of evidence to indicate that a vast majority of animal and human neoplasms arise from a single cell of origin.[15,16,23]

The clonal origins of human neoplasms have been established through the use of specific biochemical, molecular, chromosomal, and antigenic markers. Some examples of human malignant neoplasms that in all likelihood develop from a single altered cell, as well as the markers used to determine their monoclonal origin, are as follows: (1) chronic myelocytic leukemia, i.e., Philadelphia chromosome with additional chromosomal changes, X-chromosome-linked isozymes of glucose 6-phosphate dehydrogenase (G6PD), phosphogluconate dehydrogenase isozymes, Rh antigens,[15,16,23] (2) B-cell lymphomas, i.e., exclusive presence of but one immunoglobulin light-chain isotype-kappa (K) or lambda (λ), glucose 6-phosphate dehydrogenase isozymes, unique immunoglobulin-gene rearrangements,[15,24,25] (3) multiple myeloma, i.e., monoclonal gammopathy, presence of the light-chain isotype K or λ,[26] and (4) some hepatocellular carcinomas, i.e., clonal associated sites of integration of hepatitis B virus (HBV) DNA into cellular DNA.[27] A much more complete listing of human neoplasms having a single cell origin can be found in the reviews by Fialkow[15] and Nowell.[16,23]

Analysis of the clonal origin of spontaneous and chemically induced neoplasms as well as of certain preneoplastic lesions has been facilitated by the use of mosaic and chimeric rodent models. Studies employing such animal models have provided strong support for the monoclonal origin of a number of experimentally important neoplasms or preneoplasias that develop in the rat or mouse (Table I). With respect to the mouse skin carcinogenesis studies referred to in Table I, it appears that the discrepancy between the reported findings of Reddy and Fialkow[36] and those of Taguchi et al.[37] and of Iannaccone et al.[32] concerning the percentages of skin papillomas determined to be of monoclonal origin when induced by repeated applications of 7,12-dimethylbenz[a]anthracene (54% versus >90%) is related to the difference in the weekly doses of carcinogen that were applied,[37] and even more likely to the amount of host-derived dermal connective tissue present in the papilloma.[32] In addition, the results obtained by Taguchi et al.[37] are of further interest, having demonstrated that most epidermal carcinomas arising at the same sites at which preceding papillomas were observed had expressed a type of phosphoglycerate kinase-1 that was identical to that of the original papillomas. This finding suggests that malignant conversion occurs within the clone comprising a papilloma, and is quite consistent with Nowell's concept of clonal evolution in neoplastic populations.

As related to the multistage process of hepatocarcinogenesis in rodent liver, it is also relevant that most of the mouse hepatomas and their presumed precursor lesions, as well as the vast majority of atypical hepatocyte foci and nodules expressed in rat liver following initiation with diethylnitrosamine and promotion with phenobarbital, seem to be arising from a single altered cell. The single-cell origin of hepatic neoplasms is further supported by the mathematical analysis performed by Goldfarb and Pugh[31] of hyperbasophilic hepatocyte foci observed in liver at different times after a single injection of diethylnitrosamine into infant male mice. Based upon extrapolations of survival curves for the distribution of foci at 10, 20, and 28 weeks after the carcinogen administration, these investigators were able to estimate that the initial diameter of the foci emerging in livers was 36.4 μm, which is very close to the diameter of a single hepatocyte (13–30 μm). It has also been suggested that at least some metastatic neoplasms may be arising from a single cell within tumor emboli.[38] In this regard, Talmadge and Zbar[38] recently reported that when B16–BL6 mouse melanoma cell clones containing unique genetic markers (introduced into the tumor cells by transfection) were mixed and then inoculated into the footpads of normal syngeneic mice, 87% of the resulting pulmonary metastases were found to be characterized by single markers, indicating that they were clonal in origin.

*Table I. Examples of Spontaneous and Chemically Induced Neoplasms and Preneoplastic Lesions Determined to Be of Monoclonal Origin in Mosaic or Chimeric Rodents*

| Animal model | Carcinogenic treatment | Marker | Lesion | Percentage of lesions of monoclonal origin | References |
|---|---|---|---|---|---|
| Chimeric mouse | None | β-Glucuronidase | Spontaneous hepatomas | 83% | 28 |
| Mosaic mouse | Chronic feeding of 2-acetylamino-fluorene | X-linked phospho-glycerate kinase-1 isozymes | Preneoplastic hepatocyte nodules | 98% | 29 |
| Mosaic mouse | Injection of diethyl-nitrosamine into infants | X-linked carbamyl transferase iso-zymes | Hepatomas | 95% | 30, 31 |
| Chimeric rat | Initiation with diethylnitros-amine; promotion with phenobarbi-tal | Class 1 major histo-compatibility complex alloanti-gens | Preneoplastic hepatocyte foci and nod-ules | 92–98% | 32, 33 |
| Mosaic mouse | Injection of 3-methylcholan-threne | X-linked phospho-glycerate kinase-1 isozymes | Subcutaneous fibrosarcomas | 90% | 34 |
| Chimeric mouse | Initiation with 7,12-dimethylbenz(a)anthracene (DMBA) or 20-methylcholan-threne; promotion with croton oil or 12-*O*-tetradeca-noyl phorbol 13-acetate (TPA) | Glucose 6-phos-phate isomerase isozymes | Mostly skin pa-pillomas and some carci-nomas and fi-brosarcomas | 92% | 35 |
| Mosaic mouse | Initiation with DMBA; promo-tion with TPA | X-linked phospho-glycerate kinase-1 isozymes | Skin papillomas | 80% | 36 |
| Mosaic mouse | Repeated applica-tions of DMBA | X-linked phospho-glycerate kinase-1 isozymes | Skin papillomas | 54% | 36 |
| Mosaic mouse | Initiation with DMBA; promo-tion with TPA | X-linked phospho-glycerate kinase-1 isozymes | Skin papillomas | 93% | 37 |
| | | | Epidermal car-cinomas | 80% | |
| Mosaic mouse | Repeated applica-tions of DMBA | X-linked phospho-glycerate kinase-1 isozymes | Skin papillomas | 93% | 37 |
| | | | Epidermal car-cinomas | 90% | |
| Mosaic mouse | Applications of methylcholan-threne or DMBA | X-linked isozymes | Skin papillomas (epidermal portion) | 96% | 32 |
| | | | Skin papillomas (dermal core) | 42% | |

## 5. MECHANISMS OF TUMOR PROGRESSION

A variety of mechanisms have been proposed to explain tumor progression and heterogeneity within neoplasms. Some of these reflect alterations that act to influence the stability of the genome directly, such as single-cell mutations,[16] unregulated gene amplification,[39,40] gene deletions and rearrangements,[11,16] aneuploidy,[16] and other karyotypic abnormalities.[11,16] In addition, factors known to affect gene regulation including changes in DNA methylation patterns,[41,42] defects in intercellular communication,[11] alterations in the tumor microenvironment,[11,16] disruption of the normal spatial and homeostatic relations between cells and tissues,[18] changes in the expression of cellular oncogenes,[11,16] repeated or continued exposures to carcinogens and other clastogenic substances,[16] and even treatments with therapeutic agents used in cancer therapy[11,16] have been suggested to contribute in varying degrees to the evolution and progression of tumors, as well as to their phenotypic heterogeneity.

It is beyond the scope of this chapter to discuss each of these proposed mechanisms in any detail. Nevertheless, an effort is made to elaborate on the associations made between aneuploidy and oncogenes, respectively, and tumor progression, as there is increasing evidence to suggest that these factors may have important prognostic implications for certain types of human malignant neoplasms.

### 5.1. Aneuploidy and Tumor Progression

Aneuploidy refers to the acquisition or loss of chromosomes so that the cell's chromosome (and nuclear DNA) complement is no longer an exact multiple of the haploid number. Earlier studies have shown that aneuploidy is common in malignant neoplasms and is particularly characteristic of metastatic cell populations. In this regard, increasing aneuploidy has recently been shown to occur during tumor progression in a human melanocyte model,[43] as well as in the progressive neoplastic lesions that develop during chemical carcinogenesis in mouse epidermis and in rat liver (see Chapter 9). In the case of human primary and metastatic melanomas, nonrandom chromosomal abnormalities, mostly involving chromosomes 1, 6, and 7, were also found, although the abnormalities often occurred at different loci within each chromosome.[43] On the other hand, data were recently presented by Gitelman et al.[44] that suggest that amplified DNA in the form of homogeneously staining regions of chromosomes correlates with an augmented metastatic capacity in the human melanoma cell line MeWo assayed in BALB/c nude mice. Of further relevance is the observation that some tumor promoters, such as 12-O-tetradecanoylphorbol 13-acetate (TPA)[45] and select bile acids[46] could induce mitotic aneuploidy in yeast, suggesting a possible mechanism for the progression of some promoted cells to the neoplastic state.

Within recent years, flow cytometry has been used to analyze DNA aneuploidy within a variety of human neoplasms. In this regard, Kokal et al.[47] reported that patients with aneuploid colorectal carcinomas had significantly higher recurrence rates and significantly shorter disease-free and overall survival times than did patients with diploid tumors. In addition, these investigators noted that tumor DNA ploidy was an independent prognostic variable and that among other clinical and pathological variables analyzed, it was the single most important predictor of recurrent disease. Schwartz et al.[48] also found that multiple colorectal carcinomas with identical DNA aneuploidy within a single colon exhibited strikingly different histopathologic features. This finding is interesting if one assumes, as did these investigators, that the multiple tumors represent, at least in some cases, intracolonic metastases from a primary tumor with an identical aneuploid DNA index; this is because it appears to illustrate that even though the DNA content of these multiple colorectal tumors is the same, their histologic phenotypes can be markedly different.

The presence of DNA aneuploidy in such malignant neoplasms as human breast carcinomas,[49] ovarian carcinomas,[50,51] and prostate carcinomas[52,53] has also been associated with higher relapse rates and lower survival times for those patients with these respective tumors. In the case of breast carcinomas, aneuploid tumors exhibited a more extensive axillary lymph node involvement than did the diploid tumors. Also, in a limited study, only ovarian tumors that were invasive were found by flow cytometry to be aneuploid as compared to those that were diploid and which exhibited a borderline malignancy.[50] More recently, Iversen and Skarrland[51] reported that DNA aneuploidy was more frequent in ovarian carcinomas that were characterized by a low degree of differentiation, in patients with advanced stages of the disease, and in the tumors of older patients. DNA aneuploidy was also correlated with the histologic grading of human bladder carcinomas, with the frequency of occurrence of aneuploid cell populations increasing in the more poorly differentiated and invasive tumors.[54,55] On the other hand, Lundberg *et al.*[52] could find no apparent correlation between DNA ploidy and the histologic grade of human prostate carcinomas. Stephenson *et al.*[53] further noted that the DNA ploidy of lymph node metastases of prostate carcinomas had a prognostic impact that was independent of such other variables as the age of the patient, time from diagnosis to treatment, local stage, primary and metastatic grades, and number of positive lymph nodes.

This relationship between DNA aneuploidy and higher tumor recurrence rates and shorter survival times is unclear. However, this relationship is not an absolute one, since Bauer *et al.*[56] found that DNA aneuploidy was without prognostic significance for patients with diffuse large cell lymphomas, although it did appear to correlate with the development of bone marrow infiltration by this cancer. In addition, DNA aneuploidy does not appear to be a prerequisite for metastasis. For example, Stephenson *et al.*[53] reported that of 38 patients with grade-matched moderately differentiated primary carcinomas of the prostate gland, the lymph node metastases in one half of these were diploid and in the other half, aneuploid. Thus, while DNA aneuploidy appears in a number of primary tumors to be related to their biologic aggressiveness, the absence of aneuploidy in a malignant primary tumor does not necessarily mean that it lacks the ability to metastasize, nor does the development of aneuploidy per se appear to be obligatory for a conversion to the malignant neoplastic state.

## 5.2. Oncogenes and Tumor Progression

There is increasing evidence to indicate that alterations of certain cellular oncogenes or proto-oncogenes may play a role in tumor progression in addition to having clinical value as prognostic indicators of tumor aggressiveness for a number of different human cancers. This is illustrated by the following examples. Yokota *et al.*[57] recently observed that amplification of c-*myc* occurred in a variety of advanced widespread solid tumors and in aggressive primary carcinomas and sarcomas but was rare in lymphomas and leukemias. Apparent allelic deletions of c-*ras*[Ha] and c-*myb* were also reported to correlate with tumor progression and metastasis of certain carcinomas and sarcomas. For example, an altered allelic ratio of c-*myb* was noted in a metastasis of a breast carcinoma but was not observed in either the primary tumor or in homologous normal breast tissue. In addition, deletion of the c-*ras*[Ha] allele occurred in metastatic tumors, including those derived from primary carcinomas of the breast, colon, lung, and ovary, at a frequency approximately twice as high as that determined for the primary tumors.

N-*myc*, a cellular proto-oncogene with homology to c-*myc*, has also been shown to be frequently amplified in human neuroblastoma and neuroblastoma cell lines.[58,59] The amplification of N-*myc* in human neuroblastomas has further been demonstrated to correlate with a rapid tumor progression and a poorer prognosis for patients with this cancer. In this regard, the greater the degree of N-*myc* DNA amplification, the worse the patient's prognosis for all stages of the disease.[57,58] Rosen *et al.*[60] also recently demonstrated that N-*myc* expression is increased in neuroblastoma cell lines that were derived from two patients whose tumors had undergone progressive changes *in vivo*.

Amplification of the HER-2/*neu* oncogene, which is related to the *erb* B oncogene family, was demonstrated by Slamon *et al.*[61] to correlate with both the overall survival and time to relapse in humans with breast cancer. As is the case for N-*myc* amplification in human neuroblastomas, the greater the degree of amplification of HER-2/*neu*, the worse the patient's prognosis. Interestingly, HER-2/*neu* gene amplification appeared to have a greater prognostic value than other predicting factors that were examined, including age at the time of diagnosis, size of the primary tumors, and their hormone-receptor status. Moreover, there seemed to be a strong relationship between the amplification of this oncogene in the primary breast tumors and the number of axillary lymph nodes containing metastatic cells. However, it is not yet been established as to whether the HER-2/*neu* gene copy number is greater in the metastatic lesions than in the primary tumors.*

Some human primary colorectal carcinomas have been shown to exhibit amplification of the c-*myc* locus relative to adjacent normal colon tissue and, in a few cases, to manifest a deletion of an allele of c-*ras*Ha.[57,62] In addition, Rothberg et al.[63] presented evidence to suggest that tumors arising in the rectum, as well as the sigmoid and descending colon (left side), more often show an elevation in c-*myc* expression than do tumors of the cecum and ascending colon (right side). In comparison, Augenlicht et al.[64] found no changes in the expression of the *myc* gene family in differentiated human carcinoma cell lines. However, these investigators observed in the differentiated low tumorigenic lines that secrete mucin an overexpression of both c-*ras*Ha and c-Ki-*ras*, with the increase in expression being greater for c-*ras*Ha than for c-Ki-*ras*. This increase was not seen in colon carcinoma cells which are not mucin secreting. These findings are also consistent with those of Gallick et al.,[65] who reported that P21ras levels are higher in more differentiated primary carcinomas than in metastatic tumors of the human colon and rectum.

Recently, Bos et al.[66] demonstrated that 11 of 27 colorectal carcinomas contained mutations of the *ras* genes. Ten of 11 of the mutations were in the c-Ki-*ras* gene, and nine of these were at codon 12 of this gene. In a single tumor, a mutation of codon 12 of the N-*ras* gene was also found. Of particular interest was the observation that in five of six colorectal tumors with *ras* mutations, the same mutation occurred in both adenomatous and carcinomatous portions, suggesting that in most cases, such alterations may precede the development of malignancy. Mutations of *ras* were also noted in both advanced-stage and early-stage carcinomas and, like the elevated expression of c-*myc* described above, seemed to be more common in tumors of the left side than of the right side of colon. By contrast, that mutations in c-Ki-*ras* may be related to the progression of some human colorectal carcinomas was suggested by the finding that in one tumor, a mutation of this gene was exhibited by only that portion of the tumor that was diagnosed as being carcinoma but was not present in that portion that was comprised of adenoma.

At the same time, Forrester et al.[67] independently detected a high incidence of mutant c-Ki-*ras* in primary human colorectal carcinomas, particularly in those originating in pre-existing villous adenomas. These investigators also could find no significant differences between the mutation frequency at codon 12 of this gene and the degree of differentiation or stage of progression of the tumors. However, they did observe a strong correlation between the position of mutations at codon 12 of c-Ki-*ras* and the degree of invasiveness of the tumors. In this regard, 50% of mutations detected in the gene of tumors at an early stage of progression, before they invaded through the bowel wall, were present at the first position (NGT) of codon 12, while almost 90% of the mutations of the more advanced stage carcinomas were at the second position (GNT) of this codon. Activation of c-Ki-*ras* together with the inactivation of certain other c-*onc* genes has also been suggested to be related to cancer progression in cultured lines of malignant myoblasts from rat.[68]

One of the more interesting recent reports suggesting a relationship between proto-oncogene activation and tumor progression is that by Croce and Nowell and their colleagues, who employed combined cytogenetic and molecular genetic studies of a human acute B-cell leukemia cell line to suggest how the sequential activation of two proto-oncogenes might be involved in enhancing the malignancy of a B-lymphocyte neoplasm.[16,69] Analysis of the karyotype of this cell line revealed

---

*Zhou et al. more recently reported that the c-*erb* B-2 oncogene, which has been mapped to the same human chromosomal locus (17q21) as HER-2/*neu*, is amplified at least three times more frequently in breast cancer than in most other types of carcinomas examined and was not found in sarcomas, hematologic malignancies, or other types of tumors studied, including hepatoblastoma, Wilms tumor, and germ cell and neuroendocrine tumors. Amplification of c-*erb* B2 in the breast carcinomas was most evident in those of advanced stage and in which metastasis to regional lymph nodes had occurred, further suggesting a role of this oncogene in the progression and spread of breast cancers.[80] Tal et al. also demonstrated recently that the HER-2/*neu* protooncogene is sporadically amplified in adenocarcinomas of human breast and various gastrointestinal tissues and that, in one colon tumor, a rearrangement in the 3' region of the gene was revealed.[81]

that it carried both the $t$ (8;14) chromosome translocation characteristic of Burkitt lymphoma and the $t$ (14; 18) translocation most often found in the low-grade malignant follicular lymphoma. Furthermore, it was indicated that the $t$ (14; 18) translocation involves the putative oncogene *bcl*-2, while the $t$ (8;14) rearrangement results in activation of c-*myc*. On the basis of these findings, it was postulated by these investigators that if the $t$ (14;18) translocation occurs first, this leads to activation and constitutive expression of the *bcl*-2 gene, resulting in an expansion of a neoplastic B lymphocyte population of relatively low-grade malignancy. These workers further surmised that the subsequent activation of c-*myc* by the $t$ (8; 14) translocation can then lead to the development of a highly malignant neoplasm presented as an acute leukemia.

## 6. CONCLUSIONS

The importance of defining the mechanisms of tumor progression and tumor heterogeneity is obvious, for ultimately it is the emergence of new neoplastic cell populations with changing growth rates, increased invasive and metastatic capabilities, and/or developed resistance against cancer chemotherapeutic drugs which prevents the effective clinical management of many types of animal and human cancers. Also, as indicated in this chapter, while many factors are likely involved in tumor progression, some, such as aneuploidy and c-oncogene changes, have already been shown to have potential clinical value in terms of their being prognostic indicators for certain types of human malignant neoplasms. Moreover, based on currently available data, one may speculate that the increased expression of c-*myc* in some tumors is likely related to further alterations in their proliferative activities, while specific changes in the expression and/or forms of proto-oncogenes such as c-*myb*, HER-2/*neu*, and c-Ki-*ras* may be associated with the acquisition of invasive and metastatic properties by certain neoplastic cell types. However, it is also evident that there is considerable variation in oncogene and proto-oncogene expression among tumors of the same class and of different classes. Thus, the relationship between c-oncogene expression and tumor progression is not an absolute one.[11] Likewise, while aneuploidy changes have been shown to be associated with tumor progression, such changes also do not appear to be absolutely necessary for either neoplastic transformation itself or for metastasis.[53]

The management of progressive neoplastic disease will no doubt benefit by a clearer understanding at the cellular, cytogenetic, biochemical, and molecular genetic levels of those mechanisms or events that (1) permit select rare cells within given precancerous lesions to convert to the neoplastic state, and (2) govern the clonal development of invasive and metastatic cells within tumors. For a detailed discussion of invasion, metastasis, and phenotypic heterogeneity, the reader is referred to Chapters 27 and 28, respectively.

Little is actually known of the mechanisms involved in the conversion of an initiated cell to one that is neoplastic. However, recent studies have focused on the possibility that in some instances, nonrandom genetic events may be involved in this process (see also Chapters 11 and 12).* For example, the loss of genes at specific chromosomal loci has been shown to be characteristic of an number of human cancers, including retinoblastoma, Wilms' tumor, renal carcinoma, transitional cell carcinoma of the bladder, embryonal tumors, and small cell carcinoma of the lung.[70] Another well-known specific chromosomal alteration, involving the c-*abl* oncogene, is the Philadelphia chromosome observed in chronic granulocytic leukemia;[16] nonrandom chromosomal changes may also be involved in the origin or progression of malignant melanoma in the human. Becker[71] further demonstrated that the presence of the viable yellow (A$^{vy}$) gene in C57BL/6N mice, a strain that is not normally predisposed to hepatocarcinogenesis, is associated with not only a much earlier

---

*Hsu also recently reviewed data for specific genetic and cytogenetic alterations associated with malignant neoplasms in humans and has provided additional information to support the role of chromosome instability in cancer predisposition. He further suggested that persons with genetic defects that make them hypersensitive to chromosome damage by carcinogenic mutagens are more likely to develop malignant neoplasms than are those who are more resistant to such damage.[82]

appearance, but also with progression of the histotype of hepatocellular neoplasms that resulted following a single intraperitoneal injection of a low dose of diethylnitrosamine to male neonates containing this gene. Drinkwater and Ginsler[72] recently reported that the single intraperitoneal administration of diethylnitrosamine to newborn male C3H/HeJ mice resulted in the induction of hepatocellular adenomas and carcinomas with a mean number of tumors per animal approximately 20- to 50-fold higher than that for similarly treated C57B1/6J male mice. Furthermore, it was determined that allelic differences for at least two loci contributed to the higher sensitivity to hepatocarcinogenesis of the C3H/HeJ strain relative to the C57BL/6J strain and that a single locus, denoted Hcs for hepatocarcinogen sensitivity, was responsible for about 85% of the difference in susceptibility. Interestingly, newborn male C3H/HeJ mice and C57BL/6J mice injected with [1-$^{14}$C]diethylnitrosamine were found not to differ significantly with respect to the extent of ethylation of their hepatic DNA or in the relative proportions of the two ethylated bases, N-7-ethylguanine and O$^6$-ethylguanine. By contrast, data were obtained to suggest that the Hcs gene primarily affects the promotion stage of liver tumor induction during mouse hepatocarcinogenesis. Such results are interesting because they suggest that the evolution of certain malignant neoplasms may be dependent on nonrandom genetic events that can be defined.

Finally, it is now well established that cell differentiation can be induced in a number of highly malignant cell types, including mouse and/or human embryonal carcinoma cells,[73,74] some other carcinoma cell types,[75] neuroblastoma cells,[76] and various leukemia cell lines[77,78] (see also Chapter 22). These findings indicate that the genomes of such malignant cell types have not been markedly altered by the neoplastic process and that, under appropriate circumstances, the malignant phenotype can be reversed through differentiation. Thus, for at least some malignant neoplasms, tumor progression does not appear to be an irreversible phenomenon. The potential therapeutic implications were recently reviewed by Sartorelli[75,79] and are discussed further in Chapter 22.

## REFERENCES

1. Rous, P., and Beard, J. W., 1935, The progression to carcinoma of virus-induced rabbit papillomas (Shope), *J. Exp. Med.* **62**:523–548.
2. Foulds, L., 1949, Mammary tumors in hybrid mice: Growth and progression of spontaneous tumours, *Br. J. Cancer* **3**:345–375.
3. Foulds, L., 1965, Multuple etiologic factors in neoplastic development, *Cancer Res.* **25**:1339–1347.
4. Foulds, L., 1969, *Neoplastic Development* Vol. 1, Academic Press, London.
5. Farber, E., 1984, The multistep nature of cancer development, *Cancer Res.* **44**:4217–4223.
6. Heppner, G. H., 1984, Tumor heterogeneity, *Cancer Res.* **44**:2259–2265.
7. Potter, V. R., 1964, Biochemical perspectives in cancer research, *Cancer Res.* **24**:1085–1098.
8. Potter, V. R., Watanabe, M., Pitot, H. C., and Morris, H. P., 1969, Systematic oscillations in metabolic activity in rat liver and hepatomas. Survey of normal diploid and other hepatoma lines, *Cancer Res.* **29**:55–78.
9. Poste, G., and Greig, R., 1982, On the genesis and regulation of cellular heterogeneity in malignant tumors, *Invasion Metastasis* **2**:137–176.
10. Ling, V., Chambers, A. F., Harris, J. F., and Hill, R. P., 1985, Quantitative genetic analysis of tumor progression, *Cancer Metastasis Rev.* **4**:173–194.
11. Nicolson, G. L., 1987, Tumor cell instability, diversification, and progression to the metastatic phenotype: From oncogene to oncofetal expression, *Cancer Res.* **47**:1473–1487.
12. Pugh, T. D., and Goldfarb, S., 1978, Quantitative histochemical and autoradiographic studies of hepatocarcinogenesis in rats fed 2-acetylaminofluorene followed by phenobarbital, *Cancer Res.* **38**:4450–4457.
13. Pitot, H. C., Goldsworthy, T., Campbell, H. A., and Poland, A., 1980, Quantitative evaluation of the promotion by 2,3,7,8-tetrachlorodibenzo-*p*-dioxin of hepatocarcinogenesis from diethylnitrosamine, *Cancer Res.* **40**:3616–3620.
14. Peraino, C., Staffeldt, E. E., Carnes, B. A., Ludeman, V. A., Blomquist, J. A., and Vesselinovitch, S. D., 1984, Characterization of histochemically detectable altered hepatocyte foci and their relationship to hepatic tumorigenesis in rats treated once with diethylnitrosamine or benzo(a)pyrene within one day after birth, *Cancer Res.* **44**:3340–3347.

15. Fialkow, P. J., 1976, Clonal origin of human tumors, *Biochim. Biophys. Acta* **458**:283–321.
16. Nowell, P. C., 1986, Mechanisms of tumor progression, *Cancer Res.* **46**:2203–2207.
17. Nowell, P. C., 1980, Chromosomes and tumor progression, in: *Results and Problems in Cell Differentiation—Differentiation and Neoplasia*, Vol. 11 (R. C. McKinnell, M. A. DiBerardino, M. Blumenfeld, and R. D. Bergad, eds.), pp. 102–106, Springer-Verlag, Berlin.
18. Rubin, H., 1985, Cancer as a dynamic developmental disorder, *Cancer Res.* **45**:2935–2942.
19. Ashley, D. J. B., 1972, *An Introduction to the General Pathology of Tumors*, Williams & Wilkins, Baltimore.
20. Robbins, S. L., Cotran, R. S., and Kumar, V., 1984, *Pathologic Basic of Disease*, 3rd ed., W. B. Saunders, Philadelphia.
21. McDivitt, R. W., 1985, Breast in: *Anderson's Pathology*, Vol. 2, 8th ed. (J. M. Kissane, ed.), pp. 1546–1569, C. V. Mosby, St. Louis.
22. Jones, T. C., and Hunt, R. D., 1983, *Veterinary Pathology*, Lea & Febiger, Philadelphia.
23. Nowell, P. C., 1976, The clonal evolution of tumor cell populations, *Science* **194**:23–28.
24. Arnold, A., Cossman, J., Bakhshi, A., Jaffe, E. S., Waldmann, T. A., and Korsmeyer, S. J., 1983, Immunoglobulin-gene rearrangements as unique clonal markers in human lymphoid neoplasms, *N. England J. Med.* **309**:1593–1599.
25. Raffeld, M., Wright, J. J., Lipford, E., Cossman, J., Longo, D. L., Bakhshi, A., and Korsmeyer, S. J., 1987, Clonal evolution of t (14; 18) follicular lymphomas demonstrated by immunoglobulin genes and the 18 q 21 major breakpoint region, *Cancer Res.* **47**:2537–2542.
26. Rywlin, A. M., 1985, Hemopoietic system: reticuloendothelial system, spleen, lymph nodes, bone marrow and blood, in: *Anderson's Pathology* Vol. 2, 8th ed. (J. M. Kissane, ed.), pp. 1338–1340, C. V. Mosby, St. Louis.
27. Esumi, M., Aritaka, T., Arii, M., Suzuki, K., Tanikawa, K., Mizuo, H., Mima, T., and Shikata, T., 1986, Clonal origin of human hepatoma determined by integration of hepatitis B virus DNA, *Cancer Res.* **46**:5767–5771.
28. Condamine, H., Custer, R. P., and Mintz, B., 1971, Pure-strain and genetically mosaic liver tumors histochemically identified with the β-glucuronidase marker in allophenic mice, *Proc. Natl. Acad. Sci. USA* **68**:2032–2036.
29. Rabes, H. M., Bücher, T., Hartmann, A., Linke, I., and Dünnwald, M., 1982, Clonal growth of carcinogen-induced enzyme-deficient proneoplastic cell populations in mouse liver, *Cancer Res.* **42**:3220–3227.
30. Williams, E. D., Wareham, K. A., and Howell, S., 1982, Direct evidence for the single cell origin of mouse liver tumors, *Br. J. Cancer* **47**:723–726.
31. Goldfarb, S., and Pugh, T. D., 1986, Multistage rodent hepatocarcinogenesis, *Prog. Liver Dis.* **8**:597–620.
32. Iannaccone, P. M., Weinberg, W. C., and Deamant, F. D., 1987, Chemically-induced tumors and preneoplasias are clonal growths, *Proc. Am. Assoc. Cancer Res.* **28**:52.
33. Weinberg, W. C., Berkwits, L., and Iannaccone, P. M., 1987, The clonal nature of carcinogen-induced altered foci of γ-glutamyl transpeptidase expression in rat liver, *Carcinogenesis* **8**:565–570.
34. Deamant, F. D., and Iannaccone, P. M., 1985, Evidence concerning the clonal nature of chemically induced tumors: phosphoglycerate kinase-1 isozyme patterns in chemically induced fibrosarcomas, *J. Natl. Cancer Inst.* **74**:145–150.
35. Iannaccone, P. M., Gardner, R. L., and Harris, H., 1978, The cellular origin of chemically induced tumours. *J. Cell Sci.* **29**:249–269.
36. Reddy, A. L., and Fialkow, P. J., 1983, Papillomas induced by initiation-promotion differ from those induced by carcinogen alone, *Nature (Lond.)* **304**:69–71.
37. Taguchi, T., Yokoyama, M., and Kitamura, Y., 1984, Intraclonal conversion from papilloma to carcinoma in the skin of Pgk-1a/Pgk-1b mice treated by a complete carcinogenesis process or by an initiation-promotion regimen, *Cancer Res.* **44**:3779–3782.
38. Talmadge, J. E., and Zbar, B., 1987, Clonality of pulmonary metastases from the bladder 6 subline of the B 16 melanoma studied by Southern hybridization, *J. Natl. Cancer Inst.* **78**:315–320.
39. Sager, R., Gadi, I. K., Stephens, L., and Grabowy, C. T., 1985, Gene amplification: An example of accelerated evolution in tumorigenic cells, *Proc. Natl. Acad. Sci. USA* **82**:7015–7019.
40. Aldaz, C. M., Conti, C. J., O'Connell, J., Yuspa, S. H., Klein-Szanto, A. J. P., and Slaga, T. J., 1986, Cytogenetic evidence for gene amplification in mouse skin carcinogenesis, *Cancer Res.* **46**:3565–3568.
41. Frost, P., and Kerbel, R. S., 1983, On a possible epigenetic mechanism(s) of tumor cell heterogeneity—The role of DNA methylation, *Cancer Metastasis Rev.* **2**:375–378.

42. Jones, P. A., 1986, DNA methylation and cancer, *Cancer Res.* **46:**461–466.

43. Herlyn, M., Clark, W. H., Rodeck, U., Mancianti, M. L., Jambrosci, J., and Koprowski, H., 1987, Biology of disease—Biology of tumor progression in human melanocytes, *Lab. Invest.* **56:**461–474.

44. Gitelman, I., Dexter, D. F., and Roder, J. C., 1987, DNA amplication and metastasis of the human melanoma cell line MeWO, *Cancer Res.* **47:**3851–3855.

45. Parry, J. M., Parry, E. M., and Barrett, J. C., 1981, Tumor promoters induced mitotic aneuploidy in yeast, *Nature (Lond.)* **294:**263–265.

46. Ferguson, L. R., and Parry, J. M., 1984, Mitotic aneuploidy as a possible mechanism for tumour promoting activity in bile acids, *Carcinogenesis* **5:**447–451.

47. Kokal, W., Sheibani, K., Terz, J., and Harada, J. R., 1986, Tumor DNA content in the prognosis of colorectal carcinoma, *JAMA* **255:**3123–3127.

48. Schwartz, D., Banner, B. F., Roseman, D. L., and Coon, J. S., 1986, Origin of multiple "primary" colon carcinomas—A retrospective flow cytometric study, *Cancer* **58:**2082–2088.

49. Hedley, D. W., Rugg, C. A., Ng, A. B. P., and Taylor, I. W., 1984, Influence of cellular DNA content on disease free survival stage II breast cancer patients, *Cancer Res.* **44:**5395–5398.

50. Friedlander, M. L., Russell, P., Taylor, I. W., Hedley, D. W., and Tattersall, M. H. N., 1984, Flow cytometric analysis of cellular DNA content as an adjunct to the diagnosis of ovarian tumours of borderline malignancy, *Pathology* **16:**301–306.

51. Iversen, O., and Skaarland, E., 1987, Ploidy assessment of benign and malignant ovarian tumors by flow cytometry—A clinicopathologic study, *Cancer* **60:**82–87.

52. Lundberg, S., Carstensen, J., and Rundquist, I., 1987, DNA flow cytometry and histopathological grading of paraffin-embedded prostate biopsy specimens in a survival study, *Cancer Res.* **47:**1972–1977.

53. Stephenson, R. A., James, B. C., Gay, H., Fair, W. R., Whitmore, Jr., W. F., and Melamed, M. R., 1987, Flow cytometry of prostate cancer: Relationship of DNA content to survival, *Cancer Res.* **47:**2504–2509.

54. Tribukait, B., and Esposti, P. L., 1978, Quantitative flow-microfluorometric analysis of the DNA in cells from neoplasms of the urinary bladder: Correlation of aneuploidy with histological grading and the cytological findings, *Urol. Res.* **6:**201–205.

55. Badalament, R. A., Kimmel, M., Gay, H., Cibas, E. S., Whitmore, W. F., Herr, H. W., Fair, W. R., and Melamed, M. R., 1987, The sensitivity of flow cytometry compared with conventional cytology in the detection of superficial bladder carcinoma, *Cancer* **59:**2078–2085.

56. Bauer, K. D., Merkel, D. E., Winter, J. N., Marder, R. J., Hauck, W. W., Wallemark, C. B., Williams, T. J., and Variakojis, D., 1986, Prognostic implications of ploidy and proliferative activity in diffuse large cell lymphomas, *Cancer Res.* **46:**3173–3178.

57. Yokota, J., Tsunetsugu-Yokota, Y., Battifora, H., LeFevre, C., and Cline, M. J., 1986, Alterations of myc, myb, and ras$^{Ha}$ proto-oncogenes in cancers are frequent and show clinical correlation, *Science* **231:**261–265.

58. Seeger, R. C., Brodeur, G. M., Sather, H., Dalton, A., Siegel, S. E., Wong, K. Y., and Hammond, D., 1985, Association of multiple copies of the N-myc oncogene with rapid progression of neuroblastomas, *N. Engl. J. Med.* **313:**1111–1116.

59. Brodeur, G. M., Seeger, R. C., Sather, H., Dalton, A., Siegel, S. E., Wong, K. Y., and Hammond, D., 1986, Clinical implications of oncogene activation in human neuroblastomas, *Cancer* **58:**541–545.

60. Rosen, N., Reynolds, C. P., Thiele, C. J., Biedler, J. L., and Israel, M. A., 1986, Increased N-myc expression following progressive growth of human neuroblastoma, *Cancer Res.* **46:**4139–4142.

61. Slamon, D. J., Clark, G. M., Wong, S. G., Levin, W. J., Ullrich, A., and McGuire, W. L., 1987, Human breast cancer: Correlation of relapse and survival with amplification of the HER-2/neu oncogene, *Science* **235:**177–182.

62. Alexander, R. J., Buxbaum, J. N., and Raicht, R. F., 1986, Oncogene alterations in primary human colon tumors, *Gastroenterology* **91:**1503–1510.

63. Rothberg, P. G., Spandorfer, J. M., Erisman, M. D., Staroscik, R. N., Sears, H. F., Petersen, R. O., and Astrin, S. M., 1985, Evidence that c-myc expression defines two genetically distinct forms of colorectal adenocarcinoma, *Br. J. Cancer* **52:**629–632.

64. Augenlicht, L. H., Augeron, C., Yander, G., and Laboisse, C., 1987, Overexpression of ras in mucus-secreting human colon carcinoma cells of low tumorigenicity, *Cancer Res.* **47:**3763–3765.

65. Gallick, G. E., Kurzrock, P., Kloetzer, W. S., Arlinghaus, R. B., and Gutterman, J. U., Expression of P21$^{ras}$ in fresh primary and metastatic human colorectal tumors. *Proc. Natl. Acad. Sci. USA* **82:**1795–1799.

66. Bos, J. L., Fearon, E. R., Hamilton, S. R., Verlaan-de Vries, M., van Boom, J. H., van der Eb, A. J., and

Vogelstein, B., 1987, Prevalence of ras gene mutations in human colorectal cancers, *Nature (Lond.)* **327**:293–297.

67. Forrester, K., Almoguera, C., Han, K., Grizzle, W. E., and Perucho, M., 1987, Detection of high incidence of K-ras oncogenes during human colon tumorigenesis, *Nature (Lond.)* 327:298–303.

68. Leibovitch, S. A., Leibovitch, M.-P., Guillier, M., Hillion, J., and Harel, J., 1986, Differentiated expression of proto-oncogenes related to transformation and cancer progression in rat myoblasts, *Cancer Res.* **46**:4097–4013.

69. Pegoraro, L., Palumbo, A., Erikson, J., Falda, M., Giovanazzo, B., Emanuel, B. S., Rovera, G., Nowell, P. C., and Croce, C. M., 1984, A 14; 18 and an 8;14 chromosome translocation in a cell line derived from an acute B-cell leukemia, *Proc. Natl. Acad. Sci. USA* **81**:7166–7170.

70. Zbar, B., Brauch, H., Talmadge, C., and Linehan, M., 1987, Loss of alleles of loci on the short arm of chromosome 3 in renal cell carcinoma, *Nature (Lond.)* **327**:721–724.

71. Becker, F. F., 1986, Progression of tumor histotype during mouse hepatocarcinogenesis associated with the viable yellow (A$^{vy}$) gene, *Cancer Res.* **46**:2241–2244.

72. Drinkwater, N. R., and Ginsler, J. J., 1986, Genetic control of hepatocarcinogenesis in C57BL/6J and C$_3$H/HeJ inbred mice, *Carcinogenesis* **7**:1701–1707.

73. Oredsson, S. M., Billgren, M., and Heby, O., 1985, Induction of F9 embryonal carcinoma cell differentiation by inhibition of polyamine synthesis, *Eur. J. Cell Biol.* **38**:335–343.

74. Uhl, L., Kelly, M., and Schindler, J., 1986, α-Difluoromethylornithine induces differentiation of a human embryonal carcinoma cell line *in vitro*, *Biochem. Biophys. Res. Commun.* **140**:66–73.

75. Reiss, M., Gamba-Vitalo, C., and Sartorelli, A. C., 1986, Induction of tumor cell differentiation as a therapeutic approach: preclinical models for hematopoietic and solid neoplasms, *Cancer Treat. Rep.* **70**:201–218.

76. Danon, Y. L., and Kaminsky, E., 1985, Dimethyl sulfoxide-induced differentiation does not alter tumorigenicity of neuroblastoma cells, *J. Neuro-Oncol.* **3**:43–51.

77. Yun, K., and Sugihara, H., 1986, Cell differentiation and cell cycle effects on human promyelocytic leukemia cells induced by 12-O-tetradecanoylphorbol-13-acetate, *Lab. Invest.* **54**:336–344.

78. Marks, P. A., Sheffrey, M., and Rifkind, R. A., 1987, Induction of transformed cells to terminal differentiation and the modulation of gene expression, *Cancer Res.* **47**:659–666.

79. Sartorelli, A. C., 1985, The 1985 Walter Hubert Lecture—Malignant cell differentiation as a potential therapeutic approach, *Br. J. Cancer* **52**:293–302.

80. Zhou, D., Battifora, H., Yokota, J., Yamamoto, T., and Cline, M. J., 1987, Association of multiple copies of the c-erb B-2 oncogene with spread of breast cancer, *Cancer Res.* **47**:6123–6125.

81. Tal, M., Wetzler, M., Josefberg, Z., Deutch, A., Gutman, M., Assaf, D., Kris, R., Shiloh, Y., Givol, D., and Schlessinger, J., 1988, Sporadic amplification of the HER/neu protooncogene in adenocarcinomas of various tissues, *Cancer Res.* **48**:1517–1520.

82. Hsu, T. C., 1987, Genetic predisposition to cancer with special reference to mutagen sensitivity, *In Vitro Cell. Dev. Biol.* **23**:591–603.

# 11

# Cytogenetics and Human Neoplasia

## Frederick Hecht, Barbara K. Hecht, and Avery A. Sandberg

## 1. INTRODUCTION

While the exact role of chromosomal (karyotypic, cytogenetic) changes in the pathobiology of neoplasia has not been clearly defined in most conditions in which such changes have been observed, sufficient data have been accumulated in recent years to encourage cytogeneticists to examine even more closely the chromosomal changes associated with neoplasia in an effort to define karyotypically as many neoplastic entities as are possible with presently available techniques. What is becoming apparent is that a variety of neoplasias (leukemias, carcinomas, sarcomas, benign tumors) can be characterized cytogenetically and can also be further classified into a number of specific subtypes within each major class of tumor. This cytogenetic definition of neoplastic subtypes, beyond the information supplied by previously available diagnostic techniques, points not only to the limitations of earlier classifications but also to the need of using the chromosome data as a gateway to establishing (probably at the molecular level) further reliable criteria by which to distinguish and characterize such subtypes.

It is beyond the scope of this chapter to cover or speculate on the various genes (including oncogenes) affected by the large number of chromosomal changes described to date in human neoplasia (see Chapter 13). Nevertheless, through cytogenetics, the molecular biologist may be provided with further insight into the complex nature of the neoplastic process, and it is by means of such approaches that the role of chromosomal changes in the pathobiology of neoplasia will be put on firmer ground.

## 2. CHROMOSOMAL SYMBOLS, ABBREVIATIONS, AND NOMENCLATURE

The field of human cytogenetics is like other fields of science and medicine. It possesses its own symbols, abbreviations, and nomenclature. Although it may seem drab to learn the special language of cytogenetics, it is necessary in order to read or write intelligently about chromosomes and their anomalies or to do research that touches on human chromosomes.

Beginning in 1960, human cytogeneticists have met at intervals to devise and agree on a

*Frederick Hecht, Barbara K. Hecht, and Avery A. Sandberg* • The Genetics Center and The Cancer Center, Southwest Biomedical Research Institute, Scottsdale, Arizona 85251.

standard international chromosome nomenclature. The current version of the International System for Human Cytogenetic Nomenclature[1,2] was communicated in 1985 and is known as ISCN 1985. It is the official handbook on chromosome terms.

Table I presents a selection of symbols and abbreviations that are largely taken from ISCN 1985, and are of particular use in defining the nomenclature of cancer cytogenetics. In addition, Table II illustrates specific aspects of human chromosome nomenclature. The terms used here for naming normal and abnormal cytogenetic features are crucial with respect to describing chromosomal anomalies in cancer. For the most part, the examples given relate to actual findings in cancer cytogenetics, e.g., t(9;22)(q34;q11). This translocation between chromosomes 9 and 22 is due to breaks in bands 9q34 and 22q11. It is the Philadelphia (Ph) chromosome translocation, the "classic" one usually associated with chronic myelocytic leukemia (CML).

## 3. COMPUTER DATA MANAGEMENT

Since 1971, the International System for Human Cytogenetic Nomenclature has been designed to include computer storage, retrieval, and analysis of chromosome data. Although some chromosome laboratories are not yet using computers in data management, it is becoming evident that the use of such technology can provide the cancer cytogeneticist with powerful tools to sort out the many types of chromosomal alterations being observed in human malignant neoplasms.

Malignant cells from a specific type of human tumor may be (1) chromosomally abnormal; (2) complexly abnormal with a long list of structural and/or numerical chromosomal aberrations; or (3) karyotypically heterogeneous.

## 4. CONSTITUTIONAL VERSUS ACQUIRED CHROMOSOMAL ABNORMALITIES IN CANCER

A key distinction is made between constitutional and acquired chromosomal abnormalities. This distinction is pertinent to cancer cytogenetics.

*Table I. Chromosome Symbols and Abbreviations[a]*

| Symbol or abbreviation | Meaning |
|---|---|
| cen | Centromere; usually the point of spindle attachment |
| del | Deletion; loss of chromosome segment |
| DM | Double-minute chromosome; also called dmin |
| dup | Duplication; gain of chromosome segment |
| fra | Fragile site on a chromosome |
| HSR | Homogeneously staining region in a chromosome |
| i | Isochromosome formed of two identical arms |
| ins | Insertion of material into a chromosome |
| inv | Inversion of part of a chromosome |
| mar | Marker chromosome; unidentified |
| − (minus) | Loss of a chromosome or chromosome segment |
| p | Short arm of chromosome |
| Ph | Philadelphia chromosome |
| + (plus) | Extra chromosome or chromosome segment |
| q | Long arm of chromosome |
| t | Translocation; exchange of material between chromosomes |

[a]Based on ISCN (1985)[1,2]; DM and HSR are unofficial abbreviations but are widely used; Ph is unofficial but appropriate, since the superscript Ph[1] is essentially superfluous because there is no Ph[2] chromosome.

*Table II. Examples of Chromosome Nomenclature[a]*

| Type of term | Term | Meaning |
|---|---|---|
| Normal landmarks on chromo- somes | p1 | Region 1 on short arm of chromosome |
| | p14 | Band 14 on short arm |
| | p14.2 | Sub-band 14.2 on short arm |
| | 3p14.2 | Sub-band 14.2 on short arm of chromosome 3 |
| | q2 | Region 2 on long arm of chromosome |
| | q22 | Band 22 on long arm |
| | q22.3 | Sub-band 22.3 on long arm |
| | 8q22.3 | Sub-band 22.3 on long arm of chromosome 8 |
| Normal chromo- somes | 46,XX | Normal female karyotype |
| | 46,XY | Normal male karyotype |
| Abnormal struc- ture of chromo- some | del(13) | Deletion from chromosome 13 |
| | del(13)(q14) | Deletion of chromosome band 13q14 |
| | del(13)(q14q22) | Deletion from chromosome band 13q14 to 13q22 |
| | dup(1) | Duplication of chromosome 1 |
| | dup(1)(p36) | Duplication of chromosome band 1p36 |
| | dup(1)(p36p32) | Duplication of segment from 1p36 to 1p32 |
| | fra(16) | Fragile site on chromosome 16 |
| | fra(16)(q22) | Fragile site in chromosome band 16q22 |
| | i(17q) | Isochromosome of the chromosome 17 long arm |
| | ins(3) | Insertion into chromosome 3 |
| | ins(3;3)(q26;q21q26) | Insertion at chromosome band 3q26 and segment from 3q21 to 3q26 |
| | inv(16) | Inversion of part of chromosome 16 |
| | inv(16)(p13q22) | Inversion of segment from 16p13 to 16q22 |
| | t(9;22) | Translocation between chromosomes 9 and 22 |
| | t(9;22)(q34;q11) | Translocation with breakpoints in 9q34 and 22q11 |
| | 14q+ | Increased length of long arm of chromosome 14 |
| | 14q− | Decreased length of long arm of chromosome 14 |
| Abnormal number of chromosomes | 45,X, −X or −Y | 45 chromosomes including one X chromosome and loss of an X or Y |
| | 47,XY,+21 | 47 chromosomes including extra chromosome 21 |
| | 48,XXY, +8 | 48 chromosomes, including an extra X (Klinefelter syndrome) and an extra chromosome 8 |
| | 48,XY, +X, +8 | 48 chromosomes with acquisition of an extra X chromosome and an extra chromosome 8 |

[a]Based on ISCN (1985).[1,2]

## 4.1. Constitutional Chromosomal Abnormalities

Constitutional chromosomal abnormalities are present in normal cells from the patient. These chromosomal abnormalities may also be observed in neoplastic cells from the patient, but the key feature is that they are found in the normal cells.

The term germline chromosomal abnormalities is occasionally applied to designate constitutional chromosomal aberrations. This may or may not be appropriate, depending on the circumstances. Down syndrome is a good example. The extra chromosome 21 is usually present at the time of fertilization. Nondisjunction occurs in meiosis, most often in the female, but also with a fair frequency in the male. The resultant gamete is diplo-21; it has an extra chromosome 21. Upon fertilization, a trisomy 21 zygote is created and the baby is born with Down syndrome. However, some individuals with Down syndrome exhibit chromosomal mosaicism. They possess two or more cell lines with different chromosomal constitutions, e.g., trisomy 21 and normal (diploid) cells. The trisomy 21 cell line may be the original one, or it may have arisen due to nondisjunction during embryogenesis. The patient has a constitutional chromosomal abnormality, since it is present in nonmalignant cells, but it is not truly a germline chromosomal abnormality because it was not present at conception. The more accurate and inclusive term is constitutional chromosome abnormality. Some of these abnormalities have been associated in the human with a greatly increased risk for cancer development (Table III).

## 4.2. Acquired Chromosomal Abnormalities

In contrast to the chromosomal changes in constitutional disorders, which are present in all the somatic cells of affected persons (in mosaicism a population of normal cells may also be present), the cytogenetic changes in leukemia, lymphoma, and solid tumors are confined to the affected neoplastic cells only.[10] In the case of the leukemias, generally the best source of abnormal cells is the bone marrow; however, if a sufficient number of leukemic cells in division are present in the blood, they may also supply metaphases for cytogenetic analysis. In the case of lymphomas, the

### Table III. Constitutional (Germ-Line) Chromosomal Abnormalities Predisposing to Neoplasia

| Origin | Chromosomal abnormality | Neoplasia | References |
|--------|------------------------|-----------|------------|
| Inherited | Translocation between chromosomes 3 and 8 | Renal cell carcinoma | 3 |
| | Translocation involving chromosome 11 | Wilms tumor | 4 |
| | | Hepatoblastoma | 5, 6 |
| | | Rhabdomyosarcoma | 7 |
| | Translocation involving chromosome 13 | Retinoblastoma | 8 |
| | | Osteosarcoma | 9 |
| | Translocation involving chromosome 21 | Acute leukemia | 10 |
| De novo | Deletion of part of chromosome 11 | Wilms tumor | 4 |
| | | Hepatoblastoma | 5, 6 |
| | | Rhabdomyosarcoma | 7 |
| | Deletion of part of chromosome 13 | Retinoblastoma | 8 |
| | | Osteosarcoma | 9 |
| | Duplication of part of chromosome 21 | Acute leukemia | 10 |
| | 47 XXY (Klinefelter syndrome) | Germ-line-cell tumors | 10 |
| | | Breast cancer | 10 |
| | 45,X/46,XY (gonadal dysgenesis) | Gonadoblastoma | 10 |

optimal source of cytogenetically abnormal cells is lymph nodes. For solid tumors, the chromosome picture can only be established in the tumor cells per se. Stimulated with phytohemagglutinin (PHA), blood lymphocytes yield the constitutional karyotype of patients, which is often used as a control when indicated.

## 5. CYTOGENETIC DISSECTION OF A TRANSLOCATION BETWEEN CHROMOSOMES 9 AND 22: THE PHILADELPHIA TRANSLOCATION

The Philadelphia (Ph) chromosome was the opening act in the malignant play that might be called *Chromosomes and Cancer*. This opening act was written back in 1960.[11] A number of years passed before other acts and scenes were written. However, a more complete story is emerging about the Ph chromosome.[12,13] This story provides a model.

### 5.1. The Ph Translocation Occurs in Multiple Types of Leukemia and Related Disorders

The Ph chromosome was originally discovered in chronic myelocytic leukemia (CML). Most patients with CML have the Ph chromosome in their malignant cells, and it is believed by some to be a specific chromosomal marker for CML. The Ph chromosome has been encountered in multiple types of leukemia and related disorders other than CML. These include the acute nonlymphocytic leukemias, particularly of the M1 and M2 types (ANLL-M1 and ANLL-M2), acute lymphoblastic leukemia (ALL), and myelodysplastic syndromes. Thus, a number of diverse types of leukemia and related conditions have been shown to possess in common the Ph chromosome, although it is possible that some of these may be part of a single disease continuum. Studies of the Ph chromosome have already shown differences at the molecular level in some of the conditions[14] (see Section 5.3).

### 5.2. Biology of Cell Lineages

How can a single (primary) chromosomal rearrangement be found in multiple types of leukemia, especially when these leukemias display distinctive cell types that can be easily distinguished through morphology and immunology? The problem resolves itself simply by one means, i.e., to see that the various cells in these leukemias are biologically related during development. In other words, do all the leukemic cells descend from a shared precursor stem cell? This solution is supported by the clinical knowledge that patients with CML go into a blast crisis that can present as conditions resembling ANLL or ALL (of B- or T-cell variety). Moreover, Ph-positive CML can lead to the development of Ph-positive acute leukemias of the ANLL type or into Ph-positive ALL. Since these myeloid and lymphoid cells appear to share a common cell lineage, the Ph translocation serves as a chromosomal marker of neoplastic change in this cellular family.

### 5.3. Molecular Dissection of the Ph Translocation

The discussion regarding the Ph chromosome has dealt so far with the cytogenetic evidence, specifically the t(9;22)(q34;q11) translocation. Molecular studies have shown that almost all Ph translocations in CML are characterized by a break in a region named *bcr* located in band q11 of chromosome 22, to which is juxtaposed the oncogene *abl* originating at band q34 on chromosome 9.[13,15–19] Hence, expression of the new gene created, *c-abl-bcr*, on the Ph chromosome may be playing a key role in the genesis of CML.

When the molecular events just described were investigated in Ph-positive acute leukemias, exceptions were encountered, particularly in ALL.[14,20] The break on chromosome 22 resulting in the Ph chromosome was shown to be outside the *bcr*, a finding seen not infrequently in Ph-positive

ALL. Thus, it appears that the microscopically established Ph translocation may be the result of more than one type of molecular event, each possibly having unique biologic manifestations.

## 6. CYTOGENETIC DISSECTION OF THE ACUTE NONLYMPHOCYTIC LEUKEMIAS

The acute nonlymphocytic leukemias (ANLL) have long been known to be morphologically heterogeneous. Among the unifying features in ANLL, however, were the following: (1) all types of ANLL did not involve lymphocytes; and (2) all types of ANLL were acute leukemias.

The group of nonlymphocytic acute leukemias has been analyzed as to chromosomal changes and the results of such studies have revolutionized our thinking about ANLL.[21]

### 6.1. The French–American–British Classification of ANLL

In 1976 and subsequent years, a group of investigators brought order to ANLL.[22–24] The investigators were French, American, and British (FAB). They proposed a classification of ANLL, now known as the FAB system. This classification was initially based largely on morphologic cellular criteria, although cytochemical and immunologic aspects were later incorporated. The FAB classification of ANLL is briefly presented in Table IV.

As is evident in Table IV, the FAB classification of ANLL resides upon the distinctions between cell types: myeloblasts versus promyeloblasts versus monoblasts, and so forth. This was entirely logical, since morphologic features were the only ones initially available. Problems with the FAB classification included the need for considerable histopathologic expertise, the bizarre appearance of some malignant cells, and the absence of unequivocal laboratory criteria for diagnosis of the individual types of ANLL. Cancer cytogenetics provides just such unequivocal criteria.

### 6.2. Primary Chromosomal Rearrangements and Numerical Changes

Primary chromosomal rearrangements are structural changes that are due to two or more breaks in chromosomes with subsequent shuffling of chromosome material. These structural changes are primary in several senses.

The primary chromosomal change is (1) the first chromosomal abnormality detected in a malignancy; (2) the only chromosomal abnormality detected, if there is a single cytogenetic change in a malignancy; (3) a marker of all malignant cells descended from an ancestral transformed cell; and (4) the key cytogenetic event possibly related to the initiation of the malignancy.

### Table IV. Acute Nonlymphocytic Leukemias Classified by the French–American–British System[a]

| FAB class | Disease entity |
|-----------|----------------|
| M1 | Acute myeloblastic leukemia (AML) without differentiation |
| M2 | Acute myeloblastic leukemia (AML) with differentiation |
| M3 | Acute promyelocytic leukemia (APL) with hypergranularity |
| M4 | Acute myelomonocytic leukemia (AMMoL) |
| M5 | Acute monocytic leukemia (AMoL) |
| M6 | Acute erythroleukemia (AEL) |
| M7 | Acute megakaryocytic leukemia (AMeL) |

[a]Based on Bennet et al.[22]

### Table V. Common Chromosomal Changes in Acute Nonlymphocytic Leukemias Classified by the French–American–British System

| | |
|---|---|
| M1: Acute myeloblastic leukemia without differentiation | M2: Acute myeloblastic leukemia with differentiation |
| 5q−/−5; 7q−/−7; −17 | t(8;21)(q22;q22) |
| t(9;22)(q34;q11)(Ph) | 5q−/5; 7q−/−7 |
| del(3p) and t with 3 | del(3p) and inv(3) |
| +21 | t(6;9)(p22;q34)[a] |
| +8 | t(9;22)(q34;q11)(Ph) |
| | +8 |
| M3: Acute promyelocytic leukemia | M4: Acute myelomonocytic leukemia |
| t(15;17)(q22;q11) | 5q−/−5; 7q/−7 |
| i(17q) | inv(16) or 16q− or t with 16[b] |
| | t(6;9)(p22;q34) |
| | t(?;11)(?;q23)[c] |
| | +8 |
| | t(9;22)(Ph) |
| | +4 |
| M5: Acute monocytic leukemia | M6: Acute erythroleukemia |
| t(9;11)(p21;q23), M5a | 5q−/−5; 7q−/−7 |
| t(?;11)(?;q23),[c] M5a | −3 and t(3;?)[c] |
| +8 | dup(1) |
| | +8 |
| M7: Acute megakaryocytic leukemia | |
| inv or del(3) | |
| +8 | |
| +21 | |

[a]Often with marrow basophilia.
[b]With marrow eosinophilia.
[c]The chromosome involved in the translocation may vary.

## 6.2.1. Primary Chromosomal Rearrangements in ANLL

In ANLL, a sequential set of detailed studies uncovered the primary chromosomal rearrangements that are set forth in Tables V and VI. The chromosomal changes here are in order of chromosome number and were found in diverse FAB types of ANLL. All the primary chromosomal changes (Table VI) in ANLL are cytologically balanced. Balanced means that there is no loss or gain of chromosome material evident by meticulous microscopic analysis. Nearly a dozen primary chromosome rearrangements have been detected in ANLL, as of the time that this chapter was written in 1987. These chromosome changes consist primarily of translocations and, less frequently, inversions.[25]

## 6.2.2. Creation of a New DNA Continuum

We must indicate that the essential feature here is not whether a chromosome change is achieved by a particular mechanistic type of segment shuffling, e.g., by translocation versus inversion. The essential features are the locations of the chromosome breakpoints and, also, the

Table VI. Primary Chromosomal Rearrangements in Acute
Nonlymphocytic Leukemias

| Primary chromosomal rearrangement | Acute nonlymphocytic leukemias (FAB classification)[a] | | | | | | |
|---|---|---|---|---|---|---|---|
| | M1 | M2 | M3 | M4 | M5 | M6 | M7 |
| t(1;12)(p36p;p12) | | | | | + | | |
| t(1;17)(p36;q21) | | | + | | | | |
| t(1;16)(q21;q22) | | | | | | | + |
| t(3;9)(p14;q34) | | | | | | | + |
| t(3;3)(p21;q26) | + | + | | | | | |
| inv(3)(q21q26) | + | + | | | | | |
| ins(3;3)(q26;q21q26) | + | + | | | | | |
| t(6;9)(p22;q34) | + | + | | | | | |
| t(6;11)(q27;q23) | | | | | + | | |
| t(8;16)(p11;p13) | | | | | + | | |
| t(8;21)(q22;q22) | | + | | | | | |
| t(9;11)(p22;q23) | | | | | + | | |
| t(9;22)(q34;q11) | + | + | | | | | |
| t(10;11)(p15-p11;q23) | | | | | + | | |
| t(10;11)(p14;q13-q14) | | | | + | + | | |
| ins(10;11)(p11;q23q24) | | | | | + | | |
| t(11;17)(q23;q25) | | | | + | + | | |
| t(15;17)(q22;q11) | | | + | | | | |
| t(16;16)(p13;q22) | | | | + | | | |
| inv(16)(p13q22) | | | | + | | | |
| del(16)(q22) | | | | + | | | |

[a]French–American–British.

creation of a novel DNA continuum. The breaks must be in highly specific points in the chromosome. They cannot be just anywhere. Rather, they must be situated with considerable exactitude in the DNA. This permits the generation of new genetic neighborhoods.

To illustrate this general principle, in ANLL an inversion of chromosome 3 has been found.[26,27] The breakpoints leading to this inversion are in bands 3q21 and 3q26. The resultant inversion juxtaposes 3q21 and 3q26, which are normally separated by a long stretch of DNA: the region running virtually a third the length of this lengthy chromosome long arm. The precisely identical juxtaposition of 3q21 and 3q26 can be obtained and has been observed to occur by other types of chromosome mechanics, namely, by an insertion or by a translocation.[28,29] Thus, we have three chromosome mechanisms:

An inversion: inv(3)(q21q26)
An insertion: ins(3;3)(q26;q21q26)
A translocation: t(3;3)(q21;q26)

All three mechanisms produce the identical result: the creation of a new DNA continuum. Numerical changes of a primary nature are not as common as structural rearrangements in ANLL. The most common ones are −5, −7, and +8. The former two (−5 and −7) are often seen in secondary leukemia and the latter (+8) in several types of ANLL.[30]

## 6.3. *Cytogenetic Dissection: A New Perspective on ANLL*

The primary chromosome rearrangements discovered in ANLL can be utilized to gain a new view of ANLL.[31,32] This new view is presented by us in Table VII. One consequence is the fusion of the FAB M1 and M2 types of ANLL. Both M1 and M2 share most of the same primary chromosomal rearrangements. Clearly, the matter of differentiation (M1) versus lack of differentiation (M2) does not reflect a detectable difference in fundamental etiology.

However, a new morphologic feature may be emerging within the M1–M2 fusion class. This feature involves the frequent presence of bone marrow basophilia with the t(6;9) type of translocation.[33–35] Thus, this specific chromosome abnormality allows a subtype of ANLL to be split out as a particular cohesive malignant entity.

Splitting of a single type of ANLL into cohesive entities of malignant disease appears also to be feasible with M5. The splitting edge is the translocation type: t(9;11) characterizing ANLL subtype M5a and t(8;16) characterizing subtype M5b.

The total process is not yet finished with regard to the chromosomal dissection and integration of ANLL. On the other hand, it is apparent that cytogenetics has changed our view of ANLL, and it is likely that a new understanding of the pathobiology of ANLL will be forthcoming.

## 7. CYTOGENETIC DISSECTION OF ALL

Although immunologic and other approaches have been of considerable help in the characterization of ALL and have made it possible to identify the stage of differentiation of the leukemic cells in the lymphoid (and myeloid) lineages, the FAB classification has generally recognized three entities, i.e., L1–L3.[36] The need for further characterization of ALL became evident when it was shown cytogenetically that a much larger number of subtypes of ALL existed than L1–L3. As in the case of ANLL,[25] this need led to a special meeting (MIC-1 Workshop) dealing with the amalgamation with and incorporation of the chromosomal findings and the criteria of the FAB classification

*Table VII. Current Cytogenetic Perspective on Acute Nonlymphocytic Leukemias Based on Primary Chromosomal Changes*

| Primary chromosomal rearrangement | Morphology | Abbreviation | Revision of FAB classes |
|---|---|---|---|
| inv(3) t(6;9) t(9;22) t(8;21) | Myeloblastic | AML | M1 + M2 |
| t(15;17) | Promyelocytic | APL | M3 |
| inv(16) | Myelomonoblastic with marrow eosinophilia | AMMoL | M4 |
| t(9;11) | Monoblastic | AMoL, type a | M5a |
| t(8;16) | Monoblastic | AMoL, type b | M5b |
| Unknown | Erythroleukemia | AEL | M6 |
| t(1;16) t(3;9) | Megakaryocytic | AMeL | M7 |

Table VIII. Combination of Morphology, Immunology, and Cytogenetics (MIC)
Used to Classify the B-Lineage Acute Lymphoblastic Leukemias[a,b]

| Morphology (FAB) | Immunologic markers | | | | | | Cytogenetics (karyotype) | Class of B-lineage ALL |
|---|---|---|---|---|---|---|---|---|
| | HLA-DR (Ia) | TdT | B4 (CD19) | cALLA (CD10) | CyIg | SmIg | | |
| L1 or L2 | + | + | + | − | − | − | t(4;11) | Early B-precursor ALL, t(4;11) |
| | | | | | | | t(9;22) | Early B-precursor ALL, t(9;22) |
| L1 or L2 | + | + | + | + | − | − | del(6q) | Common ALL, del(6) |
| | | | | | | | Near haploid | Common ALL, near haploid |
| | | | | | | | t or del(12p) | Common ALL, t or del(12p) |
| | | | | | | | t(9;22) | Common ALL, t(9;22) |
| L1 | + | + | + | +[c] | + | − | t(1;19) | Pre-B ALL, t(1;19) |
| | | | | | | | t(9;22) | Pre-B ALL, t(9;22) |
| L3 | + | − | + | +/− | −/+ | +[d] | t(8;14) | B-cell ALL, t(8;14) |
| | | | | | | | t(2;8) | B-cell ALL, t(2;8) |
| | | | | | | | t(8;22) | B-cell ALL, t(8;22) |
| | | | | | | | del(6q) | B-cell ALL, del(6q) |

[a]Based on report of First MIC Cooperative Study Group.[32]
[b]+, ≥10% cells positive over control.
[c]cALLA may rarely be absent.
[d]Single light chain.

and other parameters. As is apparent from Tables VIII and IX, dissection of the ALL entities into a number of subtypes was accomplished and, as in the case of ANLL (MIC-2 Workshop),[25] other subtypes will undoubtedly be added to these lists in the future.

## 8. OTHER HEMATOLOGIC CONDITIONS

Although the chromosomal dissection of disease entities has been most successfully accomplished in the leukemias, a similar process has been applied to the myelodysplastic syndromes, the lymphomas, and myeloproliferative disorders. The success level in each has been variable, but the emerging findings all point in the same direction, i.e., that entities thought to be homogeneous by

Table IX. Combination of Morphology, Immunology, and Cytogenetics (MIC)
Used to Classify the T-Lineage Acute Lymphoblastic Leukemias (ALL)[a,b]

| Morphology (FAB) | Immunologic markers | | | Cytogenetics (karyotype) | Class of T-lineage ALL |
|---|---|---|---|---|---|
| | TdT | gp40 (CD7) | E-receptor (CD2) | | |
| L1 or L2 | + | + | − | t or del(9p) | Early T-precursor ALL, t or del(9p) |
| L1 or L2 | + | + | + | t(11;14) | T-cell ALL, t(11;14) |
| | + | + | + | del(6q) | T-cell ALL, del(6q) |

[a]Based on report of First MIC Cooperative Study Group.[32]
[b]+, ≥10% cells positive over controls.

previous criteria (cytology, clinical aspects, immunology, cytochemistry) are invariably shown to contain a number of cytogenetically defined subtypes.[37,38]

## 9. COMMENTS ON CHROMOSOMAL CHANGES IN HEMATOLOGIC DISORDERS

The availability of a large body of cytogenetic information on the leukemias and related disorders has led to a number of international meetings in which the clinical (diagnostic and prognostic) aspects of these diseases have been defined, or at least supplemented, in cytogenetic terms. The reader is referred to the proceedings of these meetings, as well as to other sources, for further information in this area.[25,32,39–44]

Emerging from these meetings and the literature is the crucial value of cytogenetic analysis not only in the diagnostic aspects of the leukemias, but also as independent prognostic criteria. Thus, chromosome data supply the clinician with key information useful in the evaluation of the disease, as well as a basis for molecular biologists to investigate the crucial submicroscopic events associated with each condition. The latter is related to the location of important genes (including oncogenes) within the breakpoints of chromosomal rearrangements or changes.

## 10. CHROMOSOMAL CHANGES IN CLL AND LYMPHOMA

The cytogenetic changes seen in chronic lymphocytic leukemia (CLL) have primarily consisted of trisomy 12 (+12), 14q+, and t(11;14)(q13;q32). The latter translocation may also be seen in diffuse small cell lymphoma, a disease that is sometimes difficult to differentiate from CLL. The chromosomal changes mentioned for CLL are seen in only about 50% of the cases.[31]

Although much has been learned about the cytogenetic changes in lymphoma and the associated molecular events underlying some of these conditions,[37,38,45] the karyotypic definition of the lymphomas, akin to that obtained for the acute leukemias, has lagged behind. In general terms, only t(8;14)(q24;q32) in diffuse types of lymphoma and t(14;18)(q32;q21) in the follicular variety constitute specific karyotypic anomalies related to a characteristic cell type of lymphoma. Thus, a significant portion of the lymphomas have yet to be defined cytogenetically, although the new formulation for the classification of the lymphomas was of help in this regard.[46]

More importantly, few correlations of the cytogenetic changes with the biology and clinical parameters have been described. In some cases, these indicated specificity with the additional or secondary chromosome changes occurring in relation to the cell type and course of the disease.[38] For example, patients with follicular small cleaved-cell lymphoma with t(14;18) as a single karyotypic change had a more indolent course than cases with follicular small cleaved-cell lymphoma with t(14;18) and, in addition, a deletion of chromosome 13(q32). The latter patients acquired the hematologic features of leukemia with an acceleration of the disease.[38]

A deletion of 6q (6q−) with a complete or partial trisomy 7 (+7) or trisomy 12 (+12), or both, was associated with a more aggressive follicular mixed small and large cell, or large-cell-only histologic type. A complete or partial trisomy of chromosomes 3, 18, and/or 21 correlated almost exclusively with follicular large cell lymphoma. In all follicular stages, a trisomy 2 (+2) or duplication of 2p often was associated with an accelerated clinical course and a poor response to therapy.[38]

Burkitt lymphoma and its related type of ALL have been more clearly defined cytogenetically than any other subgroup of lymphomas.[47] Most of these tumors have a t(8;14), with small subgroups having either t(2;8) or t(8;22). The molecular events underlying these tumors have been explored extensively and point to an array of such events[48–50] (i.e., see Chapter 15). It is possible that those seen in the endemic variety (e.g., in parts of Africa) may be different from those seen in the sporadic types (e.g., in the Western world).

## 11. CYTOGENETICS OF SOLID TUMORS

In a recent review of the cytogenetics of solid tumors,[51] we indicated that the practical application of chromosome results has not been as extensive or meaningful as that in the leukemias. However, the findings already applied (Table X) in the diagnosis, classification, and pathology of some tumor types, such as sarcomas and bladder cancer, augur well for the utilization of karyotypic findings in a number of solid tumors. We feel confident that the cytogenetic results obtained in both benign and malignant tumors will tell us much about their biology and may ultimately prove to be key contributors to our understanding of these tumors, including their diagnosis, therapy, and basic biology.

The finding of specific chromosome changes in sarcomas now permits differentiation of myxoid liposarcomas with a t(12;16) from other liposarcomas and myxoid tumors, the diagnosis of synovial sarcoma with t(X;18), and of Ewing sarcoma with t(11;22) (Figs. 1 and 2).

In bladder cancer (transitional cell carcinoma), we have shown[53] that cytogenetically this entity can be divided into subsets, each characterized by a primary karyotypic change, i.e., isochromosome 5p, +7, −9, and 11p−. Whether these are related to different etiologies or variability in the cell type affected remains to be demonstrated. Some correlations between the primary chromosomal changes and the clinical, pathologic, and prognostic aspects of bladder cancers are already evident[53] (see also Chapter 10), although many more cases will have to be analyzed before this correlation is put on a solid basis.

Cytogenetic experience similar to that in sarcomas and bladder cancer is being applied to a

### Table X. Specific or Primary Chromosomal Changes in Solid Tumors

| Tumors | Chromosomal changes |
|---|---|
| **Benign** | |
| Meningioma | −22,22q− |
| Mixed tumors of salivary glands | t(3;8)(p21;q12),t(9p;12)(p13-22;q13-15) |
| Lipoma | t with 12q14 |
| Colonic adenomas | 12q−,+8 |
| **Adenocarcinomas** | |
| Bladder | i(5p),+7,−9/9q−,11p− |
| Prostate | del(10)(q24) |
| Lung (SCLC) | del(3)(p14p23) |
| Colon | 12q−,+7,+8,+12,17(q11) |
| Kidney | del(3)(p21) |
| Uterus | 1q− |
| Ovary | 6q−,t(6;14)(q21;q24) |
| **Sarcomas** | |
| Liposarcoma (myxoid) | t(12;16)(q13;p11) |
| Synovial | t(X;18)(p11.2;q11.2) |
| Rhabdomyosarcoma (alveolar) | t(2;13)(q37;q14) |
| Myxoid chondrosarcoma (extraskeletal) | t(9;22)(q31;q12.2) |
| **Embryonal and other tumors** | |
| Testicular (germ cell tumors) | i(12p) |
| Retinoblastoma | del(13)(q14)[a] |
| Wilms | del(11)(p13)[a] |
| Neuroblastoma | del(1)(p32p36) |
| Malignant melanoma | del(6)(q11q27),i(6p),del(1)(p11p22), t(1;9)(q12;q13) |
| Ewing sarcoma and peripheral neuroepithelioma | t(11;22)(q24;q12) |
| Mesothelioma | del(3)(p13p23) |

[a]Associated with constitutional chromosomal change.

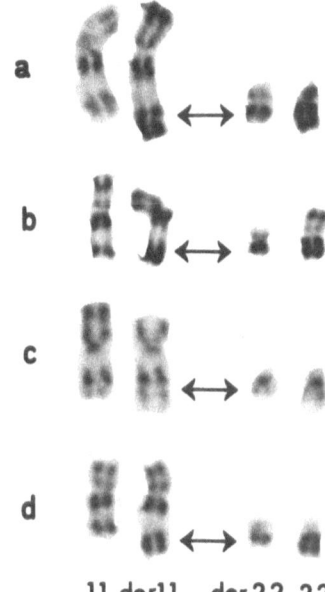

11 der11    der22 22

Figure 1. Four partial karyotypes showing the characteristic translocation t(11;22)(q24;q12) seen in Ewing sarcoma and neuroectodermal tumors (e.g., peripheral neuroepithelioma). In fact, the finding of this translocation in these disorders has led to the hypothesis that Ewing sarcoma may be of neuroectodermal origin.[51,52] The presence (or absence) of the translocation has been used diagnostically in cases where other criteria have not been clear or helpful. Thus, this figure demonstrates a primary chromosome change specific for a tumor.

number of other tumors, such as cancers of the colon, lung, and breast.[51] An interesting and intriguing development in tumor cytogenetics has been the demonstration of specific translocations and other cytogenetic changes in benign tumors, particularly lipomas and leiomyomas.[54-56] Although other apparently benign tumors (e.g., meningiomas and mixed tumors of the salivary glands) had been shown to be accompanied by nonrandom changes (Table X), the demonstration of such

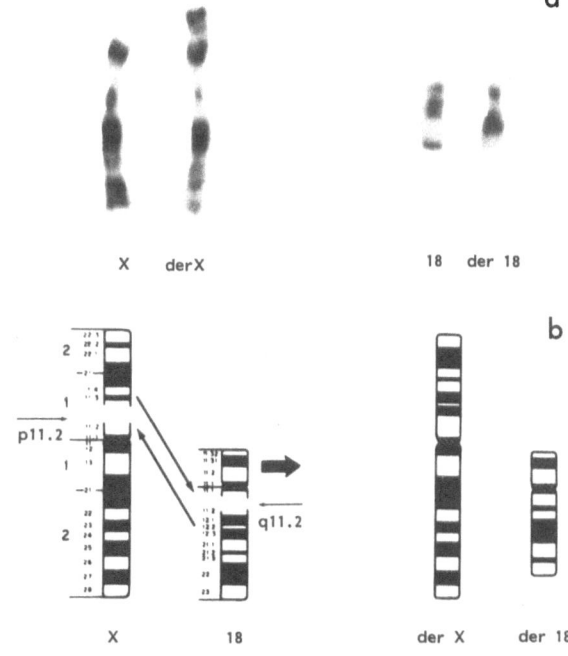

Figure 2. Partial karyotype (A) and its schematic presentation (B) of the translocation t(X;18)(p11.2;p11.2) seen in synovial sarcoma. This primary cytogenetic change appears to be the only one to date involving a sex chromosome. Again, this translocation is a demonstration of a specific (primary) chromosome change in a specific tumor (synovial sarcoma).

chromosomal changes in lipomas, particularly tumors known to almost never become malignant, places the meaning of cytogenetic abnormalities in solid tumors in a new and different light.

## REFERENCES

1. Harnden, D. G., and Linger, H. P. (eds.), 1985, *An International System for Human Cytogenetic Nomenclature (Cytogenet. Cell Genet.)*, S. Karger, Basel.
2. *Birth Defects: Original Article Series*, Vol. 21, No. 1, March of Dimes Birth Defects Foundation, New York.
3. Cohen, A. J., Li, F. P., Berg, S., Marchetto, D. J., Tsai, S., Jacobs, S. C., and Brown, R. S., 1979, Hereditary renal cell carcinoma associated with chromosomal translocation, *N. Engl. J. Med.* **301**:592–595.
4. Riccardi, V. M., Hittner, H. M., Francke, U., Yunis, J. J., Ledbetter, D., and Borges, W., 1980, The aniridia–Wilms' tumor association: The critical role of chromosome band 11p13, *Cancer Genet. Cytogenet.* **2**:131–137.
5. Koufos, A., Hansen, M. F., Lampkin, B. C., Workman, M. L., Copeland, N. G., Jenkins, N. A., and Cavenee, W. K., 1984, Loss of alleles at loci on human chromosome 11 during genesis of Wilms' tumour, *Nature (Lond.)* **309**:170–172.
6. Koufos, A., Hansen, M. F., Copeland, N. G., Jenkins, N. A., Lampkin, B. C., and Cavenee, W. K., 1985, Loss of heterozygosity in three embryonal tumours suggests a common pathogenetic mechanism, *Nature (Lond.)* **316**:330–334.
7. Scrable, H. J., Witte, D. P., Lampkin, B. C., and Cavenee, W. K., 1987, Chromosomal localization of the human rhabdomyosarcoma locus by mitotic recombination mapping, *Nature (Lond.)* **329**:645–647.
8. Vogel, F., 1979, Genetics of retinoblastoma, *Hum. Genet.* **52**:1–54.
9. Dryja, T. P., Rapaport, J. M., Epstein, J., Goorin, A. M., Weichselbaum, R., Koufos, A., and Cavenee, W. K., 1986, Chromosome 13 homozygosity in osteosarcoma without retinoblastoma, *Am. J. Hum. Genet.* **38**:59–66.
10. Sandberg, A. A., 1980, *The Chromosomes in Human Cancer and Leukemia*, Elsevier/North-Holland, New York.
11. Nowell, P. C., and Hungerford, D. A., 1960, A minute chromosome in human chronic granulocytic leukemia, *Science* **132**:1497.
12. Rowley, J. D., 1973, A new consistent chromosomal abnormality in chronic myelogenous leukaemia identified by quinacrine fluorescence and Giemsa staining, *Nature (Lond.)* **243**:290–293.
13. Sandberg, A. A., Gemmill, R. M., Hecht, B. K., and Hecht, F., 1986, The Philadelphia chromosome: A model of cancer and molecular cytogenetics, *Cancer Genet. Cytogenet.* **21**:129–146.
14. Hermans, A., Heisterkamp, N., von Lindern, M., van Baal, S., Meijer, D., van der Plas, D., Wiedemann, L. M., Groffen, J., Bootsma, D., and Grosveld, G., 1987, Unique fusion of *bcr* and c-*abl* genes in Philadelphia chromosome positive acute lymphoblastic leukemia, *Cell* **51**:33–40.
15. Heisterkamp, N., Stam, K., Groffen, J., de Klein, A., and Grosveld, G., 1985, Structural organization of the *bcr* gene and its role in the Ph[1] translocation, *Nature (Lond.)* **315**:758–761.
16. Heisterkamp, N., Stephenson, J., Grosveld, G., and Groffen, J., 1984, The involvement of human c-*abl* and *bcr* in the Philadelphia translocation, in: *Genes and Cancer* (J. M. Bishop, J. D. Rowley, and M. Greaves, eds.), pp. 547–567, Liss, New York.
17. Boehm, T. L. J., and Drahovsky, D., 1987, Application of a bcr-specific probe in the classification of human leukaemia, *J. Cancer Res. Clin. Oncol.* **113**:267–272.
18. Collins, S. J., 1986, Breakpoints on chromosomes 9 and 22 in Philadelphia chromosome-positive chronic myelogenous leukemia (CML), *J. Clin. Invest.* **78**:1392–1396.
19. Torelli, G., Selleri, L., Emilia, G., Narni, F., Colò, A., Zucchini, P., Donelli, A., Venturelli, D., and Torelli, U., 1987, Molecular study of the Philadelphia translocation in chronic myelogenous leukemia in different stages of disease, *Haematologica* **72**:201–208.
20. Rodenhuis, S., Smets, L. A., Slater, R. M., Behrendt, H., and Veerman, A. J. P., 1985, Distinguishing the Philadelphia chromosome of acute lymphoblastic leukemia from its counterpart in chronic myelogenous leukemia, *N. Engl. J. Med.* **313**:51–52.
21. Sandberg, A. A., 1987, The usefulness of chromosome analysis in clinical oncology, *Oncology* **1**:21–33.
22. Bennett, J. M., Catovsky, D., Daniel, M.-T., Flandrin, G., Galton, D. A. G., Gralnick, H. R., and Sultan, C., 1976, Proposals for the classification of the acute leukaemias, *Br. J. Haematol.* **33**:451–458.

23. Bennett, J. M., Catovsky, D., Daniel, M.-T., Flandrin, G., Galton, D. A. G., Gralnick, H. R., and Sultan, C., 1982, Proposals for the classification of the myelodysplastic syndromes, *Br. J. Haematol.* **51**:189–199.

24. Bennett, J. M., Catovsky, D., Daniel, M.-T., Flandrin, G., Galton, D. A. G., Gralnick, H. R., and Sultan, C., 1985, Criteria for the diagnosis of acute leukemia of megakaryocyte lineage (M7), *Ann. Intern. Med.* **103**:460–462.

25. Second MIC Cooperative Study Group, 1987, Morphologic, immunologic, and cytogenetic (MIC) working classification of acute lymphoblastic leukemias, *Cancer Genet. Cytogenet.* (in press).

26. Bernstein, R., Pinto, M. R., Behr, A., and Mendelow, B., 1982, Chromosome 3 abnormalities in acute nonlymphocytic leukemia (ANLL) with abnormal thrombopoiesis: Report of three patients with a "new" inversion anomaly and a further case of homologous translocation, *Blood* **60**:613–617.

27. Bernstein, R., Bagg, A., Pinto, M., Lewis, D., and Mendelow, B., 1986, Chromosome 3q21 abnormalities associated with hyperactive thrombopoiesis in acute blastic transformation of chronic myeloid leukemia, *Blood* **68**:652–657.

28. Sweet, D. L., Golomb, H. M., Rowley, J. D., and Vardiman, J. M., 1979, Acute myelogenous leukemia and thrombocythemia associated with an abnormality of chromosome No. 3, *Cancer Genet. Cytogenet.* **1**:33–37.

29. Bitter, M. A., Neilly, M. E., Le Beau, M. M., Pearson, M. G., and Rowley, J. D., 1985, Rearrangements of chromosome 3 involving bands 3q21 and 3q26 are associated with normal or elevated platelet counts in acute nonlymphocytic leukemia, *Blood* **66**:1362–1370.

30. Berger, R., Bernheim, A., Daniel, M.-T., Valensi, F., and Flandrin, G., 1981, Karyotypes and cell phenotypes in acute leukemia following other diseases, *Blood Cells* **7**:293–299.

31. Sandberg, A. A., 1986, The chromosomes in human leukemia, *Semin. Hematol.* **23**:201.

32. First MIC Cooperative Study Group, 1986, Morphologic, immunologic, and cytogenetic (MIC) working classification of acute lymphoblastic leukemias, *Cancer Genet. Cytogenet.* **23**:189–197.

33. Sandberg, A. A., Morgan, R., McCallister, J. A., Kaiser-McCaw, B., and Hecht, F., 1983, Acute myeloblastic leukemia (AML) with t(6;9)(p23;q34): A specific subgroup of AML?, *Cancer Genet. Cytogenet.* **10**:139–142.

34. Schwartz, S., Jiji, R., Kerman, S., Meekins, J., and Cohen, M. M., 1983, Translocation (6;9)(p23;q34) in acute nonlymphocytic leukemia, *Cancer Genet. Cytogenet.* **10**:133–138.

35. Vermaelen, K., Michaux, J.-L., Louwagie, A., and Van Den Berghe, H., 1983, Reciprocal translocation t(6;9)(p21;q33): A new characteristic chromosome anomaly in myeloid leukemias, *Cancer Genet. Cytogenet.* **10**:125–131.

36. Bennett, J. M., Catovsky, D., Daniel, M.-T., Flandrin, G., Galton, D. A. G., Gralnick, H. R., and Sultan, C., 1981, Morphological classification of acute lymphoblastic leukemia: Concordance among observers and clinical correlations, *Br. J. Haematol.* **47**:553–561.

37. Yunis, J. J., Oken, M. M., Theologides, A., Howe, R. B., and Kaplan, M. E., 1984, Recurrent chromosomal defects are found in most patients with non-Hodgkin's-lymphoma, *Cancer Genet. Cytogenet.* **13**:17–28.

38. Yunis, J. J., Frizzera, G., Oken, M. M., McKenna, J., Theologides, A., and Arnesen, M., 1987, Multiple recurrent genomic defects in follicular lymphoma: A possible model for cancer, *N. Engl. J. Med.* **316**:79–84.

39. First International Workshop on Chromosomes in Leukemia 1977, 1978, Chromosomes in Ph[1]-positive chronic granulocytic leukaemia, *Br. J. Haematol.* **39**:305–309.

40. First International Workshop on Chromosomes in Leukemia 1977, 1978, Chromosomes in acute non-lymphocytic leukaemia, *Br. J. Haematol.* **39**:311–316.

41. Second International Workshop on Chromosomes in Leukemia 1979, 1980: Morphological analysis of acute promyelocytic leukemia (M3) and t(8;21) cases, *Cancer Genet. Cytogenet.* **2**:97–98.

42. Third International Workshop on Chromosomes in Leukemia 1980, 1981: Chromosomal abnormalities in acute lymphoblastic leukemia, *Cancer Genet. Cytogenet.* **4**:101–110.

43. Third International Workshop on Chromosomes in Leukemia 1980, 1981: Clinical significance of chromosomal abnormalities in acute lymphoblastic leukemia, *Cancer Genet. Cytogenet.* **4**:111–137.

44. Fourth International Workshop on Chromosomes in Leukemia 1982, 1984: A prospective study of acute nonlymphocytic leukemia, *Cancer Genet. Cytogenet.* **11**:249–360.

45. Croce, C. M., 1986, Chromosome translocations in human cancer, *Cancer Res.* **46**:6019–6023.

46. The Non-Hodgkin's Lymphoma Pathologic Classification Project, 1982, National Cancer Institute-sponsored study of classification of non-Hodgkin's lymphomas, 1982, Summary and description of a working formulation for clinical usage, *Cancer* **49**:2112.

47. Sandberg, A. A., 1986, Cytogenetics of the leukemias and lymphomas, in: *The Human Oncogenic Viruses* (A. A. Luderer and H. H. Weetall, eds.), pp. 1–41, Humana Press, Clifton, New Jersey.
48. Dalla-Favera, R., Bregni, M., Erikson, J., Patterson, D., Gallo, R. C., and Croce, C. M., 1982, Human c-myc onc gene is located in the region of chromosome 8 that is translocated in Burkitt lymphoma cells, *Proc. Natl. Acad. Sci. USA* **79:**7824–7827.
49. Croce, C. M., and Nowell, P. C., 1985, Molecular basis of human B cell neoplasia, *Blood* **65:**1–7.
50. Croce, C. M., Erikson, J., Tsujimoto, Y., and Nowell, P.C., 1987, Molecular basis of human B- and T-cell neoplasia, in: *Advances in Viral Oncology*, Vol. 7 (G. Klein, Ed.), pp. 35–51, Raven, New York.
51. Sandberg, A. A., and Turc-Carel, C., 1987, The cytogenetics of solid tumors: Relation to diagnosis, classification and pathology, *Cancer* **59:**387–395.
52. Cavazzana, A., Ross, R., Miser, J. S., Triche, T. J., 1987, Experimental evidence for a neural origin of Ewing's sarcoma, *Am. J. Pathol.* **127:**507–518.
53. Sandberg, A. A., 1986, Chromosome changes in bladder cancer: Clinical and other correlations, *Cancer Genet. Cytogenet.* **19:**163–175.
54. Turc-Carel, C., Limon, J., Dal Cin, P., Rao, U., Karakousis, C., and Sandberg, A. A., 1986, Cytogenetic studies of adipose tissue tumors. I. A benign lipoma with reciprocal translocation t(3;12)(q28;q14), *Cancer Genet. Cytogenet.* **23:**283–289.
55. Turc-Carel, C., Limon, J., Dal Cin, P., Rao, U., Karakousis, C., and Sandberg, A. A., 1986, Cytogenetic studies of adipose tissue tumors. II. Recurrent reciprocal translocation t(12;16)(q13;p11) in myxoid liposarcomas, *Cancer Genet. Cytogenet.* **23:**291–299.
56. Mandahl, N., Heim, S., Johansson, B., Bennet, K., Mertens, F., Olsson, G., Rööser, B., Rydholm, A., Willén, H., and Mitelman, F., 1987, Lipomas have characteristic structural chromosomal rearrangements of 12q13–q14, *Int. J. Cancer* **39:**685–688.

# 12

# Genetics of Susceptibility to Mouse Skin Tumor Promotion

## John DiGiovanni

## 1. INTRODUCTION

### 1.1. Multistage Carcinogenesis in Mouse Skin

The protocol used in most two-stage carcinogenesis studies in mouse skin was first described by Mottram[1] and forms the basis of the operational criteria defining a promoter. Mottram elicited skin tumors by treating the backs of mice with a single subcarcinogenic dose of the polycyclic aromatic hydrocarbon (PAH) benzo(a)pyrene [B(a)P], followed by repeated applications of croton oil, obtained from the seeds of *Croton tiglium*. Subsequently, the most active tumor-promoting component of croton oil was identified as the phorbol diester, 12-*O*-tetradecanoyl-phorbol-13-acetate (TPA),[2–5] and today it is the most frequently used promoter for mechanistic studies.

Tumor promotion in mouse skin can itself be divided into at least two steps that can each be mediated by TPA. Boutwell[6] was the first to recognize an early step involving the conversion of an initiated cell into a dormant or latent tumor cell and a second step in which the propagation of that cell is promoted. These steps or stages were further defined by Slaga and co-workers.[7,8] These investigators found that mezerein, a diterpene ester similar in structure to TPA, but with little or no skin tumor-promoting activity, acts as a potent second-stage promoter if applied to initiated skin that first has been treated with TPA, even if with only a single application.[7–10] Similar experiments have defined the semisynthetic compound phorbol-12-retinoate-13-acetate as a second-stage promoter in the NMRI mouse.[11]

Although the phorbol esters have been the most widely studied skin tumor promoters to date, many other chemical compounds have been shown to possess skin tumor promoting properties. Teleocidin, isolated from *Streptomyces mediocidicus*, is an indole alkaloid composed of teleocidin a and teleocidin b and their isomers. Both teleocidin and dihydroteleocidin B, a catalytically hydrogenated derivative of teleocidin b, induce many of the same biologic and biochemical effects and have promoting activity comparable to that of TPA.[12–14] Lyngbyatoxin was first isolated from the Hawaiian seaweed *Lyngbya majuscula* by Cardellina and co-workers.[15] It was subsequently shown to be structurally identical to teleocidin a.[16]

Two polyacetates that differ in chemical structure only by the presence or absence of a bromine residue in the hydrophilic region of the molecule were isolated from the seaweed *Lyngbya gracilis*.[16] Both induce many of the same effects as TPA, but aplysiatoxin is a good promoter, whereas

*John DiGiovanni* • The University of Texas System Cancer Center, Science Park, Research Division, Smithville, Texas 78957.

debromoaplysiatoxin, which lacks the bromine residue, is a very weak promoter.[16–18] Other examples of mouse skin tumor promoters include fatty acid methyl esters,[19] anthralin,[20,21] chrysarobin,[22] iodoacetic acid,[23] the weakly acidic fraction of cigarette smoke condensate,[24–27] 7-bromomethylbenz(a)anthracene,[28] benzoyl peroxide (BzP),[29] retinoic acid (RA),[30] 2,3,7,8-tetrachlorodibenzo-*p*-dioxin (TCDD),[31] and wound healing.[32]

## 1.2. Morphologic and Biochemical Effects of Tumor Promoters in Mouse Skin

Within a few hours after application of a single effective dose of a promoter such as TPA to mouse skin, localized edema and erythema characteristic of inflammation and irritation are evident and, by 24 hr, there is leukocytic infiltration of the dermis.[33,34] At that time, there is also a 5- to 10-fold increase in the percentage of dark basal keratinocytes in the interfollicular epidermis.[35–37] These dark cells (DC) are characterized by their strong basophilia, dense chromatin, and large numbers of free ribosomes. They increase in number in TPA-induced hyperplasia to a greater extent than in hyperplasia induced by mezerein or weakly promoting hyperplastic agents.[37,38] In addition, this increase can be prevented by simultaneous treatment of the skin with tosylphenylalanine chloromethylketone (TPCK) or fluocinolone acetonide (FA),[39] inhibitors of stage I of promotion (see Section 5.1). Some investigators[7,40] consider dark cells to be primitive stem cells and an increase in their number an important component of stage I of promotion, whereas other workers question these conclusions.[41,42] It should be noted that several recent studies[43,44] have demonstrated that DC are proliferating rather than degenerating cells, supporting an important role in the process of skin tumor promotion.

Within 1–2 days after a single promoter treatment, stimulation of mitotic activity in the basal cell layer of the epidermis continues for several days and results in an increased number of nucleated cell layers.[35] This is followed by a phase of increased keratinization of the upper layers of the epidermis.[35,45,46] Without additional promoter treatments, all these responses to the promoter gradually subside and the epidermis regains its normal appearance within approximately 2–3 weeks of treatment.[47] Repeated promoter treatment, however, prevents this decrease in response, and the skin appears to be in a chronic state of irritation and regenerative hyperplasia.[48] In fact, repeated treatment with TPA leads to potentiation in the hyperplastic response in species and strains that are susceptible to skin tumor promotion by phorbol esters.[49] With repeated TPA treatment of initiated skin, benign tumors begin to appear in about 6 weeks[6] and, with some mouse stocks such as the selectively bred SENCAR, there may be an average of 20–30 papillomas per mouse after 18 weeks of promoter treatment.[50]

Phorbol diesters with promoting activity produce an initial inhibition of tritiated thymidine incorporation into skin or epidermal DNA.[35,51,52] This is soon followed by greatly increased rates of nucleic acid and protein synthesis.[51–53] Promoter-treated skin shows an increase in phospholipid turnover[54–56] and prostaglandin accumulation,[57,58] a decreased responsiveness to epidermal chalones[59,60] and β-adrenergic agonists,[61–64] and a decrease in the basal activities of epidermal superoxide dismutase (SOD) and catalase.[65] Tumor promoter treatments also lead to a decrease in epidermal histidase,[66] modification of epidermal keratins,[46,67,68] increased synthesis and phosphorylation of histones,[69–71] and a large induction of ornithine decarboxylase (ODC),[72,73] the rate-limiting enzyme in polyamine biosynthesis.

Recently, specific high-affinity phorbol ester membrane-binding sites have been demonstrated in a variety of tissues, including mouse epidermis (using either particulate fractions or whole cells).[74–82] Castagna *et al.*[83] demonstrated that phorbol esters capable of promoting skin tumors directly activated a partially purified protein kinase from rat brain, termed protein kinase C (PKC). This widely distributed protein kinase in mammalian tissues, especially brain, is cyclic nucleotide and calmodulin insensitive but $Ca^{2+}$ and phopholipid dependent.[84] Castagna *et al.*[83] also showed that low concentrations of TPA can substitute for 1,2-diacylglycerol in the activation *in vitro* of PKC. Subsequently, it was found that saturable phorbol ester receptors in particulate or cytosolic preparations from several cells and tissues copurified with PKC.[85–88] Sharkey *et al.*[89] showed that diolein and other diacylglycerols competitively inhibit specific phorbol diester binding and suggested that diacylglycerol may be the endogenous ligand for the phorbol ester receptor. It should be pointed out that TPA has been found to increase diacylglycerol levels in several cell systems, suggesting activation of phospholipase C.[90] Thus, phorbol esters may exert some of their effects by initially binding to high-affinity sites on PKC (and/or increasing membrane levels of 1,2-diacylglycerol) with a resultant increase in membrane-associated kinase activity and subsequent changes in the phosphorylation of cellular proteins.[91] Evidence has recently accumulated indicating that activation of PKC by TPA leads to the induction of ODC.[92–94]

An exciting development in the field of tumor promotion stems from observations that PKC is not a single entity but in fact represents a family of closely related proteins (i.e., isozymes).[95–101] These findings may now explain the large body of data suggesting phorbol ester receptor heterogeneity.[102] All these studies support the accumulating evidence that different isozymic forms of PKC may mediate different biologic and biochemical responses. Either the relative ability to bind or the efficacy to activate a particular form of PKC, or both, may determine the response to a particular promoting agent. In addition, since species and tissue variation have been observed in PKC isozyme content,[95–101] the response of a particular cell, tissue, strain, or species to various classes of promoters believed to work through PKC may therefore depend on a genetically determined isozymic constitution.

## 2. GENETIC DIFFERENCES IN RESPONSE TO SKIN TUMOR PROMOTERS

### 2.1. Species Differences

Classically, the mouse has been considered most sensitive to epidermal carcinogenesis by either the complete carcinogenesis protocol or the initiation–promotion protocol using TPA.[103,104] Other species such as the rat and hamster are much less sensitive.[104–108] Shubik[103] failed to demonstrate initiation–promotion in either guinea pigs or rabbits (using croton oil as the promoter). However, wound healing was an effective promoting stimulus in rabbits. Stenback[109] was able to demonstrate both complete and two-stage epidermal carcinogenesis in New Zealand rabbits. It is interesting to note that the mouse is the only species in which the major skin tumors induced after topical treatment with either initiators and promoters are papillomas and squamous cell carcinomas. In hamsters, croton oil (or TPA) is capable of promoting the development of dermal melanomas in animals that have been initiated with 7,12-dimethylbenz(a)anthracene (DMBA).[107] It should be emphasized that the above comparisons are based on only very limited data. In no cases are there in-depth studies involving dose–response relationships and treatment frequency relationships. Such comparisons must therefore be considered tentative.

With regard to human skin, there is also a paucity of information from which to draw conclusions. Nevertheless, human skin[110,111] appears to respond to phorbol esters in a manner similar to mouse and pig skin.[112] It has also been reported[113] that psoriasis patients receiving psoralen and ultraviolet A (PUVA) treatments following initial treatment with initiating agents (i.e., ionizing radiation, coal tar, UVB light) have a higher incidence of squamous cell carcinomas, suggesting that PUVA may possess promoting activity. These data further emphasize the need to explore how different species respond to other classes of tumor promoters in addition to the phorbol esters. In this regard, a two-stage initiation–promotion experiment was performed in Syrian golden hamsters using BzP as the promoter.[114] Interestingly, BzP, like TPA, enhanced the development of dermal melanotic foci and melanotic tumors, indicating its promoting activity in this species. These data suggest that the genetic difference in target tissue specificity in the Syrian hamster may apply to all classes of tumor promoters, including those that possibly work by different mechanisms.

### 2.2. Strain Differences

In addition to the marked species differences discussed, there are also marked strain differences in response to epidermal tumor promotion. Most of these studies have used various stocks and strains of mice and assessed their response to phorbol esters. Table I ranks some of the commonly

### Table I. Sensitivity to Skin Tumor Promotion by TPA in Various Strains and Stocks of Mice[a]

| Mouse strain or stock | Relative sensitivity |
| --- | --- |
| SENCAR | +++++ |
| DBA/2 | +++ |
| CD-1 | ++ |
| C3H/He | ++ |
| C57BL/6 | ± |

[a]Data are relative values and apply only to PAH used as initiators and phorbol esters (TPA) as promoter.

employed mouse stocks and strains for their sensitivity to tumor promotion using phorbol esters. The differences among SENCAR, DBA/2, CD-1, C3H/He, and C57BL/6 mice have now been reasonably well documented[115–119] (J. DiGiovanni and M. Naito, unpublished studies).

The SENCAR mice are an outbred mouse line derived by selective breeding techniques for sensitivity to the initiation–promotion regimen.[6,50] Numerous studies have demonstrated that these mice were selected primarily for their sensitivity to the tumor promotion stage using phorbol esters,[50,116–121] although it cannot be conclusively ruled out that some aspect of initiation is different in these mice as well. More recently, an inbred strain of SENCAR mice (called SSln) has been developed[122] similar to the original skin-tumor-susceptible (STS) mouse derived by Boutwell.[6] These highly sensitive inbred mice will greatly facilitate studies of the genetic factors involved in controlling susceptibility and resistance to skin tumor promotion.

The relative rankings listed in Table I apply only to the phorbol ester class of tumor promoters. It is clear that certain mouse strains are much more sensitive to one type of treatment protocol than another. For example, C57BL/6 mice are quite refractory to the initiation–promotion regimen using TPA as noted in Table I. However, this mouse strain is sensitive to complete carcinogenesis with either DMBA or B(a)P[116,118] or to skin tumor promotion by BzP[118] or chrysarobin.[123] Thus, the genetic factors that control susceptibility and/or resistance to one class of tumor promoter may not control responsiveness to other chemical classes of tumor promoters (see Section 6).

## 2.3. Inheritance of Susceptibility to Phorbol Ester Skin Tumor Promotion

DBA/2 and C57BL/6 mice are inbred mouse strains representing extremes in sensitivity to tumor promotion by TPA (see Table I). We have examined in greater detail the genetic basis for these differences by determining the sensitivity of B6D2F$_1$ mice to skin tumor promotion by TPA. In general, F$_1$ mice (both B6D2F$_1$ and D2B6F$_1$) responded in a very similar manner compared with the DBA/2 parental strain[119,121] regardless of whether DMBA or N-methyl-N'-nitro-N-nitroso guanidine (MNNG) was used as the initiator. However, upon examination of more extensive dose–response relationships in male and female B6D2F$_1$ mice, we have found them to be less sensitive than DBA/2 mice at low doses of TPA.[124] These data indicate that susceptibility to TPA promotion is inherited as an incomplete dominant trait. Furthermore, the fact that the reciprocal F$_1$ generations responded very similarly indicates that cytoplasmic genetic determinants are not involved in determining susceptibility to TPA promotion in DBA/2 mice. Finally, comparison of the responsiveness of male and female D2B6F$_1$ and B6D2F$_1$ mice indicated that there were few differences between sexes. Therefore, the X chromosome does not appear to play a role in determining susceptibility to phorbol ester promotion in DBA/2 and C57BL/6 mice.[124] These early experiments aimed at understanding the genetics of susceptibility to various promoting stimuli using inbred mouse strains demonstrate the complexity of the problem and show that much work will be needed to understand this interesting problem fully. By contrast, these studies suggest the possibility that genetic models can be developed using inbred mouse strains not only to study the underlying genetic basis for sensitivity, but also to help understand basic mechanism(s) of tumor promotion (see Section 7).

Recently, several laboratories reported genetic models for the control of chemical carcinogenesis in mouse liver,[125] rat mammary gland,[126] and mouse lung.[127] Drinkwater and Ginsler[125] proposed that allelic differences for at least two loci contribute to the sensitivity of C3H/HeJ mice to *N,N*-diethylnitrosamine-induced hepatocarcinogenesis and that these alleles display semidominance. Studies by Malkinson *et al.*,[127] using AXB and BXA recombinant inbred (RI) strains, have suggested a three-locus model for controlling the susceptibility to urethan-induced pulmonary adenomas. Finally, Gould[126] presented evidence for dominant inheritance of susceptibility to DMBA induced mammary cancer in Wistar–Furth rats with a three-locus model. The nature of the genes controlling susceptibility in all these studies is unknown, although Drinkwater and Ginsler[125] and Gould[126] provided evidence to rule out differences in metabolic and DNA binding in their respective model systems. In addition, Drinkwater and Ginsler[125] suggested that the major locus controlling susceptibility to hepatocarcinogenesis in C3H/HeJ mice affects the promotion stage of liver tumor induction. It is not known whether the genes that control sensitivity to phorbol ester skin tumor promotion are related to those proposed in the above studies. If there are similarities in the mechanism of promotion in different organs, however, this is a strong possibility. In addition, despite the complexity of these types of experiments, it would seem extremely important to continue to explore the number and nature of genes controlling sensitivity to tumor promotion in a variety of model systems. Colburn and colleagues[128] described the cloning and characterization of putative genes from preneoplastic mouse epidermal JB6 cells (pro-1 and pro-2) which transfer to insensitive cells sensitivity to tumor promoter-induced neoplastic transformation. An interesting question is whether these genes are related to the genes that control sensitivity to phorbol ester skin tumor promotion *in vivo*. In this regard, it will be very important to determine the number of genes controlling susceptibility of phorbol ester skin tumor promotion *in vivo*. This can be accomplished by examining sensitivity of appropriate $F_2$, backcross, and recombinant inbred strains.

## 3. MORPHOLOGIC CHANGES IN MOUSE SKIN POTENTIALLY IMPORTANT IN DETERMINING GENETIC DIFFERENCES IN RESPONSE TO PHORBOL ESTERS

### 3.1. Hyperplasia

The induction of epidermal hyperplasia and dark basal keratinocytes are closely associated with the promoting ability of various phorbol esters as well as other types of tumor promoters.[2–4] The epidermal hyperplasia induced by treatment of mouse skin with phorbol esters is characterized by a marked increase in nucleated interfollicular cell layers (from one to two to three to four cell layers). In addition, repetitive applications of TPA to the skin of responsive mouse strains produces a potentiated hyperplasia of greater magnitude than that induced by a single application (up to four to five nucleated cell layers). Sisskin *et al.*[49] first noted that strain differences in response to multiple, but not single, treatments of TPA could distinguish between phorbol ester sensitive versus resistant mouse strains. In their studies, C57BL/6 mice displayed only slight hyperplasia after both single and multiple treatments with TPA. On the other hand, CD-1 mice (an outbred mouse stock fairly sensitive to initiation-promotion) responded with slight hyperplasia after a single application, but with a potentiation of hyperplasia after multiple applications of TPA. BALB/c mice responded with hyperplasia to a single application but, with multiple applications, this mouse strain became refractory to the TPA-induced hyperplasia. Interestingly, in their study, DBA/2 mice responded to single and multiple applications of TPA much like the CD-1 mouse, such that multiple TPA applications gave rise to a potentiated hyperplastic response. DBA/2 mice were subsequently found to be very sensitive to skin tumor promotion by TPA[119] (see also Table I).

Work in our laboratory has extended these earlier observations by exploring in more detail the hyperplasia induced in DBA/2, C57BL/6, and B6D2F$_1$ hybrids.[124] Figure 1 shows the epidermal hyperplasia induced 48 hr after the last of 4 applications of 6.8 nmol TPA to the skins of DBA/2,

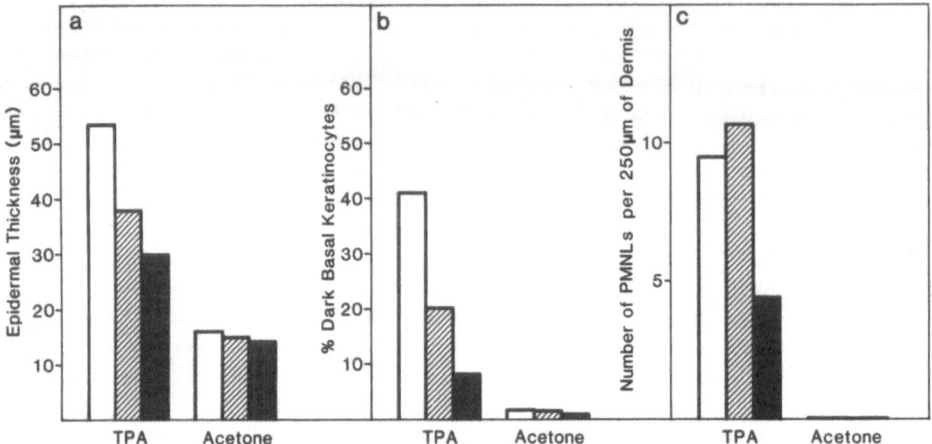

*Figure 1.* Morphologic changes in skin from female DBA/2□, B6D2F₁▨, and C57BL/6■ mice following repetitive applications of TPA. Seven week old female mice of each strain were treated twice-weekly with either 6.8 nmol TPA or acetone (0.2 ml) for 2 weeks; 48 hr after the last treatment, the mice were sacrificed and the skins removed and processed for histologic analysis. Each value shown represents an average of at least 12 observations per mouse from two mice. (a) Epidermal thickness (in µm). (b) Percentage of dark basal keratinocytes. (c) Number of polymorphonuclear leukocytes per 250 (µm) of the dermis.

C57BL/6, and B6D2F₁ mice. The dose and treatment protocol was similar to that used in tumor experiments showing dramatic differences in susceptibility to TPA promotion between DBA/2 and C57BL/6 mice.[119] C57BL/6 and DBA/2 mice differed significantly in their hyperplastic response to TPA[44,49] (see Figs. 1a, 2b,f, and 4a,b). Interestingly, the B6D2F₁ hybrid gave a hyperplasia response intermediate between the two parental strains (see Figs. 1a and 2b,d). Further dose-response experiments[124] have confirmed that B6D2F₁ mice are less sensitive over a broad dose range compared with the DBA/2 parental strain for induction of this sustained epidermal hyperplasia by TPA. These data confirm the results of tumor experiments showing the B6D2F₁ mice to be of lower sensitivity to TPA promotion than DBA/2.[124]

## 3.2. Dark Basal Keratinocytes

Raick first reported in his series of nonquantitative electron microscopic observations that the number of dark basal keratinocytes (DC) in TPA-induced hyperplasia was much higher than in epidermal hyperplasia induced by the weak tumor promoter ethyl phenyl propiolate (EPP) or by skin wounding.[38,129] DC are believed to be primitive stem cells, since they are present in high numbers in skin during embryogenesis and then decrease with age of the animal.[36] Klein-Szanto and Slaga[36] also reported, using a light microscopic technique for quantification of DC, that the first-stage tumor promoters such as 4-O-Me-TPA and calcium ionophore A23187, as well as strong complete promoters, induced the appearance of a large number of DC. The induction of DC is believed to result from the modulation of the commitment to differentiation or differentiation potential of subpopulations of basal cells, and it may be important in the expansion or accumulation of initiated cells during early stages of tumor promotion.[130] Chiba *et al.*[131] have divided TPA-induced DC into types I and II and proposed the view that type I DC are the poorly differentiated cells or dedifferentiated cells, different from type II or involuted DC. One can also see from Fig. 1b that at the 6.8-nmole dose of TPA, the percentage of DC induced in C57BL/6 mice was fivefold less than in DBA/2 mice. Again, the response of the B6D2F₁ hybrid was intermediate between the sensitive and resistant parental strains. Although we have not strictly classified the DC into type I and II, most DC observed in sections from DBA/2, C57BL/6, and B6D2F$_1$ mice corresponded to type I DC (see Fig. 2 for representative DCs in epon sections from DBA/2, C57BL/6, and B6D2F$_1$ mice).[124]

## 3.3. Inflammation

A role for inflammation and inflammatory processes in tumor promotion is supported by a variety of studies.[132,133] The inflammatory response to TPA is characterized by erythema, edema, and a marked leukocyte infiltration into the dermis, which can be readily scored.[33] Leukocyte (mainly PMN) infiltration is observed with doses of 1–2 µg TPA in SENCAR mice 24 and 48 hr after a single topical treatment.[40] After the eighth treatment in a multiple-treatment regimen with TPA, the relative number of dermal PMNs decreases markedly and that of lymphocytes and macrophages increases.[48] Lewis and Adams[134] reported that TPA treatment of C57BL/6 mice induced the dermal infiltration of a very small number of PMN compared with SENCAR mice. They also reported that inflammatory macrophages from SENCAR mice secreted four times more H$_2$O$_2$ than the corresponding cells from C57BL/6 mice and that cells from SENCAR mice required less than one third the amount of TPA to obtain 50% of the maximal response than that required by cells from C57BL/6 mice.[135] We have also demonstrated a correlation between sensitivity to TPA promotion and infiltration of PMNs in the dermis of DBA/2 and C57BL/6 mice. This can be readily seen in Fig. 1c. Furthermore, examination of skin sections from the B6D2F$_1$ hybrid demonstrated a marked dermal infiltration of PMN similar in magnitude to that observed in sections from DBA/2 mice[124] (Fig. 1c).

## 4. BIOCHEMICAL AND MOLECULAR CHANGES POTENTIALLY IMPORTANT IN DETERMINING GENETIC DIFFERENCES IN RESPONSE TO PHORBOL ESTERS

### 4.1. Receptor-Mediated Events

A number of possible mechanisms that might explain the genetic differences in response to phorbol ester skin tumor promotion have been explored. First, since the phorbol ester and phorbol esterlike compounds appear to work at least in part through interaction with PKC (see Chapter 18), genetic differences might be related to differences in number or affinity of these receptors. To date, however, significant differences in phorbol ester receptor number or affinity have not been observed in mice that differ in their response to TPA.[136,137] Furthermore, the levels of total epidermal PKC are not significantly different in SENCAR and C57BL/6 mice[138] or in other organs such as brain, spleen, lung, and heart between DBA/2 and C57BL/6 mice.[139] All of these studies are consistent with a number of additional investigations showing similar phorbol ester-binding characteristics in cultured cell variants altered in responsiveness to phorbol esters.[140] It is important to point out, however, that numerous studies have suggested the possibility of phorbol ester receptor heterogeneity.[102,140] Furthermore, in light of the recent information demonstrating different isozymes of PKC,[95–101] all the above experiments must now be re-evaluated. Until we have a better understanding of the expression and function of these different isozymes of PKC in various tissues, strains, and species, we cannot rule out the possibility that some aspect of the epidermal PKC system is involved in genetic differences in sensitivity to tumor promotion. Furthermore, recent studies have demonstrated that cell culture variants in responsiveness to TPA have been identified in which there is a defect in the translocation of PKC from cytosol to cell membrane.[141] In addition, these cells fail to downmodulate phorbol ester receptors.[82] These potential differences also remain to be explored in the various strains of mice. If inbred mouse strains show cross sensitivity/resistance to other classes of tumor promoters, that may not work through the phorbol ester receptor, this would be strong evidence against involvement of the phorbol ester receptor in genetically mediated differences to skin tumor promotion. Clearly, the C57BL/6 strain can respond to other classes of promoters.[118,123] Whether this will hold for the other stocks and strains of mice remains to be determined.

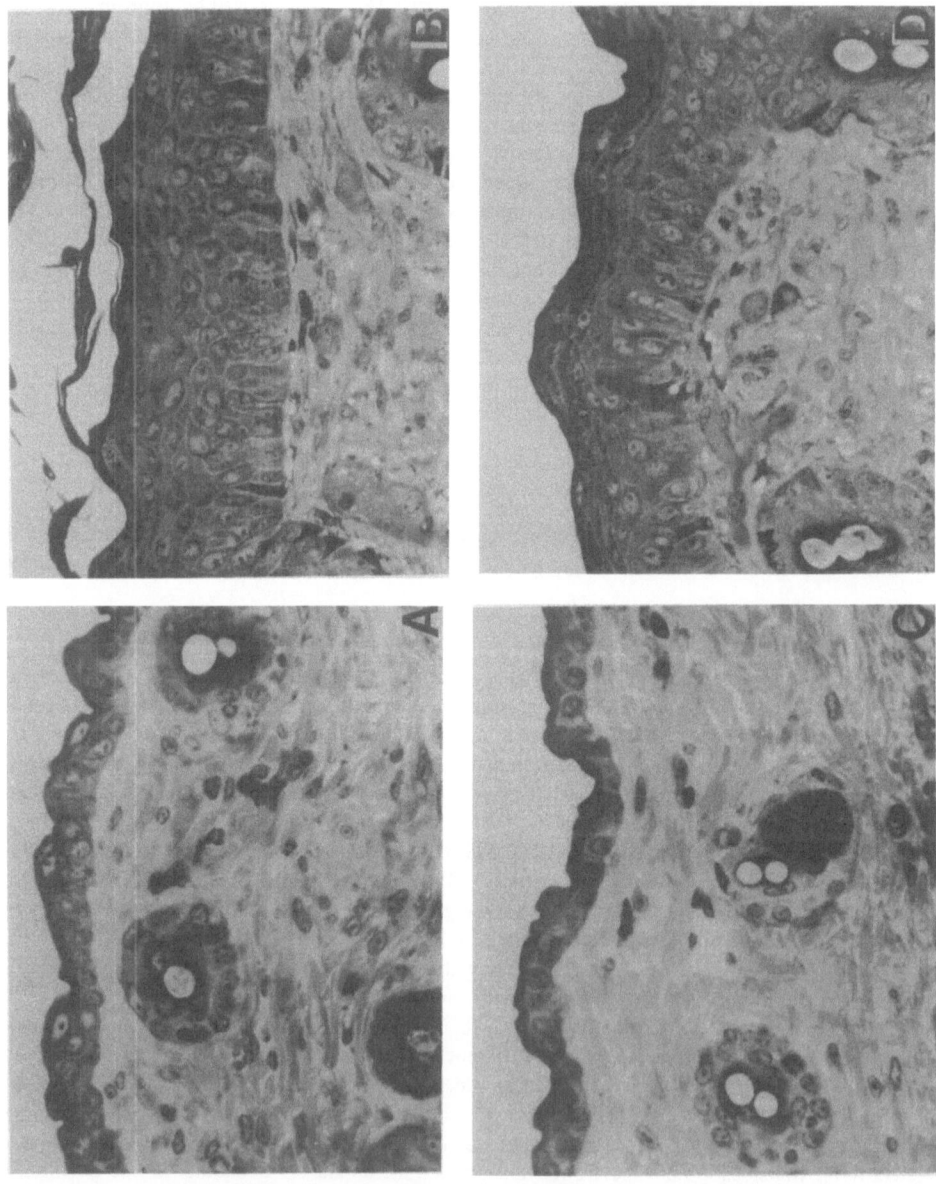

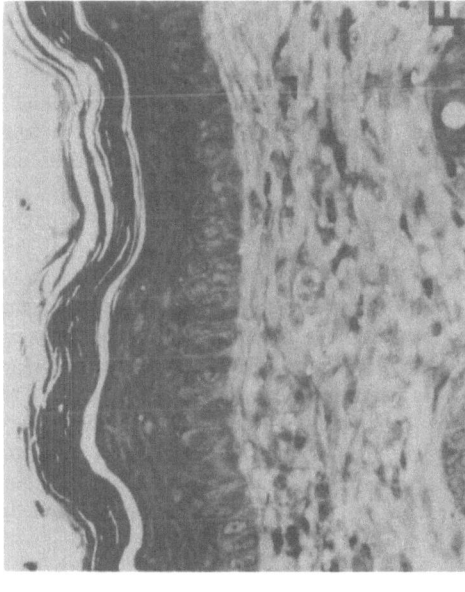

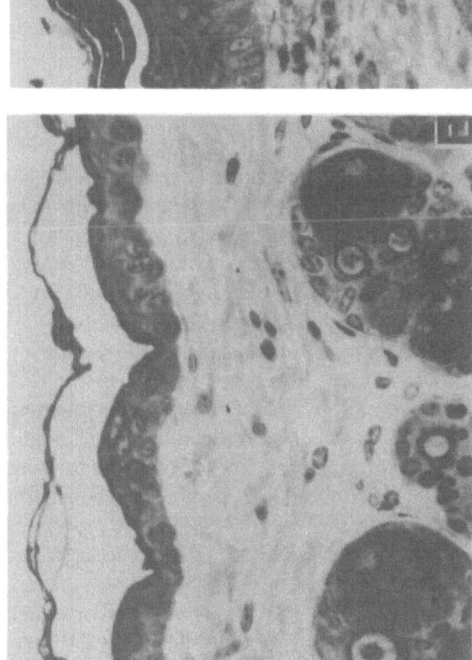

*Figure 2.* Response of the skin of female DBA/2, B6D2F₁, and C57BL/6 mice 48 hr after the last of four treatments with 6.8 nmol TPA (treatments given twice weekly): (A), (C) and (E), DBA/2, B6D2F₁, and C57BL/6 mice, respectively, acetone (0.2 ml). Note that there are only a few epidermal cell layers. (B), DBA/2 mice, TPA (6.8 nmol). Note the marked epidermal hyperplasia and large number of DCs. (D), B6D2F₁ mice, TPA (6.8 nmol). Note the significant hyperplastic response and the fairly large number of DCs. The hyperplasia (epidermal thickness) is less than that observed in DBA/2 mice. (F), C57BL/6, TPA (6.8 nmol). Note the weaker hyperplastic response and the very small number of DCs compared with DBA/2 mice. (Epon–toluidine blue, ×300)

## 4.2. Phorbol Ester Metabolism

Another possible mechanism for the strain and species differences in sensitivity to phorbol esters could reside in their ability to metabolize these compounds. It is clear that TPA does not require metabolic activation for its promoting action in mouse skin.[142–144] The major metabolic pathways for TPA in mouse skin involve formation of monoesters and the parent phorbol molecule.[142–144] Interestingly, when mouse skin is treated with TPA prior to isolation of epidermal homogenates, metabolism is enhanced.[144] To date, metabolism studies with TPA have not been performed in the skin of C57BL/6 or DBA/2 mice. Reiners et al.[118] suggested that "since the skin of CD-1 mice and Syrian hamsters are similar in their ability to clear and metabolize TPA, it is unlikely that differences in metabolism can account for differences in response to TPA promotion." Barret and co-workers[145] also provided convincing evidence that species differences in responsiveness to phorbol esters are not related to the ability or inability to deacylate TPA. It therefore appears unlikely that differences in the pharmacokinetics of TPA in mouse skin can explain the strain differences in response to TPA promotion. It should be pointed out that the differences between strains are apparent primarily after multiple applications of TPA (e.g., hyperplasia).[49] The possibility exists that some aspect of the absorption, distribution, metabolism, or elimination of TPA from the skin changes after multiple but not single treatments in the various mouse stocks and strains. Furthermore, Shoyab et al.[146] identified a tissue esterase capable of rapidly metabolizing TPA. These investigators reported that the enzyme is apparently present in skin from hamsters (a species relatively resistant to TPA), whereas it was virtually absent from the skin of mice. The extent to which this enzyme is induced or elevated after high doses or repetitive treatments with TPA on mouse skin is unknown. Finally, Segal et al.[147] reported the formation of a reduction product at the C-5 carbonyl group of TPA in mouse skin, phorbol-5-ol myristate acetate. The extent to which this and other potential metabolites[148] are formed in mouse skin and play a role in genetically determined sensitivity to phorbol ester promotion remains to be determined.

## 4.3. Other Mechanisms

Clearly, the C57BL/6 mouse displays a markedly reduced inflammatory response after exposure to TPA compared with SENCAR[44,134,135] and DBA/2 mice[44] (see also Fig. 1). It has been suggested that oxygen radicals ($O_2^-$, OH·) produced during inflammatory processes may play an important role in skin tumor promotion.[149] Lewis and Adams[134,135] recently demonstrated that the sensitivity of SENCAR and C57BL/6 mice to TPA promotion correlates with the ability of TPA to attract inflammatory cells to the skin as well as stimulate oxygen radical production in macrophages. Furthermore, the release of oxidized metabolites of arachidonic acid stimulated by TPA was greatly enhanced in macrophages from SENCAR versus C57BL/6 mice. Fischer et al.[150] showed that TPA can induce oxidant production directly in mouse epidermal cells in an in vitro system measured by the technique of chemiluminescence. When the response was compared between SSIn (the new inbred SENCAR mouse), SENCAR, and C57BL/6 mice, a good correlation was observed between sensitivity to TPA promotion and oxidant production by the isolated epidermal cells. The precise role of oxidant production by inflammatory cells and/or epidermal keratinocytes in the process of tumor promotion remains to be answered. However, these genetic differences provide support for an important role that certainly requires further investigation.

The mechanism(s) for the high sensitivity of the selectively bred SENCAR mouse to two-stage carcinogenesis with TPA remains to be determined. Hennings et al.[117] reported that SENCAR mice were more sensitive than BALB/c mice to the initiating action of both DMBA and MNNG. However, the magnitude of the difference between the two strains was greatest with DMBA as the initiator. Thus, there is uncertainty as to whether these mice are more susceptible to some aspect of tumor initiation in addition to skin tumor promotion. These authors also reported that SENCAR mice developed a higher incidence of "spontaneous" tumors following repeated applications of TPA alone. Whether this represents a truly higher incidence of "spontaneous" tumors remains to be determined. In addition, Yuspa et al.[151] demonstrated that skin grafts from SENCAR to nude mice developed papillomas at a higher frequency, whereas skin grafts from BALB/c mice developed no tumors. These results indicated that the susceptibility for skin carcinogenesis in SENCAR mice was determined by the target tissue and do not support a role of the systemic immune system in the observed genetic differences in sensitivity. In studies by Strickland et al.,[152,153] SENCAR and BALB/c mice were compared for differences with respect to DNA excision repair, endogenous virus complement, and epidermal growth factor (EGF) receptors. Although differences were found between the two mouse stocks, no clear relationship could be determined between any of the above parameters and susceptibility to two-stage skin carcinogenesis. Strickland[120] reported that SENCAR mice were more sensitive to UV-induced epidermal carcinogenesis and that SENCAR mice display an abnormal wound healing response following large doses of UV light compared with BALB/c mice.[154] It is not known whether this genetic defect plays a role in the altered sensitivity to skin tumor promotion. Finally, Weeks and Slaga[155] reported that SENCAR mice differed in their response to an inhibitor of tumor promotion, FA, as compared with CD-1 mice. They reported that FA, in a dose-dependent manner, inhibited TPA-induced ODC activity in the epidermis of SENCAR mice. However, FA had no consistent effect on TPA-induced ODC activity in the epidermis of CD-1 mice.

## 5. GENETIC DIFFERENCES IN RESPONSE TO STAGE-SPECIFIC PROMOTERS IN MOUSE SKIN

### 5.1. Two-Stage Promotion

Tumor promotion in mouse skin can itself be divided into at least two steps that can each be mediated by TPA. Boutwell[6] was the first to recognize an early step involving the conversion of an initiated cell into a dormant or latent tumor cell and a second step in which the propagation of that cell is promoted. In these early studies, Boutwell used a limited number of croton oil treatments followed by repetitive applications of turpentine[6] or skin wounding[53] on STS female mice (the progenitors of the current SENCAR outbred mouse). These steps or stages were further defined by Slaga and co-workers,[7,156] who found that mezerein, a diterpene ester similar in structure to TPA but with weak complete promoting activity, acts as a potent second-stage promoter if applied to initiated skin that first has been treated with TPA, even if with only a single application.[7,156] Furstenberger et al.,[11] using an outbred mouse called NMRI, showed that 12-O-retinoylphorbol-13-acetate (RPA) was inactive as a complete promoter but was quite effective as a second-stage promoter in this mouse strain. Using TPA and mezerein in a two-stage promotion protocol, Slaga et al.[7,156] demonstrated that compounds known to inhibit phorbol ester skin tumor promotion affect specific stages of promotion, presumably by inhibiting events that are important for those stages. For example, the protease inhibitor, TPCK, is a potent inhibitor specifically of stage I of promotion, whereas RA, an inhibitor of promoter-induced ODC activity, specifically inhibits the second stage. By contrast, FA inhibited both stages of tumor promotion. Thus, Slaga et al.[156] proposed that the induction of dark basal keratinocytes and prostaglandin biosynthesis that occur following TPA application are specific for stage 1 of promotion, while increased polyamine levels and cell proliferation are important for stage 2 promotion. A summary of two-stage promotion in SENCAR mice is illustrated in Fig. 3.

### 5.2. Genetic Differences in Response to Stage-Specific Promoters

Of interest to the present discussion is the fact that mezerein was reported to be a weak complete promoter in NMRI mice[11] but not SENCAR, whereas RPA was found to be a moderate skin tumor promoter in SENCAR mice.[157] In addition, skin wounding appeared to act as a stage 2-promoting stimulus in STS mice,[53] whereas in SENCAR[156] and NMRI[158] mice it has been reported to be a stage 1-promoting stimulus. Finally, 4-O-methyl-TPA and the calcium ionophore A23187 have been reported to be effective stage 1 promoters in SENCAR[156] mice, but they are ineffective in

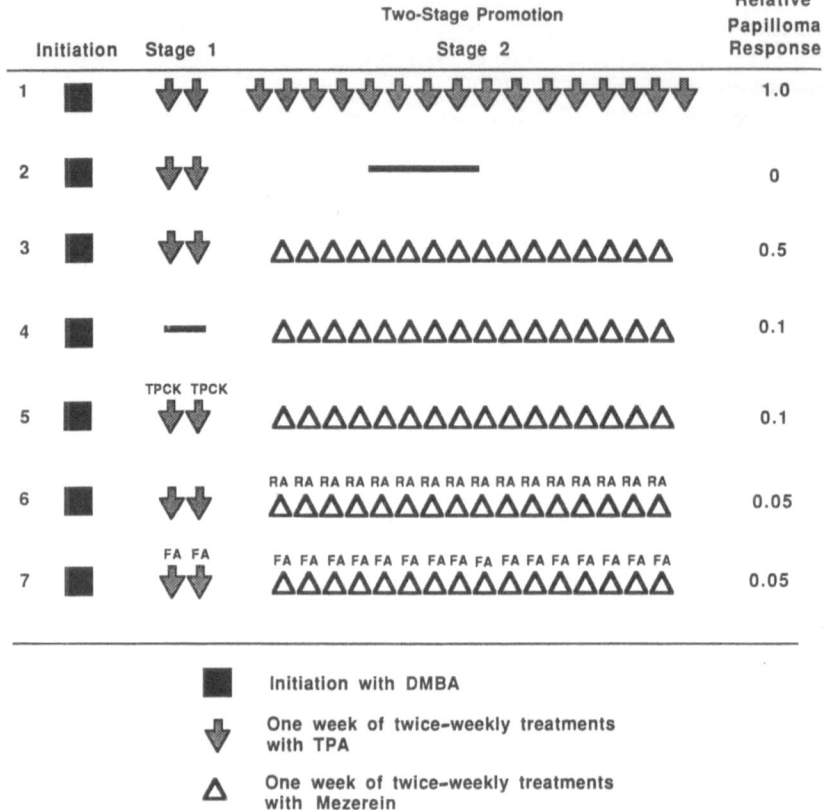

*Figure 3.* Characteristics of two-stage promotion in SENCAR mice. Each number represents an experimental group of 30 mice. Mice received a single dose of DMBA (10 nmol) at initiation followed 1 week later by twice-weekly applications of either TPA or mezerein as indicated. Group 1: the standard promotion protocol, in which TPA is given continuously during stages 1 and 2 of promotion. Group 2: stage 1 of promotion with TPA followed either by no treatment or twice-weekly treatments with 0.2 ml acetone during stage 2 of promotion. Group 3: the standard two-stage promotion protocol with TPA given during stage 1 of promotion followed by twice-weekly treatments with mezerein during stage 2 of promotion. Group 4: no stage 1 treatment or acetone (0.2 ml) twice weekly followed by twice-weekly treatments with mezerein during stage 2 of promotion. Note the weak complete papilloma-promoting activity of mezerein. Groups 5 and 6: promotion stage-specific inhibition by TPCK and RA, respectively. Group 7: inhibition of stages 1 and 2 of promotion by FA.

NMRI mice.[158] These studies indicate significant differences in the way STS, SENCAR, and NMRI mice respond to first- and second-stage promoters. The NMRI mouse is somewhat less sensitive to TPA as a complete promoter as compared with SENCAR mice.[11] Thus, higher doses of TPA are commonly used in NMRI mice. Perhaps NMRI mice are less sensitive to the toxic actions of mezerein than SENCAR mice. Hennings and Yuspa[159] suggested that mezerein is in fact a weak complete promoter in SENCAR mice, and it has been suggested that epidermal toxicity plays a role in limiting the promoting actions of this compound.[11,160] In our hands, mezerein also is a weak complete promoter of papilloma formation in SENCAR mice.[161] These differences may therefore reflect real genetic differences in responsiveness to stage 1 and 2 promoters. It would seem important to characterize further the response(s) of various strains and stocks of mice to the different types and classes of promoting agents, including putative first- and second-stage promoters (hence the underlying genetic factors controlling these differences), to understand fully the process of tumor promotion in general and the nature of multistage promotion.

## 6. GENETIC DIFFERENCES IN RESPONSE TO OTHER CLASSES OF TUMOR-PROMOTING AGENTS

### 6.1. Characteristics of the Response of Mouse Skin to Different Classes of Tumor Promoters

It is of interest to determine whether genetic factors controlling susceptibility in various inbred mouse strains to phorbol esters also control susceptibility to other classes of tumor promoters. Skin tumor promotion and the phenomenon of tumor promotion in general have been studied primarily with the phorbol esters.[2–4] Nevertheless, many other chemical classes of compounds possess skin tumor-promoting activity. In general, all skin tumor promoters must be capable of producing an epidermal hyperplasia.[34] However, it has been argued that the induction of epidermal hyperplasia is not a sufficient condition for production of epidermal tumorigenesis in mouse skin.[34,162] There are a number of substances, such as acetic acid, cantharidin, mezerein, and EPP, which apparently produce an epidermal hyperplasia similar to that produced by TPA after a single application, but unlike TPA they are poor promoters of epidermal tumorigenesis in mice. Argyris demonstrated that acetic acid was in fact a very weak hyperplasia-producing agent in multiple treatment regimens[163] and in addition multiple applications of 17 nmol mezerein could not maintain the epidermal hyperplasia it initially produced.[160]

It is also clear from other studies that the hyperplasia produced by single or multiple treatments with different chemicals on mouse skin is not the same. In this regard, Raick[129] showed that the weak tumor promoters, such as EPP and cantharidin, are capable of producing epidermal hyperplasia and an increased mitotic index but that the time sequence of these events is different from that observed with TPA. A single application of TPA induces an increase in the number of nucleated interfollicular epidermal (IFE) cell layers prior to an increase in mitotic index, whereas with EPP and cantharidin, the order of these events is reversed. We have studied in detail the anthrone derivatives, such as chrysarobin and anthralin.[164,165] The effect of a single treatment with optimal promoting doses of TPA and chrysarobin on epidermal thickness, the number of nucleated IFE cells, edema formation, DC, and dermal PMN infiltration has been studied.[164,165] The data indicate that chrysarobin is capable of inducing hyperplasia and inflammation similar in magnitude to TPA, but the time course of the response was different than that observed with TPA. With chrysarobin, a slight hyperplasia was observed at 24 and 48 hr after treatment and a greater level at 72 and 96 hr after treatment. In fact, the hyperplastic response peaked between 4 and 7 days after a single topical application. A similar result was obtained with anthralin, whereas with TPA, hyperplasia was maximal by 48–72 hr after application and by 96 hr had begun to decline significantly. Interestingly, both chrysarobin and anthralin produced edema (24 hr after application) to a greater extent than that observed with a single treatment with optimal promoting doses of TPA. Following multiple treatments with chrysarobin the epidermal changes observed were less pronounced than those with multiple treatments of TPA and correlated with the relative promoting activities of these two compounds.

With the very weak promoter EPP, the maximal increase in the number of nucleated cell layers of the IFE occurs between 72 and 120 hr.[130] Although we have not measured the mitotic index following treatment with chrysarobin (or anthralin) in SENCAR mice, the time course of hyperplasia was similar to that reported for EPP. These results suggest inherent differences in the way epidermal cells respond to TPA and chrysarobin (or EPP) treatment. Klein-Szanto and Slaga have characterized the response of SENCAR mouse skin to BzP and other free radical-generating peroxides.[166] They demonstrated that these peroxides were indeed skin irritants but that some differences existed in comparison with the phorbol esters. In this regard, BzP produced little or no inflammatory or vascular changes in the skin while at the same time producing a good hyperplasia and DC response. All the above data indicate that different types of chemicals probably produce their hyperplastic responses by different mechanisms. It would not be surprising, then, if animals resistant to tumor promotion by one class of compound were, in fact, sensitive to other classes of compounds.

## 6.2. Genetic Differences in Response to Different Classes of Promoters

C57BL/6 mice, although refractory to two-stage carcinogenesis and skin tumor promotion by TPA, are quite sensitive to complete carcinogenesis protocols with B(a)P and DMBA. Interestingly, C57BL/6 mice are sensitive to two-stage carcinogenesis if BzP is used as the promoter.[118] Anthrone tumor promoters, such as chrysarobin, are believed to work by an initial mechanism different from that of the phorbol esters for their promoting action(s).[22,123,164] We have recently shown that chrysarobin is an effective skin tumor promoter of papilloma formation in SENCAR, DBA/2, and C57BL/6 mice.[123] In light of this information, it is not totally surprising that chrysarobin induced a sustained epidermal hyperplasia and DC response of similar magnitude in all three strains of mice.[164,167] We have recently argued[123,165] that the induction of epidermal hyperplasia by anthrone derivatives results from toxicity and a subsequent regenerative response. In this regard, the sustained epidermal hyperplasia and DC response induced by chrysarobin showed a delayed time course in comparison to TPA. Furthermore, chrysarobin-treated skins had fewer nucleated cells per unit length of basement membrane (BM), and those cells had altered morphology compared to the "normal"-looking basal cells of acetone-treated control mice (Fig. 4, panels E and F).[165,167]

It should be emphasized that the current data discussed above do not allow us to ascertain whether C57BL/6 mice are of equal or lower sensitivity to organic peroxide and anthrone tumor promotion compared with SENCAR (or DBA/2) mice. This is admittedly due to the fact that in the studies using BzP[118] and in the study with chrysarobin,[123] different initiating doses of DMBA were used in SENCAR mice (10 nmoles) compared with the DBA/2 and C57BL/6 mice (400 nmoles). The reasons for using such a high initiating dose in the DBA/2 and C57BL/6 mice was to insure that initiation had taken place in these strains.[119] Bock and Burns[20] presented data suggesting that C57/st mice were less sensitive to anthralin than Swiss mice initiated with the same dose of DMBA, although small numbers of animals were used in the experimental groups of this study. Ideally, strain comparisons for sensitivity to tumor promotion by various classes of agents potentially exhibiting different mechanisms of action should use direct-acting agents such as MNNG for the initiation stage. CD-1 mice appeared to be less sensitive than SENCAR mice to the promoting effects of 7-bromomethylbenz(a)anthracene[168] and UV light.[120] These data suggest that mice less sensitive to phorbol esters also may be less sensitive to other classes of tumor promoters. The question of cross sensitivity/resistance to different classes of tumor promoters deserves further investigation in a variety of stocks and strains of mice.

To explore further the genetic differences in response of DBA/2 and C57BL/6 mice to tumor promoters, we have examined the histologic responses to additional classes of promoters other than the phorbol esters and anthrones (Figs. 4 and 5). Teleocidin, applied using a similar dose and treatment regimen as that of TPA, was very effective at producing a sustained epidermal hyperplasia and DC response in DBA/2 mice. Teleocidin is an indole alkaloid mixture (various isomers of teleocidins A+B) capable of binding to the phorbol ester receptor and with skin tumor promoting potency similar to TPA in sensitive mouse strains.[12–14] Surprisingly, C57BL/6 mice responded to multiple treatments of teleocidin exhibiting a sustained epidermal hyperplasia, DC response, and dermal PMN infiltration response similar to that of DBA/2 mice (Fig. 4C,D, respectively).[167] Although the skin tumor-promoting activity of teleocidin in DBA/2 and C57BL/6 mice has not been examined to date, our data suggest that this compound may be an effective promoter in both strains of mice. We are currently examining this possibility. It should be pointed out that there are several important differences between TPA and teleocidin that could account for the lack of a strain difference that we have observed for epidermal hyperplasia induction by the latter derivative. First, the principal metabolic pathways for TPA in mouse skin are hydrolysis of the 12 and 13 ester groups.[142,144] Teleocidin, as noted above, is an indole alkaloid whose structure contains no such ester groups and one would not expect it to be metabolized in a manner similar to TPA. The observation that teleocidin-induced hyperplasia was somewhat more persistant in DBA/2 mice than that observed following the last TPA treatment supports this hypothesis.[167] Alternatively, it has been suggested that there is heterogeneity of cellular receptors for phorbol ester and similar compounds.[102,140] This heterogeneity appears to arise from the fact that at least three isozymic forms of

PKC are known to exist in tissues.[95–101] Perhaps teleocidin is capable of interacting with a different subclass of receptors more prevalent in C57BL/6 mice than DBA/2 mice. Certainly other mechanisms could explain the relative ability of teleocidin to induce a sustained epidermal hyperplasia of similar magnitude in both DBA/2 and C57BL/6 mice, and remain to be explored.

Other promoters were also examined including mezerein, 4-O-Me-TPA, and BzP for their effects in C57BL/6 and DBA/2 mice. Interestingly, all compounds induced essentially the same histologic responses in both strains of mice[167] (see Fig. 5). Chrysarobin (Fig. 4E,F) was the only exception to this statement in that this promoter induced a slightly greater sustained hyperplasia at 48 hr after the last treatment in C57BL/6 mice compared with DBA/2, whereas dermal infiltration of PMNs was considerably greater in the latter mouse strain. These data, in conjunction with the above discussion, point to the importance of future studies to characterize fully the cross-sensitivity and resistance of different strains and species to various classes of promoting agents. If multiple mechanisms are involved in skin tumor promotion by diverse classes of chemical promoters, multiple genes are probably involved in controlling the susceptibility to these various agents.

Finally, Poland et al.[31,169] demonstrated that TCDD is capable of promoting skin tumors in certain mice. This response, however, appears only in mice that are homozygous for the hr locus (i.e., hr/hr or hairless mice) and thus capable of responding with a sustained epidermal hyperplasia following topical application of TCDD. The ability of TCDD to promote skin tumors in hairless mice is associated with the Ah locus in that the structure–activity relationships for binding to the cytosolic Ah-receptor in hairless mice (hr/hr) follows closely the ability of a given congener of TCDD to promote skin tumors in these mice. TCDD appears to promote skin tumors in hr/hr mice by first interacting with the cytosol receptor, leading to a pleiotropic response that includes the induction of a number of enzymes and also includes the induction of a sustained hyperplasia in the skin of these mice.

These findings further support the hypothesis that tumor promotion is a major determinant in genetic differences with respect to epidermal carcinogenesis. The susceptibility of C57BL/6 mice (and possibly other strains) to different classes of promoters support the hypothesis that these compounds (i.e., BzP and chrysarobin) may work through different mechanisms than the phorbol esters. A similar conclusion may be drawn from the studies with TCDD and TPA promotion in HRS/J haired versus hairless mice.[31,169] In this regard, the fact that hairless mice respond to both TCDD and TPA, whereas haired mice respond only to TPA implies different initial mechanisms for these two compounds. Finally, the data point out the importance of studies to determine the cross-sensitivity and/or resistance of various mouse strains to different classes of tumor promoters in an effort to identify both specific as well as more general genetic factors responsible for determining sensitivity to tumor-promoting agents.

# 7. USE OF GENETIC DIFFERENCES TO DEVELOP MODELS FOR STUDYING MECHANISMS OF TUMOR PROMOTION

## 7.1. In Vivo and in Vitro Models

It should be readily apparent that a knowledge of genetic differences in response to phorbol ester and other classes of tumor promoters can provide an excellent tool(s) for studying mechanisms of tumor promotion. In this regard, two major avenues are currently being explored in great detail. The first approach is the development of inbred strains of mice that are resistant/sensitive to particular types of promoting agents. In Boutwell's original experiments, he was successful in obtaining both a sensitive and resistant mouse line from the same parental stock.[6] More recently, an inbred SENCAR mouse (i.e., SSIn)[122] has become available for experimentation. The development of an inbred resistant strain from the same parental stock is currently in progress (T. J. Slaga, S. M. Fischer, and J. DiGiovanni, unpublished studies). These animals (both sensitive and resistant strains derived from the same parental stock) will greatly facilitate the elucidation of such questions as: (1) How is susceptibility inherited in offspring between resistant and sensitive parents? (2) How many

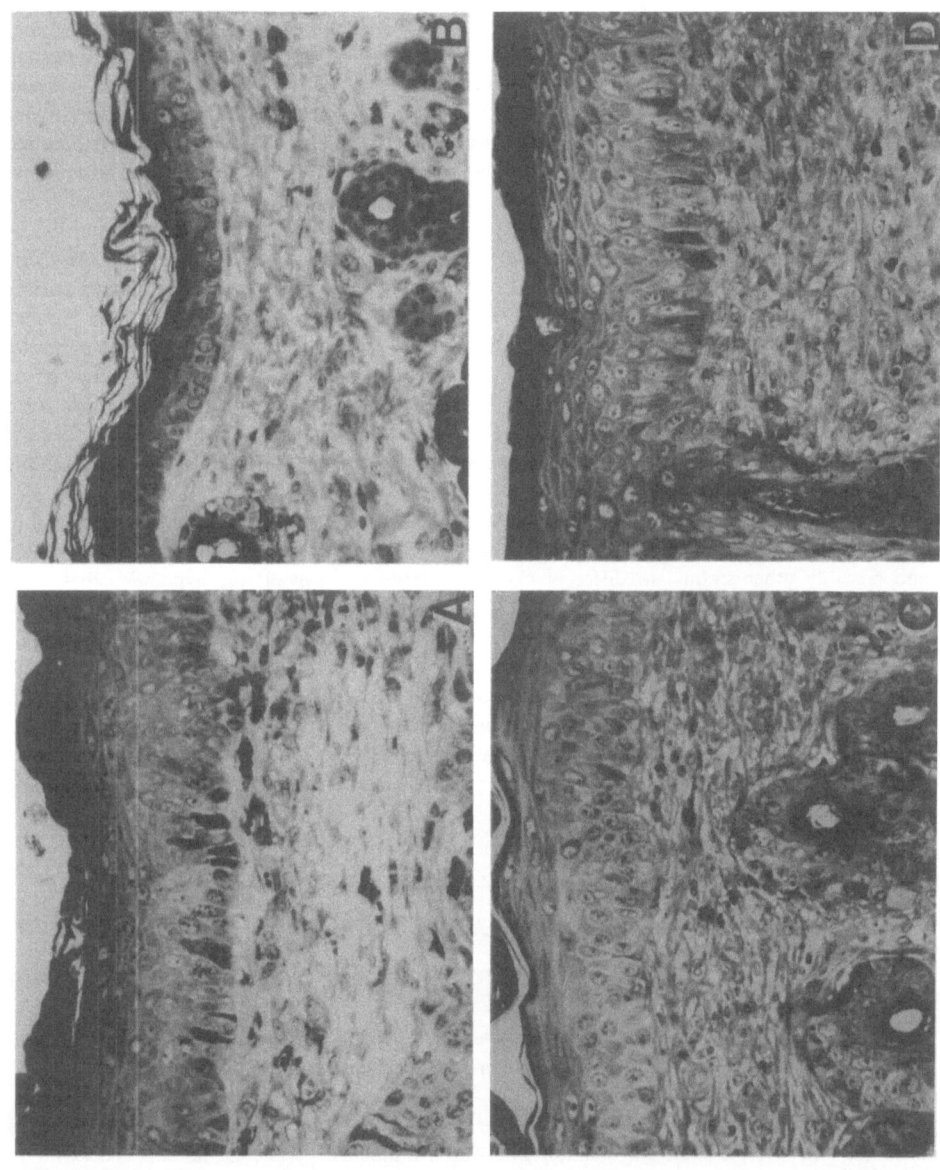

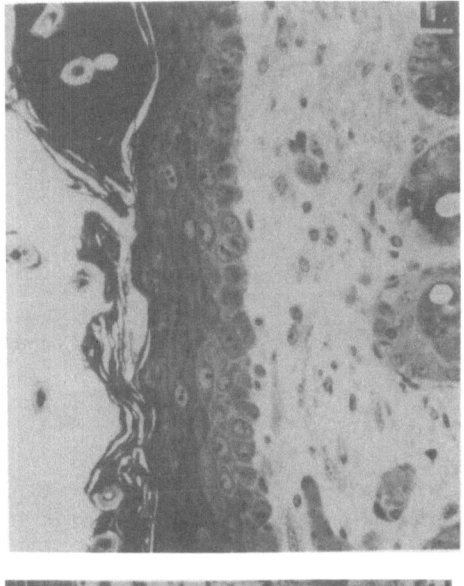

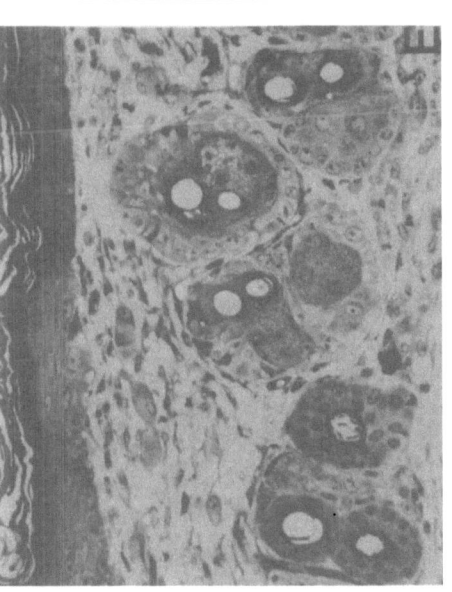

*Figure 4.* Response of the skin of DBA/2 and C57BL/6 mice 48 hr after the last of four treatments with TPA, teleocidin, or chrysarobin. TPA treatments were given twice weekly at a dose of 6.8 nmoles per mouse similar to the experiment in Fig. 2. Teleocidin treatments were given twice weekly, whereas chrysarobin treatments were given once-weekly. (A,B) DBA/2 and C57BL/6 mice, respectively, TPA (6.8 nmol). Note the marked epidermal hyperplasia and DC response in DBA/2 but not C57BL/6 mice. (C,D) DBA/2 and C57BL/6 mice, respectively, teleocidin (6.8 nmol). Note the marked epidermal hyperplasia and DC response in both DBA/2 and C57BL/6 mice. (E,F) DBA/2 and C57BL/6 mice, respectively, chrysarobin (220 nmol). Note the moderate hyperplasia and swollen basal cells compared with TPA- or teleocidin-treated skins. (Epon–toluidine blue, ×300)

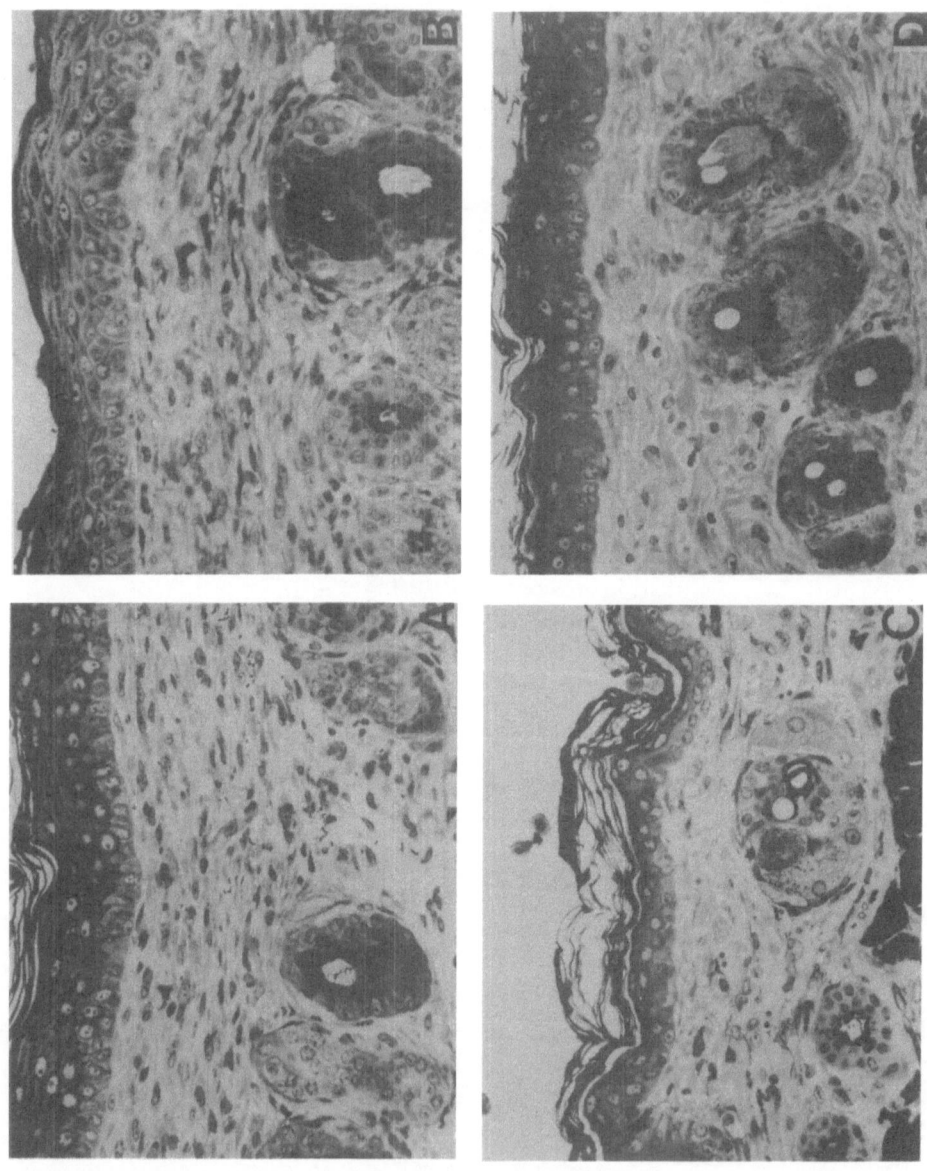

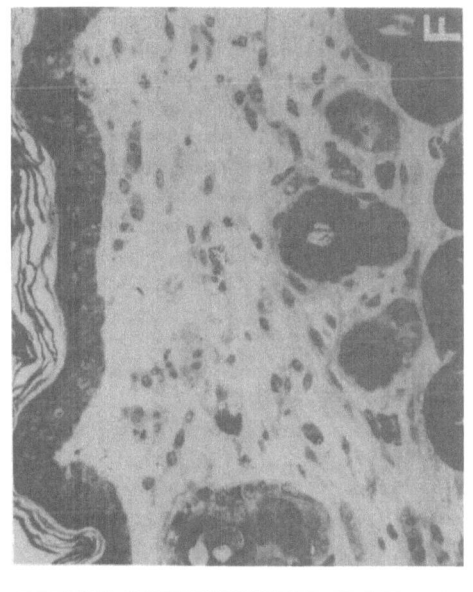

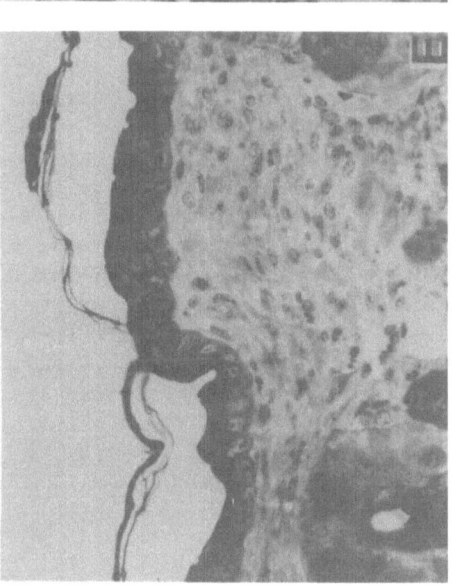

*Figure 5.* Response of the skin of DBA/2 and C57BL/6 mice 48 hr after the last of four treatments with various promoters. All compounds were applied (twice weekly. (A,B) DBA/2 and C57BL/6 mice, respectively, mezerein (6.8 nmol). Note the moderate epidermal hyperplasia and the similarity in the response of both strains. (C,D) DBA/2 and C57BL/6 mice, respectively, 4-*O*-Me-TPA (150 µg). There was only a weak epidermal hyperplasia and again no difference between strains. (E,F) DBA/2 and C57BL/6 mice, respectively, BzP (20 mg). There was only weak epidermal hyperplasia and no difference between strains. (Epon–toluidine blue, ×300)

genes control susceptibility to skin tumor promotion by various promoting agents? (3) What is the nature of the gene(s) controlling sensitivity to specific classes of tumor promoters? (4) What tumor promoter-induced biochemical and molecular effects are critical for the process of tumor promotion? and (5) Is there cross-sensitivity or resistance to different classes of tumor promoters in animals that were selectively bred for sensitivity to TPA promotion? If various classes of promoters do indeed work by different mechanism(s), then it may ultimately be possible to develop (or identify) strains of mice sensitive/resistant to individual classes of promoters.

The second approach to studying mechanisms of tumor promotion using genetic differences is to work with the large number of inbred mouse strains currently available. This approach requires that the particular inbred strain used is fully characterized in terms of its sensitivity to tumor promotion (i.e., dose–response and treatment frequency relationships). This information is available for only a few inbred strains as noted in the present chapter; nevertheless, this approach has proven useful in our laboratory since as also noted above, several inbred mouse strains are known to be either sensitive or resistant to a particular class of skin tumor promoter. The same questions outlined above can be addressed using the host of inbred mouse strains already available.

Finally, a third approach (beyond the scope of the present chapter) that deserves mentioning involves cell culture models. A considerable body of literature exists on cell culture variants that differ in their responsiveness to phorbol esters.[140] One such system is the JB6 mouse epidermal cell lines developed by Colburn and co-workers.[170] After 35 passages (JB6$_3$5$^+$) JB6 cells acquired the property of "promotion sensitivity" or the capacity to respond to phorbol esters and other tumor promoters with induction of anchorage independence and tumorigenicity (P$^+$ cells). In addition, cell lines that are resistant to TPA-induced transformation have also been developed (P$^-$ cells). Recently, it has been shown that P$^+$ cells differ from P$^-$ cells at the level of a gene that appears to specify sensitivity.[171] Colburn and colleagues[128] have now cloned and characterized these putative genes from the preneoplastic P$^+$ cells (called pro-1 and pro-2), but their nature remains to be determined. Such *in vitro* model systems may be extremely useful in identifying various genes that control sensitivity to tumor-promoting agents.

## 8. CONCLUDING REMARKS

This chapter has dealt with the subject of genetic factors controlling sensitivity to skin tumor promoters in inbred mice. It should be stressed that this is an area of research that is only in its infancy. Nevertheless, the relevance of tumor promotion to human cancer is clear, and it is most probable that genetic differences exist in the human population in response to environmental promoting agents. Therefore, further work in the area of promotion genetics is certainly warranted. It would be highly significant if a gene product(s) were identified in the mouse (or man) responsible for controlling sensitivity to tumor promoters. This along with a better understanding of the biochemical and molecular mechanisms of tumor promotion are the ultimate goals of genetic studies of tumor promotion.

ACKNOWLEDGMENTS. The author wishes to thank Ms. Joyce Mayhugh for her excellent help in preparing this manuscript. Original research was supported by grants CA 38871 and CA 37111 from the United States Public Health Service.

## REFERENCES

1. Mottram, J. C., 1944, A developing factor in experimental blastogenesis, *J. Pathol.* **56**:181–187.
2. Van Duuren, B. L., 1969, Tumor-promoting agents in two-stage carcinogenesis, *Prog. Exp. Tumor Res.* **11**:31–68.
3. Van Duuren, B. L., and Orris, L., 1965, The tumor-enhancing principles of *Croton tiglium* L., *Cancer Res.* **25**:1871–1875.

4. Hecker, E., 1968, Cocarcinogenic principles from the seed oil of *Croton tiglium* and from other Euphorbiaceae, *Cancer Res.* **28**:2338–2349.

5. Hecker, E., 1971, Isolation and characterization of the cocarcinogenic principles from croton oil, in: *Methods in Cancer Research*, Vol. 6 (H. Busch, ed.), pp. 439–484, Academic, New York.

6. Boutwell, R. K., 1964, Some biological aspects of skin carcinogenesis, *Prog. Exp. Tumor Res.* **4**:207–250.

7. Slaga, T. J., Fischer, S. M., Weeks, C. E., Nelson, K., Mamrack, M., and Klein-Szanto, A. J. P., 1982, Specificity and mechanism(s) of promoter inhibitors and multistage promotion, in: *Carcinogenesis—A Comprehensive Survey, Cocarcinogenesis and Biological Effects of Tumor Promoters*, Vol. 7 (E. Hecker, W. Kunz, N. E. Fusenig, F. Marks, and H. W. Theilman, eds.), pp. 19–34, Raven, New York.

8. Slaga, T. J., 1983, Multistage skin carcinogenesis and specificity of inhibitors, in: *Modulation and Mediation of Cancer by Vitamins* (F. L. Meyskens and K. N. Prasad, eds.), pp. 10–23, S. Karger AG, Basel.

9. Mufson, R. A., Fischer, S. M., Verma, A. K., Gleason, G. L., Slaga, T. J., and Boutwell, R. K., 1979, Effects of 12-O-tetradecanoylphorbol-13-acetate and mezerein on epidermal ornithine decarboxylase activity, isoproterenol-stimulated levels of cyclic adenosine 3':5'-monophosphate, and induction of mouse skin tumors *in vivo*, *Cancer Res.* **39**:4791–4795.

10. Slaga, T. J., Fischer, S. M., Nelson, K., and Gleason, G. L., 1980, Studies on the mechanism of skin tumor promotion: Evidence for several stages in promotion, *Proc. Natl. Acad. Sci., USA* **77**:3659–3663.

11. Furstenberger, G., Berry, D. L., Sorg, B., and Marks, F., 1981, Skin tumor promotion by phorbol esters is a two-stage process, *Proc. Natl. Acad. Sci. USA* **78**:7722–7726.

12. Fujiki, H., Mori, M., Nakayasu, M., Terada, M., Sugimura, T., and Moore, R. E., 1981, Indole alkaloids: Dihydroteleocidin B, teleocidin, and lyngbyatoxin A as members of a new class of tumor promoters, *Proc. Natl. Acad. Sci. USA* **78**:3872–3876.

13. Fujiki, H., Suganuma, M., Matsukura, N., Sugimura, T., and Takayama, S., 1982, Teleocidin from *Streptomyces* is a potent promoter of mouse skin carcinogenesis, *Carcinogenesis* **3**:895–898.

14. Suganuma, M., Fujiki, H., and Sugimura, T., 1982, Existence of an optimal dose of dihydroteleocidin B for skin tumor promotion, *Gann* **73**:531–533.

15. Cardellina, J. H. II, Marner, F.-J., and Moore, R. E., 1979, Seaweed dermatitis: Structure of lyngbyatoxin A, *Science* **204**:193–195.

16. Sugimura, T., 1982, Potent tumor promoters other than phorbol ester and their significance, *Gann* **73**:499–507.

17. Fujiki, H., Suganuma, M., Nakayasu, M., Hoshino, H., Moore, R. E., and Sugimura, T., 1982, The third class of new tumor promoters, polyacetates (debromoaplysiatoxin and aplysiatoxin), can differentiate biological actions relevant to tumor promoters, *Gann* **73**:495–497.

18. Shimomura, K., Mullinix, M. G., Kakunaga, T., Fujiki, H., and Sugimura, T., 1983, Bromine residue at hydrophilic region influences biological activity of aplysiatoxin, a tumor promoter, *Science* **222**:1242–1244.

19. Arffmann, E., and Glavind, J., 1971, Tumor-promoting activity of fatty acid methyl esters in mice, *Experientia* **27**:1465–1466.

20. Bock, F. G., and Burns, R., 1963, Tumor-promoting properties of anthralin (1,8,9-Anthratriol), *J. Natl. Cancer Inst.* **30**:393–398.

21. Van Duuren, B. L., Witz, G., and Goldschmidt, B. M., 1978, Structure-activity relationships of tumor promoters and cocarcinogens and interaction of phorbol myristate acetate and related esters with plasma membranes, in: *Carcinogenesis, Mechanisms of Tumor Promotion and Cocarcinogensis*, Vol. 2 (T. J. Slaga, A. Sivak, and R. K. Boutwell, eds.), pp. 491–507, Raven, New York.

22. DiGiovanni, J., and Boutwell, R. K., 1983, Tumor promoting activity of 1,8-dihydroxy-3-methyl-9-anthrone (chrysarobin) in female SENCAR mice, *Carcinogenesis* **4**:281–284.

23. Gwynn, R. H., and Salaman, M. H., 1953, Studies on co-carcinogenesis SH-reactors and other substances tested for co-carcinogenic action in mouse skin, *Br. J. Cancer* **7**:482–489.

24. Wynder, E. L., and Hoffman, D., 1961, A study of tobacco carcinogenesis. VIII. The role of the acidic fractions as promoters, *Cancer* **14**:1306–1315.

25. Bock, F. G., Swain, A. P., and Stedman, R. L., 1971, Composition studies on tobacco. XLIV. Tumor-promoting activity of subfractions of the weak acid fraction of cigarette smoke condensate, *J. Natl. Cancer Inst.* **47**:429–436.

26. Hecht, S. S., Thorne, R. L., Maronpot, R. R., and Hoffman, D., 1975, A study of tobacco carcinogenesis. XIII. Tumor-promoting subfractions of the weakly acidic fraction, *J. Natl. Cancer Inst.* **55**:1329–1336.

27. Hecht, S. S., Carmella, S., and Hoffman, D., 1978, Chemical studies on tobacco smoke-LIV determination of hydroxybenzyl alcohols and hydroxyphenyl ethanols in tobacco and tobacco smoke, *J. Anal. Toxicol.* **2:**56–59.

28. Scribner, N. K., and Scribner, J. D., 1980, Separation of initiating and promoting effects of the skin carcinogen, 7-bromomethylbenz(a)anthracene, *Carcinogenesis* **1:**97–100.

29. Slaga, T. J., Klein-Szanto, A. J. P., Triplett, L. L., Yotti, L. P., and Trosko, J. E., 1981, Skin tumor-promoting activity of benzoyl peroxide, a widely used free radical-generating compound, *Science* **213:**1023–1025.

30. Hennings, H., Wenk, M. L., and Donahoe, R., 1982, Retinoic acid promotion of papilloma formation in mouse skin, *Cancer Lett.* **16:**1–5.

31. Poland, A., Palen, D., and Glover, E., 1982, Tumor-promotion by TCDD in skin of HRS/J hairless mice, *Nature (Lond.)* **300:**271–273.

32. Argyris, T. S., 1982, Epidermal tumor promotion by regeneration, in: *Carcinogenesis—A Comprehensive Survey, Cocarcinogenesis and Biological Effects of Tumor Promoters*, Vol. 7 (E. Hecker, W. Kung, N. E. Fusenig, F. Marks, and H. W. Theilmann, eds.), pp. 43–48, Raven, New York.

33. Stenback, F., Garcia, H., and Shubik, P., 1974, Present status of the concept of promoting action of cocarcinogenesis in skin, in: *The Physiopathology of Cancer, Biology and Biochemistry*, Vol. 1 (P. Shubik, ed.), pp. 155–225, S. Karger AG, Basel.

34. Scribner, J. D., and Suss, R., 1978, Tumor initiation and promotion, in: *International Review of Experimental Pathology*, Vol. 18 (G. W. Richter and M. A. Epstein, eds.), pp. 137–198, Academic, New York.

35. Raick, A. N., 1973, Ultrastructural, histological, and biochemical alterations produced by 12-*O*-tetradecanoylphorbol-13-acetate on mouse epidermis and their relevance to skin tumor promotion, *Cancer Res.* **33:**269–286.

36. Klein-Szanto, A. J. P., and Slaga, T. J., 1981, Numerical variation of dark cells in normal and chemically induced hyperplastic epidermis with age of animal and efficiency of tumor promoter, *Cancer Res.* **41:**4437–4440.

37. Klein-Szanto, A. J. P., Major, S. K., and Slaga, T. J., 1980, Induction of dark keratinocytes by 12-*O*-tetradecanoylphorbol-13-acetate and mezerein as an indicator of tumor-promoting efficiency, *Carcinogenesis* **1:**399–406.

38. Raick, A. N., and Burdzy, K., 1973, Ultrastructural and biochemical changes induced in mouse epidermis by a hyperplastic agent, ethylphenylpropiolate, *Cancer Res.* **33:**2221–2230.

39. Slaga, T. J., Klein-Szanto, A. J. P., Fischer, S. M., Weeks, C. E., Nelson, K., and Major, S., 1980, Studies on mechanism of action of anti-tumor-promoting agents: Their specificity in two-stage promotion, *Proc. Natl. Acad. Sci. USA* **77:**2251–2254.

40. Klein-Szanto, A. J. P., 1984, Morphological evaluation of tumor promoter effects on mammalian skin, in: *Mechanisms of Tumor Promotion, Tumor Promotion and Skin Carcinogenesis*, Vol. II (T. J. Slaga, ed.), pp. 41–72, CRC Press, Boca Raton, Florida.

41. Parsons, D. F., Marko, M., Braun, S. J., and Wansor, K. J., 1983, Dark cells in normal, hyperplastic, and promoter-treated mouse epidermis studied by conventional and high-voltage electron microscopy, *J. Invest. Dermatol.* **81:**62–67.

42. Glaso, M., Ree, K., Inversen, O. H., and Hovig, T., 1986, The influence of different fixatives and a tumor promoter, 12-*O*-tetradecanoylphorbol-13-acetate (TPA), on the induction of so-called dark cells in mouse epidermis, *Virchows Arch.* **50:**355–372.

43. Murakami, Y., Hibino, T., Arai, M., and Kuroki, T., 1985, Appearance of dark keratinocytes following intracutaneous injection of cholera toxin in mouse skin, *J. Invest. Dematol.* **85:**115–117.

44. Naito, M., Naito, Y., and DiGiovanni, J., 1987, Comparison of the histological changes in the skin of DBA/2 and C57BL/6 mice following exposure to various promoting agents, *Carcinogenesis* **8:**1807–1815.

45. Bach, H., and Goerttler, K., 1971, Morphologische Untersuchungen zur hyper-plasiogenen Wirkung des biologisch aktiven Phorbol esters A$_1$, *Virchows Arch.* **8:**196–205.

46. Balmain, A., 1976, The synthesis of specific proteins in adult mouse epidermis during phases of proliferation and differentiation induced by the tumor promoter TPA, and in basal and differentiating layers of neonatal mouse epidermis, *J. Invest. Dermatol.* **67:**246–253.

47. Raick, A. N., 1973, Late ultrastructural changes induced by 12-*O*-tetradecanoylphorbol-13-acetate in mouse epidermis and their reversal, *Cancer Res.* **33:**1096–1103.

48. Aldaz, C. M., Conti, C. J., Gimenez, I. B., Slaga, T. J., and Klein-Szanto, A. J. P., 1985, Cutaneous changes during prolonged application of 12-*O*-tetradecanoylphorbol-13-acetate on mouse skin and residual effects after cessation of treatment, *Cancer Res.* **45:**2753–2759.

49. Sisskin, E. E., Gray, T., and Barrett, J. C., 1982, Correlation between sensitivity to tumor promotion and

sustained epidermal hyperplasia of mice and rats treated with 12-*O*-tetradecanoylphorbol-13-acetate, *Carcinogenesis* **3**:403–407.

50. DiGiovanni, J., Slaga, T. J., and Boutwell, R. K., 1980, Comparison of the tumor-initiating activity of 7,12-dimethylbenz[a]anthracene and benzo[a]pyrene in female SENCAR and CD-1 mice, *Carcinogenesis* **1**:381–389.

51. Paul, D., and Hecker, E., 1969, On the biochemical mechanism of tumorigenesis in mouse skin. II. Early effects on the biosynthesis of nucleic acids induced by initiating doses of DMBA and by promoting doses of phorbol-12,13-diester TPA, *Z. Krebsforsch.* **73**:149–163.

52. Baird, W. M., Sedgwick, J. A., and Boutwell, R. K., 1971, Effects of phorbol and four diesters of phorbol on the incorporation of tritiated precursors into DNA, RNA and protein in mouse epidermis, *Cancer Res.* **31**:1434–1439.

53. Hennings, H., and Boutwell, R. K., 1970, Studies on the mechanism of skin tumor promotion, *Cancer Res.* **30**:312–320.

54. Suss, R., Kinzel, V., and Kreibich, G., 1971, Cocarcinogenic croton oil factor $A_1$ stimulates lipid synthesis in cell cultures, *Experientia* **27**:46–47.

55. Rohrschneider, L. R., O'Brien, D. H., and Boutwell, R. K., 1972, The stimulation of phospholipid metabolism in mouse skin following phorbol ester treatment, *Biochim. Biophys. Acta* **280**:57–70.

56. Balmain, A., and Hecker, E., 1974, On the biochemical mechanism of tumorigenesis in mouse skin. VI. Early effects of growth-stimulating phorbol esters on phosphate transport and phospholipid synthesis in mouse epidermis, *Biochim. Biophys. Acta* **362**:457–468.

57. Verma, A. K., Ashendel, C. L., and Boutwell, R. K., 1980, Inhibition by prostaglandin synthesis inhibitors of the induction of epidermal ornithine decarboxylase activity, the accumulation of prostaglandins, and tumor promotion caused by 12-*O*-tetradecanoyl-phorbol-13-acetate, *Cancer Res.* **40**:308–315.

58. Furstenberger, G., and Marks, F., 1980, Early prostaglandin E synthesis is an obligatory event in the induction of cell proliferation in mouse epidermis *in vivo* by the phorbol ester TPA, *Biochem. Biophys. Res. Commun.* **92**:749–756.

59. Marks, F., 1976, Epidermal growth control mechanisms, hyperplasia, and tumor promotion in the skin, *Cancer Res.* **36**:2636–2643.

60. Marks, F., Bertsch, S., Grimm, W., and Schweizer, J., 1978, Hyperplastic transformation and tumor promotion in mouse epidermis: Possible consequences of disturbances of endogenous mechanisms controlling proliferation and differentiation. *Carcinogenesis, Mechanisms of Tumor Promotion and Cocarcinogenesis*, Vol. 2 (T. J. Slaga, A. Sivak, and R. K. Boutwell, eds.), pp. 97–116, Raven, New York.

61. Marks, F., and Grimm, W., 1972, Diurnal fluctuation and β-adrenergic elevation of cyclic AMP in mouse epidermis *in vivo*, *Nature New Biol.* **240**:178–179.

62. Grimm, W., and Marks, F., 1974, Effect of tumor-promoting phorbol esters on the normal and the isoproterenol-elevated level of adenosine 3′,5′-cyclic monophosphate in mouse epidermis *in vivo*, *Cancer Res.* **34**:3128–3134.

63. Verma, A. K., and Murray, A. W., 1974, The effect of benzo(a)pyrene on the basal and isoproterenol-stimulated levels of cyclic adenosine 3′,5′-monophosphate in mouse epidermis, *Cancer Res.* **34**:3408–3413.

64. Mufson, R. A., Simsiman, R. C., and Boutwell, R. K., 1977, The effect of the phorbol ester tumor promoters on the basal and catecholamine-stimulated levels of cyclic adenosine 3′,5′-monophosphate in mouse skin and epidermis *in vivo*, *Cancer Res.* **37**:665–669.

65. Solanki, V., Rana, R. S., and Slaga, T. J., 1981, Diminution of mouse epidermal superoxide dismutase and catalase activities by tumor promoters, *Carcinogenesis* **2**:1141–1146.

66. Colburn, N. H., Lau, S., and Head, R., 1975, Decrease of epidermal histidase activity by tumor-promoting phorbol esters, *Cancer Res.* **35**:3154–3159.

67. Schweizer, J., and Winter, H., 1982, Changes in regional keratin polypeptide patterns during phorbol ester-mediated reversible and permanently sustained hyperplasia of mouse epidermis, *Cancer Res.* **42**:1517–1529.

68. Nelson, K. G., and Slaga, T. J., 1982, Effect of inhibitors of tumor promotion on 12-*O*-tetradecanoylphorbol-13-acetate-induced keratin modification in mouse epidermis, *Carcinogenesis* **3**:1311–1315.

69. Raineri, R., Simsiman, R. C., and Boutwell, R. K., 1973, Stimulation of the phosphorylation of mouse epidermal histones by tumor-promoting agents, *Cancer Res.* **33**:134–139.

70. Raineri, R., Simsiman, R. C., and Boutwell, R. K., 1978, Stimulation of the synthesis of the H1 and H3 histone fractions of mouse epidermis by 12-*O*-tetradecanoylphorbol-13-acetate, *Cancer Lett.* **5**:277–284.

71. Link, R., and Marks, F., 1981, Histone phosphorylation in phorbol ester stimulated and β-adrenergically stimulated mouse epidermis *in vivo* and characterization of an epidermal protein phosphorylation system, *Biochim. Biophys. Acta* **675**:265–275.

72. O'Brien, T. G., Simsiman, R. C., and Boutwell, R. K., 1975, Induction of the polyamine-biosynthetic enzymes in mouse epidermis by tumor-promoting agents, *Cancer Res.* **35:**1662–1670.

73. O'Brien, T. G., Simsiman, R. C., and Boutwell, R. K., 1975, Induction of the polyamine-biosynthetic enzymes in mouse epidermis and their specificity for tumor promotion. *Cancer Res.* **35:**2426–2433.

74. Ashendel, C. L., and Boutwell, R. K., 1981, Direct measurement of specific binding of highly lipophilic phorbol diester to mouse epidermal membranes using cold acetone, *Biochem. Biophys. Res. Commun.* **99:**435–449.

75. Delclos, K. B., Nagle, D. S., and Blumberg, P. M., 1980, Specific binding of phorbol ester tumor promoters to mouse skin, *Cell* **19:**1025–1032.

76. Driedger, P. E., and Blumberg, P. M., 1980, Specific binding of phorbol ester tumor promoters, *Proc. Natl. Acad. Sci. USA* **77:**5670–5671.

77. Dunphy, W. G., Delclos, K. B., and Blumberg, P. M., 1980, Characterization of specific binding of [$^3$H]-phorbol-12,13-dibutyrate and [$^3$H]phorbol 12-myristate-13-acetate to mouse brain, *Cancer Res.* **40:**3635–3641.

78. Nagle, D. S., Jaken, S., Castagna, M., and Blumberg, P. M., 1981, Variation with embryonic development and regional localization of specific [$^3$H]phorbol 12,13-dibutyrate binding to brain, *Cancer Res.* **41:**89–93.

79. Sando, J. J., Hilfiker, M. L., Piacentini, M. J., and Laufer, T. M., 1982, Identification of phorbol ester receptors in T-growth factor-producing and nonproducing EL4 mouse thymoma cells, *Cancer Res.* **42:**1676–1680.

80. Shoyab, M., and Todaro, G. J., 1980, Specific high affinity cell membrane receptors for biologically active phorbol and ingenol esters, *Nature (Lond.)* **288:**451–455.

81. Solanki, V., and Slaga, T. J., 1981, Specific binding of phorbol ester tumor promoters to intact primary epidermal cells from SENCAR mice, *Proc. Natl. Acad. Sci. USA* **78:**2549–2553.

82. Solanki, V., Slaga, T. J., Callahan, M., and Huberman, E., 1981, Down regulation of specific binding of [20-$^3$H]phorbol-12,13-dibutyrate and phorbol ester-induced differentiation of human promyelocytic leukemia cells, *Proc. Natl. Acad. Sci. USA* **78:**1722–1725.

83. Castagna, M., Takai, Y., Kaibuchi, K., Sano, K., Kikkawa, U., and Nishizuka, Y., 1982, Direct activation of calcium activated, phospholipid-dependent protein kinase by tumor-promoting phorbol esters, *J. Biol. Chem.* **257:**7847–7851.

84. Nishizuka, Y., 1983, Phospholipid degradation and signal translation for protein phosphorylation, *Trends Biochem. Sci.* **8:**13–16.

85. Niedel, J. E., Kuhn, L. J., and Vandenbark, G. R., 1983, Phorbol diester receptor copurifies with protein kinase C, *Proc. Natl. Acad. Sci. USA* **80:**36–40.

86. Leach, K. L., James, M. L., and Blumberg, P. M., 1983, Characterization of a specific phorbol ester aporeceptor in mouse brain cytosol, *Proc. Natl. Acad. Sci. USA* **80:**4208–4212.

87. Ashendel, C. L., Staller, J. M., and Boutwell, R. K., 1983, Protein kinase activity associated with a phorbol ester receptor purified from mouse brain, *Cancer Res.* **43:**4333–4337.

88. Vandenbark, G. R., Kuhn, L. J., and Niedel, J. E., 1984, Possible mechanism of phorbol ester-induced maturation of human promyelocytic leukemia cells, *J. Clin. Invest.* **78:**448–457.

89. Sharkey, N. A., Leach, K. L., and Blumberg, P. M., 1984, Competitive inhibition by diacyglycerol of specific phorbol ester binding, *Proc. Natl. Acad. Sci. USA* **81:**607–610.

90. Mufson, R. A., 1984, The relationship of alterations in phospholipid metabolism to the mechanism of action of phorbol ester tumor promoters, in: *Mechanisms of Tumor Promotion, Cellular Responses to Tumor Promoters,* Vol. IV (T. J. Slaga, ed.), pp. 109–117, CRC Press, Boca Raton, Florida.

91. Weinstein, I. B., 1983, Protein kinase, phospholipid and control of growth, *Nature (Lond.)* **302:**750.

92. Jetten, A. M., Ganong, B. R., Vandenbark, G. R., Shirley, J. E., and Bell, R. M., 1985, Role protein kinase C in diacylglycerol-mediated induction of ornithine decarboxylase and reduction of epidermal growth factor binding, *Proc. Natl. Acad. Sci. USA* **82:**1941–1945.

93. Smart, R. C., Huang, M.-T., and Cooney, A. J., 1986, *sn*-1,2-Diacylglycerols mimic the effects of 12-*O*-tetradecanoylphorbol-13-acetate *in vivo* by inducing biochemical changes associated with tumor promotion in mouse epidermis, *Carcinogenesis* **7:**1865–1870.

94. Verma, A. K., Pong, R.-C., and Erickson, D., 1986, Involvement of protein kinase C activation in ornithine decarboxylase gene expression in primary culture of newborn mouse epidermal cells and in skin tumor promotion by 12-*O*-tetradecanoylphorbol-13-acetate, *Cancer Res.* **46:**6149–6155.

95. Ono, Y., Kurokawa, T., Kawahara, K., Nishimura, O., Marumoto, R., Igarashi, K., Sugina, Y., Kikkawa, U., Ogiba, K., and Nishizuka, Y., 1986, Cloning of rat brain protein kinase C complementary DNA, *FEBS Lett.* **203:**111–115.

96. Knopf, J. L., Lee, M.-H., Sultzman, L. A., Keiz, R. W., Loomic, C. R., Hewick, R. M., and Bell, R. M., 1986, Cloning and expression of multiple protein kinase C cDNAs, *Cell* **46**:491–502.

97. Coussens, L., Parker, P. J., Rhee, L., Yang-Feng, T. L., Chen, E., Waterfield, M. D., Franchke, V., and Ullrich, A., 1986, Multiple distinct forms of bovine and human protein kinase C suggest diversity in cellular signaling pathways, *Science* **233**:859–866.

98. Huang, K. P., Nakabayashi, H., and Huang, F. L., 1986, Isozymic forms of rat brain $Ca^{+2}$-activated and phospholipid-dependent protein kinase, *Proc. Natl. Acad. Sci. USA* **83**:8535–8539.

99. Ohno, S., Kawasaki, H., Imajoh, S., Suzuki, K., Inagaki, M., Yikokura, H., Sakoh, T., and Hidaka, H., 1987, Tissue-specific expression of three distinct types of rabbit protein kinase C, *Nature (Lond.)* **325**:161–166.

100. Housey, G. M., O'Brian, C. A., Johnson, M. D., Kirschmeier, P., and Weinstein, I.B., 1987, Isolation of c-DNA clones encoding protein kinase C: Evidence for a protein kinase C-related gene family, *Proc. Natl. Acad. Sci. USA* **84**:1065–1069.

101. Ono, Y., Kikkawa, Y., Ogita, K., Fujii, T., Kurokawa, T., Asaoka, Y., Sekiguchi, K., Ase, K., Igarashi, K., and Nishizuka, Y., 1987, Expression and properties of two types of protein kinase C: Alternative splicing from a single gene, *Science* **236**:1116–1120.

102. Blumberg, P. M., Jeng, A. Y., Konig, B., Sharkey, N. A., Leach, K. L., and Jaken, S., 1985, Receptors and endogenous analogs for the phorbol ester tumor promoters, in: *Carcinogenesis—A Comprehensive Survey, The Role of Chemicals and Radiation in the Etiology of Cancer*, Vol. 10 (E. Huberman and S. H. Barr, eds.), pp. 249–262, Raven, New York.

103. Shubik, P., 1950, Studies on the promoting phase in the stages of carcinogenesis in mice, rats, rabbits, and guinea pigs, *Cancer Res.* **10**:13–17.

104. Goerttler, K., Loehrke, H., Schweizer, J., and Hesse, B., 1982, in: Diterpene ester mediated two-stage carcinogenesis, in: *Carcinogenesis—A Comprehensive Survey, Cocarcinogenesis and Biological Effects of Tumor Promoters*, Volume 7 (E. Hecker, N. E. Fusenig, W. Kunz, F. Marks, and H. W. Thielmann, eds.), pp. 75–83, Raven, New York.

105. Goerttler, K., Loehrke, H., Schweizer, J., and Hesse, B., 1980, Positive two-stage carcinogenesis in female Sprague-Dawley rats using 7,12-dimethylbenz(a)anthracene (DMBA) as initiator and 12-*O*-tetradecanoylphorbol-13-acetate (TPA) as promoter, Results of a pilot study, *Virchows Arch.* **385**:181–186.

106. Goerttler, K., Hecker, E., Loehrke, H., Seip, H., Hesse, B., and Schweizer, J., 1982, Effect of the tumor promoter 12-*O*-tetradecanoylphorbol-13 acetate and its nonpromoting analogue 4-*O*-methyl-TPA on dorsal dermal melanocytes of the Syrian golden hamster (*Mesocricetus quratus*), *J. Cancer Res., Clin. Oncol.* **103**:305–311.

107. Goerttler, K., Loehrke, H., Schweizer, J., and Hesse, B., 1980, Two-stage tumorigenesis of dermal melanocytes in the back of the Syrian golden hamster using systemic initiation with 7,12-dimethylbenz(a)-anthracene and topical promotion with 12-*O*-tetradecanoylphorbol-13-acetate, *Cancer Res.* **40**:155–161.

108. Della Porta, G., Rappaport, H., Suffiotti, U., and Shubik, P., 1956, Induction of melanotic lesions during skin carcinogenesis in hamsters, *Arch. Pathol.* **61**:305–313.

109. Stenback, F., 1980, Skin carcinogenesis as a model system: Observations on species, strain, and tissue specificity to 7,12-dimethylbenz(a)anthracene with or without promotion with croton oil, *Acta Pharmacol. Toxicol.* **46**:89–97.

110. Yuspa, S. H., Viguera, C., and Nims, R., 1979, Maintenance of human skin on nude mice for studies of chemical carcinogenesis, *Cancer Lett.* **6**:301–310.

111. Krueger, G. G., and Shelby, J., 1981, Biology of human skin transplanted to the nude mouse. I. Response to agents which modify epidermal proliferation, *J. Invest. Dermatol.* **76**:506–510.

112. Krueger, G. G., Chamberg, D. A., and Shelby, J., 1980, Epidermal proliferation by nude mouse skin, pig skin and pig skin grafts: Failure of nude mouse skin to respond to the tumor promoter, 12-*O*-tetradecanoyl-phorbol-13-acetate (TPA), *J. Exp. Med.* **152**:1329–1359.

113. Stern, R. S., Parish, J. A., Bleuch, H. L., and Fitzpatrick, T. B., 1981, PUVA (psoralen and ultraviolet A) and squamous cell carcinoma in patients with psoriasis, *J. Invest. Dermatol.* **76**:311.

114. Schweizer, J., Loehrke, H., Edler, L., and Goerttler, K., 1987, Benzoyl peroxide promotes the formation of melanotic tumors in the skin of 7,12-dimethylbenz(a)-anthracene-initiated Syrian golden hamsters, *Carcinogenesis* **8**:479–482.

115. Slaga, T. J., and Fischer, S. M., 1983, Strain differences and solvent effects in mouse skin carcinogenesis experiments using carcinogens, tumor initiators, and promoters, *Prog. Exp. Tumor Res.* **26**:85–109.

116. Reiners, J., Davidson, K., Nelson, K., Mamrack, M., and Slaga, T. J., 1983, Skin tumor promotion: A

comparative study of several stocks and strains of mice, in: *Organ and Species Specificity in Chemical Carcinogenesis* (R. Langenbach, S. Nesnow, and J. M. Rice, eds.), pp. 173–188, Plenum, New York.

117. Hennings, H., Devor, D., Wenk, M., Slaga, T. J., Farmer, B., Colburn, N., Bowden, G. T., Elgio, K., and Yuspa, S. H., 1981, Comparison of two-stage epidermal carcinogenesis initiated by 7,12-dimethylbenz(a)anthracene or *N*-methyl-*N'*-nitro-*N*-nitroso-guanidine in newborn and adult SENCAR and Balb/c mice, *Cancer Res.* **41**:773–779.

118. Reiners, J. J., Nesnow, S., and Slaga, T. J., 1984, Murine susceptibility to two-stage skin carcinogenesis is influenced by the agent used for promotion, *Carcinogenesis* **5**:301–307.

119. DiGiovanni, J., Prichett, W. P., Decina, P. C., and Diamond, L., 1984, DBA/2 mice are as sensitive as SENCAR mice to skin tumor promotion by 12-*O*-tetradecanoylphorbol-13-acetate, *Carcinogenesis* **5**:1493–1498.

120. Strickland, P. T., 1982, Tumor induction in SENCAR mice in response to ultraviolet radiation, *Carcinogenesis* **3**:1487–1489.

121. DiGiovanni, J., Naito, M., and Chenicek, K. J., 1988, Genetic factors controlling susceptibility to skin tumor promotion in mice, in: *Tumor Promoters: Biological Approaches for Mechanistic Studies and Assay Systems* (C.J. Barrett, R. Langenbach, and E. Gilmore, eds.), Raven, New York (in press).

122. Fischer, S. M., O'Connell, J. F., Conti, C. J., Tacker, K. C., Fries, J. W., Patrick, K. E., Adams, L. M., and Slaga, T. J., 1987, Characterization of an inbred strain of the SENCAR mouse that is highly sensitive to phorbol esters, *Carcinogenesis* **8**:421–424.

123. DiGiovanni, J., Kruszewski, F. H., and Chenicek, K. J., 1987, Studies on the skin tumor promoting actions of chrysarobin (1,8-dihydroxy-3-methyl-9-anthrone), in: *Nongenotoxic Mechanisms of Carcinogenesis,* Banbury Report 25 (B. Butterworth, and T. J. Slaga, eds.), pp. 25–39, Cold Spring Harbor Press, Cold Spring Harbor, New York.

124. Naito, M., Chenicek, K. J., Naito, Y., and DiGiovanni, J., 1987, Susceptibility to phorbol ester skin tumor promotion in (C57BL/6 × DBA/2)F$_1$ mice is inherited as an incomplete dominant trait: evidence for multilocus involvement, *Carcinogenesis* **9**:639–645.

125. Drinkwater, N. R., and Ginsler, J. J., 1986, Genetic control of hepatocarcinogensis in C57BL/6 and C3H/H3J inbred mice, *Carcinogenesis* **7**:1701–1707.

126. Gould, M. N., 1986, Inheritance and site of expression of genes controlling susceptibility to mammary cancer in an inbred rat model, *Cancer Res.* **46**:1199–1202.

127. Malkinson, A. M., Nesbitt, M. N., and Skamene, E., 1985, Susceptibility to urethan-induced pulmonary adenomas between A/J and C57BL/6 mice: Use of AXB and BXA recombinant inbred lines indicating a three-locus genetic model, *J. Natl. Cancer Inst.* **75**:971–974.

128. Lerman, M. I., Hegamyer, G. A., and Colburn, N. H., 1986, Cloning and characterization of putative genes that specify sensitivity to neoplastic transformation by tumor promoters, *Int. J. Cancer* **37**:293–302.

129. Raick, A. N., 1974, Cell differentiation and tumor-promoting action in skin carcinogenesis, *Cancer Res.* **34**:2915–2925.

130. Slaga, T. J., 1985, Mechanism involved in multistage skin tumorigenesis, in: *Carcinogenesis: The Role of Chemicals and Radiation in the Etiology of Cancer,* Vol. 10 (E. Huberman and S. H. Barr, eds.), pp. 189–199, Raven, New York.

131. Chiba, M., Slaga, T. J., and Klein-Szanto, A. J. P., 1984, A morphometric study of dedifferentiated and involutional dark keratinocytes in 12-*O*-tetradecanoylphorbol-13-acetate-treated epidermis, *Cancer Res.* **44**:2711–2717.

132. Slaga, T. J., Fischer, S. M., Weeks, C. E., and Klein-Szanto, A. J. P., 1987, Cellular and biochemical mechanisms of mouse skin tumor promoters, in: *Reviews in Biochemicals Toxicology,* Vol. 3 (E. Hodgson, E. Bend, and P. M. Philpot, eds.), pp. 231–281, Elsevier/North-Holland, New York.

133. Scribner, J. D., and Suss, R., 1978, Tumor initiation and promotion, *Int. Rev. Pathol.* **18**:137–198.

134. Lewis, J. G., and Adams, D. O., 1986, Correlation between inflammation in skin, the release of H$_2$O$_2$ by macrophages (m), and sensitivity to the promotion of skin tumors by phorbol esters (PE), *Proc. Am. Assoc. Cancer Res.* **27**:146.

135. Lewis, J. G., and Adams, 1986, Enhanced release of hydrogen peroxide and metabolites of arachidonic acid by macrophages from SENCAR mice following stimulation with phorbol esters, *Cancer Res.* **46**:5696–5700.

136. Wheldrake, J. F., Marshall, J., Ramli, J., and Murray, A. W., 1982, Skin carcinogenesis and promoter binding characteristics in different mouse strains, *Carcinogenesis* **3**:805–807.

137. Blumberg, P. M., Delclos, K. B., and Jaken, S., 1983, Tissue and species specificity for phorbol ester

receptors, in: *Organ and Species Specificity in Chemical Carcinogenesis* (R. Langenbach, S. Nesnow, and J. Rice, eds.), pp. 201–220, Plenum, New York.

138. Garte, S. J., Edinger, F., and Mufson, R. A., 1985, Phorbol ester activation of epidermal protein kinase C from tumor promotion sensitive and resistant mouse strains, *Cancer Lett.* **29**:215–221.

139. Malkinson, A. M., Conway, K., Bartlett, S., Butley, M. S., and Conroy, C., 1984, Strain differences among inbred mice in protein kinase C activity, *Biochem. Biophys. Res. Commun.* **122**:492–498.

140. Blumberg, B. M., Dunn, J. A., Jaken, S., Jeng, A. Y., Leach, K. L., Sharkey, N. A., and Yeh, E., 1984, Specific receptors for phorbol ester tumor promoters and their involvement in biological responses, in: *Mechanisms of Tumor Promotion: Tumor Promotion and Carcinogenesis In Vitro*, Vol. 3 (T. J. Slaga, ed.), pp. 143–185, CRC Press, Boca Raton, Florida.

141. Homma, Y., Henning-Chubb, C. B., and Huberman, E., 1986, Translocation of protein kinase C in human leukemia cells susceptible or resistant to differentiation induced by phorbol-12-myristate-13-acetate, *Proc. Natl. Acad. Sci. USA* **83**:7316–7319.

142. Kreibich, G., Suss, R., and Kinzel, V., 1974, On the biochemical mechanism of tumorigenesis in mouse skin. V. Studies of the metabolism of tumor promoting and non-promoting phorbol derivatives *in vivo* and *in vitro*, *Z. Krebsforsch.* **81**:135–149.

143. Berry, D. L., Lieber, M. R., Fischer, S. M., and Slaga, T. J., 1977, Qualitative and quantitative separation of a series of phorbol ester tumor promoters by high-pressure liquid chromatography, *Cancer Lett.* **3**:125–132.

144. Berry, D. L., Bracken, W. M., Fischer, S. M., Viaje, A., and Slaga, T. J., 1978, Metabolic conversion of 12-*O*-tetradecanoylphorbol-13-acetate in adult and newborn mouse skin and mouse liver microsomes, *Cancer Res.* **38**:2301–2306.

145. Barrett, J. C., Brown, M. T., and Sisskin, E. E., 1982, Deacylation of 12-*O*-[$^3$H]-tetradecanoylphorbol-13-acetate and [$^3$H]-phorbol-12,13-acetate in hamster skin and hamster cells in culture, *Cancer Res.* **42**:3098–3101.

146. Shoyab, M., Warren, R. C., and Todaro, G. J., 1982, Phorbol-12,13-diester 12-ester hydrolase may prevent tumor promotion by phorbol diesters in skin, *Nature (Lond.)* **295**:152–154.

147. Segal, A., VanDuuren, B. L., and Mate, U., 1975, The identification of phorbolol myristate acetate as a new metabolite of phorbol myristate acetate in mouse skin, *Cancer Res.* **35**:2154–2159.

148. O'Brien, T. G., Saladik, D., Sina, J. F., and Mullin, J. M., 1982, Formation of a glucuronide conjugate of 12-*O*-tetradecanoylphorbol-13-acetate by LLC-Pk$_1$ renal epithelial cells in culture, *Carcinogenesis* **3**:1165–1169.

149. Cerutti, P., 1985, Prooxidant states and tumor promotion, *Science* **227**:375–381.

150. Fischer, S. M., Baldwin, J. K., and Adams, L. M., 1986, Effect of antipromoters and strain of mouse on tumor promoter-induced oxidants in murine epidermal cells, *Carcinogenesis* **7**:915–918.

151. Yuspa, S. H., Spangler, E. F., Donahoe, R., Gensz, S., Ferguson, E., Wenk, M., and Hennings, H., 1982, Sensitivity to two-stage carcinogenesis of SENCAR mouse skin grafted to nude mice, *Cancer Res.* **42**:437–439.

152. Strickland, J. E., and Strickland, A. G., 1984, Host cell reactivation studies with epidermal cells of mice sensitive and resistant to carcinogenesis, *Cancer Res.* **44**:893–895.

153. Strickland, J. E., Jetten, A. M., Kawamura, H., and Yuspa, S. H., 1984, Interaction of epidermal growth factor with basal and differentiating epidermal cells of mice resistant and sensitive to carcinogenesis, *Carcinogenesis* **5**:735–740.

154. Strickland, P. T., 1986, Abnormal wound healing in UV-irradiated skin of SENCAR mice, *J. Invest. Dermatol.* **86**:37–41.

155. Weeks, C. E., and Slaga, T. J., 1979, Inhibition of phorbol ester induced polyamine accumulation in mouse epidermis by antiinflammatory steroids, *Biochem. Biophys. Res. Commun.* **91**:1488–1496.

156. Slaga, T. J., 1984, Multistage skin tumor promotion and specificity of inhibition, in: *Mechanisms of Tumor Promotion: Tumor Promotion and Skin Carcinogenesis*, Vol. II (T. J. Slaga, ed.), pp. 189–196, CRC Press, Boca Raton, Florida.

157. Fischer, S. M., Hardin, K., Klein-Szanto, A. J. P., and Slaga, T. J., 1985, Retinoyl-phorbol-acetate is a complete skin tumor promoter in SENCAR mice, *Cancer Lett.* **27**:323–327.

158. Furstenberger, G., and Marks, F., 1983, Growth stimulation and tumor promotion in skin, *J. Invest. Dermatol.* **81**:157s–161s.

159. Hennings, H., and Yuspa, S. H., 1985, Two-stage promotion an alternative interpretation, *J. Natl. Cancer Inst.* **74**:735–740.

160. Argyris, T. S., 1983, Nature of the epidermal hyperplasia produced by mezerein, a weak tumor promoter, in initiated skin of mice, *Cancer Res.* **43**:1768–1773.

161. Ewing, M. W., Phillips, J., Slaga, T. J., and DiGiovanni, J., 1987, Influence of promoter dose, duration, and type on progression of papillomas to carcinomas in SENCAR mice, *Proc. Am. Assoc. Cancer Res.* **18**:173.

162. Boutwell, R. K., 1974, The function and mechanisms of promoters of carcinogenesis, *Crit. Rev. Toxicol.* **2**:419–443.

163. Argyris, T. S., 1983, An analysis of the epidermal hyperplasia produced by acetic acid, a poor promoter, in the skin of female mice initiated with dimethylbenzanthracene, *J. Invest. Dermatol.* **80**:430–435.

164. DiGiovanni, J., Decina, P. C., Prichett, W. P., Cantor, J., Aalfs, K. K., and Coombs, M. M., 1985, Mechanism of mouse skin tumor promotion by chrysarobin, *Cancer Res.* **45**:2584–2589.

165. Kruszewski, F. H., Naito, M., Naito, Y., and DiGiovanni, J., 1987, Histological alterations produced by the tumor promoting anthrone, chrysarobin, in SENCAR mouse skin, *J. Invest. Dermatol.* in press.

166. Klein-Szanto, A. J. P., and Slaga, T. J., 1982, Effects of peroxides on rodent skin: Epidermal hyperplasia and tumor promotion, *J. Invest. Dermatol.* **79**:30–34.

167. Naito, M., Naito, Y., and DiGiovanni, J., 1987, Comparison of the histological changes in the skin of DBA/2 and C57BL/6 mice following exposure to various promoting agents, *Carcinogenesis,* in press.

168. Scribner, J. D., Scribner, N. K., McKnight, B., and Mottet, N. K., 1983, Evidence for a new model of tumor progression from carcinogenesis and tumor promotion studies with 7-bromomethylbenz(a)anthracene, *Cancer Res.* **43**:2034–2041.

169. Poland, A., Knutson, J., Glover, E., and Kende, A., 1983, Tumor promotion in the skin of hairless mice by halogenated aromatic hydrocarbons, in: *Genes and Proteins in Oncogenesis* (I. B. Weinstein and J. H. Vogel, eds.), pp. 143–161, Academic Press, New York.

170. Colburn, N. H., 1985, Genes and membrane signals involved in neoplastic transformation, in: *Carcinogenesis—A Comprehensive Survey, The Role of Chemicals and Radiation in the Etiology of Cancer,* Volume 10 (E. Huberman, and S. H. Barr, eds.), pp. 235–248, Raven Press, New York.

171. Colburn, N. H., Talmadge, C. B., and Gindhart, T. D., 1983, Transfer of sensitivity to tumor promoters by transfection of DNA from sensitive into insensitive mouse JB6 epidermal cells, *Molec. Cell. Biol.* **3**:1182–1186.

# 13

# *Oncogenes*

## *Eric H. Westin*

## *1. INTRODUCTION*

Transformation of normal cells that compose the spectrum of tissues and organ systems of the intact organism is commonly thought to involve a multistep process ultimately reflected in genetic aberrations in the evolving tumor cell. These genetic aberrations may represent important factors that modulate both the individual tumor phenotype and the diversity evident in many tumors.[1] The spectrum of genetic alterations observed is broad but includes such events as chromosomal alterations with breakage, duplications or loss, gene amplification, mutations, and transposition-mediated events such as those associated with retroviruses. Ultimately, these genetic events must result in altered function of one or more gene products associated with control of cell proliferation and differentiation.

Recently, intense interest has been focused on a group of cellular genes termed proto-oncogenes as potentially important targets of genetic alterations leading to altered cell proliferation and transformation.[2,3] The focus of this chapter is to provide a framework within which one can tentatively group and classify the oncogenes, permitting a better understanding of their role in both normal and, when structurally altered, abnormal cell proliferation and differentiation.

## *2. RETROVIRUSES AND ONCOGENES*

### *2.1. Acute and Chronic Transforming Retroviruses*

Initial interest in the oncogenes stemmed from early work with the acutely transforming retroviruses. In 1911, Rous first described a virus, later termed Rous sarcoma virus, which was capable of causing rapid (within several weeks) induction of sarcomas when inoculated into chickens.[4] From these initial observations, the number and variety of tumor-associated retroviruses has been rapidly expanding.[5,6] Tumor-causing retroviruses can be divided into two broad groups.[6,7] The first group, representing that found most frequently outside the laboratory, are the chronic transforming viruses. These viruses, in general, are characterized as being replication competent but causing tumors in only a minority of infected animals and, then, only after long latency periods. In general, these viruses are also incapable of causing cell transformation *in vitro*, although exceptions such as HTLV-1 do exist.[8]

Unlike the chronic transforming retroviruses, the acute transforming viruses rapidly cause

*Eric H. Westin* • Department of Medicine, Division of Hematology/Oncology, Medical College of Virginia, Virginia Commonwealth University, Richmond, Virginia 23298.

tumors that are multifocal in origin.[5,6] These viruses can also transform a variety of primary cells in culture, which are then found to be tumorigenic when inoculated into the appropriate animal host strain. With the exception of Rous sarcoma virus, these viruses are also replication deficient and therefore require a replication-competent chronically transforming helper virus for sustained virus production. Thus, most infectious acutely transforming retroviruses are actually mixtures of the defective retrovirus along with the helper virus.

## 2.2. Acute Transforming Retroviruses and Viral Oncogenes

With the advent of improved retroviral growth and purification procedures, along with molecular cloning, it became possible for the first time to investigate the relation of the acute and chronic transforming retroviruses to each other and determine, in part, the mechanism by which a chronically transforming retrovirus strain can rapidly develop an acutely transforming component following its serial passage through host animals.

Initial studies of the acutely transforming retroviruses demonstrated the presence of additional genetic material within the retrovirus that had substituted for a part of the retroviral encoded sequences necessary for replication. In this way, the virus became dependent on a helper virus to provide the functions lost during this substitution of genetic material.

The origin of the additional genetic material present in the acutely transforming virus and shown experimentally to be required for acute transformation also became apparent. In these viruses, genetic material obtained from the host species genome had become incorporated or transduced directly into the virus.[9–11] Although the precise mechanism underlying this transduction process remains unknown, with only a few exceptions,[12] the entire group of retroviruses found to be acutely transforming contain transduced cellular genes that have been modified during the transduction process. Based on the properties of these genes to cause rapid transformation of cells *in vitro* and *in vivo*, they have been termed v-*onc* genes to connote both their viral origin and oncogenic potential.[13]

Since these v-*onc* genes were derived from presumably normal cellular genes that have a normal function other than transformation, the cellular homologues of these genes were termed c-*onc* genes or cellular proto-oncogenes to connote their cellular origin and presumed oncogenic potential if altered in a structural fashion.[13]

A list of known v-*onc* genes is presented in Table I. The viral oncogenes are categorized according to either a known function or by some other specific biochemical properties. As can be seen, the viral oncogenes can be divided into several large groups, including those coding for either tyrosine or serine-threonine kinases, GTP-binding proteins with GTPase activity, growth factors, and DNA-binding nuclear proteins of unknown function. Activation of these oncogenes on transduction into a retrovirus can be accompanied by a variety of changes in the protein product.[6,7] These include truncation of either the amino- or carboxy-terminal as well as point mutation within the protein and fusion to other viral-derived proteins such as the *gag* or group-specific antigen gene of the retrovirus. In addition, incorporation of the v-*onc* gene brings expression of this gene under the transcriptional control of the retrovirus long terminal repeat,[6] which can then cause unregulated and in some instances extremely high-level expression of the v-*onc* gene product. In this way, transduction of a cellular proto-oncogene into an acutely transforming retrovirus can be associated with multiple changes in that gene product.

This wide variety of simultaneous changes, each representing a relatively rare genetic event in the intact cell, may explain in part the ability of the acutely transforming retrovirus to transform primary cells in culture without requiring additional genetic steps or events. However, as will be seen for transformational activation of cellular proto-oncogenes, for some retroviruses, two oncogenes may be transduced simultaneously by the same virus, both of which are required for expression of the malignant cell phenotype induced by the virus. This has been found to be the case in particular in the avian erythroblastosis virus, which contains both the v-*erbA* and v-*erbB* oncogenes,[14,15] as well as the MH2 virus containing both v-*myc* and v-*raf* genes.[16] Thus, the transforming retroviruses themselves provided some of the early evidence that alteration in function of more than one gene product may be required to produce the complete transformed phenotype in

*Table I.  Viral Oncogenes*

| Viral gene | Product[a] | Biochemical function or enzymatic activity |
|---|---|---|
| erbA | p75gag-erbA | No enzymatic activity known[b] |
| ets | p135gag-myb-ets | No enzymatic activity known |
| rel | p56env-rel | No enzymatic activity known |
| sis | p28sis | No enzymatic activity known[c] |
| ski | p125gag-ski | No enzymatic activity known |
| mil | p100gag-mil | Serine-threonine kinase |
| mos | p37mos | Serine-threonine kinase |
| raf | p90gag-raf | Serine-threonine kinase |
| Ha-ras | p21Ha-ras | GTP binding, GTPase |
| Ki-ras | p21Ki-ras | GTP binding, GTPase |
| abl | p120gag-abl | Tyrosine kinase |
| erbB | gp74erbB | Tyrosine kinase[b] |
| fes | p85gag-fes | Tyrosine kinase |
| fgr | p70gag-actin-fgr | Tyrosine kinase |
| fms | gp170gag-fms | Tyrosine kinase[b] |
| fps | p140gag-fms | Tyrosine kinase |
| ros | p68gag-ros | Tyrosine kinase |
| yes | p90gag-yes | Tyrosine kinase |
| fos | p55fos | DNA binding, RNA transcription activation |
| myb | p48gag-myb | DNA binding |
| myc | p110gag-myc | DNA binding |
| jun | p55gag-jun | DNA binding, RNA transcription activation |

[a]p 75, etc. refers to molecular weight of the protein produced.
[b]Cellular homologue is a known growth factor receptor.
[c]Cellular homologue is a known peptide growth factor.

certain tissue types. If the cellular proto-oncogenes were to be implicated in human tumorigenesis, cooperation among altered functions of several cellular genes would also be most consistent with the broad experimental literature, suggesting a multistep nature to carcinogenesis (see Chapters 6 and 20).

## 3. CELLULAR PROTO-ONCOGENES

### 3.1. Conservation among Species

With the finding that viral oncogenes were derived from the cellular counterparts of these genes, research focused rapidly on examining the structure and function of the cellular proto-oncogenes. Early studies showed the cellular counterparts of the viral oncogenes to be highly conserved over a broad range of species.[2] Thus, probes derived from murine or avian v-onc-containing retroviruses could be used to examine structure and expression of these genes from yeast to humans. This close sequence conservation, and ultimately even greater protein conservation, offered initial support to the hypothesis that these genes were involved in important aspects of normal cell function. Examination of the sequences transduced by the retrovirus and the cellular counterpart from which it was derived demonstrated that the viral gene lacked the normal intron–exon structure of the cellular gene.[2] During the transduction process, intron sequences are removed. Therefore the v-onc sequences represent a spliced form of the cellular proto-oncogene. In addition, truncation of cellular gene-coding sequences has occurred frequently in the transduction process, as well as fusion of the onc sequences to viral-encoded sequences.

### 3.2. Cellular Proto-Oncogenes as Control Elements in Normal Cell Growth and Differentiation

A list of the cellular homologues of the viral oncogenes, along with their presumed function, where known, and their chromosomal localization is shown in Table II.[16a] With the cloning and sequencing of the viral and cellular oncogenes, data rapidly accumulated to implicate these genes and their protein products in the control of the normal proliferative response of cells, such as occurs with wound healing and regeneration of tissues or in normal hematopoiesis. The first such evidence was obtained with the sequencing of the v-*sis* oncogene from the simian sarcoma virus. This virus, derived from a woolly monkey with multiple fibrosarcomas, can transform fibroblasts on infection *in vitro*.[17] The v-*sis* oncogene was found to be highly homologous to the protein sequence for the β-

### Table II. Cellular Homologues of Retroviral Oncogenes[a]

| Cellular proto-oncogene | Biochemical function or enzymatic activity | Chromosomal localization[b] |
|---|---|---|
| c-*abl* | Tyrosine kinase | 9q34 |
| c-*erbA* | Thyroid hormone receptor | 17q11-q21 |
| c-*erbB*-1 | Epidermal growth factor Receptor, tyrosine kinase | 7p14-p12 |
| c-*erbB*-2 | Tyrosine kinase related to EGF receptor | 17q21-q22 |
| c-*ets*-1 | Not known | 11q13.3 |
| c-*ets*-2 | Not known | 21q22 |
| c-*fes* | Tyrosine kinase | 15q25-q26 |
| c-*fgr* | Tyrosine kinase | 1p36.1-36.2 |
| c-*fms* | Colony-stimulating factor-1 receptor, tyrosine kinase | 5q33-q34 |
| c-*fos* | DNA binding | 14q21-q31 |
| c-*Ha-ras*-1 | GTP binding, GTPase | 11p15.5 |
| c-*Ha-ras*-2 | Not known | Xpter-q28 |
| c-*int*-1 | Not known | 12pter-q14 |
| c-*int*-2 | Not known | 11q13 |
| c-*Ki-ras*-1 | Not known | 6p23-q12 |
| c-*Ki-ras*-2 | GTP binding, GTPase | 12p12.1 |
| c-*L-myc* | Presumed DNA binding | 1p32 |
| c-*mos* | Serine-threonine kinase | 8q11-q22 |
| c-*myb* | DNA binding | 6q21-q23 |
| c-*myc* | DNA binding | 8q24 |
| c-*N-ras* | GTP binding, GTPase | 1p22 |
| c-*N-myc* | Presumed DNA binding | 2p25-p23 |
| c-*raf*-1 | Serine threonine kinase | 3p25-p24 |
| c-*raf*-2 | Not known | 4 |
| c-*rel* | Not known | 2p13-cen |
| c-*ros* | Tyrosine kinase | 6q16-q22 |
| c-*sis* | β-chain platelet-derived growth factor | 22q12.3-q13.1 |
| c-*ski* | Not known | 1q22-qter |
| c-*src* | Tyrosine kinase | 20q12-q13 |
| c-*yes*-1 | Tyrosine kinase | 18q21.3 |
| c-*yes*-2 | Tyrosine kinase | 6 |

[a]Abstracted from LeBeau and Rowley[16a] and from the Yale University/Howard Hughes Medical Institute human gene mapping on-line database.
[b]Localization on human chromosomes.

chain of human platelet-derived growth factor (PDGF) by comparison with protein sequence databases.[18-20] Subsequent cloning and sequencing of the human homologue of this gene confirmed that the c-*sis* gene encoded the β-chain of human PDGF.[21,22]

Additional work rapidly implicated other cellular proto-oncogenes in the growth factor/growth factor-receptor signaling pathway (see also Chapter 17). The c-*erbB* proto-oncogene was shown to encode the epidermal growth factor receptor and the c-*erbA* gene encoded a high-affinity receptor for thyroid hormone.[23-25] The c-*fms* gene, the chromosomal localization of which has led to the suspicion that it is involved in the production of a variety of hematopoietic neoplasms,[26-28] has also been found to code for the receptor for colony-stimulating factor-1 (CSF-1).[29]

Additional support for the role of the proto-oncogenes in a signal cascade controlling normal cell proliferation and differentiation has come from studies of the *ras* family of proto-oncogenes that includes c-Ha-*ras*, c-Ki-*ras*, and c-N-*ras*.[30-32] These genes have been found to code for membrane-associated proteins that have GTP binding and GTPase activity.[33-36] In this way, they are remarkably similar to, but nevertheless distinct from, the G proteins that couple hormone–receptor interactions to cytoplasmic signals in a variety of cells.[37,38] However, data showing that these proteins do function in signal transduction from growth factor–growth factor-receptor interactions have been obtained from a variety of sources, including microinjection studies with monoclonal antibodies that bind the *ras* GTP-binding domain. These studies have indicated that this activity is required for the proliferation of a variety of cells stimulated with growth factors or transformed by altered growth-factor receptors.[39,40] Also, altered growth-factor dependency or responsiveness has been found in cells transformed by altered c-*ras* genes in which mutations have occurred that alter GTP binding or GTPase activity.[41,42]

The membrane-associated tyrosine kinases such as those coded for by c-*src*[43] and the serine-threonine kinase such as coded for by c-*raf*[44,45] also represent potential growth or differentiation factor signal-coupling mechanisms. These may function to alter by their phosphorylation reactions a large number of membrane and cytoplasmic proteins, such as those of the cytoskeleton.[46,47]

Definition of the biochemical activity of the nuclear localized cellular proto-oncogenes remains elusive. Genes such as c-*myc*,[48-50] c-*fos*,[51,52] and c-*myb*[53-56] have all been shown to exhibit DNA-binding activity *in vitro*. Studies of c-*myc* have strongly implicated this gene in the control of cell cycle-mediated events. Recent support for studies that have associated expression of this gene with cell proliferation comes from the direct demonstration with antibody inactivation that c-*myc* is required for DNA synthesis.[57] Similar studies have implicated c-*myb* in messenger RNA (mRNA) processing.[58] A definitive role for c-*fos* has not been demonstrated; however, rapid transient induction of c-*fos* has been shown to occur in response to a wide variety of growth and differentiation stimuli.[59] In addition, a requirement for the expression of c-*fos* in normal fibroblast proliferation has been demonstrated using an inducible antisense c-*fos* RNA expression construct to block expression of this gene.[60]

Thus, the cellular proto-oncogenes might be viewed as a group of gene products involved in the control of normal cell proliferation and function. This occurs through the action of a variety of growth and differentiation factors, their receptors, signal-coupling proteins such as GTP-binding proteins as well as tyrosine and serine-threonine kinases, and ultimately nuclear proteins responsible for control of events such as the entrance of a cell into the cell cycle. Altered function or expression of these gene products through genetic events, including retroviral insertion, mutations, chromosomal translocations, and gene amplification (discussed in Section 4), can then lead to altered cell proliferation or differentiation as manifested in carcinoma, sarcoma, or leukemia.

## 4. TUMOR FORMATION AND MECHANISMS OF ACTIVATION OF CELLULAR PROTO-ONCOGENES

### 4.1. Overview of Mechanisms of Activation

Alteration in the normal function of a gene and its protein product can take place through a variety of mechanisms. These include mutation of specific bases leading to an altered amino acid composition, as well as small deletions or insertions of genetic material. Gene structure and expression may also be altered by chromosomal translocation with or without structural alteration of the encoded protein products. Finally, gene expression can be quantitatively altered through the amplification of its locus and increased expression based on this amplification. That retroviruses have been implicated in the causation of tumors in a wide variety of lower animal model systems has also focused attention on the fact that proviral insertion, in a manner analogous to chromosomal translocation, is an important factor in the genesis of these viral-induced neoplasms. Each of the mechanisms described above has been implicated in a variety of neoplastic states. The only exception to date is lack of evidence of proviral insertion as a mechanism of proto-oncogene activation in humans. A representative list of frequently activated oncogenes in human neoplasms is shown in Table III.[60a]

## 4.2. Activation of Cellular Proto-Oncogenes by Retroviral Insertion

Studies of tumors caused by chronically transforming retroviruses, without evidence for production of an acutely transforming virus, pointed to viral integration as a possible mechanism leading to the genetic changes associated with the development of neoplasia.[61] An early observation was integration of the avian leukosis virus (ALV) into the c-*myc* locus in virtually all bursal neoplasms (B-cell lymphomas) induced by this virus in chickens.[12,62–64] The integration event occurred in sequences upstream from the 5' end or within the first (noncoding) exon of the c-*myc* gene and led to high-level expression of the c-*myc* gene product in these neoplasms. This, in turn, is most likely a necessary but not wholly sufficient event in the genesis of viral-induced bursal neoplasms of chickens. Other events, such as additional mutations or alterations of other gene products, also appear to be required for full expression of the transformed phenotype exhibited by these B-cell neoplasms.

Following the demonstration of frequent integration of avian leukosis virus into the c-*myc* gene locus in B-cell tumors, other models were examined for evidence of common integration sites that were tumor specific. These have been subsequently demonstrated in viral oncogenic models as diverse as avian erythroblastosis and mouse mammary tumor virus-induced mammary neoplasms.[65] In the case of avian erythroblastosis, viral integration is found in proximity to the *erbB* gene in the induced neoplasms. In the case of mouse mammary tumor virus, a total of three common integration sites termed *int*-1, -2, and -3 have been identified in tumor tissues.[66–68]

Retroviral integration events are generally believed to occur on a relatively random basis. Thus, the finding of common integration sites in specific tumor types is thought to represent an important event in the genetic causation of the tumor. This event may be associated with altered

### Table III. Oncogene Alterations Frequently Associated with Specific Human Neoplasms[a]

| Tumor type | Oncogene association | Mechanism of activation |
|---|---|---|
| Acute leukemias | c-*N-ras* | Mutation |
| Acute lymphoid leukemia | c-*ets*-1 | Translocation |
| Acute myeloid leukemia | c-*ets*-2 | Translocation |
| Breast carcinoma | c-*erbB*-2 | Amplification |
| Burkitt lymphoma | c-*myc* | Translocation and mutation |
| Cervical carcinoma | c-*myc* | Amplification and rearrangement |
| Chronic myeloid leukemia | c-*abl* | Translocation |
| Colonic carcinoma | c-*Ki-ras*-1 | Mutation |
| Embryonal carcinoma | c-*Ki-ras*-2 | Amplification and rearrangement |
| Neuroblastoma | c-*N-myc* | Amplification |
| Small cell lung carcinoma | c-*L-myc* | Amplification |

[a]Abstracted from Aaronson and Tronick.[60a]

function or expression of a proto-oncogene, leading to altered cell proliferation. Additional genetic events might culminate in expression of the fully transformed phenotype in cells that possess this specific viral integration.

By contrast, there is now increasing evidence indicating that retroviral integration may not be a truly random event.[69] Certain sites, particularly areas of open chromatin structure that may represent actively transcribed genes, have been associated with enhanced probability of integration. Thus, although a retrovirus may integrate in a wide variety of sites, this integration may not be truly random throughout the genome. However, calculations of the probability of specific integration events leading to alteration of a particular genetic locus cannot be made simply on the basis of the number of base pairs contained in the infected species genome.

## 4.3. Mutations Activating Proto-Oncogenes

Initial studies examining mutations as a mechanism of activation of proto-oncogenes were derived from studies searching for dominantly acting transforming genes that could be detected in tumors by using the NIH 3T3 transfection/transformation assay.[70–76] Table IV presents a partial list of activated dominant transforming genes either related or unrelated to known retroviral oncogenes discovered by this technique (see also Chapters 14 and 20).

Early studies focused on members of the *ras* family of oncogenes. Cloning and sequencing of multiple transforming and nontransforming alleles of this gene family have shown that its transforming potential can be activated by single point mutations leading to single amino acid substitutions. In particular, changes in codons 12 and 61 of all three *ras* family members appear to activate this gene.[77–85] Associated with these mutations are alterations in GTP binding and GTPase activity that appear specific for the activation of transforming potential.[36,86,87]

Detection by transfection methods of mutated and therefore activated proto-oncogenes such as *ras* gene family members has led to the estimate that only 10–15% of a given tumor type contain detectable dominantly acting transforming genes. However, depending on the tumor type examined, some specificity, particularly among the *ras* gene family members, has been observed. Examples in humans include tumors of hematopoietic origin that most frequently display activation of N-*ras* and colonic neoplasms, which have mutational activation of Ki-*ras*.[88] Despite this specificity, however, the low apparent frequency of detection of activated genes by transfection techniques has led at least one observer to speculate that because the frequency is so low, these findings may be irrelevant to

### Table IV. Activated Proto-Oncogenes Detected by Transfection Techniques[a]

| Oncogene detected | Source from which DNA was obtained |
| --- | --- |
| c-*dbl* | Diffuse poorly differentiated lymphocytic lymphoma |
| c-*erbB*-2/*neu* | Brain tumors |
| c-*Ha-ras*-1 | Large variety of tumor types |
| c-*hst* | Stomach cancer |
| c-*Ki-ras*-2 | Large variety of tumor types |
| c-*lca* | Hepatocellular carcinoma |
| c-*mas* | Epidermoid carcinoma |
| c-*mcf*-2 | Mammary carcinoma |
| c-*mel* | Melanoma |
| c-*met* | Transformed osteosarcoma cell line |
| c-N-*ras* | Large variety of tumor types |
| c-*ret* | T-cell lymphoma |
| c-*trk* | Colon carcinoma |

[a]Abstracted from Aaronson and Tronick.[60a]

the pathogenesis of these tumors. However, recently developed techniques that permit the detection of specific mutations within a gene using either oligonucleotide probes or direct sequencing of genomic DNA without a need to resort to a cumbersome biologic assay for detection have increased the incidence of mutational activation of the Ki-*ras* gene to at least 40%.[89,90] Future work to elucidate other mutations outside of positions 12 and 61 that can activate these *ras* family members may increase this incidence still further. Thus, point mutations as potential mechanisms of activation of proto-oncogenes may represent frequent events in a variety of tumors. However, only a restricted number of members of the proto-oncogene family of genes appear to have point mutation as the primary mechanism of activation. This has been observed extensively, however, in all members of the *ras* family. With other genes, such as c-*myc*, other mechanisms of activation assume a greater importance.

## 4.4. Amplification of Proto-Oncogenes

One mechanism by which expression of a gene can be altered is by increasing the gene dosage through amplification of the gene. Many tumor cells contain evidence of gene amplification based on cytogenetic findings.[91–94] These include the presence of abnormal karyotypic markers such as homogeneously staining regions, double minutes, and abnormally banded regions. In several instances, oncogene amplification has been associated with these changes, leading to increased expression of the amplified gene product.

Initial evidence for oncogene amplification came from examination of c-*myc* in the human promyelocytic leukemia cell line HL-60. Initial studies of differential oncogene expression showed this line to be unusual in that a high-level c-*myc* expression was present in contrast with other similar leukemic cell lines.[95] Subsequent studies have shown that the c-*myc* locus is amplified 16- to 32-fold in this cell line.[96,97] Other studies have now also shown that c-*myc* is amplified in a colon carcinoma cell line[98] as well as in human small cell lung carcinoma cell lines and in a non-small cell lung carcinoma cell line.[99]

Not only c-*myc* is amplified in tumor cells. A gene closely related to c-*myc*, termed N-*myc*, has been found to be frequently amplified in human neuroblastomas and neuroblastoma-derived cell lines.[100,101] Amplification and high-level expression of this gene has been associated with more aggressive tumor histology and clinical behavior.[102,103] Other examples of oncogene amplification include the *abl* proto-oncogene in a cell line derived from a patient with chronic myelogenous leukemia,[104] as well as amplification of the *erbB*/EGF receptor gene in a variety of human tumor cell lines.[105,106] Recently, amplification of an EGF receptor-related oncogene was also found in primary breast tumor cells. This proto-oncogene has been designated c-*erbB*-2 (also termed HER-2/neu) and is found amplified at high frequency in primary breast tumors.[107–110] The high frequency suggests relevance of the amplification in the development of breast tumors. In addition, the amplification of the c-*erbB*-2 gene in breast tumors may provide a valuable prognostic marker of aggressive tumor behavior based on preliminary studies of amplification of this gene and correlation with clinical disease outcome.[111]

Thus, amplification of a variety of oncogenes has been found in a broad spectrum of tumor types. However, the actual mechanism by which increased expression of a gene product can lead to cell transformation in the instances examined remains unknown. The high frequency at which amplification of genes such as N-*myc* in neuroblastomas, L-*myc* in small cell lung carcinomas,[112] and *erbB*-2 in primary breast tumors occurs would suggest that this amplification is important in controlling at least some aspects of tumor cell behavior. This hypothesis is further supported by the finding of correlation of amplification of both N-*myc* and *erbB*-2 with more aggressive clinical tumor behavior (see Chapter 10).

## 4.5. Chromosomal Translocations in the Activation of Cellular Proto-Oncogenes

Specific chromosomal alterations have for many years been associated with specific tumor types. This has in particular been true for Burkitt lymphoma with the t(8;14) translocation and chronic myelogenous leukemia with the Philadelphia chromosome, which represents a t(9;22) reciprocal translocation.[113] The localization of the proto-oncogenes to specific chromosomal sites (see Table II) led to the hypothesis that these genes may become specifically altered during the course of tumorigenesis by chromosome translocation.

Initial studies focused on the c-*myc* gene, which was localized to the distal portion of the long arm of chromosome 8 in humans since the breakpoint in Burkitt lymphoma involved this specific site. Data from these studies showed that the c-*myc* gene was specifically translocated into an immunoglobulin locus during generation of the t(8;14) or variant t(2;8) and t(8;22) translocations associated with Burkitt lymphoma.[114–117] During the course of these translocations, several important alterations occur in the c-*myc* gene analogous to those induced by ALV proviral insertion in avian bursal lymphomas. The sequences upstream of the c-*myc* gene, including in some cases the first exon of this three-exon gene, are removed and immunoglobulin gene sequences are substituted.[118,119] In this way, sequences important to proper transcriptional control of the c-*myc* gene are removed. This in turn can lead to inappropriate, although not necessarily high-level, c-*myc* expression. In addition, mutations generated either during the course of, or immediately following, the translocation event in the terminal portion of the first exon may be important in altering c-*myc* gene function.[120–122]

The importance of the c-*myc* translocation and involvement of the translocation in the pathogenesis of Burkitt lymphoma can be demonstrated directly *in vitro*.[123] Human umbilical cord blood B lymphocytes can be immortalized and grown readily in culture by infection with Epstein–Barr virus (EBV). Infection with this virus has also been shown to be an important contributing factor in the development of the African form of Burkitt lymphoma. However, B cells immortalized with EBV are not tumorigenic in a variety of mouse transplantation models. Using DNA transfection techniques, a cloned translocated c-*myc* allele has been introduced into EBV-immortalized B cells. Upon introduction into nude mice, these cells are fully tumorigenic, with a tumor histology consistent with Burkitt lymphoma. Thus, the translocated c-*myc* allele can function directly in the tumorigenic conversion of B cells. These experiments also show that the c-*myc* translocation alone may not be sufficient for tumorigenesis but requires concomitant infection with EBV. This requirement for more than a single genetic event is further supported by experiments using transgenic mice containing a translocated c-*myc* allele, which over time develop fatal B-cell lymphomas.[124]

Other tumor-specific translocations have now been shown to alter proto-oncogenes. The Philadelphia translocation has been shown to lead to rearrangement of the c-*abl* oncogene with fusion of both the *abl* transcript as well as the *abl* protein to a gene designated *bcr*.[125–127] This translocation and gene rearrangement has been associated with virtually all cases of chronic myelogenous leukemia. The specific changes in the c-*abl* protein induced in this translocation are analogous to those induced through production of a *gag–abl* fusion protein when this gene was transduced into the Abelson murine leukemia virus. Finally, in acute myelogenous leukemia, a t(8;21) translocation has frequently been observed. In this instance, translocation of yet another proto-oncogene, c-*ets*-2, has also been shown to occur.[128,129] Thus, tumor-specific translocations have been demonstrated frequently to involve rearrangement of proto-oncogenes.

## 5. COOPERATION AMONG ACTIVATED ONCOGENES IN CELL TRANSFORMATION

The process of transformation has been shown to involve multiple definable steps. Thus, it would be expected that if each of these stages in the transformation process were to involve genetic events, multiple genetic changes would be required before a cell could be considered fully transformed. Studies of mechanism of transformation by activated proto-oncogenes have provided direct evidence supporting this hypothesis. These studies initially involved examination of the requirements for transformation of primary rat embryo fibroblasts.[130,131] Using this system, proto-oncogenes such as c-*myc*, when transcriptionally activated, provide an immortalization function to transfected cells. However, these cells are otherwise contact inhibited and cannot form tumors in nude mice. Other activated proto-oncogenes, such as c-Ha-*ras*, when introduced into these cells, lead to loss of contact inhibition but not immortalization and only abortive tumor formation. By contrast, transfection of both genes together results in a population of rat embryo fibroblasts that are both immortalized as well as transformed in culture and tumorigenic in nude mice. Thus, cooperation in the action of several oncogenes by alteration of either their expression or protein product function may be required for complete cell transformation.

Evidence for cooperation among altered proto-oncogenes has come from work with transgenic mice containing a mouse mammary tumor virus-linked c-*myc* gene that develop mammary tumors at a high rate.[132] However, considering latency periods and tumor behavior, these tumors must also undergo additional genetic changes before tumors can develop and become independent of estrogen.

Work with transgenic mice has also provided the first evidence for specific alterations in a proto-oncogene at time of initiation in a model of skin tumor initiation and promotion.[133] Initial observations suggested that the c-Ha-*ras* proto-oncogene was mutated as an early event in skin tumorigenesis. Transgeneic mice were subsequently created that carried a mutated form of the c-Ha-*ras* gene that was transforming in NIH 3T3 cells. That this activation event is not in itself sufficient for cell transformation in the intact animal is indicated by the fact that mice carrying these genes did not uniformly develop tumors. However, the use of this engineered mouse strain in initiation–promotion assays of skin tumorigenesis has demonstrated that mice carrying a mutated *ras* gene no longer require the initiation event. Therefore, at least in a skin tumor model system, mutation of c-Ha-*ras* appears to be a critical genetic event associated with tumor initiation. Additional genetic events must then be required during tumor-promotion steps before the cell can become fully transformed.

Thus, alteration of multiple proto-oncogene functions may be required before a cell can become fully transformed. Future work in this area should provide further definition of the genetic events that form each stage in the complex process of carcinogenesis, as well as the specific target genes for each tumor cell type.

## 6. SUMMARY

Multiple genetic mechanisms can be used to alter the structure, function, or expression of individual proto-oncogene products. These mechanisms can be used either singly or in combination to create changes in the structure of the oncogene that may be specific to an individual tumor type and able to cause transformation in specific *in vitro* and *in vivo* model systems. Alterations of more than one proto-oncogene may also be required for complete transformation of normal cells. Despite the complexity of these changes however, a common theme exists throughout these alterations, that is, the activation of proto-oncogenes.

The proto-oncogene products themselves represent proteins involved in the normal proliferation and differentiation process. Some represent growth factors such as c-*sis*/PDGF-2, which is a growth and proliferation factor specific for cells of mesenchymal origin. Inappropriate expression of this gene in cells possessing the PDGF receptor can lead directly to transformation. Thus, deregulation of c-*sis* expression in tumors such as sarcomas may lead to autocrine stimulation of cell proliferation that, coupled with other genetic events, may produce cells that behave neoplastically. Genes such as the *erbB* gene, which encodes the EGF receptor, can be altered as a result of truncation of the extracellular domain of the receptor. This leads to activation and uncontrolled expression, thereby resulting in a constant growth stimulation. Other proto-oncogenes, such as c-*src* and c-Ha-*ras*, when mutated during transformational activation, have altered biochemical properties. In the case of *ras*, specific alterations lead to increased GTP binding and decreased GTPase activity. These changes closely mimic the effect on this gene when a growth factor receptor-mediated signal is coupled to the cytoplasm and nuclear response of the cell. In the case of c-*src*, a similar phenomenon may be operative when the tyrosine kinase activity of the gene product is altered during the process of transformation by this gene. Finally, genes such as c-*myc*, the expression of which is closely related to DNA synthesis and proliferation, can undergo alterations in genetic elements required for control of its expression through translocation or gene amplification. Alteration in this control can lead to changes in the manner whereby this gene is regulated either as a function of the cell cycle or stage of differentiation. These changes can then be responsible, in part, for the inability of a cell to undergo terminal differentiation, and thus continue to proliferate. Therefore, although multiple mechanisms of activation can be involved and changes in several genes may be required for cells to become fully transformed, these changes revolve around alteration in the function and action of genes that represent normal components of the pathway of cell differentiation and proliferation. Future studies of the proto-oncogenes should continue to provide useful data on the mechanisms of normal cell proliferation and differentiation as well as lead to increased understanding of how these mechanisms may be subverted during the process of tumorigenesis.

## REFERENCES

1. Nicolson, G. L., 1987, Tumor cell instability, diversification, and progression to metastatic phenotype: From oncogene to oncofetal expression, *Cancer Res.* **47:**1473–1487.
2. Varmus, H. E., 1984, The molecular genetics of cellular oncogenes, *Annu. Rev. Genet.* **18:**553–612.
3. Bishop, J. M., 1987, The molecular genetics of cancer, *Science* **235:**305–311.
4. Rous, P., 1911, A sarcoma of the fowl transmissible by an agent separable from the tumor cells, *J. Exp. Med.* **13:**397–411.
5. Klein, G. (ed.), 1980, *Viral Oncology,* Raven, New York.
6. Bishop, J. M., 1981, Retroviruses, *Annu. Rev. Biochem.* **47:**35–88.
7. Weiss, R., Teich, N., Varmus, H., and Coffin, J., 1984, *RNA Tumor Viruses,* Vol. 1, Cold Spring Harbor Laboratory, Cold Spring Harbor, New York.
8. Popovic, M., Lange-Wantzin, G., Sarin, P. S., Mann, D., and Gallo, R. C., 1983, Transformation of human umbilical cord blood T cells by human T-cell leukemia/lymphoma virus (HTLV), *Proc. Natl. Acad. Sci. USA* **80:**5402–5406.
9. Stehelin, D., Varmus, H. E., and Bishop, J. M., 1976, DNA related to the transforming gene(s) of avian sarcoma virus is present in normal avian DNA, *Nature (Lond.)* **260:**170–172.
10. Spector, D. H., Baker, B., Varmus, H. E., and Bishop, J. M., 1978, Characteristics of cellular RNA related to the transforming gene of avian sarcoma virus, *Cell* **13:**381–386.
11. Wang, L. H., Halpern, C. C., Nadel, M., and Hanafusa, H., 1978, Recombination between viral and cellular sequences generates transforming sarcoma virus, *Proc. Natl. Acad. Sci. USA* **12:**5812–5816.
12. Robinson, H. L., and Gagnon, G. C., 1986, Patterns of proviral insertion and deletion in avian leukosis virus-induced lymphomas, *J. Virol.* **57:**26–36.
13. Coffin, J. M., Varmus, H. E., Bishop, J. M., Essex, M., Hardy, W. D., Martin, G. S., Rosenberg, N. E., Scolnick, E. M., Weinberg, R. A., and Vogt, P. K., 1981, Proposal for naming host cell-derived inserts in retrovirus genomes, *J. Virol.* **40:**953–957.
14. Lai, M. M. C., Neil, J. C., and Vogt, P. K., 1980, Cell-free translation of avian erythroblastosis virus RNA yields two specific and distinct proteins with molecular weights of 75,000 and 40,000, *Virology* **100:**475–483.
15. Vennstrom, B., and Bishop, J. M., 1982, Isolation and characterization of chicken DNA homologous to the two putative oncogenes of avian erythroblastosis virus, *Cell* **28:**135–143.
16. Kan, N. C., Flordellis, C. S., Mark, G. E., Deusberg, P. H., and Papas, T. S., 1984, A common onc gene sequence transduced by avian carcinoma virus MH2 and by murine sarcoma virus 3611, *Science* **223:**813–816.
16a. LeBeau, M. M., and Rowley, J. D., 1986, Chromosomal abnormalities in leukemia and lymphoma: Clinical and biological significance, *Adv. Hum. Genet.* **15:**1–54.
17. Wolfe, L. G., Deinhardt, F., Theilen, G. H., Rabin, H., Kawakami, T., and Bustad, L. K., 1971, Induction of tumors in marmoset monkeys by simian sarcoma virus, type 1 (Lagothrix): A preliminary report, *J. Natl. Cancer Inst.* **47:**1115–1120.
18. Waterfield, M. D., Scrace, G. T., Whittle, N., Stroobant, P., Johnson, A., Wasteson, A., Westermark, B., Heldin, C. H., Huang, J. S., and Deuel, T. F., 1983, Platelet-derived growth factor is structurally related to the putative transforming protein p28 sis of simian sarcoma virus, *Nature (Lond.)* **304:**35–39.
19. Doolittle, R. F., Hunkapiller, M. W., Hood, L. E., Devare, S. G., Robbins, K. C., Aaronson, S. A., and

Antoniades, H. N., 1983, Simian sarcoma virus onc gene, v-sis, is derived from the gene (or genes) encoding a platelet-derived growth factor, *Science* 221:275–277.

20. Robbins, K. C., Antoniades, H. N., Devare, S. G., Hunkapiller, M. W., and Aaronson, S. A., 1983, Structural and immunological similarities between simian sarcoma virus gene product(s) and human platelet-derived growth factor, *Nature (Lond.)* 305:605–608.

21. Josephs, S. F., Ratner, L., Clarke, M. F., Westin, E. H., Reitz, M. S., and Wong-Staal, F., 1984, Transforming potential of human c-sis nucleotide sequences encoding platelet-derived growth factor, *Science* 225:636–639.

22. Chiu, I. M., Reddy, E. P., Givol, D., Robbins, K. C., Tronick, S. R., and Aaronson, S. A., 1984, Nucleotide sequence analysis identifies the human c-sis proto-oncogene as a structural gene for platelet-derived growth factor, *Cell* 37:123–129.

23. Downward, J., Yarden, Y., Mayes, E., Scrace, G., Totty, N., Stockwell, P., Ullrich, A., Schlessinger, J., and Waterfield, M. D., 1984, Close similarity of epidermal growth factor receptor and v-erb-B oncogene protein sequences, *Nature (Lond.)* 307:521–527.

24. Sap, J., Munoz, A., Damm, K., Goldberg, Y., Ghysdael, J., Leutz, A., Beug, H., and Vennstrom, B., 1986, The c-erb-A protein is a high-affinity receptor for thyroid hormone, *Nature (Lond.)* 324:635–640.

25. Weinberger, C., Thompson, C. C., Ong, E. S., Lebo, R., Gruol, D. J., and Evans, R. M., 1986, The c-erb-A gene encodes a thyroid hormone receptor, *Nature (Lond.)* 324:641–646.

26. Roussel, M. F., Scherr, C. J., Barker, P. E., and Ruddle, F. H., 1983, Molecular cloning of the c-fms locus and its assignment to human chromosome 5, *J. Virol.* 48:770–773.

27. Neinhuis, A. W., Bunn, H. F., Turner, P. H., Gopal, T. V., Nash, W. G., O'Brien, S. J., and Scherr, C. J., 1985, Expression of the human c-fms proto-oncogene in hematopoietic cells and its deletion in the 5q- syndrome, *Cell* 42:421–426.

28. Le Beau, M. M., Westbrook, C. A., Diaz, M. O., Larson, R. A., Rowley, J. D., Gasson, J. C., Golde, D. W., and Sherr, C. J., 1986, Evidence for the involvement of GM-CSF and fms in the deletion (5q) in myeloid disorders, *Science* 231:984–987.

29. Sherr, C. J., Rettenmier, C. W., Sacca, R., Roussel, M. F., Look, A. T., and Stanley, E. R., 1985, The c-fms proto-oncogene product is related to the receptor for the mononuclear phagocyte growth factor, CSF-1, *Cell* 41:665–676.

30. Chang, E. H., Gonda, M. A., Ellis, R. W., Scolnick, E. M., and Lowy, D. R., 1982, Human genome contains four genes homologous to transforming genes of Harvey and Kirsten murine sarcoma viruses, *Proc. Natl. Acad. Sci. USA* 79:4848–4852.

31. Hall, A., Marshall, C. J., Spurr, N. K., and Weiss, R. A., 1983, Identification of transforming gene in two human sarcoma cell lines as a new member of the ras gene family located on chromosome 1, *Nature (Lond.)* 303:396–400.

32. Taparowsky, E., Shimizu, K., Goldfarb, M., and Wigler, M., 1983, Structure and activation of the human N-ras gene, *Cell* 34:581–586.

33. Scolnick, E. M., Papageorge, A. G., and Shih, T. Y., 1979, Guanine nucleotide-binding activity as an assay for src protein of rat-derived murine sarcoma viruses, *Proc. Natl. Acad. Sci. USA* 76:5355–5359.

34. Papageorge, A., Lowy, D., and Scolnick, E. M., 1982, Comparative biochemical properties of p21 ras molecules coded for by viral and cellular ras genes, *J. Virol.* 44:509–519.

35. Manne, V., Yamazaki, S., and Kung, H., 1984, Guanosine nucleotide binding by highly purified Ha-ras-encoded p21 protein produced in *Escherichia coli*, *Proc. Natl. Acad. Sci. USA* 81:6953–6957.

36. Sweet, R., Yokoyama, S., Kamata, T., Feramisco, J. R., Rosenberg, M., and Gross, M., 1984, The product of ras is a GTPase and the T24 oncogenic mutant is deficient in this activity, *Nature (Lond.)* 311:273–275.

37. Gilman, A. G., 1984, G proteins and dual control of adenylate cyclase, *Cell* 36:577–579.

38. Hurley, J. B., Simon, M. I., Teplow, D. B., Robishaw, J. D., and Gilman, A. G., 1984, Homologies between signal transducing G proteins and ras gene products, *Science* 226:860–862.

39. Mulcahy, L. S., Smith, M. R., and Stacey, D. W., 1985, Requirement for ras proto-oncogene function during serum-stimulated growth of NIH 3T3 cells, *Nature (Lond.)* 318:241–243.

40. Smith, M. R., DeGudicibus, S. J., and Stacey, D. W., 1986, Requirement for c-ras proteins during viral oncogene transformation, *Nature (Lond.)* 320:540–543.

41. Fleischman, L. F., Chahwala, S. B., and Cantley, L., 1986, Ras-transformed cells: Altered levels of phosphatidylinositol-4,5-bisphosphate and catabolites, *Science* 231:407–410.

42. Wolfman, A., and Macara, I. G., Elevated levels of diacylglycerol and decreased phorbol ester sensitivity in ras-transformed fibroblasts, *Nature (Lond.)* 325:359–361.

43. Parker, R. C., Varmus, H. E., and Bishop, J. M., 1981, Cellular homologue (c-src) of the transforming

gene of Rous sarcoma virus: Isolation, mapping, and transcriptional analysis of c-src and flanking regions, *Proc. Natl. Acad. Sci. USA* **78**:5842–5846.

44. Bonner, T. I., Oppermann, H., Seeburg, P., Kerby, S. B., Gunnell, M. A., Young, A. C., and Rapp, U. R., 1986, The complete nucleotide sequence of the human raf oncogene and the corresponding structure of the c-raf-1 gene, *Nucleic Acids Res.* **14**:1009–1015.

45. Moelling, K., Heimann, B., Beimling, P., Rapp, U. R., and Sander, T., 1984, Serine- and threonine-specific protein kinase activities of purified gag-mil and gag-raf proteins, *Nature (Lond.)* **312**:558–561.

46. Chen, W. T., Chen, J. M., Parsons, S. J., and Parsons, J. T., 1985, Local degradation of fibronectin at sites of expression of the transforming gene product pp60src, *Nature (Lond.)* **316**:156–158.

47. Hamaguchi, M., and Hanafusa, H., 1987, Association of p60src with Triton X-100 resistant cellular structure correlates with morphological transformation, *Proc. Natl. Acad. Sci. USA* **84**:2312–2316.

48. Dalla Favera, R., Gelmann, E. P., Martinotti, S., Franchini, G., Papas, T. S., Gallo, R. C., and Wong-Staal, F., 1982, Cloning and characterization of different human sequences related to the onc gene (v-myc) of avian myelocytomatosis virus (MC29), *Proc. Natl. Acad. Sci. USA* **79**:6497–6501.

49. Watt, R., Stanton, L. W., Marcu, K. B., Gallo, R. C., Croce, C. M., and Rovera, G., 1983, Nucleotide sequence of cloned cDNA of human c-myc oncogene, *Nature (Lond.)* **303**:725–728.

50. Alitalo, K., Ramsay, G., Bishop, J. M., Pfeifer, S. O., Colby, W. W., and Levinson, A. D., 1983, Identification of nuclear proteins encoded by viral and cellular myc genes, *Nature (Lond.)* **306**:274–277.

51. Straaten, F., Muller, R., Curran, T., Beveren, C. V., and Verma, I. M., 1983, Complete nucleotide sequence of a human c-onc gene: Deduced amino acid sequence of the human c-fos protein, *Proc. Natl. Acad. Sci. USA* **80**:3183–3187.

52. Sambucetti, L. C., and Curran, T., 1986, The fos protein complex is associated with DNA in isolated nuclei and binds to DNA cellulose, *Science* **234**:1417–1419.

53. Leprince, D., Saule, S., de Taisne, C., Gegonne, A., Begue, A., Righi, M., and Stehelin, D., 1983, The human DNA locus related to the oncogene myb of avian myeloblastosis virus (AMV): Molecular cloning and structural characterization, *EMBO J.* **2**:1073–1078.

54. Slamon, D. J., Boone, T. C., Murdock, D. C., Keith, D. E., Press, M. F., Larson, R. A., and Souza, L. M., 1986, Studies of the human c-myb gene and its product in human acute leukemias, *Science* **233**:347–351.

55. Majello, B., Kenyon, L. C., and Dalla Favera, R., 1986, Human c-myb protooncogene: Nucleotide sequence of cDNA and organization of the genomic locus, *Proc. Natl. Acad. Sci. USA* **83**:9636–9640.

56. Boyle, W. J., Lampert, M. A., Li, A. C., and Baluda, M. A., 1985, Nuclear compartmentalization of the v-myb oncogene product, *Mol. Cell. Biol.* **5**:3017–3023.

57. Studzinski, G. P., Brelvi, Z. S., Feldman, S. C., and Watt, R. A., 1986, Participation of c-myc protein in DNA synthesis of human cells, *Science* **234**:467–470.

58. Ishikura, H., Honma, Y., Honma, C., Hozumi, M., Black, J. D., Kieber-Emmons, T., and Bloch, A., 1987, Inhibition of messenger RNA transcriptional activity in ML-1 human myeloblastic leukemia cell nuclei by antiserum to a c-myb-specific peptide, *Cancer Res.* **47**:1052–1057.

59. Gilman, M. Z., Wilson, R. N., and Weinberg, R. A., 1986, Multiple protein binding sites in the 5′-flanking region regulate c-fos expression, *Mol. Cell. Biol.* **6**:4305–4316.

60. Holt, J. T., Venkat Gopal, T., Moulton, A. D., and Nienhuis, A. W., 1986, Inducible production of c-fos antisense RNA inhibits 3T3 cell proliferation, *Proc. Natl. Acad. Sci. USA* **83**:4794–4798.

60a. Aaronson, S. A., and Tronick, S. R., 1987, Oncogenes, in: *Medical Genetics: 1987* (D. Camerini-Otero, J. J. Mulvihill, and A. N. Schechter, eds.), pp. 101–132, Foundation for Advanced Education in the Sciences, Bethesda, Maryland.

61. Groudine, M., and Weintraub, H., 1980, Activation of cellular genes by avian RNA tumor viruses, *Proc. Natl. Acad. Sci. USA* **77**:5351–5354.

62. Neel, B. J., Hayward, W. S., Robinson, H. L., Fang, J., and Astrin, S. M., 1981, Avian leukosis virus-induced tumors have common proviral integration sites and synthesize discrete new RNAs: Oncogenesis by promoter insertion, *Cell* **23**:323–334.

63. Hayward, W. S., Neel, B. G., and Astrin, S. M., 1981, Activation of a cellular onc gene by promoter insertion in ALV-induced lymphoid leukosis, *Nature (Lond.)* **290**:475–480.

64. Fung, Y. K. T., Fadly, A. M., Crittenden, L. B., and Kung, H. J., 1981, On the mechanism of retrovirus-induced avian lymphoid leukosis: Deletion and integration of the proviruses, *Proc. Natl. Acad. Sci. USA* **78**:3418–3422.

65. Raines, M. A., Lewis, W. G., Crittenden, L. B., and Kung, H. J., 1985, c-erbB activation in avian leukosis virus-induced erythroblastosis: Clustered integration sites and the arrangement of provirus in the c-erbB alleles, *Proc. Natl. Acad. Sci. USA* **82**:2287–2291.

66. Nusse, R., and Varmus, H. E., 1982, Many tumors induced by the mouse mammary tumor virus contain a provirus integrated in the same region of the host genome, *Cell* **31**:99–109.

67. Dickson, C., Smith, R., Brookes, S., and Peters, G., 1984, Tumorigenesis by mouse mammary tumor virus: Proviral activation of a cellular gene in the common integration region int-2, *Cell* **37**:529–536.

68. van Ooyen, A., and Nusse, R., 1984, Structure and nucleotide sequence of the putative mammary oncogene int-1; Proviral insertions leave the protein-encoding domain intact, *Cell* **39**:233–240.

69. Rhodewohld, H., Weiher, H., Reik, W., Jaenisch, R., and Breindl, M., 1987, Retrovirus integration and chromatin structure: Moloney murine leukemia proviral integration sites map near DNase I-hypersensitive sites, *J. Virol.* **61**:336–343.

70. Shih, C., Shilo, B. Z., Goldfarb, M. P., Dannenberg, A., and Weinberg, R. A., 1979, Passage of phenotypes of chemically transformed cells via transfection of DNA and chromatin, *Proc. Natl. Acad. Sci. USA* **76**:5714–5718.

71. Blair, D. G., Cooper, C. S., Oskarsson, M. K., Eader, L. A., and Vande Woude, G., 1982, New method for detecting cellular transforming genes, *Science* **218**:1122–1125.

72. Shih, C., Padhy, L. C., Murray, M., and Weinberg, R. A., 1981, Transforming genes of carcinomas and neuroblastomas introduced into mouse fibroblasts, *Nature (Lond.)* **290**:261–264.

73. Krontiris, T. G., and Cooper, G. M., 1981, Transforming activity of human tumor DNAs, *Proc. Natl. Acad. Sci. USA* **78**:1181–1184.

74. Murray, M. J., Shilo, B. Z., Shih, C., Cowing, D., Hsu, H. W., and Weinberg, R. A., 1981, Three different human tumor cell lines contain different oncogenes, *Cell* **25**:355–361.

75. Perucho, M., Goldfarb, M., Shimizu, K., Lama, C., Fogh, J., and Wigler, M., 1981, Human tumor derived cell lines contain common and different transforming genes, *Cell* **27**:467–476.

76. Goldfarb, M., Shimizu, K., Perucho, M., and Wigler, M., 1982, Isolation and preliminary characterization of a human transforming gene from T24 bladder carcinoma cells, *Nature (Lond.)* **296**:404–409.

77. Parada, L. F., Tabin, C. J., Shih, C., and Weinberg, R. A., 1982, Human EJ bladder carcinoma oncogene is homologue of Harvey sarcoma virus ras gene, *Nature (Lond.)* **297**:474–478.

78. Taparowsky, E., Suard, Y., Fasano, O., Shimizu, K., Goldfarb, M., and Wigler, M., 1982, Activation of the T24 bladder carcinoma transforming gene is linked to a single amino acid change, *Nature (Lond.)* **300**:762–765.

79. Shimizu, K., Birnbaum, D., Ruley, M. A., Fasano, O., Suard, Y., Edlund, L., Taparowsky, E., Goldfarb, M., and Wigler, M., 1983, Structure of the Ki-ras gene of the human lung carcinoma cell line Calu-1, *Nature (Lond.)* **304**:497–500.

80. Capon, D. J., Seeburg, P. H., McGrath, J. P., Hayflick, J. S., Edman, U., Levinson, A. D., and Goeddel, D. V., 1983, Activation of Ki-ras2 gene in human colon and lung carcinomas by two different point mutations, *Nature (Lond.)* **304**:507–513.

81. Sukumar, S., Notario, V., Martin-Zanca, D., and Barbacid, M., 1983, Induction of mammary carcinomas in rats by nitrosomethylurea involves malignant activation of H-ras-1 locus by single point mutations, *Nature (Lond.)* **306**:658–661.

82. Taparowsky, E., Shimizu, K., Goldfarb, M., and Wigler, M., 1983, Structure and activation of the human N-ras gene, *Cell* **34**:581–586.

83. Yuasa, Y., Gol, R. A., Chang, A., Chiu, I. M., Reddy, E. P., Tronick, S. R., and Aaronson, S. A., 1984, Mechanism of activation of an N-ras oncogene of SW-1271 human lung carcinoma cells, *Proc. Natl. Acad. Sci. USA* **81**:3670–3674.

84. Santos, E., Martin-Zanca, D., Reddy, E. P., Pierotti, M. A., Porta, G. D., and Barbacid, M., Malignant activation of a K-ras oncogene in lung carcinoma but not in normal tissue of the same patient, *Science* **223**:661–664.

85. Kraus, M., Yuasa, Y., and Aaronson, S. A., 1984, A position 12-activated H-ras oncogene in all HS578T mammary carcinosarcoma cells but not normal mammary cells of the same patient, *Proc. Natl. Acad. Sci. USA* **81**:5384–5388.

86. McGrath, J. P., Capon, D. J., Goeddel, D. V., and Levinson, A. D., Comparative biochemical properties of normal and activated human ras p21 protein. *Nature (Lond.)* **310**:644–649.

87. Srivastava, S. K., Yuasa, Y., Reynolds, S. H., and Aaronson, S. A., 1985, Effects of two major activating lesions on the structure and conformation of human ras oncogene products, *Proc. Natl. Acad. Sci. USA* **82**:38–42.

88. Barbacid, M., 1987, ras Genes, *Annu. Rev. Biochem.* **56**:779–827.

89. Bos, J. L., Fearon, E. R., Hamilton, S. R., Verlaan-de Vries, M., van Boom, J. H., van der Eb, A. J., and Vogelstein, B., Prevalence of ras gene mutuations in human colorectal cancers, *Nature (Lond.)* **327**:293–297.

90. Forrester, K., Almoguera, C., Han, K., Grizzle, W. E., and Perucho, M., Detection of high incidence of K-ras oncogenes during human colon tumorigenesis, *Nature (Lond.)* **327**:298–303.

91. Alitalo, K., and Schwab, M., 1986, Oncogene amplification in tumor cells, *Adv. Cancer Res.* **47**:235–281.

92. Biedler, J. L., Henson, L., and Spengler, B. A., 1973, Morphology and growth, tumorigenicity, and cytogenetics of human neuroblastoma cells in continuous culture, *Cancer Res.* **33**:2643–2652.

93. Biedler, J. L., and Spengler, B. A., 1976, Metaphase chromosome anomaly: Association with drug resistance and cell-specific products, *Science* **191**:185–187.

94. Sandberg, A. A., Sakurai, M., Holdsworth, R. N., 1972, Chromosomes and causation of human cancer and leukemia I: DMS chromosomes in a neuroblastoma, *Cancer* **29**:1671–1678.

95. Westin, E. H., Wong-Staal, F., Gelmann, E. P., Dalla Favera, R., Papas, T. S., Lautenberger, J. A., Eva, A., Reddy, E. P., Tronick, S. R., Aaronson, S. A., and Gallo, R. C., 1982, Expression of the cellular homologues of retroviral onc genes in human hematopoietic cells, *Proc. Natl. Acad. Sci. USA* **79**:2490–2494.

96. Collins, S., and Groudine, M., 1982, Amplification of endogenous myc related DNA sequences in a human myeloid leukemia cell line, *Nature (Lond.)* **298**:679–681.

97. Dalla Favera, R., Wong-Staal, F., and Gallo, R. C., 1982, Onc gene amplification in promyelocytic leukemia cell line HL-60 and primary leukemic cells of the same patient, *Nature (Lond.)* **299**:61–63.

98. Alitalo, K., Schwab, M., Lin, C. C., Varmus, H. E., and Bishop, J. M., 1983, Homogeneously staining chromosomal regions contain amplified copies of an abundantly expressed cellular oncogene (c-myc) in malignant neuroendocrine cells from a human colon carcinoma, *Proc. Natl. Acad. Sci. USA* **80**:1707–1711.

99. Little, C. D., Nau, M. M., Carney, D. N., Gazdar, A. F., and Minna, J. D., 1983, Amplification and expression of the c-myc oncogene in human lung cancer cell lines, *Nature (Lond.)* **306**:194–196.

100. Schwab, M., Alitalo, K., Klempnauer, K. H., Varmus, H. E., Bishop, J. M., Gilbert, F., Brodeur, G., Goldstein, M., and Trent, J., 1983, Amplified DNA with limited homology to myc cellular oncogene is shared by human neuroblastoma cell lines and a neuroblastoma tumour, *Nature (Lond.)* **305**:245–248.

101. Kohl, N. E., Legouy, E., DePinho, R. A., Nisen, P. D., Smith, R. K., Gee, C. E., and Alt, F. W., 1986, Human N-myc is closely related in organization and nucleotide sequence to c-myc, *Nature (Lond.)* **319**:73–77.

102. Brodeur, G. M., Seeger, R. C., Schwab, M., Varmus, H. E., and Bishop, J. M., 1984, Amplification of N-myc in untreated human neuroblastomas correlate with advanced disease stage, *Science* **224**:1121–1124.

103. Schwab, M., Ellison, J., Busch, M., Rosenau, W., Varmus, H. E., and Bishop, J. M., 1984, Enhanced expression of the human gene N-myc consequent to amplification of DNA may contribute to malignant progression of neuroblastoma, *Proc. Natl. Acad. Sci. USA* **81**:4940–4944.

104. Collins, S. J., and Groudine, M., 1983, Rearrangement and amplification of c-abl sequences in the human chronic myelogenous leukemia cell line K-562, *Proc. Natl. Acad. Sci. USA* **80**:4813–4817.

105. Libermann, T. A., Nusbaum, H. R., Razon, N., Kris, R., Laz, I., Soreg, H., Whittle, N., Waterfield, M. D., Ullrich, A., and Schlessinger, J., 1985, Amplification, enhanced expression and possible rearrangement of EGF receptor gene in primary human brain tumours of glial origin, *Nature (Lond.)* **313**:144–147.

106. King, C. R., Kraus, M. H., Williams, L. T., Merlino, G. T., Pastan, I. H., and Aaronson, S. A., 1985, Human tumor cell lines with EGF receptor gene amplification in the absence of aberrant sized mRNAs, *Nucleic Acids Res.* **13**:8477–8486.

107. Akiyama, T., Sudo, C., Ogawara, H., Toyoshima, K., and Yamamoto, T., 1986, The product of the human c-erb B-2 gene: A 185-kilodalton glycoprotein with tyrosine kinase activity, *Science* **232**:1644–1646.

108. Yamamoto, T., Ikawa, S., Akiyama, T., Semba, K., Nomura, N., Miyajima, N., Saito, T., and Toyoshima, K., 1986, Similarity of protein encoded by the human c-erbB-2 gene to epidermal growth factor receptor, *Nature (Lond.)* **319**:230–234.

109. Kraus, M. H., Popescu, N. C., Amsbaugh, S. C., and King, C. R., 1987, Overexpression of the EGF receptor-related proto-oncogene erbB-2 in human mammary tumor cell lines by different molecular mechanisms, *EMBO J.* **6**:605–610.

110. van de Vijver, M., van de Bersselaar, R., Devilee, P., Cornelisse, C., Peterse, J., and Nusse, R., 1987, Amplification of the neu (c-erbB-2) oncogene in human mammary tumors is relatively frequent and is often accompanied by amplification of the linked c-erbA oncogene, *Mol. Cell. Biol.* **7**:2019–2023.

111. Slamon, D. J., Clarke, G. M., Wong, S. G., Levin, W. J., Ullrich, A., and McGuire, W. L., 1987,

Human breast cancer: Correlation of relapse and survival with amplification of the HER-2/neu oncogene, *Science* **235**:177–182.

112. Nau, M. M., Brooks, B. J., Battey, J., Sausville, E., Gazdar, A. F., Kirsch, I. R., McBride, O. W., Bertness, V., Hollis, G. F., and Minna, J. D., 1985, L-myc, a new myc-related gene amplified and expressed in human small cell lung cancer, *Nature (Lond.)* **318**:69–73.

113. Yunis, J. J., 1983, The chromosomal basis of human neoplasia, *Science* **221**:227–236.

114. Dalla Favera, R., Bregni, M., Erikson, J., Patterson, D., Gallo, R. C., and Croce, C. M., 1982, Human c-myc onc gene is located on the region of chromosome 8 that is translocated in Burkitt lymphoma cells, *Proc. Natl. Acad. Sci. USA* **79**:7824–7827.

115. Hayday, A. C., Gillies, S. D., Saito, H., Wood, C., Wiman, K., Hayward, W. S., and Tonegawa, S., 1984, Activation of a translocated human c-myc gene by an enhancer in the immunoglobulin heavy-chain locus, *Nature (Lond.)* **307**:334–340.

116. Showe, L. C., Moore, R. C., Erikson, J., and Croce, C. M., 1987, MYC oncogene involved in a t(8;22) chromosome translocation is not altered in its putative regulatory regions, *Proc. Natl. Acad. Sci. USA* **84**:2824–2828.

117. ar-Rushdi, A., Nishikura, K., Erikson, J., Watt, R., Rovera, G., and Croce, C. M., 1983, Differential expression of the translocated and the untranslocated c-myc oncogene in Burkitt lymphoma, *Science* **222**:390–393.

118. Davis, M., Malcolm, S., and Rabbitts, T. H., 1984, Chromosome translocation can occur on either side of the c-myc oncogene in Burkitt lymphoma cells, *Nature (Lond.)* **308**:286–288.

119. Lanfrancone, L., Pelicci, P. G., and Dalla Favera, R., 1986, Structure and expression of translocated c-myc oncogenes: Specific differences in endemic, sporadic and AIDS-associated forms of Burkitt lymphomas, *Curr. Topics Microbiol. Immunol.* **125**:257–265.

120. Rabbitts, T. H., Hamlyn, P. H., and Baer, R., 1983, Altered nucleotide sequences of a translocated c-myc gene in Burkitt lymphoma, *Nature (Lond.)* **306**:760–765.

121. Murphy, W., Sarid, J., Taub, R., Vasicek, T., Battey, J., Lenoir, G., and Leder, P., 1986, A translocated human c-myc oncogene is altered in a conserved coding sequence, *Proc. Natl. Acad. Sci. USA* **83**:2939–2943.

122. Pelicci, P. G., Knowles, D. M., Magrath, I., and Dalla Favera, R., 1986, Chromosomal breakpoints and structural alterations of the c-myc locus differ in endemic and sporadic forms of Burkitt lymphoma, *Proc. Natl. Acad. Sci. USA* **83**:2984–2988.

123. Lombardi, L., Newcomb, E. W., and Dalla Favera, R., 1987, Pathogenesis of Burkitt lymphoma: Expression of an activated c-myc oncogene causes the tumorigenic conversion of EBV-infected human B lymphoblasts, *Cell* **49**:161–170.

124. Adams, J. M., Harris, A. W., Pinkert, C. A., Corcoran, L. M., Alexander, W. S., Cory, S., Palmiter, R. D., and Brinster, R. L., 1985, The c-myc oncogene driven by immunoglobulin enhancers induces lymphoid malignancy in transgenic mice, *Nature (Lond.)* **318**:533–538.

125. De Klein, A., van Kessel, A. G., Grosvelg, G., Bartram, C. R., Hagemeiger, A., Bootsma, D., Spurr, N. K., Heisterkamp, N., Groffen, N., and Stephenson, J. R., 1982, A cellular oncogene is translocated to the Philadelphia chromosome in chronic myelocytic leukemia, *Nature (Lond.)* **300**:765–767.

126. Shtivelman, E., Lifshitz, B., Gale, R. P., and Canaani, E., 1985, Fused transcript of abl and bcr genes in chronic myelogenous leukaemia, *Nature (Lond.)* **315**:550–554.

127. Davis, R. L., Konopka, J. B., and Witte, O. N., 1985, Activation of the c-abl oncogene by viral transduction or chromosomal translocation generates altered c-abl proteins with similar in vitro kinase properties, *Mol. Cell. Biol.* **5**:204–213.

128. Sacchi, N., Watson, D. K., van Kessel, A. H. M., Hagemeijer, A., Kersey, J., Drabkin, H. D., Patterson, D., and Papas, T. S., 1986, Hu-ets-1 and Hu-ets-2 genes are transposed in acute leukemias with (4;11) and (8;21) translocations, *Science* **231**:379–382.

129. Diaz, M. O., Le Beau, M. M., Pitha, P., and Rowley, J. D., 1986, Interferon and c-ets-1 genes in the translocation (9;11)(p22;q23) in human acute monocytic leukemia, *Science* **231**:265–267.

130. Land, H., Parada, L. F., and Weinberg, R. A., 1983, Tumorigenic conversion of primary embryo fibroblasts requires at least two cooperating oncogenes, *Nature (Lond.)* **304**:596–602.

131. Ruley, H. E., 1983, Adenovirus early region 1A enables viral and cellular transforming genes to transform primary cells in culture, *Nature (Lond.)* **304**:602–606.

132. Stewart, T. A., Pattengale, P. K., and Leder, P., 1984, Spontaneous mammary adenocarcinomas in transgenic mice that carry and express MTV/myc fusion genes, *Cell* **38**:627–637.

133. Brown, K., Quintanilla, M., Ramsden, M., Kerr, I. B., Young, S., and Balmain, A., 1986, v-ras Genes from Harvey and BALB murine sarcoma viruses can act as initiators of two-stage mouse skin carcinogenesis, *Cell* **46**:447–456.

# 14

# Activation of Oncogenes by Chemical Carcinogens

## Marshall W. Anderson and Steven H. Reynolds

## 1. INTRODUCTION

Increasing evidence suggests that a small set of cellular genes appear to be targets for genetic alterations that contribute to the neoplastic transformation of cells. These genes, termed proto-oncogenes, appear to play a crucial role in normal cellular growth or differentiation since they are highly conserved in nature, being detected in species as divergent as yeast, *Drosophila,* and humans. Recent identification of a number of these genes as encoding for putative growth factors (*sis, hst, int-2*), growth factor receptors (*neu, erb B, fms*), proteins involved in the regulation of transmembrane signal transduction (*ras*), nuclear regulatory proteins (*myc, myb, fos, jun*), tyrosine kinases (*src*) and serine/threonine kinases (*raf, mos*) has served to substantiate this idea.

The proto-oncogenes were initially discovered as the transduced oncogenes of acute transforming retroviruses.[1-4] Retroviral transduction has been shown to result in the acquisition of point mutations, deletions, or gene fusions within the coding sequences of the transduced proto-oncogenes.[2,3] These types of genetic damage are thought to interfere with the normal functions of the proto-oncogenes by a variety of mechanisms such as the alteration of enzymatic activities or substrates and changes in subcellular localizations or levels and schedules of expression of their protein products.[1-4] Retroviruses are also able to affect the expression of proto-oncogenes via insertional mutagenesis. In these instances the retroviral DNA integrates into the host cell DNA adjacent to or within the coding sequence of a proto-oncogene and the retroviral promoters then drive transcription of the normal or truncated gene product.[5]

Recent studies have established that proto-oncogenes can also be activated as oncogenes by mechanisms independent of retroviral involvement. These mechanisms include point mutations or gross DNA rearrangements such as translocation or gene amplification.[2,5] The activation of proto-oncogenes by these types of genetic alterations results in altered levels or schedules of expression of the normal protein product, or in normal or altered levels of expression of an abnormal protein.

The activation of proto-oncogenes in spontaneous and chemically induced tumors has been studied in great detail during the past several years. Investigations in rodent models for chemical carcinogenesis imply that certain types of oncogenes are activated by carcinogen treatment and that this activation process is an early event in tumor induction.[6-9] Alternatively, analysis of some human and rodent tumors suggests that oncogene activation is involved in neoplastic progres-

*Marshall W. Anderson and Steven H. Reynolds* • Laboratory of Biochemical Risk Analysis, National Institute of Environmental Health Sciences, Research Triangle Park, North Carolina 27709.

sion.[10-13] The number of proto-oncogenes that must be activated in the multistep process of neoplasia is also unclear at present. The concerted, low level expression of at least two oncogenes, *ras* and *myc*, is needed for the partial transformation of primary rodent cells *in vitro*.[14] Other *in vitro* experiments indicate that high level expression of a single oncogene, *ras*, is sufficient to transform primary rodent cells.[15] Furthermore, in addition to the activation of proto-oncogenes, the loss of specific regulatory functions such as tumor suppressor genes may be a distinct step in neoplastic transformation.[16]

## 2. ACTIVATION OF PROTO-ONCOGENES BY GENE AMPLIFICATION AND CHROMOSOMAL TRANSLOCATION

The induction of aberrant expression of proto-oncogenes by gene amplification or chromosomal translocation has been observed in a variety of human and rodent tumors (Tables I and II). Amplification of a proto-oncogene usually results in overexpression or deregulated cell-cycle expression of the affected gene. Elevated levels of proto-oncogene expression have also been noted when no apparent gene-amplification or chromosomal rearrangements were observed,[17,18] indicating that other, perhaps more subtle, types of mechanisms can also induce aberrant expression. One example listed in Table I involved the deletion of a region upstream from the c-*myb* locus, which resulted in increased c-*myb* messenger RNA (mRNA) levels.[19]

Proto-oncogene amplification is observed as both a low frequency event in diverse tumor types and as a high-frequency event in specific tumor types (Table I). From the available evidence, it appears as if proto-oncogene amplification is usually associated with neoplastic progression rather

#### Table I. Activation of Proto-Oncogenes by Gene Amplification[a]

| Gene | Tumor type[b] | Tumors showing gene involvement (%) | References |
|------|---------------|:---:|:---:|
| c-*myc*[c] | Breast carcinoma | 32 | 18 |
| c-*myc* | Uterine cervix carcinomas | >90 | 57 |
| c-*myc* | Epithelial tumors and sarcomas | 11–22 | 58 |
| c-*myc* | Morphologic variant cell lines from small cell lung cancer | 89[d] | 17 |
| N-*myc* | Cell lines from small cell lung cancer | — | 59 |
| L-*myc* | Small cell lung cancer and cell lines from small cell lung cancer | — | 60 |
| c-*myc* or N-*myc* | Small cell lung cancer | 11 | 61 |
| N-*myc* | Neuroblastoma | >50 | 10 |
| HER-2/*neu* | Breast carcinoma | 30 | 20,62 |
| | Salivary gland carcinoma | — | 63 |
| c-*myb* | Acute myelogenous leukemias | — | 64,65 |
| c-*myb*[e] | Leukemias and lymphomas | — | 19 |
| c-*myc*[f] | Rat skin tumors | 83 | 46 |
| c-H-*ras* | Mouse skin tumors | — | 42 |
| c-K-*ras* | Embryonal carcinomas | >50 | 66 |
| | Bladder carcinomas | 5 | 67 |

[a]Aberrant proto-oncogene expression was observed in all cases examined. Examples are also included when no gene amplification was observed but elevated levels of mRNA were detected.
[b]Human neoplasia except where noted.
[c]Some tumors showed elevated levels of mRNA, even though no gene amplification was observed.
[d]Seven of nine cell lines had c-*myc* amplification and one line had N-*myc* amplification.
[e]Elevated levels of mRNA resulted from a deletion upstream from the c-*myb* locus.
[f]Gene rearrangement was also observed in some of the tumors.

*Table II. Activation of Proto-Oncogenes by Chromosomal Translocations[a]*

| Gene | Tumor type[b] | Tumors showing gene involvement (%) | References |
|------|---------------|-------------------------------------|------------|
| c-*myc* | Burkitt lymphoma | >95 | 68–70 |
| c-*myc* | Murine plasmacytoma | >95 | 71–73 |
| c-*myc* | Acute T-cell leukemia | 10–20 | 74 |
| c-*myc* | Woodchuck hepatocellular carcinoma | 33 | 75 |
| bcl-1 | Chronic lymphocytic leukemia | 10–30 | 76 |
| bcl-2 | Follicular lymphoma | 85–95 | 24 |
| c-*abl* | Chronic myelogenous leukemia | >90 | 77 |
| c-*abl* | Acute lymphocytic leukemia | 10 | 78 |

[a]Translocation resulted in aberrant expression of the normal proto-oncogene, except for the c-*abl* translocation, which resulted in a hybrid c-*abl-bcr* protein product in chronic myelogenous leukemias and acute myelogenous leukemias and additional novel hybrids in acute myelogenous leukemias.
[b]Human neoplasia, except where noted.

than with the initiation of tumorigenesis (see also Chapter 10). For example, N-*myc* amplification correlates with the stage classification of neuroblastoma, and the degree of gene amplification is a better predictor of survival time than any other clinical data.[10,11] Similarly, the degree of *neu* amplification is inversely related to survival and time to relapse in women with breast cancer.[20]

Chromosome translocations have been shown to affect either the expression or enzymatic activity, or both, of proto-oncogenes. For instance, increased expression of c-*myc* is observed in Burkitt lymphoma and mouse plasmacytomas where c-*myc* is joined to various immunoglobulin genes (Table II). The mechanism of increased c-*myc* expression in these instances is not clear. The Philadelphia chromosome, found in over 90% of chronic myelogenous leukemias, creates a fusion protein where an undefined genetic locus termed *bcr* is joined to the tyrosine kinase domain of the c-*abl* protein (Table II). The enzymatic activity of the *bcr-abl* fusion protein is substantially higher than that of the normal c-*abl* protein,[21] but the effect of the fusion on gene expression is unclear.[22,23] Chromosome translocations may also elucidate the presence and chromosomal location of unknown putative oncogenes. *Bcl*-1 and *bcl*-2 are loci frequently involved in chromosomal translocations of human leukemias (Table II). *Bcl*-2 has been cloned, and its protein products have been identified.[24] Other consistent chromosome translocations in human or rodent neoplasms may yield further putative oncogenes.

## 3. DETECTION OF ONCOGENES BY GENE TRANSFER (DNA TRANSFECTION ASSAY)

The NIH 3T3 cell line, derived from mouse embryo fibroblasts, is very efficient at the uptake and expression of exogenous DNA sequences. Shih *et al.*[25] were the first to show that DNA from carcinogen transformed cell lines could cause morphologic transformation of NIH 3T3 cells after DNA transfection. This morphologic transformation was further characterized by an increase in refractility of the transformed cells and by their ability to exhibit anchorage-independent growth. Using this technique, other investigators were then able to demonstrate that oncogenes were present in a variety of human tumors and in carcinogen-induced animal tumors.

Members of the *ras* gene family were the first and most frequently activated proto-oncogenes detected by the NIH 3T3 transfection assay. H-, K-, and N-*ras* have been shown to acquire transforming activity by a single point mutation within their coding sequences, usually at codon 12, 13, or 61.[2] Early studies using the NIH 3T3 assay detected *ras* gene activation in only 10–20% of human tumors. However, more recent studies using site-directed DNA amplification in conjunction with oligonucleotide hybridization[26,27] and the RNase A mismatch cleavage method[28] have detected activated *ras* genes at a much higher frequency in some human tumor types (Table III). For example, Verlaan-deVries *et al.*[27] detected activated *ras* genes in 27% of the acute myeloid leukemias examined, and Bos *et al.*[26] and Forrester *et al.*[28] detected activated K-*ras* in 33–40% of human colon tumors. Other oncogenes have also been detected in human tumors by DNA transfection, including *lca*,[29] *hst*,[30] *trk*,[31] and a transforming gene in human thyroid carcinomas.[32] The prevalence of these non-*ras*-transforming genes in human tumors is unclear at present, but it appears that they occur much less frequently than do activated *ras* genes.

A variety of animal tumors derived from model systems have also been examined for oncogenes using the NIH 3T3 assay. These include spontaneous tumors in rats and mice, tumors that arise after single or multiple doses of carcinogen, and tumors that arise after long-term exposure to carcinogen. Examples of the detectable oncogenes in the different tumor model systems are shown in Table IV. As in human tumors, the majority of oncogenes detected in animal tumors are members of the *ras* gene family, but other classes of oncogenes do appear at low frequency (Table IV). One example is the *neu* oncogene found in nervous tissue tumors induced in rats by transplacental exposure to *N*-methyl-*N'*-nitrosourea (MNU)[33] or *N*-ethyl-*N'*-nitrosourea (ENU).[34] In both instances, the activation of the *neu* proto-oncogene occurred by a single point mutation in a region of the gene which encodes a putative transmembrane segment of the protein product. *Neu* and the *ras* genes are the only examples of activated proto-oncogenes detected in animal or human tumors where the demonstrated mechanism of activation was by point mutation. The non-*ras* transforming genes detected in rodent and human tumors by DNA transfection assays are presented in Table V. For most of these oncogenes, the mechanism of activation of the proto-oncogene is unknown.

The NIH 3T3 cell line has been frequently criticized as being limited in value for detection of various classes of oncogenes. NIH 3T3 cells appear to be refractory to morphologic transformation by nuclear oncogenes such as *myc*, and even some activating mutations in *ras* genes are unable to induce efficient morphologic transformation. Consequently, the nude mouse tumorigenicity assay, an extension of the NIH 3T3 transfection assay that affords greater sensitivity, was developed. This assay involves cotransfection of NIH 3T3 cells with tumor DNA and a selectable marker gene.[35]

## Table III.  Activated Oncogenes Detected in Human Tumors by DNA Transfection Assay[a]

| Tumor | Number positive/ number tested | Oncogene | Reference |
|---|---|---|---|
| Colon | 26/66 | K-*ras* (26),[b] N-*ras* (2)[c] | 28 |
| Colon | 11/27 | K-*ras* (10), N-*ras* (1) | 26 |
| Lung | 2/19 | K-*ras* (2) | 79 |
| Acute myeloid leukemia | 12/45 | N-*ras* (10), K-*ras* (2) | 80 |
| Bladder carcinoma | 3/38 | H-*ras* (3) | 67 |
| Squamous cell carcinoma | 4/6 | H-*ras* (4) | 37 |
| Myelodysplastic syndrome and acute myeloid leukemia[d] | 3/8 | N-*ras* (3) | 81 |
| Thyroid papillary carcinoma | 5/20 | Unknown (5) | 32 |
| Hepatocellular carcinoma | 2/11 | lca (2) | 29 |
| Stomach carcinoma | 3/58 | hst (3) | 30 |
|  | 1/3 | raf (1) | 82 |
| B-cell lymphoma | — | dbl | 83 |
| Colon carcinoma | — | trk | 31 |

[a]The basis for detection of the oncogenes listed in this table is the DNA transfection assay. Biochemical methods have enhanced the sensitivity to detect mutations in the *ras* genes.
[b]Numbers in parentheses indicate the number of positive samples with that oncogene.
[c]Two tumors contained both K-*ras* and N-*ras*.
[d]Activated N-*ras* was detected in DNA from bone marrow cells before patients developed acute myeloid leukemia.

Table IV. Activated Oncogenes Detected in Rodent Tumor Models by DNA Transfection Assay

| Model | Tumor | Number positive/ number tested | Oncogene | Reference |
|---|---|---|---|---|
| Spontaneous | Mouse liver tumor | 17/27 | H-ras (15),[a] raf (1), unknown (1) | 38,43 |
| | Rat tumors | 1/37 | H-ras (1) | 43.(S. W. Reynolds and M. W. Anderson, unpublished results) |
| | Mouse reticulum cell sarcoma | 3/3 | Unknown (3) | 84 |
| Single dose | | | | |
| MNU[b] | Rat mammary tumor | 61/71 | H-ras (61) | 40 |
| DMBA[b] | Rat mammary tumor | 6/29 | H-ras (6) | 8 |
| Single dose, neonatal | | | | |
| HO-AAF[b] | Mouse liver tumor | 10/10 | H-ras (10) | 50 |
| HO-DHE[b] | Mouse liver tumor | 11/11 | H-ras (10), K-ras (1) | 50 |
| VC[b] | Mouse liver tumor | 10/10 | H-ras (10) | 50 |
| DEN[b] | Mouse liver tumor | 14/33 | H-ras (14) | 89 |
| Multiple doses | | | | |
| DMN-OME[b] | Rat renal tumors | 11/35 | K-ras (10), N-ras (1) | 85 |
| Aflatoxin B$_1$ | Rat liver tumors | 10/11 | K-ras (2), unknown (8) | 86 |
| Continuous doses | | | | |
| TNM[b] | Rat and mouse lung tumors | 18/19,10/10 | H-ras (18), K-ras (10) | 49 |
| Furan | Mouse liver tumor | 13/29 | H-ras (10), raf (1), K-ras (2) | 38 |
| Furfural | Mouse liver tumor | 13/16 | H-ras (9), K-ras (1), unknown (3) | 38 |
| Benzidine-derived dyes | Rat tumors[c] | 34/58 | H-ras (31), N-ras (3) | (S. W. Reynolds and M. W. Anderson, unpublished results) |
| DEN | Rat liver tumors | 1/12 | Unknown | 89 |
| DMBA | Mouse skin tumors | 4/4 | H-ras (3), unknown (1) | 9 |

(continued)

## Table IV. (Continued)

| Model | Tumor | Number positive/ number tested | Oncogene | Reference |
|---|---|---|---|---|
| Initiation-promotion | | | | |
| DEN–Farber protocol | Rat liver tumors | 0/20 | — | 87 |
| Den + PB[b] | Rat liver tumors | 0/12 | — | 89 |
| DMBA + TPA[b] | Mouse skin tumors | 33/37 | H-ras | 51 |
| DB[c,h]ACR[b] + TPA | Mouse skin tumors | 6/6 | H-ras (5), unknown (1) | 9 |
| Transplacental dose | | | | |
| ENU[b] | Rat neuroblastomas | 3/3 | neu (3) | 33 |
| MNU | Rat schwannomas | 10/13 | neu (10) | 34 |
| Radiation | | | | |
| Gamma | Mouse lymphomas | 4/4 | K-ras | 7 |
| Ionizing | Rat skin tumors | 1/10 | K-ras | 46 |

[a]Numbers in parentheses indicate the number of positive samples with that oncogene.

[b]MNU, N-methyl-N'-nitrosourea; DMBA, 7,12-dimethylbenz(a)anthracene; HO-AAF, N-hydroxy-2-acetylaminofluorene; HO-DHE, 1'-hydroxy-2',3'-dehydroestragole; VC, vinyl carbamate; DEN, diethylnitrosamine; DMN-OME, methyl(methoxymethyl)nitrosamine; TNM, tetranitromethane; PB, phenobarbital; EE$_2$, ethynylestradiol; TPA, phorbol 12-myristate 13-acetate; DB[c,h]ACR, dibenz[c,h]acridine; ENU, N-ethyl-N'-nitrosourea.

[c]Benzidine derived dye-induced rat tumors include preputial gland tumors, squamous cell carcinomas, basal cell tumors, clitoral gland tumors, and mammary tumors.

Table V. Non-ras Oncogenes Detected in Human and Rodent Tumors
by DNA Transfection Assay

| Tumor | Treatment | Oncogene | | Reference |
|---|---|---|---|---|
| Neuroblastomas (R)[a] | N-Ethyl-N'-nitrosourea | neu | 33 | |
| Schwannomas (R) | N-Methyl-N'-nitrosourea | neu | 34 | |
| Stomach carcinomas (H) | — | hst | 30 | |
| | | raf | 82 | |
| Colon carcinomas (H) | — | trk | 31 | |
| Hepatocellular carcinomas (M) | Spontaneous | raf | 38 | |
| Hepatocellular carcinoma (H) | — | lca | 29 | |
| Hepatocellular carcinoma (R) | Aflatoxin $B_1$ | ? | 86 | |
| Hepatocellular carcinoma (M) | Spontaneous | ? | 38 | |
| Hepatocellular carcinomas (M) | Furfural | ? | 38 | |
| Pulmonary adenocarcinoma (M) | Spontaneous | ? | (U. Candrian, S. H. Reynolds and M. W. Anderson, unpublished results) | |
| Nasal squamous carcinomas (R) | Methylmethanesulfonate | ? | 88 | |
| Skin carcinoma (M) | 7,12-Dimethylbenz(a)anthracene | ? | 9 | |
| Skin carcinoma (M) | Dibenz[c,h]acridine | ? | 9 | |
| Thyroid carcinoma (H) | — | ? | 32 | |
| B-Cell lymphoma (H) | — | dbl | 83 | |
| Reticulum cell sarcoma (M) | — | ? | 84 | |

[a]Letters in parentheses ( ) indicate species in which tumors occur. R, rat; M, mouse; H, human.

The selected cell populations are then subcutaneously injected into immunocompromised mice, and tumor formation is monitored. The tumors that develop in the nude mice are then analyzed to characterize the transfected oncogene. The tumorigenicity assay provides an advantage for oncogene detection in that it is not dependent on morphologic transformation. Using this technique, Bos et al.[36] detected codon 13-activated N-ras genes in four of five human acute myeloid leukemias, and Ananthaswamy et al.[37] detected activated H-ras genes in four out of six human squamous cell carcinomas examined.

The identification of new classes of putative oncogenes, as well as the detection of novel mutations in ras genes,[36,38] should be enhanced by the extension of the NIH 3T3 transfection methodology to the nude mouse tumorigenicity assay and by development of recipient cell lines other than fibroblasts for gene-transfer assays.[39]

## 4. ACTIVATION OF PROTO-ONCOGENES BY CARCINOGENS

Studies in animal tumor model systems suggest that chemicals or radiation can activate a proto-oncogene by induction of a point mutation. Point mutations resulting in the activation of ras proto-oncogenes in several chemically induced rodent tumors have been consistent with the known alkylation patterns of the carcinogens. For example, the mutation at codon 12 of the H-ras gene detected in rat mammary tumors induced by MNU[40] is consistent with the formation of the O-6 methylguanine adduct. The activating mutation in codon 61 of the H-ras gene found in rat mammary tumors and mouse skin tumors induced by 7,12-dimethylbenz(a)anthracene (DMBA) is consistent with DMBA binding to adenosine residues.[41] Moreover, selectivity for activating mutations in ras oncogenes has been observed in chemical-induced tumors. For example, the GGT or GGA → GAT or GAA mutation observed in codon 12 of H-ras oncogenes detected in MNU-induced tumors is always at the second G of this codon, even though a similar mutation at the first G could also produce an activated ras oncogene. Another striking example of selectivity was observed in rat tumors induced by either dimethoxybenzidine or dimethylbenzidine. $GGC \rightarrow CGC$ transversions occurred in codon 13 of H-*ras* in dimethoxybenzidine-induced tumors, whereas $GGA \rightarrow GAA$ or $GGA \rightarrow AGA$ transitions were found in codon 12 of H-*ras* in dimethylbenzidine-induced tumors (S. H. Reynolds and M. W. Anderson, unpublished results). The slight change in structure shifted the selectivity for the activating mutation. Thus, in at least some cases, the *ras* oncogene observed in the tumor was a direct consequence of chemical-induced damage to the proto-oncogene.

Mutations in several codons of the *ras* oncogenes have been observed in primary tumors.[2,36,38] *In vitro* mutagenesis studies have shown that point mutations in codon 12, 13, 59, 63, 116, or 119 can also activate the *ras* proto-oncogene to a transforming gene. Our laboratory recently reported codon 117 mutations in H-*ras* detected in furan-induced mouse liver tumors.[38] Also, two K-*ras* and one H-*ras* oncogene with unknown mutations, but distinct from any of the known activating lesions, were detected in mouse liver tumors. Thus, numerous sites on this gene are possible targets for chemicals or radiation. If a sequence of specificity for the binding of a chemical to DNA corresponds to a biologically significant lesion in a proto-oncogene, then this chemical has the potential to be a very potent carcinogen.

Evidence in several animal studies suggests that activation of the *ras* proto-oncogene is an early event. The activated *ras* gene has been detected in many benign tumors, including mouse skin papillomas,[42] mouse lung and liver adenomas,[38,43,49] and basal cell and clitoral gland tumors of the rat (S. H. Reynolds and M. W. Anderson, unpublished results). This implies that the activated *ras* was present in the cell that clonally expanded to these benign tumors. In addition, it was recently shown that mouse epidermal cells infected *in vivo* with the viral H-*ras* gene can be promoted with TPA to form papillomas.[44] Thus, activation of the *ras* proto-oncogene may be the "initiation" event in some model systems. Moreover, dormant initiated cells with the activated *ras* gene can survive surrounded by normal cells until stimulated to proliferate by some endogenous or exogenous agent.

Activated *neu* oncogenes were detected in gliomas and schwannomas induced by ENU and MNU, respectively.[33,41] The activating mutation in each case was a $T \rightarrow A$ transversion in the transmembrane region of the *neu* proto-oncogene, which encodes a putative growth factor receptor. This mutation apparently alters the receptor specificity and/or receptor–ligand interactions such that cell transformation results.[45] The $T \rightarrow A$ mutation is not a consequence of a major premutagenic lesion of ENU or MNU. However, the mutation can be explained by $N^3$-alkylated adenines, a minor DNA adduct observed with these chemicals. Thus, activation of *neu* could be a direct consequence of the interaction of these chemicals with DNA.

Although gene amplification and chromosomal translocation have been observed in several types of human tumors, these activating mechanisms have not been extensively observed or studied in spontaneous or chemically induced rodent tumors. Sawey *et al.*[46] did observe c-*myc* gene amplification and restriction polymorphisms in addition to activated K-*ras* genes in rat skin tumors induced by ionizing radiation. Quintanilla *et al.*[42] suggested that amplification of the mutated H-*ras* gene may be involved in the progression of mouse skin papillomas to carcinomas. Further studies are required to determine the possible role of chemicals and radiation in the activation of proto-oncogenes by gene amplification, chromosomal translocation, or other mechanisms that can alter gene expression.

# 5. ONCOGENE ACTIVATION IN LONG-TERM RODENT CARCINOGENIC STUDIES

Determination of the origin of an activated oncogene detected in a rodent tumor generated by a long-term (i.e., 2 years) rodent carcinogenic study is often complicated by spontaneously occurring tumors. Species- and strain-specific spontaneously occurring tumors have been observed in rodents maintained under normal laboratory conditions.[47] For example, the B6C3F1 mouse hybrid exhibits a high incidence of spontaneous hepatocellular adenoma (10%) and carcinoma (21%) in males and a lower but significant incidence of adenoma (4%) and carcinoma (4%) in females. Moreover, activated *ras* oncogenes have been detected in a high percentage of these spontaneous mouse liver tumors.[43,48] More recently, our laboratory has detected oncogenes in spontaneous lung tumors of the B6C3F1 and A/J mice strains and in several other tumor types of the B6C3F1 mouse (U. Candrian, S. H. Reynolds, and M. W. Anderson, unpublished results). Initial attempts to identify oncogenes in spontaneous tumors of the Fischer 344 rat have been unsuccessful except for the detection of an activated H-*ras* in a clitoral gland carcinoma (S. H. Reynolds and M. W. Anderson, unpublished results). The presence of activated oncogenes in spontaneous tumors suggest that in some cases the chemical may not have directly activated the oncogenes detected in the chemical-induced tumors. The chemical may have increased the background tumor incidence by a mechanism such as cytotoxicity or receptor-mediated promotion.

Comparison of proto-oncogene activation between spontaneous and chemical-induced tumors may help determine the mechanism of tumor induction by the chemical. A recent study in our laboratory illustrates this approach.[38] Furan and furfural caused an increased incidence in mouse liver tumors in a 2-year carcinogenicity study. These compounds tested negative in *Salmonella* assays. Analysis of oncogene activation showed weakly activating mutations in the H-*ras* genes detected in the chemical-induced tumors.[38] Also, several activated K-*ras* genes were detected in the chemical-induced tumors. K-*ras* oncogenes have not been detected in spontaneous mouse liver tumors. More than 60% of the *ras* oncogenes detected in furan-induced tumors are distinct from those seen in spontaneous mouse liver tumors.[38] Thus, these chemicals appear to have caused an increase in mouse liver tumors at least in part by a genotoxic mechanism.

Another example in which the role of the chemical in oncogene activation is unclear is the activated K-*ras* oncogene detected in tetranitromethane (TNM)-induced rat and mice lung tumors. In a recent long-term carcinogenic study conducted by the National Toxicology Program, chronic exposure to TNM resulted in a high incidence of primary lung tumors in Fischer 344 rats and B6C3F1 mice.[49] K-*ras* oncogenes with a GGT $\rightarrow$ GAT mutation in codon 12 were observed in 18 of 19 rat lung tumors and 10 of 10 mouse lung tumors.[49] The activation of the K-*ras* oncogene in these TNM-induced lung tumors may be the result of one or more actions of the chemical:

1. A direct consequence of TNM-induced DNA damage
2. Spontaneously occurring
3. An enhancement of spontaneously occurring K-*ras* by TNM-induced cell replication
4. A combination of 1 and 3

It is possible that these activated K-*ras* oncogenes with GC $\rightarrow$ AT transitions in the second base of codon 12 are spontaneous, since an activated K-*ras* with the same mutation was observed in a spontaneously occurring pulmonary adenocarcinoma in the B6C3F1 mouse (U. Candrian *et al.*, unpublished results). Even though spontaneous lung tumors in the Fischer 344 rat are rare, it is still possible that TNM could have promoted cells which contain the activated K-*ras* or enhanced the spontaneously occurring K-*ras*. The reproducible detection of the K-*ras* in lung tumors of mice and rats suggests that TNM could have directly induced the mutation. In support of this conclusion, mutagenicity studies have shown that TNM causes mutant bacterial strains to revert to the wild type by the same GC $\rightarrow$ AT transition. Studies on the possible interactions of TNM with DNA are required to determine precisely the origin of the activated K-*ras* oncogenes in these TNM-induced lung tumors.

## 6. TISSUE- AND CARCINOGEN-SPECIFIC ACTIVATION OF PROTO-ONCOGENES

Selectivity for activation of a specific oncogene has been observed in some tissues. We will discuss this issue for the oncogenes detected by transfection since selectivity for activation by amplification and translocation is illustrated in Tables I and II, respectively. The H-*ras* oncogene has been frequently detected in mouse liver hepatocellular carcinomas,[38,43,50] mouse skin tumors,[51] and rat mammary tumors.[40,41] Activated K-*ras* has been observed in lung tumors of rats and mice[49] and in colon tumors of humans.[26,28] Activated N-*ras* has been observed in acute myeloid leukemias.[36]

Although a specific oncogene may be the most prevalent one observed in tumors arising from a cell type, other types of oncogenes are also observed in some cases. A good example is hepatocellular carcinomas. In addition to activated H-*ras*, activated K-*ras*, *raf*, and uncharacterized oncogenes have been detected in mouse liver tumors.[38] The *lca* oncogene was detected in several human liver tumors.[29] K-*ras* and uncharacterized oncogenes were observed in rat liver tumors.[52] Thus, numerous hepatocellular tumors are associated with the activation of different types of proto-oncogenes (see also Chapter 20).

The nature of the oncogene involved in tumor induction in a tissue may depend as much, or more, on the carcinogen than on the cell type. For example, thymic lymphomas induced by MNU contain predominantly activated N-*ras*,[53,54] whereas activated K-*ras* genes are observed in this tumor type when induced by radiation[7] or by methylcholanthrene.[55] However, it should be noted that a chemical can activate more than one type of oncogene in a specific tissue. This is illustrated by 3,3'-dimethoxybenzidine-induced tumors in the clitoral gland of rats. Both N-*ras* and H-*ras* were detected and several types of activating mutations were observed in the H-*ras* gene (S. H. Reynolds and M. W. Anderson, unpublished results). Thus, the type of proto-oncogene activated is a complex function of both the tissue type and the carcinogenic agent.

## 7. EXTRAPOLATION FROM RODENTS TO HUMANS

The transformation of a normal cell into a turmorigenic cell involves the activation and concerted expression of several proto-oncogenes as well as, perhaps, the inactivation of suppressor genes. The activation of *ras* proto-oncogenes represents one step in the multistep process of carcinogenesis for a variety of rodent and human tumors. This activation is probably an early event in tumorigenesis and may be the initiation event in some cases. Thus, a chemical that induces rodent tumors by activation of *ras* proto-oncogenes can potentially invoke one step of the neoplastic process in humans exposed to the chemical. Dominant transforming oncogenes other than *ras* have also been detected in chemically-induced rodent tumors (Table V). The involvement of these oncogenes in the development of human tumors is unclear at present, as well as whether the non-*ras* genes detected in human tumors (Tables I–III and V) can be activated by chemicals or radiation.

Most chemicals are classified as potentially hazardous to humans on the basis of long-term carcinogenesis studies in rodents. While these rodent carcinogenesis studies are often designed to mimic the route of human exposure in the environment or workplace, the dose of a given chemical is usually higher than that which actually occurs in human exposure. Coupled with the appearance of species- and strain-specific spontaneously occurring tumors in vehicle-treated rodents, this complicates the extrapolation of rodent carcinogenic data to human risk. Oncogene analysis of tumors from spontaneous origin and from long-term carcinogenesis studies should help determine the mechanisms of tumor formation at a molecular level. For instance, the finding of activating mutations in different codons of the H-*ras* gene in furan-induced liver tumors versus finding activating mutations in only one codon of the H-*ras* gene in spontaneous liver tumors suggest that the chemical itself activated the H-*ras* proto-oncogene by a genotoxic event.[38] In general, comparison of patterns of oncogene activation in spontaneous versus chemically induced rodent tumors, together with cytotoxic information, should be helpful in determining whether the chemical in question is mutagenic, cytotoxic, has a receptor-mediated mechanism of promotion, or some combination of these (and other) modes of action. This type of analysis might be of particular importance for compounds negative for mutagenicity on short-term tests but which are positive for carcinogenicity in long-term bioassays.[56] Species-to-species extrapolation of risk from carcinogenic data may become more reliable from examination of oncogene activation and expression. For example, K-*ras* oncogenes with the same activating lesion in codon 12 were observed in both rat and mouse lung tumors induced by tetranitromethane.[48] Although little is known about the DNA-damaging properties of this chemical, these data suggest that this compound is acting in the same manner to induce tumors in both rats and mice.

The role of chemicals and radiation in activating proto-oncogenes by gene amplification, chromosomal translocation, and other mechanisms capable of altering gene expression is currently being investigated by several groups. Also, as human life span increases, it becomes more important to study chemical-induced enhancement of the progression of benign to malignant tumors. These and similar approaches to explore the mechanisms by which chemicals induce tumors in animal model systems may remove some of the uncertainty in risk analysis of rodent carcinogenic data.

## REFERENCES

1. Land, H., Parada, L., and Weinberg, R. A., 1983, Cellular oncogenes and multistep carcinogenesis, *Science* **44**:771–778.
2. Varmus, H. E., 1984, The molecular genetics of cellular oncogenes, *Annu. Rev. Genet.* **18**:553–612.
3. Bishop, J. M., 1985, Viral oncogenes, *Cell* **42**:23–38.
4. Weinberg, R. A., 1985, The action of oncogenes in the cytoplasm and nucleus, *Science* **230**:770–776.
5. Bishop, J. M., 1987, The molecular genetics of cancer, *Science* **235**:305–311.
6. Balmain, A., Ramsden, M., Bowden, G. T., and Smith, J., 1984, Activation of the mouse cellular Harvey-*ras* gene in chemically induced benign skin papillomas, *Nature (Lond.)* **307**:658–660.
7. Guerrero, I., Villasante, A., Corces, V., and Pellicer, A., 1984, Activation of the c-K-*ras* oncogene by somatic mutation in mouse lymphomas induced by gamma radiation, *Science* **225**:1159–1162.
8. Zarbl, H., Sukumar, S., Arthur, A. V., Martin-Zanca, D., and Barbacid, M., 1985, Direct mutagenesis of H-*ras*-1 oncogenes by nitroso-methylurea during initiation of mammary carcinogenesis in rats, *Nature (Lond.)* **315**:382–385.
9. Bizub, D., Wood, A. W., and Skalka, A. M., 1986, Mutagenesis of the Ha-*ras* oncogene in mouse skin tumors induced by polycyclic aromatic hydrocarbons, *Proc. Natl. Acad. Sci. USA* **83**:6048–6052.
10. Brodeur, G. M., Seeger, R. C., Schwab, M., Varmus, H. E., and Bishop, J. M., 1984, Amplification of N-*myc* in untreated neuroblastomas correlates with advanced disease stage, *Science* **224**:1121–1124.
11. Seeger, R. C., Brodeur, G. M., Sather, H., Dalton, A., Siegel, S. E., Wong, K. Y., and Hammond, D., 1985, Association of multiple copies of the N-*myc* oncogene with rapid progression of neuroblasts, *N. Engl. J. Med.* **313**:1111–1116.
12. Vousden, K. H., and Marshall, C. J., 1984, Three different activated *ras* genes in mouse tumors; evidence for oncogene activation during progression of a mouse lymphoma, *EMBO J.* **3**:913–917.
13. Tainsky, M. A., Cooper, C. S., Giovanella, B. C., and Vande Woude, G. F., 1984, An activated N-*ras* gene: Detected in late but not early passage human PA1 teratocarcinoma cells, *Science* **225**:643–645.
14. Land, H., Parada, L. F., and Weinberg, R. A., 1983, Tumorigenic conversion of primary embryo fibroblasts requires at least two cooperating oncogenes, *Nature (Lond.)* **304**:596–602.
15. Spandidos, D. A., and Wilkie, N. M., 1984, Malignant transformation of early passage rodent cells by a single mutated oncogene, *Nature (Lond.)* **310**:469–475.
16. Barrett, J. C., Oshimura, M., and Koi, M., 1987, Role of oncogenes and tumor supressant genes in a multistep model of carcinogenesis, in: *Symposium on Fundamental Cancer Research*, Vol. 38 (F. Becker, ed.), pp. 45–56.
17. Gazdar, A. F., Carney, D. N., Nau, M. M., and Minna, J. D., 1985, Characterization of variant subclasses of cell lines derived from small cell lung cancer having distinctive biochemical, morphological, and growth properties, *Cancer Res.* **45**:2924–2930.
18. Escot, C., Theillet, C., Lidereau, R., Spyratos, F., Champema, M. H., Gest, J., and Callahan, R., 1986, Genetic alteration of the c-*myc* proto-oncogene (MYC) in human primary breast carcinomas, *Proc. Natl. Acad. Sci. USA* **83**:4834–4838.
19. Barletta, C., Pelicci, P-G., Kenyon, L. C., Smith, S. D., and Dalla-Favera, R., 1987, Relationship between the c-*myb* locus and the 6q-chromosomal aberration in leukemias and lymphomas, *Science* **235**:1064–1067.
20. Slamon, D. J., Clark, G. M., Wong, S. G., Levin, W. J., Ullrich, A., and McGuire, W. L., 1987, Human breast cancer: correlation of relapse and survival with amplification of the HER-2/*neu* oncogene, *Science* **235**:177–182.
21. Konopka, J. B., Watanabe, S. M., and Witte, O. N., 1984, An alteration of the human c-*abl* protein in K562 leukemia cells unmasks associated tyrosine kinase activity, *Cell* **37**:1035–1042.

22. Shtivelman, E., Lifshitz, B., Gale, R. P., and Canaani, E., 1985, Fused transcript of *abl* and *bcr* genes in chronic myelogenous leukaemia, *Nature (Lond.)* **315**:550–554.

23. Konopka, J. B., Clark, S., McLaughlin, J., Nitta, M., Kato, Y., Strife, A., Clarkson, B., and Witte, O. N., 1986, Variable expression of the translocated c-*abl* oncogene in Philadelphia-chromosome-positive B-lymphoid cell lines from chronic myelogenous leukemia patients, *Proc. Natl. Acad. Sci. USA* **83**:4049–4052.

24. Tsujimoto, Y., and Croce, C. M., 1986, Analysis of the structure, transcripts, and protein products of *bcl*-2, the gene involved in human follicular lymphoma, *Proc. Natl. Acad. Sci. USA* **83**:5214–5218.

25. Shih, C., Shilo, B., Goldfarb, M. P., Dannenberg, A., and Weinberg, R. A., 1979, Passage of phenotypes of chemically transformed cells via transfection of DNA and chromatin, *Proc. Natl. Acad. Sci. USA* **76**:5714–5718.

26. Bos, J. L., Fearon, E. R., Hamilton, S. R., Verlaan-deVries, M., van Boom, J. H., van der Eb, A. J., and Vogelstein, B., 1987, Prevalence of *ras* gene mutations in human colorectal cancers, *Nature (Lond.)* **327**:293–297.

27. Verlaan-deVries, M., Boggard, M., van den Elst, H., van Boom, J. H., van der Eb, A. J., and Bos, J. L., 1986, A dot-blot screening procedure for mutated *ras* oncogenes using synthetic oligonucleotides, *Gene* **50**:313–320.

28. Forrester, K., Almoguera, C., Han, K., Grizzle, W. E., and Perucho, M., 1987, Detection of high incidence of K-*ras* oncogenes during human colon tumorigenesis, *Nature (Lond.)* **327**:298–303.

29. Ochiya, T., Fujiyama, A., Fukushige, S., Hatada, I., and Matsubara, K., 1986, Molecular cloning of an oncogene from a human hepatocellular carcinoma, *Proc. Natl. Acad. Sci. USA* **83**:4993–4997.

30. Sakamoto, H., Mori, M., Taira, M., Yoshida, T., Matsukawa, S., Shimizu, K., Sekiguchi, M., Terada, M., and Sugimura, T., 1986, Transforming gene from human stomach cancers and a noncancerous portion of stomach mucosa, *Proc. Natl. Acad. Sci. USA* **83**:3997–4001.

31. Martin-Zanca, D., Hughes, S. H., and Barbacid, M., 1986, A human oncogene formed by the fusion of truncated tropomyosin and protein kinase sequences, *Nature (Lond.)* **319**:743–748.

32. Fusco, A., Arieco, M., Santoro, M., Berlingieri, M. T., Pilotti, S., Pierotti, M. A., Della Porta, G., and Vecchio, G., 1987, A new oncogene in human thyroid papillary carcinomas and their lymph-nodal metastases, *Nature (Lond.)* **328**:170–172.

33. Schechter, A. L., Stern, D. F., Vaidyanathan, L., Decker, S. J., Drebin, J. A., Greene, M. I., and Weinberg, R. A., 1984, The *neu* oncogene: An *erb*-B-related gene encoding a 185,000-$M_r$ tumour antigen, *Nature (Lond.)* **312**:513–516.

34. Sukumar, S., 1987, Involvement of oncogenes in carcinogenesis, in: *Cellular and Molecular Biology of Experimental Mammary Cancer* (D. Medina, W. Kidwell, G. Heppnar, and E. Anderson, eds.), pp. 381–398, Plenum, New York.

35. Fasano, O., Birnbaum, D., Edlund, L., Fogh, J., and Wigler, M., 1984, New human genes detected by a tumorigenicity assay, *Mol. Cell. Biol.* **4**:1695–1705.

36. Bos, J. L., Toksoz, D., Marshall, C. J., Verlaan-deVries, M., Veeneman, G. H., van der Eb, A. J., van Boom, J. H., Janssen, J. W. G., and Steenvoorden, C. M., 1985, Amino-acid substitutions at codon 13 of the N-*ras* oncogene in human acute myeloid leukaemia, *Nature (Lond.)* **315**:726–730.

37. Ananthaswamy, H. N., Price, J. E., Goldberg, L. H., and Straka, C., 1987, Simultaneous transfer of tumorigenic and metastatic phenotypes by transfection with genomic DNA from a human cutaneous squamous cell carcinoma, *Proc. Am. Assoc. Cancer Res.* **28**:69.

38. Reynolds, S. H., Stowers, S. J., Patterson, R., Maronpot, R. R., Aaronson, S. A., and Anderson, M. W., 1987, Activated oncogenes in B6C3F1 mouse liver tumors: Implications for risk assessment, *Science* **237**:1309–1316.

39. Tainsky, M. A., Shamanski, F. L., Blair, D., and Vande Woude, G., 1987, Human recipient cell for oncogene transfection studies, *Mol. Cell. Biol.* **7**:1280–1284.

40. Sukumar, S., Notario, V., Martin-Zanca, D., and Barbacid, M., 1983, Induction of mammary carcinomas by nitroso-methyl-urea involves malignant activation of H-*ras*-1 locus by single point mutations, *Nature (Lond.)* **306**:658–661.

41. Barbacid, M., 1987, *ras* Genes, *Annu. Rev. Biochem.* **56**:780–813.

42. Quintanilla, M., Brown, K., Ramsden, M., and Balmain, A., 1986, Carcinogen-specific mutation and amplification of Ha-*ras* during mouse skin carcinogenesis, *Nature (Lond.)* **322**:78–80.

43. Reynolds, S. H., Stowers, S. J., Maronpot, R. R., Anderson, M. W., and Aaronson, S. A., 1986, Detection and identification of activated oncogenes in spontaneously occurring benign and malignant hepatocellular tumors of the B6C3F1 mouse, *Proc. Natl. Acad. Sci. USA* **83**:33–37.

44. Brown, K., Quintanilla, M., Ramsden, M., Kerr, I. B., Young, S., and Balmain, A., 1986, v-*ras* Genes

from harvey and balb murine sarcoma viruses can act as initiators of two-stage mouse skin carcinogenesis, *Cell* **46**:447–456.

45. Bargmann, C. I., Hung, M. C., and Weinberg, R. A., 1986, Multiple independent activations of the *neu* oncogene by a point mutation altering the transmembrane domain of p185, *Cell* **45**:649–657.

46. Sawey, M. J., Hood, A. T., Burns, F. J., and Garte, S. J., 1987, Activation of *myc* and *ras* oncogenes in primary rat tumors induced by ionizing radiation, *Mol. Cell. Biol.* **7**:932–935.

47. Haseman, J. K., Huff, J., and Boorman, G. A., 1984, Use of historical control data in carcinogenicity studies in rodents, *Toxicol. Pathol.* **12**:126–135.

48. Fox, T. R., and Watanabe, P. G., 1985, Detection of a cellular oncogene in spontaneous liver tumors of B6C3F1 mice, *Science* **228**:596–597.

49. Stowers, S. J., Glover, P. L., Boone, L. R., Maronpot, R. R., Reynolds, S. H., and Anderson, M. W., 1987, Activation of the K-*ras* proto-oncogene in rat and mouse lung tumors induced by chronic exposure to tetranitromethane, *Cancer Res.* **47**:3212–3219.

50. Wiseman, R. W., Stowers, S.J., Miller, E. C., Anderson, M. W., and Miller, J. A., 1986, Activating mutations of the c-Ha-*ras* proto-oncogene in chemically induced hepatomas of the male B6C3F1 mouse, *Proc. Natl. Acad. Sci. USA* **83**:5285–5289.

51. Balmain, A., and Pragnell, I. B., 1983, Mouse skin carcinomas induced *in vivo* by chemical carcinogens have a transforming Harvey-*ras* oncogene, *Nature (Lond.)* **303**:72–74.

52. McMahon, G., Hanson, L., Lee, J., and Wogan, G. N., 1986, Identification of an activated c-Ki-*ras* oncogene in rat liver tumors induced by aflatoxin $B_1$, *Proc. Natl. Acad. Sci. USA* **83**:9418–9422.

53. Guerrero, I., Calzada, P., Mayer, A., and Pellicer, A., 1984, A molecular approach to leukemogenesis: mouse lymphomas contain an activated c-*ras* gene, *Proc. Natl. Acad. Sci. USA* **81**:202–205.

54. Guerrero, I., Villasante, A., Corces, V., and Pellicer, A., 1985, Loss of the normal N-*ras* allele in a mouse thymic lymphoma induced by a chemical carcinogen, *Proc. Natl. Acad. Sci. USA* **82**:7810–7814.

55. Eva, A., and Trimmer, R. W., 1986, High frequency of c-K-*ras* activation in 3-methylcholanthrene-induced mouse thymomas, *Carcinogenesis* **7**:1931–1933.

56. Tennant, R. W., Margolin, B. H., Shelby, M. D., Zeiger, E., Haseman, J. K., Spalding, J., Caspary, W., Resnick, M., Stasiewicz, S., Anderson, B., and Minor, R., 1987, Prediction of chemical carcinogenicity in rodents from *in vitro* genetic toxicity assays, *Science* **236**:933–941.

57. Ocadiz, R., Sauceda, R., Cruz, M., Graef, A. M., and Gariglio, P., 1987, High correlation between molecular alterations of the c-*myc* oncogene and carcinoma of the uterine cervix, *Cancer Res.* **47**:4173–4177.

58. Yokota, J., Tsunetsugu-Yakota, Y., Battifora, H., Le Fevre, C., and Cline, M. J., 1986, Alterations of *myc*, *myb*, and Ha-*ras* proto-oncogenes in cancers are frequent and show clinical correlation, *Science* **231**:261–265.

59. Nau, M. M., Carney, D. N., Battey, J., Johnson, B., Little, C., Gazdar, A., and Minna, J. D., 1984, Amplification, expression and rearrangement of c-*myc* and N-*myc* oncogenes in human lung cancer, *Curr. Topics Microbiol. Immunol.* **113**:172–177.

60. Nau, M. M., Brooks, B. J., Battey, J., Sausville, E., Gazdar, A. F., Kirsch, I. R., McBride, O. W., Bertness, V., Hollis, G. F., and Minna, J. D., 1985, L-*myc*, a new *myc*-related gene amplified and expressed in human small cell lung cancer, *Nature (Lond.)* **318**:69–73.

61. Wong, A. J., Ruppert, J. M., Eggleston, J., Hamilton, S. R., Baylin, S. B., and Vogelstein, B., 1986, Gene amplification of c-*myc* and N-*myc* in small cell carcinoma of the lung, *Science* **233**:461–464.

62. King, C. R., Kraus, M. H., and Aaronson, S. A., 1985, Amplification of a novel V-*erbB*-related gene in a human mammary carcinoma, *Science* **229**:974–976.

63. Semlea, K., Kamata, N., Toyoshima, K., and Yamamoto, T., 1985, A v-*erbB*-related protooncogene, e-*erbB*-2, is distinct from the c-*erbB*-1/epidermal growth factor-receptor gene and is amplified in a human salivary gland adenocarcinoma, *Proc. Natl. Acad. Sci. USA* **82**:6497–6501.

64. Pelicci, P.-G., Lanfrancone, L., Brathwaite, M. D., Wolman, S. R., and Dalla-Favera, R., 1984, Amplification of the c-*myb* oncogene in a case of human acute myelogenous leukemia, *Science* **224**:1117–1121.

65. Slamon, D. J., deKernion, J. B., Verma, I. M., and Cline, M. J., 1984, Expression of cellular oncogenes in human malignancies, *Science* **224**:256–262.

66. Wang, L.-C., Vass, W., Gao, C., and Chang, K. S. S., 1987, Amplification and enhanced expression of the c-Ki-*ras*-2 protooncogene in human embryonal carcinomas, *Cancer Res.* **47**:4192–4198.

67. Fujita, J., Srivastava, S. K., Kraus, M. H., Rhim, J. S., Tronick, S. R., and Aaronson, S. A., 1985, Frequency of molecular alterations affecting *ras* protooncogenes in human urinary tract tumors, *Proc. Natl. Acad. Sci. USA* **82**:3849–3853.

68. Croce, C. M., Thierfelder, W., Erikson, J., Nishikura, K., Finan, J., Lenoir, G. M., and Nowell, P. C.,

1983, Transcriptional activation of an unrearranged and untranslocated c-*myc* oncogene by translocation of a cλ locus in Burkitt lymphoma cells, *Proc. Natl. Acad. Sci. USA* **80**:6922–6926.

69. Dalla-Favera, R., Bregni, M., Erikson, J., Patterson, D., Gallo, R. C., and Croce, C. M., 1982, Human c-*myc* oncogene is located on the region of chromosome 8 that is translocated in Burkitt lymphoma cells, *Proc. Natl. Acad. Sci. USA* **79**:7824–7827.

70. Erikson, J., Nishikura, K., Ar-Rushdi, A., Finan, J., Emanuel, B., Lenoir, G., Nowell, P. C., and Croce, C. M., 1983, Translocation of an immunoglobulin κ locus to a region 3' of a unnrearranged c-*myc* oncogene enhances c-*myc* transcription, *Proc. Natl. Acad. Sci. USA* **80**:7581–7585.

71. Cory, S., Gerondakis, S., and Adams, J. M., 1983, Interchromosomal recombination of the cellular oncogene c-*myc* with the immunoglobulin heavy chain locus in murine plasmacytomas is a reciprocal exchange, *EMBO J.* **2**:697–703.

72. Shen-Ong, G. L. C., Keath, E. J., Piccoli, S. P., and Cole, M., 1982, Novel *myc* oncogene RNA from abortive immunoglobulin-gene recombination in mouse plasmacytomas, *Cell* **31**:443–452.

73. Stanton, L. W., Watt, R., and Marcu, K. B., 1983, Translocation, breakage, and truncated transcripts of c-*myc* oncogene in murine plasmacytomas, *Nature (Lond.)* **303**:401–406.

74. Erikson, J., Finger, L., Sun, L., Ar-Rushdi, A., Nishikura, K., Minowada, J., Finan, J., Emanuel, B. S., Nowell, P. C., and Croce, C. M., 1986, Deregulation of c-*myc* by translocation of the α-locus of the T-cell receptor in T-cell leukemias, *Science* **232**:884–886.

75. Moroy, T., Marchio, A., Etiemble, J., Trepo, C., Tiollais, P., and Buendia, M-A., 1986, Rearrangement and enhanced expression of c-*myc* in hepatocellular carcinoma of hepatitis virus infected woodchucks, *Nature (Lond.)* **324**:276–279.

76. Tsujimoto, H., Yunis, J., Onovato-Showe, L., Erikson, J., Nowell, P. C., and Croce, C. M., 1984, Molecular cloning of the chromosomal breakpoint of B-cell lymphomas and leukemias with the t(11;14) chromosome translocation, *Science* **224**:1403–1406.

77. Groffen, J., Stephenson, J. R., Heisterkamp, N., de Klein, A., Bartram, C. R., and Grosveld, G., 1984, Philadelphia chromosomal breakpoints are clustered within a limited region, *bcr*, on chromosome 22, *Cell* **36**:93–99.

78. Clark, S. S., McLaughlin, J., Crist, W. M., Champlin, R., and Witte, O. N., 1987, Unique forms of the *abl* tyrosine kinase distinguish Ph[1]-positive CML from Ph[1]-positive ALL, *Science* **235**:85–88.

79. Stanton, V. P., and Cooper, G. M., 1987, Activation of human *raf* transforming genes by deletion of normal amino-terminal coding sequences, *Mol. Cell. Biol.* **7**:1171–1179.

80. Bos, J. L., Verlaan-deVries, M., van der Eb, A. J., Janssen, J. W. G., Delwel, R., Lownberg, B., and Colly, L. P., 1987, Mutations in N-*ras* predominate in acute myeloid leukemia, *Blood* **69**:1237–1241.

81. Hirari, H., Kobayashi, Y., Mano, H., Hagiwara, K., Maru, Y., Omine, M., Mizoguchi, H., Nishida, J., and Takaku, F., 1987, A point mutation at codon 13 of the N-*ras* oncogene in myelodysplastic syndrome, *Nature (Lond.)* **327**:430–432.

82. Shimizu, K., Nakatsu, Y., Sekiguchi, M., Hokamura, K., Tanaka, K., Terada, M., and Sugimura, T., 1985, Molecular cloning of an activated human oncogene, homologous to v-*raf*, from primary stomach cancer, *Proc. Natl. Acad. Sci. USA* **82**:5641–5645.

83. Eva, A., and Aaronson, S. A., 1985, Isolation of a new human oncogene from a diffuse B-cell lymphoma, *Nature (Lond.)* **316**:273–275.

84. Pulciani, S., Sakano, T., Ohnishi, K., Anastasi, A. M., Pecorelli, A., Fiorucci, G., Oppi, C., Rossi, G. B., and Bonavida, B., 1987, Detection of a transforming gene in spontaneous reticulum cell sarcoma of SJL/J mice: Genetically linked and host-dependent neoplasia, *Cancer Res.* **47**:523–526.

85. Sukumar, S., Peroantoni, A., Reed, C., Rice, J. M., and Wenk, M. L., 1986, Activated K-*ras* and N-*ras* oncogenes in primary renal mesenchymal tumors induced in F344 rats by methyl(methoxymethyl)nitrosamine, *Mol. Cell. Biol.* **6**:2716–2720.

86. McMahon, G., Hanson, L., Lee, J., and Wogan, G. N., 1986, Identification of an activated c-Ki-*ras* oncogene in rat liver tumors induced by aflatoxin $B_1$, *Proc. Natl. Acad. Sci. USA* **83**:9418–9422.

87. Farber, E., 1984, Cellular biochemistry of the stepwise development of cancer with chemicals. *Cancer Res.* **44**:5463–5474.

88. Garte, S. J., Hood, A. T., Hochwait, A. E., D'Eustachio, P., Snyder, C. A., Segal, A., and Albert, R. E., 1985, Carcinogen specificity in the activation of transforming genes by direct-acting alkylating agents, *Carcinogenesis* **6**:1709–1712.

89. Stowers, S. J., Wiseman, R. W., Ward, J. M., Miller, C. M., Miller, J. A., Anderson, M. W., and Eva, A., 1988, Detection of activated proto-oncogenes in *N*-nitrosodiethylamine-induced liver tumors: A comparison between B6C3F₁ mice and Fischer 344 rats, *Carcinogenesis* **9**:271–276.

# 15

# Alterations in Biochemical Control Mechanisms of Neoplastic Cells

## Charles E. Wenner and Anthony Cutry

## 1. INTRODUCTION

An alteration in the regulation of cell growth underlies the basic defect in the transformed state. A primary goal is to understand the molecular mechanisms by which control of cell-cycle proliferation differs in normal versus neoplastic cells. Much attention is being paid to several areas in an effort to develop knowledge of the molecular processes involved in these changes: (1) regulation of gene expression and their messenger RNA (mRNA); (2) growth factor–receptor interactions and their subsequent messenger processes; (3) alteration in biochemical control mechanisms, including the role of ion transport in signal transduction mechanisms; and (4) changes in the bioenergetics or metabolism of the cell that contribute to the maintenance of an active proliferative cycle. Considerable data have been obtained from experiments with cell culture, and attempts to integrate findings in relationship to the classic periods of cell cycle have been made.

The demonstration of transforming genes, so-called *oncogenes*, has led to intensive study of their function and role in immortalization and cell transformation. The question as to how oncogene products are involved in the activation and progression of cell cycle is of pivotal interest. The discovery of cellular proto-oncogenes in this altered form has led to the search for biochemical correlations associated with oncogene expression. Some viral oncogenes (v-*myc*, v-*ras*, and v-*sis*) have contributed to our understanding of growth control, as their cellular counterparts (proto-oncogenes) are implicated in tumorigenesis. When certain proto-oncogenes are expressed at high levels, transformation of established cell lines can be observed.[1,2] Furthermore, in some cases, c-*myc* and c-H-*ras* transform primary as well as established cultures when induced with viral vectors.[2,3]

One mechanism by which some transformed or malignant cells escape normal growth control is presumed to involve the release of growth-promoting hormones or hormonelike agents that resemble known polypeptide growth factors (cf 2). Transformation by retroviruses, as well as by chemical carcinogenesis, involves in some cases the production of transforming growth factors. Transforming growth factor α (TGF-α), which is structurally and functionally related to epidermal growth factor (EGF), is expressed in a variety of human and animal cell tumors[4] and is thought to be involved in the malignant process. Although TGF-α produces certain changes in cellular properties that are analogous to those observed in transformed cells, it is unable to produce other changes associated with the transformed phenotype. However, TGF-α together with transforming growth factor β

*Charles E. Wenner and Anthony Cutry* • Biological Chemistry Division, Roswell Park Memorial Institute, Buffalo, New York 14263

(TGF-β) has been shown to provide the requisite anchorage-independent growth—a property in cell culture that correlates with tumorigenicity *in vivo*.[4]

Since growth factors and other mitogenic agents initiate the signal that prompts quiescent cells to enter the $G_1$ phase with subsequent progression through the cell cycle, a key question is how the mediating signal triggers the RNA and protein synthetic machinery. When a net gain in the rate of macromolecular synthesis is achieved, the cell can then ready itself for the replicative period. Some of the changes induced by growth factors, presumably including TGFα, are elevation of intracellular $Ca^{2+}$; changes in ion fluxes across cell membranes, such as sodium and potassium ions; and increased rate of glycolysis. These biochemical features are also found in many transformed cells. Thus, examination of changes induced by growth factors, including TGFα, should offer insight into the mechanism by which these biochemical processes are coupled, as well as how signals are transduced to the nucleus. An understanding of the coupling processes may also contribute clues leading to an understanding of those changes that influence the channeling of deoxy- and ribonucleotide precursors into the requisite substrates for DNA replication.

## 2. ALTERATIONS OF MEMBRANE TRANSPORT IN NEOPLASIA

### 2.1. Acceleration of Amino Acid Uptake by Transformed Cells— Relationship to (Na+/K+)ATPase Activity

Foster and Pardee[5] first reported that the system A* amino acid analogue aminoisobutyrate (AIB) accumulated to a greater extent in nonconfluent 3T3 cells than in confluent cells and to an even greater extent in polyoma virus-transformed 3T3 nonconfluent cells. Many transformed cell lines have also been reported to take up this Na+-dependent amino acid at an appreciably faster rate than their parent cells.[5–9] The activity of system A appears to be continuously elevated in transformed cells.[10] In addition, the uptake of methylaminoisobutyrate via system A by NRK-49F cells was shown to be stimulated by either TGFβ or EGF.[11] The possibility therefore arises that this system is subject to growth regulatory mechanisms critical for expression of the transformed state.

Although it is widely accepted that a primary source of energy for the active accumulation of amino acids is by cotransport of Na+ down its electrochemical potential gradient, it may be questioned as to whether this mechanism suffices to explain the steady-state accumulation of amino acids, especially in cells such as the Ehrlich ascites, in which high cell to medium distribution of amino acids is observed.[12] The effects of Na+-coupled solute transport on (Na+/K+)ATPase activity in intact cells have been studied; one determinant of cation pumping was found to be the transport of Na+-dependent amino acids.[13] Evidence was presented to indicate that "system A is able to exert profound effects on both the short-term and on long-term activity of the (Na+/K+)ATPase."[13]

The loss of regulatory mechanisms that act on system A in transformed cells is further reflected by a decreased responsiveness of cells such as the Ehrlich ascites carcinoma and Yoshida ascites hepatoma to regulation of transport of amino acid substrates mediated by system A.[14] The increased transport via system A may possibly be attributed to an increased driving force related to enhanced activity of the electrogenic (Na+/K+)ATPase.

What is needed is a better understanding of the interrelationship between Na+-dependent solute transport such as system A and ASC† amino acid transport for alanine, serine, and cysteine and (Na+/K+)ATPase-mediated cation pumping in the intact cell. Pump activity is regulated (at least partly) by Na+ influx and/or the concentration of intracellular (Na+),[15] as well as by changes in membrane potential.[16] However, it is not clear whether the increased system A activity is due to

---

*System A is a ubiquitous Na+ transport system which serves for most zwitterionic amino acids.

†System ASC is also a ubiquitous Na+ amino acid transport system, so named since alanine, serine, and cysteine were found to be capable of transport by this system. It also is accessible to other certain zwitterionic amino acids but excludes *N*-methyl amino acids.

an increase in the number of active carriers at the cell surface or whether the regulation of amino acid transport is dependent on coupling to the $(Na^+/K^+)$ATPase activity, or both.[17] For example, evidence has been obtained that the electrogenic properties of the $(Na^+/K^+)$ATPase may be the driving force for system A transport[18] (K. J. Leister, personal communication). Graves and Wheeler[19] also reported that after treatment of fibroblasts with low $K^+$, there was an increase in α-AIB active transport and ouabain-sensitive $K^+$ uptake, which is in accord with an adaptive regulation to restore ion gradients and amino acid levels.

## 2.2. Alterations in $(Na^+/K^+)$ATPase in Neoplasia

The $(Na^+/K^+)$ATPase activity of transformed cells has been found to be higher than that in nontransformed cells.[20] Similar results were obtained by other investigators,[15] although it has been argued that the absolute magnitude of the total and active component of $K^+$ influx during exponential growth is not directly related to maintenance of growth control.[21] Tupper[21] stated that in 3T3 cells in which growth control can be manifested at either low or high saturation densities,

> The $K^+$ influx may be less, greater, or equivalent to that of transformed cells. However, when 3T3 cells become quiescent there is an associated drop in the active component of $K^+$ influx relative to that observed during exponential growth. This would appear to be associated with growth regulation.

What these studies point out is that actively growing cells, whether normal or transformed, are associated with an active $(Na^+/K^+)$ATPase. The difference in pump rates between normal and transformed cells observed under experimental conditions, during the exponential phase of growth may reflect, in part, either differing amino acid conditions or metabolic states at the time of sampling. Since measurements of $(Na^+/K^+)$ATPase activity in buffer solution differ from those for which amino acids are present,[13] it becomes necessary to compare pump activities under states that imitate culture conditions. Amino acid transport was reported to be a major determinant of pump activity in exponentially growing cells.[13] Conversely, the driving force for amino acid transport may be $(Na^+/K^+)$ATPase activity.

In our view, enhanced $(Na^+/K^+)$ATPase activity appears to be required for advancement in the cell cycle in both normal and neoplastic cells; this requirement is seen in the $G_1$–S progression. The experimental evidence supports the development of a transient ouabain-insensitive state in $G_1$ that is approximately 2 hr prior to entry of the cells into S phase.[22] The question as to why $(Na^+/K^+)$ATPase is required prior to S-phase entry may depend on the following considerations: (1) the $(Na^+/K^+)$ATPase pump has been implicated in volume control, i.e., cells may need to reach a volume threshold level before S-phase entry can proceed; (2) this ATPase pump is presumed to be responsible for the plasma membrane potential of several animal cell types,[17] and the transmembrane potential may have a critical regulatory role in transport activity needed for advancement of cells through the cell cycle. For example, the accumulation of nutrients such as amino acids may be dependent on an electrogenic $(Na^+/K^+)$ATPase pump[18] (K. J. Leister, personal communication); (3) the ionic environment would also be expected to influence enzymatic activity and, as the $(Na^+/K^+)$ATPase pump activity is tightly coupled to the glycolysis pathway, the activity of the pump may be necessary in maintaining the proper bioenergetics of the cell; and (4) the ionic environment may have a critical role in either translational or transcriptional processes, or both, which may act individually or in concert with respect to influencing cell-cycle progression.

Simply increasing cell volume or even cell mass is in itself insufficient to trigger the division cycle.[23] Early experiments showed that under conditions of sufficient nutrients, when DNA biosynthesis is blocked with excess thymidine (which inhibits nucleotide biosynthesis), cells in S phase that are progressing through the DNA division cycle are arrested.[23] The growth cycle (as measured by protein and RNA synthesis) continued despite the block in nucleotide biosynthesis. In some cases, this resulted in the formation of abnormally large cells. Upon removal of the block, consecutive division did not occur. However, cell-cycle periods were observed but were shortened.

With respect to the aforementioned consideration,[2] evidence was obtained with Ehrlich ascites tumor cells indicating that ouabain caused a rapid depolarization in the absence of measurable changes in intracellular $Na^+$ or $K^+$, suggesting that this pump generates the plasma membrane potential in this cell type. Furthermore, Hacking, and Eddy[24] obtained data compatible with the idea that amino acids such as glycine, L-leucine, and aminoisobutyrate were accumulated electrogenically by mouse ascites tumor cells. The link between system A amino acid transport and $(Na^+/K^+)$ATPase activity is strongly supported by parallel alterations in amino acid transport and pump activity induced by long-term treatment with ouabain.[18] Although a highly malignant cell type, such as Ehrlich ascites tumor cells, might be considered abnormal in its membrane properties, this would not appear to be the case. As pointed out by Bashford and Pasternak,[17] human neutrophils also set their membrane potential by a mechanism like that described above. The question then arises as to what is controlling pump activity and whether it differs in transformed cells. The answer to this question will depend, in our view, on how activation of the relevant genes induces the introduction of ion channels that modulate the activity of the pump. In the case of cells that produce transforming growth factors, is it a sodium–proton antiport system that is turned on? The key to these questions must await further understanding of the role of ion channels and characterization of antiport or other transport systems.

In addition to the pump having a role in transport processes, there is also the possibility that ion movements may directly influence macromolecular synthesis. It should be noted that Pestka reported that protein biosynthesis was linearly dependent on $(K^+)$ in prokaryotic cell-free lysates.[25] Similar potassium concentrations are required for eukaryotic systems.[26] In this regard, potassium is an essential requirement for peptide bond synthesis, with concentrations of 100 mM or greater giving optimal results. This requirement has been localized to the $(K^+)$ dependency of peptidyltransferase A.[25] Potassium in high concentration is also required for nucleotide biosynthesis notably in the formation of 5'-phosphoribosyl-5-aminoimidazole by the $K^+$-dependent and 5-amino-4-imidazolecarboxamide ribotide transformylase.

Potassium ion pumping involves a major expenditure of energy that results in large part in the high aerobic glycolysis of some transformed cells. Although inhibitors of energy-using processes have been used to evaluate the contribution of energy expenditures to the respiration and glycolysis of cells,[27] the use of ouabain as an inhibitor of $(Na^+/K^+)$ATPase activity is subject to the constraint that its ability to inhibit is related to the extracellular potassium, $(K^+)_o$, since ouabain is competitive with $(K^+)$. It should also be pointed out that ouabain sensitivity is dependent on other parameters. For example, transformed cells in many instances are more sensitive to ouabain inhibition,[28] and Lelievre *et al.*[29] found removal of tropomyosin from plasma membranes to increase ouabain sensitivity. Since many transformed cells exhibit a loss of two forms of tropomyosin,[30] and suppression of tropomyosin synthesis is a common property of the oncogenic process induced by structurally diverse retroviral oncogenes,[31] it is conceivable that this decreased level of tropomyosin confers increased ouabain sensitivity to transformed cells.[28] The differential expression of tropomyosin isoforms might further play a significant role in the reorganization of microfilaments upon cell transformation.[31] The mechanism by which tropomyosins influence actin bundling is currently under study.[32]

# 3. ALTERATIONS IN METABOLIC PATHWAYS IN TRANSFORMED CELLS—ENHANCED GLYCOLYSIS

## 3.1. (Na⁺/K⁺)ATPase as a Major Contributor of ADP and Pᵢ Rate-Limiting Factors of Glycolysis

A high rate of aerobic glycolysis, the so-called Warburg effect, is common to a wide variety of tumors. Exceptions to this generalization are the slow-growing minimal deviation hepatomas. It would appear that the enhanced glycolysis is a consequence of the loss of growth control. This loss of growth control with its reduced dependency on growth factors may, in part, be due to the ability of transformed cells to make their own growth factors.[4] The administration of growth factors to quiescent cells in many cases induces enhanced $K^+$ uptake and, in view of the major expenditure of energy for pumping monovalent cations, it might be expected that this would contribute to an enhanced glycolysis. In accord with this idea, there are numerous examples in which ouabain was shown to inhibit glycolysis.[27,33] A major question is: Does the control of the $(Na^+/K^+)ATPase$ differ in transformed cells? Although it has been proposed that the pump may operate inefficiently,[34] there has not been unequivocal proof of this.[35] Rather, it would appear that factors that influence this equilibrium enzyme are altered in the transformed phenotype. As yet, ion channels that modulate sodium and potassium movements have not been systematically studied with regard to related $(Na^+/K^+)ATPase$ activity. The availability of patch-clamp techniques offers new promise in this direction.

## 3.2. Role of Transforming Growth Factors in Increased Glycolysis of Transformed Cells

Relatively little is known concerning the role of transforming growth factors in the metabolism of tumor cells. In view of the structural and functional similarity of TGF-$\alpha$ to EGF, and since EGF has been observed to enhance $(Na^+/K^+)ATPase$ activity, it might be expected that TGF-$\alpha$ would enhance glycolysis as well as ion pumping. TGF-$\alpha$ also induces cytoskeletal changes such as decreased expression of tropomyosin forms (H. L. Cooper, personal communication). Thus, it would be important to determine whether these alterations are related to the altered ouabain sensitivity displayed by some tumor cells.

## 3.3. Metabolic Alterations Induced by Specific Oncogenes

Racker *et al.*[33,34] reported a study of metabolic alterations induced by specific oncogenes. Rat-1 fibroblasts transfected with either *myc* or *ras* were used for measurements of glycolysis and amino acid transport. The most striking change was a fourfold increase in glycolysis in the *ras* cells, while in *myc* cells, glycolysis was similar to that in the parental Rat-1 cells. These findings are of interest in that *ras* transfection is frequently associated with decreased tropomyosin synthesis and altered ouabain sensitivity. By contrast, glycolysis or amino acid transport was unaffected in *myc*-transfected cells, but these cells were more susceptible to treatment with TGF-$\beta$ than were the parent cells.[34] These observations of specific oncogenes inducing different metabolic effects may contribute to the understanding of their cooperative response in tumorigenicity.

Of particular interest is the role played by the *ras* gene product, a GTP-binding protein with a molecular weight of $21,000 M_r$,[36] in the altered glycolysis of transformed cells. It is likely that the *ras* gene product is capable of influencing system A transport, since Racker *et al.*[33] reported that this gene product induces methionine-sensitive amplification of glycolysis.

The uptake of labeled methylaminoisobutyrate or 1-methionine via system A was also observed to be accelerated after treatment of these cells with TGF-$\beta$, with *myc*-transformed cells most sensitive and *ras*-transformed cells somewhat less sensitive.[33] These findings suggest that *myc* induces a change in either the TGF-$\beta$ receptor or the system A transporter. The further finding by these investigators that cycloheximide prevented the TGF-$\beta$ stimulation of system A transport is in agreement with the idea that newly synthesized protein is required. The elucidation of the role of oncogene products in influencing glycolysis and amino acid transport awaits a clearer understanding of the coupling between these metabolic events and the role of G proteins in signal transduction. What remains to be investigated is the association between G proteins of membrane receptor systems and GTP-binding gene products of the *ras* oncogene family that share homology with the $\alpha$-subunit of G proteins.[36]

## 4. CYTOSKELETAL ALTERATIONS IN TRANSFORMED CELLS

The transformed state is characterized by changes in the cytoskeleton, which in turn result in striking morphologic changes. When cells are infected with retroviruses, such as the Rous sarcoma virus, or injection of pp60[src] tyrosine kinase, phosphorylations of membrane-associated proteins appear to be involved in cytoskeletal architecture that presumably give rise to altered morphology. Whether the changes are due to phosphorylation of soluble or plasma membrane protein(s) that affects the assembly of the cytoskeleton is not clear, but it is conceivable that cytoskeletal changes influence functional expression of growth factor responses. Vinculin has been reported to be phosphorylated at a tyrosine residue, but it should be noted that this represents a small fraction of the total vinculin pool.[34]

If we accept the hypothesis suggested by Sporn and Todaro[4] that autocrine growth factors contribute to the transformed state, examination of the interactions of growth factors with their receptors and associated relationships to actin-cable networks will be of particular interest. Study of the early events accompanying growth factor–receptor interaction has implicated actin in at least two ways in the responses that lead to cell-cycle proliferation. First, actin mRNA is representative of the immediate early genes transcriptionally activated by growth factor interaction with its receptor.[37] With regard to actin as an early gene, much evidence has accumulated to suggest that growth factors cause disorganization of the actin–microfilament network very rapidly (possibly involving phosphorylation). Since the rate of actin polymerization is due in large part to $(actin)_{sol}$,[38] this early activation of actin gene transcription may be critical to increased $(actin)_{sol}$, and thereby triggering actin microfilament polymerization to cause eventual downregulation of growth response.

Second, cytoskeletal disrupting agents such as cytochalasin B potentiate chemoattractant-induced superoxide production in human granulocytes suggesting that receptor–cytoskeleton interactions are integral to regulation of signal transduction in this system.[39] Such mechanisms could apply to other receptor systems. Microfilament-mediated control may be at the level of regulation of the expression of the receptor at the cell surface; alternatively, it could be at the level of receptor desensitization or downregulation.[38] In light of such studies, the question arises as to whether the transformed state with its altered cytoskeletal characteristics favors ligand–receptor maintenance in the activated state. The extensive network involved in transmembrane signaling with the involvement of phosphatidylinositol pathways and endoplasmic $Ca^{2+}$ release, as well as the many possible feedback mechanisms, makes it difficult to give a definitive response to these considerations.

## 5. ALTERATIONS IN MITOCHONDRIAL CITRIC ACID CYCLE

Although the early findings by Warburg and subsequent workers provided evidence for altered qualitative or quantitative respiration in transformed cells, the generalization that the malignant state has a defective Pasteur effect has been challenged by Weinhouse and colleagues.[40,41] For example, Ehrlich ascites tumor cells have one of the highest rates of aerobic glycolysis, but they also have actively phosphorylating mitochondria capable of suppressing glycolysis under aerobic conditions. However, the rate of anaerobic glycolysis is so high that oxygen is incapable of completely suppressing lactate formation. Furthermore, few or no differences have been observed in the rate of glycolysis or respiration of minimal deviation hepatomas compared with their normal counterpart. In contrast to these findings, mitochondria from rapidly growing, poorly differentiated Morris hepatomas have been found to export citrate derived from pyruvate at a rate fourfold greater than that of normal liver preparations.[42] These findings have been interpreted to imply that these cholesterol-rich hepatoma mitochondria have a functionally truncated Krebs cycle [also known as the citric acid or tricarboxylic acid (TCA) cycle], as well as having a mechanism for providing higher cytoplasmic levels of precursor metabolite intermediates that help sustain deregulated cholesterogenesis in these and other types of malignant neoplasms.[42] Since mitochondrial $NAD(P)^+$-dependent malic enzyme is progression linked in Morris hepatomas,[43] it is possible that the high $NAD(P)H/NAD(P)^+$ ratio maintained by the activity of this enzyme would favor inhibition of isocitrate dehydrogenase and could explain the apparent buildup of citrate observed with rapidly growing tumor cells.[42] The activity of this malic enzyme in rapidly growing tumor cells and other proliferative nonmalignant cells such as jejunal epithelium may also favor the pyridine nucleotides in a reduced state and thus allow for anabolic reactions, such as cholesterol biosynthesis.[44]

Data have accumulated to demonstrate that glutamine is a major respiratory fuel of tumor cells.[45] The increased malic enzyme activity and progression-linked phosphate-dependent glutaminase of some transformed cells may stimulate a high rate of oxidation of this amino acid. The malic enzyme contributes to the relatively reduced oxidation–reduction state of tumor cells.[44] Reduced pyridine nucleotides maintained by the malic enzyme could result in inhibition of glutamic dehydrogenase. Glutamate formation via glutaminase with consequent conversion of glutamate via transamination to $\alpha$-ketoglutarate may then give rise to malate.[44] Thus, reduced pyridine nucleotide would be regenerated along with pyruvate and carbon dioxide by the malic enzyme. It is also conceivable that reduced pyridine nucleotide derived via the malic enzyme of tumor cells would contribute to the available supply of reduced cofactor for the lactic dehydrogenase reaction and glycolysis.

Despite a preference for glutamine as substrate for mitochondrial energy, it is our view that a truncated citric acid cycle is not responsible for the high aerobic glycolysis of tumor cells. The fact that normal respiratory control and moderate rates of oxidation occur and that oxygen suppresses glycolysis in large part, albeit not completely, implies that the Pasteur effect is operative. However, a normal rate of oxidation cannot suppress the high rates of tumor cell glycolysis.

## 6. ALTERATIONS IN PROTO-ONCOGENES IN NEOPLASIA

Oncogenes, which are often thought to be associated exclusively with neoplastic transformation, is somewhat of a misnomer. In their normal cellular form (proto-oncogenes), these genes perform functions relevant to the survival of the cell and the performance of its duties. For example, normal p21*ras* appears to play a crucial role in the proliferative responses of normal cells to agents which stimulate phospholipase C.[46] The c-*fms* proto-oncogene codes for the receptor for macrophage colony stimulating factor-1 (CSF-1). The proto-oncogenes of the tyrosine kinase family, such as c-*abl*, c-*src*, and c-*ros* have been implicated for having a role in the phosphatidylinositol cycle.[47] The c-*erb*-A proto-oncogene encodes a member of the thyroid hormone receptor family.[48] These examples illustrate the importance of the normal oncogene counterparts in cellular function.

These oncogenes have been incontrovertibly associated with various neoplasias, however, and although most associations have been conceived through experiments with cell-culture systems, it appears likely that they are also involved in some human neoplasias. Consequently, elucidation of the function and regulation of oncogene protein products, particularly at the level of the gene itself, can shed considerable light onto the process of carcinogenesis. More than 40 proto-oncogenes and oncogenes are known[1] (Chapter 13), but this section is restricted to discussion of two oncogenes considered important in neoplasia: the *ras* oncogene family and the *myc* oncogene family.

An important point to be considered is how changes in the normal regulation of proto-oncogenes enables these genes to then become capable of causing malignant transformation. The following possibilities come to mind. First, mutations within a gene may cause a significant alteration in the function of the protein product of that gene. This could be relevant to functions such as proteolytic activities, hydrolysis, binding activities, and substrate specificities. Some evidence points to this type of alteration as being a causal event in *ras* transformation. Second, genetic damage within a proto-oncogene may render it free of its normal regulation; i.e., it may allow for unchecked transcription of the gene by stripping the gene of its normal regulatory elements. Conversely, chromosomal translocations involving proto-oncogenes may juxtapose them to the regulatory elements of a gene that has far greater activity than the proto-oncogene itself. The result is an abnormally high rate of transcription of the proto-oncogene, or transcription of the proto-oncogene at inappropriate times in the cell cycle, which could then give rise to transformation. We must be able to integrate such changes in the function or regulation of proto-oncogenes into a working model that results in significant alterations in the replicative functions of the affected cells.

How do these alterations perturb the normal signal transduction pathways within the cell that govern the responses of the cell to various polypeptide hormones and growth factors? While the models presented here represent speculation, we believe they are nonetheless possibilities of how such alterations in proto-oncogene function or regulation may be involved in the carcinogenic process. Such insights are necessary for one to be able to subsequently design experiments to test the hypotheses and advance our understanding of fundamental biochemical regulatory alterations responsible for neoplasia.

## 6.1. The ras Oncogene, G Proteins, and Transforming Growth Factors

The *ras* oncogene family consists of several members: Kirsten (K-*ras*-1 and K-*ras*-2), Harvey (H-*ras*-1 and H-*ras*2), N-*ras*, and the recently identified R-*ras* genes.[49] The protein products are immunologically related, and all code for a protein of 21,000 $M_r$, hence the designation p21. H-*ras*-2 and K-*ras*-1 are nonfunctional pseudogenes. p21 shares some homology to the α-subunits of the GTP-binding proteins ($G_s$ and $G_i$) of the cAMP second-messenger system, as well as other G proteins not associated with the adenylate cyclase system. A concise introduction to the function of the cAMP system will aid in understanding the forthcoming section.

Upon binding of β-adrenergic agents to their membrane receptors, the activated receptor (in the case of a stimulatory agent) interacts with a G protein ($G_s$) that is stimulatory to the adenylate cyclase system. This interaction causes the dissociation of bound GDP from $G_s$ and allows it to now bind GTP. $G_s$ is a trimer of α-, β-, and γ-subunits, and it is believed that the binding of GTP to the α-subunit allows it to dissociate reversibly from the other two subunits so as to act as the positive effector of adenylate cyclase. This latter enzyme is then responsible for the synthesis of cAMP, which then can bind to the regulatory subunits of protein kinase A, causing them to dissociate from the catalytic subunits of the kinase. This, in turn, frees the catalytic subunits to phosphorylate substrate proteins and elicit cellular responses. Here, the $G_s$ protein plays a central role, since its α-subunit possesses a GTPase activity that hydrolyzes bound GTP to GDP, allowing for the reassociation of the $G_s$ trimer, and relieving the stimulus on adenylate cyclase. Thus, by this action, the activity of the entire system can be terminated. It should be noted, however, that the existence of an inhibitory G protein ($G_i$), which is nearly identical to $G_s$ in structure and function, except that it inhibits adenylate cyclase, also acts to attenuate the activity of the system. The role of G proteins in this system is more completely covered by Gilman.[50]

From the similarities between *ras* p21 and the G proteins of the above system, it is tempting to speculate that transformation by *ras* is a consequence of a perturbation of this second messenger system. There are established links between adenylate cyclase activity and cell growth, particularly in yeast, where in some cases this activity is essential for growth. Interestingly, *ras* gene products have been identified as necessary components of this system in yeast;[51] thus, we see a connection between *ras* and cell growth. However, in higher eukaryotes, the picture is not nearly as clear. Boynton and Whitfield[52] proposed a multifaceted role for cAMP, in which it is stimulatory for cell growth in a substage of $G_1$ and inhibitory at two other points in the cell cycle. The major obstacle in connecting *ras* transformation to an alteration in regulation of the cAMP system lies in associating the *ras* proteins with key regulatory elements of this system. First, let us consider the alterations in cellular *ras* proteins, which may account for its transforming ability. The p21 gene product has, as do G proteins, an intrinsic ability to bind and hydrolyze GTP.[53] There are reports that the normal *ras* proteins differ from the transforming *ras* proteins in that the transforming protein is severely deficient in its ability to hydrolyze bound GTP.[53,54] The nature of this defect appears to be associated with amino acid substitutions at or near positions 12 and 61 of the 189-amino acid protein, and a recent report indicates that mutations at these positions inhibit the interaction of *ras* with a GTPase-activating protein.[55] Mutation at amino acid position 12 and/or 61 is sufficient to cause transformation of cells in culture; these mutations have also been observed in human tumors associated with *ras* transformation.[56-60] The nature of these amino acid substitutions results from single point mutations within the codons specifying the proper amino acids. Indeed, it has been shown that tumors resulting from 7,12-dimethylbenz(a)anthracene (DMBA) treatment of mouse skin contain a specific A-T transversion at the second nucleotide of codon 61 of Harvey *ras*.[61] Given the decreased GTPase activity of such mutant proteins, it is tempting to speculate that loss or impairment of this activity could lead to unchecked stimulation of the cAMP system, with the end result being an enhanced proliferative capacity for the cell. Cholera toxin, which ADP ribosylates the $G_s$ protein causing a dramatic decrease in the GTPase activity of $G_s$, has been shown to exert a strong proliferative stimulus on some cell-culture systems.[62] It is still unclear, however, whether normal or oncogenic *ras* proteins are associated with the cAMP system. Some reports[63] discount the *ras* proteins as being regulatory components of adenylate cyclase, while others[64] have demonstrated that oncogenic K-*ras* p21 does indeed stimulate adenylate cyclase activity. However, it must be kept in mind that *ras* proteins need not be limited to a stimulatory role with regard to adenylate cyclase to elicit a proliferative stimulus. An inhibitory function could serve to lift the negative proliferative effects of cAMP at one of two points within the cell cycle. Indeed, as outlined by Beckner *et al.*,[63] the membranes of many transformed cells have a lowered capacity for synthesis of cAMP. Nevertheless, even though alterations in the GTPase activity of transforming *ras* proteins have been documented, it remains unclear as to how such changes can give rise to neoplasia.

There are other possible modes in which *ras* proteins may act to transform cells besides interactions with the cAMP second-messenger system. G proteins distinct from those associated with adenylate cyclase have been shown to couple activated membrane receptors to phospholipase C[65,66] to activate phosphatidylinositol (PI) breakdown with an eventual stimulation of protein kinase C, which is often stimulatory to cell proliferation. Indeed, NIH 3T3 cells transformed by either Harvey or Kirsten *ras* appear to possess increased levels of diacylglycerol (a product of PI turnover that is the endogenous activator of protein kinase C) as well as increases in phosphorylation levels of an $80,000\text{-}M_r$ substrate for protein kinase C.[67] This suggests that *ras* proteins may be a key regulatory component of PI turnover. Again, as with attempts to associate *ras* with adenylate cyclase, it is unclear whether *ras* is truly exerting transformation through perturbation of the PI turnover system or, if it is, whether this can be linked to an alteration in the GTPase activity of p21. Furthermore, the transforming potential of H-*ras* p21 appears to be dependent on protein kinase C activity, which may again implicate *ras* in PI turnover, or perhaps *ras* interacts directly with kinase C, resulting in its activation.[68] Finally, G proteins have been shown to activate calcium channels in some cell types,[69] and it will be of interest to see whether *ras* is capable of performing this function.

Two studies have claimed that deregulation of *ras* at the level of the gene is responsible for transformation.[70,71] It is interesting to note that ionizing radiation was used in both cases to induce malignant neoplasms; in one case, skin cancers in rats,[70] and in the other, lymphomas in mice.[71] Both studies demonstrated a specific activation of K-*ras*, and it appears that this activation was due to either amplification of the gene, increased transcription of the gene, or a combination of both. It is well documented that ionizing radiation causes strand breaks in DNA, which may lead to chromosomal translocation. This, in turn, can activate an oncogene by placing it under the influence of powerful promoter and/or enhancer sequences. A third report[72] showed that H-*ras* genes transform via truncation of a newly identified upstream exon, termed exon −1. This report did imply, however, that the point mutations previously described can, in some cases, aid the transformation efficiency of this gene. The three-dimensional structure of c-Ha-*ras* p21 has recently been determined by X-ray crystallographic methods,[73] which should allow for determination of structure–function relationships of normal *ras* proteins and transforming *ras* proteins. Such studies have potential to allow for a far greater understanding of the mechanisms by which both normal and oncogenic *ras* proteins function.

Perhaps a more important issue in the process of *ras* transformation is the production of transforming growth factors. Initially termed sarcoma growth factor, since they were isolated from murine sarcoma virus-transformed cells,[74] these growth factors are able to induce profound morphologic change on cells in culture (including the induction of anchorage-independent growth, a property that correlates with tumorigenesis *in vivo*). It was initially believed that sarcoma growth factor was a single entity, but more extensive work showed that the preparations were actually a mix of the structurally unrelated peptides TGF-α and TGF-β.[75] It was subsequently demonstrated that the profound morphologic changes exerted by the crude preparations were due to the synergistic action of the two individual growth factors.[76] What is of particular interest with regard to *ras* transformation is the observation that v-K-*ras* transformed cells release TGF-α.[77] Later experiments showed that NIH 3T3 cells transformed with any of the mutant *ras* genes (those with amino acid substitutions at position 12 or 61) previously discussed produced TGF-α.[78] Therefore, when considering transformation by *ras*, it may be crucial to consider the effects of TGF-α production. It should be noted that both TGF-α and TGF-β are necessary to induce anchorage-independent growth. However, it appears that TGF-β is a ubiquitous growth factor present in normal as well as transformed cells,[79] while TGF-α production is more closely linked to the transformed state. (Recent evidence[80] has demonstrated, however, that α is produced in a few normal cells.) Therefore, the induction of TGF-α synthesis by the malignant cell may be an important consideration in tumor outgrowth and maintanence.

TGF-α is a small polypeptide of 50 amino acids,[81] which binds to the EGF receptor.[74] TGF-α is synthesized during early fetal development but is not detectable after birth in murine systems, indicating that this particular growth factor may serve as an embryonal form of EGF and related growth factors.[82,83] It was shown that TGF-α was synthesized in a variety of solid tumors or cell lines derived from these,[84] indicating that its synthesis is reactivated during malignant transformation. Indeed, the autocrine function of TGF-α on cells was demonstrated by Marshall *et al.*,[78] where it was shown that cells transformed with *ras* genes did not grow as rapidly when their media was changed more frequently. It may be that TGF-α secretion by tumor cells is a reason why transformed cells in culture can continue to grow and be maintained at low concentrations of serum that would not support the growth of normal cells.

In a detailed review of TGF-α, Derynck[75] compared the effects of TGF-α with EGF. Since both use the same membrane receptor, at first glance it would appear that they should have nearly identical biologic effects. While this is true in some cases, there is an expanding body of literature showing major differences between the responses elicited by the two growth factors for some parameters. To quote Derynck, "In many cases, TGF-α is much more potent than EGF and seems to act as a superagonist," but the basis of the differential effects of α and EGF remain obscure. At any rate, the finding that *ras*-transformed cells secrete TGF-α may be quite significant in terms of attempting to understand the events of *ras*-mediated transformation. First, it may represent an answer for the apparent paradox of how a membrane-associated G protein, whose involvement in any signal transduction pathway has not been conclusively proved, can serve to enhance the proliferative capacity of the cell. Second, it provides a link for a membrane-associated *ras* oncogene product with a nuclear event. Proliferation centers around unregulated cell-cycle progression involving constant passes through S phase in which DNA is replicated. The question arises as to how a membrane-bound protein such as *ras* can effect a nuclear event such as DNA replication. TGF-α may be a vital link here, since a common feature of growth factors is their ability to induce cell-cycle progression. Finally, the role of TGF-α in *ras* transformation may require that researchers reevaluate the alterations associated with *ras* transformation. While mutations within *ras* genes or deregulation of the genes may be an initial step toward malignant transformation, it may be that TGF-α synthesis is a critical variable that may be responsible, in part, for the acquisition and maintenance of the transformed phenotype. If so, one must consider how TGF-α is regulated and then attempt to correlate changes in this to changes in *ras* for a more lucid picture of the alterations in these biochemical control mechanisms that lead to neoplasia.

## 6.2. The myc Oncogene in Burkitt Lymphomas and Murine Plasmacytomas

The c-*myc* oncogene is composed of three exons and two introns and codes for a protein of 439 amino acids with a molecular weight of 48,812,[85] which is post-translationally modified to a 62,000- to 64,000-$M_r$ nuclear protein.[86] The first exon of the mature mRNA is noncoding, as all three of its reading frames (in mice) contain stop codons. c-*myc* does not represent the only gene in the *myc* oncogene family. There are also other tissue-specific homologues, such as N-*myc* and L-*myc*.

The protein product of c-*myc* has been associated with DNA replication[87] (although the antibody to c-*myc* used in this study may cross-react with a DNA polymerase, which would tend to lessen the significance of this finding) and components involved in RNA processing.[88] These observations, coupled with earlier studies that showed that c-*myc* mRNA levels increased dramatically in response to mitogens,[89] seem to indicate an integral role for c-*myc* in proliferation of cells. Thus, neoplasia has been associated with deregulated or altered c-*myc* expression.

There are now several types of neoplasias in which an alteration of c-*myc* has been reported. For example, amplification (an increase in the number of genes associated with the appearance of double minute chromosomes) of c-*myc* has been linked to small cell lung carcinomas and carcinomas of the breast.[1,90] L-*myc* amplification has also been observed in small cell lung carcinomas, and amplification of N-*myc* has been seen in neuroblastomas, as well as small cell lung carcinomas.[90] However, the changes in c-*myc* that have been studied in greatest detail and that involve alterations in the control of c-*myc*, are those neoplasias involving chromosomal translocations at or near the c-*myc* gene locus. Such translocations are thought to be causal aberrations in Burkitt lymphomas and murine plasmactyomas.[91,92]

The chromosomal translocations involving c-*myc* in Burkitt lymphomas[90] and murine plasmacytomas[91] involve the joining of the c-*myc* locus to various immunoglobulin genes. This joining creates several situations in which the expression of c-*myc* can be altered, and it should be noted that a consensus of the exact modality of alteration has not been reached, since it is entirely possible that the various translocations and truncations of c-*myc* may allow for alterations in its expression by a variety of mechanisms. There are several possible modes for altering the levels of c-*myc* mRNA levels are: First, an alteration may render the normal control mechanisms inoperative so that c-*myc* can be expressed at inappropriate times. This is related to the cell-cycle specificity of c-*myc*, which has been reported to be activated during early $G_1$ shortly after mitogenic stimulation.[89,93] As noted by Campisi *et al.*,[93] a change in the cell-cycle specificity of an oncogene may contribute to the transformed phenotype. However, others[94] report that c-*myc* expression is not cell-cycle specific, which would in this case tend to make this hypothesis less plausible. Second, the translocated c-*myc* gene juxtaposed to an immunoglobulin gene may be subject to regulation by the immunoglobulin control elements, which can drive the expression of c-*myc* mRNA to higher than normal levels. Third, during the process of translocation, the c-*myc* gene is often truncated; i.e., the breakpoint of translocation occurs within the c-*myc* gene. The result is that c-*myc* minus a good deal of its 5' region (i.e., 5' flanking sequences, the first exon and/or some or all of the first intron) is joined to the immunoglobulin gene(s). The lack of these sequences in the subsequently transcribed truncated c-*myc* mRNA may increase the half-life time of c-*myc* mRNA, having a stabilizing effect. This can then give rise to abnormally high levels of c-*myc* mRNA.[1]

We will now examine these possibilities in the cases of Burkitt lymphomas and murine plasmacytomas. Three chromosomal translocations have been identified in Burkitt lymphomas. The most prevalent is t(8;14)(q24;q32), while variants of lower frequency, t(8;22)(q24;q11) and t(2;8)(p11;q24), have also been described.[95] Chromosomes 2, 14, and 22 all carry an immunoglobulin locus,[96–99] while the c-*myc* locus is at band q24 on chromosome 8, the region of chromosome 8 involved in all the aforementioned translocations.[100] In the first two translocations noted, the c-*myc* gene breaks at the noncoding 5' end or at various points upstream of that, so that either a truncated or intact c-*myc* is juxtaposed in a head-to-head fashion with an immunoglobulin locus.[95,101] The third translocation involves the breakage of an immunoglobulin light-chain gene, which then translocates to the normal c-*myc* locus in such a manner that the constant region of the light-chain locus is attached to c-*myc* in a head-to-tail fashion.[101–104] Even in translocations in which c-*myc* is broken within its 5' region, the protein product remains normal, since only the second and third exons of the gene code for the c-*myc* protein. What is the end result of these translocations? In the case of Burkitt lymphoma, it appears that the critical alteration in c-*myc* is a change in the transcriptional activity of the gene. c-*myc* is placed under the control of the constitutively active immunoglobulin regions, which results in constitutive expression of c-*myc* mRNA.[101] It is interesting to note that when the translocated allele is expressed at a high titer, the normal c-*myc* allele is expressed at very low levels or is transcriptionally silent.[105] Evidence has suggested that the critical alteration of c-*myc* in Burkitt lymphomas is due to the deletion or alteration of its first exon during breakage and subsequent translocation,[106] but the fact remains that in many Burkitt lymphomas, the c-*myc* gene remains completely intact upon translocation. Furthermore, truncated c-*myc* genes are not expressed at abnormally high levels, unless they are adjacent to one of the previously mentioned immunoglobulin loci.[105,107,108] It also appears that translocated c-*myc* genes in Burkitt lymphomas are more susceptible to mutations within the first exon of the gene, and these mutations have been reported to alter the transcription of c-*myc*.[109]

The murine plasmacytomas represent another system in which alterations in the control of c-*myc* have been closely studied. This neoplasm contains a translocation analogous to one of those found in human Burkitt lymphomas; c-*myc* is translocated to the immunoglobulin heavy-chain locus. c-*myc* resides on murine chromosome 15 and the murine heavy-chain immunoglobulin locus is on chromosome 12.[110] In the case of this neoplasia, it has been postulated by some that the critical alteration in the control of c-*myc* does not arise from a change in the transcriptional rate, but from a change in the stability of the c-*myc* mRNA. One study that concurs with this viewpoint[111] demonstrated that in various plasmacytoma cell lines, only those with a truncated c-*myc* gene code for a more stable mRNA, while those with an intact c-*myc* gene have a more labile c-*myc* mRNA. Transcriptional rates were nearly the same in all the plasmacytoma cell lines tested. This finding suggests a critical role for post-transcriptional processes in the regulation of c-*myc* mRNA levels. This mode of regulation has also been hypothesized to be a critical factor in normal Chinese hamster lung fibroblasts, which have been shown to have a relatively constant level of c-*myc* transcription, with the increase in c-*myc* mRNA following growth factor stimulation attributed to post-transcriptional mechanisms.[112]

An interesting finding is that in the case of the truncated c-*myc* gene, mRNA transcription is initiated from a little-used promoter within the first intron of the gene.[111] c-*myc* transcripts usually initiate from one of two promoters 160 base pairs apart at the 5' end of exon 1. One hypothesis attempting to explain the increased stability of the truncated c-*myc* mRNA is that the deletion of exon 1 and/or the presence of intron 1 sequences in the mature message confer extra stability on the mRNA. A recent report by Ray *et al.*[113] concurs with this viewpoint. These investigators showed that in Friend erythroleukemia cells, which do not have a rearranged c-*myc* gene, c-*myc* mRNA initiated from this promoter located in intron 1, known as P3, is more stable than those transcripts initiated from promoters within exon 1. These studies would apparently lend support to the idea that transcripts of c-*myc* initiated from promoters within the first intron, either naturally (no evidence of c-*myc* rearrangement) or as an artifact of truncation of the gene, exhibit significantly greater half-life times than do c-*myc* mRNA initiated from the usual promoter sites at the 5' end of exon 1.

From these studies, it becomes clear that the regulation of c-*myc* expression is subject to extremely complex control mechanisms that may vary from cell type to cell type or from mitogen to mitogen. For example, in BALB/cA31 fibroblasts, serum induction of c-*myc* is due both to changes in transcriptional rates and to post-transcriptional mechanisms. In the same cells, c-*myc* mRNA accumulation in response to EGF and effectors of cAMP is attributed to abrogation of a transcriptional block near the 3' end of exon 1.[114] New transcription per se and post-transcriptional mechanisms do not appear to be involved in this EGF response. Furthermore, this report also demonstrates that in F9 embryonal carcinoma cells control of c-*myc* occurs only at the post-transcriptional level.

It is important to give consideration to all models presented as being applicable when postulating how an alteration in the control of c-*myc* brings about neoplastic transformation. It must be stressed that the models are not mutually exclusive; i.e., deregulation of c-*myc* may be associated with changes in both transcriptional activity of the gene, as well as changes in the stability of c-*myc* mRNA half-lives. Indeed, it must first be answered whether the alteration in c-*myc* is the sole event precipitating the neoplasm in these tumors. There is evidence[115] that c-*myc* driven by immunoglobulin-enhancer elements may not in itself be capable of inducing neoplasia in transgenic mice. Rather, the constitutively high levels of c-*myc* mRNA may favor self-renewal or proliferation of the affected cell rather than allowing the cell to follow its normal maturation pathway, i.e., differentiation. This may then produce an expanded subject of immature cells (in this case, pre-B cells), which are, in turn, more vulnerable to a second genetic accident that can lead to neoplasia.

Control mechanisms involving the 3' end of c-*myc* mRNA have recently been uncovered. One report suggests that 3' untranslated sequences of c-*myc* are necessary for the normal rapid turnover of the mRNA.[116] Another report[117] demonstrates that polyadenylated c-*myc* mRNA turns over at a faster rate than does nonpolyadenylated c-*myc* mRNA. These observations may eventually become more significant with regard to alterations in c-*myc* that can lead to neoplastic changes as they are investigated more fully.

## 7. CONCLUSIONS

Although much work has been done concerning the alterations in biochemical controls that contribute to the malignant phenotype, the diverse etiologies of transformed cells require the consideration of multiple mechanisms for what results in the malignant cell. What has been presented here is only a concise discussion of some of the changes characteristic of neoplasias. We must elucidate control mechanisms at the levels of transcription and translation; we must further characterize the differences between normal and transformed cells; we need to determine, through in-depth analysis, which of the changes in neoplastic cells are causal changes and which are noncausal alterations. It must also be determined whether neoplasia results from a series of alterations in the cell that converge on a single point, that of the malignant phenotype, or whether a single event, be it at the level of the gene or the cell membrane, diverges into a multitude of changes collectively responsible for transformation.

Despite the identification of more than 40 oncogenes, a pattern of cooperation among two or more oncogenes is apparent. We consider the proposal by Weinberg,[2] that relatively few pathways are involved in the control of cell proliferation. Weinberg[2] grouped some of the oncogenes into two functional classes: cytoplasmic gene products such as that elicited by *ras*, which may be involved in second-messenger responses, and nuclear gene products such as *myc*-like proteins, which may be involved in transcriptional processes and nuclear functions. The patterns by which oncogene proteins may function are beginning to emerge in that the growth-control pathways may be altered by various mechanisms. Transduction of growth signals via altered receptor(s) or changes in signal-transducing proteins that are farther along in the pathway(s) but critical to $G_1/S$ transition are possibilities, as is autocrine stimulation of tumor cell growth. In the future, the interrelationships between the effectors that pass the signals from the cell surface to the nucleus and vice versa will be studied to dissect the mechanisms by which transformed cells are able to manifest their autonomous behavior.

The contribution of anti-oncogene (or tumor suppressor gene) inactivation in the development of neoplasia is presently undergoing active study. The role of negative regulatory functions in maintenance of the normal phenotype remains for further investigation. The contributions provided by anti-oncogenes, such as the retinoblastoma (RB) gene, whose loss results in neoplastic transformation in some cell types,[118,119] may be as important a consideration in tumorigenesis as is activation of some of the aforementioned oncogenes. This is an exciting field of cancer research that holds promise to further our understanding of the molecular events leading to neoplastic transformation.

## REFERENCES

1. Bishop, J. M., 1987, The molecular genetics of cancer, *Science* **235**:305–311.
2. Weinberg, R., 1985, The action of oncogenes in the cytoplasm and nucleus, *Science* **230**:770–776.
3. Baumbach, W. R., Keath, E. J., and Cole, M. D., 1986, A mouse c-myc retrovirus transforms established fibroblast lines *in vitro* and induces monocyte–macrophage tumors *in vivo*, *J. Virol.* **59**:276–283.
4. Sporn, M. B., and Todaro, G., 1986, Autocrine secretion and malignant transforming of cells, *N. Engl. J. Med.* **303**:878–880.
5. Foster, D. O., and Pardee, A. B., 1969, Transport of amino acids by confluent and nonconfluent 3T3 and polyoma virus-transformed 3T3 cells growing on glass cover slips, *J. Biol. Chem.* **244**:2675–2681.
6. Cunningham, D. D., and Pardee, A. B., 1969, Transport changes rapidly initiated by serum additions to "contact inhibited" 3T3 cells, *Proc. Natl. Acad. Sci. USA* **64**:1049–1056.

7. Isselbacher, K. J., 1972, Increased uptake of amino acids and 2-deoxy-*d*-glucose by virus-transformed cells in culture, *Proc. Natl. Acad. Sci. USA* **69**:585–589.

8. Boerner, P., and Saier, M., 1982, Growth regulation and amino acid transport in epithelial cells: Influence of culture conditions and transformation on A, ASC, L transport activities, *J. Cell. Physiol.* **113**:240–246.

9. Boerner, P., and Racker, E., 1985, Methionine-sensitive glycolysis in transformed cells, *Proc. Natl. Acad. Sci. USA* **82**:6750–6754.

10. Boerner, P., and Saier, M. H., Jr., 1985, Adaptive regulatory control of system A transport activity in a kidney epithelial cell line (MDCK) and in a transformed variant (MDCK-T$_1$), *J. Cell Physiol.* **122**:308–315.

11. Boerner, P., Resnick, R., and Racker, E., 1985, Stimulation of glycolysis and amino acid uptake in NRK-49F cells by transforming growth factor, *Proc. Natl. Acad. Sci. USA* **82**:1350–1353.

12. Heinz, A., Jackson, J. W., Richey, B. E., Sachs, G., and Schaefer, J. A., 1981, Amino acid active transport and stimulation by substrates in the absence of a Na$^+$ electrochemical potential gradient, *J. Membrane Biol.* **62**:149–160.

13. Zibirre, R., Poronnik, P., and Koch, G., 1986, Na$^+$-dependent amino transport is a major factor determining the rate of (Na$^+$/K$^+$)-ATPase mediated cation transport in intact HeLa cells, *J. Cell. Physiol.* **129**:85–93.

14. Guidotti, G. G., Gazzola, G. C., Borghetti, A. F., and Franchi-Gazzola, R., 1975, Adaptive regulation of amino acid transport across the cell membrane in avian and mammalian tissues, *Biochim. Biophys. Acta* **406**:264–275.

15. Mendoza, S. A., Wigglesworth, N. M., Pohjanpelto, P., and Rozengurt, E., 1980, Na entry and Na–K pump activity in murine, hamster, and human cells—Effect of monensin, serum, platelet extract, and viral transformation, *J. Cell. Physiol.* **103**:17–27.

16. Gadsby, D. C., Kimura, J., and Noma, A., 1985, Voltage dependence of Na/K pump current in isolated heart cells, *Nature (Lond.)* **315**:63–65.

17. Bashford, C. L., and Pasternak, C. A., 1986, Plasma membrane potential of some animal cells is generated by ion pumping, not by ion gradients, *Trends Biol. Sci.* **11**:113–116.

18. Leister, K. J., Schenerman, M. A., and Racker, E., 1988, Energetic mechanisms of System A transport in normal and transformed fibroblasts, *J. Cell. Physiol.* **135**:163–168.

19. Graves, J. S., and Wheeler, D. D., 1982, Increase in K$^+$ and a-AIB active transport after low (K$^+$) treatment, *Am. J. Physiol.* **243**:C124–130.

20. Kimelberg, H., and Mayhew, E., 1975, Increased ouabain-sensitive $^{86}$Rb$^+$ uptake and sodium and potassium ion-activated adenosine triphosphatase activity in transformed cell lines, *J. Biol. Chem.* **250**:100–104.

21. Tupper, J. T., 1977, Variation in potassium transport properties of mouse 3T3 cells as a result of subcultivation, *J. Cell. Physiol.* **93**:303–308.

22. Leister, K. J., Tomei, L. D., and Wenner, C. E., 1985, Correlation of ion movements with cell cycle activation, *Proc. Natl. Acad. Sci. USA* **82**:1599–1603.

23. Mitchison, J. M., 1971, *The Biology of the Cell Cycle*, Cambridge University Press, England.

24. Hacking, C., and Eddy, A. A., 1981, The accumulation of amino acids by mouse ascites-tumour cells, *Biochem. J.* **194**:415–426.

25. Pestka, S., 1971, Protein biosynthesis: Mechanism, requirements and potassium-dependency, in: *Membranes and Ion Transport* (E. E. Bittar, ed.), pp. 279–296, Wiley, New York.

26. Moldave, K., 1985, Eukaryotic protein synthesis, *Annu. Rev. Biochem.* **54**:1109–1149.

27. Suolinna, E-M., Lang, D., and Racker, E., 1974, Quercetin, an artificial regulator of the high aerobic glycolysis of tumor cells, *J. Natl. Cancer Inst.* **53**:1515–1519.

28. Benade, L. E., Talbot, N., Tagliaferri, P., Hardy, C., Card, J., Noda, M., Najam, N., and Bassin. R., 1986, Ouabain sensitivity is linked to ras-transformation in human HOS cells, *Biochem. Biophys. Res. Commun.* **136**:807–814.

29. Lelievre, L. G., Potter, J. D., Piascik, M., Wallick, E. T., Schwartz, A., Charlemagne, D., and Geny, B., 1985, Specific involvement of calmodulin and non-specific effect of tropomyosin in the sensitivity to ouabain of Na$^+$,K$^+$-ATPase in murine plasmacytoma cells, *Eur. J. Biochem.* **148**:13–19.

30. Lin, J. J., Yamashiro-Matsumura, S., and Matsumura, F., 1984, Microfilaments in normal and transformed cells: Changes in the multiple forms of tropomyosin, in: *Cancer Cells/The Transformed Phenotype* (A. Levine, G. Vande Woude, W. Topp, and J. D. Watson, eds.), pp. 57–65, Cold Spring Harbor Laboratory, New York.

31. Cooper, H. L., Feuerstein, N., Noda, M., and Bassin, R., 1985, Suppression of tropomyosin synthesis, a

common biochemical feature of oncogenesis by structurally diverse retroviral oncogenes, *Mol. Cell. Biol.* **5:**972–983.

32. Matsumura, F., and Yamashiro-Matsamura, S., 1986, Modulation of actin-bundling activity of 55-kDa protein by multiple isoforms of tropomyosin, *J. Biol. Chem.* **261:**4655–4659.

33. Racker, E., Resnick, R. J., and Feldman, R., 1985, Glycolysis, and methylaminoisobutyrate uptake in rat-1 cells transfected with ras or myc oncogenes, *Proc. Natl. Acad. Sci. USA.* **82:**3535–3538.

34. Racker, E., 1985, *Reconstitution of Transporters, Receptors, and Pathological States*, Academic, New York.

35. Balaban, B. S., and Bader, J. P., 1983, The efficiency of $(Na^+/K^+)$-ATPase in tumorigenic cells, *Biochim. Biophys. Acta* **730:**271–275.

36. Gibbs, J. B., Ellis, R. W., and Scolnick, E. M., 1979, Autophosphorylation of v-Ha-ras p21 is modulated by amino acid residue 12, *Proc. Natl. Acad. Sci. USA* **81:**2674–2678.

37. Lau, L. F., and Nathans, D., 1987, Expression of a set of growth-related immediate early genes in BALB/3T3 cells: Coordinate regulation with c-fos or c-myc, *Proc. Natl. Acad. Sci. USA* **84:**1182–1186.

38. Pollard, T. D., and Craig, S. W., 1982, Mechanism of actin polymerization, *Trends Biol. Sci.* **7:**55–58.

39. Jesaitis, A. J., Tolley, J. O., and Allen, R. A., 1986, Receptor–cytoskeleton interactions and membrane traffic may regulate chemoattractant-induced superoxide production in human granulocytes, *J. Biol. Chem.* **261:**13662–13669.

40. Weinhouser, S., 1956, On respiratory impairment in cancer cells, *Science* **124:**267–268.

41. Wenner, C. E., 1975, Regulation of energy metabolism in normal and tumor tissue, in: *Cancer: A Comprehensive Treatise*, Vol. 3 (F. F. Becker, ed.), pp. 389–401, Plenum, New York.

42. Parlo, R. A., and Coleman, P. S., 1984, Enhanced rate of citrate export from cholesterol-rich hepatoma mitochondria, *J. Biol. Chem.* **259:**9997–10003.

43. Sauer, L., Dauchy, R. T., Nagel, W. O., and Morris, H., 1980, Mitochondrial malic enzymes, *J. Biol. Chem.* **255:**3844–3848.

44. Fiskum, G., and Pease, A., 1986, Hydroperoxide-stimulated release of calcium from rat liver and AS-30D hepatoma mitochondria, *Cancer Res.* **46:**3459–3463.

45. Moreadith, R. W., and Lehninger, A. L., 1984, The pathways of glutamate and glutamine oxidation by tumor cell mitochondria, *J Biol. Chem* **259:**6215–6221.

46. Yu, C-L., Tsai, M-H., and Stacey, D. W., 1988, Cellular ras activity and phospholipid metabolism, *Cell* **52:**63–71.

47. Macara, I., 1985, Oncogenes, ions and phospholipids, *Am. J. Physiol.* **249:**C3–C11.

48. Weinberger, C., Thompson, C. C, Ong, E. S., Lebo, R., Gruol, D. J., and Evans, R. M., 1986, The c-erb-A gene encodes a thyroid hormone receptor, *Nature (Lond.)* **324:**641–646.

49. Loew, D. G., Capon, D. J., Delwart, E., Sakaguchi, A. Y., Naylor, S. L., and Goeddel, D. V., 1987, Structure of the human and murine R-ras genes, novel genes closely related to ras proto-oncogenes, *Cell* **48:**137–146.

50. Gilman, A. G., 1984, G proteins and dual control of adenylate cyclase, *Cell* **36:**577–579.

51. Robinson, C. L., Gibbs, J. B., Marshall, M. S., Sigal, I. S., and Tatchell, K., 1987, CDC25: A component of the RAS-adenylate cyclase pathway in *Saccharomyces cerevisiae, Science* **235:**1218–1221.

52. Boynton, A. L., and Whitfield, J. F., 1983, The role of cyclic AMP in cell proliferation: A critical assessment of the evidence, *Adv. Cyclic Nucleotides Res.* **15:**193–294.

53. Sweet, R. W., Yokoyama, S., Kamata, T., Feramisco, J. R., Rosenberg, M., and Gross, M., 1984, The product of ras is a GTPase and the T24 oncogenic mutant is deficient in this activity, *Nature (Lond.)* **311:**273–275.

54. Gibbs, J. B., Sigal, I. S., Poe, M., and Scolnick, E. M., 1984, Intrinsic GTPase activity distinguishes normal and oncogenic ras p21 molecules, *Proc. Natl. Acad. Sci. USA* **81:**5704–5708.

55. McCormick, F., Trahey, M., Rubinfeld, B., Wong, G., and Adari, H., 1988, Control of ras p21 GTPase activity by a cellular protein, *J. Cell. Biochem.* Suppl. 12A, Abstracts of the UCLA Symposia on Molecular and Cellular Biology, abst. C732, p. 170.

56. Taparowsky, E., Shimizu, K., Goldfarb, M., and Wigler, M., 1983, Structure and activation of the human N-ras gene, *Cell* **34:**581–586.

57. Santos, E., Tronick, S. R., Aaronson, S. A., Pulciani, S., and Barbacid, M., 1982, T24 human bladder carcinoma oncogene is an activated form of the normal human homologue of BALB- and Harvey-MSV transforming genes, *Nature (Lond.)* **298:**343–347.

58. Tabin, C. J., Bradley, S. M., Bargmann, C. I., Weinberg, R. A., Papageorge, A. G., Scolnick, E. M.,

Dahr, R., Lowy, D. R., and Chang, E. H., 1982, Mechanism of activation of a human oncogene, *Nature (Lond.)* **300:**143–149.

59. Yuasa, Y., Srivastava, S. K., Dunn, C. Y., Rhim, J. S., Reddy, E. P., and Aaronson, S. A., 1983, Acquisition of transforming properties by alternative point mutations within c-bas/has human proto-oncogene, *Nature (Lond.)* **303:**775–779.

60. Capon, D. J., Seeburg, P. H., McGrath, J. P., Hayflick, J. S., Edman, U., Levinson, A. D., and Goeddel, D. V., 1983, Activation of Ki-ras2 gene in human colon and lung carcinomas by two different point mutations, *Nature (Lond.)* **304:**507–513.

61. Quintanilla, M., Brown, K., Ramsden, M., and Balmain, A., 1986, Carcinogen-specific mutation and amplification of Ha-ras during mouse skin carcinogenesis, *Nature (Lond.)* **322:**78–80.

62. Newbold, R., 1984, Mutant ras proteins and cell transformation, *Nature (Lond.)* **310:**628–629.

63. Beckner, S. K., Hattori, S., and Shih, T. Y., 1985, The ras oncogene product is not a regulatory component of adenylate cyclase, *Nature (Lond.)* **317:**71–72.

64. Franks, D. J., Whitfield, J. F., and Durkin, J. P., 1985, The mitogenic/oncogenic p21 Ki-ras protein stimulates adenylate cyclase activity early in the $G_1$ phase of NRK rat kidney cells, *Biochem. Biophys. Res. Commun.* **132:**780–786.

65. Litosch, I., Wallis, C., and Fain, J. N., 1985, 5-Hydroxytryptamine stimulates inositol phosphate production in a cell-free system from blowfly salivary glands, *J. Biol. Chem.* **260:**5464–5471.

66. Houslay, D. A., Bojanic, D., and Wilson, A., 1986, Platelet activating factor and U44069 stimulate a GTPase activity in human platelets which is distinct from the guanine nucleotide regulatory proteins, $N_s$ and $N_i$, *Biochem. J.* **234:**737–740.

67. Wolfman, A., and Macara, I. G., 1987, Elevated levels of diacylglycerol and decreased phorbol ester sensitivity in ras-transformed fibroblasts, *Nature (Lond.)* **325:**359–361.

68. Lacal, J. C., Fleming, T. P., Warren, B. S., Blumberg, P. M., and Aaronson, S. A., 1987, Involvement of functional protein kinase C in the mitogenic response to the H-ras oncogene product, *Mol. Cell. Biol.* **7:**4146–4149.

69. Yatani, A., Codina, J., Imoto, Y., Reeves, J. P., Birnbaumer, L., and Brown, A. M., 1987, A G protein directly regulates mammalian cardiac calcium channels, *Science* **239:**1288–1292.

70. Sawey, M. J., Hood, A. T., Burns, F. J., and Garte, S. J., 1987, Activation of c-myc and c-K-ras oncogenes in primary rat tumors induced by ionizing radiation, *Mol. Cell. Biol.* **7:**932–935.

71. Guerrero, I., Calzada, P., Mayer, A., and Pellicer, A., 1984, A molecular approach to leukemogenesis: Mouse lymphomas contain an activated c-ras oncogene, *Proc. Natl. Acad. Sci. USA* **81:**202–205.

72. Cichutek, K., and Duesberg, P. H., 1986, Harvey ras genes transform without mutant codons, apparently activated by truncation of a 5′ (exon-1), *Proc. Natl. Acad. Sci. USA* **83:**2340–2344.

73. deVos, A. M., Tong, L., Milburn, M. V., Matias, P. M., Jancarik, J., Noguchi, S., Nishimura, S., Miura, K., Ohtsuka, E., and Kim, S-H., 1988, Three-dimensional structure of an oncogene protein: Catalytic domain of human c-H-ras p21, *Science* **239:**888–893.

74. DeLarco, J. E., and Todaro, G. J., 1978, Growth factors from murine sarcoma virus-transformed cells, *Proc. Natl. Acad. Sci. USA* **75:**4001–4005.

75. Derynck, R., 1986, Transforming growth factor-α: Structure and biological activities, *J. Cell. Biochem.* **32:**293–304.

76. Anzano, M. A., Roberts, A. B., Smith, J. M., Sporn, M. B., and DeLarco, J. E., 1983, Sarcoma growth factor from conditioned medium of virally transformed cells is composed of both type and transforming growth factors, *Proc. Natl. Acad. Sci. USA* **80:**6264–6268.

77. Kaplan, P. L., Anderson, M., and Ozanne, B., 1982, Transforming growth factor(s) production enables cells to grow in the absence of serum: An autocrine system, *Proc. Natl. Acad. Sci. USA* **79:**485–489.

78. Marshall, C. J., Vousden, K., and Ozanne, B., 1985, The involvement of activated ras genes in determining the transformed phenotype, *Proc. R. Soc. Lond.* **226:**99–106.

79. Massague, J., 1987, The transforming growth factors, in: *Oncogenes and Growth Factors* (R. A. Bradshaw and S. Prentis, eds.), pp. 157–163, Elsevier, New York.

80. Coffey, R. J., Jr., Derynck, R., Wilcox, J. N., Bringman, T. S., Goustin, A. S., Moses, H. L., and Pittelkow, M. R., 1987, Production and auto-induction of transforming growth factor alpha in human keratinocytes, *Nature (Lond.)* **328:**817–820.

81. Marquardt, H., Hunkapiller, M. A., Hood, L. E., and Todaro, G. J., 1984, Rat transforming growth factor type 1: Structure and relation to epidermal growth factor, *Science* **223:**1079–1082.

82. Twardzik, D. R., Kimball, E. S., Sherwin, S. A., Ranchalis, J. E., and Todaro, G. J., 1985, Comparison of growth factors functionally related to epidermal growth factor in the urine of normal and human tumor bearing athymic mice, *Cancer Res.* **45:**1934–939.

83. Lee, D. C., Rose, T. M., Webb, N. R., and Todaro, G. J., 1985, Cloning and sequence analysis of a cDNA for rat transforming growth factor-α, *Nature (Lond.)* **313**:489–491.

84. Derynck, R., Goeddel, D. V., Ullrich, A., Gutterman, J. U., Williams, R. D., Bringman, T. S., and Berger, W. H., 1987, Synthesis of messenger RNAs for transforming growth factors and the epidermal growth factor receptor by human tumors, *Cancer Res.* **47**:707–712.

85. Watt, R., Stanton, L. W., Marcu, K. B., Gallo, R. C., Croce, C. M., and Rovera, G., 1983, Nucleotide sequence of cloned cDNA of human c-myc oncogene, *Nature (Lond.)* **303**:725–728.

86. Marcu, K. B., 1987, Regulation of expression of the c-myc proto-oncogene, *BioEssays* **6**:28–32.

87. Studzinski, G. P., Brelvi, Z. S., Feldman, S. C., and Watt, R. A., 1986, Participation of c-myc protein in DNA synthesis of human cells, *Science* **234**:467–470.

88. Spector, D. L., Watt, R. A., and Sullivan, N. F., 1987, The v- and c-myc oncogene proteins colocalize *in situ* with small nuclear ribonucleoprotein particles, *Oncogene* **1**:5–12.

89. Kelly, K., Cochran, B. H., Stiles, C. D., and Leder, P., 1983, Cell-specific regulation of the c-myc gene by lymphocyte mitogens and platelet-derived growth factor, *Cell* **35**:603–610.

90. Varmus, H. E., 1984, The molecular genetics of cellular oncogenes, *Annu. Rev. Genet.* **18**:553–612.

91. Klein, G., 1983, Specific chromosomal translocations and the genesis of B-cell derived tumors in mice and men, *Cell* **32**:311–315.

92. Marcu, K. B., Harris, L. J., Stanton, L. W., Erikson, J., Watt, R., and Croce, C. M., 1983, Transcriptionally active c-myc oncogene is contained within NIARD, a DNA sequence associated with chromosomal translocations in B-cell neoplasia, *Proc. Natl. Acad. Sci. USA* **80**:519–523.

93. Campisi, J., Gray, H. E., Pardee, A. B., Dean, M., and Sonenshein, G. E., 1984, Cell-cycle control of c-myc but not c-ras expression is lost following chemical transformation, *Cell* **36**:241–247.

94. Thompson, C. B., Challoner, P. B., Neiman, P. E., and Groudine, M., 1985, Levels of c-myc oncogene mRNA are invariant throughout the cell cycle, *Nature (Lond.)* **314**:363–366.

95. Croce, C. M., 1986, Chromosomal translocations and human cancer, *Cancer Res.* **46**:6019–6023.

96. Croce, C. M., Shander, M., Martinis, J., Cicurel, L., D'Ancona, G. G., Dolby, T. W., and Koprowski, H., 1979, Chromosomal location of the genes for human immunoglobulin heavy chains, *Proc. Natl. Acad. Sci. USA* **76**:3416–3419.

97. Erikson, J., Martinis, J., and Croce, C. M., 1981, Assignment of the genes for human immunoglobulin chains to chromosome 22, *Nature (Lond.)* **294**:173–175.

98. McBride, O. W., Hieter, P. A., Hollis, G. F., Swan, D., Otey, M. C., and Leder, P., 1982, Chromosomal location of human kappa and lambda immunoglobulin light chain constant regions, *J. Exp. Med.* **155**:1480–1490.

99. Erikson, J., ar-Rushdi, A., Drwinga, H. L., Nowell, P. C., and Croce, C. M., 1983, Transcriptional activation of the translocated c-myc oncogene in Burkitt lymphoma, *Proc. Natl. Acad. Sci. USA* **80**:810–824.

100. Dalla-Favera, R., Martinotti, S., Gallo, R. C., Erikson, J., and Croce, C. M., 1983, Translocation and rearrangements of the c-myc oncogene locus in human undifferentiated B-cell lymphomas, *Science* **219**:963–967.

101. Klein, G., and Klein, E., 1985, Evolution of tumors and the impact of molecular oncology, *Nature (Lond.)* **315**:190–195.

102. Croce, C. M., Thierfelder, W., Erikson, J., Nishikura, K., Finan, J., Lenoir, G. M., and Nowell, P. C., 1983, Transcriptional activation of an unrearranged and untranslocated c-myc oncogene by translocation of a C locus in Burkitt lymphoma cells, *Proc. Natl. Acad. Sci. USA* **80**:6922–6926.

103. Erikson, J., Nishikura, K., ar-Rushdi, A., Finan, J., Emanuel, B., Lenoir, G., Nowell, P. C., and Croce, C. M., 1983, Translocation of an immunoglobulin k locus to a region 3' of an unrearranged c-myc oncogene enhances c-myc transcription, *Proc. Natl. Acad. Sci. USA* **80**:7581–7585.

104. Emanuel, B. S., Selden, J. R., Chaganti, R. S. K., Jhanwar, S., Nowell, P. C., and Croce, C. M., 1984, The 2p breakpoint of a 2;8 translocation in Burkitt lymphoma interrupts the $V_k$ locus, *Proc. Natl. Acad. Sci. USA* **81**:2444–2446.

105. Nishikura, K., ar-Rushdi, A., Erikson, J., Watt, R., Rovera, G., and Croce, C. M., 1983, Differential expression of the normal and of the translocated human c-myc oncogenes in B cells, *Proc. Natl. Acad. Sci. USA* **80**:4822–4826.

106. Leder, P., Battey, J., Lenoir, G., Moulding, C., Murphy, W., Potter, H., Stewart, T., and Taub, R., 1983, Translocations among antibody genes in human cancer, *Science* **222**:765–771.

107. Nishikura, K., ar-Rushdi, A., Erikson, J., DeJesus, E., Dugan, D., and Croce, C. M., 1984, Repression of rearranged gene and translocated c-myc in mouse 3T3 cells × Burkitt lymphoma cell hybrids, *Science* **224**:399–402.

108. Feo, S., Harvey, R., Showe, L., and Croce, C. M., 1986, Regulation of translocated c-myc genes transfected into plasmacytoma cells, *Proc. Natl. Acad. Sci. USA* **83:**706–709.

109. Cesarman, E., Dalla-Favera, R., Bentley, D., and Groudine, M., 1987, Mutations in the first exon are associated with altered transcription of c-myc in Burkitt lymphoma, *Science* **238:**1272–1275.

110. Stanton, L. W., Watt, R., and Marcu, K. B., 1983, Translocation, breakage and truncated transcripts of c-myc oncogene in murine plasmacytomas, *Nature (Lond.)* **303:**401–406.

111. Piechaczyk, M., Yang, J. Q., Blanchard, J. M., Jeanteur, P., and Marcu, K. B., 1985, Posttranscriptional mechanisms are responsible for accumulation of truncated c-myc RNAs in murine plasma cell tumors, *Cell* **42:**589–597.

112. Blanchard, J. M., Piechaczyk, M., Dani, C., Chambard, J. C., Franchi, A., Pouyssegur, J., and Jeanteur, P., 1985, c-myc gene is transcribed at high rate in $G_0$-arrested fibroblasts and is post-transcriptionally regulated in response to growth factors, *Nature (Lond.)* **317:**443–445.

113. Ray, D., Meneceur, P., Tavitian, A., and Robert-Lezenes, J., 1987, Presence of a c-myc transcript initiated in intron 1 in Friend erythroleukemia cells and in other murine cell types with no evidence of c-myc gene rearrangement, *Mol. Cell. Biol.* **7:**940–945.

114. Nepveu, A., Levine, R. A., Campisi, J., Greenberg, M. E., Ziff, E. B., and Marcu, K. B., 1987, Alternative modes of c-myc regulation in growth factor-stimulated and differentiating cells, *Oncogene* **1:**243–250.

115. Langdon, W. Y., Harris, A. W., Cory, S., and Adams, J. M., 1986, The c-myc oncogene perturbs B lymphocyte development in Eμ-*myc* transgenic mice, *Cell* **47:**11–18.

116. Jones, T. R., and Cole, M. D., 1987, Rapid cytoplasmic turnover of c-myc mRNA: Requirement of the 3′ untranslated sequences, *Mol. Cell. Biol.* **7:**4513–4521.

117. Swartwout, S. G., Preisler, H., Guan, W., and Kinniburgh, A. J., 1987, Relatively stable population of c-myc RNA that lacks long poly(A), *Mol. Cell. Biol.* **7:**2052–2058.

118. Friend, S. H., Dryja, T. P., and Weinberg, 1988, Oncogenes and tumor-suppressing genes, *N. Engl. J. Med.* **318:**618–622.

119. Harbour, J. W., Lai, S., Whang-peng, J., Gazdar, A. F., Minna, J. D., and Kaye, F. J., 1988, Abnormalities in structure and expression of the human retinoblastoma gene in SCLC, *Science* **241:**353–357.

# 16

# Membrane Alterations in Neoplasia

## D. James Morré

## 1. INTRODUCTION

Since the 1960s, considerable attention has been paid to alterations of cellular membranes associated with cell transformation and malignancy. Many studies have been directed at a search for significant alterations particularly at the cell surface* and, more specifically, in the plasma membrane. However, during malignancy, membrane alterations are not limited to the plasma membrane. They have also been demonstrated in intracellular membranes. Nevertheless, since the plasma membrane plays a key role in cellular growth control, differentiation, invasion, and metastasis, it continues to be the focus of much attention in cancer research.

For membrane alterations to be expressed at the cell surface, it is most likely that they arise through biosynthetic or processing modifications directed through the ultimate action of altered genetic information but expressed through membrane-associated enzymes of the cell's internal endomembranes (Golgi apparatus, endoplasmic reticulum, and nuclear envelope). Furthermore, organelles such as mitochondria, lysosomes, and peroxisomes also show modifications, especially during the more advanced stages of tumor progression. Thus, the alterations associated with cell transformation and malignancy have been observed to be both numerous and varied. It is the aim of this chapter to review some of the more important membrane alterations associated with cell transformation and malignancy and to provide the reader with an appreciation of those changes most often expressed as part of the cancer phenotype.

## 2. ULTRASTRUCTURAL MEMBRANE PATHOLOGY OF NEOPLASIA

It follows from a considerable number of observations that functional changes in membranes are frequently expressed in terms of ultrastructural alterations and vice versa. Thus, much can be appreciated about the extent of membrane changes associated with neoplasia from a careful survey of known ultrastructural membrane pathology. It is important that only observations of well-fixed and well-preserved material be considered. What may appear as an ultrastructural alteration under

---

*The cell surface is defined here as the plasma membrane plus associated glycoconjugate molecules at the cell's exterior, which form a surface coat.

*D. James Morré* • Department of Medicinal Chemistry and Pharmacognosy, Purdue University, West Lafayette, Indiana 47907.

certain circumstances may only be a response to fixation or some pathologic change resulting from a delay perhaps between tissue collection and actual fixation.

In addition, it is clear that in certain tumors or transformed cell types, one particular type of change may be manifest but will be absent from another tumor of the same type or from a tumor of a different tissue of origin. The following sections emphasize the ultrastructural changes that occur with relative frequency in transformed cells and tissues. Among the more widely studied experimental tumors are rat hepatomas.

For purpose of analysis, the cellular membranes are grouped broadly into four categories[1]: (1) the internal endomembranes, chiefly the nuclear envelope with its extensions continuous with a system of rough (with ribosomes) and smooth (lacking ribosomes) endoplasmic reticulum (the endoplasmic reticulum is coupled via various transition membranes and vesicles to the Golgi apparatus, which in turn delivers membrane to the cell surface by a system of secretory vesicles); (2) a second pathway extends from the cell surface inward and is involved in endocytosis and intracellular digestion (membrane types of this pathway include the endosomes and lysosomes and their associated carrier vesicles and tubules); (3) a third major category of membranous cell components are the respiratory organelles, mitochondria, and peroxisomes; and (4) the final cell component is the plasma membrane itself.

## 2.1. Endomembranes

### 2.1.1. Nuclei and Nuclear Envelopes

The nucleus of malignant neoplastic cells is characterized by alterations in the structure of the chromatin, nuclear membrane, and nucleolus.[2] The shape of the nucleus is frequently irregular with sharp projections jutting into the cytoplasm together with indentations and deep angular folds (Fig. 1). The marked irregularities of shape presented by nuclei are well known to pathologists. Even more dramatic are the complex, extreme, and bizarre shapes of tumor nuclei seen in the electron microscope. However, the severity of the alterations in nuclear shape appears to be linked more or less to tumor progression, and certain minimum deviation hepatomas have been found to exhibit quite normal-appearing nuclei. Abnormal mitoses, such as tripolar or quadripolar figures, provide a better indication of neoplasia than do simply the mere presence of mitoses. Multinucleation with variation between daughter nuclei also occurs in malignant neoplasia and aids in its identification. Also related to malignancy is the nuclear to cytoplasmic ratio, which increases in malignancy. In most normal cell types, the nuclear volume as percent of cell volume ranges from about 2 to 25%, depending on the cell type, but in cells from malignant solid tumors this percentage generally increases to 20–40%.[3,4]

The well-known hyperchromasia of the neoplastic nucleus is now attributed to polyploidy.[5] Such hyperchromatic nuclei contain large and numerous heterochromatin masses. However, among tumors one also finds pale nuclei with a paucity of heterochromatin and a preponderance of active euchromatin. In many instances, the tumor nucleus is large and pale, with only scant small aggregates of heterochromatin.

Nucleolar form also is irregular. Nucleoli are sometimes enlarged, although size is not a discriminating criterion. They may be at the nuclear periphery and often have abnormal arrangements of their major components. Their larger size, when it occurs, is indicative of rapid RNA turnover, perhaps reflecting a heightened rate of cell replication. In some Morris hepatomas, the nucleoli have been shown to more nearly resemble those of embryonic rat liver than those of adult rat hepatocytes.[6]

The nuclear envelope per se is little changed in neoplasia. Nuclear pore diameter of nuclear envelopes of rat hepatomas also is unchanged. Values range from 92 to 109 nm outer diameter (depending on the method of specimen preparation) compared with 92–114 nm outer diameter for normal rat liver.[7] Parallel sets of lamellar structures known as annulate lamellae, resembling and sometimes continuous with the nuclear envelope, are usually seen in tumor cells with greater frequency than in normal cells. Annulate lamellae are essentially nuclear envelope material that exists in the cytoplasm and, as such, are characterized by regularly spaced nuclear pore structures.

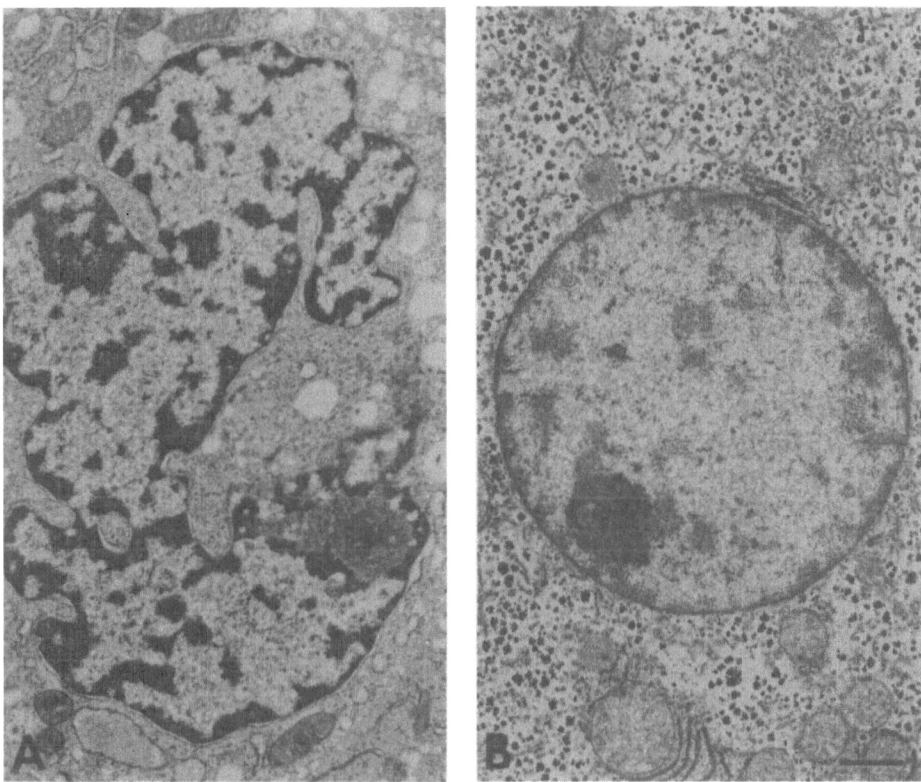

*Figure 1.* (A) Nuclear irregularity in a rat hepatoma cell culture. (B) A nucleus of a parenchyma cell from rat liver is shown on the right for comparison. These two views represent the extremes of nuclear morphology likely to be encountered in, for example, a series of hepatomas of varying growth rates.

## 2.1.2. Rough Endoplasmic Reticulum

The main functions of the rough endoplasmic reticulum with its attached polyribosomes are the synthesis of membrane proteins as well as the elaboration of secretory or export proteins. Other proteins required for endogenous cellular needs, along with some additional membrane proteins, are translated on free polyribosomes located within the cytoplasm.

A well-developed rough endoplasmic reticulum with regularly arranged cisternae running parallel to one other (so-called stacked configuration) is primarily an expression of cells differentiated for protein export. Immature or undifferentiated cells such as stem, blast, or embryonal cells, or even cells in culture, have a much more sparse and less well-ordered complement of rough endoplasmic reticulum.

By contrast, growing cells have a larger abundance of free polyribosomes in the cytoplasm. Thus, it is not surprising that one of the hallmarks of the transformed cell cytoplasm, which is associated with rapid rates of cell proliferation, is a decrease in the ratio of polyribosomes bound to the endoplasmic reticulum to the polyribosomes free in the cytoplasm.[8,9] Within the range of Morris hepatomas, for example, rough endoplasmic reticulum may range from well-ordered and near-normal appearance in minimum deviation tumors to only occasional irregularly spaced cisternae in the more poorly differentiated invasive tumors. Less commonly observed, but frequently associated with late stages of tumor development, are bizarre endoplasmic reticulum forms, such as whorls or tightly coiled arrangements.

### 2.1.3. Smooth Endoplasmic Reticulum

Smooth endoplasmic reticulum, endoplasmic reticulum lacking ribosomes, is most evident in such cell types as hepatocytes, in which it can be induced. Smooth endoplasmic reticulum is formed in large quantities through the administration of xenobiotic substances. These substances are subjected in smooth endoplasmic reticulum to mixed-function oxidation as an initial step in the detoxification process or as occurs during the metabolism of chemical procarcinogens to their active forms (see Chapter 2). While such endoplasmic reticulum forms are encountered in preneoplastic livers following administration of high doses of many types of chemical carcinogens, they appear not to persist as a general characteristic of the cytoplasm of malignant hepatic tumors. In most malignant tumors, the smooth endoplasmic reticulum is restricted to transition regions in association with the Golgi apparatus or other organelles in which ribosomes may be naturally sparse or absent. However, in tumors producing steroid hormones, smooth endoplasmic reticulum is typically abundant.

### 2.1.4. Golgi Apparatus

The Golgi apparatus is a cell component of membrane biogenesis[10] and also has as a major function the secretion of materials for export to the cell surface.[11] It is involved in the processing of membrane proteins and glycoproteins [12-14] as well as in the formation of lysosomes.[12,15] Its role in cell transformation and cancer is less well understood, although several authors have noted that a relationship must exist.[1,16-18]

Evidence for an altered Golgi apparatus in the transformed state has come both from morphologic and from biochemical investigations. A change in the dimensions of Golgi apparatus in hepatomas compared with host liver was noted by McCarthy et al.[19] Similarly, in a series of 35 Morris hepatomas of differing growth rates, Hruban et al.[20,21] found an effect on the lengths or number of cisternae of the Golgi apparatus that was largely independent of hepatoma growth rate. Compared with normal liver, hepatomas have also lost to varying degrees the ability to elaborate specific secretory proteins into serum.[22] These, and other observations, led Reutter and Bauer[16] to suggest that, in transformed cells, the Golgi apparatus may shift from a secretory to a membrane-generating mode of functioning (see also Hudgin et al.[23] for a similar interpretation).

The Golgi apparatus of tumor cells does not appear grossly altered, although the dictyosomal stacks have been found to be of a smaller diameter relative to tissues of origin. For the most part, the tumor Golgi apparatus seems to acquire a morphology similar to that ascribed to Golgi apparatus forms in juvenile or dividing cells.[1]

## 2.2. Lysosomes and Endocytic Compartments

There appears to be no consistent correlation between the number and distribution of lysosomes and transformation. Lysosomes may occur in various types of neoplastic cells, and their numbers may either be increased or decreased relative to normal. Autophagosomes occur frequently in some instances, but not in others. Using protein A-colloidal gold immunoelectron microscopy and monospecific antibodies to the weak base primaquine, HEP G-2 cells were found to contain a normal spectrum of endocytic compartments.[24]

Lysosomal changes in tumor cells include an increased number in several carcinogen-induced [7,12-dimethylbenz[a]anthracene (DMBA)] and transplanted (renal, Guérin, Walker, mammary, hepatoma) tumors and in the livers of tumor-bearing animals (see Leighton and Morré[25] for specific examples). Yet size, heterogeneity, and extreme pleomorphism exhibited by normal lysosomes make it difficult to evaluate the lysosomal characteristics that may be altered in response to malignant transformation.

Targeting of lysosomal enzymes to lysosomes is thought to involve a mannose 6-phosphate signal recognized by specific membrane-located receptors. In Morris hepatoma 7777 cells, in contrast to normal rat hepatocytes, synthesis of mannose 6-phosphate receptors was found to be below the limits of detection.[26] Apparently, transfer of cathepsin C and perhaps other lysosomal enzymes to lysosomes in Morris hepatoma 7777 cells occurs by mechanisms independent of the mannose 6-phosphate-specific receptors.

## 2.3. Mitochondria and Peroxisomes

### 2.3.1. Mitochondria

There is abundant information to suggest that tumor cells contain fewer mitochondria than their normal counterparts.[27] Tumor mitochondria generally display pleomorphism and are often smaller and electron lucent, but their contents can be electron dense.[28] Those mitochondria that are present in transformed malignant neoplastic cells are more heterogeneous in size and appearance than are those of their nontransformed counterparts (Fig. 2). The mitochondria may be larger or smaller than normal, with differences in the amount and organization of the cristae. Rapidly growing tumors

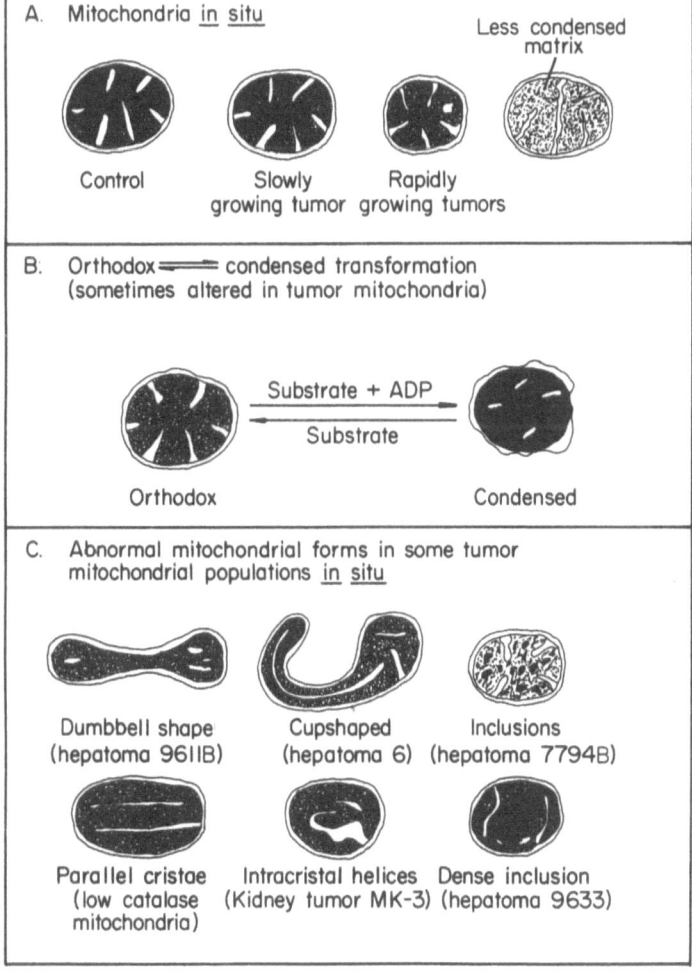

*Figure 2.* Diagram illustrating changes in mitochondria associated with transformation. (Adapted from Pedersen.[27])

generally have smaller mitochondria with fewer cristae. In slow-growing tumors, mitochondria may be larger with more normal appearing characteristics or may even contain a number of cristae that is greater than normal. Tumor mitochondria exhibit such a wide range of variation that it may be that each type of tumor exhibits a mitochondrial population of characteristic size, shape, and number. Yet, despite consistent quantitative changes and numerous differences between tumor and normal mitochondria in terms of size, length, diameter, morphology, and distribution,[29] most tumors are characterized by a relatively normal appearing population of mitochondria. The abnormal or bizarre mitochondrial forms (Fig. 2) that may occur in some tumors, i.e., those with either unusual shapes (dumbbell or cup) or with unusual cristae or inclusions appear to be more the exception than the rule. Even less common are alterations in mitochondrial morphology, such as pyknotic mitochondria or rodlike, C-shaped, or ring-shaped mitochondrial profiles with longitudinal rather than transverse cristae.[27]

Mitochondria appear to be among the most pleomorphic of all cell components in regard to sensitivity to transformation. Despite this wide range of variation *in situ,* tumor mitochondria when isolated from the cell are relatively normal in respiration, ATP synthesis, P/O ratio, and other basic properties related to energy.[27] The high aerobic glycolysis generally characteristic of poorly differentiated tumors may result partly from low respiratory activity (due perhaps only to the reduced numbers of mitochondria rather than any particular functional defect). Equally important, however, are the high levels of glycolytic transphosphorylating enzymes of the cytoplasm, the overall elevation of glycolytic enzymes, the predominance of fetal isozymes of key glycolytic enzymes, and the overall reduction of gluconeogenesis that seem to accompany tumor progression (see Chapters 15 and 21).

### 2.3.2. Peroxisomes

Peroxisomes, cell components containing oxidases that generate hydrogen peroxide and use it to oxidize various compounds, are ubiquitous among normal cells. Identification is often based solely on the biochemical or histochemical detection of catalase. Nevertheless, data suggest that peroxisomes from transformed cells are biochemically and morphologically heterogeneous[30–32] and perhaps even absent from some malignant neoplasms. Because of their small size in some neoplasms, lack of nucleoids, and frequent connections with endoplasmic reticulum, they are sometimes identified as microperoxisomes.[33]

Dalton[8] observed that the size of peroxisomes (microbodies) is related inversely to growth rate of hepatomas (see also refs. 9 and 34). This is shown in Fig. 3 for a series of Morris hepatomas. In rapidly growing hepatomas, peroxisomes were swollen or absent and frequently lacked nucleoids.[36,37] Microbody crystalloid size decreased in Morris hepatomas compared with normal liver.[20] Thus, the loss of morphologic organization of peroxisomes in hepatomas[38] leads to the conclusion that in highly differentiated hepatomas, the control mechanism for formation of peroxisomes is impaired.[39] Even though peroxisomes may disappear completely from certain poorly differentiated hepatomas, their presence in other tumors suggests that their loss is a result of the transformation process rather than a causal factor in neoplastic development.[20]

### 2.4. Plasma Membrane

Scanning electron microscopy (SEM) studies have suggested that the surface of malignant cells is generally more irregular than normal, with a relative increase in the number of surface microvilli and cytoplasmic lamellipodia suggestive of a retention in tumors of those features characteristic of rapidly dividing cells (Table I). Other changes may be more functionally related to the loss of contact inhibition or the failure of cancer cells to adhere (i.e., thicker cytoplasm, tendency to round up).

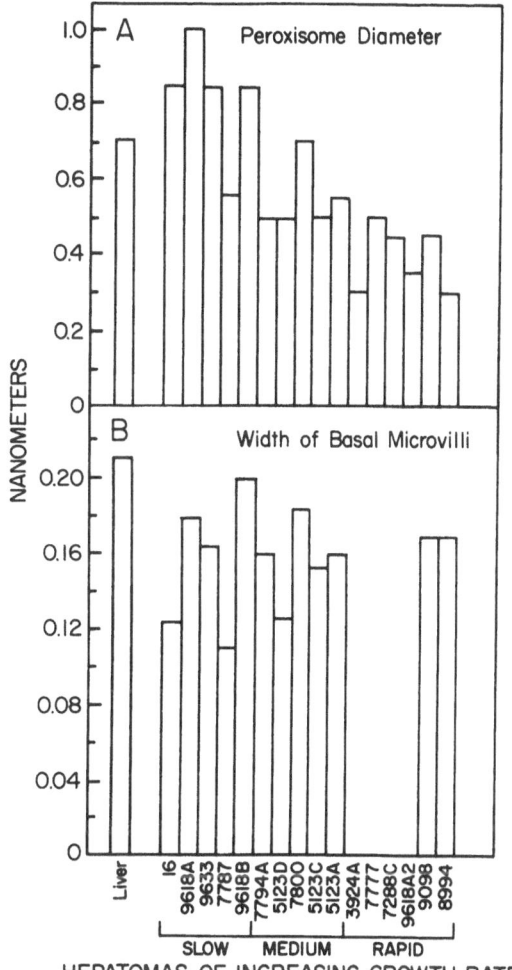

*Figure 3.* Comparison of two morphological parameters, peroxisome diameter (a) and width of microvilli at the basal cell surface (b) for a series of Morris hepatomas of increasing growth rate. Morphologic measurements are from Hruban *et al.*[20] Hepatoma growth rates were ranked according to Weber.[35] (a) Peroxisome diameter decreases progressively with increasing hepatoma growth rate, suggesting that this parameter is progression linked. (b) A 10–40% decrease (average 25%) in the width of basal microvilli, when significantly different from normal liver, shows characteristics of being a transformation-linked alteration. The reduction was observed in all hepatomas whether slow, medium, or rapidly growing.

With cancer cells growing in organized tissues, important surface features have to do with cell junctions. Normal cells *in vivo* form cell–cell junctions that are ultrastructurally complex.[40] Cells of tumors are often found to be deficient in the formation of junctional complexes. In carcinomas, the number of junctions may be reduced compared with the normal tissue of origin, and those junctions that are present may be modified (i.e., attenuation of desmosomes, "opening up" of tight junctions). In some benign tumors of epithelial origin (e.g., warts, keratoacanthomas), however, junctions and especially desmosomes, may actually increase in frequency.[41,42] Despite some rather dramatic examples, Weinstein *et al.*[43] concluded, after an extensive review of the literature, that no consistent pattern of junctional deficiencies existed in reference to malignancy as a whole.

The occurrence of cell junctions nevertheless continues to serve as an important criterion in tumor diagnosis. Tight junctions and desmosomes, characteristic of epithelia, denote a carcinoma when found in tumor tissue, whereas the complete absence of junctions is typically a characteristic of sarcomas.

Some tumor plasma membranes may exhibit desmosomelike structures (paired subplasma

Table I. External Surface Features of Normal and Malignant Cells in Culture[a]

| Feature | Description | Location | Internal structure | Appearance on transformed cells |
|---|---|---|---|---|
| Microvilli | Filamentous 0.1-$\mu$m diameter and up to 2 $\mu$m length | Mostly on top surface | Longitudinal, parallel 6-nm microfilaments | Varying in number, length, and distribution, often exhibiting distorted shapes |
| Filopodia | Filamentous 0.1-$\mu$m diameter up to 30 $\mu$m or longer in length | Often from margin, may be from top surface; extends to substrate and other cells | May contain microfilaments | Occur in unusual numbers and may be distorted |
| Ruffles | Sheetlike, 0.1-$\mu$m thick, up to 10 $\mu$m long, may be as wide as the cell | Mostly marginal at leading edge of migrating cell; occasionally on top surface | Microtrabecular lattice that is actin rich | On margins and top surfaces, possibly several on a cell |
| Blebs (knobs) | Spherical and hemispherical; 0.2–5–10 $\mu$m in diameter | May appear anywhere on cell surface not adherent to substrate | Any cytoplasmic material | May appear in large numbers and persist for long duration, especially on unspread cells |
| Retraction fibers and attachment fibers | Filamentous, 0.1-$\mu$m diameter, and wider, as long as 30 $\mu$m | From surface of spherical and highly convex cells; extend to substrate and other cells | May contain microfilaments | May be reduced in number; usually absent on poorly spread cells |
| Lobopodia | Peninsular strands of cytoplasm, cross section may be flat or round | From margin of flat cells or from spherical mass of mitotic cells | May contain filaments of cytoskeleton (e.g., stress fibers) | Perhaps fewer on mitotic cells; absent on poorly spread cells |

[a]Adapted from Hynes.[54]

membrane densities) or hemidesmosomelike structures (subplasma membrane densities).[5] Desmosomelike structures are not just poorly differentiated desmosomes; they are entirely different structures. Franke et al.[44] reported that antibodies to desmoplakins (peptides found in plaques of desmosomes) bind specifically to surfaces of tumor types that contain desmosomes but not to those that lack true desmosomes or attenuated desmosomes, but that may contain desmosomelike structures (e.g., rhabdomyosarcoma, hemangioma, malignant fibrous histocytoma). In this regard, it has been proposed that these specific desmosomal proteins may serve as new markers for the identification and classification of tumors.[45]

## 3. FUNCTIONAL ALTERATIONS OF ENDOMEMBRANES AND THE PLASMA MEMBRANE IN NEOPLASIA

### 3.1. Endoplasmic Reticulum

Membrane proteins are assembled on polyribosomes. A portion is synthesized on membrane-bound polyribosomes, and others are synthesized on cytoplasmic polyribosomes. Proteins exported from the cell are synthesized predominantly on membrane-bound polyribosomes, whereas proteins synthesized by free polyribosomes are most often involved with maintenance of cellular function. The shift from membrane-bound to free polyribosomes in many types of tumors is consistent with the emphasis in tumors on synthesis of cellular proteins needed for cell growth and division.

Fast growth rate is often, but not always, associated with a paucity of rough endoplasmic reticulum. Rapid cellular division, reduction of rough-surfaced endoplasmic reticulum, and abundance of free polysomes in fast growing tumors are highly correlated.[46] Yet, endoplasmic reticulum that remains in tumor cells appears to carry out functions similar to those of endoplasmic reticulum in normal cells, including the co-translational addition of asparagine-linked high-mannose oligosaccharides to nascent polypeptide chains and their transport to Golgi apparatus for processing and delivery to the cell surface.[47]

Abnormal endoplasmic reticulum forms do occur and seem to be produced in excess in some rat hepatomas.[48] These abnormal intracellular membranes are recognized in normal liver cells and removed by autophagy and focal degradation. Hruban *et al.*[48] suggested that tumor cells may not readily recognize the abnormal endoplasmic reticulum structures or possess defects that limit the autophagic system.

## 3.2. Golgi Apparatus

Biochemical evidence for a functionally altered Golgi apparatus in transformation has been more inferred from the known subcellular localization of glycoconjugate processing enzymes in various parts of the Golgi apparatus rather than from direct measurements either *in situ* or with isolated fractions. Glycoproteins and glycolipids that are altered in tumorigenesis frequently have L-fucose or *N*-acetylneuraminic acid as terminal sugars.[16] While well-studied examples are lacking, many authors have reached the conclusion that at least some of the glycoproteins so modified may be involved in changes in cellular adhesion and communication that contribute to the aberrant social behavior characteristic of the transformed phenotype.[18,49–54] Thus, the Golgi apparatus appears to function not only as a shipping and receiving center for membrane quanta, but it may be responsible as well for imparting to the membranes some of the specific characteristics important to their postulated roles in control of growth and cell adhesion.[10–12]

Variability in transport rates of secretory glycoproteins through the endoplasmic reticulum and Golgi apparatus from both rodent and human hepatoma cells were noted,[47,55] but it is not known to what extent they are influenced by transformation. The overall pattern of processing and movement through the Golgi apparatus appears to be similar to that for nontransformed cells and tissues. Thus, functional alterations in Golgi apparatus currently are being sought in terms of more subtle changes such as alterations in transit times[56] and in the activities of specific glycosyltransferases.[57]

Fucosyltransferase activity is located in the Golgi apparatus and is involved in the formation of both fucoproteins[16] and fucolipids.[58,59] That this enzyme along with sialyltransferase is altered in transformed cells points to a central role of the Golgi apparatus in affecting altered patterns of cell-surface glycosylation that occur during tumorigenesis. However, many of the precise mechanisms whereby the Golgi apparatus may contribute to an altered glycosylation of cell surface glycoproteins and glycolipids are presently not known. In Morris hepatoma 7777, the pool size of GDP-L-fucose was found to be 12.8 nmoles/g wet weight compared with 6.5 nmoles/g wet weight for normal liver (Table II). Furthermore, specific activities of GDP-fucose : glycoprotein fucosyltransferase were determined to be increased in a number of rat hepatomas at least two- to threefold over that of normal liver,[16] whereas the specific activities of sialyltransferase generally were decreased in these tumors.[16] Galactosyltransferase-specific activity remained unchanged. During hepatocarcinogenesis induced in the rat by 2-acetylaminofluorene, CMP-sialic acid : glycoprotein sialyltransferase activity was found to be unchanged or decreased during tumor progression,[60] while that of galactosyltransferase was unchanged.[61]

Buck *et al.*[62] described a fucose-containing sialoprotein that is increased in the plasma membrane of Rous sarcoma virus-transformed hamster cells, and Bryant *et al.*[63] demonstrated that lung tumor cells synthesize elevated amounts of fucoproteins. Various measurements have shown that both fucose metabolism[17,64] and sialic acid metabolism[62,65,66] were altered in a number of experimental cancers.

Table II. Alterations of Glycoprotein Metabolism in Morris Hepatoma 7777 Compared with Normal Rat Liver[a]

| Terminal or subterminal sugar | Plasma membrane-bound sugars[b] | | Nucleotide sugar | Nucleotide sugar pool[c] | | Glycosyltransferase | Glycosyltransferase-specific activity[d] | |
|---|---|---|---|---|---|---|---|---|
| | Liver | Hepatoma 7777 | | Liver | Hepatoma 7777 | | Liver | Hepatoma 7777 |
| L-Fucose | 6 | 27 | GDP-fucose | 6 | 12 | Fucosyltransferase | 0.2 | 0.4 |
| N-Acetylneuraminic acid (sialic acid) | 50 | 60 | CMP-N-acetylneuraminic acid (-sialic acid) | 41 | 62 | Sialyltransferase | 5.3 | 3.3 |
| D-Galactose | 81 | 100 | UDP-galactose | 145 | 69 | Galactosyltransferase | 7.0 | 6.1 |

[a] Adapted from Reutter et al.[17]
[b] Nanomoles per milligram protein.
[c] Nanomoles per gram wet weight of tissue.
[d] Nanomoles sugar transferred/mg protein/hr.

### 3.3. Membrane Dynamics and Membrane Recycling

The kinetics of synthesis and secretion of apolipoprotein B-100 were studied in a human hepatoma line.[56] The times needed for transfer between endoplasmic reticulum and Golgi apparatus (10 min) and for transfer through the Golgi apparatus to the extracellular space (20 min) were very similar to transit times estimated for other secretory and membrane protein through the endoplasmic reticulum–Golgi apparatus–cell surface export route of normal liver.[10]

Other opportunities for membrane trafficking in normal and tumor cells as outlined in Fig. 4 have been less well studied. The capacity to interiorize and recycle plasma membranes was retained by pancreatic acinar carcinoma cells when they were supplied with radiolabeled cationic ferritin.[67] In undifferentiated granule-deficient cells, the tracer was internalized primarily to lysosomes as determined by electron microscopic autoradiography.

### 3.4. Role of Endomembranes in Oncogene Expression

To the extent that oncogene products functioning at the cell surface are translated on membrane-associated polyribosomes and delivered to the plasma membrane via the Golgi apparatus and other endomembrane components, endomembranes play an essential role in oncogene expression. Examples include the v-*sis* oncogene of Simian sarcoma virus, which has strong sequence homology with platelet-derived growth factor (PDGF). Lacking an obvious stop-transfer sequence or membrane anchor, it might be secreted to stimulate growth in an autocrine fashion.[68] Another example is the receptor for epidermal growth factor (EGF), which has homology with the v-*erb*-B oncogene of avian erythroblastosis virus. The v-*erb*-B protein appears to be a truncated form of the EGF receptor, which lacks most of the external EGF binding domain, but which retains the proposed membrane anchor domain. It, too, is synthesized on polyribosomes of endoplasmic reticulum, is glycosylated in Golgi apparatus, and is delivered to the cell surface.[69,70] Doubtless other examples will emerge as new information is generated in this rapidly expanding and important area of cancer research (see Chapter 17).

### 3.5. Plasma Membranes

The plasma membranes of malignant cells and/or that of transformed cells in culture exhibit a variety of biochemical and physical alterations that have been proposed to be either directly or indirectly related to an altered growth control or to invasion and metastasis. Many of these alterations are summarized in Fig. 5.

Modified protein, glycoprotein, phospholipid, and fatty acid patterns have been observed, but no consistent patterns of change have emerged due in part to a surprisingly small number of definitive studies.[18,51–54] Plasma membranes of hepatomas are enriched in cholesterol compared with plasma membranes of normal hepatocytes. However, comparable cholesterol changes have not been observed in other neoplasms.[51] Fluidity and other physical changes observed in plasma membranes of tumor cells emerge as highly dependent on tumor type and may differ widely, e.g., between solid hepatomas and single-cell (leukemias and lymphomas) neoplasms.[71]

Among the more consistent alterations in plasma membrane composition due to malignant changes have been the glycolipids.[72] These constituents represent a small fraction (about 1%) of the total lipids and may undergo extensive alterations upon cell transformation to include both early increases and late reductions and/or simplifications in carbohydrate chains.[73] These changes have been implicated as important to both metastasis[74] and growth control.[75]

Despite the lack of emergence of a detailed understanding of the molecular lesions characteristic of a wide range of tumor types required to explain altered social behavior critical to the transformed phenotype, both loss of growth control and malignant behavior must involve fundamental alterations in the properties of the cell surface. Undoubtedly, the cell-surface alterations associated with cancer must somehow interact to affect one or more of the transducing mechanisms for generating mitogenic signals as well as surface properties affecting invasive ability and adhe-

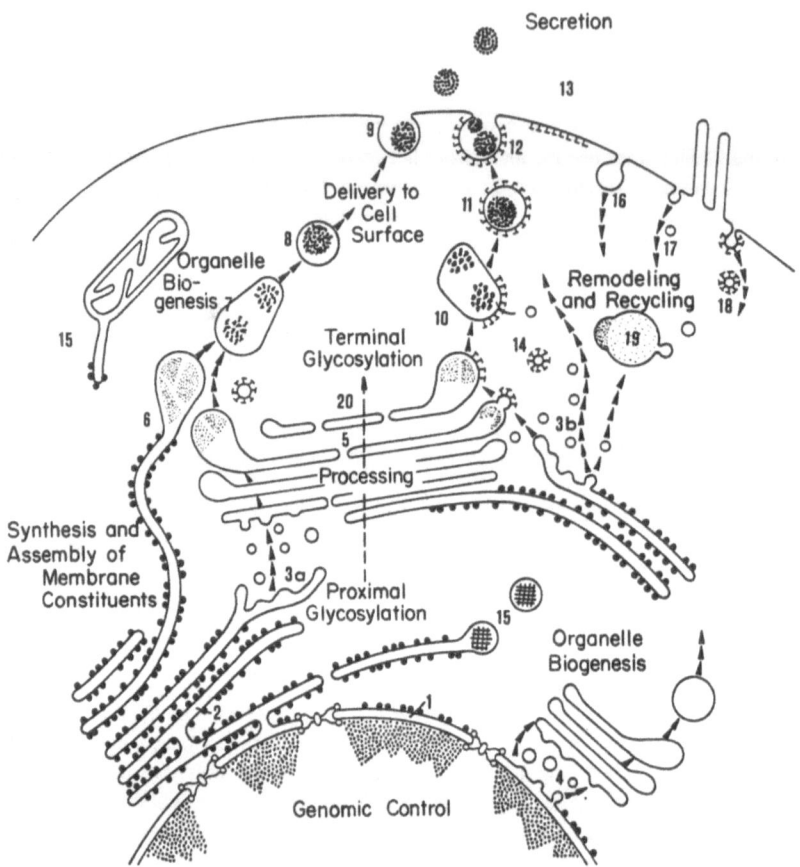

*Figure 4.* Schematic representation of the role of endomembranes (and organelles) in membrane biogenesis and renewal essential for the expression of the neoplastic phenotype. The major processes indicated appear to occur normally in cancer cells but, through altered genomic control, become reprogrammed to generate an altered cell surface. Numbers refer to some of the many different compartments involved as follows: (1) nuclear envelope, which frequently exhibits continuity with (2) rough endoplasmic reticulum. Together with smooth endoplasmic reticulum (3), these membranes serve as major sites of membrane biogenesis as well as drug metabolism important to carcinogen activation. (3a) Transition vesicles bud from specialized endoplasmic reticulum regions to form new Golgi apparatus cisternae. This process emerges as a critical control point to regulate delivery of newly synthesized membrane quanta to the plasma membrane modified to keep pace with accelerated growth of transformed cells. (3b) Other transition vesicles may contribute in other routes of membrane trafficking. (4) In cells with Golgi apparatus adjacent to the nucleus, the nuclear envelope can replace endoplasmic reticulum in the formation of transition vesicles. (5) Golgi apparatus are major sites of processing of membrane and secretory proteins preparatory to their delivery to the cell surface. Modified in transformed cells, the Golgi apparatus emerges as a second critical control point, where tumor cell modification, i.e., altered glycosylation, is expressed. (6) Direct delivery of membrane material to the cell surface bypassing the Golgi apparatus. Strong evidence for such a pathway is indicated from experiments where the Golgi apparatus route is blocked with monensin and incompletely processed proteins and glycoproteins are still delivered to the cell surface. (7) Complex secretory vesicle (condensing vacuole) where materials for export are collected and perhaps further modified. (8) Mature secretory vesicle in transit to the cell surface. (9) Fusion of the secretory vesicle with the plasma membrane to complete exocytosis. (10–13) As in (7) except secretory vesicles are partly or entirely covered by a clathrin coat. In most transformed cells and many normal cells, delivery to the cell surface does not involve a separate condensing vacuole as an obligatory step. Rather, the secretory vesicles bud directly from the Golgi apparatus periphery. Coated vesicles are found both at the Golgi apparatus (14) and at the cell surface (18). (15) Associations of rough endoplasmic reticulum with organelles including direct continuities. (16) Endocytosis of large material (phagocytosis) and (17) of small material (pinocytosis). (18) As in (16) and (17) except involving clathrin-coated membranes (or coated pits). (19) Secondary lysosomes. (20) Distal cisternae of the Golgi apparatus (trans-Golgi apparatus reticulum) sometimes separated from the stack as a cisternal fragment or as a thick cisternae. The latter may also be an important site of terminal glycosylation reactions although its relationship to cell surface formation remains to be investigated. (Modified from Morré *et al.*[10])

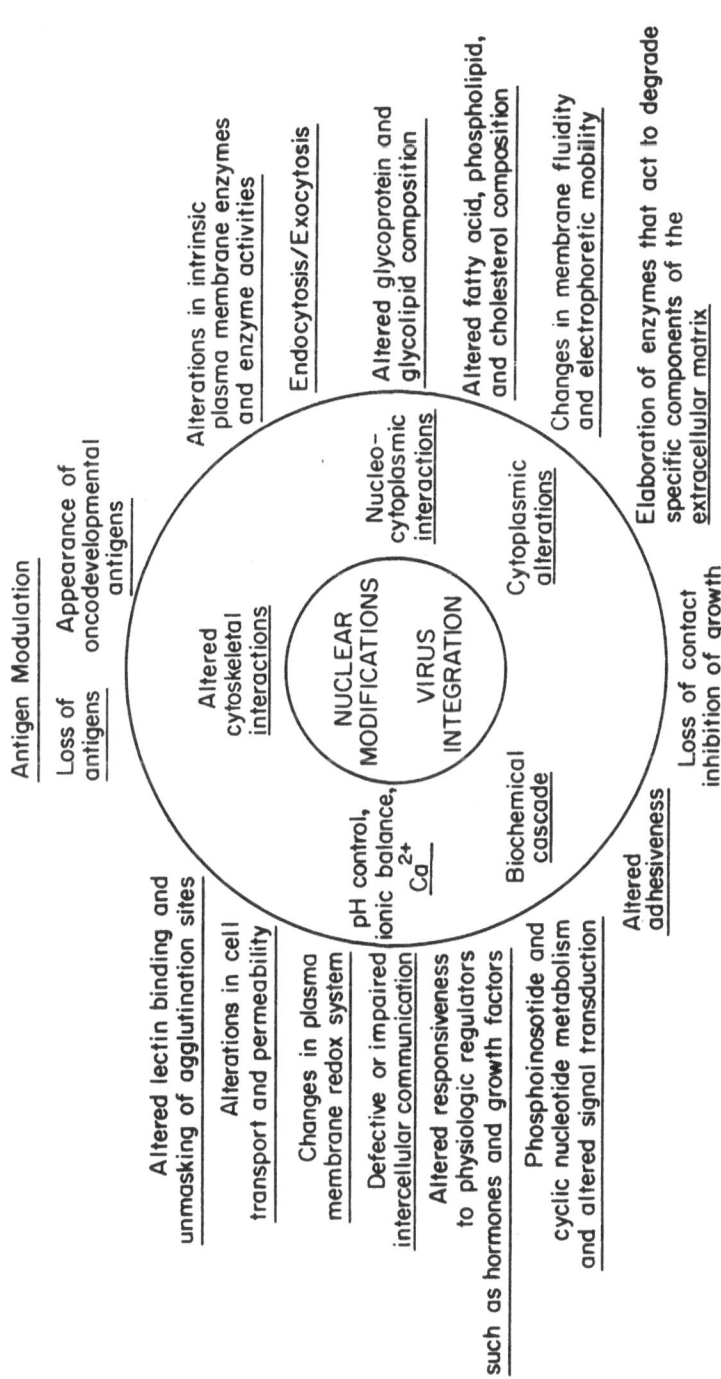

*Figure 5.* Properties of tumor cell surfaces. (Modified and redrawn from Nicolson[52] and Wallach.[105])

sion. (See Chapters 15, 17, 18, and 27, in particular, for more complete discussion of growth regulation, membrane signal transduction, membrane transport, invasion, and metastasis.)

## 3.6. Intercellular Communication

Among the functional alterations in plasma membrane function associated with malignancy is a defect or impairment in intercellular communication. Lowenstein and associates[76] pioneered the demonstration of defects in the ionic intercellular communication in a variety of malignant epithelial cell types. Subsequently, such cell types were found to be impaired with respect to the intercellular passage of small-molecular-weight dye molecules and this could be correlated, in most instances, with either a deficiency in gap junctions or with defects in gap junction structure.

Tumor promoters of the phorbol ester type cause disruption of epithelial junctions in confluent monolayers of cell lines grown in culture.[77] The increased leakiness results in breakdown of transepithelial gradients similar to that observed in frank neoplasms by Lowenstein and associates.[76] This, in turn, could allow for a greater access to mitogenic factors and nutrients important to growth control. In addition, using different methods to measure intercellular communication such as metabolic cooperation, electrical coupling, and dye transfer, exchanges among contiguous cells were found to be inhibited.[78,79] Thus, transfer of growth-controlling molecules from cell to cell via gap junctions also would be diminished. Such alterations in the fluid composition surrounding and within cells in which the tumorigenesis transformation has been initiated may be important to tumor promotion or to tumor progression *in vivo*.

## 4. THE CYTOSKELETON IN CELL TRANSFORMATION AND MALIGNANT NEOPLASIA

All cells contain a network of microtubules and micro- and intermediate filaments[80,81] (Table III). The network extends from the nucleus to the cell surface and is expected to play an important

*Table III. Comparison of Cytoskeletal Components*

| Feature | Microfilaments | Microtubules | Intermediate filaments |
|---|---|---|---|
| Diameter | 6 nm | 24 nm | 7-11 nm |
| Major protein | F-actin | $\alpha$- and $\beta$-tubulin | At least five major groups |
| Mode of occurrence | Bundles (stress fibers) Fine net under PM (plasma membrane) | Cytoplasmic scaffold Mitotic spindle | As highly insoluble cytoplasmic filaments Junctional complexes |
| Associated proteins | Contractile apparatus (myosin, tropomyosin, $\alpha$-actinin, filamin) Cytoplasmic gelation (gelsolin, fragmin, villin, fimbrin, calmodulin) Linkage to PM (vinculin, talin) | MAPs (microtubule-associated proteins); $\tau$ | |
| Structural associations | Linked to PM intermediate filaments (IF), microtubules (MT), glycolytic enzymes | Linked to IF, F-actin, mitochondria | Linked to PM, desmosomes, nucleus, mitochondria, polyribosomes, MT, and F-actin |
| Suggested functions | Control of cell shape; guide elements | Control of cell shape; guide elements; mitotic spindle | Possible mechanical integrators of cellular space |

role in the nucleocytoplasmic phenotypic expression of transformation as well as in growth control and metastasis.

Generally the cytoskeletons of transformed cells appear less ordered than normal cytoskeletons.[81] Fewer stress fibers are present, and cells are more rounded with few contacts with the substratum and with adjacent cells.

The cell–substratum contacts that became reduced with transformation are mediated by focal adhesions such as adhesion plaques.[82] Evidence now points to the regions of actin–membrane contact at focal adhesions as one of the prime loci of transformation-induced changes in tissue culture cells and a potential target for the action of the products of the Rous sarcoma virus (RSV) oncogene v[src] (see also Chapter 15).

In cells transformed by RSV, altered growth characteristics have been attributed to effects of a single gene product, pp60[src], a 60,000-$M_r$ phosphoprotein possessing an ability to phosphorylate proteins on tyrosine residues.[83,84] In cells transformed in culture by RSV, the organization of actin, α-actinin, and vinculin is altered dramatically.[85–87] Focal adhesions are clustered and are not oval shaped. They are not dispersed under the ventral cell surface as in normal cells. This latter characteristic leads to a general loss of the typical spread-out cell morphology and a tendency of the transformed cells to round up. As it turns out, vinculin is among the few proteins phosphorylated by pp60[src].[87–89] Other cytoskeletal proteins, such as filamin, myosin, α-actinin, and vimentin, appeared not to be phosphorylated on tyrosines.

Evidence that vinculin may, in fact, be one of the cellular targets of pp60[src] was provided by Shriver and Rohrschneider,[87] who showed that pp60[src] itself was concentrated within the adhesion plaques of infected fibroblasts with a distribution that coincided with that of vinculin. Since the distribution of α-actinin was also altered in RSV-infected cells, it may be that the organization of α-actinin, or even of actin itself, may be affected by changes in the degree of vinculin phosphorylation. One difficulty with the interpretation that vinculin phosphorylation by pp60[src] is related causally to transformation comes from the calculation that even with the elevated phosphorylation associated with transformation, there would be only about 0.01 phosphotyrosines/vinculin. Certainly not all the vinculin of the cell is associated with adhesion plaques, and that portion phosphorylated may exhibit rapid turnover of phosphate. It may also be that other intracellular changes contribute to the cytoskeletal alterations associated with RSV transformation.

Vinculin was more recently shown to contain a covalently attached fatty acid.[90] Such a covalent modification of vinculin, which is apparently sensitive to transformation, could be important in its reversible association with membranes to facilitate its proposed function as a possible linker between the plasma membrane and microfilament bundles.

The significance of focal adhesions rests, at least in part, on the importance of transmembrane contacts with proteins of the extracellular matrix. There is some relationship between actin filaments associated with focal adhesions and the ability of these focal contacts to bind fibronectin. Whether fibronectin is present at all focal adhesions on the ventral cell surface is still the subject of some controversy.[82] Observations from immunofluorescence microscopy have established close proximity between actin fibers on the inside of the cell and fibronectin at the cell surface. Evidence for the transmembrane connection has come from electron microscopic examination.[91] This junction between fibronectin and actin fibers has been termed the fibronexus. While some focal adhesions appear to lack fibronectin in certain instances, close contacts (regions of 30- to 50-nm spacing between membrane and substrate) normally do contain fibronectin.[92] Virtanen *et al.*[93] reported that cells blocked from secreting fibronectin fail altogether to form focal adhesions. Thus, close associations, such as those afforded by focal adhesions between cytoskeletal components and oncogene products, adhesion proteins, and cell-surface membranes, likely play an important role in maintaining normal cell adhesion, cell spatial configurations, and polarity, in addition to contributing to growth control.

Cell-attachment (cell-adhesion) proteins must interact with the plasma membrane of cells in order to facilitate cell attachment. This requires a receptor or binding site for each attachment protein. Such cell-surface sites for fibronectin have been identified on cells and include a glycoprotein of estimated 140,000 $M_r$,[94] a glycoprotein of estimated molecular weight 47,000,[95] and certain, gangliosides containing two or more sialic acids (see Matyas *et al.*[74] and references cited therein.)

The organization of microtubules in transformed cells is still a subject of controversy.[81] Early studies suggested an involvement,[96] and contemporary investigations continue to show both quantitative and qualitative differences in microtubules and microtubule-associated proteins between normal and transformed cells.

In contrast to microfilaments and microtubules, there is general agreement that the ultrastructural and immunological characteristics of intermediate filaments are maintained during transformation into malignant neoplastic cells. This fact, plus their different antigenic properties related to their tissues of origin, has led to the use of intermediate filament proteins as a molecular basis for tumor diagnostics using monoclonal antibodies.[97] Carcinomas are characterized by cytokeratins, sarcomas of muscle by desmin, nonmuscle sarcomas by vimentin, gliomas by glial fibrillary acidic proteins, and tumors from sympathetic nervous systems by neurofilament proteins.

## 5. MEMBRANES AND CARCINOGENESIS

In addition to phenotypic expression of genetic alterations accompanying neoplasia, membranes carry out additional roles important to tumorigenesis concerned with carcinogen activation and carcinogenesis generally. The best studied example is that of the well-established role of the endoplasmic reticulum in carcinogen metabolism. Other examples include potential roles for the peroxidative metabolism of peroxisomes and other membranes and for lysosomal enzymes.

### 5.1. Endoplasmic Reticulum and Carcinogen Activation

Endoplasmic reticulum, both rough and smooth, as well as nuclear envelope, are the major loci of the mixed-function oxidation reactions of xenobiotic detoxification and carcinogen activation. The enzymatic reactions involved constitute a major pathway of microsomal electron transport in which an atom of molecular oxygen is introduced into a hydrophobic substrate molecule with the concomitant oxidation of reduced pyridine nucleotide (see also Chapter 2). The enzyme systems are inducible in certain tissues such as liver to include an obligatory overall increase in smooth endoplasmic reticulum and the unique cytochrome constituent P-450.[98] Alterations in drug metabolism enzymes in endoplasmic reticulum have been implicated as well in the survival of preneoplastic lesions induced in response to administration of chemical carcinogens.[99]

A second important mechanism of drug metabolism and detoxification related to chemical carcinogenesis and carried out by endoplasmic reticulum is the formation of glucuronic acid derivatives or sulfate esters. A great many drugs and xenobiotics, as well as natural products, are excreted in the bile or urine as glucuronides by direct esterification after prior hydroxylation through the action of the mixed function oxidases. Other enzymes of carcinogen activation present in endoplasmic reticulum include oxygenases capable of inserting both oxygen atoms of $O_2$ to cleave alicyclic or aromatic rings, for example, and epoxide hydrolase.

Highly purified nuclear envelope from rat liver contains most of the same biologic activities found in endoplasmic reticulum, including all the enzymes, for example, necessary to activate the polycyclic aromatic hydrocarbons (PAH). The activities include cytochrome P-450, epoxide hydrolase, and NADH-cytochrome P-450 oxidoreductase in forms immunologically indistinguishable from their counterparts in the endoplasmic reticulum.[100]

### 5.2. Peroxisomes and Carcinogenesis

Several structurally dissimilar drugs related by the property of a capability of lowering plasma triglyceride levels are regularly associated with a marked proliferation of peroxisomes in liver parenchyma.[101] Prolonged treatment of rodents with such peroxisome proliferators leads to the development of hepatomas. Yet these drugs of themselves do not appear to interact directly with DNA either before or after activation by hepatic microsomal mixed function oxidases. Thus, some more indirect route must contribute to their carcinogenicity.

One possibility that has been suggested is that the excessive amounts of $H_2O_2$ generated by peroxisomal oxidases resulting from the increased peroxisomal numbers leads to DNA damage and the initiation of carcinogenesis. Included among the agents eliciting the peroxisomal proliferation response are the hyperlipidemic drug chlofibrate and the widely used industrial phthalate ester plasticizers, e.g., di(2-tehylhexyl)phthalate. Alternatively, these chemicals might constitute a prototype to investigate alternative mechanisms of carcinogenesis such as activation or amplification of cellular oncogenes that would not depend directly on the interaction of the inducing chemical or its active metabolites with DNA.

## 5.3. Lipid Peroxidation and Carcinogenesis

An extensive literature suggests that peroxidation of membrane lipids is a significant factor in the production of cellular damage by drugs, chemicals, radiation, and natural aging.[102,103] Lipid peroxidation causes deleterious effects directly through modification of membrane function and indirectly through production of reactive products that may alter DNA. Either through overproduction or a diminished ability to destroy them, activated forms of oxygen lead to lipid peroxidation. These include the superoxide anion, $O_2^-$, and the hydroperoxy radical, $HO_2\cdot$, singlet oxygen, the hydroxy radical $-OH\cdot$, and hydrogen peroxide, $H_2O_2$.[102] These result in the initiation of autoxidation chain processes; addition to double bonds; hydrogen abstractions; and oxidation of sulfhydryl, thioether, and amino functions. Biologic consequences include genetic damage, cytotoxicity, and carcinogenesis. Antioxidants [e.g., vitamins A, E, and C, butylated hydroxytoluene (BHT)], free radical scavengers, and antioxidant enzymes (superoxide dismutase, glutathione peroxidase, and catalase) are frequently anticarcinogenic. The lipid peroxidation reactions involve membrane-located substrates, but the damage leading to carcinogenesis is usually considered to occur elsewhere, most likely at the level of the DNA.

## 5.4. Lysosomes and Carcinogenesis

Less widely studied is the role of lysosomes in carcinogenesis. Allison[104] reviewed evidence for participation of lysosomes in mutagenesis, including the possibility that lysosomal DNAse from selectively damaged lysosomes might enter the nuclei and contribute to chromosomal breaks. Lipid peroxidation and resultant labilization of the lysosome membrane provide a mechanism to achieve such selective lysosomal damage.[25]

## 6. CONCLUSIONS

Cancer cells exhibit characteristic membrane changes involving the cell surface and intracellular membranes and organelles as well. Some, like decreases in peroxisome and mitochondrial numbers and in the proportion of membrane-associated ribosomes to ribosomes free in the cytoplasm, are clearly linked to tumor progression and become most evident in either poorly differentiated or rapidly growing tumors, or both. Other changes observed with the Golgi apparatus and at the plasma membrane emerge as being potentially transformation linked, and appear to be basic to the expression of malignant neoplasia.

The major impetus for membrane research in cancer is the need to determine mechanisms of how the transformed state is expressed phenotypically in terms of the regulation of cell proliferation and surface characteristics important to growth control. Here, contemporary research focuses not only on surface alterations but on various transducing and signaling mechanisms responsible for growth control and the generation of mitogenic stimuli as well. These growth-related cellular functions normally occur within the context of an organized cytoskeleton and a complex cell membrane–cytoskeleton interface. Finally, for membrane alterations to be expressed at the cell surface, biosynthesis and processing are directed by a complex system of internal endomembranes (e.g., nuclear envelope, endoplasmic reticulum, Golgi apparatus, vesicles) all ultimately under genetic control.

A major limitation to the design of effective strategies of cancer control is the overall lack of understanding of basic mechanisms of loss of growth control and adhesive properties manifest in most clinical malignancies. Knowledge of the types of changes that take place in cell-surface membranes and of how these changes result from coordinated activities of the endomembrane system may open the way to the rational design of new cancer control strategies as well as provide a better understanding of the nature of the surface lesions responsible for the neoplastic phenotype and the ultimate underlying genomic alterations.

## REFERENCES

1. Morré, D. J., and Ovtracht, L., 1977, Dynamics of Golgi apparatus: Membrane differentiation and membrane flow, *Int. Rev. Cytol. Suppl.* **5:**61–188.
2. Frost, J. K., 1969, *The Cell in Health and Disease,* Williams & Wilkins, Baltimore.
3. David, H., 1977, *Quantitative Ultrastructural Data of Animal and Human Cells,* Gustav Fischer Verlag, Stuttgart.
4. David, H., 1978, Cellular pathology, in: *Electron Microscopy in Human Medicine,* Vol. 2: *Cellular Pathology, Metabolic and Storage Diseases* (J. V. Johannessen, ed.), pt. I, pp. 1–148, McGraw-Hill, New York.
5. Ghadially, F. N., 1985, *Diagnostic Electron Microscopy of Tumors,* 2nd ed., Butterworths, London.
6. Unuma, T., Morris, H. P., and Busch, H., 1967, Comparative studies of the nucleoli of Morris hepatomas, embryonic liver, and aflatoxin $B_1$-treated liver of rats, *Cancer Res.* **27:**2221–2233.
7. Harris, J. R., Price, M. R., and Willison, M., 1974, A comparative study on rat liver and hepatoma nuclear membranes, *J. Ultrastruct. Res.* **48:**17–32.
8. Dalton, A. J., 1964, An electron microscopic study of a series of chemically induced hepatomas, in: *Cellular Control Mechanisms and Cancer* (P. Emmelot and O. Muhlbock, eds.), pp. 211–225, Elsevier, Amsterdam.
9. Hruban, Z., Swift, H., and Rechcigl, M., Jr., 1965, Fine structure of transplantable hepatomas of the rat, *J. Natl. Cancer Inst.* **35:**459–495.
10. Morré, D. J., Kartenbeck, J., and Franke, W. W., 1979, Membrane flow and interconversions among endomembranes, *Biochim. Biophys. Acta* **559:**71–152.
11. Farquhar, M. G., and Palade, G. F., 1981, The Golgi apparatus (complex)—1954–1981: From artefact to center stage, *J. Cell Biol.* **91:**77s–103s.
12. Farquhar, M. G., 1985, Progress in unraveling pathways of Golgi traffic, *Annu. Rev. Cell Biol.* **1:**447–488.
13. Kornfeld, R., and Kornfeld, S., 1985, Assembly of asparagine-linked oligosaccharides, *Annu. Rev. Biochem.* **54:**631–664.
14. Dunphy, W. G., and Rothman, J. E., 1985, Compartmental organization of the Golgi stack, *Cell* **42:**13–21.
15. Creek, K. E., and Sly, W. S., 1984, The role of the phosphomannosyl receptor in the transport of acid hydrolases to lysosomes, in: *Lysosomes in Biology and Pathology* (J. T. Dingle, R. T. Dean, and W. Sly, eds.), pp. 63–82, Elsevier/North-Holland, New York.
16. Reutter, W., and Bauer, C., 1978, Terminal sugars in glycoconjugates: Metabolism of free and protein-bound L-fucose, *N*-acetylneuraminic acid and D-galactose in liver and Morris hepatomas, in: *Morris Hepatomas. Mechanisms of Regulation* (H. P. Morris and W. E. Criss, eds.), pp. 405–437, Plenum, New York.
17. Reutter, W., Tauber, R., Vischer, P., Harms, E., Grunholz, H.-J., and Bauer, C., 1978, Turnover of proteins and glycoproteins of plasma membranes in liver, regenerating liver and Morris hepatoma, in: *Protein Turnover and Lysosome Function* (H. L. Segal and D. J. Doyle, eds.), pp. 779–790, Academic, New York.
18. Nicolson, G. L., 1984, Cell surface molecules and tumor metastasis, *Exp. Cell Res.* **150:**3–22.
19. McCarthy, P., Richardson, C. L., Merritt, W. D., Morré, D. J., and Mollenhauer, H. H., 1974, Altered Golgi apparatus architecture in animal and plant tumors, *Proc. Ind. Acad. Sci.* **84:**179–185.
20. Hruban, Z., Mochizuki, Y., Slesers, A., and Morris, H. P., 1972a, A comparative study of cellular organelles of Morris hepatomas, *Cancer Res.* **32:**853–867.
21. Hruban, Z., 1979, Ultrastructure of hepatocellular tumors, in: *Liver Carcinogenesis* (K. Lapis and J. V. Johannessen, eds.), pp. 403–431, McGraw-Hill, New York.

22. Redman, C. M., Yu, S., Bannerjee, D., and Morris, H. P., 1979, In vitro synthesis and secretion of albumin by Morris hepatoma 5123C and 7800, *Cancer Res.* **39**:101–111.

23. Hudgin, R. L., Murray, R. K., Pinteric, L., Morris, H.P., and Schachter, H., 1971, The use of nucleotide-sugar: Glycoprotein glycosyl-transferases to assess Golgi apparatus function in Morris hepatomas, *Can. J. Biochem.* **49**:61–70.

24. Schwartz, A. L., Strous, G. J. A. M., Slot, J. W., and Geuze, H. J., 1985, Immunoelectron microscopic localization of acidic intracellular compartments in hepatoma cells, *EMBO J.* **4**:899–204.

25. Leighton, F., and Morré, D. M., 1982, Lysosomes of tumors: Function, properties and isolation, in: *Cancer-Cell Organelles* (E. Reid, G. Cook, and D. J. Morré, eds.), pp. 239–248, Wiley, New York.

26. Maniferme, F., Wattiaux, R., and Von Figura, K., 1985, Synthesis, transport and processing of cathespin C in Morris hepatoma 7777 cells and rat hepatocytes. *Eur. J. Biochem.* **153**:211–216.

27. Pedersen, P. L., 1978, Tumor mitochondria and the bioenergetics of cancer cells, in: *Progress in Experimental Research,* Vol. 22 (F. Homburger, ed.), pp. 190–274, S. Karger, Basel.

28. Trump, B. F., Jesudason, M. L., and Jones, R. T., 1978, Ultrastructural features of diseased cells, in: *Diagnostic Electron Microscopy,* Vol. 1 (B. L. Trump and R. T. Jones, eds.), pp. 1–88, Wiley, New York.

29. Chen, L. B., Summerhayes, I. C., Nadakavukaren, K. K., Lampidis, T. J., Bernal, S. D., and Shepard, E. L., 1984, Mitochondria in tumor cells: Effects of cytoskeleton on distribution and as targets for selective killing. in: *Cancer Cells,* Vol. 1: *The Transformed Phenotype* (A. J. Levine, G. G. Van de Woude, W. C. Topp, and J. D. Watson, eds.), pp. 75–86, Cold Spring Harbor Laboratory, Cold Spring Harbor, New York.

30. Leighton, F., 1982, Peroxisomes of cancer cells, in: *Cancer-Cell Organelles* (E. Reid, G. Cook, and D. J. Morré, eds.), pp. 257–259, Wiley, New York.

31. Hruban, Z., and Rechcigl, M., 1969. Microbodies in neoplastic cells, *Int. Rev. Cytol. (Suppl.)* **1**:122–125.

32. Reddy, J. K., and Svoboda, D., 1972, Microbodies in Leydig cell tumors of rat testis, *J. Histochem. Cytochem.* **20**:793–803.

33. Novikoff, A. B., Novikoff, P. M., Davis, C., and Quintana, N., 1973, Studies on microperoxisomes. V. Are microperoxisomes ubiquitous in mammalian cells? *J. Histochem. Cytochem.* **21**:737–755.

34. Rechcigl, M., Jr., Hruban, Z., and Morris, H. P., 1969, The roles of synthesis and degradation in the regulation of catalase levels in the neoplastic tissues, *Enzymol. Biol. Clin.* **10**:161–180.

35. Weber, G., 1983, Biochemical strategy of cancer cells and the design of chemotherapy: G. H. A. Clowes Memorial Lecture, *Cancer Res.* **43**:3466–3492.

36. Mochizuki, Y., Hruban, Z., Morris, H. P., Slegers, A., and Vigil, E. L., 1971, Microbodies of Morris hepatomas, *Cancer Res.* **31**:763–773.

37. Itabashi, M., Mochizuki, K., and Tsukada, H., 1975, Peroxisomes in liver tumors of rats induced by 3′-methyl-4-(dimethylamino)azobenzene, *Gann* **66**:463–472.

38. Malick, L. E., 1972, Ultrastructure of transplantable mouse hepatomas with different growth rates, *J. Natl. Cancer Inst.* **49**:1039–1055.

39. Tsukada, H., Mochizuki, Y., Habashi, M., Gotoh, M., and Morris, H. P., 1975, Response of microbodies in Morris hepatoma 9618A to chlofibrate, *J. Natl. Cancer Inst.* **55**:153–158.

40. Staehelin, L. A., 1974, Structure and function of intracellular junctions, *Int. Rev. Cytol.* **39**:191–278.

41. Fisher, E. R., McCoy, M. M., and Wechsler, H. L., 1972, Analysis of histopathologic and electron microscopic determinants of keratoacanthoma and squamous cell carcinoma, *Cancer* **29**:1387–1397.

42. Takaki, Y., Masuiani, M., Kawada, A., 1971, Electron microscopic study of keratoacanthoma, *Arch. Derm.* (Stockh) **51**:21–31.

43. Weinstein, R. S., Merk, F. B., and Alroy, J., 1976, The structure and function of intercellular junctions in cancer, *Adv. Cancer Res.* **23**:23–79.

44. Franke, W. W., Moll, R., Mueller, H., Schmid, E., Kuha, C., Krepler, B., Artlieb, U., and Dowk, H., 1983, Immunocytochemical identification of epithelium-derived human tumors with antibodies to desmosomal plague proteins, *Proc. Natl. Acad. Sci. USA* **80**:543–547.

45. Moll, R., Cowin, P., Kapprell, H.-P., and Franke, W. W., 1986, Desmosomal proteins: New markers for identification and classification of tumors. *Lab. Invest.* **54**:4–25.

46. Becker, F. F., 1970, The normal hepatocyte in division: regeneration of the mammalian liver, in: *Progress in Liver Diseases,* Vol. III (H. Popper and F. Schaffner, eds.), pp. 60–78, Grune & Stratton, New York.

47. Yeo, K., Partent, J. B., Yeo, T.-K., and Olden, K., 1985, Variability in transport rates of secretory glycoproteins through the endoplasmic reticulum and Golgi in human hepatoma cells, *J. Biol. Chem.* **260**:7896–7902.

48. Hruban, Z., Mochizuki, Y., Slesers, A., and Morris, H. P., 1972, Endoplasmic reticulum, lipid and glycogen of Morris hepatomas, *Lab. Invest.* **26**:86–99.
49. Kemp, R. B., 1968, Effects of the removal of cell surface sialic acids on cell aggregation *in vitro, Nature (Lond.)* **218**:1255–1256.
50. Roth, S., McGuire, E. J., and Roseman, S., 1971, Evidence for cell-surface glycosyltransferases. Their potential role in cellular recognition, *J. Cell Biol.* **51**:536–547.
51. Wallach, D. F. H., 1979, *Plasma membranes and Disease,* Academic, New York.
52. Nicolson, G. L., 1976, Trans-membrane control of the receptors on normal and tumor cells, II. Surface changes associated with transformation and malignancy, *Biochim. Biophys. Acta* **458**:1–72.
53. Hynes, R. O., 1976, Cell surface proteins and malignant transformation, *Biochim. Biophys. Acta* **458**:73–107.
54. Hynes, R. O., 1979, *Surfaces of Normal and Malignant Cells,* Wiley, New York.
55. Lodish, H. F., Kong, N., Snider, M., and Strous, J. A. M., 1983, Hepatoma secretory proteins migrate from rough endoplasmic reticulum to Golgi at characteristic rates, *Nature (Lond.)* **304**:80–83.
56. Bostrom, K., Wettesten, M., Boren, J., Bondjuers, G., Wiklund, O., and Olofsson, S.-O, 1986, Pulse-chase studies of the synthesis and intracellular transport of apolipoprotein B-100 in Hep-G-2 cells, *J. Biol. Chem.* **261**:13800–13804.
57. Ikehara, Y., and Takahashi, K., 1983, Glycosyltransferases of the Golgi complex in relation to cell surface changes in rat hepatoma, *Gann Monog. Cancer Res.* **29**:221–229.
58. Bosmann, H. B., 1969, Glycolipid biosynthesis: Biosynthesis of mannose and fucose-containing glycolipids of HeLa cells, *Biochim. Biophys. Acta* **187**:122–132.
59. Steiner, S., Brennan, P. J., and Melnick, J. L., 1973, Fucosylglycolipid metabolism in oncoRNA virus-transformed cell lines, *Nature New Biol.* **245**:19–21.
60. Creek, K. E., Walter, V. P., Evers, D., Yeo, E., Elliott, W. L., Heinstein, P. F., Morré, D. M., and Morré, D. J., 1984, Sialoglycoconjugate changes during 2-acetylaminofluorene-induced hepatocarcinogenesis in the rat, *Biochim. Biophys. Acta* **793**:133–144.
61. Elliott, W. L., Sawick, D. P., Creek, K. E., Walter, V. P., Deutscher, S. L., Quinn, J. F., Yeo, E., Morré, D. M., Heinstein, P. F., Cassady, J. M., and Morré, D. J., 1984, Early biochemical alterations induced by acetylaminofluorene in rat liver, *Int. J. Biochem.* **16**:947–956.
62. Buck, C. A., Glick, M. C., and Warren, L., 1970, A comparative study of glycoproteins from the surface of control and Rous sarcoma virus transformed hamster cells, *Biochemistry* **9**:4567–4576.
63. Bryant, M. L., Stoner, G. D., and Metzger, R. P., 1974, Protein-bound carbohydrate content of normal and tumorous lung tissue, *Biochim. Biophys. Acta* **343**:226–231.
64. Buck, C. A., Fuhrer, J. P., Soslau, G., and Warren, L., 1974, Membrane glycopeptides from subcellular fractions of control and virus-transformed cells, *J. Biol. Chem.* **249**:1541–1550.
65. Grimes, W. J., 1970, Sialic acid transferases and sialic acid levels in normal and transformed cells, *Biochemistry* **9**:5083–5092.
66. Harms, E., Kreisel, W., Morris, H. D., and Reutter, W., 1973, Biosynthesis of *N*-acetylneuraminic acid in Morris hepatoma, *Eur. J. Biochem.* **32**:254–262.
67. Kanwar, Y. S., Rosenzweig, L. J., Jakubowstri, M. L., and Reddy, J. K., 1983, Plasma membrane retrieval in neoplastic pancreatic acinar cells, *Proc. Natl. Acad. Sci. USA* **80**:6877–6881.
68. Hunter, T, 1985, Oncogenes and growth control, *TIBS* **10**:275–280.
69. Hayman, M. J., and Beug, H., 1984, Identification of a form of the avian erythroblastosis virus erb-B gene product at the cell surface, *Nature (Lond.)* **309**:460–462.
70. Schatzman, R. C., Evan, G. I., Privalsky, M. L., and Bishop, J. M., 1986, Orientation of the v-erb-B gene product in the plasma membrane, *Mol. Cell Biol.* **6**:1329–1333.
71. Shinitzky, M., 1984, Membrane fluidity in malignancy. Administrative and recuperative, *Biochim. Biophys. Acta* **738**:251–261.
72. Hakomori, S.-I., 1981, Glycosphingolipids in cellular interaction; Differentiation and oncogenes, *Annu. Rev. Biochem.* **50**:733–764.
73. Morré, D. J., Kloppel, T. M., Merritt, W. D., and Keenan, T. W., 1978, Glycolipids as indicators of tumorigenesis, *J. Supramol. Struct.* **9**:157–177.
74. Matyas, G. R., Evers, D. C., Radinsky, R., and Morré, D. J., 1986, Fibronectin binding to gangliosides and rat liver plasma membranes, *Exp. Cell Res.* **162**:296–318.
75. Spiegel, S., and Fishman, P. H., 1987, Gangliosides as bimodal regulators of cell growth, *Proc. Natl. Acad. Sci. USA* **84**:141–145.
76. Lowenstein, W. R., 1978, The cell-to-cell membrane channel in development and growth, in: *Differention*

*and Development, Miami Winter Symposium,* Vol. 15 (F. Ahmad, J. Schultz, T. R. Russell, and R. Wermer, eds.), pp. 399–409, Academic, New York.

77. Mullin, J. M., and O'Brien, T. G., 1986, Effects of tumor promoters on LLC-PK₁ renal epithelial tight junctions and transepithelial fluxes, *Am. J. Physiol.* **251**:C597–C602.

78. Yancey, S. B., Edens, J. E., Trosko, J. E., Chang, C. C., and Revel, J. P., 1982, Decreased gap junctions between Chinese hamster V79 cells upon exposure to the tumor promoter 12-o-tetradecanoyl-phorbol-13-acetate. *Exp. Cell Res.* **139**:329–340.

79. Mesnil, M., Montesano, R., and Yamasaki, H., 1986, Intracellular communication of transformed and non transformed rat liver epithelial cells, *Exp. Cell Res.* **165**:391–402.

80. Weatherbee, J. A., 1981, Membranes and cell movement: Interactions of membranes with the proteins of the cytoskeleton, *Int. Rev. Cytol. (Suppl.)* **12**:113–176.

81. Ben-Zeev, A., 1985, The cytoskeleton in cancer cells, *Biochim. Biophys. Acta* **780**:197–232.

82. Cohen, C. M., and Smith, D. K., 1985, Associations of cytoskeletal proteins with plasma membranes, in: *The Enzymes of Biological Membranes,* Vol. 1: *Membrane Structure and Dynamics,* 2nd ed. (A. N. Martonosi, ed.), pp. 29–80, Plenum, New York.

83. Collett, M. S., and Erikson, R. L., 1978, Protein kinase activity associated with ovarian sarcoma virus src gene product, *Proc. Natl. Acad. Sci. USA* **75**:2021–2024.

84. Hunter, T. and Sefton, B. M., 1980, The transforming gene product of Rous sarcoma virus phosphorylates tyrosine, *Proc. Natl. Acad. Sci. USA* **77**:1311–1315.

85. David-Pfeuty, T., and Singer, S. J., 1980, Altered distributions of the cytoskeletal proteins vinculin and α-actinin in cultured fibroblasts transformed by Rous sarcoma virus, *Proc Natl. Acad. Sci. USA* **77**:6687–6691.

86. Carley, W. W., Barak, L. S., and Webb, W. W., 1981, F-actin aggregates in transformed cells, *J. Cell Biol.* **90**:797–802.

87. Shriver, K., and Rohrschneider, L., 1981, Organization of pp60src and selected cytoskeletal proteins within adhesion plaques and junctions of Rous sarcoma virus-transformed cells, *J. Cell Biol.* **89**:525–533.

88. Sefton, B. M., Hunter, T., Ball, E. H., and Singer, S. J., 1981, Vinculin: A cytoskeletal target of the transforming protein of Rous sarcoma virus, *Cell* **24**:165–174.

89. Hynes, R. O., 1982, Phosphorylation of vinculin by pp60src: What might it mean?, *Cell* **28**:437–438.

90. Burger, B. P., 1987, The cytoskeletal protein vinculin contains transformation sensitive, covalently bound lipid, *Science* **235**:476–479.

91. Singer, I. I., and Paradiso, P. R., 1981, A transmembrane relationship between fibronectin and vinculin (130 kd protein): Serum modulation in normal and transformed hamster fibroblasts, *Cell* **24**:481–492.

92. Norton, E. K., and Issard, C. S., 1982, Fibronectin promotes formation of the close cell-to-substrate contact in cultured cells, *Exp. Cell Res.* **139**:463–467.

93. Virtanen, I., Vartio, T., Badley, R. A., and Lehto, V. P., 1982, Fibronectin in adhesion spreading and cytoskeletal organization of cultured fibroblasts, *Nature (Lond.)* **298**:660–663.

94. Pytela, R., Pierschbacher, M. D., and Ruoslahti, E., 1985, Identification and isolation of a 140 kd cell surface glycoprotein with properties expected of a fibronectin receptor, *Cell* **40**:191–198.

95. Oppenheimer-Marks, N., and Grinnell, F., 1984, Calcium ions protect cell-substratum adhesion receptors against proteolysis. Evidence from immunoabsorption and electroblotting studies, *Exp. Cell Res.* **152**:467–475.

96. Puck, T. T., 1977, Cyclic AMP, the microtubule-microfilament system, and cancer, *Proc. Natl. Acad. Sci. USA* **74**:4491–4495.

97. Benz, E. W., 1985, Intermediate filament proteins: A molecular basis for tumor diagnostics, *BioTechniques* **3**:412–420.

98. Fouts, J. R., and Gram, T. E., 1969, The metabolism of drugs by subfractionations of hepatic microsomes: The case for microsomal heterogeneity, in: *Microsomes and Drug Oxidations* (J. R. Gillete, A. H. Conney, G. J. Cosmides, R. W. Estabrook, J. R. Fouts, and G. J. Mannering, eds.), pp. 81–91, Academic, New York.

99. Farber, E., and Cameron, R., 1980, The sequential analysis of cancer development, *Adv. Cancer Res.* **31**:125–226.

100. Kasper, C. B., and Henton, D., 1980, in: *Enzymatic Basis of Detoxification,* Vol. 2 (W. B. Jakoby, ed.), pp. 4–27, Academic, New York.

101. Reddy, J. K., and Lalwani, N. D., 1983, Carcinogenesis by hepatic peroxisome proliferators: Evaluation of the risk of hypolipedemic drugs and industrial plasticizers to humans, *CRC Crit. Rev. Toxicol.* **12**:1–58.

102. Cerutti, P. A., 1985, Peroxidant states and tumor promotion, *Science* **227**:375–381.

103. Comporti, M., 1985, Biology of disease. Lipid peroxidation and cellular damage in toxic liver injury, *Lab. Invest.* **53:**599–623.
104. Allison, S. C., 1969, Lysosomes and cancer, in: *Lysosomes in Biology and Pathology*, Vol. 2 (J. T. Dingle and H. B. Fell, eds.), pp. 178–204, North-Holland, Amsterdam.
105. Wallach, D. F. H., 1972, *The Plasma Membrane: Dynamic Perspectives, Genetics and Pathology*, Springer-Verlag, New York.

# 17

# Growth Factors and Neoplasia

## George K. Michalopoulos

## 1. INTRODUCTION

Function and growth are two interrelated aspects of life in all organisms. Whereas function permits manifestation of the specific aspects and life patterns of all organisms, growth is the essential process that guarantees the continuity of life. Growth occurs at the level of organismal populations or cell populations within an organism. Regulation of the phenomenon of growth has been a central point of scientific investigation since ancient times. The rapidity of embryonic growth has always fascinated investigators in the biologic sciences. Whereas regulated normal growth is essential for maintenance of life, aberrations of growth characterize several aspects of disease. Aberrant growth is a hallmark of the neoplastic process. The foundations of modern research in oncology were laid down on the premise that the cause of neoplasia could be shown by comparing the growth of normal and neoplastic tissues. Comparisons were made of the growth between regenerating liver and hepatocellular carcinomas as well as of the growth of normal skin and skin papillomas and squamous cell carcinomas. These studies have now expanded to many normal and neoplastic cell systems and have received added impetus with the realization that the growth of normal cells is a highly regulated process. The essential regulatory controls have been intensely investigated during the past 15 years. As a result of these investigations, we understand that cells are stimulated to grow in response to specific chemical messages. These messages are produced by other cells located remotely or adjacent to the responding cell. Occasionally, these messages are produced by the growing cells themselves. The term Growth Factors has been coined to describe collectively the chemical substances that constitute the signals that regulate in a positive or negative manner the growth of cells.

The role of the growth factors in the development of the neoplastic phenotype was highlighted by early observations of the behavior of neoplastic cells in tissue culture. Using cell culture models, it was found that (1) neoplastic cells have reduced requirements for substances commonly used to stimulate growth of cells in culture, such as serum; (2) neoplastic cells in culture often produce substances released in the tissue culture medium that stimulate growth of normal cells; and (3) whereas normal cells in culture need to be anchored to a substrate in order to grow, neoplastic cells tend to be anchorage independent and may grow in the absence of a definitive substrate support.

Recent developments in growth factor research have done much to help us understand the above differences between the normal and the neoplastic phenotype. It is now known that the products of many of the genes (oncogenes) associated with neoplasia turned out to be abnormal or supernumerary copies of growth factors or their receptors. These findings are summarized in

*George K. Michalopoulos* • Department of Pathology, Duke University Medical Center, Durham, North Carolina 27710.

relationship to the specific growth factors. The relationship between many growth factors and their receptors and specific oncogene products has strengthened the notion that abnormalities in the regulation of growth of normal cells are not an epiphenomenon but that they are causally associated with the development of the neoplastic process.

This chapter summarizes recent knowledge on some of the better studied and understood growth factors and their receptors. An attempt is made to integrate the mode of action of these factors using specific tissue models and to describe the abnormal relationship among some of these growth factors, their receptors, and specific examples of neoplastic growth.

## 2. EPIDERMAL GROWTH FACTOR

Of the several growth factors known to date, epidermal growth factor (EGF) is probably the best studied. EGF was first described by Cohen in 1962 and was isolated based on its capacity to accelerate the opening of the eyelids of newborn mice and kittens.[1] The active molecule was called EGF because it was found to induce proliferation of epidermal cells. Human EGF was first isolated from urine in 1975 under the name β-urogastrone by Gregory[2] and was later shown to be identical to human EGF.[3] Subsequent studies have resulted in complete elucidation of the aminoacid sequence of EGF in several species. The EGF molecule is a 6000-$M_r$ polypeptide. The mouse EGF contains 53 amino acids. Its structure is shown in Fig. 1. The polypeptide chain is linked to form loops by the presence of three disulfide bridges.[4] The structure of the molecule is highly conserved between species. A 92% homology is seen between rat and human EGF, and a 70% homology is seen between mouse and human EGF. The most conserved feature of the EGF molecule is the positioning of the cysteine residues. These residues determine the three-dimensional structure of the molecule. The EGF molecule and its 53 amino acids are derived from a precursor of a larger molecular weight.[5-7] The EGF precursor (pre-pro-EGF) is a protein of 1217 amino acid residues and 133,000 $M_r$. There is only one sequence on the pre-pro-EGF molecule, which is identical to the final structure of EGF. That sequence is close to the carboxy terminal. It is of interest, however, that in the region between the EGF sequence and the amino terminus, seven other regions have been found that were composed of amino acid sequences closely related but not identical to the amino acid sequence of EGF itself. Another point of interest in the structure of the EGF precursor is a sequence

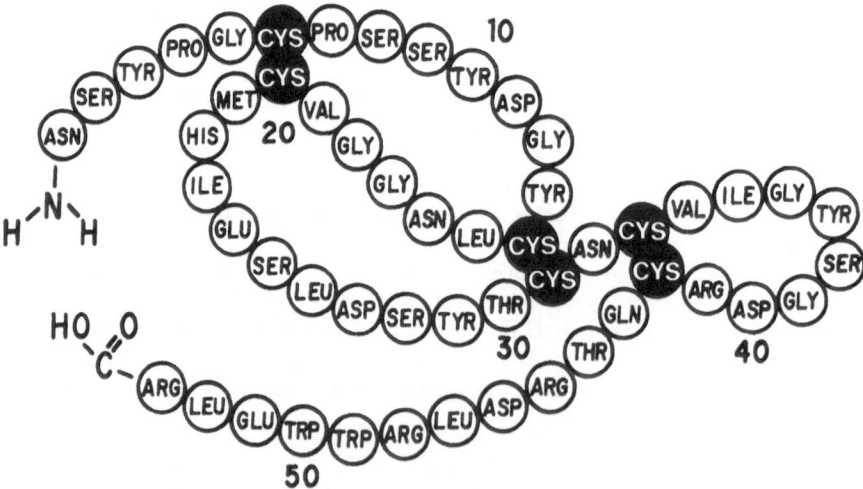

Figure 1. Amino acid sequence of the molecule of epidermal growth factor (EGF) as defined by Savage et al.[4] The numbers indicate the amino acid position from the terminal amino group. The cysteine residues that participate in the formation of the cystine S–S bonds are shown in black.

of approximately 400 amino acid residues in the mid-portion of the molecule, which show substantial homology to a portion of the low-density lipoprotein receptor. A short hydrophobic region is also present in the molecule of the EGF precursor, suggesting that part of the function of the molecule of EGF precursor may involve intercalation through cell membranes. Conceivably, the EGF precursor may play a role as a receptor or as an important molecule located on the plasma membrane of specific cell types. The function of this molecule, however, in its intact form remains entirely unknown at the present time. It should also be pointed out that the functional significance of short hydrophobic transmembrane sequences is much better understood for transforming growth factor alpha (TGF-$\alpha$) precursor, in which the short transmembrane sequence plays a role in the proper positioning of the molecule for the proteolytic cleavage step employed in the generation of mature TGF-$\alpha$. It is not certain whether such a step of transmembrane positioning of the receptor occurs in the case of EGF precursor. In salivary glands, the EGF precursor is cleaved to release mature EGF by an arginine esteropeptidase. This is in contrast to the peptidase employed in the generation of TGF-$\alpha$ that has a different molecular specificity and recognizes the hydrophobic sequence alanine–valine.

Epidermal growth factor is present in most biologic fluids of mammalian organisms. Its concentration is relatively low in plasma[8] (less than 1 ng/ml), whereas much higher concentrations are found in saliva (more than 10 ng/ml) and urine. Perhaps the highest concentrations of EGF have been found so far in prostatic fluid (more than 100 ng/ml). High concentrations are also found in the precolostrum from the mammary gland. The use of complementary DNA (cDNA) probes has shown that the precursor form of EGF is actively synthesized in many tissues. The sites of the most active synthesis of EGF are the granular convoluted tubules of the submaxillary gland, Brunner's glands of the duodenum, and the cells of the distal convoluted tubules of the kidney. The processing of the precursor molecule, however, differs between the salivary gland and the kidney. Whereas in the salivary gland the precursor is cleaved by an arginine peptidase to form the final 53-amino acid EGF molecule, the EGF precursor molecule in the kidney is not further processed and is used intact.[9] EGF is found in high concentrations in the urine. It is not clear whether the urinary EGF is produced by the kidneys or merely excreted through the kidneys but derived from plasma. In the human, the concentration of the urinary EGF increases gradually from birth to the second year of life, gradually declining thereafter to about one half the value of the 2-year mark at old age.[10] EGF is not found in fetal tissues or in fetal urine, despite the fact that EGF can cross the placenta. Most of the EGF in adult male mice is produced in the salivary glands. Removal of the salivary glands in these animals causes a dramatic decline of the circulating EGF and a decrease in spermatogenesis,[11] suggesting that the circulating EGF is important in maintaining spermatogenesis in these animals. EGF stimulates mitogenesis in many cell types in culture and has been implicated in stimulating DNA synthesis in many tissues. Injection of EGF stimulates DNA synthesis in liver,[12] suggesting that EGF is involved in liver regeneration. This is reinforced by the findings that the EGF receptor numbers in hepatocytes decline during liver regeneration,[13] presumably due to EGF binding and receptor internalization. In addition to the mitogenic effects of EGF, other functional effects of EGF have also been noted. Addition of EGF to hepatocytes in culture often results in cellular cytoplasmic enlargement and stimulation of amino acid uptake. Injection of EGF into animals is associated with inhibition of gastric secretion. EGF stimulates wound healing. It is also of interest that despite the presence of EGF in many biological fluids and the identification of the messenger RNA responsible for the synthesis of EGF precursor in many tissues, EGF has not so far been found to be produced by tumor cells. The insertion of EGF expression vectors in normal cells, however, was recently shown to cause neoplastic transformation in culture.[14]

The actions of EGF on its target cells are mediated by the binding of EGF to a specific receptor molecule on the plasma membrane of responsive cell types. This molecule is called the EGF receptor.[7] The EGF receptor is a glycoprotein of 170,000-$M_r$ that binds EGF with high affinity and has been found in most cell types. In fact, of all cells of mammalian species, only the circulating cells of the blood appear not to contain EGF receptors. Specific EGF binding has been reported in fish, and the receptor has been cloned from *Drosophila* DNA. Mitogenic effects of EGF and specific binding of EGF have also been reported in primary cultures of frog (*Xenopus*) hepatocytes.

The structure and function of the EGF receptor are better understood than those of any other growth factor receptor.[15,16] The polypeptide backbone of the EGF receptor has a molecular weight of 130,000. The additional 40,000 in molecular weight is attributable to the addition of N-linked oligosaccharides. Three domains are recognized on the EGF receptor. The extracellular domain comprises half of the molecule and contains most of the oligosaccharide residues. This is approximately the portion from the middle of the molecule to the amino terminus. It contains the site for the binding of EGF. A short transmembrane region composed of 23 amino acids composes the portion that connects the extracellular to the intracellular domain. The intracellular domain contains several potential sites of phosphorylation and is made up of approximately 40% of the polypeptide backbone.

The intracellular domain of the EGF receptor has tyrosine kinase activity.[15,16] Binding of EGF to its receptor results in phosphorylation of tyrosine residues of the intracellular domain of the receptor by the tyrosine kinase activity of the receptor itself (autophosphorylation).[17] Binding of EGF to its receptor also appears to promote formation of EGF receptor dimers.[18,19] Recent evidence suggests that the formation of receptor dimers following EGF binding is essential for the activation of the kinase activity of the intracellular domain. If the receptors are bound to solid surfaces so that the dimerization is prevented, the activation of the tyrosine kinase function is inhibited. Kinetic analyses of the binding of EGF to its receptor suggest the presence of high-affinity and low-affinity classes of EGF receptors. Despite extensive evidence for the presence of two affinity classes of EGF receptors, no specific changes in the receptor molecule have been found associated with high affinity. The rate of degradation of the EGF receptor is enhanced approximately 10-fold after binding with EGF. Groups of [EGF–(EGF receptor)] complexes enter into clathrin-coated pits of the plasma membrane of cells. These pits form vesicles that fuse with lysosomes inside the cytoplasm. The [EGF–(EGF receptor)] complexes in lysosomes are degraded by proteolytic enzymes, and the EGF receptor molecule is not recirculated.[20] Another, minor, pathway exists in hepatocytes, in which the [EGF–(EGF receptor)] complex is maintained intact, does not enter into lysosomes, and is excreted into the bile.[21]

Concomitant with the autophosphorylation of the EGF receptor, other effects are seen to occur rapidly after the EGF binds to its receptor. These include stimulation of sodium–hydrogen exchange (hydrogen ions are excreted from the cell and sodium ions are taken up by the cell), resulting in elevation of the intracellular pH value.[22] There is also a rapid calcium mobilization (within 30–50 sec) that results in increase of intracellular calcium. The increase in breakdown of inositol phospholipids as a result of stimulation by EGF is described in some cell types but not in others. The phosphorylation of specific protein substrates within the cell has also been noted. Some of these proteins are phosphorylated on a tyrosine residue, and other are phosphorylated on a serine or threonine position. It is not clear whether the tyrosine phosphorylated cytoplasmic proteins are phosphorylated by the EGF receptor itself or other kinases. Although these events occur in most cell types after EGF binding to its receptor, there is no understanding about the mechanism of the transmission of the mitogenic signal from the [EGF–(EGF receptor)] complex to the cell nucleus. It does not appear that the internalization per se of the [EGF–(EGF receptor)] complex is associated with the transmission of the mitogenic signal. The finding that the oncogene *v-erb-B* causes cell transformation suggests that the tyrosine kinase function of the EGF receptor must play a role in the transmission of the mitogenic signal by mechanisms which are as yet not clearly understood. Most of the above described effects seen after the binding of EGF are fairly rapid, whereas the stimulation of cells to enter the DNA synthesis and replicate usually requires prolonged (6–8 hr) exposure to EGF.

A strong homology in sequence has been found between the intracellular domain of the EGF receptor and the protein encoded by the oncogene *v-erb-B*.[7] In fact, it is now accepted that the *v-erb-B* oncogene is in fact a slightly truncated version of the intracellular domain of the EGF receptor. The tyrosine residue most commonly phosphorylated in the EGF receptor autophosphorylation is missing in the protein encoded by the *v-erb-B* oncogene. This is consistent with the fact that phosphorylation of the *v-erb-B* protein has not been demonstrated. It is believed that the genetic alteration that results in a gene coding for a truncated intracellular domain of the EGF receptor (resulting in the formation of the *v-erb-B* protein) also results in a constitutive activation of the kinase function in the absence of binding of the EGF to any extracellular domain. However, when a chimeric construct consisting of *v-erb-B* protein and an extracellular ligand-binding portion was inserted into cells, the transforming properties of the *v-erb-B* oncogene were still maintained.[23] Thus, it appears that even if the extracellular portion of the receptor were to be attached to the *v-erb-B* oncogene, it would not modify its transforming effects. In addition to the formation of the truncated form of the intracellular domain (*v-erb-B*), portions of the EGF receptor comprising the extracellular and transmembrane domain, without including the intracellular domain, have also been found in some specific tumor cell types. In other tumor cell lines, one occasionally finds very large numbers of intact functional EGF receptors. This is seen especially in some squamous cell carcinoma cells (e.g., A431 cells, from which the EGF receptor was originally isolated) and in cells from gliomas.

Although it is clear that phosphorylation of the EGF receptor by its own kinase function is an essential step in the action of the molecule, it is also evident that phosphorylation of the EGF receptor can occur at other sites, catalyzed by other protein kinases present in the plasma membrane. Protein kinase C (PKC) activation leads to phosphorylation of the threonine residue at position 654 of the EGF receptor molecule.[24] This phenomenon may be the reason for the often demonstrated modulation of EGF binding after activation of PKC, seen after the addition of PDGF, phorbol esters, bombesin, or norepinephrine (see Section 8, under heterologous regulation). The decrease in EGF binding after PKC activation has been variably described to cause a decrease in EGF receptor number or affinity to the ligand EGF. The mechanism may vary with different cell types. In all of these instances, however, the responsiveness of EGF is enhanced as the number of EGF receptors appears to decline. This paradox may reflect higher rates of internalization of the EGF receptor in situations in which the cells become hyperresponsive to EGF.

In summary EGF, a low-molecular-weight growth factor, binds to specific receptors on the plasma membrane of most cells. The binding is essential to transmit mitogenic signals to the cell through mechanisms of action that are not clear. Although EGF has not been shown to be produced by tumors, the kinase portion of the EGF receptor is homologous to the protein synthesized by the *v-erb-B* oncogene.

## 3. TRANSFORMING GROWTH FACTOR-α

Transforming growth factor-alpha is a polypeptide composed of 50 amino acids, which is produced by many tumor cell lines. It was initially discovered by Todaro *et al.*[25] as a component of an activity that stimulated growth of normal cells in soft agar. The capacity to grow in soft agar, in the absence of anchorage to a firm substrate, is usually characteristic of transformed neoplastic cells. The induction of the transformed phenotype on normal cells by extracts produced by neoplastic cells was the first evidence of abnormal growth factor production in neoplasia. Production of TGF-α has since been demonstrated in other examples of neoplasia, such as chemically transformed cells[26] and human solid tumors.[27] It was subsequently found that the activity responsible for this effect was in part due to TGF-α and in part to another growth factor, TGF-β. There are several similarities between EGF and TGF-α.[28,29] Several amino acids (30–40% of the total, depending on the species) are present in identical locations in the two molecules. Three disulfide bridges are present in the same locations on TGF-α as they are present on EGF, imparting on the TGF-α molecule a three-dimensional structure similar to that of the EGF molecule. TGF-α binds to the EGF receptor. In fact, it is accepted today that EGF and TGF-α share the same receptor and that there is no other receptor that is specific for TGF-α.

Comparison of the biologic effects of EGF and TGF-α shows qualitative similarities with occasional quantitative differences. In most systems examined, TGF-α and EGF will elicit the same effects. The systems range from stimulation of growth of normal cells in culture, to colony formation of normal cells in soft agar in the presence of TGF-β, to eyelid opening and tooth eruption in mice,[30] to vascularization in animals.[31] In several of these systems, TGF-α appears to be more effective than EGF, whereas in other systems both factors appear equally effective. The differences in the magnitude of induced response are puzzling in view of the fact that both of these substances bind to the same receptor.

Epidermal growth factor is found in many biologic fluids, including plasma. Whereas EGF is present in most biologic fluids, TGF-α has not been found in biologic fluids (except urine) or other locations in the body of adult mammalian organisms. TGF-α activity, consisting of several molecular species, has been found in the urine of normal individuals and cancer patients.[32] In humans, kidney carcinomas are the most frequent producers of TGF-α, followed by hepatocellular carcinomas, mammary carcinomas and other cell types. Production of messenger RNA (mRNA) for TGF-α precursor is seen only in fetuses and in the adjacent decidua[33] (hyperplastic uterine endometrium during pregnancy). The expression of TGF-α mRNA in the fetus peaks on the ninth day of gestational development in the mouse. This finding suggests that TGF-α may in fact be a fetal form of EGF. This is consistent with earlier observations which demonstrate the acquisition of fetal properties by neoplasms. According to this dogma, first expressed by Potter as "oncogeny is blocked ontogeny"[34] (see also Chapter 21), the production of TGF-α by neoplasms would be one more manifestation of the capability of tumors of producing fetal markers. Despite the presence of TGF-α in many tumors, its role in the induction of neoplastic phenotype is debated. The addition of antibodies against the EGF receptor (which is also the TGF-α receptor) in cultures of tumor cells producing TGF-α did not appreciably slow down the growth of these neoplastic cells, suggesting that TGF-α did not play a role in the formation of the malignant phenotype.[35] In other experiments, however, normal cells were transformed when infected with a retrovirus carrying a TGF-α gene.[36] The high frequency with which TGF-α is expressed by neoplastic cells, especially carcinomas, suggests that TGF-α must have a important role to play in the regulation of the growth of the neoplastic cells. A corollary question relates to the biologic role of TGF-α in fetal development or in the adult organism. Despite the fact that TGF-α is not found in the tissues or biologic fluid of adult mammalian organisms, the application of TGF-α has been shown to induce several effects characteristic of EGF.

Similar to EGF, TGF-α is also derived from a precursor of much higher molecular weight.[28,37] The TGF-α precursor contains 160 amino acids (compared with EGF precursor with 1200 amino acids). Analysis of the amino acid sequence of the precursor shows that TGF-α is produced by proteolytic cleavage of a short hydrophobic sequence (at an alanine–valine site). Currently no protease enzymes are known to have such a specificity, with the exception of elastase. Other studies have shown that the precursor is produced intact by several neoplastic cell lines and is biologically active.[38, 39] The precursor, in contrast to TGF-α, is glycosylated, and it also contains palmitic acid.[40] A hydrophobic sequence of 23 amino acids long is present distal to the carboxy terminus of TGF-α. Its extremely hydrophobic structure suggests that it may function as a transmembrane sequence to anchor the TGF-α precursor to the plasma membrane. This has led to speculations that TGF-α precursor may in some cell types play the role of a membrane receptor. Similar questions have also been raised about the EGF precursor. Such a function, however, for either the EGF or the TGF-α precursor has not yet been demonstrated. Recent findings[41] have also shown that the presence of the hydrophobic sequences is required for the transmembrane insertion of the TGF-α precursor in such a way that the portion of the precursor molecule that constitutes the final mature product protrudes into the lumen of the endoplasmic reticulum. There, the mature TGF-α is freed by proteolytic cleavage by an unusual protease recognizing the sequence alanine–valine. The role of the short transmembrane sequence should thus be seen as being that of positioning the TGF-α precursor molecule for orderly processing of the precursor into the mature form.

TGF-α can stimulate resorption of bone and the release of calcium in organ cultures of long bone or calvarium.[42] It is more potent in stimulating bone resorption than EGF. Clinical observations have also shown that the presence of TGF-α correlates well with hypercalcemia, often seen in the presence of malignancy. The findings strongly suggest that TGF-α is the factor responsible for many of the cases of hypercalcemia associated with malignancy (see also Chapter 23).

## 4. PLATELET-DERIVED GROWTH FACTOR

Platelet-derived growth factor (PDGF) is a protein of 28,000–35,000 $M_r$ that is responsible for most of the stimulation of growth of cells in culture by serum.[43,44] The existence of a range of molecular weights of PDGF is probably due to different degrees of glycosylation. The discovery of PDGF was preceded by the observation that serum stimulates the growth of cells in culture more than plasma. These studies led to the search for growth factors in platelets and to the discovery of PDGF.[45] We know today that PDGF is present in the α-granules of platelets, from which it was originally isolated. We also know, however, that PDGF is found or produced by many other cell types besides platelets.

Analysis of the molecular structure of PDGF reveals the presence of two polypeptide chains held together by disulfide bridges.[44] These chains, called A and B, have extensive homology in their amino acid sequence, suggesting that they arose in the remote past from identical genes. Typically, a molecule of PDGF consists of one A-chain and one B-chain. Homodimers of either A- or B-chain are also produced by some cell types, especially neoplastic cells, or selectively in some species (e.g., the porcine PDGF is a homodimer of B-chains). These homodimers have been shown to be biologically active. The PDGF molecule is very cationic and readily attaches to hydrophobic surfaces such as tissue culture substrates and connective tissue proteins.

In a recent study of the phylogenetic distribution of PDGF by Stiles *et al.*,[46] it was found that the PDGF molecule first appeared with the evolution of the chordates. PDGF molecules were not found in animals that had evolved before the chordates or in animals such as arthropods, which diverged into a different evolutionary line before the appearance of chordates. It is also of interest that PDGF appeared before the appearance of organisms with platelets in their blood. Thus, animals such as fish and amphibians, which do not have platelets in their blood, do have PDGF nonetheless, in a noncompartmentalized form.

In addition to its presence in platelets, evidence for presence or production of PDGF has accumulated from studies with other cell types. PDGF (or expression of the *sis* gene, the gene for the B-chain of PDGF) is produced by macrophages,[47] endothelial cells,[48] and smooth muscle cells.[49] Biological material identical to intact PDGF or B-chain homodimer is produced by neoplastic cells transformed by the simian sarcoma virus. Of interest are studies in AKR-2B cells that can be stimulated to grow by TGF-β. After entry into the cell cycle following TGF-β stimulation, these cells produce intact PDGF as part of their proliferative response. The production of PDGF in these cells and in other cells is considered a normal phenomenon associated with their cell cycle. Production of PDGF is also seen in the cytotrophoblast of the placental villi.

Evidence exists from studies with human osteosarcoma cell lines that each of the chains of PDGF is the final product of processing from a larger molecule.[50] In one of these cell lines, precursor molecules of 180,000 were found to be synthesized. It is not clear whether these precursors form dimers, which are then cleaved to the final PDGF molecule, or whether the processing of the individual chains to their final size occurs before the formation of the dimers. In either case, the evidence is clear that the original larger molecules are first synthesized and cleaved by several proteolytic steps. This, in turn, results in intermediate products, some of which are larger than the standard PDGF and are being secreted by the cells. The gene for the A-chain has been localized on chromosome 7 in humans.

The effects of PDGF on target cells are mediated by its binding to a specific plasma membrane receptor.[51] The PDGF receptor is a glycoprotein that extends from outside to inside of the plasma membrane, in a manner analogous to that previously described for the EGF receptor. The molecular weight of the receptor is 185,000. It has an extracellular part that contains the domain that binds PDGF, a transmembrane portion, and an intracellular domain containing a tyrosine kinase activity. It is worth noting the structural similarity and the presence of tyrosine kinase activity in both the EGF and PDGF receptor. The theme of an extracellular portion with the ligand binding domain, transmembrane portion, and intracellular domain with tyrosine kinase activity has been found on EGF, PDGF, insulin, and other receptors. In some cells, the PDGF receptor is processed to a smaller molecule of 130,000 $M_r$ by an endogenous calcium-dependent SH-protease. The smaller form of the receptor also retains the kinase activity. Furthermore, the tyrosine kinase activity of the receptor results in autophosphorylation after binding of the ligand (PDGF) in an analogous manner to that observed for the EGF receptor. The primary structure of the PDGF receptor was determined from a complementary (cDNA) sequence. It is closely related to that of an oncogene product called *v-kit*.[52] Homologies were also found to the receptor for macrophage colony-stimulating factor (CSF-1). This suggests that these two receptors may have arisen from a common ancestral molecule. The PDGF receptor is present mainly in cells derived from mesenchymal tissues. Approximately 400,000 receptors per cell are present in human fibroblasts. PDGF receptors are not seen in general in epithelial cells. They are seen, however, in the placental cytotrophoblasts.[53] In view of the findings that these cells also produce the ligand for this receptor (i.e., PDGF), it has been speculated that PDGF is responsible for some properties of these cells that are similar to the neoplastic phenotype (i.e., the capacity to invade adjacent tissues and to permeate vasculature).

The addition of PDGF to susceptible cells results in stimulation of mitogenesis. Studies by Pledger *et al.*[54] with BALB/c-3T3 cells have shown that PDGF renders these cells competent to enter into DNA synthesis. These cells, however, do not actually enter into DNA synthesis unless factors such as IGF or EGF are added subsequent to their exposure to PDGF. These studies have led to the notion that the entry of cells into the cell cycle is associated with a state of competence followed by a state of progression. By contrast, studies with other cell types have shown that PDGF alone or EGF alone are capable of stimulating all aspects associated with entry of the cells into the cell cycle, including DNA synthesis and mitosis. Although the notion of competence and progression through the cell cycle is a valid one, the delineation of specific factors which are individually responsible for each one of these two states may be possible only for particular cell types (e.g. BALB/c-3T3 fibroblasts). In most other cell types, various mitogenic growth factors, including PDGF, may elicit the full spectrum of events associated with the cell cycle.

Stimulation of cells to proliferate by PDGF is associated with a series of well-characterized events.[55] The first event is the autophosphorylation of tyrosine moieties of the PDGF receptor itself.[56] The tyrosine kinase activity of the receptor is also associated with phosphorylation of a small number of specific protein substrates. In addition, activation of the receptor is associated with enhanced turnover of plasma membrane inositol lipids. This results, by mechanisms to be described below, in mobilization of calcium from intracellular stores and activation of PKC. Shortly after binding of PDGF to its receptor, there is enhanced production of proteins encoded by *myc* and *fos* cellular proto-oncogenes.[56a] These events are rapid, all of them occurring within less than 1 hr after addition of PDGF, and precede the entry of the responding cells into S phase (DNA synthesis). Other genes are also involved, some characteristic to stimulation by PDGF. This includes the JE-3 and KC-1 gene. It is not clear whether the enhanced expression of these genes is due to direct effects of the activated PDGF receptor or to effects of activated PKC. Some of these events, including enhanced expression of *fos* and *myc* genes are seen after direct activation of PKC alone by phorbol esters. In addition to the mobilization of calcium, other ions such as $Na^+$ and $H^+$ are quickly mobilized through the plasma membrane.

Less is known about the actions of PDGF within the context of the homeostasis of the whole organism. PDGF is found mainly in serum but is absent in plasma, suggesting that platelets are the main source of circulating PDGF in the blood. Activation of platelets and release of the platelet granules in sites of endothelial injury or tissue injury results in release of PDGF. PDGF has chemotactic effects on connective tissue cells, including fibroblasts and macrophages. Several models have been proposed, suggesting that PDGF-induced chemotaxis of connective tissue cells and subsequent stimulation of their proliferation is associated with wound healing and maintenance of vascular integrity. Studies by Ross *et al.*[44] also suggested that PDGF may be involved in the pathogenesis of atherosclerosis. The presumed mechanism is based on the fact that cholesterol deposits start on smooth muscle cells in close proximity to the endothelial surface. These deposits serve as the focus of accumulation of platelets that release PDGF to stimulate smooth muscle cells to proliferate. Increased numbers of smooth muscle cells then result in more cells that can accumulate cholesterol, leading to further accumulation of cholesterol at the site of the plaque.

The importance of PDGF in the context of neoplasia was highlighted by the finding that the *sis* oncogene is identical to the gene for the B-chain of PDGF.[43,55,57] It was originally observed that the amino acid sequence of the B-chain of PDGF had extensive homology to the product of *sis* oncogene. The originally defined structure of PDGF was that of the human molecule, whereas the *sis* oncogene was considered as having been derived from the woolly monkey. Further studies have shown that the human *c-sis* gene, the counterpart to the cellular *sis* of the woolly monkey, has a structure identical to that of the gene for the B-chain of PDGF, thereby establishing the identity of these two genes. These studies were the first ones to link a specific growth factor with a specific oncogene product. The transforming activity of the simian sarcoma virus (SSV) is now understood to derive from stimulation of production of an altered PDGF-like molecule consisting of a homo dimer of the B-chain of PDGF. The production of PDGF-like molecules or native PDGF molecules, however, has been also shown in association with other forms of neoplasia. In many of the cells the production of PDGF contrasts with the absence of PDGF receptors. It is presumed that the secreted PDGF binds to the plasma membrane receptor and this results in the internalization of the ligand–receptor complex. When antibodies against PDGF are added to cells transformed by the *sis* oncogene, the growth of the cells was arrested despite the absence of measurable PDGF receptors.[57a] This proved that the secreted B-chain homodimer, the *sis* oncogene product, was required for the abnormal growth and the maintenance of the transformed phenotype of these cells. By contrast, in other neoplastic cell lines, such as the U-20S osteosarcoma cell line, smaller amounts of PDGF are produced and occasionally PDGF receptors on the plasma membrane can be found. In these cells, addition of the antibody against PDGF to the medium did not arrest growth. Thus, it is possible that in some neoplastic cell types the production of PDGF is causally related to the presence of the transformed phenotype, whereas in other neoplastic cells, the production of PDGF is not causally related to their neoplastic state but rather represents an epiphenomenon.

The elegant studies of PDGF, its receptor and the relationship of PDGF to the *sis* oncogene have served as the framework for many similar studies in neoplasia with other growth factors. They have further strengthened the notion that growth factors and their receptors, while being essential links in the chain of events that leads to proliferation of normal cells, can also alter this chain of events and lead to permanent stimulation of growth and the establishment of the neoplastic phenotype.

## 5. BOMBESIN

Bombesin is a peptide of 14 amino acids, originally isolated from frog skin.[58] Since its original isolation, the peptide was shown to have many physiological functions in mammalian organisms. Antibodies against bombesin demonstrated the existence in mammalian organisms of bombesin immunoreactivity. The molecules responsible were purified and shown to be identical to the so-called gastrin release peptide (GRP). The two molecules responsible for bombesin immunoreactivity in mammalian organisms are a peptide with 27 amino acids and a peptide with 10 amino acids. The 27-amino-acid peptide contains a sequence of 10 amino acids, starting from the carboxy terminal, which is homologous to the bombesin sequence with the exception of one amino acid. The decapeptide also has strong homology to bombesin and is responsible for most of the bombesin immunoreactivity seen in mammalian tissues. These peptides are most abundant in gastrointestinal (GI) mucosa, pancreas, and the CNS. Immunolocalization studies in the GI tract and pancreas showed that these peptides are exclusively localized in nerve cells present in these organs in sites such as the myenteric plexus of the intestinal wall. The peptides are produced by the nerve cells and function in a paracrine manner for the adjacent cells of the intestinal mucosa or pancreas. When the connections of the myenteric plexus to spinal cord are severed, bombesin persists in the nerve cells of the intestine, a finding that demonstrates that bombesin is produced locally by the peripheral nerve cells and not from cells of the spinal cord. The only cells other than nerve cells that produce bombesin are cells in fetal lung and several tumor cell lines.

Injection of bombesin has a variety of physiologic effects in the GI tract, of which the most prominent is the release of gastrin, followed by secretion of gastric fluid.[59] Bombesin is also a stimulator of growth of tracheobronchial cells and 3T3 cells in culture. The interest in bombesin in the context of studies of neoplasia originally derived from the demonstration that bombesin is one of several peptides produced by small cell carcinoma of the lung (SCCL).[60] Other such peptides include calcitonin, ACTH, MSH, vasopressin, and the beta chain of chorionic gonadotropin (see Chapter 23). When bombesin-producing SCCL cells were grown in culture or in nude mice, their growth was arrested when exposed to monoclonal antibodies against bombesin.[61] This demonstrated that production of bombesin, a growth stimulator for tracheobronchial cells, was not a mere epiphenomenon, but was necessary to stimulate growth of the neoplastic SCCL cells themselves. The inhibition of tumor growth in the presence of antibombesin antibodies, analogous to the blockade of the SSV-transformed cells in the presence of antibody against PDGF (see Section 4, on PDGF), is a further clear example of the importance of the autocrine growth stimulation by growth factors produced by neoplastic cells.

Cells susceptible to bombesin stimulation respond to the addition of bombesin with a series of intracellular events that are similar to those seen when sensitive cells are stimulated by PDGF.[62] These phenomena include rapid mobilization of ions (exchange of hydrogen and sodium, calcium mobilization from intracellular stores), increased expression of the genes c-*fos* and c-*myc*, and eventually DNA synthesis and mitosis. Enhanced breakdown of inositol phospholipids after bombesin simulation is also seen, in analogy to the PDGF model. Despite the apparent similarity in mode of action between bombesin and PDGF, differences may exist as to the molecular details. Administration of pertussis toxin to cells sensitive to both PDGF and bombesin blocks the enhancement of c-*myc* expression induced by bombesin, but did not effect the enhancement of c-*myc* induced by PDGF or the protein kinase C stimulator, phorbol ester phorbol myristate acetate (PMA).[63] Pertussis toxin is an enzyme which transfers ADP-ribose moieties to specific receptor-associated proteins, including G proteins of the plasma membrane. The data from these experiments show that the G proteins associated with the function of PDGF and bombesin receptors in these cells are different. The bombesin receptor has recently been characterized. It has an approximate molecular weight of 115,000 and it is present on the cell surface. Binding with bombesin results in phosphorylation of a tyrosine moiety on the receptor,[64] in analogy to the receptors for EGF and PDGF.

## 6. FIBROBLAST GROWTH FACTOR(S)

The term fibroblast growth factor (FGF) is used to describe two growth factors with extensive amino acid sequence homology and differing physical chemical properties.[65,66] The basic FGF has a pI of 9.6, while the acidic form has a pI of 5.6–6.0. Acidic FGF has so far been found only in brain and retina, whereas basic FGF has been found in several tissues, including kidney, placenta, pituitary, corpus luteum, adrenal gland, macrophages, prostate, and thymus. The effects of these two factors are similar in terms of cell targets but different in terms of potency. In general, the basic FGF is much more potent than acidic FGF. Both factors stimulate proliferation of endothelial cells and also stimulate proliferation and differentiation of many cell types derived from mesoderm or neuroectoderm. So far epithelial cells, and especially cells derived from the endoderm (including cells of GI tract, pancreas, and liver), are not affected by the presence of FGF. The acidic FGF on average is 30- to 100-fold less potent than the basic FGF. The basic FGF is a single chain polypeptide composed of 146 amino acids. Electrophoretic studies have revealed a microheterogeneity of structure that may be related to differing degrees of degradation or processing of the molecule. In fact, a form of FGF missing the first 15 amino acids from the NH$_2$ terminal has been characterized. Some of the organs in which FGF is found appear to contain the intact form, and some contain the form missing the 15 amino acids. Detailed analysis of the amino acid structure of the basic and acidic FGF shows that they are very closely related[67,68]: 55% of the amino acids that make up these two molecules are homologous. The amino acids that are different are in many instances derived from changes resulting from single base substitution. The similarity also extends to the tertiary structure of the molecules. For example, both acidic and basic FGF contain potential binding domains for heparin in similar locations. Basic FGF (and not acidic FGF) contains a sequence similar to one present in fibronectin called the intense minimal cellular recognition site. This site allows fibronectin to interact with characteristic cell-surface recognition sites. The extensive homology between the acidic and basic FGF suggests that they are derived from a single ancestral gene. Their genes have been localized on chromosome 4 for the basic FGF and chromosome 5 for the acidic FGF. Molecular processing from a larger form, as seen with other growth factors, appears to be true as well in the case of the FGF, but the precursor form is larger by only 9 amino acids for the basic FGF and 15 amino acids for the acidic FGF.

Receptors for the basic and acidic FGF are found in the cell types that appear to respond to these growth factors.[69] Two receptors exist, with molecular weights of 145,000 and 125,000. It appears that both basic and acidic FGF bind to both of these receptors with differences in affinity proportional to the differences in potency manifested between these two growth factors. In contrast to the receptors for PDGF, EGF, and insulin, binding of basic or acidic FGF to their receptors does not appear to result in autophosphorylation of the receptors.[67] Incubation of FGF with the receptors, however, results in downregulation of the receptors, as also seen with the other receptor models.

In general, the cellular effects observed after adding the FGF are similar to the effects seen after adding PDGF. The similarities extend to induced movements of ions, stimulation of turnover of inositol phospholipids in the plasma membrane, activation of PKC from the diacylglycerols that result from the breakdown of the inositol phospholipids, enhanced expression of the genes for c-*fos* and c-*myc*, stimulation of DNA synthesis, and mitosis. In systems in which the effect of PDGF can be shown to be purely that of inducing mitotic competence, FGF can be shown to have similar competence-inducing effects. Though the underlying cellular events following stimulation of FGF and PDGF appear similar, FGF tends to have strong effects on the differentiation of some of its cellular targets. These effects encompass aspects of cell morphology and function and may be either directly due to the effect of FGF or indirectly due to the stimulation of production of components of extracellular matrix by these cells. An interesting effect of FGF is their capability of prolonging the life of many mesodermal and neuroectodermal cell lines in tissue culture, postponing the senescence which most of the cell lines from these tissues normally manifest in culture.[70,71]

Both basic and acidic FGF have strong affinities for heparin and heparan sulfate.[65,66] Exposure to heparin results in binding of the FGF. Heparin and heparan sulfate also compete with binding of FGF to the FGF receptors. However, the presence of heparin and heparan results in either a decrease or sometimes an increase of effect on FGF. These effects of heparin on the action of FGF have been explained as due either to competition with binding to the FGF receptor or to stabilization of the FGF molecule. Both FGF are highly susceptible to denaturing influences, and binding to heparin could lead to stabilization of the molecule.

Several studies have focused on the relationship between FGF and the extracellular matrix. FGF stimulate production of extracellular matrix in different cell types. In addition, FGF, especially basic FGF, bind to the extracellular matrix of many tissues. This has led to the notion that the extracellular matrix can act as a reservoir of bound FGF, which could then be released in many processes in which breakdown of connective tissue is observed, such as invasion of tissues by neoplasms or embryonic development. Despite the attractiveness of the notion that the extracellular matrix may act as a reservoir of FGF, there is no direct experimental evidence to support this concept.[65,67]

A physiologic role for FGF has been shown in many situations related to tissue growth and regeneration. The amphibian blastema growth is enhanced by the addition of FGF, and FGF has been shown to be able to replace the neural trophic influences that regulate the growth of this tissue.[72] Similar trophic effects of FGF have been shown in regeneration of the lens from the dorsal iris.[73] In many instances, the cells that are targets for FGF also appear to produce it. This is true for both endothelial cells and adrenal cortex cells. The latter have been shown to produce but not to release FGF. When FGF is added to adrenal cortex cells, however, it stimulates their proliferation.[74] Furthermore, it is of interest that adrenal cortex carcinoma cell lines have been shown not only to produce FGF, but also to release them into the medium.

Perhaps the best studied property of FGF is their ability to stimulate angiogenesis[75] (see Chapter 26). FGF were demonstrated to be the endothelial cell mitogens present in corpus luteum, adrenal gland, kidney, and retina. The stimulation of angiogenesis is an integral part of the growth or regeneration of these tissues, and strong evidence exists that the production of FGF plays a defining role in this matter. The angiogenic effects of FGF may be relevant in influencing tumor growth. Previous studies showed that the growth of tumors is associated with release of factors in the tumor microenvironment that stimulates growth and formation of small blood vessels. These angiogenesis factors have not yet been fully identified. However, it has been demonstrated that many tumors produce FGF and, in view of the strong angiogenic effect of the FGF's, it is very likely that in many instances tumor angiogenesis factors may be identical to the two FGF.

Despite the production of the two FGF by many normal and neoplastic tissues, a clear-cut role for these substances in the development of neoplasia has not yet been demonstrated. Such a role has been shown for PDGF, the EGF receptor, and so forth. It is highly likely that the genes producing these factors and their receptors will in the future be associated with cellular proto-oncogenes. Such a relationship, however, has not been demonstrated as yet.

## 7. INTERLEUKIN-2

Interleukin is the name given collectively to a set of molecules that are produced from lymphocytes or macrophages and mediate some aspects of the immune response. This section focuses on interleukin-2 (IL-2). Other interleukins are considered to play a role in the growth and function of cells of the immune or the hematopoietic system. However, we will focus on IL-2 because the effects of this molecule on growth regulation are better understood and they may be of relevance in understanding the pathogenesis of some types of human neoplasia.

The production of IL-2 and the expression of the IL-2 receptor both play a significant role in control of the expansion of clones of T cells during the process of immune response to specific antigenic stimuli.[76] The first step in this process involves the presentation of the specific antigen by macrophages to resting T cells. The macrophages display appropriate and specific major histocompatibility antigens. The foreign antigen presented by macrophages binds to specific receptors present on the surface of resting T cells. This event, in the presence of IL-1, stimulates production and secretion of IL-2 by the T lymphocytes. The production of IL-2 takes place in a small subset of T lymphocytes, variably called T-helper cells (or L3T4+ T-helper subset). Other types of T lymphocytes including suppressor and cytotoxic T lymphocytes do not produce IL-2 following antigenic stimulation. Whereas the production of IL-2 and its secretion is limited to a small subset of T lymphocytes, a larger population of T lymphocytes expresses IL-2 receptors following the secretion of IL-2 by the helper cells. The IL-2 receptors are expressed also in the helper cells themselves, resulting in expansion of the antigenically responsive clone of the T-helper cells in a fashion that can be best characterized as autocrine stimulation of growth of T-helper cells by IL-2. The process is self-limited. In the presence of IL-2, studies have shown that the IL-2 receptor is changed from a high-affinity to a low-affinity form. The kinetics of expression of the IL-2 receptor and the affinity types of receptors expressed do not seem to differ between the different T-cell subsets. This process is maintained in the presence of antigen, resulting in prolonged expansion of the immune responsive clone. In the absence of antigen the IL-2 production gradually declines, thus limiting the whole process. The final result of the coordinated production of IL-2 and IL-2 receptor by T cells is the generation of populations of effector cells with helper, suppressor, and cytotoxic T-cell functions. IL-2 receptor is expressed not only on T cells but also on activated B cells. Thus, the expansion of the clones of cells that participate in the immune response to a specific antigen, eventually involving the production of humoral antibodies by B cells, involves IL-2 and its receptor in all aspects of the response.

Both the human and the mouse IL-2 have been purified to homogeneity and cloned by introduction of plasmids in bacterial organisms. The mouse IL-2 has a molecular weight of 30,000 with a pI in the acidic range, whereas the human IL-2 has a molecular weight of 15,000 with a pI in the neutral range. The human IL-2 consists of 133 amino acids and is produced from a precursor form that is 153 amino acid residues long. The mouse and human IL-2 share an extensive homology

(70%) despite the difference in molecular weight. Analysis of the cDNA structure for the two molecules shows 153 amino acids for the human IL-2 precursor, as mentioned, and 169 amino acids for the mouse. These data strongly suggest that the mouse IL-2 is a dimer.

The IL-2 receptor has been purified from several sources, normal and transformed.[79–81] It exists in two states of activation, a high-affinity and a low-affinity state. They differ in their binding affinity for IL-2 by approximately 1000- to 2000-fold. The effective form that transmits the signal for growth is the high-affinity IL-2 receptor. Recent evidence suggests that the high-affinity state is imparted by the binding of another protein. After IL-2 binds to its receptor, the complex is internalized, and the receptor is degraded in lysosomes, analogous to what was described for the [EGF–(EGF receptor)] complex. The molecular structure of the IL-2 receptor is interesting. Both the human and mouse IL-2 receptors have been purified to homogeneity, sequenced, and cloned.[80] These studies have shown that they are glycoproteins of 55,000 $M_r$. Precursor molecules of lower molecular weight have been found intracellularly. These precursors range from 30,000 to 40,000 $M_r$. The IL-2 receptor is extensively glycosylated, and it is very likely that the precursor forms of lower molecular weight represent molecules with different amounts of glycosylation. The studies of IL-2 receptor in both human and mouse have revealed an unexpected degree of complexity in terms of the control mechanisms for the production of this molecule. Two mRNAs have been found in the human, and five mRNAs have been identified in the mouse.[81] The differences for the proteins encoded by these differing mRNAs are not known. The structure of the receptor consists of an extracellular domain, heavily glycosylated, attached onto a transmembrane portion, followed by a very small portion of intracellular domain. The structure of the intracellular domain is so limited that it practically precludes the possibility of the presence of a tyrosine kinase function, analogous to that seen for PDGF, EGF, and bombesin receptors. The gene for the IL-2 receptor in humans is located on the short arm of chromosome 10. When the gene is transcribed, at least two families of messenger RNAs appear. Sequence analysis of the cDNA shows that the receptor is composed of 270 amino acids. These include a 19-amino acid transmembrane domain and a short intracytoplasmic domain composed of 13 amino acids. Of interest is the fact that the intracytoplasmic domain does not contain tyrosine, but it does contain serine and threonine. These findings are consistent with the suggestion that the intracytoplasmic domain does not function as a protein kinase.

A set of characteristic intracellular events has been described following binding of IL-2 to its receptor.[82] These events are analogous to the events described after binding of EGF and PDGF to their receptors. They include rapid ionic fluxes, stimulation of turnover of inositol phospholipids, mobilization of calcium from intracellular stores, and increased expression of the proto-oncogenes c-fos, c-myc, and c-myb. Direct measurements of GTPase activity of membrane preparations shows that IL-2 binding stimulates a GTP-ase function in the membrane, suggesting that G proteins are involved in mediation of the intracellular events following activation of the IL-2 receptor. PKC is also activated following these events.

The role of the production of IL-2 and/or expression of the IL-2 receptor by leukemic cell lines has been extensively studied. Particularly intriguing is the role of IL-2 and its receptor in the transformation of T cells by the HTLV virus (for review, see ref. 80). An unregulated IL-2 receptor expression in several leukemic T cells has been described. Some of these cell lines are infected with the human T lymphotropic virus types 1 and 2 (HTLV-I HTLV-II). The available evidence suggests that these retroviruses contain a gene with transactivating capabilities (i.e., encoding for products that affect expression of genes present on other chromosomes). The product of this gene induces the expression of the genes both for IL-2 and also for the IL-2 receptor, resulting in a situation where growth can be stimulated in an autocrine fashion by IL-2. Several T cell lines infected by the HTLV-I have been studied and they all express higher levels of IL-2 receptor (5–10-fold greater) than those levels seen when T cells are activated by the T-cell mitogen phytohemagglutinin. Most of these cell lines do not produce or secrete IL-2 despite the fact that they produce and express high levels of the IL-2 receptor. HTLV-I is a transforming virus for T cells. Extensive analysis of its structure, however, has not shown the presence of a recognized oncogene. The genes regularly seen in retroviruses, such as gag, pol, env, and the typical retroviral LTR segments are present. An additional region, called pX, has also been found that has been described as a transactivator gene and named *tat* (transactivation of transcription). It appears that this gene is the gene with the transactivating capabilities whose existence was previously postulated. The transactivator gene was inserted into an established T-cell line. The presence of the gene was associated with increased expression of the IL-2 receptor as well as increased expression of the IL-2 gene. Although this suggests that the two molecules can be involved in a model of autocrine stimulation of neoplasia, it should also be mentioned that most of the HTLV-I transformed cell lines do not produce or secrete IL-2. In addition, when IL-2 is administered to these cell lines, it does not stimulate their growth. It is possible that the independence of these cell lines from IL-2 reflects a progression of tumor growth from early IL-2 dependent cells to later stages of IL-2 independence. These interesting results establish again a correlation between the molecular biology of a characteristic growth factor and its receptor and the molecular biology underlying the events associated with a specific neoplastic transformation, in this case the transformation of T cells by HTLV-I.

## 8. INSULINLIKE GROWTH FACTORS: IGFS AND SOMATOMEDINS

This category encompasses essentially two polypeptides described under several names, resulting in a confusing terminology. It is now accepted that $IGF_1$ corresponds to activities in the past described under the names somatomedin C and somatomedin A, whereas $IGF_2$ corresponds to the activity identified as rat multiplication-stimulating activity. These substances have been called insulinlike growth factors because of their structural homologies to insulin and similarity of the biologic effect.[83,84] In the adult rat and human, the main IGF is $IGF_1$, whereas $IGF_2$ appears to be the main IGF of the fetal rat serum. The amino acid sequence of $IGF_1$ and $IGF_2$ is fairly similar, with a 62% sequence homology between the two molecules. Each of these molecules consists of a single-chain polypeptide with molecular weights of approximately 7500. The polypeptide chain is separated into A, B, C, and D domains. The A and B domains are extensively homologous to the A and B chain of the human proinsulin (approximately 40% homology). This extensive homology suggests that the IGF and insulin have emerged from a common ancestral gene which diverged into a gene for human proinsulin and a gene for a common IGF peptide sometime before the appearance of the first vertebrates. A second gene duplication led to the appearance of separate peptides for $IGF_1$ and $IGF_2$ and that probably took place approximately three hundred million years ago (before the appearance of mammals).

Both IGF are present in the plasma, not as free polypeptides but rather bound in a noncovalent manner to specific carrier proteins.[85] The complexed polypeptides are not biologically active and the presence of the bound carrier prevents the molecule from diffusing through capillaries or accessing membrane receptors. Several forms of the binding proteins have been identified in human serum with molecular weights of 24,000–42,000. The complexed IGF can be released from the carrier molecules by acid treatment. The released IGF is biologically active. IGF are synthesized from larger precursors, after proteolytic removable of amino acids toward both the carboxy- as well as the amino-terminal. The IGF-gene is located on the long arm of chromosome 12 in humans.[86]

The term *somatomedin* originated from the finding that these molecules are produced following the stimulation of several tissues by growth hormone. The implication of the term was that the effects of growth hormone (also known as somatotropic hormone) are mediated by the production and secretion of these molecules. Of the tissues affected by growth hormone, liver[87,88] seems the most responsive and it appears that most IGF are produced in that organ. IGF production, however, has been shown in many different cell types in culture[89] and IGF in biologically inactive form have been extracted from many organs. The biologic effects[83,84] of IGF mimic those of insulin in several respects, including the effects on glucose regulation and amino acid transport. In addition, the IGF have long-term effects that seem to promote growth. $IGF_1$ is more potent than $IGF_2$ in most of the assays. $IGF_1$ in particular has been associated with the rapid onset of growth during puberty. It has been shown that there is a complex interrelationship between the increased levels of sex steroids, growth hormone production, and levels of $IGF_1$ that results in a surge of $IGF_1$ during the years of the rapid growth in puberty.[90] Measurements of $IGF_1$ in Pygmies have also shown that these people lack the surge of $IGF_1$ during puberty and it has been postulated that this is responsible for the short stature of these people compared with the other human races. Although the correlation between $IGF_1$ and body growth is now well accepted, other studies have also shown that occasionally, infusion of growth hormone alone can result in stimulation of body growth in the absence of measurable increase in $IGF_1$ levels.

Two types of receptor for IGF have been found.[91,92] Type 1 receptor binds strongly to $IGF_1$ and weakly to insulin. The type 2 IGF receptor binds strongly to $IGF_2$ and does not interact with insulin. The type 1 receptor has structural similarity and sequence homology to the insulin receptor. Like the insulin receptor, it consists of two types of glycoprotein subunits, $\alpha$- and $\beta$-subunits, linked by disulfide bonds to form complexes, probably composed of a structure that contains two of each of these subunits ($\alpha_2$-$\beta_2$). The $\alpha$-subunits contain the IGF-binding site. The $\beta$-subunits contain the intracellular domain and manifest tyrosine-specific protein kinase activity as well as a tyrosine residue that can be autophosphorylated. These functions and the structure of the receptor are strikingly similar to the insulin receptor. It should be emphasized, however, that despite their similarities, these two molecules (IGF receptor type 1 and insulin receptor) are different. The type 2 IGF receptor is distinct from both the type 1 IGF receptor and the insulin receptor. It consists of a glycoprotein of 260,000 $M_r$ that contains interchain disulfate bridges. The type 2 receptor does not have a tyrosine-specific protein kinase activity. Although the type 1 IGF receptor and the type 2 IGF receptor tend to bind predominantly the corresponding IGF, it should also be emphasized that both IGF can bind to either receptor, and it appears likely that both receptors are responsible for mediating the events associated with $IGF_1$ and $IGF_2$. The affinity of insulin for the IGF receptor type 1 is probably responsible for many of the so-called growth-stimulatory effects of insulin on cells in culture in which insulin, added at supraphysiologic concentrations, occasionally stimulates cell growth in conjunction with other growth factors.

IGF are produced by several tumors. Fibrosarcoma tumor cell lines produce $IGF_2$. $IGF_1$ is a secretion product from many tumor cell lines, including osteosarcoma cells and mammary tumor cells. The latter cell lines, while frequently producing $IGF_1$, also occasionally exhibit receptors for $IGF_1$. It is not known whether this relationship is responsible for the growth of the tumors in autocrine fashion, as has been postulated with other growth factors and tumor models. Currently, the two IGF have not as yet been associated with any particular transforming oncogene. By contrast, the presence of a tyrosine kinase function on the receptor suggests the possibility that such oncogenes related to the receptors will probably be identified in the future. It has been shown that many oncogene proteins have tyrosine kinase function, including the protein produced by the oncogene v-erb-B and the members of the src family of oncogene proteins.

## 9. NERVE GROWTH FACTOR

Nerve growth factor (NGF) is perhaps the first described and fully characterized growth factor. It was isolated from snake venom and male mouse submaxillary glands by R. Levi-Montalchini and S. Cohen[93] (prior to the isolation of EGF by the same team from the same sources). This factor is of relatively high molecular weight and consists of three noncovalently linked subunits. The subunits are called $\alpha$, $\beta$, and $\gamma$ and compose the NGF molecule in the proportion 2:2:1. The NGF activity resides with the $\beta$-subunit, which consists of two identical peptide chains, each of 13,000 $M_r$.[94,95] The role of the associated $\alpha$- and $\gamma$-subunits is not entirely clear. Studies with the pheochromocytoma cell line PC12[96] have shown that complexes of the $\beta$-subunit to either the $\alpha$- or the $\gamma$-subunit inhibit binding of the $\beta$-subunit to its receptor. Other studies have shown that the $\gamma$-subunit is an arginine esteropeptidase and, as such, it may be involved in processing of the $\beta$-subunit from a larger precursor by proteolysis. Such a precursor for the $\beta$-subunit has been recently demonstrated; it appears to be a dimer with 307 amino acids per chain, of which the NGF final molecule is present in residues 188–305.

Although NGF is included in the category of growth factors, it has functional characteristics that set it aside from the other growth factors considered thus far. The primary demonstrated function of NGF is on the differentiation of sympathetic ganglia and the formation of sympathetic and sensory neurons.[94,97] When NGF is added to organ cultures of chicken embryo sympathetic ganglia, it induces profuse outgrowth of neurite axons. Injections of NGF to developing organisms also lead to profuse outgrowth of sympathetic neurons in the target organs. These neurons grow in tangles and are seen to invade smooth muscle and vessels. Conversely, lack of NGF is associated with different degrees of malformation or lack of development of the autonomic nervous system. It appears that the presence and secretion of NGF is required during embryonic development to prevent the death of the cells that lead to the formation of sympathetic and dorsal root ganglia. Injection of antibodies against NGF to developing animals or neonates leads to atrophy of the sympathetic nervous system, a procedure described as *immunosympathectomy*. Despite such strong trophic effects on the development of the peripheral nervous system, the addition of NGF is generally not associated with stimulation of DNA synthesis in most cell types. An exception to this finding is the PC12 pheochromocytoma cell line, in which the addition of NGF stimulates a transient wave of DNA synthesis followed by differentiation of cells and formation of neurite axons. These differentiated cells manifest no more DNA synthesis. At the time that DNA synthesis is stimulated there is a transient increase in the expression of the c-*fos* gene.[98] The strong trophic effects of NGF and the abundance of embryonic and neonatal animal studies have amply documented that NGF is essential for normal development of the peripheral nervous system. In fact, recent studies have shown that the production of NGF correlates well with the density of sympathetic innervation of the peripheral tissues. The timing of the production of NGF and the appearance of NGF receptors in neurons or in other susceptible targets is also well correlated with the embryogenic establishment of different events that relate to peripheral innervation. Studies with developing skin[99] have shown that NGF synthesis starts at a time when the sensory neurons approach the epidermal cells. At that time, the epidermal cells as well as the mesenchyme of the dermis synthesize NGF, and NGF receptors appear in the sensory neurons when the fibers of these neurons reach their skin targets.

The structure of the NGF receptor is well characterized from many different cell lines and species. The human NGF-receptor[100–102] consists of 399 amino acids organized in an extracellular domain with 40 amino acids, a transmembrane domain, and a cytoplasmic domain with 155 amino acids. The extracellular domain is glycosylated with multiple residues of sialic acid. The receptor can exist in high- and low-affinity states. The available evidence with PC12 cells indicates that the NGF receptor is not associated with a tyrosine kinase activity.[103] Numerous studies, however, have shown that the addition of NGF to cells causes an increase in levels of intracellular cyclic adenosine monophosphate (cAMP). It is not clear whether this is exclusively due to stimulation of NGF–receptor or whether additional mechanisms may be involved. In general, the molecular events that mediate the signals for differentiation generated by the NGF receptor are not clear. Multiple components of the plasma membrane and cytoplasm, however, may be involved, including the products of *fos* and *ras* proto-oncogenes.

The relationship of NGF or its receptor to neoplastic transformation is not clear. NGF is produced by several glioma cell lines. It has also been found in mammary adenocarcinomas, fibrosarcomas, melanomas, neuroblastomas, and human glioblastoma cell lines. Some of the neuroblastoma cell lines that secrete NGF also possess high-affinity receptors for NGF,[104] although they do not appear to respond to NGF with cell differentiation. Strong differentiation-related effects are stimulated by NGF in several other neuroblastoma cell lines not producing NGF. In these cell lines, the addition of NGF is associated with production of long neuritelike processes and cessation of cell proliferation. The relationship between this phenomenon and the often observed maturation of neuroblastomas into ganglioneuromas in humans, associated with tumor regression and benign behavior, is quite probable but not proven.

## 10. MACROPHAGE COLONY-STIMULATING FACTOR-1

Colony-stimulating factor-1 (CSF-1) is a polypeptide of 14,500 $M_r$ that, in its final configuration, exists as a dimeric glycoprotein of approximately 45,000–90,000 $M_r$. The discrepancy between the projected molecular weight of the dimeric form (29,000) and the actual recorded molecular weight is due to heavy degree of glycosylation. Approximately 40–60% of the molecule consists of glycosylation residues.[105,106] CSF-1 stimulates the proliferation or increased survival of macrophages and macrophage precursors in cell culture. A long range of monocyte–macrophage precursors can be stimulated by CSF-1. The final differentiated cell (adherent macrophage) is not further stimulated into DNA synthesis, but its survival is enhanced in culture. The earliest hemo-poietic precursor stimulated to proliferate by CSF-1 alone is a cell type identified as bone marrow CFU/C. Other, earlier, hematopoietic precursors, can also be stimulated by CSF-1 but only in the presence of two other unidentified factors, called hematopoietin-2 and hematopoietin-1. CSF-1 is produced by specific fibroblastlike cells in the bone marrow. It is present in the circulation, and it binds specifically to macrophages. The major mechanism of clearance of CSF-1 involves the binding to a specific receptor, which is then cleared by endocytosis in the macrophages. The endocytosed [receptor–ligand] complex is taken into lysosomes and degraded.

Recent studies[105] have shown that binding of CSF-1 to its receptor results in stimulation of a tyrosine kinase function in the receptor, resulting in phosphorylation of tyrosine residues of the receptor itself. Other substrates in macrophages also appear to be phosphorylated by the stimulated CSF-1 receptor. It has now been established that the CSF-1 receptor is very similar to the product of the *fms* oncogene.[107] The product of the *fms* oncogene contains the ligand-binding portion of the CSF-1 receptor and differs from the receptor by changes in the extreme carboxy terminal end of the molecule. Whereas the receptor for the CSF-1 is phosphorylated only in the presence of the ligand, the viral *fms* gene product is consistently phosphorylated in the absence of the CSF-1 factor. In addition to the expression of the CSF-1 receptor in transformed fibroblasts, this receptor is also expressed in high levels in human placenta[108] as well as in choriocarcinoma cell lines. The function of CSF-1 in placenta formation and function has not yet been fully investigated. From limited studies available, it appears that transformation by *fms* oncogene is associated with increased turnover of PIP-2 (Fig. 2). Stimulation of the CSF-1 receptor in normal cells, however, is not associated with increased breakdown of PIP-2.

## 11. TRANSFORMING GROWTH FACTOR-β

TGF-β is a polypeptide growth factor that can be best characterized as a growth modu-lator.[109,110] It was originally discovered along with TGF-α, in the conditioned medium of cell cultures of sarcoma cells. The combined biologic activity was initially called sarcoma growth factor.[25] This was subsequently shown to be composed of TGF-α and TGF-β. The combination of TGF-α and TGF-β stimulated the growth of certain normal fibroblast cell lines in soft agar, without any anchorage to a substratum. This finding, considered characteristic of the neoplastic phenotype, was imparted to normal cells by the combined action of TGF-α and TGF-β. This led to the nomenclature of these polypeptides as transforming growth factors (TGF). While TGF-α uniformly stimulates DNA synthesis in cells that carry the EGF receptor, TGF-β stimulates growth only in a small number of mesenchymal cell types, while it inhibits the proliferation of most cells, especially epithelial cells. In addition, unlike TGF-α, TGF-β does not bind to the EGF receptor, but rather to a novel receptor characteristic and specific for TGF-β.

Platelets are a rich source of TGF-β,[111] from which it is currently prepared. TGF-β is pre-sent in the α-granules of platelets (which also contain PDGF) and is released after platelet rupture during blood coagulation. TGF-β mRNA, however, has been identified in many cell types,[112] including most tumor cell lines as well as some normal cell and tissue sources (i.e., lymphocytes, placenta). In addition, high sources of TGF-β protein material have been extracted from bone.[109] The concentration of TGF-β in bone is the highest than from any other source, excluding platelets.

The precise biologic effects of TGF-β are not thoroughly understood. It appears to be acting more as a growth inhibitor than as a growth stimulator. It inhibits the growth of most epithelial cells in which it has been tested, including keratinocytes, hepatocytes,[113] mammary epithelial cells, and bronchial epithelial cells. Whereas the normal cells are inhibited in their growth by TGF-β, the

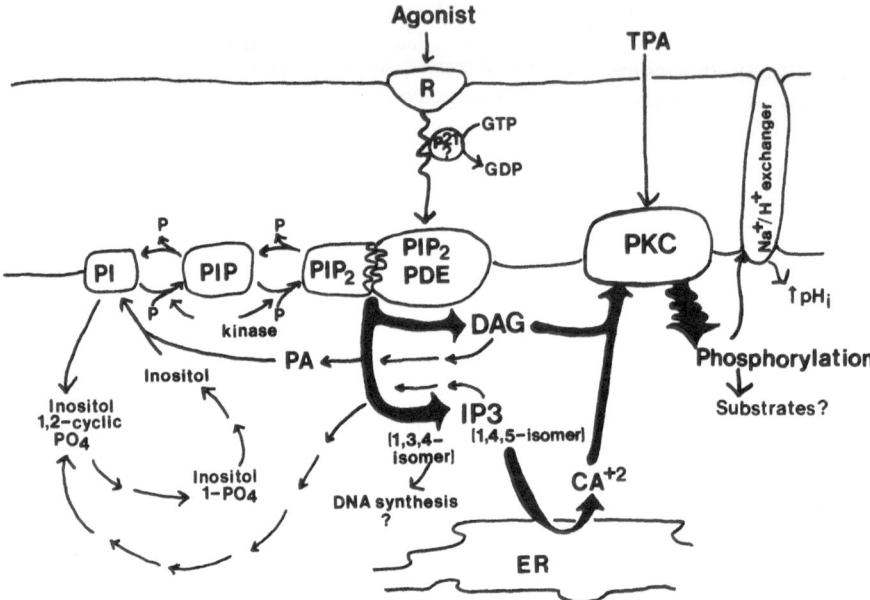

*Figure 2.* Schematic diagram of the pathways of interchange of phosphatidyl inositol derivatives and their effects on intracellular events. PI, phosphatidylinositol; PIP, phosphatidylinositol-4-phosphate; PIP-2, phosphatidylinositol-4,5-bisphosphate; IP3, inositol-1,4,5-triphosphate (note the existence of two isomers); DAG, diacylglycerol; PDE, phosphodiesterase; p21, protein belonging to the *ras* gene family of proteins; PKC, protein kinase C; R, receptor for growth factor; TPA, tetradecanoylphorbol ester; P, phosphate moiety; GTP, guanosine triphosphate. Binding of a growth factor (agonist, in classic pharmacologic terminology) to its receptor stimulates a sequence of events hitherto undetermined and mediated by unknown GTP binding proteins (of which p21 is a potential candidate). These events lead to the activation of PIP-2 phosphodiesterase (PIP-2 PDE), which catalyzes breakdown of PIP-2 to DAG and IP3. (*Note:* The phosphate moiety attached to phosphatidic acid is now attached to the inositol moiety to form IP3.) IP3 exists as two isomers. One of the isomers is now generally accepted to be responsible for calcium mobilization from intracellular stores. The role of the other isomer is not understood and it has been speculated that it may be involved in the mediation of the signal that leads to DNA synthesis. DAG (there are potentially many different types, depending on the fatty acids attached to the glycerol) allosterically activate PKC. The effect of DAG is mimicked by the phorbol ester TPA. PKC exists as membrane and as cytoplasmic form. The latter form is translocated to the former under the influence of calcium, thus resulting in an increased concentration of PKC on the plasma membrane. PKC phosphorylates a variety of substrates on the plasma membrane (including some growth factor receptors) in serine and threonine positions.

neoplastic cell counterparts (carcinoma cell lines produced from the above sources) tend to be entirely or completely resistant to the inhibitory effect of TGF-β.[109,114] The reason for this differential performance between normal and neoplastic cells is not clear.

TGF-β is a dimer with a molecular weight of 25,000. It is composed of two identical chains, each chain containing 112 amino acids.[115] The molecule is extremely stable and contains nine disulfide bridges. The amino acid sequence of human and mouse TGF-β have been identified and the two molecules differ by only one amino acid. Futhermore, variants of this molecule have recently been purified.[116] These were described as TGF-β₁ (the originally described molecule) and TGF-β₂. There is also ample evidence to indicate that TGF-β is synthesized from a larger precursor, which has now been characterized.[117] Although each of the chains in the final molecule contains 112 amino acids, it appears to be synthesized from an original precursor containing 391 amino acids, with the final product located toward the carboxyl-terminal portion of the precursor molecule. Studies with other growth factors suggest that TGF-β may be part of a family of peptides with growth-modulating or inhibitory activity. One such peptide is *inhibin*,[118] which inhibits secretion of

FHS from pituitary. Another such molecule is the Mullerian inhibitory substance (MIS),[119] which is produced by the testes and results in regression of the Mullerian ducts in the male embryo. These peptides have structures similar to TGF-β and substantial amino acid sequence homology.

Although the structure of TGF-β is completely understood, it appears that treatment with acid is required to render the molecule active for most of the *in vitro* studies. The effect of acidification on the molecule and the mechanism of this bioactivation are not clear. It has been shown in some instances, however, that a number of tumor cell lines that produce TGF-β are also incapable of activating the molecule, although they do respond (by growth inhibition) to the acid-activated form of TGF-β.[109]

A large receptor exists for TGF-β. This receptor is specific for this molecule and does not bind to any other molecule known at this point, including MIS and inhibin. Other molecules besides the main TGF-β receptor may also exist in cells that bind TGF-β with high affinity. The main TGF-β receptor is a large molecule of approximately $600,000 M_r$ and is composed of two subunits linked by disulfide bridges.[120] It does not have any tyrosine kinase activity nor does it stimulate increased turnover of PIP-2. Binding of TGF-β to its receptor does not result in a decrease in receptor concentration on the membrane (downregulation), a phenomenon that is commonly seen with the binding of ligands to specific receptors, as in the case of EGF, PDGF, and most other growth factors. Recently,[116] smaller types of TGF-β receptors have also been described, and it has been suggested that there may be several types of TGF-β receptors, often coexisting in single cell types. The nature or the properties of the smaller TGF-β receptors are not at all understood at this time.

The functions of TGF-β in fetal development are not very clear (for review, see ref. 110). TGF-β has been localized in mesenchymal embryonal tissues during embryonic development, and it may be of biologic importance for the optimal development of mesenchymal connective tissues. Injection of TGF-β in animals also results in vascularization and collagen deposition at the site of injection, suggesting that TGF-β may have a role in stimulating the production of connective tissue proteins. The high concentration of TGF-β in the bone was mentioned above.

## 12. OTHER GROWTH FACTORS

The above-described growth factors are better characterized and the cellular responses to them are well understood. Numerous other growth-stimulatory activities have been characterized for many tissues. Several of these activities have been shown to be identical to either the final products or to precursors of the above-mentioned growth factors. Other growth factors, however, undoubtedly exist that have not yet been characterized and which must play a role for the optimal growth and differentiation of target tissues. Tissues with strong regenerative potential or high rate of cell replication appear to be influenced by complex interplays of numerous known and unknown growth factors. Research is being done to further identify growth factors involved in the regeneration of liver, as well as replication of bone marrow hematopoietic cells and intestinal and pancreatic cells, among others. Considering the fact that most of the known growth factors are produced from precursors and that some of these precursors are biologically active (e.g., TGF-α), it is important to establish the relationship of newly discovered growth factors to precursor molecules of known growth factors. It is also important to characterize whether the new growth factors will share receptors with existing growth factors or have receptors of their own. In parallel with the studies on identification of more growth factors, other molecules are also being characterized which may play a more complex role in cell growth regulation. These substances may modulate or inhibit the effect of other growth factors. The complex effects of TGF-β (growth inhibition or stimulation, depending on cell type) were mentioned above. Another molecule called tumor necrosis factor (TNF) has been recently characterized and shown to inhibit the growth of several neoplastic cell lines. TNF has lipolytic activity when given to whole animals and exhibits other complex effects.

Another example of the role of a substance whose function strains the definition of a growth factor is norepinephrine, the neurotransmitter of the sympathetic nervous system. Norepinephrine does not stimulate growth of hepatocytes by itself, but it modulates the growth stimulatory effect of

EGF on hepatocytes.[122,123] When norepinephrine binds to the $\alpha_1$-adrenergic receptor, the latter, either directly or through the mediation of other plasma membrane components, modifies the EGF receptor in ways that enhance the effectiveness of EGF. This phenomenon whereby one substance modifies indirectly (through its own receptor) the receptor of another substance is called heterologous regulation of receptors. Conversely, in a similar manner, norepinephrine also diminishes the growth inhibitory effect of TGF-$\beta$ on hepatocyte DNA synthesis. Given the fact there is substantial evidence to suggest that liver regeneration in the whole animal depends on proper function of the $\alpha_1$-adrenergic receptor, it is likely that a prolonged and sustained pulse of norepinephrine could trigger the early events associated with liver regeneration by altering the balance of responses of the quiescent parenchymal hepatocytes to these two growth-modulating substances. In this instance, norepinephrine, although not a growth factor by itself, could be viewed as being a growth trigger. Within this context, cell replication is initiated by one substance (the trigger) and driven to proceed by the effect of another substance (the growth factor). The original definition of the term growth factor included the notion that the substances covered under that term enhanced the rate of growth of the responder cells. As the pathways of organization and interaction of the complex signals that regulate cellular growth become elucidated, this definition may need to be reconsidered to encompass all molecules whose role is crucial, either in a stimulatory or an inhibitory mode, in orchestrating the events that regulate growth of cells or tissues. In many instances, a substance may not be a growth factor by itself, but it might modulate the effects of other growth-related substances.

## 13. SECOND MESSENGERS MEDIATING GROWTH FACTOR EFFECTS

Although the nature of the messages generated by growth factors is not very clear, many phenomena have been described after the addition of growth factors to susceptible cells. Many of these phenomena are common between different cell types and are seen in these susceptible cells regardless of the fact that the cells may be responding to different growth factors. Some of these phenomena[62] include ionic fluxes of Na$^+$ and H$^+$ (see Chapter 15), as well as calcium mobilization. Calcium in most instances appears to be mobilized from intracellular stores such as mitochondria. A phenomenon elicited by many growth factors (GF) is the stimulation of enhanced turnover of inositol phospholipids (Fig. 2). This is seen with many GF very soon (less than 1 min) after the GF binds to its receptor. The detailed discussion of the chemistry of the substances involved and the pathways of the resynthesis of the molecules broken down are beyond the scope of this chapter and are discussed in many recent reviews.[124–126] Only a diagrammatic presentation is attempted in this section. In general, all the events that eventually result in the formation of these secondary messenger molecules are triggered by the binding of the GF to their receptors. Binding between GF and GF receptors results in increase of the breakdown of phosphatidylinositol-4,5-bisphosphate (PIP-2) to inositol 1,4,5-triphosphate (IP3) and diacylglycerol(s). This reaction is catalyzed by a specific PIP-2 phosphodiesterase. The latter is activated by several receptors and the activation is mediated by as yet unidentified protein(s) catalyzing breakdown of GTP, collectively called G proteins. IP3 is believed to lead to rapid influx of calcium into the cell or mobilize intracellular calcium from the mitochondria. In either case, the concentration of intracellular calcium is increased following the effect of IP3. An increase in calcium affects several other enzymes directly or by its interaction with calmodulin. Diacylglycerols (resulting from the breakdown of PIP-2) and calcium ions (mobilized from the effects of IP3) can activate PKC. The latter enzyme, in the presence of increased levels of cytoplasmic calcium, is translocated from the cytoplasm to the plasma membrane. The substrates of this enzyme are currently under study. It can phosphorylate several targets, including GF receptors such as the EGF receptor mentioned earlier. Phosphorylation takes place usually on serine or threonine residues. The interaction among the G proteins, GF, receptors, and PKC on the plasma membrane, mediated by the different species of inositol phospholipids, is shown diagrammatically in Fig. 2. This complex set of events, in addition to the tyrosine phosphorylation that is stimulated when many GF bind to their receptors, is considered to somehow lead to the generation of a mitogenic signal. The distribution of tyrosine kinase activities and the capability to stimulate PIP-2

*Table I. Tyrosine Kinase Activity and PIP-2*
*Turnover Stimulation in Relationship to*
*Specific Growth Factor Receptors* <sup>a</sup>

| Receptor for | Tyrosine kinase | PIP-2 turnover increase |
|---|---|---|
| EGF | + | + / − |
| PDGF | + | + |
| FGF | − | + |
| Bombesin | + | + |
| IL-2 | − | + |
| Insulin | + | + / − |
| IGF (type 1) | + | − |
| IGF (type 2) | − | − |
| NGF | − | − |
| Norepinephrine (A1) | − | + |
| CSF1 | + | − |
| TGF-β | − | − |

<sup>a</sup> TGFα shares the same receptor with EGF.

turnover in target cells for the receptors of several GF is shown in Table I. A rather limited set of substrates is currently known to be phosphorylated after GF (whose receptors have a tyrosine kinase function) are added to susceptible cells. Probably more substrates of modification (phosphorylation?) will be discovered in the near future that will be found to be involved in this process. Of interest for the field of tumor biology, the well-known tumor promoters phorbol esters were found to be potent activators of PKC, and the role of this molecule in tumor promotion needs to be further understood. In addition, the products of the *ras* family of genes (which in mutated or overexpressed form can function as oncogenes) are G proteins (they can bind GTP and catalyze its hydrolysis). It is not very clear at this point whether any of the *ras* proteins are associated with a specific receptor, although such an association is considered most likely. Recent studies suggest that the *ras* proteins may be involved in mediating the effects of insulin on oocyte maturation in the frog.[127]

## REFERENCES

1. Cohen, S., 1962, Isolation of a mouse submaxillary gland protein accelerating incisor eruption and eyelid opening in the new-born animal. *J. Biol. Chem.* **237:**1555–1562.
2. Gregory, H., 1975, Isolation and structure of urogastrone and its relationship to epidermal growth factor, *Nature (Lond.)* **257:**325–327.
3. Cohen, S., and Carpenter, G., 1975, Human epidermal growth factor: Isolation and chemical and biological properties, *Proc. Natl. Acad. Sci. USA* **72:**1317–1321.
4. Savage, R. C., Hash, J. H., and Cohen, S., 1973, Epidermal growth factor: Location of disulfide bonds, *J. Biol. Chem.* **248:**7669–7672.
5. Gray, A., Dull, T. J., and Ullrich, A., 1983, Nucleotide sequence of epidermal growth factor cDNA predicts a 128,000-molecular weight precursor, *Nature (Lond.)* **303:**722–725.
6. Scott, J., Urdea, M., Quiroga, M., Sanchez-Pescador, R., Fong, N., Selby, M., Rutter, W. J., and Bell, G. I., 1983, Structure of a mouse submaxillary messenger RNA encoding epidermal growth factor and seven related proteins, *Science* **221:**236–240.
7. Carpenter, G., and Xendegui, J. G., 1986, Epidermal growth factor, its receptor and related proteins, *Exp. Cell Res.* **164:**1–10.
8. Perheentupa, J., Lakshmanan, J., Hoath, S. B., and Fisher, D. A., 1984, Hormonal modulation of mouse plasma concentration of epidermal growth factor, *Acta Endocrinol. (Copenh.)* **107:**571–576.
9. Rall, L. B., Scott, J., and Bell, G. I., 1985, Mouse prepro-epidermal growth factor synthesis by the kidney and other tissues, *Nature (Lond.)* **313:**228–231.

10. Mattila, A.-L., Perheentupa, J., Pesonen, K., and Viinikka, L., 1985, Epidermal growth factor in human urine from birth to puberty, *J. Clin. Endocrinol. Metab.* **61**:997–1000.

11. Tsutsumi, O., Kurachi, H., and Oka, T., 1986, A physiological role of epidermal growth factor in male reproductive function, *Science* **233**:975–977.

12. Bucher, N. R. L., Patel, U., and Cohen, S., 1978, Hormonal factors and liver growth, *Adv. Enzyme Regul.* **16**:205–213.

13. Earp, H. S., and O'Keefe, E. J., 1981, Epidermal growth factor receptor number decreases during rat liver regeneration, *J. Clin. Invest.* **67**:1580–1583.

14. Stern, D. F., Hare, D. L., Cecchini, M. A., and Weinberg, R. A., 1987, Construction of a novel oncogene based on synthetic sequences encoding epidermal growth factor, *Science* **235**:321–324.

15. Ushiro, H., and Cohen, S., 1980, Identification of phosphotyrosine as a product of epidermal growth factor-activated protein kinase A431 cell membranes, *J. Biol. Chem.* **255**:8363–8365.

16. Cohen, S., Ushiro, H., Stoscheck, C., and Chinkers, M. A., 1982, A native 170,000 epidermal growth factor receptor kinase complex from shed membrane vesicles, *J. Biol. Chem.* **257**:1523–1531.

17. Schlessinger, J., 1986, Allosteric regulation of the epidermal growth factor receptor kinase, *J. Cell Biol.* **103**:2067–2072.

18. Yarden, Y., and Schlessinger, J., 1987, Self-phosphorylation of epidermal growth factor receptor: Evidence for a model of intermolecular allosteric activation, *Biochemistry* **26**:1434–1442.

19. Yarden, Y., and Schlessinger, J., 1987, Epidermal growth factor induces rapid, reversible aggregation of the purified epidermal growth factor receptor, *Biochemistry* **26**:1443–1451.

20. St. Hilaire, R. J., and Jones, A. L., 1982, Epidermal growth factor: its biologic and metabolic effects with emphasis on the hepatocyte, *Hepatology* **2**:601–613.

21. Bursen, S. J., Barker, M. E., Goldman, I. S., Hradek, G. T., Raper, S. E., and Jones, A. L., 1984, Transport of epidermal growth factor by rat liver: Evidence for a nonlysosomal pathway, *J. Cell. Biol.* **99**:1259–1265.

22. DeLaat, S. W., Moolenaar, W. H., Defize, L. H. K., Boonstra, J., and van der Saag, P. T., 1986, Ionic signal transduction growth factor action, *Biochem. Soc. Symp.* **50**:205–220.

23. Riedel, H., Schlessinger, J., and Ullrich, A., 1987, A chimeric, ligand-binding v-erbB/EGF receptor retains transforming potential, *Science* **236**:197–236.

24. Hunter, T., Ling, N., and Cooper, J. A., 1984, Protein kinase C phosphorylation of the EGF receptor at a threonine residue close to the cytoplasmic face of the plasma membrane, *Nature (Lond.)* **311**:480–483.

25. DeLarco, J. E., and Todaro, G. J., 1978, Growth factors from murine sarcoma virus transformed cells, *Proc. Natl. Acad. Sci. USA* **75**:4001–4005.

26. Moses, H. L., Branum, E. L., Proper, J. A., and Robinson, R. A., 1981, Transforming growth factor production by chemically transformed cells, *Cancer Res.* **41**:2842–2848.

27. Nickell, K. A., Halper, J., and Moses, H. L., 1983, Transforming growth factors solid human malignant neoplasms, *Cancer Res.* **43**:1966–1971.

28. Derynck, R., 1986, Transforming growth factor-alpha:structure and biological activities, *J. Cell. Biochem.* **32**:293–304.

29. Marquardt, H., Hunkapiller, M. W., Hood, L. E., Twardzik, D. R., DeLarco, J. E., Stephenson, J. R., and Todaro, G. J., 1983, Transforming growth factors produced by retrovirus-transformed rodent fibroblasts and human melanoma cells: Amino acid sequence homology with epidermal growth factor, *Proc. Natl. Acad. Sci. USA* **80**:4684–4688.

30. Tam, J. P., 1985, Physiological effects of transforming growth factor in the newborn mouse, *Science* **229**:673–675.

31. Schreiber, A. B., Winkler, M. E., and Derynck, R., 1986, Transforming growth factor-alpha: A more potent angiogenic mediator than epidermal growth factor, *Science* **232**:1250–1253.

32. Kimball, E. S., Bohn, W. H., Cockley, K. D., Warren, T. C., and Sherwin, S. A., 1984, Distinct high-performance liquid chromatography pattern of transforming growth factor activity urine of cancer patients as compared with that of normal individuals, *Cancer Res.* **44**:3613–3619.

33. Lee, D. C., Rochford, R., Rodaro, G. J., and Villarreal, L. P., 1985, Developmental expression of rat transforming growth factor-alpha mRNA, *Mol. Cell. Biol.* **5**:3644–3646.

34. Potter, V. R., 1969, Recent trends in cancer biochemistry: The importance of studies on fetal tissue, *Can. Cancer Conf.* **8**:9–30.

35. Kudkow, J. E., Khosravi, M. J., Kobrin, M. S., and Mak, W. W., 1984, Inability of anti-epidermal growth factor receptor monoclonal antibody to block ''autocrine'' growth stimulation transforming growth factor-secreting melanoma cells, *J. Biol. Chem.* **19**:11895–11900.

36. Watanabe, S., Lazar, E., and Sporn, M. B., 1987, Transformation of normal rat kidney (NRK) cells by an

infectious retrovirus carrying a synthetic rat type alpha transforming growth factor gene, *Proc. Natl. Acad. Sci. USA* **84:**1258–1262.

37. Lee, D. C., Rose, T. M., Webb, N. R., and Todaro, G. J., 1985, Cloning and sequence analysis of a cDNA for rat transforming growth factor-alpha, *Nature (Lond.)* **313:**489–491.

38. Luetteke, N. C., and Michalopoulos, G. K., 1985, Partial purification and characterization of a hepatocyte growth factor produced by rat hepatocellular carcinoma cells, *Cancer Res.* **45:**6331–6337.

39. Halper, J., and Moses, H. L., 1983, Epithelial tissue-derived growth factor-like polypeptides, *Cancer Res.* **43:**1971–1979.

40. Bringman, T. S., Lindquist, P. B., Derynck, R., 1987, Different transforming growth factor-alpha species are derived from a glycosylated and palmitoylated transmembrane precursor, *Cell* **48:**429–440.

41. Teixido, J., Gilmore, R., Lee, D. C., and Massague, J., 1987, Integral membrane glycoprotein properties of the prohormone pro-transforming growth factor-alpha, *Nature (Lond.)* **326:**883–885.

42. Ibbotson, K. J., D'Souza, S. M., Ng, K. W., Osborne, C. K., Naill, M., Martin, T. J., and Mundy, G. R., 1983, Tumor-derived growth factor increases bone resorption in a tumor associated with humoral hypercalcemia of malignancy, *Science* **221:**1292–1294.

43. Heldin, C.-H., Wasteson, A., and Westermark, B., 1985, Platelet-derived growth factor, *Mol. Cell. Endocrinol.* **39:**169–187.

44. Ross, R., Raines, E. W., and Bowen-Pope, D. F., 1986, The biology of platelet-derived growth factor, *Cell* **46:**155–169.

45. Antoniades, H. N., Scher, C. D., and Stiles, C. D., 1979, Purification of human platelet-derived growth factor, *Proc. Natl. Acad. Sci. USA* **76:**1809–1813.

46. Stiles, C. D., 1985, The biological role of oncogenes—Insights from platelet-derived growth factor: Rhoads Memorial Award Lecture, *Cancer Res.* **45:**5215–5218.

47. Shimokado, K., Raines, E. W., Madtes, D. K., Barrett, T. B., Benditt, E. P., and Ross, R., 1985, A significant part of macrophage-derived growth factor consists of at least two forms of PDGF, *Cell* **43:**277–286.

48. DiCorleto, P. E., and Bowen-Pope, D. F., 1983, Cultured endothelial cells produce a platelet-derived growth factor-like protein, *Proc. Natl. Acad. Sci. USA* **80:**1919–1923.

49. Seifert, R. A., Schwartz, S. M., and Bowen-Pope, D. F., 1984, Developmentally regulated production of platelet-derived growth factor-like molecules, *Nature (Lond.)* **311:**669–671.

50. Graves, D. T., Owen, A. J., Williams, S. R., and Antoniades, H. N., 1986, Identification of processing events in the synthesis of platelet-derived growth factor-like proteins by human osteosarcoma cells, *Proc. Natl. Acad. Sci. USA* **83:**4636–4640.

51. Heldin, C.-H., Westermark, B., and Wasteson, A., 1981, Specific receptors for platelet-derived growth factor on cells derived from connective tissue and glia, *Proc. Natl. Acad. Sci USA* **78:**3664–3668.

52. Yarden, Y., Escobedo, J. A., Kuang, W. J., Yang-Feng, T. L., Daniel, T. O., Tremble, P. M., Chen, E. Y., Ando, M. E., Harkins, R. N., and Francke, U., 1986, Structure of the receptor for platelet-derived growth factor helps define a family of closely related growth factor receptors, *Nature (Lond.)* **323:**226–232.

53. Goustin, A. S., Betsholtz, C., Pfeifer-Ohlsson, S., Persson, H., Rydnert, J., Bywater, M., Holmgren, G., Heldin, C.-H., Westermark, B., and Ohlsson, R., 1985, Coexpression of the sis and myc protooncogenes in developing human placenta suggests autocrine control of trophoblast growth, *Cell* **41:**301–312.

54. O'Keefe, E. J., and Pledger, W. J., A model of cell cycle control: Sequential events regulated by growth factors, *Mol. Cell. Endocrinol.* **31:**167–186.

55. Heldin, C. H., Btesholtz, C., Johnsson, A., Nister, M., Ek, B., Ronnstrand, L., Wasteson, A., and Westermark, B., 1985, Platelet-derived growth factor: Mechanism of action and relation to oncogenes, *J. Cell Sci. (Suppl)* **3:**65–76.

56. Ek, B., Westermark, B., Wasteson, A., and Heldin, C.-H., 1982, Stimulation of tyrosine-specific phosphorylation by platelet-derived growth factor, *Nature (Lond.)* **295:**419–420.

56a. Huang, J. S., and Huang, S. S., 1985, Role of growth factors in oncogenesis: Growth factor-protoon-cogene pathways of mitogenesis, *Ciba Found. Symp.* **116:**46–65.

57. Williams, L. T., 1986, The sis gene and PDGF, *Cancer Surv.* **5:**233–241.

57a. Kelly, K., Cochran, B. H., Stiles, C. D., and Leder, P., 1983, Cell-specific regulation of the c-myc gene by lymphocyte mitogens and platelet-derived growth factor, *Cell* **35:**603–610.

58. Walsh, J. H., and Reeve, J. R., 1985, Mammalian bombesin-like peptides: Neuromodulators of gastric function and autocrine regulators of lung cancer growth, *Peptides* **6**(suppl. 3):63–68.

59. Varner, A., Modlin, I., and Walsh, J., 1981, High potency of bombesin for stimulation of human gastric release and gastric acid secretion, *Regul. Peptides* **1:**289–296.

60. Dorreen, M. S., 1986, Role of biological markers and probes in lung carcinomas, *Bull. Eur. Physiopathol. Respir.* **22**(2):137–146.

61. Cuttitta, F., Carney, D. N., Mulshine, J., Moody, T. W., Fedorko, J., Fischler, A., and Minna, J. D., 1985, Bombesin-like peptides can function as autocrine growth factors in human small-cell lung cancer, *Nature (Lond.)* **316**:823–826.

62. Rozengurt, E., 1986, Early signals of the mitogenic response, *Science* **234**:161–166.

63. Letterio, J. J., Coughlin, S. R., and Williams, L. T., 1986, Pertussis toxin-sensitive pathway for the stimulation of c-myc expression and DNA synthesis by bombesin, *Science* **234**:1117–1119.

64. Cirillo, D. M., Gaudino, G., Naldini, L., and Comoglio, P. M., 1986, Receptor for bombesin with associated tyrosine kinase activity, *Mol. Cell. Biol.* **6**:4641–4649.

65. Gospodarowicz, D., Neufeld, G., and Schweigerer, L., 1986, Fibroblast growth factor, *Mol. Cell. Endocrinol.* **46**:187–204.

66. Baird, A., Esch, F., Mormede, P., Ueno, N., Ling, N., Bohlen, P., Ying, S.-Y., Wehrenberg, W. B., and Guillemin, R., 1986, Molecular characterization of fibroblast growth factor: Distribution and biological activities in various tissues, *Rec. Prog. Horm. Res.* **42**:143–205.

67. Gospodarowicz, D., Neufeld, G., and Schweigerer, L., 1986, Molecular and biological characterization of fibroblast growth factor, an angiogenic factor which also controls the proliferation and differentiation of mesoderm and neuroectoderm derived cells, *Cell Diff.* **19**:1–17.

68. Esch, F., Ueno, N., Baird, A., Hill, F., Denoroy, L., Ling, N., Gospodarowicz, D., and R. Guillemin, 1985, Primary structure of bovine brain acidic fibroblast growth factor (FGF), *Biochem. Biophys. Res. Commun.* **133**:554–562.

69. Neufeld, G., and Gospodarowicz, D., 1985, The identification and partial characterization of the fibroblast growth factor receptor of baby hamster kidney cells, *J. Biol. Chem.* **260**:13860–13868.

70. Gospodarowicz, D., and Bialecki, H., 1978, The effects of the epidermal and fibroblast growth factor on the replicative lifespan of bovine granulosa cells in culture, *Endocrinology* **103**:854–858.

71. Simonian, M. H., Hornsby, P. J., Ill, C. R., O'Hare, M. J., and Gill, O., 1979, Characterization of cultured bovine adrenal cortex and derived clonal lines: Regulation of steroidogenesis and cultured life span, *Endocrinology* **105**:99–108.

72. Mescher, A. L., and Gospodarowicz, D., 1979, Mitogenic effect of a growth factor derived from myelin on denervated regenerates of newt forelimbs, *J. Exp. Zool.* **207**:497–503.

73. Gospodarowicz, D., Mescher, A. L., Brown, K., and Birdwell, C. R., 1977, The role of fibroblastic growth factor and epidermal growth factor in the proliferative response of the corneal and lens epithelium, *Exp. Eye Res.* **25**:631–649.

74. Gospodarowicz, D., Ill, C. R., Hornsby, P. J., and Gill, G. N., 1977, Control of bovine adrenal cortical cell proliferation by fibroblast cell growth factor. Lack of effect of epidermal growth factor, *Endocrinology* **100**:1080–1089.

75. Folkman, J., and Klagsbrun, M., 1987, Angiogenic factors, *Science* **235**:442–447.

76. Larsson, E.-L., 1986, Interleukin-2 (IL-2) and its receptor, *Med. Oncol. Tumor Pharmacother.* **3**:231–236.

77. Mier, J. W., and Gallo, R. C., 1982, The purification and properties of human T cell growth factor, *J. Immunol.* **128**:1122–1126.

78. Watson, J., Gillis, S., Marbrook, J., Mochizuki, D., and Smith, K. A., 1979, Biochemical and biological characterization of lymphocyte regulatory molecules. I. Purification of a class of murine lymphokines, *J. Exp. Med.* **150**:849–878.

79. Leonard, W. J., Depper, J. M., Crabtree, G. F., Rudikoff, S., Pumphrey, J., Robb, R. J., Kronke, M., Svetlik, P. B., Peffer, N. J., Waldmann, T. A., and Greene, W. C., 1984, Molecular cloning and expression of cDNAs for the human interleukin 2 receptor, *Nature (Lond.)* **311**:626–628.

80. Greene, W. C., Depper, J. M., Kronke, M., and Leonard, W. J., 1986, The human interleukin-2 receptor: Analysis of structure and function, *Immunol. Rev.* **92**:29–48.

81. Urdal, D. L., March, C. J., Gillis, S., Larsen, A., and Dower, S. R., 1984, Purification and chemical characterization of the receptor for interleukin 2 from activated human T lymphocytes and from a human T-cell lymphoma line, *Proc. Natl. Acad. Sci. USA* **81**:6481–6485.

81. Miller, J., Malek, T. R., Leonard, W. J., Greene, W. C., Shevach, E. M., and Germain, R. N., 1985, Nucleotide sequence and expression of a mouse interleukin-2 receptor cDNA, *J. Immunol.* **134**:4212–4217.

82. Farrar, W. L., Cleveland, J. L., Beckner, S. K., Bonvini, E., and Evans, S. W., 1986, Biochemical and

molecular events associated with interleukin 2 regulation of lymphocyte proliferation, *Immunol. Rev.* **92**:49–65.

83. Zapf, J., and Foresch, E. R., 1986, Insulin-like growth factors/somatomedins: Structure, secretion, biological actions and physiological role, *Hormone Res.* **24**:121–130.

84. van Wyk, J. J., 1984: Somatomedins: Biological actions and physiologic control mechanisms: in: *Hormonal Proteins and Peptides* Vol. 12 (C. H. Li, ed.), pp. 82–128, Academic, Orlando, Florida.

85. Binoux, M., Hossenlopp, P., Hardouin, S., Seurin, D., Lassarre, C., and Gourmelen, M., 1986, Somatomedin (insulin-like growth factors)-binding proteins: Molecular forms and regulation, *Hormone Res.* **24**:141–151.

86. Van den Brande, J. L., Jansen, M., Hoogerbrugge, C. M., de Pagter-Holthuizen, P., van Buul-Offers, S. C., van Schaik, F. M. A., and Sussenbach, J. S., 1986, Molecular aspects of the human somatomedins, *Hormone Res.* **24**:131–140.

87. Nissley, S. B., and Rechler, M. M., 1984, Insulin-like growth factors: Biosynthesis, receptors, and carrier proteins: in: *Hormonal Proteins and Peptides*, Vol. 12, (C. H. Li, ed.) pp. 128–205, Academic, Orlando, Florida.

88. Schwander, J. C., Hauri, C., Zapf, J., and Foresch, E. R., 1983, Synthesis and secretion of insulin-like growth factor and its binding protein by the perfused rat liver: Dependence on growth hormone status, *Endocrinology* **113**:297–305.

89. Adams, S. O., Nissley, S. P., Handwerger, S., and Rechler, M. M., 1983, Developmental patterns of insulin-like growth factor-I and -II synthesis and regulation rat fibroblasts, *Nature (Lond.)* **302**:150–153.

90. Merimee, T. J., Zapf, J., Hewlett, B., and Cavalli-Sforza, L. L., 1987, Insulin-like growth factors in pygmies: The role of puberty in determining final stature, *N. Engl. J. Med.* **316**:906–911.

91. Rechler, M. M., and Nissley, S. P., 1986, Insulin-like growth factor (IGF)/somatomedin receptor subtypes: Structure, function, and relationships to insulin receptors and IGF carrier proteins, *Hormone Res.* **24**:152–159.

92. Nissley, P. S., Haskell, J. F., Sasaki, N., deVroede, M. A., and Rechler, M. M., Insulin-like growth factor receptors, *J. Cell. Sci. (Suppl)* **3**:39–51.

93. Levi-Montalchini, R., and Cohen, S., 1960, Effects of extracts of mouse submaxillary glands on the sympathetic system of mammals, *Ann. NY Acad. Sci.* **85**:324–341.

94. Smith, A. P., Varon, S., and Shooter, E. M., 1968, Multiple forms of nerve growth factor protein and its subunits, *Biochemistry* **7**:3259–3268.

95. Vinores, A. K., and Perez-Polo, J. R., 1983, Nerve growth factor and neural oncology, *J. Neurosci. Res.* **9**:81–100.

96. Woodruff, N. R., and Neet, K. E., 1986, Inhibition of beta nerve growth factor binding to PC12 cells by alpha nerve growth factor and gamma nerve growth factor, *Biochemistry* **25**:7967–7974.

97. Crutcher, K. A., 1986, The role of growth factors in neuronal development and plasticity, *CRC Crit. Rev. Clin. Neurobiol.* **2**:297–333.

98. Milbrandt, J., 1986, Nerve growth factor rapidly induces c-fos mRNA PC12 in rat pheochromocytoma cells, *Proc. Natl. Acad. Sci. USA* **83**:4789–4793.

99. Davies, A. M., Bandtlow, C., Heumann, R., Korsching, S., Rohrer, H., and Thoenen, H., 1987, Timing and site of nerve growth factor synthesis developing skin relation to innervation and expression of the receptor, *Nature (Lond.)* **326**:353–358.

100. Johnson, D., Lanahan, A., Buck, C. R., Sehgal, A., Morgan, C., Mercer, E., Bothwell, M., and Chao, M., 1986, Expression and structure of the human NGF receptor, *Cell* **47**:545–554.

101. Buxser, S., Puma, P., and Johnson, G. L., 1985, Properties of the nerve growth factor receptor. Relationship between receptor structure and affinity, *J. Biol. Chem.* 1917–1926.

102. Hosang, M., and Shooter, E. M., 1985, Molecular characteristics of nerve growth factor receptors on PC12 cells, *J. Biol. Chem.* **260**:655–662.

103. Boonstra, J., van der Saag, P. T., Feijen, A., Bisschop, A., and de Laat, S., 1985, Epidermal growth factor, but not nerve growth factor, stimulates tyrosine-specific protein-kinase activity in pheochromocytoma (PC12) plasma membranes, *Biochimie* **67**:1177–1183.

104. Bradshaw, R. A., and Young, M., 1976, Nerve growth factor—Recent developments and perspectives, *Biochem. Pharmacol.* **25**:1445–1449.

105. Das, S. K., and Stanley, E. R., 1982, Structure-function studies of a colony stimulating factor (CSF-1), *J. Biol. Chem.* **257**:13679–13684.

106. Stanley, E. R., 1986, Action of the colony-stimulating factor, CSF-1, *Ciba Found. Symp.* **118**:29–41.

107. Sherr, C. J., and Rettenmier, C. W., 1986, The fms gene and the CSF-1 receptor, *Cancer Surv.* **5:**221–232.

108. Muller, R., Slamon, D. J., Adamson, E. D., Tremblay, J. M., Muller, D., Cline, M. J., and Verma, I. M., 1983, Transcription of c-onc genes c-ras and c-fms during mouse development, *Mol. Cell. Biol.* **3:**1062–1069.

109. Sporn, M. B., Roberts, A. B., Wakefield, L. M., and Assoian, R. K., 1986, Transforming growth factor-beta: Biological function and chemical structure, *Science* **233:**532–534.

110. Roberts, A. B., Anzano, M. A., Wakefield, L. M., Roche, N. S., Stern, D. F., and Sporn, M. B., 1985, Type beta transforming growth factor: A bifunctional regulator of cellular growth, *Proc. Natl. Acad. Sci. USA* **82:**119–123.

111. Assoian, R. K., Komoriya, A., Meyers, C. A., Miller, D. M., and Sporn, M. B., 1983, Transforming growth factor-beta human platelets. Identification of a major storage site, purification, and characterization, *J. Biol. Chem.* **258:**7155–7160.

112. Derynck, R., Jarrett, J. A., Chen, E. Y., Eaton, D. H., Bell, J. R., Assoian, R. K., Roberts, A. B., Sporn, M. B., and Goeddel, D. V., 1985, Human transforming growth factor-beta complementary DNA sequence and expression in normal and transformed cells, *Nature (Lond.)* **316:**701–705.

113. Carr, B. I., Hayashi, I., Branum, E. L., and Moses, H. L., 1986, Inhibition of DNA synthesis in rat hepatocytes by platelet-derived type beta transforming growth factor, *Cancer Res.* **46:**2330–2334.

114. Goustin, A. S., Leof, E. B., Shipley, G. D., and Moses, H. L., 1986, Growth factors and cancer, *Cancer Res.* **46:**1015–1029.

115. Roberts, A. B., Anzano, M. A., Meyers, C. A., Wideman, J., Blacher, R., Pan, Y.-C.E., Stein, S., Lehrman, S. R., Smith, J. M., Lamb, L. C., and Sporn, M. B., 1983, Purification and properties of a type beta transforming growth factor from bovine kidney, *Biochemistry* **22:**5692–5698.

116. Cheifetz, S., Weatherbee, J. A., Tsang, M.L.-S., Anderson, J. K., Mole, J. E., Lucas, R., and Massague, J., 1987, The transforming growth factor-beta system, a complex pattern of cross-reactive ligands and receptors, *Cell* **48:**409–415.

117. Derynck, R., Jarret, J. A., Chen, E. Y., and Goeddel, D. V., 1986, The murine transforming growth factor-beta precursor, *J. Biol. Chem.* **261:**4377–4379.

118. Mason, A. J., Hayflick, J. S., Ling, N., Esch, F., Ueno, N., Ying, S.-Y., Guillemin, R., Niall, H., and Seeburg, P. H., 1985, Complementary DNA sequences of ovarian follicular fluid inhibin show precursor structure and homology with transforming growth factor-beta, *Nature (Lond.)* **318:**659–663.

119. Cate, R. L., Mattaliano, R. J., Hession, C., Tizard, R., Farber, N. M., Cheung, A., Ninfa, E. G., Frey, A. Z., Gash, D. J., and Chow, E. P., 1986, Isolation of the bovine and human genes for Mullerian inhibiting substance and expression of the human gene in animal cells, *Cell* **45:**685–698.

120. Massague, J., 1985, Subunit structure of a high affinity receptor for type beta transforming growth factor. Evidence for a disulfide-linked glycosylated receptor complex, *J. Biol. Chem.* **260:**7059–7066.

121. Old, L. J., 1985, Tumor necrosis factor (TNF), *Science* **230:**630–632.

122. Cruise, J. L., Houck, K. A., and Michalopoulos, G. K., 1985, Induction of DNA synthesis in cultured rat hepatocytes through stimulation of alpha-1 adrenoreceptor by norepinephrine, *Science* **227:**749–751.

123. Cruise, J. L., Cotecchia, S., and Michalopoulos, G., 1986, Norepinephrine decreased EGF binding primary rat hepatocyte cultures, *J. Cell. Physiol.* **127:**39–44.

124. Berridge, M. J., 1985, Phosphoinositides and signal transductions, *Rev. Clin. Basic Pharmacol.* **5**(suppl):5S–13S.

125. Berridge, M. J., 1986, Inositol trisphosphate and calcium mobilization, *J. Cardiovasc. Pharmacol.* **8**(suppl.):S85–S90.

126. Nishizuka, Y., 1986, Studies and perspectives of protein kinase C, *Science* **233:**305–312.

127. Korn, L. J., Siebel, C. W., McCormick, F., and Roth, R. A., 1987, Ras p21 as a potential mediator of insulin action in xenopus oocytes, *Science* **236:**840–843.

# 18

# Biochemical Mechanisms of Action of the Phorbol Ester Class of Tumor Promoters

## Arco Y. Jeng and Peter M. Blumberg

## 1. INTRODUCTION

The discovery by Driedger and Blumberg[1] that the phorbol esters functioned through specific receptors, followed by the finding of Castagna et al.[2] that the tumor-promoting phorbol esters activated the $Ca^{2+}$- and phospholipid-dependent protein kinase (protein kinase C), suggesting its identity with the phorbol ester receptor, has had major impact on the understanding of the molecular mechanisms of tumor promotion. Following the initial convergence of these two previously independent research areas, phorbol ester tumor promotion and protein kinase C, a host of related fields such as signal transduction, phosphatidylinositol turnover, growth factors, and oncogenes have also been found to involve the phorbol ester receptor significantly. Hundreds of publications appearing in the literature yearly demonstrate the emphasis on the interactions among these systems.

The objective of this chapter is to evaluate critically the current understanding of biochemical mechanisms of action of the phorbol ester tumor promoters. In the interest of brevity, original work regarding generally accepted findings that have been reviewed elsewhere is not cited; representative reviews are used instead. For further documentation, the interested reader should consult the cited reviews. Recent original articles are emphasized to make the chapter as timely as possible. Complementary perspectives are those of phorbol ester tumor promotion and of protein kinase C. This chapter emphasizes the former.

## 2. EFFECTS OF PHORBOL ESTERS

The phorbol esters initially became the objects of intense research interest on account of their activity as potent tumor promoters in the mouse skin system. As characterized in this system, tumor

*Abbreviations used in this chapter:* EGF, epidermal growth factor; PDBu, phorbol 12,13-dibutyrate; 4α-PDD, 4α-phorbol 12,13-didecanoate; PDGF, platelet-derived growth factor; PMA, phorbol 12-myristate 13-acetate; protein kinase C, $Ca^{2+}$- and phospholipid-dependent protein kinase; TLCK, N-p-tosyl-L-lysine chloromethyl ketone; TPCK, N-tosyl-L-phenylalanine chloromethyl ketone.

---

*Arco Y. Jeng* • Research Department, Pharmaceuticals Division, Ciba-Geigy Corporation, Summit, New Jersey 07901. *Peter M. Blumberg* • Molecular Mechanisms of Tumor Promotion Section, Laboratory of Cellular Carcinogenesis and Tumor Promotion, National Cancer Institute, National Institutes of Health, Bethesda, Maryland 20892.

promoters are agents that, by themselves, are not carcinogenic. However, if the animals are first treated with a single subeffective dose of a carcinogen termed an *initiator,* subsequent chronic treatment with a tumor promoter results in the appearance of numerous skin tumors.[3,4] Critical characteristics of the tumor promoters are that (1) the treatment must follow that with the initiator, (2) it must be chronic, and (3) the application must not be at time intervals spaced too far apart. By contrast, a very long interval between treatment with the initiator and the beginning of the promotion phase has little effect, since the promoter probably is not acting to regulate carcinogen metabolism or repair of carcinogen-induced DNA damage.

In the classic experiments of Berenblum and co-workers, croton oil was used as the tumor promoter. Hecker and co-workers isolated the active constituents in croton oil and identified them as derivatives of the tetracyclic diterpene phorbol, esterified in the 12 and 13 positions.[5] The most potent derivative was identified as phorbol 12-myristate 13-acetate, whereas its 4α-isomer was inactive. Other nonphorbol ester tumor promoters were also isolated and identified.[5]

Tumor promoters are generally skin irritants. Animal models used in the essays of inflammation and promotion were mouse ear reddening and mouse skin tumor formation, respectively. For phorbol esters, the inflammatory potencies generally correlated well with the promoting activities.[5,6] A number of derivatives that are potent inflammatory agents but only weak promoters have been identified, however. Noninflammatory but potent tumor promoters related to the phorbol esters have not been found.

In addition to their effects on whole animals, the phorbol esters exert a variety of actions at the cellular level. Examples include altered cell morphology, interaction with other cellular effectors, inhibition of cell–cell communication, protein phosphorylation, induction of protein synthesis, gene amplification, and cell differentiation. In contrast to conflicting outcomes in different cell types (e.g., induction or inhibition of terminal differentiation), the structure–activity relationships obtained from these studies (see Blumberg[3] and Diamond[7] and references cited therein), in general, correlated with those from the whole animal experiments.

# 3. RECEPTORS FOR PHORBOL ESTERS

## 3.1. Identification of Receptors

The similarity in the structure–activity requirements observed for tumor promotion and for cellular responses, the stereospecificity of phorbol esters for activity, and their high potencies strongly suggested the existence of specific receptors for the phorbol esters. Initial attempts in the measurement of receptor binding by [³H]-PMA were unsuccessful due to a high level of nonspecific binding of this lipophilic derivative.[6,8] In certain cases, harsh conditions such as a cold acetone wash procedure were employed to minimize nonspecific binding to membranes. This problem was finally overcome by Driedger and Blumberg, who used a less lipophilic derivative, PDBu,[1] with which they could demonstrate specific binding of phorbol esters to chick embryo fibroblasts. Subsequent studies showed specific [³H]-PDBu binding in virtually all mouse tissues examined.[6] Brain was found to have the highest level of binding followed by spleen and skin.

The phorbol ester receptors are highly conserved. Not only were receptors identified in all vertebrates examined, but invertebrates such as sea urchins, fruit flies, and nematodes were found to have specific binding sites for the phorbol esters.[6] The observed dissociation constant for PDBu, in general, ranged between 5 and 50 nM. Occasional, significantly different values have also been reported. The number of binding sites per cells is generally on the order of $10^5$.

Binding of phorbol esters to their receptors requires $Ca^{2+}$ and phospholipids. Leach *et al.*[9] reconstituted phorbol ester binding in mouse brain cytosol using these cofactors. Phosphatidylserine, phosphatidic acid, and phosphatidylinositol were effective, whereas phosphatidylcholine and phosphatidylethanolamine were inactive. In membrane preparations and intact cells these cofactors were not needed. Presumably, the $Ca^{2+}$ and phospholipids associated with the membranes sufficed.

The structure–activity relationships obtained from the displacement of [³H]-PDBu binding by nonradioactive derivatives correlated well with those from the mouse skin irritancy and tumor-promotion experiments[4,6]; PMA possessed the highest affinity, whereas phorbol and 4α-PDD were inactive. Likewise, this approach provided evidence that the binding of phorbol esters to their receptors in specific cell types mediated the subsequent biologic effects. Of particular interest was the [3H]-PDBu binding to particulate preparations of mouse skin. Using a three-site model to analyze the curvilinear Scatchard plots for [3H]-PDBu binding, Dunn and Blumberg[10] found the structure–activity relationships at site 2 yielded good correlation with the potencies obtained for mouse ear inflammation while that at site 3 appeared to correlate better with tumor-promoting activity.

## 3.2. Similarities between Phorbol Ester Receptors and Protein Kinase C

The phorbol ester receptors bore striking similarities to protein kinase C, an enzyme discovered by Nishizuka and co-workers[11,12]:

1. *Tissue distribution:* Protein kinase C, similar to phorbol ester receptors, was found in all tissues of the rat.[13] In addition, brain tissue had the highest absolute level of protein kinase C. Both light microscopic autoradiography using [3H]-PDBu[14,15] and immunocytochemical studies using polyclonal antisera to protein kinase C[16] yielded similar discrete localization in hippocampus and cerebral cortex in murine brain.
2. *Evolutionary conservation:* Like the phorbol ester receptors, protein kinase C was found to be highly conserved over evolution. The occurrence of protein kinase C was shown in all vertebrates surveyed as well as in invertebrates such as earthworms and snails.[13]
3. *Developmental variation:* An increase in the level of phorbol ester binding was reported in embryonic chicken brain and mouse brain during development.[6] Likewise, protein kinase C activity in particulate preparations of gray and white matter of rat brain also increased markedly during development and reached the highest level after 30 days,[17] a time course consistent with that of PDBu binding in murine brain.
4. *Ca²⁺ and phosphatidylserine dependence:* $Ca^{2+}$ and phospholipids were required for optimal activity for both phorbol ester binding and protein kinase C, especially for proteins obtained from the cytosolic compartment.[9,11] Phosphatidylserine was found to be the most active phospholipid for both activities.
5. *Interaction with phorbol esters:* Protein kinase C could be stimulated by the phorbol esters.[2] The structure–activity relationships for the phorbol esters in the stimulation of protein kinase C were similar to those of phorbol ester binding.

## 3.3. Evidence That Protein Kinase C Is the Major Phorbol Ester Receptor

The co-elution of both phorbol ester binding and protein kinase C activities upon gel filtration[9,18] and ion-exchange column chromatography[18] strongly suggested that these two activities might be associated with the same protein molecule. Studies with electrophoretically homogeneous preparations of protein kinase C confirmed this hypothesis. Protein kinase C was purified by techniques including various column chromatography,[19] gel filtration in the absence and presence of phosphatidylserine,[20] polyacrylamide–phosphatidylserine affinity column chromatography,[21] and specific ligand elution on fast protein liquid chromatography.[22] In all cases, the purified enzyme displayed both phorbol ester binding and protein kinase C activity.

Pasti *et al.*[23] reported that microinjection of purified protein kinase C into Swiss 3T3 fibroblasts pretreated with PDBu could restore the mitogenic response of the cells to PDBu. This direct approach corroborates the strong but indirect evidence that protein kinase C is the major functional receptor for phorbol esters. Methodologically, the equivalence of these activities permits quantitation of the level of protein kinase C either by phorbol ester binding or by protein kinase assay depending on the needs. In crude cell or tissue homogenates, in which endogenous inhibitors of protein kinase C enzymatic activity may exist, phorbol ester binding typically offers a more reliable measurement.

## 4. CHARACTERIZATION OF PROTEIN KINASE C IN VITRO

### 4.1. Domains

Protein kinase C contains at least two distinct domains: a catalytic domain for the kinase activity and a regulatory domain interacting with $Ca^{2+}$, phospholipids, and phorbol esters. In addition, there are two sites of autophosphorylation.[24]

In the presence of phosphatidylserine, submillimolar concentrations of $Ca^{2+}$ were required to activate protein kinase C. The addition of diacylglycerols or PMA not only yielded higher protein kinase activity but also reduced the requirement of $Ca^{2+}$ for activation to submicromolar concentrations.[11] Diacylglycerols inhibited phorbol ester binding in a competitive manner,[25] with a stoichiometry of 1:1.[26] The activation of diacylglycerols was shown to be stereospecific; only *sn*-1,2-diacylglycerols were active.[27] Using a Triton X-100 and phosphatidylserine mixed micellar system, Hannun and Bell[28] demonstrated that the activated complex contained a molecule of monomeric protein kinase C, $Ca^{2+}$, and 4 molecules of phosphatidylserine. Phospholipid bilayers were not necessary for activation. With the same micellar system, Ganong *et al.*[29] found that, in the presence of diacylglycerols, the activated complex contained 1 molecule each of $Ca^{2+}$, *sn*-1,2-diacylglycerol, and protein kinase C, and 4 molecules of phosphatidylserine.

Upon limited proteolysis by a $Ca^{2+}$-dependent neutral protease, a lower-molecular-weight (50,000) catalytic fragment of protein kinase C could be generated.[30] This fragment did not require $Ca^{2+}$, phospholipids, or diacylglycerol for activity. Subsequent studies using limited tryptic digestion led to the purification of the phorbol ester binding (32,000 $M_r$)[31,32] and the catalytic[31,33] fragments. Whether the binding fragment still requires $Ca^{2+}$ for activity is not certain. Lee and Bell[32] reported that PDBu binding to this fragment was absolutely $Ca^{2+}$ dependent, while Huang and Huang[31] presented isolation of a $Ca^{2+}$-independent PDBu binding fragment. The proposed $Ca^{2+}$-binding site of protein kinase C is very close to the site of trypsin cleavage.[34] Possibly, minor variations in the conditions of tryptic digestion yielded varying protection of this $Ca^{2+}$-binding site. The catalytic domain, located at the carboxyl terminal, showed substantial homology to sequences of other protein kinases.[34]

The role of autophosphorylation in the regulation of the activity of protein kinase C was investigated by Mochly-Rosen and Koshland.[24] These investigators found that the catalytic and regulatory domains each had a site of autophosphorylation. Autophosphorylation appeared to increase the affinity of protein kinase C for the substrate.

### 4.2. Molecular Cloning

The heterogeneity in biologic responses to phorbol esters is well documented.[6] Different structure–activity relationships made it possible to subdivide skin tumor promotion into multiple stages.[35] Furthermore, antagonistic, rather than additive, effects on tumor yield were noted in some instances when different phorbol esters were co-applied.[36] Similarly, heterogeneity was also observed in some binding studies, in which the phorbol ester binding data gave curvilinear Scatchard plots, indicating the existence of more than one binding site.[6] Detailed analysis of PDBu binding to mouse skin particulate preparations at different binding sites generated different structure–activity relationships.[10] These results strongly suggested that receptor isoforms might exist. Consistent with this hypothesis, Kikkawa *et al.*[37] found double bands in the purified protein kinase C, and Huang *et al.*[38] observed three isoforms of protein kinase C activity using hydroxylapatite column chromatography.

Recent advances in molecular biology led to the cloning of protein kinase C complementary DNA (cDNA). Coussens *et al.*[39] identified three types of protein kinase C clones in human brain and demonstrated distinct chromosomal loci of the human genome for the corresponding genes. Three different protein kinase C-related cDNA clones were also isolated from rabbit brain[40] and rat brain[41] cDNA libraries, independently. Tissue specificity in the expression of the messenger RNA (mRNA) for these three distinct types of protein kinase C were reported.[40] These different isoforms of protein kinase C might be useful for elucidating the differences in the structure–activity relationships observed in phorbol ester binding and biologic responses.

## 4.3. Substrate Specificity

The protein kinase C has a broad substrate specificity. In addition to histone H1, the substrate commonly used in the enzyme assay, protein kinase C phosphorylates a variety of receptors, cytosolic and membrane-bound proteins and enzymes.[12] The $K_m$ values of protein kinase C for these substrates are mostly in the micromolar range, and the physiologic consequence of these phosphorylations is generally unknown.

Several groups of investigators have selected specific substrates of protein kinase C and probed the substrate-recognition requirements using synthetic peptides analogous to the physiologic sites of phosphorylation. In examining the phosphorylation site of chick muscle lactate dehydrogenase, Woodgett et al.[42] concluded that a phosphorylatable residue, Ser/Thr, followed by an uncharged residue and then a basic residue C-terminal to Ser/Thr, constituted a preferred sequence for phosphorylation by protein kinase C. With an undecapeptide mimicking the phosphorylation site of ribosomal protein S6 by protein kinase C, House et al.[43] came to the same conclusion of substrate-recognition requirements. The $K_m$ value of this undecapeptide was 0.5 µM, making it one of the most potent peptide substrates reported so far. Additional basic residues, both N- and C-terminal to the substrate recognition sequence, enhanced the $V_{max}$ and $K_m$ values of phosphorylation.[42,44] Interestingly, if the basic residue in the substrate recognition sequence for protein kinase C was moved to the mirror-symmetric position N-terminal to the phosphorylatable residue (Ser/Thr), the new sequence became a preferred site of phosphorylation by the cAMP-dependent protein kinase.[44]

## 4.4. Activators of Protein Kinase C

$Ca^{2+}$, phospholipids, phorbol esters, and diacylglycerols are well documented as activators of protein kinase C. The ion requirement is rather specific. At millimolar ranges, $Sr^{2+}$ and $Ba^{2+}$ could only partially substitute for $Ca^{2+}$.[45] Other activators of protein kinase C can be categorized as phorbol ester type or phospholipid type.

The phorbol ester-type activators of protein kinase C include phorbol esters,[2] nonphorbol ester tumor promoters,[45] and diacylglycerols.[11] In general, they compete for [$^3$H]-PDBu-binding competitively in a stoichiometric fashion. These three classes of structurally dissimilar compounds all have their own requirements for stereospecificity in activating protein kinase C. An understanding of the common structural features of these activators may provide a basis for rational design of new analogues. Jeffrey and Liskamp[46] used computer modeling to compare the spatial relationships of three chemical classes of tumor promoters and concluded that the oxygens in PMA at the 3, 4, 9, and 20 positions corresponded to the O-11, N-13, N-1, and O-24 positions in teleocidin and the oxygens at the 27, 3, 11, and 30 positions in aplysiatoxin. Using the same technique, Wender et al.[47] examined five families of biologically active compounds and concluded that the oxygens at the 4, 9, and 20 positions of phorbol as well as a spatially defined hydrophobic group were crucial for activity. Diacylglycerols were also found to fit this model. On the basis of these observations, a novel class of activators of protein kinase C possessing a simplified ring structure were synthesized.[47] These compounds inhibited phorbol ester binding to protein kinase C specifically and induced some biologic responses characteristic of phorbol esters.[47] Recently, bryostatin, an antineoplastic macrocyclic lactone, was found to be an activator of protein kinase C via specific binding to the same site of phorbol ester binding.[48] The spatial relationships of bryostatin and other phorbol ester-type activators are in the process of being compared.

Among the phospholipid-type activators of protein kinase C, phosphatidylserine is most effective. Other activators of this class include unsaturated fatty acids[49] and eicosanoids.[50] In contrast to the phospholipids, the unsaturated fatty acid could activate protein kinase C in the absence of $Ca^{2+}$.[51]

## 4.5. Inhibitors of Protein Kinase C

The inhibitors of protein kinase C discovered so far can be classified into three categories: agents interacting with the phospholipids, compounds inhibiting ATP binding, and endogenous inhibitors. The phospholipid-interacting type of inhibitors include anesthetics, antipsychotics, fatty acid metabolites, calmodulin antagonists, and others.[45] These agents, in general, inhibited protein kinase C in micromolar concentrations and the inhibitory effects could be reversed by the addition of phospholipids. A group of calmodulin antagonists, exemplified by the naphthalenesulfonamides, showed interesting properties. While most derivatives of this class were inhibitors of protein kinase C, the derivatives with a hydrophobic residue at the end of the hydrocarbon chain, such as N-(6-phenylhexyl)-5-chloro-1-naphthalenesulfonamide, stimulated protein kinase C activity.[52] As expected, this stimulatory effect could also be reversed by the addition of phosphatidylserine.[52]

The isoquinolinesulfonamides[53] represent a class of inhibitors that interact with the ATP-binding site of protein kinase C. With isoquinoline replacing the naphthalene ring in the naphthalenesulfonamides, these new derivatives were no longer calmodulin antagonists. The apparent $K_i$ (inhibition constant) value of the most potent isoquinolinesulfonamide was in the low micromolar range, and the compound was not selective among the cyclic nucleotide-dependent protein kinases and the protein kinase C, although it was selective relative to the myosin light-chain kinase. Another group of compounds are the K-252 compounds obtained from the culture broth of the microorganism *Nocardiopsis* sp. K-290.[54] The inhibition of protein kinase C by this class of compounds was of the competitive type with respect to ATP. K-252b inhibited protein kinase C with a $K_i$ value of 20 nM and was about five-fold more potent for protein kinase C than for the cyclic nucleotide-dependent protein kinases.[54] A structure-related compound, staurosporine, is the most potent inhibitor of protein kinase C discovered so far, with an $IC_{50}$ (concentration for 50% inhibition) value of 2.7 nM.[55] Staurosporine did not compete for PDBu binding, nor did it compete with $Ca^{2+}$, substrate, diacylglycerol, and ATP.[55] The precise mechanism of action of this compound has to be determined.

Among the endogenous inhibitors of protein kinase C are a heat-labile 20,000-$M_r$ protein from rat brain,[56] a heat-stable 17,000-$M_r$ low-affinity $Ca^{2+}$-binding protein from bovine brain,[57] and some complex lipids and their metabolites.[58,59] Whether the two protein inhibitors are related is not known. The 20,000-$M_r$ protein seemed to compete for the substrate,[56] whereas the mechanism of inhibition of the 17,000-$M_r$ protein has not been determined. The observations that some lipids or lipid metabolites could function as inhibitors of protein kinase C complement the already documented findings that diacylglycerols, metabolites of phosphatidylinositol, could function as activators in the same system. Lysosphingolipids[58] and sphingosine[59] were reported to inhibit both protein kinase C and PDBu binding activities. Using a phosphatidylserine and Triton X-100 mixed micellar assay, Hannun et al.[59] found that a 50% inhibition of protein kinase C activity occurred when sphingosine was equimolar with sn-1,2-dioleoylglycerol.

## 5. REGULATION OF PHORBOL ESTER RECEPTOR/PROTEIN KINASE C IN VIVO

## 5.1. Translocation and Proteolytic Processing

Kraft and Anderson[60] first reported that, in parietal yolk sac (PYS-2) cells, treatment with PMA resulted in a decrease of protein kinase C activity in cytosol and a concomitant increase in the activity of the membrane fraction. The maximal effects were seen within 5 min at 37°C. This translocation of protein kinase C upon phorbol ester treatment was also detected in many other systems.[61] Experiments performed in human neutrophils demonstrated that, subsequent to the translocation, a $Ca^{2+}$- and phospholipid-independent protein kinase was generated by a $Ca^{2+}$-activated protease and was released to the cytosolic compartment.[62] This $Ca^{2+}$- and phospholipid-independent protein kinase had properties similar to those of the proteolytically generated catalytic fragment of protein kinase C characterized by Kishimoto et al.[30] in *in vitro* studies. When preloaded with inhibitors of the $Ca^{2+}$-activated protease, the production of the $Ca^{2+}$- and phospholipid-independent protein kinase was prevented, but the translocation of protein kinase C was still observed in PMA-treated neutrophils.[62] Similar results were also obtained in human platelets treated with PMA.[63]

It is not clear whether the translocation of protein kinase C from the cytosol to membrane fraction in cells treated with PMA is absolutely necessary in mediating the subsequent biologic effects. In human neutrophils treated with mezerein, the translocation of protein kinase C was not observed. However, the generation of superoxide anion and the release of lysosomal enzymes into the extracellular medium were detected in neutrophils treated with mezerein,[64] effects similar to that of phorbol ester treatment.

## 5.2. Modulation of the Affinity of Receptor for Phorbol Esters

Since diacylglycerols, which inhibit phorbol ester-binding competitively,[25] are thought to be the endogenous activators of protein kinase C, an elevation of the intracellular level of diacylglycerols should produce phorbol esterlike biologic effects. Jeng *et al.*[65] examined primary mouse epidermal cells exposed to phospholipase C (*C. perfringens*), a treatment expected to generate enzymatically a sustained level of intracellular diacylglycerols from the endogenous phospholipids. The phospholipase C treatment not only led to morphologic changes but also resulted in the reduction of EGF binding and the induction of ornithine decarboxylase and of transglutaminase in a fashion characteristic of phorbol ester treatment. In addition, the binding affinity of PDBu for its receptors was substantially suppressed without a reduction in the total number of binding sites, consistent with the production of a competitive inhibitor of phorbol ester binding.[65] Similar results were reported in rat tracheal epithelial 2C5 cells.[66] Two other methods have also been used to achieve an elevated level of intracellular diacylglycerols: addition of appropriate synthetic diacylglycerols in the culture medium,[65,66] and perturbation of glyceride metabolism, e.g., inhibition by 2-bromooctanoate of diacylglycerol acyltransferase, which synthesizes triacylglycerols from the diacylglycerols.[67]

*In vitro* experiments showed that the composition of the phospholipids used in the reconstitution of phorbol ester binding had dramatic effects on the affinity of phorbol esters for their receptors.[68] It is predicted that similar results could also be obtained in mutant cells with variations in phospholipid composition.

## 5.3. Modulation of the Number of Receptors

The kinetics of [$^3$H]-PDBu binding to whole cells is complicated. In some cells (e.g., mouse thymoma cells, rat embryo fibroblasts, and rat pituitary cells), specific binding increased to maximal levels within 15 min at 37°C followed by a decrease, the rate and the extent of which varied from cell type to cell type.[6,8] This phenomenon is referred to as downmodulation (or downregulation) of receptors. The decrease in phorbol ester binding was shown to be due to a decrease in the number of receptors rather than to a decrease in the binding affinity. At 4°C, this downmodulation of receptors did not usually occur. In other cells, such as human polymorphonuclear leukocytes, downmodulation of receptors was not observed within 1 hr.[6] Whether downmodulation could occur at a later time remains to be clarified.

Chida *et al.*[69] reported that in fetal rat skin keratinocytes, downmodulation of [$^3$H]-PDBu binding could be prevented by the addition of the protease inhibitors TPCK or TLCK. The same protease inhibitors could also prevent the generation, from membrane-associated intact protein kinase C, of cytosolic $Ca^{2+}$- and phospholipid-independent protein kinase after translocation in cells treated with PMA. It seems likely that a proteolytic degradation of protein kinase C is involved in the downmodulation of receptors for the phorbol esters. *In vitro* studies demonstrated that the regulatory domain generated by a limited tryptic digestion was still able to bind the phorbol esters.[31–33] It is thus not clear why the regulatory domain produced by the $Ca^{2+}$-activated protease lost its phorbol ester binding activity in the whole cell experiments.

In contrast to the downmodulation of receptors, Dunn et al.[70] found an increase of [³H]-PDBu binding in primary mouse keratinocytes exposed to millimolar $Ca^{2+}$ concentrations. This up-modulation of receptors was due to an increase in receptor number and was apparent after 6 hr of exposure to $Ca^{2+}$. $Ca^{2+}$ is known to induce differentiation in these cells. The results suggest that the state of maturation of the keratinocytes can modulate the level of phorbol ester receptors.

## 6. FEEDBACK OF PROTEIN KINASE C ON OTHER PATHWAYS

### 6.1. Signal Transduction

Research on the signal transduction pathway of the hormone- or neurotransmitter-sensitive adenylate cyclase system has advanced considerably in recent years. A detailed review of this subject is beyond the scope of this chapter (see Chapters 15 and 17). It is generally accepted that the guanine nucleotide-binding proteins (G proteins)[71] couple to this system to generate an integrated response from information received by the appropriate receptors upon the interaction with various agonists or antagonists. The stimulatory receptors, exemplified by those for β-adrenergic agonists, interact with the $G_s$ proteins that mediate a stimulation of the adenylate cyclase activity while the inhibitory receptors, including those for $α_2$-adrenergic and muscarinic agonists, interact with the $G_i$ proteins, which then exert an inhibition of the adenylate cyclase activity.

Katada et al.[72] reported that the phosphorylation of the α subunit of $G_i$ by protein kinase C inhibited the coupling between $G_i$ and the adenylate cyclase of cyc⁻ S49 lymphoma cells. By contrast, Kelleher et al.[73] observed that phosphorylation of the β-adrenergic receptor by protein kinase C-induced desensitization of the adenylate cyclase due to an inhibition of receptor–$G_s$ coupling in turkey erythrocytes. Protein kinase C thus exerts positive or negative control on the adenylate cyclase depending on the specific system employed.

### 6.2. Phosphatidylinositol Turnover

The effects of hormone- or neurotransmitter-stimulated phosphatidylinositol breakdown by phospholipase C is well documented.[74] The activation of phospholipase C is probably mediated by an unknown GTP-binding protein. Unlike the receptor-mediated activation of the adenylate cyclase, which generates cAMP as the sole second messenger, the receptor-mediated phosphatidylinositol 4,5-bisphosphate turnover produces two second messengers with different functions. One product is the diacylglycerol, which activates protein kinase C. The other is the inositol-1,4,5,-trisphosphate, which is shown to be able to mobilize $Ca^{2+}$ from a nonmitochondrial intracellular $Ca^{2+}$ pool, such as endoplasmic reticulum.[75]

A recent study by Connolly et al.[76] demonstrated that the phosphatase activity of inositol trisphosphate 5′-phosphomonoesterase in human platelets increased after the phosphorylation of the enzyme by protein kinase C. This enzyme hydrolyzes the 5-phosphate from inositol-1,4,5-trisphos-phate, to form inositol 1,4-bisphosphate, which is unable to mobilize intracellular $Ca^{2+}$, thereby terminating the signal for $Ca^{2+}$ mobilization. These results can only partially account for the observation on the effects of phorbol esters in cultured astrocytoma cells[77] and human platelets[78] in which the agonist-induced formation of *all* inositol phosphates (inositol mono-, bis-, and trisphos-phate) were inhibited. It is thus likely that other negative feedback mechanism(s) on ligand-stimulated phosphatidylinositol turnover may exist.

### 6.3. Cellular Responses to Growth Factors

The growth factors can be subdivided into several groups depending on the mechanisms by which the subsequent signals are transduced upon binding of the growth factors to the appropriate receptors. One group of growth factors such as EGF and insulin exert their actions through ligand-stimulated tyrosine phosphorylation. The effects of phorbol esters on the cellular response to EGF have been studied in some detail. The EGF receptor from A431 human epidermoid carcinoma cells was shown to be phosphorylated by protein kinase C with a concomitant decrease in EGF stimulated-tyrosine protein kinase activity[79,80] and the conversion of high-affinity EGF-binding to a lower affinity state without a change in the total number of binding sites.[80] Similar regulation by protein kinase C of insulin receptors was also noted. Takayama *et al.*[81] showed that PMA stimulated the phosphorylation of the β-subunit of the insulin receptor, inhibited the insulin-induced receptor phosphorylation, and suppressed the insulin-stimulated glycogen synthase activity in cultured rat hepatoma cells.

Another group of the growth factors, such as PDGF and bombesin, were shown to stimulate the phosphatidylinositol turnover.[82] Protein kinase C has not been demonstrated to interact with the receptors of these growth factors directly, but it can have negative feedback on these growth factor-stimulated pathways through the phosphorylation of the inositol trisphosphate 5'-phosphomonoesterase.

## 6.4. Activation of Oncogenes

Recent studies established close relationships between some oncogene products and the growth factors. For example, the *sis* and *erbB* genes encode PDGF and a fragment of the EGF receptor, respectively.[82] It is possible that some oncogenes, growth factors, and protein kinase C share the same pathway for signal transduction. As mentioned before, PDGF could stimulate the phospholipase C activity and thereby enhance phosphatidylinositol turnover. In addition, elevated levels of *sn*-1,2-diacylglycerols were detected in *ras*- or *sis*-transformed normal rat kidney cells.[83] These observations suggested that the expression of certain oncogenes could result in an activation of protein kinase C which, in turn, could have direct feedback on the expression of other oncogenes. In fact, Ran *et al.*[84] showed that the phorbol esters induced the expression of c-*fos* and c-*myc* proto-oncogenes in density-arrested BALB/c 3T3 cells. Similar results were also reported in human peripheral blood lymphocytes treated with PMA and Ca$^{2+}$ ionophore.[85]

Many oncogene products were examined as substrates for protein kinase C. The middle-sized tumor antigen partially purified from polyoma virus-infected 3T6 cells had enhanced tyrosine-specific kinase activity after being phosphorylated by protein kinase C.[86] The pp60[v-src] and the pp21[v-H-ras] were found to be substrates of protein kinase C.[87,88] The functional consequences of these phosphorylations have yet to be examined.

## 7. CONCLUDING REMARKS

The phorbol ester receptor/protein kinase C has become a major focus for the study of receptor binding, effectors, signal transduction, and cellular and molecular biology. Despite considerable progress during the past few years, specific answers for many important questions remain to be determined. Receptor heterogeneity is an issue of particular interest because of its relevance for selective intervention in the protein kinase C pathway. Whether the multiple forms of protein kinase C detected by the molecular biologic methods correspond to receptors of distinct structure–activity relationship is unknown. The physiologic significance of protein phosphorylation is yet to be determined. Many substrates for protein kinase C are also substrates for the cAMP-dependent protein kinase. Specific inhibitors for protein kinase C would be useful in order to distinguish the effects of phosphorylation by these two protein kinases. The role of diacylglycerols in tumor promotion remains to be investigated. Furthermore, the interactions between protein kinase C and other cellular pathways need to be examined more closely. From an initial focus on tumor promotion in mouse skin, the study of the mechanism of phorbol ester action has broadened dramatically to impinge on many aspects of cancer research.

ACKNOWLEDGMENTS. We thank Dr. Stuart H. Yuspa and Dr. Lawrence P. Wennogle for critical reading of the manuscript.

## REFERENCES

1. Driedger, P. E., and Blumberg, P. M., 1980, Specific binding of phorbol ester tumor promoters, *Proc. Natl. Acad. Sci. USA* **77:**567–571.
2. Castagna, M., Takai, Y., Kaibuchi, K., Sano, K., Kikkawa, U., and Nishizuka, Y., 1982, Direct activation of calcium-activated, phospholipid-dependent protein kinase by tumor-promoting phorbol esters, *J. Biol. Chem.* **257:**7847–7851.
3. Blumberg, P. M., 1980, *In vitro* studies on the mode of action of the phorbol esters, potent tumor promoters, *CRC Crit. Rev. Toxicol.* **8:**153–234.
4. Diamond, L., O'Brien, T. G., and Baird, W. M., 1980, Tumor promoters and the mechanism of tumor promotion, *Adv. Cancer Res.* **32:**1–74.
5. Hecker, E., 1978, Structure-activity relationships in diterpene esters irritant and cocarcinogenic to mouse skin, in: *Carcinogenesis*, Vol. 2 (T. J. Slaga, A. Sivak, and R. K. Boutwell, eds.), pp. 11–48, Raven, New York.
6. Blumberg, P. M., Dunn, J. A., Jaken, S., Jeng, A. Y., Leach, K. L., Sharkey, N. A., and Yeh, E., 1984, Specific receptors for phorbol ester tumor promoters and their involvement in biological responses, in: *Mechanisms of Tumor Promotion*, Vol. 3 (T. J. Slaga, ed.), pp. 143–184, CRC Press, Boca Raton, Florida.
7. Diamond, L., 1984, Tumor promoters and cell transformation, *Pharmacol. Ther.* **26:**89–145.
8. Ashendel, C. L., 1985, The phorbol ester receptor: A phospholipid-regulated protein kinase, *Biochim. Biophys. Acta* **822:**219–242.
9. Leach, K. L., James, M. L., and Blumberg, P. M., 1983, Characterization of a specific phorbol ester aporeceptor in mouse brain cytosol, *Proc. Natl. Acad. Sci. USA* **80:**4208–4212.
10. Dunn, J. A., and Blumberg, P. M., 1983, Specific binding of [20-$^3$H]12-deoxyphorbol 13-isobutyrate to phorbol ester receptor subclasses in mouse skin particulate preparations, *Cancer Res.* **43:**4632–4637.
11. Nishizuka, Y., 1984, The role of protein kinase C in cell surface signal transduction and tumour promotion, *Nature (Lond.)* **308:**693–698.
12. Nishizuka, Y., 1986, Studies and perspectives of protein kinase C, *Science* **233:**305–312.
13. Kuo, J. F., Andersson, R. G. G., Wise, B. C., Mackerlova, L., Salomonsson, I., Brackett, N. L., Katoh, N., Shoji, M., and Wrenn, R. W., 1980, Calcium-dependent protein kinase: Widespread occurrence in various tissues and phyla of the animal kingdom and comparison of effects of phospholipid, calmodulin, and trifluoperazine, *Proc. Natl. Acad. Sci. USA* **77:**7039–7043.
14. Nagle, D. S., and Blumberg, P. M., 1983, Regional localization by light microscopic autoradiography of receptors in mouse brain for phorbol ester tumor promoters, *Cancer Lett.* **18:**35–40.
15. Worley, P. F., Baraban, J. M., and Snyder, S. H., 1986, Heterogeneous localization of protein kinase C in rat brain: Autoradiographic analysis of phorbol ester receptor binding, *J. Neurosci.* **6:**199–207.
16. Wood, J. G., Girard, P. R., Mazzei, G. J., and Kuo, J. F., 1986, Immunocytochemical localization of protein kinase C in identified neuronal compartments of rat brain, *J. Neurosci.* **6:**2571–2577.
17. Turner, R. S., Raynor, R. L., Mazzei, G. J., Girard, P. R., and Kuo, J. F., 1984, Developmental studies of phospholipid-sensitive Ca$^{2+}$-dependent protein kinase and its substrates and of phosphoprotein phosphatases in rat brain, *Proc. Natl. Acad. Sci. USA* **81:**3143–3147.
18. Niedel, J. E., Kuhn, L. J., and Vandenbark, G. R., 1983, Phorbol diester receptor copurifies with protein kinase C, *Proc. Natl. Acad. Sci. USA* **80:**36–40.
19. Kikkawa, U., Takai, Y., Minakuchi, R., Inohara, S., and Nishizuka, Y., 1982, Calcium-activated, phospholipid-dependent protein kinase from rat brain. Subcellular distribution, purification, and properties, *J. Biol. Chem.* **257:**13341–13348.
20. Le Peuch, C. J., Ballester, R., and Rosen, O. M., 1983, Purified rat brain calcium- and phospholipid-dependent protein kinase phosphorylates ribosomal protein S6, *Proc. Natl. Acad. Sci. USA* **80:**6858–6862.
21. Uchida, T., and Filburn, C. R., 1984, Affinity chromatography of protein kinase C-phorbol ester receptor on polyacrylamide-immobilized phosphatidylserine, *J. Biol. Chem.* **259:**12311–12314.
22. Jeng, A. Y., Sharkey, N. A., and Blumberg, P. M., 1986, Purification of stable protein kinase C from mouse brain cytosol by specific ligand elution using fast protein liquid chromatography, *Cancer Res.* **46:**1966–1971.
23. Pasti, G., Lacal, J.-C., Warren, B. S., Aaronson, S. A., and Blumberg, P. M., 1986, Loss of mouse fibroblast cell response to phorbol esters restored by microinjected protein kinase C, *Nature (Lond.)* **324:**375–377.
24. Mochly-Rosen, D., and Koshland, D. E., Jr., 1987, Domain structure and phosphorylation of protein kinase C, *J. Biol. Chem.* **262:**2291–2297.
25. Sharkey, N. A., Leach, K. L., and Blumberg, P. M., 1984, Competitive inhibition by diacylglycerol of

specific phorbol ester binding, *Proc. Natl. Acad. Sci. USA* **81**:607–610.

26. Blumberg, P. M., Jeng, A. Y., Konig, B., Sharkey, N. A., Leach, K. L., and Jaken, S., 1985, Receptors and endogenous analogues for the phorbol ester tumor promoters, in: *Carcinogenesis—A Comprehensive Survey*, Vol. 10 (E. Huberman and S. H. Barr, eds.), pp. 249–262, Raven, New York.

27. Rando, R. R., and Young, N., 1984, The stereospecific activation of protein kinase C, *Biochem. Biophys. Res. Commun.* **122**:818–823.

28. Hannun, Y. A., and Bell, R. M., 1986, Phorbol ester binding and activation of protein kinase C on Triton X-100 mixed micelles containing phosphatidylserine, *J. Biol. Chem.* **261**:9341–9347.

29. Ganong, B. R., Loomis, C. R., Hannun, Y. A., and Bell, R. M., 1986, Specificity and mechanism of protein kinase C activation by sn-1,2-diacylglycerols, *Proc. Natl. Acad. Sci. USA* **83**:1184–1188.

30. Kishimoto, A., Kajikawa, N., Shiota, M., and Nishizuka, Y., 1983, Proteolytic activation of calcium-activated, phospholipid-dependent protein kinase by calcium-dependent neutral protease, *J. Biol. Chem.* **258**:1156–1164.

31. Huang, K.-P., and Huang, F. L., 1986, Immunochemical characterization of rat brain protein kinase C, *J. Biol. Chem.* **261**:14781–14787.

32. Lee, M.-H., and Bell, R. M., 1986, The lipid binding, regulatory domain of protein kinase C, *J. Biol. Chem.* **261**:14867–14870.

33. Nakadate, T., Jeng, A. Y., and Blumberg, P. M., 1987, Effect of phospholipid on substrate phosphorylation by a catalytic fragment of protein kinase C, *J. Biol. Chem.* **262**:11507–11513.

34. Parker, P. J., Coussens, L., Totty, N., Rhee, L., Young, S., Chen, E., Stabel, S., Waterfield, M. D., and Ullrich, A., 1986, The complete primary structure of protein kinase C—the major phorbol ester receptor, *Science* **233**:853–859.

35. Slaga, T. J., Fischer, S. M., Nelson, K., and Gleason, G. L., 1980, Studies on the mechanism of skin tumor promotion: Evidence for several stages in promotion, *Proc. Natl. Acad. Sci. USA* **77**:3659–3663.

36. Schmidt, R., and Hecker, E., 1982, Simple phorbol esters as inhibitors of tumor promotion by TPA in mouse skin, in: *Cocarcinogenesis and Biological Effects of Tumor Promoters* (E. Hecker, N. E. Fusenig, W. Kunz, F. Marks, and H. W. Thielmann, eds.), pp. 57–63, Raven, New York.

37. Kikkawa, U., Go, M., Koumoto, J., and Nishizuka, Y., 1986, Rapid purification of protein kinase C by high performance liquid chromatography, *Biochem. Biophys. Res. Commun.* **135**:636–643.

38. Huang, K.-P., Nakabayashi, H., and Huang, F. L., 1986, Isozymic forms of rat brain $Ca^{2+}$-activated and phospholipid-dependent protein kinase, *Proc. Natl. Acad. Sci. USA* **83**:8535–8539.

39. Coussens, L., Parker, P. J., Rhee, L., Yang-Feng, T. L., Chen, E., Waterfield, M. D., Francke, U., and Ullrich, A., 1986, Multiple, distinct forms of bovine and human protein kinase C suggest diversity in cellular signaling pathways, *Science* **233**:859–866.

40. Ohno, S., Kawasaki, H., Imajoh, S., and Suzuki, K., 1987, Tissue-specific expression of three distinct types of rabbit protein kinase C, *Nature (Lond.)* **325**:161–166.

41. Knopf, J. L., Lee, M.-H., Sultzman, L. A., Kriz, R. W., Loomis, C. R., Hewick, R. M., and Bell, R. M., 1986, Cloning and expression of multiple protein kinase C cDNAs, *Cell* **46**:491–502.

42. Woodgett, J. R., Gould, K. L., and Hunter, T., 1986, Substrate specificity of protein kinase C. Use of synthetic peptides corresponding to physiological sites as probes for substrate recognition requirements, *Eur. J. Biochem.* **161**:177–184.

43. House, C., Wettenhall, R. E. H., and Kemp, B. E., 1987, The influence of basic residues on the substrate specificity of protein kinase C, *J. Biol. Chem.* **262**:772–777.

44. Kishimoto, A., Nishiyama, K., Nakanishi, H., Uratsuji, Y., Nomura, H., Takeyama, Y., and Nishizuka, Y., 1985, Studies on the phosphorylation of myelin basic protein by protein kinase C and adenosine 3':5'-monophosphate-dependent protein kinase, *J. Biol. Chem.* **260**:12492–12499.

45. Turner, R. S., and Kuo, J. F., 1985, Phospholipid-sensitive $Ca^{2+}$-dependent protein kinase (protein kinase C): The enzyme, substrates, and regulation, in: *Phospholipids and Cellular Regulation*, Vol. 2 (J. F. Kuo, ed.), pp. 75–110, CRC Press, Boca Raton, Florida.

46. Jeffrey, A. M., and Liskamp, R. M. J., 1986, Computer-assisted molecular modeling of tumor promoters: Rationale for the activity of phorbol esters, teleocidin B, and aplysiatoxin, *Proc. Natl. Acad. Sci. USA* **83**:241–245.

47. Wender, P. A., Koehler, K. F., Sharkey, N. A., Dell'Aquila, M. L., and Blumberg, P. M., 1986, Analysis of the phorbol ester pharmacophore on protein kinase C as a guide to the rational design of new classes of analogs, *Proc. Natl. Acad. Sci. USA* **83**:4214–4218.

48. Kraft, A. S., Smith, J. B., and Berkow, R. L., 1986, Bryostatin, an activator of the calcium phospholipid-dependent protein kinase, blocks phorbol ester-induced differentiation of human promyelocytic leukemia cells HL-60, *Proc. Natl. Acad. Sci. USA* **83**:1334–1338.

49. Leach, K. L., and Blumberg, P. M., 1985, Modulation of protein kinase C activity and [³H]phorbol 12,13-dibutyrate binding by various tumor promoters in mouse brain cytosol, *Cancer Res.* **45:**1958–1963.

50. Hansson, A., Serhan, C. N., Haeggstrom, J., Ingelman-Sundberg, M., Samuelsson, B., and Morris, J., 1986, Activation of protein kinase C by lipoxin A and other eicosanoids. Intracellular action of oxygenation products of arachidonic acid, *Biochem. Biophys. Res. Commun.* **134:**1215–1222.

51. Murakami, K., Chan, S. Y., and Routtenberg, A., 1986, Protein kinase C activation by cis-fatty acid in the absence of $Ca^{2+}$ and phospholipids, *J. Biol. Chem.* **261:**15424–15429.

52. Ito, M., Tanaka, T., Inagaki, M., Nakanishi, K., and Hidaka, H., 1986, *N*-(6-Phenylhexyl)-5-chloro-1-naphthalene sulfonamide, a novel activator of protein kinase C, *Biochemistry* **25:**4179–4184.

53. Hidaka, H., Inagaki, M., Kawamoto, S., and Sasaki, Y., 1984, Isoquinolinesulfonamides, novel and potent inhibitors of cyclic nucleotide dependent protein kinase and protein kinase C, *Biochemistry* **23:**5036–5041.

54. Kase, H., Iwahashi, K., Nakanishi, S., Matsuda, Y., Yamada, K., Takahashi, M., Murakata, C., Sato, A., and Kaneko, M., 1987, K-252 compounds, novel and potent inhibitors of protein kinase C and cyclic nucleotide-dependent protein kinases, *Biochem. Biophys. Res. Commun.* **142:**436–440.

55. Tamaoki, T., Nomoto, H., Takahashi, I., Kato, Y., Morimoto, M., and Tomita, F., 1986, Staurosporine, a potent inhibitor of phospholipid/Ca⁺⁺ dependent protein kinase, *Biochem. Biophys. Res. Commun.* **135:**397–402.

56. Schwantke, N., and Le Peuch, C. J., 1984, A protein kinase C inhibitory activity is present in rat brain homogenate, *FEBS Lett.* **177:**36–40.

57. McDonald, J. R., and Walsh, M. P., 1985, $Ca^{2+}$-binding proteins from bovine brain including a potent inhibitor of protein kinase C, *Biochem. J.* **232:**559–567.

58. Hannun, Y. A., and Bell, R. M., 1987, Lysosphingolipids inhibit protein kinase C: Implications for the sphingolipidoses, *Science* **235:**670–674.

59. Hannun, Y. A., Loomis, C. R., Merrill, A. H., Jr., and Bell, R. M., 1986, Sphingosine inhibition of protein kinase C activity and of phorbol dibutyrate binding *in vitro* and in human platelets, *J. Biol. Chem.* **261:**12604–12609.

60. Kraft, A. S., and Anderson, W. B., 1983, Phorbol esters increase the amount of $Ca^{2+}$, phospholipid-dependent protein kinase associated with plasma membrane, *Nature (Lond.)* **301:**621–623.

61. Hirota, K., Hirota, T., Aguilera, G., and Catt, K. J., 1986, Gonadotropin release and redistribution of calcium-activated, phospholipid-dependent protein kinase in phorbol-stimulated rat pituitary cells, *Arch. Biochem. Biophys.* **249:**557–562.

62. Melloni, E., Pontremoli, S., Michetti, M., Sacco, O., Sparatore, B., and Horecker, B. L., 1986, The involvement of calpain in the activation of protein kinase C in neutrophils stimulated by phorbol myristic acid, *J. Biol. Chem.* **261:**4101–4105.

63. Tapley, P. M., and Murray, A. W., 1985, Evidence that treatment of platelets with phorbol ester causes proteolytic activation of $Ca^{2+}$-activated, phospholipid-dependent protein kinase, *Eur. J. Biochem.* **151:**419–423.

64. Balazovich, K. J., Smolen, J. E., and Boxer, L. A., 1986, $Ca^{2+}$ and phospholipid-dependent protein kinase (protein kinase C) activity is not necessarily required for secretion by human neutrophils, *Blood* **68:**810–817.

65. Jeng, A. Y., Lichti, U., Strickland, J. E., and Blumberg, P. M., 1985, Similar effects of phospholipase C and phorbol ester tumor promoters on primary mouse epidermal cells, *Cancer Res.* **45:**5714–5721.

66. Jetten, A. M., Ganong, B. R., Vandenbark, G. R., Shirley, J. E., and Bell, R. M., 1985, Role of protein kinase C in diacylglycerol-mediated induction of ornithine decarboxylase and reduction of epidermal growth factor binding, *Proc. Natl. Acad. Sci. USA* **82:**1941–1945.

67. Mayorek, N., and Bar-Tana, J., 1985, Inhibition of diacylglycerol acyltransferase by 2-bromooctanoate in cultured rat hepatocytes, *J. Biol. Chem.* **260:**6528–6532.

68. Blumberg, P. M., Sharkey, N. A., Konig, B., Jaken, S., Leach, K. L., and Jeng, A. Y., 1984, Membrane and cytosolic receptors for the phorbol ester tumor promoters, in: *Cancer cells*, Vol. 1 (A. J. Levine, G. F. Vande Woude, W. C. Topp, and J. D. Watson, eds.), pp. 245–251, Cold Spring Harbor Laboratory, Cold Spring Harbor, New York.

69. Chida, K., Kato, N., and Kuroki, T., 1986, Down regulation of phorbol diester receptors by proteolytic degradation of protein kinase C in a cultured cell line of fetal rat skin keratinocytes, *J. Biol. Chem.* **261:**13013–13018.

70. Dunn, J. A., Jeng, A. Y., Yuspa, S. H., and Blumberg, P. M., 1985, Heterogeneity of [³H]phorbol 12,13-dibutyrate binding in primary mouse keratinocytes at different stages of maturation, *Cancer Res.* **45:**5540–5546.

71. Gilman, A. G., 1984, G proteins and dual control of adenylate cyclase, *Cell* **36:**577–579.
72. Katada, T., Gilman, A. G., Watanabe, Y., Bauer, S., and Jakobs, K. H., 1985, Protein kinase C phosphorylates the inhibitory guanine-nucleotide-binding regulatory component and apparently suppresses its function in hormonal inhibition of adenylate cyclase, *Eur. J. Biochem.* **151:**431–437.
73. Kelleher, D. J., Pessin, J. E., Ruoho, A. E., and Johnson, G. L., 1984, Phorbol ester induces desensitization of adenylate cyclase and phosphorylation of the β-adrenergic receptor in turkey erythrocytes, *Proc. Natl. Acad. Sci. USA* **81:**4316–4320.
74. Abdel-Latif, A. A., 1986, Calcium-mobilizing receptors, polyphosphoinositides, and the generation of second messengers, *Pharmacol. Rev.* **38:**227–272.
75. Berridge, M. J., 1986, Regulation of ion channels by inositol trisphosphate and diacylglycerol, *J. Exp. Biol.* **124:**323–335.
76. Connolly, T. M., Lawing, W. J., Jr., and Majerus, P. W., 1986, Protein kinase C phosphorylates human platelet inositol trisphosphate 5'-phosphomonoesterase, increasing the phosphatase activity, *Cell* **46:**951–958.
77. Orellana, S. A., Solski, P. A., and Brown, J. H., 1985, Phorbol ester inhibits phosphoinositide hydrolysis and calcium mobilization in cultured astrocytoma cells, *J. Biol. Chem.* **260:**5236–5239.
78. Watson, S. P., and Lapetina, E. G., 1985, 1,2-Diacylglycerol and phorbol ester inhibit agonist-induced formation of inositol phosphates in human platelets: Possible implications for negative feedback regulation of inositol phospholipid hydrolysis, *Proc. Natl. Acad. Sci. USA* **82:**2623–2626.
79. Cochet, C., Gill, G. N., Meisenhelder, J., Cooper, J. A., and Hunter, T., 1984, C-kinase phosphorylates the epidermal growth factor receptor and reduces its epidermal growth factor-stimulated tyrosine protein kinase activity, *J. Biol. Chem.* **259:**2553–2558.
80. Downward, J., Waterfield, M. D., and Parker, P. J., 1985, Autophosphorylation and protein kinase C phosphorylation of the epidermal growth factor receptor. Effect on tyrosine kinase activity and ligand binding affinity, *J. Biol. Chem.* **260:**14538–14546.
81. Takayama, S., White, M. F., Lauris, V., and Kahn, R., 1984, Phorbol esters modulate insulin receptor phosphorylation and insulin action in cultured hepatoma cells, *Proc. Natl. Acad. Sci. USA* **81:**7797–7801.
82. Berridge, M. J., 1986, Growth factors, oncogenes and inositol lipids, *Cancer Surv.* **5:**413–430.
83. Preiss, J., Loomis, C. R., Bishop, W. R., Stein, R., Niedel, J. E., and Bell, R. M., 1986, Quantitative measurement of sn-1,2-diacylglycerols present in platelets, hepatocytes, and ras- and sis-transformed normal rat kidney cells, *J. Biol. Chem.* **261:**8597–8600.
84. Ran, W., Dean, M., Levine, R. A., Henkle, C., and Campisi, J., 1986, Induction of c-fos and c-myc mRNA by epidermal growth factor or calcium ionophore is cAMP dependent, *Proc. Natl. Acad. Sci. USA* **83:**8216–8220.
85. Grausz, J. D., Fradelizi, D., Dautry, F., Monier, R., and Lehn, P., 1986, Modulation of c-fos and c-myc mRNA levels in normal human lymphocytes by calcium ionophore A23187 and phorbol ester, *Eur. J. Immunol.* **16:**1217–1221.
86. Hirata, F., Matsuda, K., Notsu, Y., Hattori, T., and Del Carmine, R., 1984, Phosphorylation at a tyrosine residue of lipomodulin in mitogen-stimulated murine thymocytes, *Proc. Natl. Acad. Sci. USA* **81:**4717–4721.
87. Purchio, A. F., Gentry, L., and Shoyab, M., 1986, Phosphorylation of pp60[v-src] by the TPA receptor kinase (protein kinase C), *Virology* **150:**524–529.
88. Jeng, A. Y., Srivastava, S. K., Lacal, J. C., and Blumberg, P. M., 1987, Phosphorylation of ras oncogene product by protein kinase C, *Biochem. Biophys. Res. Commun.* **145:**782–788.

# 19

# Biochemical Marker Alterations in Hepatic Preneoplasia and Neoplasia

## Snorri S. Thorgeirsson and Peter J. Wirth

## 1. INTRODUCTION

Beginning with the first demonstration of chemically induced hepatocarcinogenesis in 1935,[1] the liver has been, and continues to be, a major focus of investigation for many experimental oncologists. Although early studies in chemical hepatocarcinogenesis provided only indirect evidence for the multistage process involved in the neoplastic development in this organ, recent work by Peraino and others has now clearly established the existence of the initiation–promotion–progression phenomenon in the liver.[2,3] Since numerous and voluminous reviews have been written in recent years discussing the histology, time course, markers, and the putative characteristics of the different stages of hepatocarcinogenesis, we make no attempt to deal comprehensively with all the markers associated with chemically induced tumors in the rat liver. Rather, we focus our discussion on the relevance of new markers recently identified during early stages of hepatocarcinogenesis in the authors' laboratory and provide references to more extensive reviews whenever appropriate. Furthermore, the issue of the occurrence of stage-specific markers during hepatocarcinogenesis is addressed.

### 1.1. Relationship of Markers to Different Stages in Neoplasia

The development of cancer in the liver, and most probably all other organs and tissues, is a long process with many steps that ultimately lead to frank development of hepatocellular carcinoma. The operational division of this process into the stages of initiation, promotion, and progression is clearly justified,[2-6] although the molecular mechanisms responsible for these stages of carcinogenesis are far from being adequately defined. Nevertheless, the initiation–promotion–progression concept has both stimulated and challenged the experimental oncologist to identify and define the critical steps in neoplastic development. Within the context of the initiation–promotion–progression concept, Farber and co-workers[4] delineated a minimum of 10 steps during hepatocarcinogenesis. The experimental model used in these studies is the resistant hepatocyte model in the

---

*Snorri S. Thorgeirsson and Peter J. Wirth* • Laboratory of Experimental Carcinogenesis, National Cancer Institute, National Institutes of Health, Bethesda, Maryland 20892.

rat.[4,7] Since most of the following discussion involves the analysis of the resistant hepatocyte model, some background information seems appropriate.

The resistant hepatocyte model or the Solt–Farber model[7] is based on the hypothesis that many chemical carcinogens induce resistance to toxic injury in the initiated cell population.[7,8] This resistant cell population can then be stimulated to develop into focal proliferations and nodules by brief exposure to low noninitiating doses of a second carcinogen coupled with a mitogenic stimulus (i.e., partial hepatectomy). The noninitiating carcinogen (most often 2-acetylaminofluorene) inhibits proliferation of most normal hepatocytes, whereas the rare initiated and resistant cells respond to the proliferation stimulus. In this model, the selection pressure is intense; consequently, the initiated hepatocytes proliferate, at least in the beginning, in a synchronous manner.[4] The fate of these early initiated cells has been extensively described by Farber (for review, see refs. 4 and 6), and only a brief outline is given here. By far most of the early focal and nodular lesions in the resistant hepatocyte model revert back to (remodel or redifferentiate) apparently normal liver. However, a small percentage, possibly less than 5% of the original lesions, progress toward primary tumors.[4] In this respect, the resistant hepatocyte model differs from a number of other models currently used in studying the mechanisms of chemical hepatocarcinogenesis.[2,4] The advantage offered by the resistant hepatocyte model beyond all the other models currently being used in hepatocarcinogenesis research is the synchrony of lesion formation. This makes it possible to analyze the sequence of events readily in a precursor–product fashion.

Although the initiation stage cannot be precisely defined, we offer a variation on a common theme as follows: initiation is a permanent and heritable change in a target tissue or organ, induced by exposure to a carcinogen, that can be promoted to develop into focal lesions composed of clonally expanded cell populations capable of developing into malignant neoplasms. This definition is only operative in experimental systems in which cancer development can be observed to follow the initiation–promotion–progression model.

There are no markers that specifically and exclusively characterize the initiation stage in chemical hepatocarcinogenesis or for that matter in any other experimental tumor model.[2,4,9] In spite of this, the liver model, as well as the mouse skin model of carcinogenesis, provides a tremendous advantage in having available assays for initiation. Scherer et al.[10] were the first to demonstrate that the appearance of histochemically altered foci of hepatocytes could be used to assay for initiation; most importantly, they were able to show that the number of these enzyme-altered islands was positively correlated with the dose of the carcinogen used.[10] This principle has since been used to identify islands or foci of altered hepatocytes with many different carcinogens and in several model systems employing different sets of histochemical and other types of markers.[4] The most commonly used markers in these assays for initiated cell populations include both negative markers such as ATPase and glucose 6-phosphatase (G6P) and positive markers such as γ-glutamyltranspeptidase, epoxide hydrolase, and glutathione S-transferase (GST).[4] Although capable of identifying the initiated cell population, these markers are not specific for the initiation stage. A number of recent and excellent reviews have dealt with the possible significance of these markers in the neoplastic development in the liver; that issue is not discussed further here.[2,4,9]

The promotional stage in hepatocarcinogenesis, as is the case in all experimental systems that conform to the initiation–promotion–progression concept of carcinogenesis, involves expansion of the initiated cell population. In the case of the liver, this would be the transition from the enzyme-altered foci to the hyperplastic nodule stage. We may therefore define the promotional stage operationally as focal expansions of initiated cells (possibly a clonal expansion) into such structures as nodules, polyps, and papillomas having a definite, albeit small, probability of developing into malignant neoplasms.

Although no markers are available that are strictly characteristic of the promotional stage, there is a distinct difference in the pattern of markers observed in the foci and in the nodules. As contrasted with the foci, the nodules have a much more uniform metabolic pattern, both among nodules within the same liver and between different models.[4] As emphasized by Farber and coworkers,[4] this commonality extends to most nodules that remodel by differentiation and to the few that persist as precursors for further neoplastic development. This is a particularly important observation, since there must be a fundamental difference(s) between those nodules that differentiate into apparently normal and functional hepatocytes and those that persist and ultimately may advance into frank neoplasms. The fact that commonality is observed among these nodular lesions implies that relatively few but important differences must exist among the nodules that have the capacity to differentiate into normal hepatocytes and those persisting and developing into neoplasia. A marker(s) capable of discriminating between these two lesions would obviously be of tremendous value in defining the essential steps in the promotion stage.

The transition from the promotion stage to that of progression is not well defined. Nevertheless, a number of definitions have been proposed.[3,4] If one considers in hepatocarcinogenesis that the promotion stage involves expansion of the early focal lesions (possibly from a single initiated cell) to the appearance of the nodular lesions, it is possible to define progression as the process by which certain hyperplastic liver nodules (and some foci) evolve into malignant neoplasms capable of invading surrounding tissues and metastasizing.

The progression stage is almost certainly composed of a number of steps. However, the central characteristic of this process is the slowness by which this cellular evolution to malignancy takes place.[4] One of the most attractive features of the resistant hepatocyte model is the ability to differentiate between the remodeling and persistent nodules, thereby making it possible to analyze the sequence or steps leading from the early nodular lesions to the formation of cancer. This analytic approach has already been embarked upon by Farber and co-workers,[4,6] particularly with respect to control of cell proliferation, cell death, and altered shutoff of cell cycle in the nodule-to-cancer sequence. Although several steps have been proposed in this sequence, no characteristic markers have so far been identified.[4] Furthermore, the existence of some of these steps in the evolution of cancer from the nodular lesions remains speculative at best.[4,6]

## 1.2. Approaches to Evaluation of Markers

Neoplastic markers provide important tools to the study the process of neoplastic development. These markers have historically been grouped under the general term oncofetal proteins (for review, see ref. 11 and Chapter 21) as most are expressed during fetal development. These observations have generated two main hypotheses regarding neoplastic development. The first of these involves the retrodifferentiation of the tumor cell,[11,12] while the second is the stem cell hypothesis.[13-15] Both hypotheses are discussed in detail in Chapter 21.

The approach we have taken to identify new markers associated with the development of chemically induced hepatoma involves the application of a pattern recognition system capable of identifying both qualitative and quantitative changes in gene expression at the protein synthesis level during the neoplastic process. The analysis system involves the computer-based two-dimensional polyacrylamide gel electrophoresis (2D-PAGE) of total cellular polypeptides.[16-19] 2D-PAGE can separate thousands of polypeptides on a single polyacrylamide gel, and the gel pattern can be used to characterize the cell type and the metabolic state of the cell under a given set of environmental and/or experimental conditions.[20-23] The remainder of this chapter reports recent data obtained from analyzing the early preneoplastic and neoplastic liver lesions with the 2D-PAGE system.

## 2. MARKER ALTERATIONS IN PRENEOPLASTIC AND NEOPLASTIC LIVER LESIONS

The identification of specific cellular markers at each stage of hepatocarcinogenesis (e.g., pre- and neoplastic) and the relationship of these markers to specific biologic changes exhibited at these stages would obviously be of great importance in understanding the multistep process of carcinogenesis. One would expect that the acquisition of either the preneoplastic or neoplastic phenotype would bring about both qualitative and quantitative changes in cellular functions distinctly different from those observed under normal and/or preneoplastic conditions. It is furthermore expected that these changes would be reflected at both the cellular DNA and protein level. From polysomal messenger RNA (mRNA)–DNA hybridization studies, estimates have been made indicating that 7000–15,000 mRNA sequences are present in polysomes from mammalian cells and that the typical mammalian cell may contain 5000–20,000 proteins.[24] Moreover, the number of structural genes for differentiated cells may approach 50,000–100,000.[25,26] Obviously, what is needed is an analytic technique that permits simultaneous separation and quantitation of the greatest number of genes or their products (i.e., proteins) as possible. The only technique capable of this is 2D-PAGE of total cellular proteins.[16,27] With this powerful analytic technology in hand, our laboratory has undertaken the study of the sequential changes in polypeptide expression during the multistep process of hepatocarcinogenesis, asking two basic questions concerning the development of chemically induced rat hepatomas: (1) What are the polypeptide differences between normal liver and preneoplastic and neoplastic liver nodules?, and (2) What are the differences between the early preneoplastic and neoplastic nodules within the same liver?

## 2.1. Two-Dimensional Polyacrylamide Gel Electrophoresis

The technique of 2D-PAGE combines two relatively simple electrophoretic procedures, i.e., isoelectric focusing (IEF) and sodium dodecyl sulfate (SDS)-polyacrylamide gel electrophoresis, into a single technique. Proteins, actually polypeptides, are separated on the basis of their isoelectric point (pI) in the first dimension and then on the basis of their molecular weight ($M_r$) in the second dimension. Since each separation technique is based on independent physicochemical parameters (e.g., pI and $M_r$) and, since each technique has a resolving power of approximately 100–150 proteins, the overall resolution in theory is approximately 10,000–20,000 proteins. In practice, however, depending on the polypeptide spot-detection procedures used (e.g., Coomassie blue, silver staining, metabolic labeling with radioactive amino acids), one can easily separate and analyze 1000–1500 polypeptides from a typical 2D-PAGE electrophoretogram. Figure 1 illustrates a typical 2D-PAGE separation of cytosolic polypeptides from a normal liver (Fig. 1A) and from a preneoplastic liver nodule (Fig. 1B) generated using the Solt–Farber initiation–promotion protocol.[7,28] Polypeptides have been visualized using an ultrasensitive silver stain.[29] As might be expected, the polypeptide patterns are quite complex; as a result, our laboratory has also developed a computer system to aid in the analysis of such 2D-PAGE patterns. A detailed description of the analysis system is, however, beyond the scope of this review. Suffice it to say, our computer system is capable of finding all spots (at least those visible to the eye) separated on a 2D-PAGE gel and is also capable of an accurate quantitation of each individual polypeptide spot.[17–19]

## 2.2. Known Markers of Hepatocarcinogenesis

Work in our laboratory[21,22,30] and by others[31–37] has demonstrated that 2D-PAGE can be used to detect and quantitate changes in known markers for hepatocarcinogenesis reliably. Table I lists some of the classic liver enzymes and proteins, both membrane-associated and cytosolic, which are modulated during various stages of rat hepatocarcinogenesis. It should be emphasized that Table I is by no means complete and lists only those markers routinely used in our laboratory. The arrows indicate the generally associated changes of each marker during the course of hepatocarcinogenesis. With the exception of G6P, all these markers have been identified on 2D-PAGE gels.

### 2.2.1. Identification of Markers on 2D-PAGE Gels

*2.2.1.a. γ-Glutamyltranspeptidase.* Initial work was directed toward demonstrating that 2D-PAGE could be used to detect and quantitate changes in known markers of hepatocarcinogenesis reliably. Protein markers were identified on 2D-PAGE gels using three criteria: (1) co-migration on gels with highly purified marker protein preparations; (2) Western transfer and immunoblot analysis of markers with antibody preparations to the purified marker proteins; and (3) comparison with published 2D-PAGE pattern of known marker proteins, if possible. The 2D-PAGE separation of two of the more widely used markers, i.e., GGT and the Y subunits, of the GST are shown in Figs. 2 and 3, respectively.

One-dimensional SDS-PAGE previously showed that GGT, one of the most reliable markers

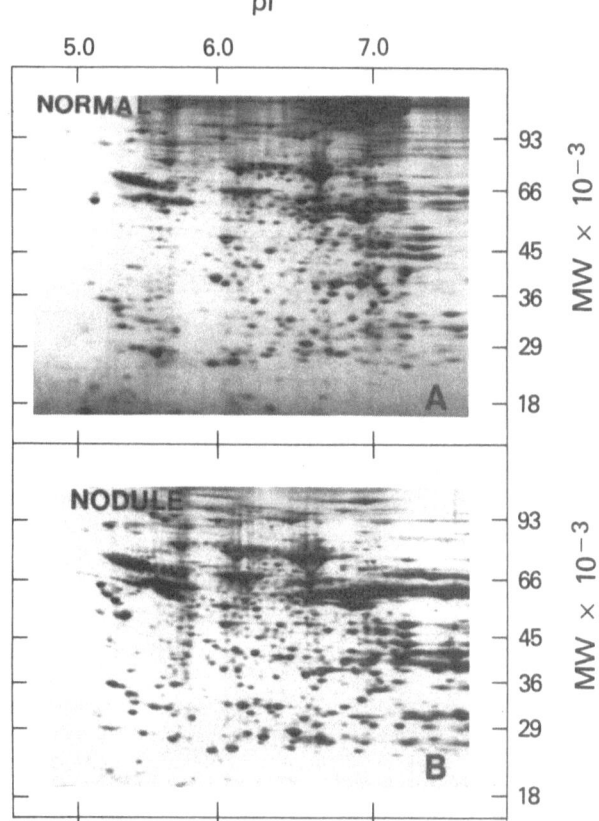

*Figure 1.* 2D-PAGE separation of cytosolic polypeptides from a normal untreated rat liver (A) and a preneoplastic liver nodule (B). Polypeptides were separated in the first dimension by isoelectric focusing between the pH range of 5 (left) and 8 (right). Abscissa, pH range; ordinate, molecular weight $\times 10^{-3}$. (From Wirth *et al.*[21])

for preneoplastic liver transformation,[38–40] is composed of two subunit chains, a light and a heavy chain. 2D-PAGE shows that these subunit chains are extensively modified and are composed of multiple isoforms. Seven polypeptides (pI 7.0–5.4, 23,000–26,000 $M_r$) comprise the light chain and 11 polypeptides (pI 7.1–5.8, 59,000–66,000 $M_r$) comprise the heavy chain. The 2D-PAGE

*Table I. Some Known Biochemical Markers of Preneoplastic and Neoplastic Hepatocellular Lesions in the Rat*[a,b]

| Membrane | | | Cytosolic | | |
|---|---|---|---|---|---|
| | Direction of change | Lesion | | Direction of change | Lesion |
| γ-Glutamyltranspeptidase | ↑ | EAF,HN,HC | Glutathione S-transferase | ↑ | EAF,HC |
| Epoxide hydrolase | ↑ | EAF,HN,HC | DT-Diaphorase | ↑ | EAF,HN |
| 5'-Nucleosidase | ↓ | EAF,HN,HC | Aldehyde dehydrogenase | ↑ | EAF,HN,HC |
| Cytochrome P-450(s) | ↓ | EAF,HN,HC | α-Fetoprotein | ↑ | HC |
| Asialoglycoprotein receptor | ↓ | EAF,HN,HC | Tyrosine aminotransferase | ↓ | HN,HC |
| Glucose 6-phosphatase | ↓ | EAF,HN,HC | Albumin | ↓ | EAF,HN,HC |

[a]( ↑ ) increased expression; ( ↓ ) decreased expression, during hepatocarcinogenesis.
[b]EAF, enzyme-altered foci; HN, hyperplastic liver nodule; HC, hepatocellular carcinoma.

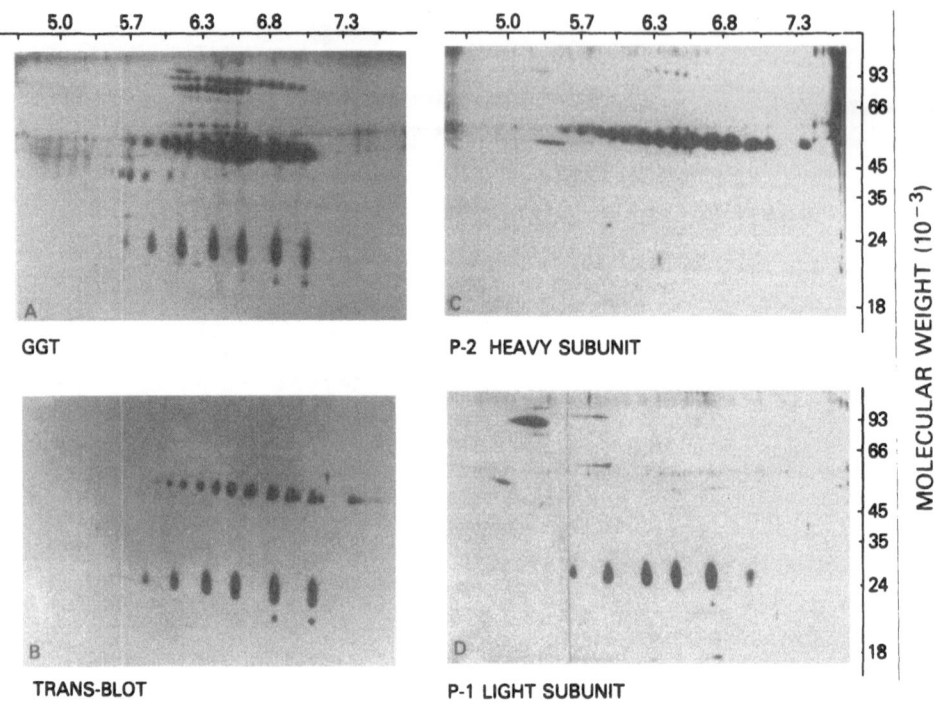

*Figure 2.* 2D-PAGE pattern of purified γ-glutamyltranspeptidase for rat kidney. (A,C,D) Polypeptides visualized with silver staining. (B) Polypeptides transblotted to nitrocellulose, treated with rabbit antirat GGT, then treated with peroxidase-conjugated goat antirabbit antiserum and visualized with 4-chloro-1-naphthol/hydrogen peroxide staining. P1 and P2 refer to the HPLC-purified light and heavy subunit chains of GGT, respectively. (From Cone *et al.*[30])

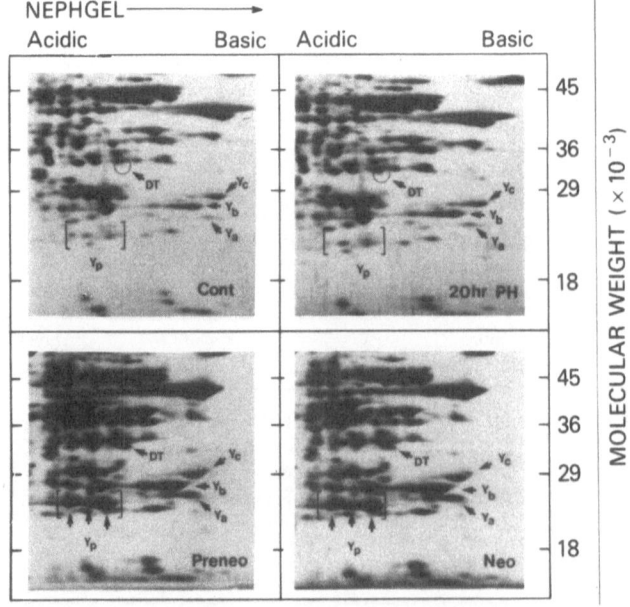

*Figure 3.* 2D-PAGE separation of the Yc, Yb, Ya, and Yp subunits of GST-A, GST-B, ligandin and GST-P, and DT-diaphorase (DT) from normal rat liver (cont), 20 hr postpartial hepatectomized rat liver (20 hr PH), preneoplastic resistant hepatocyte nodule (Preneo), and a neoplastic RH nodule (Neo).

patterns of partially purified GGT (concanavalin-A selected) from neoplastic liver nodules are electrophoretically similar, nearly identical to GGT from normal rat kidney (gel not shown) and are immunoreactive with a mixture of two antibodies raised separately against the light and heavy subunit chains of rat kidney GGT.[30]

*2.2.1.b. Glutathione S-Transferases and DT-Diaphorase.* Certain isoenzymes of GST have also been proposed as useful markers for early changes during hepatocarcinogenesis.[33,34,41] The GST(s) are a group of multifunctional predominantly cytosolic proteins, each composed of two subunits, ranging in molecular weight from 26,000 to 30,000. Because of the basic nature of the individual subunits of the GST(s), it is necessary to perform the first dimension isoelectric focusing step under nonequilibrium pH conditions (NEpHGEL).[42] Under NEpHGEL conditions, the individual Yc ($28,500$-$M_r$), Yb ($27,500$-$M_r$), and Ya ($26,000$-$M_r$) subunits of GST-A (YbYb), GST-B (YaYc), and ligandin (YaYa), as well as the Yp ($26,000$-$M_r$) subunit of the recently described placental form of GST (GST-P),[34] are readily separated on 2D-PAGE gels (Fig. 3). Previous work has demonstrated that the enzymatic activity of particular isoforms of GST is preferentially increased during early preneoplastic stages of chemical hepatocarcinogenesis in the rat. These isozymic activities then decrease during the progression of hepatocarcinogenesis from well-differentiated to poorly differentiated hepatomas.[33,43] The activities of GST-A, ligandin, GST-B, and GST-P are markedly increased in hyperplastic nodules as compared with normal liver. The expression of the Ya subunit (fourfold) of GST-B (and/or ligandin), the Yb subunit (threefold) of GST-A, and the three isoelectric point variants (Yp)(15-fold) of GST-P are markedly increased in both preneoplastic and neoplastic nodules as compared with either normal liver or regenerating liver 20 hr after a two-thirds hepatectomy.[21,22] The expression of DT-diaphorase ($32,000$ $M_r$)[44,45] is also increased two- to threefold in both preneoplastic and neoplastic nodules as compared with either normal or regenerating rat liver (Fig. 3).[21]

## 2.3. New Markers for Hepatocarcinogenesis

There are apparently no markers that specifically and exclusively characterize either the initiation, promotion, or progression stages of hepatocarcinogenesis.[2,4,10] We have therefore used 2D-PAGE analysis of total cellular polypeptides from early preneoplastic and neoplastic liver nodules to search for potential stage-specific marker proteins. The resistant hepatocyte (RH) hepatocarcinogenesis model developed by Solt and Farber[7] offers certain advantages not provided by any of the other models currently in use, i.e., the synchrony of lesion formation. This feature permits analysis of the stepwise sequence of events in a precursor–product manner. We have therefore used the resistant hepatocyte hepatocarcinogenesis model for the generation of hyperplastic liver nodules composed of preneoplastic and neoplastic cell populations in the adult male Fischer rat. Individual nodules were removed and, as an aid for polypeptide analysis, tissue samples were fractionated into cytosolic and crude membrane (particulate) associated polypeptides. 2D-PAGE analysis of cytosolic and particulate polypeptides from individual preneoplastic and neoplastic nodules demonstrated that polypeptide expression within individual nodules as compared with normal liver is not altered extensively during early stages of hepatocarcinogenesis, although both qualitative and quantitative differences were noted.[21] Analysis of approximately 800–1000 cytosolic and 1200–1400 polypeptides showed only four qualitative polypeptide differences. One cytosolic (polypeptide A; 6.80/57) (designated $pI/M_r \times 10^{-3}$) and three particulate (polypeptide B: 6.25/41; polypeptide C: 6.75/24; polypeptide D: 6.05/21) polypeptides are expressed in both preneoplastic and neoplastic nodules but are not detected in normal control liver or in regenerating liver following a two-thirds hepatectomy. These are illustrated in Fig. 4. Quantitatively, polypeptides A–D are expressed in similar concentrations in both preneoplastic and neoplastic nodules. No qualitative polypeptide differences were noted among either individual preneoplastic or neoplastic nodules. Similarly, no qualitative differences were noted between individual preneoplastic and neoplastic nodules.

In addition to these changes, comparison of 500–800 cytosolic and 750–1000 particulate polypeptides showed that 4–10% of the polypeptides analyzed were undergoing quantitative changes of at least fourfold during the preneoplastic and neoplastic stages of hepatocarcinogenesis.

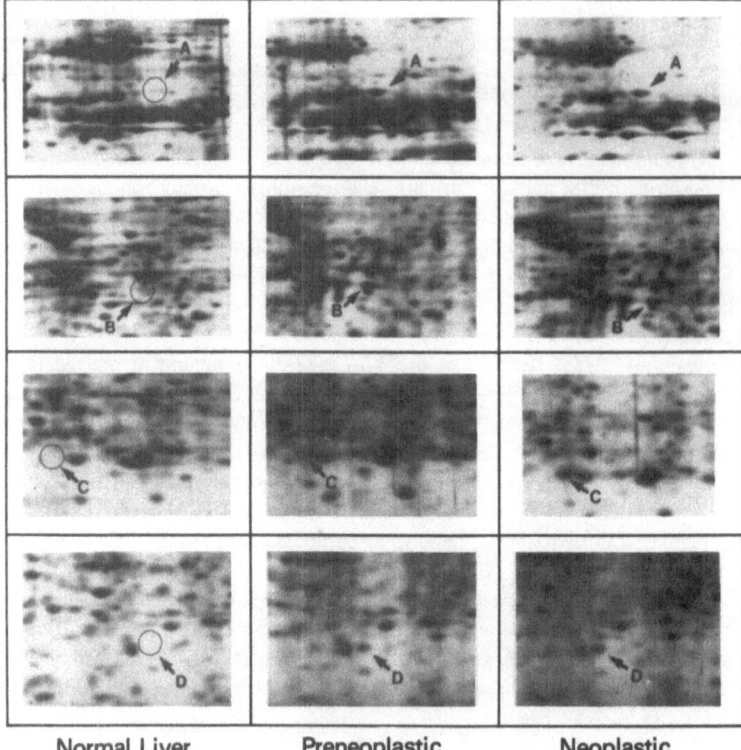

| Normal Liver | Preneoplastic | Neoplastic |

*Figure 4.* Mosaic enlargements of areas of 2D-PAGE gels from normal liver, preneoplastic, and neoplastic RH nodules illustrating polypeptides A, B, C, and D. Open circles have been placed at the expected pI and molecular-weight regions on control gels for missing polypeptides. (From Wirth *et al.*[21])

Thirty (10 cytosolic and 20 particulate) polypeptides were significantly downregulated, while 22 (7 cytosolic and 15 particulate) polypeptides were upregulated in both preneoplastic and neoplastic nodules. In all cases, the direction and magnitude of change were the same for both preneoplastic and neoplastic nodules, with the exception of three particulate polypeptides. Two polypeptides (6.58/33 and 7.25/27) remained unchanged in preneoplastic nodules but decreased in neoplastic nodules, while one polypeptide (6.55/65) increased in preneoplastic nodules but returned to normal levels in neoplastic nodules.

## 2.4. Specific Markers for the Neoplastic Stage

It has become evident that the pattern of multistage carcinogenesis in the rat liver shows remarkable similarities to the multistep development of cancer in the mouse skin and in other systems as well (e.g., urinary bladder, colon, pancreas, respiratory tract, and breast[3,6] (see Chapter 6). Furthermore, the hepatocyte nodules induced in several different hepatocarcinogenesis models show a phenotype that is remarkably similar regardless of the nature of the carcinogen used to induce cancer development.[46–48] Recently, Reddy *et al.*[49] demonstrated that exposure of rats and mice to certain apparently nongenotoxic hypolipidemic agents, including ciprofibrate (CP), results in a very high incidence of hepatocellular carcinoma formation. In addition, the liver tumors induced by these hypolipidemic agents are histologically indistinguishable from tumors induced by a variety of carcinogens, including those induced in the Solt–Farber RH model, which uses the very potent genotoxic agent, diethylnitrosamine (DEN), as the initiating carcinogen.[50]

In order to determine the specificity of the markers initially observed in the RH nodules, we next compared the 2D-PAGE patterns of polypeptide expression in early preneoplastic and neoplastic liver nodules induced using the nongenotoxic carcinogen, CP, and with those changes observed in nodules generated using the genotoxic carcinogen, DEN (RH model).

The electrophoretic patterns of both cytosolic and particulate polypeptides from normal liver, CP-induced nodules, and RH nodules were found to be very similar with respect to the total number of polypeptides detected and the overall 2D-PAGE patterns, although both qualitative and quantitative differences were observed among the different tissues. Seven polypeptide markers were observed to be highly associated with CP-induced hepatocarcinogenesis In addition, three cytosolic polypeptides ($6.90/47,000\ M_r$, $6.90/46,000\ M_r$, and $6.50/28,000\ M_r$) were expressed in both preneoplastic and neoplastic CP-induced nodules (gel not shown) but were not detected in either normal liver or RH nodules. Furthermore, the constitutive expression of one cytosolic polypeptide ($6.00/38,000\ M_r$) and one particulate polypeptide ($6.30/16,000\ M_r$) found in both normal liver and RH nodules was absent in all CP-induced nodules. Although polypeptides A and C were not detected in CP-induced nodules, polypeptides B and D were expressed in both preneoplastic and neoplastic CP-induced nodules.[22]

Quantitatively, three cytosolic and eight particulate polypeptides were observed to be coordinately modulated in both CP-induced and RH nodules as compared with normal liver. One of the cytosolic and seven of the particulate polypeptides are downregulated in both CP-induced and RH nodules, while two cytosolic and one particulate polypeptide were upregulated during early stages of carcinogenesis in both CP-induced and RH nodules. Figure 5 illustrates computer-drawn composite maps highlighting those polypeptides that are significantly altered during chemically induced hepatocarcinogenesis by both DEN and CP.

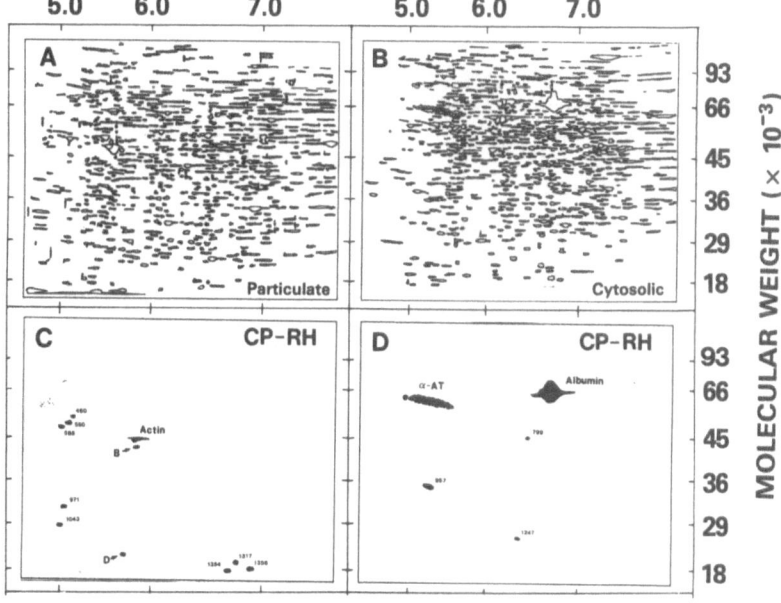

*Figure 5.* Computer-drawn composite maps highlighting polypeptides significantly altered during rat hepatocarcinogenesis. (A,B) Contour maps of commonly expressed particulate and cytosolic polypeptides, respectively, in normal liver, CP-induced, and RH nodules. (C) Particulate. (D) Cytosolic. These polypeptides are under coordinate modulation during hepatocarcinogenesis initiated by DEN and CP. As an aid for polypeptide location and orientation, actin (particulate) and the cytosolic proteins, albumin and $\alpha_1$-antitrypsin ($\alpha$-AT), have been illustrated. (From Wirth *et al.*[22])

## 2.4.1. Glutathione S-Transferase P

One of the phenotypic characteristics of initiated hepatocytes is their resistance to the mitoinhibitory effects of various chemical carcinogens including 2-acetylaminofluorene.[7] This resistant phenotype is characterized in the rat by large decreases in the enzymatic activities of some of the phase I metabolizing enzymes (e.g., P-450, cytochrome $b_5$) and concomitant increases in certain phase II enzymes such as GST(s), DT-diaphorase, epoxide hydrolase, UDP-glucuronyltransferase, and GGT. One of the GST(s), i.e., GST-P, was recently shown to be increased 10-fold in nodules generated using four independent model systems[51] and was proposed as a new marker for hepatocarcinogenesis.[34] Recently, a similar pattern of biochemical changes has been associated with multidrug resistance in human MCF-7 breast cancer cells and xenobiotic resistance induced by carcinogens.[52] A 23,000-$M_r$ GST was isolated from these cells, tentatively identified as GST-P.[53] In RH nodules, GST-P is increased from almost undetectable levels in normal and partial hepatectomized liver to one of the most abundantly expressed polypeptides (1–2% of the total cytosolic protein) in both preneoplastic and neoplastic nodules. In normal liver and in CP-induced nodules, numerous polypeptides appear at the pI and molecular-weight coordinates corresponding to the expected location of the Yp subunit (enclosed box in Fig. 6). However, Western transfer and immunoblot analysis of transferred polypeptides with rabbit anti-GST-P antibody failed to detect significant expression of the Yp subunits in either normal liver or in CP-induced nodules. Similar to GST-P, GGT staining activity is markedly increased in RH nodules, while CP-induced nodules are negative for GGT activity. Therefore, GST-P and GGT, which may be good markers for premalignant changes in RH nodules, are poor markers for identifying altered hepatic foci and neoplastic nodules induced by peroxisome proliferators during the early premalignant phase of hepatocarcinogenesis.[54,55]

## 3. CONCLUDING COMMENTS

The identification of specific cellular markers at each stage of hepatocarcinogenesis (initiation, promotion, and progression) and the relationship of these markers to specific biologic changes exhibited at each of these stages would obviously be of great importance to understanding the process of carcinogenesis. To this end, considerable effort has been made by numerous investigators to identify and characterize stage-specific markers during chemically induced hepatocarcinogenesis. Unfortunately, no such single stage-specific marker has been identified to date. The approach that we have taken involves the 2D-PAGE analysis of total cellular polypeptides from early preneoplastic and neoplastic nodules to identify those polypeptides or groups of polypeptides that control and maintain the initiated phenotype and how these polypeptides change during the course of hepatocarcinogenesis (preneoplastic to neoplastic to malignant metastasizing tumors). This approach enables us to study simultaneously the coordinate modulation of roughly 10–20% of the total number of estimated cellular proteins[24] under a relatively defined set of experimental conditions. Using this approach, we have identified two groups of polypeptides that appear to be under coordinate modulation during hepatocarcinogenesis induced by two markedly different experimental models. Two particulate polypeptides (B and D) are expressed in both preneoplastic and neoplastic nodules generated using either the genotoxic carcinogen, DEN, or the nongenotoxic peroxisome proliferator, CP, and not, or at least in very small amounts, in normal liver. In addition to these qualitative differences, three cytosolic and eight particulate polypeptides are expressed quantitatively in a coordinate manner in both CP-induced and RH nodules as compared with normal liver.

Neither the identity nor the biologic function of any of these polypeptides is known. In somewhat related studies we have demonstrated the coordinate regulation of the expression of specific polypeptides during the neoplastic transformation of Syrian hamster fetal cells by both genotoxic (benzo[a]pyrene) and nongenotoxic carcinogens (bisulfite).[20] These observations further extend the results from our liver model. The commonality of changes observed to occur in both CP-

NEPHGEL ───────────→    WESTERN TRANSFER

Acidic                Basic

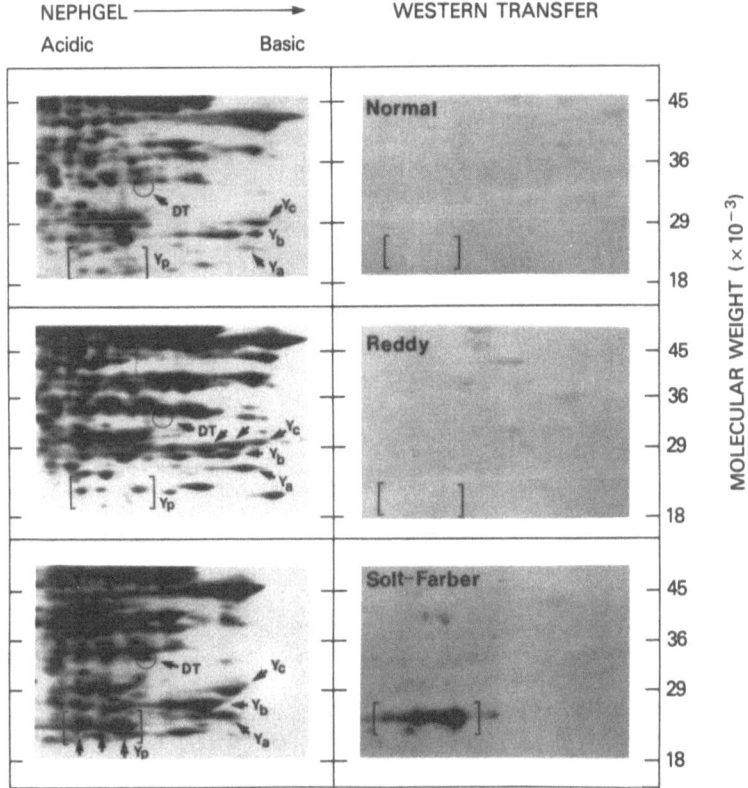

*Figure 6.* Western-blot transfer of polypeptides from normal liver, CP-induced nodule (Reddy), and a RH nodule (Solt–Farber) and immunoblot analysis of corresponding regions of transferred polypeptides with antibody to GST-P. The positions of DT-diaphorase (DT), the Yc, Yb, Ya, and the Yp GST subunits have been indicated with the lettered arrows. Open brackets have been positioned at expected regions for the Yp subunits of GST-P. (From Wirth *et al.*[22])

induced and RH nodules suggest that carcinogens with either epigenetic or genetic effects may affect similar changes in cellular polypeptide expression during carcinogenesis independent of the nature of initiation.[20]

## REFERENCES

1. Sasaki, T., and Yoshida, T., 1935, Experimentelle erzeugung des lebercarcinoma durch futterung mit o-amidoazotoluol, *Arch. Pathol. Anat. Physiol.* **295**:175–181.
2. Peraino, C., Richards, W. L., and Stevens, F. J., 1984, Multistage hepatocarcinogenesis, in: *Mechanisms of Tumor Promotion: Tumor Promotion in the Internal Organs* (T. J. Slaga, ed.), pp. 1–53, CRC Press, Boca Raton, Florida.
3. Pitot, H. C., and Sirica, A. E., 1980, The stages of initiation and promotion in hepatocarcinogenesis, *Biochim. Biophys. Acta* **605**:191–215.
4. Farber, E., and Sarma, D. S. R., 1987, Biology of disease. Hepatocarcinogenesis: A dynamic cellular perspective., *Lab. Invest.* **56**:1–22.
5. Schulte-Herman, R., 1985, Tumor promotion in the liver, *Arch. Toxicol.* **57**:147–158.
6. Farber, E., and Cameron, R., 1980, The sequential analysis of cancer development. *Adv. Cancer Res.* **31**:125–226.

7. Solt, D., and Farber, E., 1976, New principles for the analysis of chemical carcinogenesis, *Nature (Lond.)* **263:**701–703.

8. Haddow, A., 1938, Cellular inhibition and origin of cancer, *Acta Unio Int. Contra Cancrum* **3:**342–353.

9. Scherer, E., and Emmelot, P., 1980, The first relevant cell stage in rat liver carcinogenesis: A quantitative approach, *Biochim. Biophys. Acta* **605:**247–304.

10. Scherer, E., Hoffmann, M., Emmelot, P., and Friedrich-Freska, H., 1972, Quantitative study of foci of altered liver cells induced in the rat by a single dose of diethylnitrosamine and partial hepatectomy, *J. Natl. Cancer Inst.* **49:**93–106.

11. Ibsen, K. H., and Fishman, W. H., 1979, Developmental gene expression in cancer, *Biochim. Biophys. Acta* **560:**243–280.

12. Uriel, J., 1976, Cancer, retrodifferentiation and the myth of Faust, *Cancer Res.* **36:**4269–4275.

13. Sell, S., and Leffert, H. L., 1982, An evaluation of cellular lineages in the pathogenesis of experimental hepatocellular carcinoma, *Hepatology* **2:**74–86.

14. Buick, R. N., and Pollak, M. N., 1984, Perspectives on clonogenic tumor cells, stem cells, and oncogenes, *Cancer Res.* **44:**4909–4918.

15. Pierce, G. B., and Cox, W. F., 1978, Neoplasms as caricatures of tissue renewal, in: *Cell Differentiation and Neoplasia* (G. F. Saunders, ed.), pp. 57–66, Raven, New York.

16. O'Farrell, P. H., 1975, High resolution two-dimensional electrophoresis of proteins, *J. Biol. Chem.* **250:**4007–4021.

17. Vo, K. P., Miller, M. J., Geiduschek, E. P., Nielson, C., Olson, A. D., and Xuong, N. H., 1981, Computer analysis of two-dimensional gels, *Anal. Biochem.* **112:**258–271.

18. Miller, M. J., Olson, A. D., and Thorgeirsson, S. S., 1984, Computer analysis of two-dimensional gels: Automatic matching, *Electrophoresis* **5:**297–303.

19. Miller, M. J., 1986, Quantitative analysis of two-dimensional gel electrophoretograms: Strategies and requirements for computerized analysis, in: *Experimental Biology and Medicine* (A. Wolsky, ed.), pp. 235–260, S. Karger, Basel.

20. Wirth, P. J., Doniger, J., Thorgeirsson, S. S., and DiPaolo, J. A., 1986, Altered gene expression after neoplastic transformation of Syrian hamster cells by bisulfite ($NaHSO_3$), *Cancer Res.* **46:**390–399.

21. Wirth, P. J., Benjamin, T., Schwartz, D. M., and Thorgeirsson, S. S., 1986, Sequential analysis of chemically induced hepatoma development by two-dimensional electrophoresis, *Cancer Res.* **46:**400–413.

22. Wirth, P. J., Rao, M. S., and Evarts, R. P., 1987, Coordinate polypeptide expression during hepatocarcinogenesis: Comparison of the Solt–Farber and Reddy models, *Cancer Res.* **47:**2839–2851.

23. Wirth, P. J., Yuspa, S. J., Thorgeirsson, S. S., and Hennings, H., 1987, Induction of common patterns of polypeptide synthesis and phosphorylation by calcium and 12-*O*-tetradecanoylphorbol-13-acetate in mouse epidermal cell culture, *Cancer Res.* **47:**2831–2838.

24. Duncan, R., and McConkey, E. H., 1982, How many proteins are there in a typical mammalian cell?, *Clin. Chem.* **28:**749–755.

25. O'Brien, S. J., 1973, On estimating functional gene number in eukaryotes, *Nature New Biol.* **242:**52–54.

26. Bishop, J. O., 1974, The numbers game, *Cell* **2:**81–86.

27. Scheele, G. A., 1975, Two-dimensional gel analysis of soluble proteins, *J. Biol. Chem.* **250:**5375–5385.

28. Solt, D. B., Medline, A., and Farber, E., 1977, Rapid emergence of carcinogen induced hyperplastic lesions in a new model for the sequential analysis of liver carcinogenesis, *Am. J. Pathol.* **88:**595–618.

29. Morrissey, J. H., 1981, Silver stain for proteins in polyacrylamide gels: A modified procedure with enhanced uniform sensitivity, *Anal. Biochem.* **117:**307–310.

30. Cone, J. L., Glowinski, I. B., Wirth, P. J., Grantham, P. H., and Roller, P. P., 1986, Structural studies and two-dimensional gel electrophoresis of γ-glutamyl transpeptidase, *Arch. Biochem. Biophys.* **247:**165–170.

31. Rahimi-Pour, A., Wellman-Bednawska, M., Galteau, M-M., and Siest, G., 1986, Identification of gamma-glutamyltranspeptidase in rat liver plasma membranes after two-dimensional electrophoresis, *Electrophoresis* **7:**83–88.

32. Ramagli, L. S., Capetillo, S., Becker, F. F., and Rodriguez, L. V., 1985, Alterations in nonhistone chromatin proteins during hepatocarcinogenesis induced by diverse acting carcinogens, *Carcinogenesis* **6:**367–375.

33. Kitahara, A., Satoh, K., Nichimura, K., Ishikawa, T., Ruike, K., Sato, K., Tsuda, H., and Ito, N., 1984, Changes in molecular forms of rat hepatic glutathione-S-transferase during chemical hepatocarcinogenesis, *Cancer Res.* **44:**2698–2703.

34. Satoh, K., Kitahara, A., Soma, Y., Inaba, Y., Hatayama, I., and Sato, K., 1985, Purification, induction,

and distribution of placental glutathione transferase: A new marker enzyme for preneoplastic cells in the rat chemical hepatocarcinogenesis, *Proc. Natl. Acad. Sci. USA* **82**:3964–3968.

35. Sugioka, Y., Fujii-Kuriyama, Y., Kitagawa, T., and Muramatsu, M., 1985, Changes in polypeptide pattern of rat liver cells during chemical hepatocarcinogenesis, *Cancer Res.* **45**:365–378.

36. Vlasuk, G. P., and Walz, F. G., 1980, Liver endoplasmic reticulum polypeptides resolved by two-dimensional gel electrophoresis, *Anal. Biochem.* **105**:112–120.

37. Franke, W. W., Mayer, D., Schmid, E., Denk, H., and Borenfreund, E., 1981, Differences of expression of cytoskeleton proteins in cultured rat hepatocytes and hepatoma cells, *Exp. Cell Res.* **134**:345–365.

38. Fiala, S., Mohindru, A., Kettering, W. G., Fiala, A. E., and Morris, H. P., 1976, Glutathione and gamma glutamyltranspeptidase in rat liver during chemical carcinogenesis, *J. Natl. Cancer Inst.* **57**:591–599.

39. Hanigan, M. H., and Pitot, H. C., 1985, Gamma-glutamyl transpeptidase—its role in hepatocarcinogenesis, *Carcinogenesis* **6**:165–172.

40. Cameron, R., Kellen, J., Kolin, A., Malkin, A., and Farber, E., 1978, γ-glutamyltranspeptidase in putative premalignant liver cell populations during hepatocarcinogenesis, *Cancer Res.* **38**:823–829.

41. Tatematsu, M. N., Mera, Y., Ito, N., Satoh, K., and Sato, K., 1985, Relative merits of immunohistochemical demonstrations of placental, A, B, and C forms of glutathione-S-transferase and histochemical demonstrations of γ-glutamyltransferase as markers of altered foci during liver carcinogenesis in rats, *Carcinogenesis* **6**:1621–1626.

42. O'Farrell, P. Z., Goodman, H. M., and O'Farrell, P. H., 1977, High resolution two-dimensional electrophoresis of basic as well as acidic proteins, *Cell* **12**:1133–1142.

43. Sato, K., Kitahara, A., Satoh, K., Ishikawa, T., Tatematsu, M., and Ito, N., 1984, The placental form of glutathione-S-transferase as a new marker protein for preneoplasia in rat chemical hepatocarcinogenesis, *Gann* **75**:199–202.

44. Schor, N., Ogawa, K., Lee, G., and Farber, E., 1978, The use of the D-T diaphorase for the detection of foci of early neoplastic transformation in rat liver, *Cancer Lett.* **5**:167–171.

45. Pickett, C. B., Williams, J. B., Lu, A. Y. H., and Cameron, R. G., 1984, Regulation of glutathione transferase and DT-diaphorase mRNAs in persistent hepatocyte nodules during chemical hepatocarcinogenesis, *Proc. Natl. Acad. Sci. USA* **81**:5091–5095.

46. Farber, E., 1984, The biochemistry of preneoplastic liver: A common metabolic pattern in hepatocyte nodules, *Can. J. Biochem. Cell Biol.* **62**:486–494.

47. Farber, E., 1984, Cellular biochemistry of the stepwise development of cancer with chemicals: G. H. A. Clowes Memorial Lecture, *Cancer Res.* **44**:5463–5474.

48. Roomi, M. W., Ho, R. K., Sarma, D. S. R., and Farber, E., 1985, A common biochemical pattern in preneoplastic hepatocyte nodules generated in four different models in the rat, *Cancer Res.* **45**:564–571.

49. Reddy, J. K., Azarnoff, D. L. and Hignite, C. E., 1980, Hypolipidaemic hepatic peroxisome proliferators form a novel class of chemical carcinogens, *Nature (Lond.)* **283**:397–398.

50. Reddy, J. K., and Lalwani, N. D., 1983, Carcinogenesis by hepatic peroxisome proliferators: Evaluation of the risk of hypolipidemic drugs and industrial plasticizers to humans, *CRC Crit. Rev. Toxicol.* **12**:1–58.

51. Eriksson, L. C., Sharma, R. N., Roomi, M. W., Ho, R. K., Farber, E., and Murray, R. K., 1983, A characteristic electrophoretic pattern of cytosolic polypeptides from hepatocyte nodules generated during liver carcinogenesis in several models, *Biochem. Biophy. Res. Commun.* **117**:740–745.

52. Tulpule, A., Batist, G., Sinha, B., Katki, A., Myers, C. E., and Cowan, K. H., 1986, Similar biochemical changes associated with pleotropic drug resistance (PDR) in human MCF-7 breast cancer cells and xenobiotic resistance induced by carcinogens, *Proc. Am. Assoc. Cancer Res.* **27**:271.

53. Batist, G., de Muys, J-M., Cowan, K. H. and Meyers, C. E., 1986, Purification and characterization of a novel glutathione-S-transferase (GST) in multi-drug resistant (MDR) human breast cancer cells, *Proc. Am. Assoc. Cancer Res.* **27**:270.

54. Rao, M. S., Takematsu, M., Subbarao, V., Ito, N., and Reddy, J. K., 1986, Analysis of peroxisomal proliferator induced preneoplastic and neoplastic lesions of rat liver for placental form of glutathione-S-transferase and γ-glutamyltranspeptidase, *Cancer Res.* **46**:5287–5290.

55. Glauert, H. P., Beer, D., Rao, M. S., Schwarz, M., Xu, Y-D., Goldsworthy, T. L., Coloma, J., and Pitot, H. C., 1986, Induction of altered hepatic foci in rats by the administration of hypolipidemic peroxisome proliferators alone or following a single dose of diethylnitrosamine, *Cancer Res.* **46**:4601–4606.

# 20

# Oncogene Activation and Expression during Carcinogenesis in Liver and Pancreas

## James D. Yager and Joanne Zurlo

## 1. INTRODUCTION

### 1.1. Activated Oncogenes versus Proto-Oncogenes

Knowledge of the carcinogenic process has been dramatically increased by the application of recombinant DNA technology and the discovery that mutated cellular genes capable of causing neoplastic transformation can be isolated from spontaneously appearing and carcinogen-induced human and experimental animal tumors. That single genes can cause neoplastic transformation was first demonstrated in studies conducted on acutely transforming retroviruses.[1,2] Such viruses, the first being the Rous sarcoma virus, were shown to carry single genes, termed oncogenes (see Chapter 13), that were responsible for their transforming ability. It was also clearly shown that these retroviral oncogenes had homology to cellular genes and were in fact initially derived from cellular genes by retroviral transduction. The cellular homologs of the retroviral oncogenes are referred to as cellular oncogenes or proto-oncogenes. To date, about 20 retroviral oncogenes, each originating from a cellular precursor proto-oncogene, have been identified.[3]

While the existence of cellular proto-oncogenes had been clearly demonstrated, their potential role in human neoplasia and in experimental chemical and physical carcinogenesis was unknown. Evidence for the role of mutations in the carcinogenic process, especially in the initiation stage, continued to be confined to correlations between the development of cancer and (1) the mutagenicity of carcinogens or their metabolites, (2) the presence of DNA repair deficiencies and consequent increased sensitivity to induced mutagenesis in cells derived from individuals showing genetically determined increased predisposition to cancer, or (3) the association of aneuploidy with progression of the neoplastic process. The real breakthrough that implicated a role for proto-oncogene activation in the carcinogenic process came when the application of gene-transfer techniques showed that DNA derived from human tumor cell lines and primary tumors was capable of causing neoplastic transformation as revealed by focus formation in the immortalized NIH 3T3 mouse fibroblast cell line.[4] The first cellular gene, derived from the T24/EJ human bladder carcinoma cell line, to be identified as

*James D. Yager* • Department of Anatomy, Dartmouth Medical School, Hanover, New Hampshire 03756. *Joanne Zurlo* • Department of Pharmacology and Toxicology, Dartmouth Medical School, Hanover, New Hampshire 03756.

having transforming activity in the NIH 3T3 focus formation assay was shown to be homologous to the transforming gene carried in the Harvey murine sarcoma (Ha-MSV) retrovirus.[5] The activated cellular Harvey *ras* (c-H-*ras*) oncogene was subsequently shown to differ from its proto-oncogene counterpart by a point mutation in the 12th codon.[6,7] Subsequent studies demonstrated that 10–20% of the DNA samples derived from human tumor cell lines or primary human tumor tissue possess transforming activity in the NIH 3T3 cell assay. More recent studies employing new approaches that do not involve transfection of tumor DNA into NIH 3T3 cells have demonstrated that, at least for human colon tumors, *ras* activation may be a very frequent event.[8,9] To date, about 40 cellular genes that are altered through point mutation or other changes such as rearrangement or amplification leading to enhanced or inappropriate expression have been detected in various tumors.[1] Cellular oncogenes generally show evolutionary conservation, and many have been shown to function at critical points in signal transduction pathways in the control of normal tissue growth and differentiation.

Exciting new information is continually being reported concerning the molecular genetics of the various cellular oncogenes and their roles in the signal transduction pathways of growth and differentiation control in various cell and tissue types. However, fundamental questions continue to exist pertaining to their causal role in neoplasia and to the molecular events leading to their activation.[10]

The concept that the carcinogenic process is multistage, reviewed in Chapters 6 and 10, originated from the studies on tumor formation in skin.[11,12] The now classic terms "initiation" and "promotion" were first coined by Peyton Rous. The process of initiation was shown to be a persistent if not irreversible event caused by carcinogen treatment. Under appropriate conditions, it can be shown to result in the production of cells with neoplastic potential which, without further treatment, will for the most part remain quiescent. We now know that this process can involve mutation of cellular proto-oncogenes. By contrast, promotion requires chronic exposure to agents that ultimately enhance tumor incidence and number. Promoters are not mutagenic and, at least initially, their overall effects are reversible. However, the process of promotion has also been shown to consist of at least two stages, the first of which requires only a short treatment with a stage I promoter.[12] Finally, a third stage in the carcinogenic process is progression. This stage can be considered to encompass the period beginning when promotion becomes irreversible.

Acutely transforming retroviruses have the ability to mediate neoplastic transformation without need for mutation of other genes.[3] On the other hand, except in a few instances, activated cellular oncogenes alone cannot transform cells in primary culture.[13] The work of Weinberg and co-workers[13] has facilitated integration of the oncogene and multistage carcinogenesis hypotheses. It is clear from recent studies that mutation of the c-H-*ras* gene or introduction into cells of an activated c-H-*ras* gene is associated with initiation of carcinogenesis. In a recent study, Dotto *et al.*[14] introduced an activated c-H-*ras* gene into rat 1 cells, but this alone did not result in their transformation. However, introduction of the c-*myc* oncogene into these activated c-H-*ras* containing cells caused the cells to become transformed. Furthermore, the role of the c-*myc* gene could be replaced by treatment of the c-H-*ras* containing cells with the tumor promoter 12-*O*-tetradecanoylphorbol-13-acetate (TPA). These results demonstrate that, at least in this system, a two-stage transformation process can be mimicked by the presence and presumably expression of an activated c-H-*ras* oncogene together with inappropriate expression of c-*myc* or treatment with TPA. The findings that transformation of primary cultures requires pairs of activated cellular oncogenes, while not without exception,[15] suggests the existence of oncogene complementation groups.[16] This is an attractive finding since it fits into the multistage model, i.e., initiation, promotion, and progression, of carcinogenesis. However, the oncogene concept pertaining to the mechanisms through which cellular oncogenes are activated and the role of this process in carcinogenesis, whether causal or secondary, continues to be questioned.[4] It is clear that it will be difficult, if not impossible, to determine definitively the causal role of oncogene activation and/or aberrant expression in neoplasia when starting with the tumor for the isolation and study of activated cellular oncogenes. Rather, insight into this question will more likely be derived from the use of the well-defined animal and cell-culture model systems and of transgenic animals.

## 1.2. Proto-Oncogene Activation by Chemical Carcinogens and Ionizing Radiation

Induction of tumors by carcinogenic agents in six animal model systems has provided important, although still somewhat limited knowledge on the role of oncogene activation in the carcinogenic process. These model systems are mouse skin, rat skin and nasal cavity, mouse thymus, rat neuro/glioblastomas, and rat mammary gland.

### 1.2.1. Mouse Skin

The induction of skin tumors in mice has served as a classic experimental model in studies on the cellular and biochemical mechanisms of carcinogenesis.[11,12] Data obtained using this model have formed the major basis for the development of the initiation/promotion/progression multistage concept of carcinogenesis. Several laboratories have recently reported the results of experiments designed to explore the role of proto-oncogene activation in the development of mouse skin tumors. In one of these studies, Balmain and Pragnell[17] reported that transfection of DNA from three of three transplanted mouse squamous cell carcinomas, originating from primary skin carcinomas that developed after initiation by treatment with dimethylbenzanthracene (DMBA) and subsequent promotion by chronic treatment with TPA, caused transformation of NIH 3T3 cells. Upon transfection of DNA from the mouse tumors into the NIH 3T3 cells of the same species, activated oncogenes were detected by the appearance of additional restriction fragments and/or amplification of the oncogene responsible for the appearance of transformed foci. Subsequent analysis of DNA from the foci transformed by the mouse skin tumor DNA revealed the presence of an additional amplified c-H-*ras* gene in some of the foci. A polymorphism of the c-H-*ras* gene was detected in one of the carcinoma DNA samples, which was also seen in NIH 3T3 transformants arising after transfection with this DNA sample. These data were the first to show the presence of an activated proto-oncogene in chemically induced tumors in an experimental model system.

In the mouse skin system, as in other experimental model carcinogenesis systems such as liver and pancreas, as well as in many human tissues, preneoplastic lesions precede the appearance of malignant tumors (see Chapter 9). An important question is whether oncogene activation is an early or late event in the carcinogenic process. Balmain and co-workers[18] investigated the stage of the carcinogenic process at which they could first detect an activated oncogene. In this study, SENCAR mice were initiated by treatment with DMBA and promoted by repetitive treatment with TPA. Individual benign papillomas and carcinomas were obtained and their DNA purified and used to transfect NIH 3T3 cells. DNA from four of five papillomas and two of three carcinomas was positive for transforming activity. Since the efficiency of transformation, as represented by numbers of transformed foci per microgram DNA, was stated to be similar for papilloma and carcinoma DNA, it is unlikely that the transforming activity of the papilloma DNA was due to a small contaminating population of carcinoma cells. Subsequent analysis of DNA from the NIH 3T3 transformants to determine the identity of the transforming activity indicated the presence of an activated c-H-*ras* oncogene. Since an activated c-H-*ras* oncogene was detected in both papillomas, which represent precancerous lesions, and in carcinomas that arise later from papillomas, it appears that the activation of this oncogene represents an early stage in the carcinogenic process.[18] In a more recent paper from Balmain's laboratory,[19] it was reported that in the majority of tumors, both papillomas and carcinomas, arising following DMBA initiation and TPA promotion, the c-H-*ras* oncogene has been activated by an A to T transversion in codon 61. This mutation was specific for initiation by a single dose of DMBA since none of the tumors initiated with *N*-methyl-*N'*-nitro-*N*-nitrosoguanidine and promoted with TPA appeared to possess a mutation at this site. These results were confirmed by the studies reported by Bizub *et al.*[20] Thus, the initiator, not the promotor, determines the initiating mutagenic event. This argues against the possibility that the tumors arise from a mutation preexisting in this gene in this strain of mice. Finally, the potential of an altered H-*ras* oncogene to initiate skin carcinogenesis was demonstrated in a novel experimental approach used by Balmain and co-workers.[21] They applied a solution containing HaMSV to the backs of

SENCAR mice, followed by promotion with TPA. Tumors, consisting of papillomas at 4–6 weeks and a few carcinomas at >12 weeks were observed in these mice, but did not appear in controls that received virus but not TPA. These results clearly show that introduction of an activated viral H-*ras* oncogene into epidermal cells can replace treatment with a chemical carcinogen in the initiation of carcinogenesis in this model system. In addition, this represents an instance in which an acutely transforming retrovirus alone was not sufficient to complete the neoplastic process.

### 1.2.2. Rat Skin and Nasal Cavity

In another skin carcinogenesis model system, Garte *et al.*[22] determined the transforming activities in the NIH 3T3 cell assay of DNA from rat nasal and mouse skin tumors induced by various alkylating agents. DNA from rat nasal squamous carcinomas and mouse skin squamous carcinomas and fibrosarcomas produced by dimethylcarbamyl chloride failed to cause transformation. By contrast, DNA from similar rat nasal tumors induced by methylmethane sulfonate (MMS) and from mouse skin tumors initiated by B-propriolactone (BPL) did cause the appearance of transformed foci. Selected foci were isolated and their cells were found to form colonies in soft agar and tumors in nude mice. The transforming activities were maintained through successive rounds of transfection. Screening of the transformant DNA from MMS-induced tumors with probes for the c-H-, c-Kirsten (K)-, or N-*ras*, c-*abl*, c-*sis*, c-*myc*, c-*src*, or c-*erb* B oncogenes failed to reveal the identity of the transforming activity. However, an activated c-H-*ras* oncogene was identified as the transforming activity in DNA from a BPL-induced mouse skin squamous cell carcinoma. Recently, Hochwalt and Garte[23] reported that the activation of this c-H-*ras* oncogene was a result of an A to T transversion at the second nucleotide of codon 61.

Ionizing radiation is also able to cause tumors in rat skin. Recently, Garte and co-workers[24] reported that DNA from 6 of 12 radiation-induced rat skin tumors caused transformation of NIH 3T3 cells and that this was due to the presence of activated c-K-*ras* sequences. Ten of the 12 tumors also showed amplification and restriction fragment length polymorphism of the c-*myc* gene. In five of these tumors, it was found that the steady-state level of c-*myc* expression increased two- to sixfold when compared with that seen in normal rat cells.[24]

### 1.2.3. Mouse Thymus

As indicated in the experiments described for rat skin, treatment with ionizing radiation, as well as chemical carcinogens, can also result in the activation of cellular oncogenes. In AKR × RF/J $F_1$ mice, N-nitroso-N-methylurea (NMU) and ionizing radiation result in a high incidence of thymomas.[25,26] However, the chemical carcinogen-induced tumors were shown to have an activated N-*ras* oncogene,[25] whereas the radiation-induced tumors had an activated c-K-*ras*.[26] In the former case, activation was shown to be due to a C to A transversion in the first nucleotide of codon 61,[27] and in the latter instance, the mutation was shown to be a G to A transition in the second nucleotide of codon 12.[26] A similar mutation was detected in three of four radiation-induced thymomas.

### 1.2.4. Rat Neuroblastomas and Glioblastomas

Treatment of pregnant BDIX rats at 15 days of gestation with the carcinogen ethylnitrosourea (ENU) results in the appearance of neuro/glioblastomas. Weinberg and co-workers[28] reported that DNA from four neuroblastoma cell lines established from 4 independent ENU-induced tumors caused transformation in NIH 3T3 cells. Subsequent studies by this group resulted in the identification of a new cellular oncogene later named neu.[29] This gene was found to code for a 185,000-$M_r$ transmembrane protein related to, but distinct from, the epidermal growth factor receptor. Furthermore, in the four cell lines, this cellular oncogene was found to be activated by the same T to A transversion that results in the substitution of a glutamic acid for the normal valine at position 664, located within the transmembrane domain of the protein.

Taken together, the results summarized above clearly show that activation of cellular oncogenes through point mutation, i.e., the c-*ras* genes and *neu*, and rearrangement and/or overexpression, i.e. c-*myc*, are associated with tumors induced in rat and mouse skin, neuroblastomas and glioblastomas, rat nasal cavity, and thymomas induced by chemical carcinogens and ionizing radiation. The frequency of detection of the activation of the *ras* genes may be related to the NIH 3T3 cell assay, which has a bias for detecting activation of members of this gene family. The fact that different carcinogens cause activation of different members of this family and that the specific mutation induced is carcinogen dependent indicates that the carcinogens are directly causing these mutations. In addition, the fact that oncogene activation can be detected in some premalignant lesions suggests that this may be an early event in the carcinogenic process.

## 1.2.5. Rat Mammary Gland

The question of the role of oncogene activation in the carcinogenic process has been perhaps best addressed to date by the studies of Barbacid and co-workers.[30,31] Mammary carcinomas can be induced in female Buf/N rats by a single injection of the direct-acting carcinogen NMU at 50 days of age, a time when mammary gland maturation is occurring. Tumors typically appear within 6–12 months. NMU has two properties which make it attractive for use to answer the question of whether it plays a direct role in the activation of a cellular oncogene. First, it is highly reactive and thus is only present in a reactive state for several hours following treatment. Thus, initiation of the carcinogenic process by NMU must occur within a short time of treatment. Second, NMU causes alkylation at the O-6 position of G and the predominant mutation observed after NMU treatment is a G to A transition.

In an initial study, Sukumar *et al.*[30] found that DNA from nine of nine NMU-induced mammary tumors caused transformation in the NIH 3T3 cell assay and that in each case, the transforming activity was due to an activated rat c-H-*ras* oncogene. DNA from one of the transformants was isolated and the activated rat c-H-*ras* gene cloned. Sequence analysis of the first exon of the c-H-*ras* oncogene revealed the presence of a G to A transition in the second nucleotide of the 12th codon. This is the type of mutation predicted to occur with high frequency in cells following treatment with NMU. In addition, given the short half life of this direct acting carcinogen these results support the hypothesis that mutation of the c-H-*ras* oncogene is an early event in the carcinogenic process in this rat mammary tumor model system.

A second study by Barbacid and co-workers[31] reported the results of the detailed analysis of oncogene activation in additional tumors produced by NMU in this system and of several mammary tumors induced by DMBA. The normal rat c-H-*ras* nucleotide sequence at codons 12 and 13, GGAGGC, contains the MnlI restriction endonuclease site GAGG. Thus, a G to A transition at nucleotide 2 of codon 12 or at nucleotides 1 and 2 of codon 13 would eliminate this restriction site. Zarbl *et al.*[31] found that 31 of 38 DNAs obtained from NMU-induced mammary tumors showed the presence of this MnlI restriction fragment length polymorphism (RFLP) revealing the presence of a mutation at one of these two codons. Similar results were seen with DNA from mammary tumors induced by NMU in Sprague Dawley and Fischer 344 rats. Thus, 83% of all the mammary tumors examined showed the presence of the MnlI RFLP. Of these 48 tumors, DNA from 36 (75%) also caused transformation in the NIH 3T3 cell assay. Additional studies with the NIH 3T3 transformants from the 36 mammary tumors, in which oligonucleotide probes were used to identify the actual base change, showed that, in all cases, the mutation was a G to A transition at position 2 of the 12th codon. This was not the case for mammary tumors induced by DMBA. DNA from 3 of 14 of these tumors caused transformation in the NIH 3T3 cell assay mediated by an activated c-H-*ras* gene. However, a mutation was not detected in codons 12 or 13. Rather, the mutation was confined to the two adenosines found in codon 61 (CAA).

The results reported in these two papers are quite clear. Single-dose chemical carcinogen induction of rat mammary carcinogenesis is associated almost exclusively with the activation of the c-H-*ras* oncogene. The site of the mutation is dependent on the carcinogen. In addition, since, particularly for NMU, the carcinogen has a short half life, the results suggest that c-H-*ras* activation represents the initiating event for this model system.

## 2. MULTISTAGE CARCINOGENESIS IN LIVER AND PANCREAS

### 2.1. Initiation and Promotion in Liver

In animal models for carcinogenesis, the processes of initiation, promotion, and progression can be demonstrated in colon, mammary gland, liver, and pancreas, in addition to skin. In liver, the first definitive evidence that hepatocarcinogenesis is multistage came from studies by Peraino and co-workers, in which initiation was accomplished by short-term feeding of diet containing the carcinogen 2-acetylaminofluorene and promotion by subsequent continuous feeding of diet containing 0.05% phenobarbital (PB).[32] Various initiation-promotion protocols have been developed to facilitate mechanistic studies of the process of hepatocarcinogenesis in both mice and rats. Numerous chemicals have been shown to be capable of causing initiation and prolonged treatment with agents in addition to PB, including choline-deficient diet[33] and synthetic estrogens,[34] have been shown to cause promotion of hepatocarcinogenesis. Initiation and promotion in liver have been discussed in Chapter 6 and are not considered further here.

### 2.2. Initiation and Promotion in Pancreas

It is not as well recognized that the pancreas represents an excellent tissue in which to study the processes of initiation and promotion. Several animal models for pancreatic cancer have been developed with the best characterized being the azaserine-rat model[35,36] and the N-nitrosobis(2-oxopropyl)amine (BOP)-hamster model.[36,37] Studies with the azaserine-rat model have shown that single or multiple doses of this carcinogen result in the induction of atypical acinar cell foci, atypical acinar cell nodules, adenomas, carcinomas *in situ*, and adenocarcinomas.[35,36] It is generally accepted that the cell of origin in azaserine-induced tumors is the acinar cell. In the Syrian golden hamster, treatment with oxidized derivatives of dipropylnitrosamine results in the induction of pancreatic adenocarcinomas, the majority of which have a ductlike appearance.[37] However, the various carcinogens used in these animal model studies show clear species specificities related to different levels of metabolic conversion to their ultimate carcinogenic forms. Pancreatic carcinogenesis in animal models has been shown to be modulated by diet.[38–40] In the rat, azaserine-induced pancreatic carcinogenesis has been shown to be enhanced by prolonged feeding of a defined diet high in unsaturated fat, i.e., 20% corn oil, in the post-initiation phase.[38,39] This high unsaturated fat diet induces growth of preneoplastic pancreatic lesions in azaserine-treated rats and causes an increase in the incidence and number of pancreatic neoplasms. In this model, feeding of the defined diet AIN-76A itself results in a higher incidence of pancreatic cancer than seen with animals fed standard laboratory chow.[35] Concurrent studies have also demonstrated that a diet high in unsaturated fat enhances pancreatic carcinogenesis in BOP-treated hamsters.[40] More recent studies suggest that a high saturated fat diet (20% lard) can also enhance carcinogenesis in the BOP-hamster model.[41] Pancreatic carcinogenesis can also be enhanced by feeding raw soy flour[42] or purified soybean isolate[43,44] to azaserine-treated rats. The enhancement by raw soy flour appears to be attributable to the presence of both soybean trypsin inhibitor and high levels of unsaturated fat,[43,44] whereas the effect of the soybean isolate is due solely to the presence of the trypsin inhibitor, which causes pancreatic hypertrophy and hyperplasia. These results were confirmed using the synthetic trypsin inhibitor camostate (FOY-305).[45] Recent studies have suggested that the enhancing effect of soy flour/trypsin inhibitor may be mediated by the gastrointestinal hormone, cholecystokinin.[44,46] However, as in most other model experimental systems, while initiation and promotion can be readily demonstrated in the pancreas, the mechanisms of these processes and the role of altered oncogene expression and/or mutation has not been well studied.

## 3. PROTO-ONCOGENE ACTIVATION IN LIVER AND PANCREATIC NEOPLASMS

### 3.1. Transforming Genes Associated with Human Liver and Pancreatic Neoplasms

Human liver cancer is the most prevalent cancer in certain parts of the world such as southeast Asia and Africa. Its incidence is associated with exposure of humans to aflatoxin and hepatitis B virus.[47] However, despite its prevalence in these parts of the world, relatively little has been published on the search for and detection of activated oncogenes in human hepatomas. Table I shows a summary of the data published to date. While DNA from 15 liver carcinomas and cell lines has been tested,[48–50] 13 were evaluated in the same laboratory.[48] Of these 15 samples, two were cell lines and the remaining primary tumors. Both cell lines, 7402[48] and Hep G2[50] (J. E. Mignano, J. Zurlo, and J. D. Yager, unpublished), were shown to contain activated N-*ras* genes as revealed in the NIH 3T3 cell transformation assay. The remaining 13 samples were from primary hepatocellular carcinomas. DNA from eight of these samples caused transformation of NIH 3T3 cells and in four, the activated oncogene was identified as N-*ras*, whereas in the remainder, the transforming activity was not identified. However, of these remaining four, the possibility of activated N-*ras* involvement was ruled out in only one.[48] The specific site of the activating mutation for the N-*ras* gene in these individual liver carcinomas has not yet been reported. In addition to the detection of oncogene mutation, Gu *et al.*[48] also found N-*ras* amplification and rearrangement in two primary liver carcinomas. DNA from one of these, but not the other, had transforming activity in NIH 3T3 cells due to an activated N-*ras* gene. Although limited in scope, the results obtained to date are interesting in that an N-*ras* oncogene has been found in 60% of the human liver carcinomas analyzed for its presence. However, larger numbers of liver tumors will have to be analyzed before a strong correlation between N-*ras* mutation and human liver cancer can be established.

In addition to detection of oncogene activation, reports from several laboratories have described the level of expression, as represented by steady state mRNA levels, of various oncogenes in a few human primary hepatomas and hepatoma cell lines.[48,51–54] Results of studies on the levels of oncogene expression are generally difficult to interpret for the following reasons. First, changes in oncogene expression accompany changes in the proliferative state of cells within a tissue. This is not unexpected since a number of oncogenes have been shown to code for proteins involved in growth regulatory and differentiation signal transduction pathways. However, this poses the problem of selecting or even obtaining the appropriate control tissue. For liver, is RNA obtained from normal liver an appropriate control for hepatoma tissue, or should the control RNA come from a growing

*Table I. Oncogene Activation in Human Liver and Pancreatic Carcinomas and Cell Lines*

| Carcinoma | Number reported | Number positive in NIH3T3 assay | Oncogene detected | Reference |
|---|---|---|---|---|
| Liver | 15 | 10 | N-*ras*-6 | 48,50 |
| | | | UI-4[a] | 48,49 |
| Pancreas | 6 | 6 | c-K-*ras*-4 | 57,60–63 |
| | | | UI-2 | 58,64 |

[a]UI, unidentified.

liver and, if so, what would the source of such tissue be? Another problem is the selection of other genes to use as a base line for expressing the extent of changes observed. Such a base line should also be reflective of the proliferative state of the tissue. In a study by Calabretta et al.,[55] where the expression of c-*myc* and two other cell-cycle-dependent genes was evaluated in colon tumors and normal colon tissue, their level of expression was compared to that of the S-phase specific gene, histone H3. The rationale was that deviation from the normal ratios of cell-cycle dependent gene expression may be important in neoplastic transformation. What Calabretta et al.[55] found was that in the tumors, increased expression of c-*myc* was accompanied by increased expression of other cell-cycle-dependent genes. Thus c-*myc* was not being overexpressed. Rather, its increased expression was a reflection of a greater fraction of cycling cells in the tumor tissue. These limitations must be kept in mind when evaluating the results of studies done on oncogene expression in any tissue or cell culture system.

Correction for the fraction of cycling cells was not done in any of the reported studies on the expression of oncogenes in human liver tumors. Gu et al.[48] reported that N-*ras* and c-*myc* were expressed at higher levels than in normal liver tissue in six of nine and in seven of eight primary hepatocellular carcinomas (PHC), respectively. While these expression data were presented in the same report describing detection of activated N-*ras* in a liver tumor cell line and in three PHCs, it is not clear whether they were included in the same group of PHCs analyzed for expression. In addition, it is not evident that the expression data were corrected for the amount of RNA per lane and/or transferred during the Northern blotting procedure. Thus, while the authors concluded that N-*ras* and c-*myc* were activated in most cases of PHC, additional experiments with better quantitation, and more samples are necessary. In another study,[51] it was found that clone HLD$_2$-6 derived from the HepG2 human hepatoma cell line expressed c-*myc* at elevated levels compared with normal human liver. In addition, N-*ras* expression was elevated in HLD$_2$-6 cells growing as tumors in nude mice but not when the cells were growing in culture. While these experiments were adequately controlled to rule out the possibilities that the differences could be accounted for by different amounts of RNA in each sample, they did not deal with possible differences in the number of cycling cells. Several additional reports have also presented results of studies on oncogene expression in human hepatoma, fetal and adult liver tissue.[52–54] However, these studies suffer from lack of adequate controls to allow correction for the amounts of RNA and/or lack of indication of the reproducibility of the findings and will not be discussed. Thus, it is clear that well-designed studies to determine the patterns of oncogene expression in human hepatoma tissue are appropriate.

The incidence and mortality of pancreatic cancer in the human population has been increasing, and yet, to date, relatively little is known about its etiology. In human males, pancreatic cancer ranks fourth as the cause of death due to cancer, largely due to the lack of early detection.[56] Oncogene activation has not been addressed to any great extent either in human pancreatic tumors or in animal models for pancreatic carcinogenesis. Genetic analyses of pancreatic carcinomas have been reported in a limited number of studies. Table I summarizes the results of studies on oncogene activation in human pancreatic carcinomas and tumor cell lines reported to date. Pulciani et al.[57] used DNA from a primary human pancreatic carcinoma in the NIH 3T3 transfection/transformation assay, and analysis of the resulting transformant DNA samples revealed the presence of sequences homologous to the c-K-*ras* oncogene. In contrast to these findings, Der and Cooper[58] reported that the transforming gene in the human pancreatic tumor cell line PaCa-2 had no homology to c-K-*ras* and remained unidentified.

Hirai et al.[59] reported the establishment of the T3M-4 cell line from a primary pancreatic exocrine adenocarcinoma and that the DNA from this line had a high transformation efficiency in the NIH 3T3 cell assay. These investigators found that the T3M-4 cells contained an amplified c-K-*ras* gene and that this gene had undergone an A to C transversion mutation in codon 61, resulting in the substitution of histidine for glutamine in the protein. These investigators also examined the expression, by dot blot analysis, of c-K-, c-H-, and N-*ras* in poly (A)$^+$RNA from this cell line. As controls, they used poly (A)$^+$RNA from normal pancreas and placenta. Their results indicated that expression of the amplified c-K-*ras* was increased four- to eightfold, whereas no differences were seen for c-H-, and N-*ras*. This represents the only report to date wherein oncogene expression in human pancreatic normal and tumor tissue was analyzed.

Two studies[60,61] reported the characterization of transforming activity of DNA from the A165 subclone of PANC-1 cells, an epithelioid cell line derived from a human pancreatic carcinoma of ductal cell origin. This cell line was found to have an activated K-*ras* gene arising from a G to A transition in the 12th codon, which results in the substitution of aspartic acid for glycine. It is not known, however, whether this alteration was present in the original tumor.

Two reports by Yamada *et al.*[62,63] showed the amplification of the c-*myc* and c-K-*ras* oncogenes in both a primary human pancreatic carcinoma and in a cell line, PSN-1, derived from it. These investigators determined that the c-K-*ras* oncogene, in addition to being amplified, had also been activated by a G to C transversion mutation in the 12th codon, which results in the substitution of arginine for glycine in the c-K-*ras* protein. Similar changes were also found in lymph node metastases from this tumor suggesting that the changes in c-K-*ras* and c-*myc* had occurred early in the development of the tumor. These results support the hypothesis that at least two oncogenes from different complementation groups are necessary for neoplastic transformation of normal cells.

Finally, Hollingsworth *et al.*[64] reported that the transforming activity of DNA from HPAF, a cell line derived from the ascitic fluid of a patient with advanced metastatic pancreatic adenocarcinoma, had no homology to sixteen known oncogenes. However, monoclonal antibodies raised against the transformants detected proteins not found in untransformed NIH 3T3 cells or in normal pancreas, but that were antigenically identical to proteins found in the parent HPAF cell line as well as in other pancreatic tumor cells.

The evidence presented in the above studies indicates that an activated c-K-*ras* gene may be associated with a significant number of human pancreatic carcinomas. More data exist for human pancreatic tumors than for liver. However, as with human liver tumors, a larger number of human pancreatic tumors will have to be analyzed for oncogene activation before a strong correlation between c-K-*ras* mutation and pancreatic cancer can be established. The possible involvement of c-*myc* amplification also deserves further study.

## 3.2. Transforming Genes in Spontaneous and Chemically Induced Liver and Pancreatic Neoplasms

There are two reports in the literature describing the results of experiments designed to determine whether oncogene activation is associated with the appearance of spontaneously occurring liver tumors. B6C3F$_1$ mice are used in long-term bioassays for evaluation of the carcinogenicity of various compounds. Males of this strain of mice show a high incidence of spontaneously appearing hepatocellular adenomas (10%) and carcinomas (21%).[65] In one study, Fox and Watanabe[66] conducted experiments designed to determine whether activated oncogenes could be detected in spontaneous hepatic tumors arising in these mice. The results of their study are summarized in Table II. In two separate experiments with tissue from the same mice, they found that DNA from the liver tumors of 6 and 7, respectively, of 11 mice caused transformation of NIH 3T3 cells. Between the two experiments, DNA from 9 of 11 mice was shown to cause transformation. Normal liver tissue from 3- to 5- or 24-month-old mice did not. These results indicate that in 82% of B6C3F$_1$ mice bearing spontaneously appearing tumors, the tumors contained activated oncogenes detectable in the NIH 3T3 focus assay. Furthermore, since control liver DNA did not demonstrate transforming activity, one can conclude that the mutations resulting in oncogene activation occurred in somatic cells and were not in the germ line. However, what is inherited is the predisposition to develop liver tumors, a high percentage of which are associated with activation of an oncogene(s) not identified in this study.

In the second report,[67] the oncogene activated in spontaneously appearing liver adenomas and carcinomas in B6C3F$_1$ mice was identified as c-H-*ras*. These investigators analyzed the DNA from spontaneous tumors appearing in both B6C3F$_1$ mice and Fischer 344 rats for transforming activity in

Table II. Detection of Oncogene Activation in DNA from Control Liver
and Spontaneously Arising Liver Tumors[a,b]

| DNA source | Age (mo.) | Number of cultures transfected | Number of foci | Number of samples with trans. act. |
|---|---|---|---|---|
| | | Experiment 1 | | |
| Hepatic tumors | 24 | 44 | 10 | 6/11 |
| Liver | 3 | 4 | 0 | 0/1 |
| | | Experiment 2 | | |
| Hepatic tumors | 24 | 44 | 14 | 7/11 |
| Liver | 3–5 | 43 | 0 | 0/2 |
| Liver | 24 | 40 | 0 | 0/10 |

[a]Adapted from Fox and Watanabe.[66]
[b]DNA was isolated from spontaneous liver tumor tissue from 11 animals. The DNA was transfected into NIH3T3 cells in two separate experiments. In the first, control DNA was derived from the nontumorous liver of one 3-month-old mouse. In the second experiment, more control liver DNA samples were tested in a greater number of NIH 3T3 cultures. In addition, control liver was obtained from both 3- to 5-month- and 24-month-old animals.

NIH 3T3 cells. Interestingly, DNA from spontaneous tumors from various Fischer 344 rat tissues, not including liver but including mammary adenomas, a pancreatic acinar adenoma, fibrosarcomas, a mammary adenocarcinoma, and others, failed to exhibit transforming activity. This is in contrast to finding that 77% of the B6C3F$_1$ mouse spontaneous hepatocellular carcinomas and 30% of the hepatocellular adenomas were positive in the NIH 3T3 assay.[67] The transforming activity of DNA from the adenomas was probably not due to the presence of a few carcinoma cells, since the transformation efficiency of adenoma and carcinoma DNA was similar, ranging between 0.25 and 0.79. In addition, the presence of transforming activity in adenoma DNA supports the concept that at least in some early lesions, oncogene activation is an early event in the carcinogenic process, as discussed above for skin and mammary carcinogenesis. It is not known whether the adenomas containing an activated oncogene represent precursor lesions at greater risk for developing into carcinomas.

Southern blot analysis of DNA from the NIH 3T3 transformants revealed that the transforming activity of DNA from 3 of the adenomas and 8 of the 10 carcinomas was due to an activated c-H-*ras* oncogene. The transforming activity of DNA from the other two carcinomas was not due to c-H-, c-K-, or N-*ras*. The precise identification of the mutation in the activated mouse c-H-*ras* genes was not determined. However, analysis of the electrophoretic mobilities of the p21 ras proteins in the NIH 3T3 cell transformants by immunoprecipitation of $^{35}$S-labeled cellular extracts with p21 monoclonal antibody Y13-259 showed the presence of a p21 with greater mobility. This indicates that the mutations most likely reside in the 61st codon.[67] These results confirmed and extended the findings of Fox and Watanabe.[66] This mouse strain is predisposed to the development of spontaneous liver tumors, most of which contain a c-H-*ras* oncogene activated by mutation in codon 61.

Several laboratories have begun to study oncogene activation in liver tumors induced by various hepatocarcinogenic chemicals. From the Millers' laboratory, Wiseman et al.[68] recently reported the activation of c-H-*ras* in most hepatomas induced in B6C3F$_1$ mice by treatment with three hepatocarcinogens, i.e., N-hydroxy-2-acetylaminofluorene (N-OH-AAF), vinyl carbamate (VC) and 1'-hydroxy-2',3'-dehydroestragole (HO-DHE). Of the 25 DNA samples tested from hepatomas induced by these three chemicals, all induced transformation of NIH 3T3 cells, indicating the presence of an activated oncogene. Southern blot analysis of DNA from the NIH 3T3 transformants showed that an activated c-H-*ras* oncogene was responsible for the transforming activity of all but one of the hepatomas. The exception was one of 11 hepatomas induced by HO-DHE. The transforming activity of its DNA was found to be due to an activated c-K-*ras* oncogene. Experiments were done to define the mutations present in the hepatomas in order to relate specific mutations to the predominate DNA adducts known to be formed by these three carcinogens. Three types of experiments were conducted. NIH 3T3 transformants induced by DNA from hepatomas which had been induced by the three carcinogens were analyzed for the electrophoretic mobility of their ras p21 proteins. Thus, the cells were labeled with [$^{35}$S]methionine and immunoprecipates formed using the Y13-259 p21 monoclonal antibody were analyzed by sodium dodecyl sulfate polyacrylamide gel electrophoresis (SDS-PAGE). The results showed the presence of p21 proteins with a faster electrophoretic mobility in the c-H-*ras* transformants indicating the presence of a mutation in the 61st codon of the oncogene. This suggested that all three carcinogens had caused activation of the c-H-*ras* oncogene through mutations at this site. Two approaches were then used to identify the specific base change induced by each carcinogen. In the first, NIH 3T3 transformant DNA was analyzed for the presence of an XbaI restriction fragment length polymorphism. An AT to TA transversion in the second nucleotide of codon 61 would create a new XbaI site that could be detected by Southern blot analysis. In the second approach, 20-mer oligonucleotides complementary to the wild type sequence and various possible mutations within the 61st codon were used as probes to identify the specific base changes. The results of this study are shown in Table III. On the basis of other studies, the predicted mutation caused by N-OH-AAF in most cases is a CG to AT transversion which is what was seen in 7 of 7 hepatomas caused by this carcinogen. VC adducts have not been completely characterized but, based on the adducts caused by the closely related vinyl chloride, one would expect mutations involving G. However, the two mutations observed for VC induced hepatomas were AT to TA transversions in 6/7 cases and an AT to GC transition in one case. Finally, most adducts caused by OH-DHE occur with G. However, all the mutations in the DNA of the hepatomas caused by this carcinogen occurred at the AT base pair in the second position of the 61st codon. Thus, the mutations in hepatoma DNA c-H-*ras* oncogenes, while not necessarily what would have been predicted from what is known about the adducts caused by two of the three carcinogens used in this study, clearly indicate that there is carcinogen specificity and that the activation of the c-H-*ras* genes in these tumors was not a spontaneous event. Furthermore, since the hepatoma induction protocol used a single carcinogen dose, these results also support the hypothesis that c-H-*ras* gene mutation leading to its activation was an early event in the carcinogenic process. An additional study reported recently extended these results to seven more carcinogens.[69] Again, the c-H-*ras* oncogene was most frequently activated and the mutations were in the 61st codon. c-K-*ras* activation was also detected in some of the carcinogen-induced hepatomas. These recent results lend further support to the observations that carcinogen treatment results in specific mutations in the c-H-*ras* oncogene in hepatomas of B6C3F$_1$ mice.

Aflatoxin B$_1$ (AFB$_1$) is a potent hepatocarcinogen which has been shown to form predominately a 2,3-dihydro-2-(*N*$^7$-guanyl)-3-hydroxyaflatoxin adduct with guanine in rat liver DNA.[70] In a recent study,[70] DNA from 11 individual tumors present at 52 weeks in eight Fischer 344 rats, treated beginning at weaning with 40 intraperitoneal injections of AFB$_1$, was analyzed for transforming activity in NIH 3T3 cells. Ten of 11 tumor DNAs were positive in the transformation

*Table III. Codon 61 Mutations in the c-H-ras Gene of B6C3F$_1$ Hepatomas$^a$*

| Chemical treatment | Position on codon 61 | | |
|---|---|---|---|
| | 1st | 2nd | |
| | CG → AT | AT → TA | AT → GC |
| N-OH-AAF$^b$ | 7/7 | 0/7 | 0/7 |
| VC$^c$ | 0/7 | 6/7 | 1/7 |
| HO-DHE$^d$ | 0/10 | 5/10 | 5/10 |

$^a$From Wiseman *et al.*[68]
$^b$N-OH-AAF, *N*-hydroxy-2-acetylaminofluorene.
$^c$VC, vinyl carbamate.
$^d$HO-DHE, 1'-hydroxy-2',3'-dehydroestragole.

assay. Southern blot analysis was used to screen the mouse cell transformants for the presence of an activated rat c-H,- c-K-, or N-*ras* oncogene. Transformants caused by transfection of DNA from two separate tumors from each of two individual rats contained rat c-K-*ras* oncogene sequences. Thus, of the 10 tumors positive in the transformation assay, four contained an activated c-K-*ras* oncogene. The transforming activity of the other 6 tumors was not due to c-H-, c-K-, or N-*ras* and remains unidentified.

In a more recent report, McMahon *et al.*,[71] using DNA from the c-K-*ras* NIH 3T3 transformants described in the preceding paragraph, used hybridization with 20-mer oligonucleotides specific for the 12th and 61st codons of the wild type and possible single base mutants of the rat c-K-*ras* oncogene to determine the site of the mutation. Their results revealed the presence of two activated c-K-*ras* alleles containing a GC to AT transition in the first and second positions of the 12th codon. This suggests that both activated alleles were present in DNA from a single liver tumor. The mutation caused by $AFB_1$ is the predicted one based on the predominant adduct formed with DNA. However, the reason for the presence of two alleles within the same tumor is not clear but could be a result of the multiple dose protocol required to produce liver tumors with this carcinogen.

One other group has described studies on liver oncogene activation in tumors appearing following carcinogen treatment.[72–74] DNA from several rat hepatocellular carcinomas induced by 2-amino-3-methylimidazo(4,5-f)quinoline (IQ) was assayed for transforming activity in the NIH 3T3 cell assay. An activated rat c-H-*ras* gene was detected in one of the transformants[72] and an activated c-*raf* oncogene in another.[73] However, subsequent studies revealed the rat c-*raf* oncogene was activated by truncation during the transfection process and thus it had not been present in an activated form in the original hepatoma.[74,75]

There have been several studies in which the expression of oncogenes in chemically induced liver tumors and/or tumor cell lines has been measured. The problems of assessing the relevance of changes in levels of oncogene expression in animal tumors include determining the proper controls for comparison and in the correction for expression due to the increased number of proliferating cells in the tumors. These considerations must be taken into account in interpreting the following data.

Yaswan *et al.*[76] examined the expression of c-K-*ras*, c-H-*ras*, and c-*myc* in the livers from rats fed the carcinogenic choline-deficient diet containing 0.1% ethionine. These workers found that the steady-state levels of mRNA of all three oncogenes had increased by 2 weeks after first feeding the diet and that at 35 weeks, c-K-*ras* and c-*myc* expression was still elevated, but that the increase in c-H-*ras* expression was transient. Analysis of RNA from a primary tumor at 35 weeks revealed an enhancement of c-K-*ras* and c-*myc* expression. They also found that the expression of c-*src* did not change during carcinogenesis, and that levels of c-*abl* and c-*mos* were undetectable. The results of other studies have shown an increased expression of c-*myc* and c-H-*ras* in rat hepatocellular carcinomas induced by (1) diethylnitrosamine and promoted by phenobarbital[77]; (2) aflatoxin $B_1$;[78] and (3) 3'-methyl-4-dimethylaminoazobenzene (MDAB).[79,80] Makino *et al.*,[79] in addition to assessing the expression of these two genes in the MDAB-induced tumors, also examined nontumorous portions of the livers from the same rats and found that expression of c-H-*ras* was elevated to similar levels as in the tumors, but that c-*myc* expression was not increased in comparison to control liver. In a study by Corcos *et al.*,[81] the expression of the *ras* genes was examined in nodules and in perinodular hepatocytes from rats that had been treated with diethylnitrosamine. These investigators found that expression of c-H-, c-K-, and N-*ras* was increased in both the nodules and in the surrounding hepatocytes when compared with normal liver, and that in two rats, there was higher *ras* expression in the perinodular hepatocytes than in tumor tissue from the same animals.

There are two reports in which the expression of oncogenes in Morris hepatomas was assessed. Hayashi *et al.*[82] reported that c-*myc* was overexpressed in three Morris hepatomas (5123D, 7136A, and 7794A). In addition Morris hepatoma 7794A was shown to exhibit a 5- to 10-fold amplification of the c-*myc* gene. Cote *et al.*[80] found an increase in the steady state mRNA levels of c-H-*ras*, c-K-*ras*, and c-*myc* in Morris hepatomas 7800, 7777, 7288c, and 8994 over the levels of these transcripts in normal liver. However, these types of studies are difficult to interpret as to the role of these oncogenes in the development and maintenance of these tumors. It is difficult to separate their functions as transforming genes from those involved in cell proliferation.

To date, there are no published studies that address the question of oncogene activation in spontaneous or chemically induced pancreatic tumors in animal models, although there are several laboratories including our own (in conjunction with D. S. Longnecker) where studies of this nature are currently in progress. However, the induction of pancreatic neoplasia has been accomplished using the novel approach offered by transgenic mice.[83] Quaife *et al.* constructed vectors containing the rat elastase I gene regulatory region linked to either the normal or activated human c-H-*ras* gene, or the c-*myc* gene, and microinjected them separately into fertilized mouse ova. The presence of the elastase promotor and enhancer region ensured the acinar cell-specific expression of the genes. Most of the transgenic mice that carried the construct containing the mutated c-H-*ras* gene developed massive exocrine pancreatic tumors during fetal pancreatic development. No tumors developed in those transgenic mice bearing the normal c-H-*ras* or c-*myc* constructs. These results clearly indicate that in this system, the expression of an activated c-H-*ras* gene during fetal growth is sufficient to cause transformation of the exocrine pancreatic cells, in which the expression is induced. This study represents an important new approach to the study of the role of specific oncogenes in transformation in specific tissues.

## 4. MODULATION OF PROTO-ONCOGENE EXPRESSION DURING LIVER AND PANCREATIC GROWTH

### 4.1. Growth in the Liver

Proto-oncogene expression has been studied during the stimulation of liver proliferation in animals in order to determine which of these genes play a role in normal liver growth. The most comprehensive studies thus far have been done by Fausto and co-workers, who, in a series of reports,[84-87] addressed the expression of proto-oncogenes following 2/3 partial hepatectomy in the rat. They have reported a sequential, transient expression of several nuclear and cytoplasmic proto-oncogenes and have related their induction to the maximal levels of DNA synthesis, which occurs 24 hr after partial hepatectomy. A summary of their results on the expression of c-*fos*, c-*myc*, p53, c-H-*ras*, and c-K-*ras* are depicted in Fig. 1.[87]

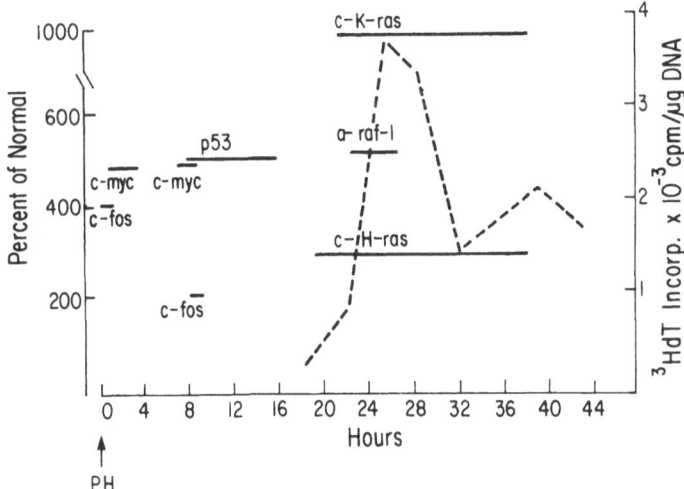

*Figure 1.* Peak expression of six proto-oncogenes following partial hepatectomy (PH) of rats relative to the peak of DNA synthesis (----), which was measured as [³H]d-Thd incorporation into DNA. (From Thompson *et al.*[86] except for a-*raf*-1, which represents the re-expression of data from Silverman *et al.*[88])

The results of these studies show that steady state levels of the nuclear oncogenes, c-*fos*, c-*myc*, and p53 increase during liver regeneration, and reach peak levels prior to the maximum DNA synthetic response. This increase is sequential, with a fourfold induction of c-*fos* expression occurring within 15 min following partial hepatectomy, and preceding the first peak of c-*myc* expression that occurs at 30–120 min. Furthermore, a second phase of increased c-*fos* and c-*myc* expression occurs at 8 hr after partial hepatectomy. The increased expression of these genes is transient. Studies on the expression of p53 during liver regeneration showed that p53 mRNA levels increase fivefold between 8 and 12 hr. In addition, immunoprecipitation and immunoblot analyses of the p53 protein using the monoclonal antibody PAb421 revealed that its steady-state level was maximal between 12 and 15 hr. The results on the regulation of expression of these nuclear oncogenes as well as the time of their maximal induction before the peak of DNA synthesis support their proposed role in cellular events which occur prior to entry into the S phase.

In contrast to the nuclear proto-oncogenes, whose peak induction precedes the time of maximal DNA synthesis following partial hepatectomy, elevated expression of c-H- and c-K-*ras* as well as their products, the p21 proteins, coincides with DNA replication. In addition, studies in our laboratory have shown that expression of the a-*raf*-1 gene also increases with a fivefold induction at 24 hr[88] (Fig. 1). In subsequent studies using nuclear runoff analysis, we have found that the regulation of expression of a-*raf*-1 is transcriptional while that of c-*myc* occurs post-transcriptionally. While it is known that the cytoplasmic oncogenes are involved in signal transduction pathways, their exact role in cellular proliferation has not been elucidated.

In addition to *in vivo* liver studies, proto-oncogene expression has also been studied in cultures of primary rat hepatocytes which can be stimulated to proliferate by mitogens such as epidermal growth factor (EGF).[89] Cell cultures were placed into a medium with or without dialyzed normal rat serum, together with the hormones insulin, glucagon, and EGF. The results of these studies showed that maximal stimulation of c-*fos* expression occurred within 30 min and required the presence of 10% serum and all three hormones. A maximal DNA synthetic response also occurred when both serum and hormones were included in the medium. The authors suggest that induction of c-*fos* may represent a transition from $G_0$ to $G_1$. They also examined the expression of c-H-*ras* following mitogen stimulation and found that its expression was increased between 6 and 24 hr, simulating the delayed increase in c-H-*ras* expression exhibited by liver *in vivo* following partial hepatectomy.

The types of studies represented in this section are important prototypes in determining the role of proto-oncogenes in cell proliferation and may serve to aid in elucidating the mechanisms by which inappropriate expression of at least some of these genes can lead to the loss of control of proliferation.

## 4.2. Growth in the Pancreas

As in the case of oncogene activation in experimentally induced pancreatic tumors, there are no published reports on proto-oncogene expression during pancreatic growth except for our own.[90] We examined the steady-state levels of mRNA for several proto-oncogenes during the initial period of pancreatic regeneration following partial pancreatectomy. A summary of our preliminary results appears in Fig. 2. Using dot-blot hybridization analysis of total RNA isolated from rat pancreas at 3, 12, and 24 hr following partial pancreatectomy, we determined that expression of amylase did not change during this time period. Expression of c-H-*ras* and c-K-*ras* showed a gradual increase up to 24 hr, while c-*myc* expression reached peak levels at 3 hr and then rapidly decreased to normal levels. Our results with c-*myc* were consistent with those observed by Fausto and colleagues in regenerating liver (see Section 4.1), supporting the idea that there is a common sequence of proto-oncogene expression following a growth stimulus. However, knowledge of this pathway in pancreas is limited compared to the extensive studies which have been done in liver. Reasons for the lack of studies with the pancreas may include problems in obtaining intact RNA because of the presence of high levels of RNase, the small size of the tissue, and lack of appreciation for the excellent animal models of pancreatic carcinogenesis that are available. There is clearly a need to continue experimentation in this area on the pancreas.

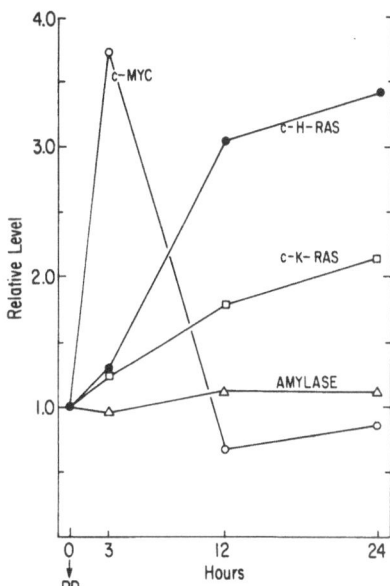

*Figure 2.* Expression of proto-oncogenes in rat pancreas during the initial 24 hr following partial pancreatectomy (PP).

## 5. CONCLUDING REMARKS

The discovery that cellular oncogenes, activated by point mutation, amplification, and/or rearrangement leading to inappropriate expression, are associated with many human neoplasms has led to dramatic increases in our knowledge of human cancer. Since these cellular genes are normally involved in signal transduction pathways regulating cellular growth and differentiation, current research efforts are focusing on the elucidation of these pathways in various cell types. However, finding activated oncogenes in tumors which are the end products of the neoplastic process does not provide much information on whether their activation is an initial obligatory event. This type of information can best be obtained from studies using the animal and cell culture models developed for the study of the specific carcinogenic events. Most of the published reports on studies of this nature in several animal model systems were discussed with a focus on liver and pancreas. It is clear that work on oncogene activation and altered expression in the animal model systems is in its initial stages, and that, particularly in pancreas, there should be a greater focus on these types of studies. The results obtained to date clearly show that the activation of a member of the cellular *ras* gene family occurs frequently in various tissues and that the mutation that is present depends on the carcinogen used. In addition, since most of the studies used single carcinogen dose protocols to initiate the carcinogenic process, the detection of an activated *ras* gene in such high percentages of the tumors is consistent with the hypothesis that *ras* mutation is an early event. The NIH 3T3 cell transformation assay used to detect the presence of activated oncogenes in most of these studies has a bias toward detection of mutated *ras* genes. Assays for activation of other oncogenes are clearly required in order to permit studies aimed to determine whether and when during the carcinogenic process multiple oncogenes become activated. In addition, definitive studies on the causal role for expression of activated oncogenes in the carcinogenic process might require novel approaches, such as introduction into appropriate cells of recombinant constructs containing the oncogene of interest under the transcriptional control of inducible promoters, or the use of transgenic mice. Many laboratories are now beginning to apply molecular genetics technology to cancer research, and we can look forward to the development of considerable new insight into the molecular mechanisms of the carcinogenic process over the next several years.

*Note added in proof*: A recent study by Almoguera *et al.* (*Cell* **53**:549–554, 1988) has shown that 21 of 22 human pancreatic carcinomas tested contained an activated c-K-*ras* gene, with mutations occuring at codon 12.

ACKNOWLEDGMENTS. We wish to acknowledge support from USPHS grant CA 36713 from the National Cancer Institute, which supports our work on oncogene activation and expression in the liver, and grant 83-11 from the Milheim Foundation, which supported the preliminary studies on oncogene expression during pancreatic growth. Norris Cotton Cancer Center Support grant USPHS CA 23108 from the National Cancer Institute has also contributed to the support of our work. We wish to thank Dr. V. F. Ferm, Dr. D. S. Longnecker, and Dr. J. A. Silverman for critical review of the manuscript and Linda Conrad for help with the word processing.

## REFERENCES

1. Bishop, J. M., 1987, The molecular genetics of cancer, *Science* **235**:305–311.
2. Bishop, J. M., 1983, Cellular oncogenes and retroviruses, *Annu. Rev. Biochem.* **52**:301–354.
3. Bishop, J. M., 1985, Viral oncogenes, *Cell* **42**:23–38.
4. Barbacid, M., 1986, Oncogenes and human cancer: cause or consequence?, *Carcinogenesis* **7**:1037–1042.
5. Santos, E., Tronick, S. R., Aaronson, S. A., Pulciani, S., and Barbacid, M., 1982, T24 human bladder carcinoma oncogene is an activated form of the normal human homologue of BALB- and Harvey-MSV transforming genes, *Nature (Lond.)* **298**:343–347.
6. Tabin, C. J., Bradley, S. M., Bargmann, C. I., Weinberg, R. A., Papageorge, A. G., Scolnick, E. M., Dhar, R., Lowy, D. R., and Chang, E. H., 1982, Mechanism of activation of a human oncogene, *Nature (Lond.)* **300**:143–149.
7. Reddy, E. P., Reynolds, R. K., Santos, E., and Barbacid, M., 1982, A point mutation is responsible for the acquisition of transforming properties by the T24 human bladder carcinoma oncogene, *Nature (Lond.)* **300**:149–152.
8. Bos, J. L., Fearon, E. R., Hamilton, S. R., Verlaan-de Vries, M., van Boom, J. H., van der Eb, A. J., and Vogelstein, B., 1987, Prevalence of ras gene mutations in human colorectal cancers, *Nature (Lond.)* **327**:293–297.
9. Forrester, K., Almoguera, C., Han, K., Grizzle, W. E., and Perucho, M., 1987, Detection of high incidence of K-ras oncogenes during human colon tumorigenesis, *Nature (Lond.)* **327**:298–303.
10. Duesberg, P. H., 1987, Cancer genes: Rare recombinants instead of activated oncogenes: A review, *Proc. Natl. Acad. Sci. USA* **84**:2117–2124.
11. Boutwell, R. K., 1974, The function and mechanism of promoters of carcinogenesis, *Crit. Rev. Toxicol.* **2**:419–443.
12. Slaga, T. J., 1983, Overview of tumor promotion in animals, *Environ. Health Perpect.* **50**:3–14.
13. Land, H., Parada, L. F., and Weinberg, R. A., 1983, Tumorigenic conversion of primary embryo fibroblasts requires at least two cooperating oncogenes, *Nature (Lond.)* **304**:596–606.
14. Dotto, G. P., Parada, L. F., and Weinberg, R. A., 1985, Specific growth response of ras-transformed embryo fibroblasts to tumour promoters, *Nature (Lond.)* **318**:471–475.
15. Spandidos, D. A., and Wilkie, N. M., 1984, Malignant transformation of early passage rodent cells by a single mutated human oncogene, *Nature (Lond.)* **310**:469–475.
16. Weinberg, R. A., 1985, The action of oncogenes in the cytoplasm and nucleus, *Science* **230**:770–776.
17. Balmain, A., and Pragnell, I. B., 1983, Mouse skin carcinomas induced in vivo by chemical carcinogens have a transforming Harvey-ras oncogene, *Nature (Lond.)* **303**:72–74.
18. Balmain, A., Ramsden, M., Bowden, G. T., and Smith, J., 1984, Activation of the mouse cellular Harvey-ras gene in chemically induced benign skin papillomas, *Nature (Lond.)* **307**:658–660.
19. Quintanilla, M., Brown, K., Ramsden, M., and Balmain, A., 1986, Carcinogen-specific mutation and amplification of Ha-ras during mouse skin carcinogenesis, *Nature (Lond.)* **322**:78–80.
20. Bizub, D., Wood, A. W., and Skalka, A. M., 1986, Mutagenesis of the Ha-ras oncogene in mouse skin tumors induced by polycyclic aromatic hydrocarbons, *Proc. Natl. Acad. Sci. USA* **83**:6048–6052.
21. Brown, K., Quintanilla, M., Ramsden, M., Kerr, I. B., Young, S., and Balmain, A., 1986, v-ras genes from Harvey and BALB murine sarcoma viruses can act as initiators of two-stage mouse skin carcinogenesis, *Cell* **46**:447–456.
22. Garte, S. J., Hood, A. T., Hochwalt, A. E., D'Eustachio, P., Snyder, C. A., Segal, A., and Albert, R. E.,

1985, Carcinogenesis specificity in the activation of transforming genes by direct-acting alkylating agents, *Carcinogenesis* **6:**1709–1712.

23. Hochwalt, A. E., and Garte, S. J., 1987, An H-ras oncogene from a beta-propriolactone-induced mouse skin tumor is activated by a specific point mutation, *Proc. Am. Assoc. Cancer Res.* **28:**146.

24. Sawey, M. J., Hood, A. T., Burns, F. J., and Garte, S. J., 1987, Activation of c-myc and c-K-ras oncogenes in primary rat tumors induced by ionizing radiation, *Mol. Cell. Biol.* **7:**932–935.

25. Guerrero, I., Villasante, A., D'Eustachio, P., and Pellicer, A., 1984, Isolation, characterization, and chromosome assignment of mouse N-ras gene from carcinogen-induced thymic lymphoma, *Science* **225:**1041–1043.

26. Guerrero, I., Villasante, A., Corces, V., and Pellicer, A., 1984, Activation of a c-K-ras oncogene by somatic mutation in mouse lymphomas induced by gamma radiation, *Science* **225:**1159–1162.

27. Guerrero, I., Villsante, A., Corces, V., and Pellicer, A., 1985, Loss of the normal N-ras allele in a mouse thymic lymphoma induced by a chemical carcinogen, *Proc. Natl. Acad. Sci. USA* **82:**7810–7814.

28. Schechter, A. L., Stern, D. F., Vaidyanathan, L., Decker, S. J., Drebin, J. A., Greene, M. I., and Weinberg, R. A., 1984, The neu oncogene: An erb-B-related gene encoding a 185,000-$M_r$ tumour antigen, *Nature (Lond.)* **312:**513–516.

29. Bargmann, C. I., Hung, M.-C., and Weinberg, R. A., 1986, Multiple independent activations of the neu oncogene by a point mutation altering the transmembrane domain of p185, *Cell* **45:**649–657.

30. Sukumar, S., Notario, V., Martin-Zanca, D., and Barbacid, M., 1983, Induction of mammary carcinomas in rats by nitroso-methylurea involves malignant activation of H-ras-1 locus by single point mutation, *Nature (Lond.)* **306:**658–661.

31. Zarbl, H., Sukumar, S., Arthur, A. V., Martin-Zanca, D., and Barbacid, M., 1985, Direct mutagenesis of Ha-ras-1 oncogenes by N-nitroso-N-methylurea during initiation of mammary carcinogenesis in rats, *Nature (Lond.)* **315:**382–385.

32. Peraino, C., Fry, R. J. M., and Staffeldt, E., 1971, Reduction and enhancement by phenobarbital of hepatocarcinogenesis induced in the rat by 2-acetylaminofluorene, *Cancer Res.* **31:**1506–1512.

33. Lombardi, B., and Shinozuka, H., 1979, Enhancement of 2-acetylaminofluorene liver carcinogenesis in rats fed a choline-devoid diet, *Int. J. Cancer* **23:**565–570.

34. Yager, J. D., Campbell, H. A., Longnecker, D. S., Roebuck, B. D., and Benoit, M. C., 1984, Enhancement of hepatocarcinogenesis in female rats by ethinyl estradiol and mestranol but not estradiol, *Cancer Res.* **44:**3862–3869.

35. Longnecker, D. S., Roebuck, B. D., Yager, J. D., Lilja, H. S., and Siegmund, B., 1981, Pancreatic carcinoma in azaserine-treated rats: Induction, classification and dietary modulation of incidence, *Cancer* **47:**1562–1572.

36. Longnecker, D. S., 1986, Experimental models of exocrine pancreatic tumors, in: *The Exocrine Pancreas: Biology, Pathobiology and Diseases* (V. L. W. Go, J. D. Gardner, F. P. Brooks, E. Lebenthal, E. P. DiMagno, and G. A. Scheele, eds.), pp. 443–458, Raven, New York.

37. Pour, P. M., Runge, R. G., Birt, D., Gingell, R., Lawson, T., Nagel, D., Wallcave, L., and Salmasi, S. Z., 1981, Current knowledge of pancreatic carcinogenesis in the hamster and its relevance to the human disease, *Cancer* **47:**1573–1587.

38. Roebuck, B. D., Yager, J. D., Jr., and Longnecker, D. S., 1981, Dietary modulation of azaserine-induced pancreatic carcinogenesis in the rat, *Cancer Res.* **41:**888–893.

39. Roebuck, B. D., Yager, J. D., Jr., Longnecker, D. S., and Wilpone, S. A., 1981, Promotion by unsaturated fat of azaserine-induced pancreatic carcinogenesis in the rat, *Cancer Res.* **41:**3961–3966.

40. Birt, D. F., Salmasi, S., and Pour, P. M., 1981, Enhancement of experimental pancreatic cancer in Syrian golden hamsters by dietary fat, *J. Natl. Cancer Inst.* **67:**1327–1332.

41. Woutersen, R. A., van Garderen-Hoetmer, A., and Longnecker, D. S., 1987, Characterization of a 4-month protocol for the quantitation of BOP-induced lesions in hamster pancreas and its application in studying the effect of dietary fat, *Carcinogenesis* **8:**833–837.

42. Morgan, R. G. H., Levinson, D. A., Hopwood, D., Saunders, J. H. B., and Wormsley, K. G., 1979, Potentiation of the action of azaserine on the rat pancreas by raw soya bean flour, *Cancer Lett.* **3:**87–90.

43. Roebuck, B. D., Kaplita, P. V., and MacMillan, D. L., 1985, Interaction of dietary fat and soybean isolate (SBI) on azaserine-induced pancreatic carcinogenesis, *Qual. Plant Foods. Hu. Nutr.* **35:**323–329.

44. Roebuck, B. D., Kaplita, P. V., Edwards, B. R., and Praissman, M., 1987, Effects of dietary fats and soybean protein on azaserine-induced pancreatic carcinogenesis and plasma cholecystokinin in the rat, *Cancer Res.* **47:**1333–1338.

45. Longnecker, D., Lhoste, E., and Roebuck, B. D., 1987, Enhancement of growth and conversion of phenotype in azaserine induced acinar cell foci of rats fed FOY-305, *Fed. Proc.* **46:**586.

46. Lhoste, E. F., and Longnecker, D. S., 1987, Effect of bombesin and caerulein on early stages of carcinogenesis induced by azaserine in the rat pancreas, *Cancer Res.* **47**:3273–3277.

47. Harris, C. C., and Sun, T.-t., 1984, Multifactoral etiology of human liver cancer, *Carcinogenesis* **5**:697–701.

48. Gu, J.-R., Hu, L.-F., Cheng, Y.-C., and Wan, D.-F., 1986, Oncogenes in human primary hepatic cancer, *J. Cell. Physiol. (Suppl.)* **4**:13–20.

49. Ochiya, T., Fujiyama, A., Fukushige, S., Hatada, I., and Matsubara, K., 1986, Molecular cloning of an oncogene from a human hepatocellular carcinoma. *Proc. Natl. Acad. Sci. USA* **83**:4993–4997.

50. Notario, V., Sukumar, S., Santos, E., and Barbacid, M., 1984, A common mechanism for the malignant activation of ras oncogenes in human neoplasia and in chemically induced animal tumors, in: *Cancer Cells, Oncogenes and Viral Genes* (G. F. Vande Woude, A. J. Levine, W. C. Topp, and J. D. Watson, eds.), pp. 425–432, Cold Spring Harbor Laboratory, Cold Spring Harbor, New York.

51. Huber, B. E., Dearfield, K. L., Williams, J. R., Heilman, C. A., and Thorgeirsson, S. S., 1985, Tumorigenicity and transcriptional modulation of c-myc and N-ras oncogenes in a human hepatoma cell line, *Cancer Res.* **45**:4322–4329.

52. Su, T.-S., Lin, L.-H., Lui, W.-Y., Chang, C., Chou, C.-K., Ting, L.-P., Hu, C.-P., Han, S.-H., and P'eng, F.-K., 1985, Expression of c-myc gene in human hepatoma, *Biochem. Biophys. Res. Commun.* **132**:264–268.

53. Motoo, Y., Mahmoudi, M., Osther, K., and Bollon, A. P., 1986, Oncogene expression in human hepatoma cells PLC/PRF/5, *Biochem. Biophys. Res. Commun.* **135**:262–268.

54. Zhang, X.-K., Huang, D.-P., Chiu, D.-K., and Chiu, J.-F., 1987, The expression of oncogenes in human developing liver and hepatomas, *Biochem. Biophys. Res. Commun.* **142**:932–938.

55. Calabretta, B., Kaczmarek, L., Ming, P.-M. L., Au, F., and Ming, S.-C., 1985, Expression of c-myc and other cell cycle-dependent genes in human colon neoplasia, *Cancer Res.* **45**:6000–6004.

56. Mack, T. M., 1982, Pancreas, in: *Cancer Epidemiology and Prevention* (D. Schottenfeld and J. F. Fraumeni, Jr., eds.), pp. 638–667, W. B. Saunders, Philadelphia.

57. Pulciani, S., Santos, E., Lauver, A. V., Long, L. K., Aaronson, S. A., and Barbacid, M., 1982, Oncogenes in solid human tumors, *Nature (Lond.)* **300**:539–542.

58. Der, C. J., and Cooper, G. M., 1983, Altered gene products are associated with activation of cellular ras$^k$ genes in human lung and colon carcinomas, *Cell* **32**:201–208.

59. Hirai, H., Okabe, T., Anraku, Y., Fujisawa, M., Urabe, A., and Takaku, F., 1985, Activation of the c-K-ras oncogene in a human pancreas carcinoma, *Biochem. Biophys. Res. Commun.* **127**:168–174.

60. Cooper, C. S., Blair, D. G., Oskarsson, M. K., Tainsky, M. A., Eader, L. A., and Vande Woude, G. F., 1984, Characterization of human transforming genes for chemically transformed, teratocarcinoma, and pancreatic carcinoma cell lines, *Cancer Res.* **44**:1–10.

61. O'Hara, B. M., Oskarsson, M., Tainsky, M. A., and Blair, D. G., 1986, Mechanism of activation of human ras genes cloned from a gastric adenocarcinoma and a pancreatic carcinoma cell line, *Cancer Res.* **46**:4695–4700.

62. Yamada, H., Sakamoto, H., Taira, M., Nishimura, S., Shimosato, Y., Terada, M., and Sugimura, T., 1986, Amplifications of both c-Ki-ras with a point mutation and c-myc in a primary pancreatic cancer and its metastatic tumors in lymph nodes, *Jpn. J. Cancer Res. (Gann)* **77**:370–375.

63. Yamada, H., Yoshida, T., Sakamoto, H., Terada, M., and Sugimura, T., 1986, Establishment of a human pancreatic adenocarcinoma cell line (PSN-1) with amplifications of both c-myc and activated c-Ki-ras by a point mutation, *Biochem. Biophys. Res. Commun.* **140**:167–173.

64. Hollingsworth, M. A., Rebellato, L. M., Moore, J. W., Finn, O. J., and Metzgar, R. S., 1986, Antigens expressed on NIH 3T3 cells following transformation with DNA from a human pancreatic tumor, *Cancer Res.* **46**:2482–2487.

65. Maronpot, R. R., Haseman, J. K., Boorman, G. A., Eustis, S. E., Rao, G. N., and Huff, J. E., 1987, Liver lesions in B6C3F1 mice: The National Toxicology Program, experience and position, *Arch. Toxicol. (Suppl.)* **10**:10–26.

66. Fox, T. R., and Watanabe, P. G., 1985, Detection of a cellular oncogene in spontaneous liver tumors of B6C3F1 mice, *Science* **228**:596–597.

67. Reynolds, S. H., Stowers, S. J., Maronpot, R. R., Anderson, M. W., and Aaronson, S. A., 1986, Detection and identification of activated oncogenes in spontaneously occurring benign and malignant hepatocellular tumors of the B6C3F1 mouse, *Proc. Natl. Acad. Sci. USA* **83**:33–37.

68. Wiseman, R. W., Stowers, S. J., Miller, E. C., Anderson, M. W., and Miller, J. A., 1986, Activating mutations of the c-Ha-ras protooncogene in chemically induced hepatomas of the male B6C3F$_1$ mouse, *Proc. Natl. Acad. Sci. USA* **83**:5825–5829.

69. Wiseman, R. W., Stewart, B. C., Grenier, D., Miller, E. C., and Miller, J. A., 1987, Characterization of c-Ha-ras proto-oncogene mutations in chemically induced hepatomas of the B6C3F$_1$ mouse, *Proc. Am. Assoc. Cancer Res.* **28:**147.

70. McMahon, G., Hanson, L., Lee, J.-J., and Wogan, G. N., 1986, Identification of an activated c-Ki-ras oncogene in rat liver tumors induced by aflatoxin B$_1$, *Proc. Natl. Acad. Sci. USA* **83:**9418–9422.

71. McMahon, G., Davis, E., and Wogan, G. N., 1987, Characterization of c-Ki-ras oncogene alleles by direct sequencing of enzymatically amplified DNA from carcinogen-induced tumors, *Proc. Natl. Acad. Sci. USA* **84:**4974–4978.

72. Ishikawa, F., Takaku, F., Nagao, M., Ochiai, M., Hayashi, K., Takayama, S., and Sugimura, T., 1985, Activated oncogenes in a rat hepatocellular carcinoma induced by 2-amino-3-methylimidazo[5,4-f]quinoline, *Jpn. J. Cancer Res. (Gann)* **76:**425–428.

73. Ishikawa, F., Takaku, F., Ochiai, M., Hayashi, K., Hirohashi, S., Terada, M., Takayama, S., Nagao, M., and Sugimura, T., 1985, Activated c-raf gene in a rat hepatocellular carcinoma induced by 2-amino-3-methylimidazo[4,5-f]quinoline, *Biochem. Biophys. Res. Commun.* **132:**186–192.

74. Ishikawa, F., Takaku, F., Hayashi, K., Nagao, M., and Sugimura, T., 1986, Activation of rat c-raf during transfection of hepatocellular carcinoma DNA, *Proc. Natl. Acad. Sci. USA* **83:**3209–3212.

75. Ishikawa, F., Takaku, F., Nagao, M., and Sugimura, T., 1987, Rat c-raf oncogene activation by a rearrangement that produces a fused protein, *Mol. Cell. Biol.* **7:**1226–1232.

76. Yaswen, P., Goyette, M., Shank, P. R., and Fausto, N., 1985, Expression of c-Ki-ras, c-Ha-ras, and c-myc in specific cell types during hepatocarcinogenesis, *Mol. Cell. Biol.* **5:**780–786.

77. Beer, D. G., Schwarz, M., Sawada, N., and Pitot, H. C., 1986, Expression of H-ras and c-myc protoon-cogenes in isolated γ-glutamyl transpeptidase-positive rat hepatocytes and in hepatocellular carcinomas induced by diethylnitrosamine, *Cancer Res.* **46:**2435–2441.

78. Tashiro, F., Morimura, S., Hayashi, K., Makino, R., Kawamura, H., Horikoshi, N., Nemoto, K., Ohtsubo, K., Sugimura, T., and Ueno, Y., 1986, Expression of the c-Ha-ras and c-myc genes in aflatoxin B$_1$-induced hepatocellular carcinomas, *Biochem. Biophys. Res. Commun.* **138:**858–864.

79. Makino, R., Hayashi, K., Sato, S., and Sugimura, T., 1984, Expressions of the c-Ha-ras and c-myc genes in rat liver tumors, *Biochem. Biophys. Res. Commun.* **119:**1096–1102.

80. Cote, G. J., Lastra, B. A., Cook, J. R., Huang, D.-P., and Chiu, J.-F., 1985, Oncogene expression in rat hepatomas and during hepatocarcinogenesis, *Cancer Lett.* **26:**121–127.

81. Corcos, D., Defer, N., Raymondjean, M., Paris, B., Corral, M., Tichonicky, L., Kruh, J., Glaise, D., Saulnier, A. and Guguen-Guillouzo, C., 1984, Correlated increase of the expression of the c-ras genes in chemically induced hepatocarcinomas, *Biochem. Biophys. Res. Commun.* **122:**259–264.

82. Hayashi, K., Makino, R., and Sugimura, T., 1984, Amplification and over-expression of the c-myc gene in Morris hepatomas, *Gann* **75:**475–478.

83. Quaife, C. J., Pinkert, C. A., Ornitz, D. M., Palmiter, R. D., and Brinster, R. L., 1987, Pancreatic neoplasia induced by expression in acinar cells of transgenic mice, *Cell* **48:**1023–1034.

84. Goyette, M., Petropoulos, C. J., Shank, P. R., and Fausto, N., 1983, Expression of a cellular oncogene during liver regeneration, *Science* **219:**510–512.

85. Fausto, N., and Shank, P. R., 1983, Oncogene expression in liver regeneration and hepatocarcinogenesis, *Hepatology* **3:**1016–1023.

86. Goyette, M., Petropoulos, C. J., Shank, P. R., and Fausto, N., 1984, Regulated transcription of c-Ki-ras and c-myc during compensatory growth of rat liver, *Mol. Cell. Biol.* **4:**1493–1498.

87. Thompson, N. L., Mead, J. E., Braun, L., Goyette, M., Shank, P. R., and Fausto, N., 1986, Sequential protooncogene expression during rat liver regeneration, *Cancer Res.* **46:**3111–3117.

88. Silverman, J. A., Zurlo, J., and Yager, J. D., 1988, Mechanisms of regulation of a-raf-1, c-raf-1, c-myc, and c-H-ras during regenerative growth of the rat liver (submitted).

89. Kruijer, W., Skelly, H., Botteri, F., van der Putten, H., Barber, J. R., Verma, I. M., and Leffert, H. L., 1986, Proto-oncogene expression in regenerating liver is simulated in cultures of primary adult rat hepatocytes, *J. Biol. Chem.* **261:**7929–7933.

90. Zurlo, J., and Yager, J. D., 1985, Oncogene expression during pancreatic regeneration and in chemically induced pancreatic and liver carcinomas in the rat, *Fed. Proc.* **44:**1943.

# 21

# Oncodevelopmental Expression and Neoplasia

## Alphonse E. Sirica

## 1. INTRODUCTION

One of the earliest investigators to associate neoplasia with development was Julius Cohnheim,[1] who in 1877 first proposed his embryonal rest theory of malignant neoplasia. Thirty-two years later, Adami provided one of the best known attempts to classify neoplasms on an embryologic basis.[2] Although these earlier efforts are now best accepted more for their historic value than for their scientific merit, they do serve to demonstrate that the developmental approach toward attempting to understand the neoplastic process is not new. However, it has only been within the past 20 years or so that the biochemical and molecular aspects of development as related to neoplasia have come to be appreciated. In this context, it is not surprising that in recent years neoplasia has come to be referred to as being a problem in developmental biology.[3–5] Perhaps even more relevant is the fact that malignant neoplasia is now frequently described as being a disease of differentiation.[6,7]

Oncodevelopmental expression relates to the production of cellular substances common to both developmental and neoplastic cells.[8] Here, developmental cells include those of the embryo, fetus, and placenta. Such substances are found for the most part not to be produced at all, or are produced at very low levels, by normal differentiated cells of the adult organism. In this regard, specific antigens, proteins, and enzymes elaborated by particular developmental cells either disappear or decrease to low levels at or shortly after birth, to be replaced within a defined period of time by a postnatal or "adult" pattern of phenotypic expression. By contrast, it is common for such developmental substances to reappear in neoplastic cells, particularly in those of malignant neoplasms.

## 2. ONCODEVELOPMENTAL ANTIGENS, PROTEINS, AND ENZYMES IN MALIGNANT NEOPLASMS

Table I lists diverse examples of oncodevelopmental substances, including antigens, proteins, enzymes, and isozymes that have been demonstrated to be produced by various types of human or rodent malignant neoplasms derived from adult somatic tissues.[9–67] In addition, studies of human neoplasms have shown α-fetoprotein (AFP), which is produced predominantly by hepatocellular carcinoma and germinal neoplasms, to also be expressed in some gastric, pancreatic, and pulmonary

*Alphonse E. Sirica* • Department of Pathology, Medical College of Virginia, Virginia Commonwealth University, Richmond, Virginia 23298.

Table I. Examples of Oncodevelopmental Antigens, Proteins, and Enzymes Expressed by Malignant Neoplasms of Adult Human and Rodent Somatic Tissues

| Oncodevelopmental substance | Classification | Species | Developmental tissues | Malignant neoplasms | References |
|---|---|---|---|---|---|
| α-Fetoprotein | Glycoprotein antigen | Mouse, rat, human | Fetal liver, yolk sac | Hepatocellular carcinomas | 9,10 |
| Carcinoembryonic antigen | Glycoprotein antigen | Human | Fetal alimentary tract, fetal pancreas, fetal liver | Colorectal carcinomas and a variety of other types of carcinomas | 11–13 |
| Large external antigen | Glycoprotein antigen | Human | Fetal colon, fetal biliary epithelium | Colorectal carcinomas | 14 |
| $M_1$ antigens | Mucin antigens | Human, rat | Fetal colon | Colorectal carcinomas | 15,16 |
| 660 antigen | Mucin-type glycoprotein antigen | Rat | Fetal goblet cells | Colonic and duodenal carcinoma | 73 |
| Stage-specific embryonic antigen 1 | Carbohydrate differentiation antigen | Human | Fetal colon, mouse embryo | Colorectal carcinomas | 17,18 |
| Second-trimester fetal antigen | — | Human | Second-trimester embryo organ extracts | Colorectal carcinomas | 19,20 |
| Tumor-associated glycoprotein-72 | Glycoprotein antigen | Human | Fetal colon, fetal stomach, fetal esophagus | A variety of carcinomas, including colorectal carcinomas, ovarian carcinomas, breast ductal carcinomas, pancreatic, gastric, and esophageal carcinomas | 21 |
| β-Oncofetal antigen | Protein antigen | Human | Various fetal organs and tissues | A number of different carcinoma cell types, including those of colorectal and pancreatic carcinomas | 22,23 |
| Pancreatic oncofetal antigen | Glycoprotein antigen | Human | Fetal pancreas | Pancreatic carcinomas | 24,25 |
| 58,000- and 80,000-$M_r$ pancreatic fetal acinar antigens | Glycoprotein antigens | Hamster | Fetal pancreas | Chemically induced pancreatic carcinomas | 26 |
| Fetal sulfoglycoprotein antigen | Sulfoglycoprotein antigen | Human | Fetal stomach | Gastric carcinomas | 23 |

| | | | | | |
|---|---|---|---|---|---|
| Oncofetal antigen-1 | Cell membrane antigen | Human | Fetal brain | Malignant melanomas and a wide variety of histologic types of malignant neoplasms, particularly those of ectodermal and mesodermal origin | 27 |
| Murine γ-fetal antigen | Protein antigen | Mouse | Fetal trunk and a number of fetal organs, including spleen, lung, and liver | A number of histologically diverse malignant neoplasms, and in particular, certain fibrosarcomas | 28–31 |
| Fibroblast oncofetal antigen | Glycoprotein antigen | Human | Fetal connective tissue cells | Histologically diverse sarcomas | 32 |
| Fetal thymocyte antigen FT-1 | Glycoprotein antigen | Mouse | Fetal thymocytes | T leukemia cells | 33 |
| Carcinofetal isoferritins | β-Globulin | Human | Fetal liver | Hepatocellular carcinoma and some other types of carcinomas | 34 |
| Oncofetal keratins | Cytokeratin antigens | Human | Non-stratified fetal epidermis | SV40-transformed keratinocytes | 35 |
| Oncofetal domain of fibronectin | Antigenic region | Human | Fetal connective tissue, fetal fibroblasts, placenta | Hepatocellular and colon carcinomas; some hepatoma and sarcoma cell lines | 36 |
| "Oncofetal" basic non-histone phosphoprotein | DNA-binding phosphoprotein | Rat | Fetal liver | Rat hepatocellular carcinomas and two human tumor cell lines | 37 |
| γ-Glutamyl transpeptidase | Enzyme | Rat, human | Fetal liver | Hepatocellular carcinomas | 38,39 |
| Aldolase A | Isozyme | Rat, human | Fetal liver | Hepatocellular carcinomas | 40–43 |
| Pyruvate kinase K, $M_2$, or III | Isozyme | Rat, human | Fetal liver | Hepatocellular carcinomas | 44–48 |
| Glycogen phosphoylase F | Isozyme | Rat | Fetal liver | Hepatocellular carcinomas | 48 |
| Hexokinase I, II, III | Isozyme | Rat | Fetal liver | Hepatocellular carcinomas | 49,50 |
| Branched-chain amino acid transaminase 1 | Isozyme | Rat | Fetal liver | Hepatocellular carcinomas | 51,52 |

(continued)

Table I. (Continued)

| Oncodevelopmental substance | Classification | Species | Developmental tissues | Malignant neoplasms | References |
|---|---|---|---|---|---|
| Glutaminase (fetal/kidney) | Isozyme | Rat | Fetal liver | Hepatocellular carcinomas | 53 |
| UDP-glucuronyltransferase-oGT form | Isozyme | Rat | Late fetal liver | Hepatocellular carcinomas | 54,55 |
| Glutathione S-transferase-A | Isozyme | Rat | Fetal liver | Hepatocellular carcinomas | 55,56 |
| Thymidine kinase F | Isozyme | Human | Fetal liver | A number of diverse malignant neoplasms, including those of breast and colon, as well as some carcinoma cell lines and SV40-transformed fibroblasts | 57–59 |
| Creatine kinase BB | Isozyme | Rat | Neonatal prostate | Prostatic carcinomas | 60 |
| Alkaline phosphatase (Regan) | Isozyme | Human | Placenta | A number of different nontrophoblastic carcinoma cell types | 61,62 |
| Glutathione S-transferase-P | Isozyme | Rat, human | Placenta | Rat hepatocellular carcinomas, human colonic carcinoma | 56,63,64 |
| Human chorionic gonadotropin | Glycoprotein hormone | Human | Placenta | A number of histologically diverse, nontrophoblastic malignant neoplasms | 65,66 |
| $SP_1$ | Pregnancy-specific $\beta_1$-glycoprotein | Human | Placenta | Some types of nontrophoblastic malignant neoplasms | 67 |

carcinomas,[65] as well as in a rare case of rectal carcinoma.[68] Oncoplacental substances, such as human chorionic gonadotropin (hCG) and placental alkaline phosphatase, are further found to be associated with trophoblastic neoplasms and with teratocarcinomas.[8] Other reported examples of oncodevelopmental expression by human malignant neoplasms not listed in Table I include the elaboration of carcinoembryonic antigenlike substances,[69] other placental and fetal isozymes of alkaline phosphatase,[8] and some embryonic or fetal nucleolar antigens.[70] Furthermore, complementary DNA (cDNA) have been cloned for proteins specifically expressed in rat embryo and in a chemically induced rat pancreatic β-cell tumor.[71]

Oncodevelopmental expression has also been determined to be associated with specific preneoplastic conditions, as well as shown to occur during the early stages of experimental chemical carcinogenesis. For example, in the rat, preneoplastic hepatocellular lesions have been found to exhibit relatively high activities of the fetal liver enzyme γ-glutamyl transpeptidase,[38] of the late fetal liver isozymic form of UDP-glucuronyltransferase,[55,72] and of the fetal liver and placental isozymic forms of glutathione S-transferase.[55,63,72] In addition, in the human, the expression of specific oncodevelopmental antigens, including oncofetal mucin M1 antigens,[16] stage-specific embryonic antigen 1,[17] and second-trimester fetal antigen,[20] have been reported to be associated with preneoplastic conditions of the colon, while oncofetal M1 antigens have also been demonstrated to be produced in rat colonic mucosa during the early stages of 1,2-dimethylhydrazine-induced colon carcinogenesis.[15] More recently, a novel mucin-associated antigen, termed 660 antigen, has been identified in precancerous epithelial lesions that were induced in rat colon during chemical carcinogenesis with dimethylhydrazine.[73] Furthermore, a 60,000-$M_r$ oncofetal protein has been shown to be induced early in rats treated with a number of different chemical carcinogens, as well as to be present in the plasma of tumor-bearing animals.[74–76]

As is the case with other markers of neoplasia, malignant neoplasms are also characterized by phenotypic heterogeneity with respect to their expression of oncodevelopmental substances. This heterogeneity can be clearly seen in terms of the patterns of AFP production and fetal liver enzymes exhibited by human and rodent hepatocellular carcinomas. Human hepatocellular carcinomas have been demonstrated to produce AFP in widely differing amounts, with the highest levels of production tending to be associated with the more poorly differentiated tumors.[12] Also, aneuploid, more rapidly growing rat hepatocellular carcinomas were found, in general, to produce higher levels of AFP than those which were near diploid and more slowly growing.[10,76] However, obvious exceptions were also noted. In addition, immunohistochemical studies of AFP production by both human and rodent hepatocellular carcinomas showed that only a fraction of the neoplastic cells within given tumors were positively stained for this antigen.[78,79] The production of AFP during hepatocarcinogenesis in rodents was further shown not to be linked to expression of the fetal liver enzyme γ-glutamyl transpeptidase in preneoplastic and neoplastic hepatocytes,[80,81] and as yet, no clear-cut correlations have been made between patterns of AFP production and fetal liver isozymes expressed by hepatocellular carcinomas.

Sato and associates[48,82] have investigated the patterns of fetal liver isozymes, including those of pyruvate kinase, aldolase, and hexokinase, expressed by rat primary hepatocellular carcinomas of different histologic grades. In general, the more anaplastic and poorly differentiated hepatocellular carcinomas showed the highest levels of the various fetal liver isozymes when compared with well- and moderately differentiated tumors, but there was considerable variation as indicated by large standard deviations in the individual fetal isozyme activities exhibited by each class of tumor. Messenger RNA (mRNA) levels for the fetal liver form of aldolase were also reported to be higher in poorly differentiated hepatocellular carcinomas.[83] In comparison, carcinogen-induced hyperplastic liver nodules of the rat have been found to possess measurable, but lower, activities of fetal liver isozymes than those of hepatocellular carcinomas.[48,82] By contrast, such preneoplastic liver lesions have been shown in most cases to express a γ-glutamyl transpeptidase activity comparable in amount to that of malignant hepatocellular neoplasms[82,84] but, unlike the malignant tumors, hyperplastic liver nodules have been found, for the most part, not to contain AFP.[85–87] Furthermore, while the expression of γ-glutamyl transpeptidase and the placental form of glutathione S-transferase has been demonstrated to be common in preneoplastic liver foci and nodules and in hepatocellular neoplasms induced in the rat by various types of hepatocarcinogenic regimens,[63,84,88] it was recently found that the majority of such lesions resulting from treatments with several forms of hepatocarcinogenic peroxisome proliferators were devoid of both oncodevelopmental marker enzymes.[89]

Evidence for heterogeneity in the expression of oncodevelopmental substances can also be found for other types of neoplasms. For example, carcinoembryonic antigen (CEA) and stage-specific embryonic antigen 1 have been demonstrated to be heterogeneously expressed in human colorectal carcinomas.[18] The secretion of human chorionic gonadotropin by specific types of human nontrophoblastic neoplasms has also been shown to be variable.[66] Also, human colon and breast carcinomas were observed to contain different percentages of cells, ranging from 0 to >90%, which were positive for oncofetal antigen tumor-associated glycoprotein-72.[21]

## 3. CONCEPTS OF STEM CELLS, BLOCKED AND PARTIALLY BLOCKED ONTOGENY, AND RETRODIFFERENTIATION IN NEOPLASTIC CELL DEVELOPMENT

Three relevant concepts have been developed over the past 18 years or so, each compatible in descriptive terms with both oncodevelopmental expression and phenotypic heterogeneity in neoplasia. These are the stem cell concept of neoplastic cell development, growth, and differentiation advocated by Pierce[4,90] and more recently by others,[91,92] the concepts of oncogeny as blocked ontogeny and as partially blocked ontogeny developed by Potter,[93,94] and retrodifferentiation in neoplasia formulated by Uriel.[95,96]

The stem cell concept proposes that the target cell in carcinogenesis is the stem cells present in normal tissue and their partially differentiated progeny. According to Pierce et al.,[4] the state of differentiation characterizing a particular neoplasm is dependent on the stage of stem cell maturation at which the carcinogenic event occurred. For example, if the undifferentiated stem cell is the target, a more anaplastic and less differentiated neoplasm would be expected to develop. On the other hand, a benign neoplasm would be the result if the stem cell target is one at an almost terminal stage of differentiation. Malignant neoplasms exhibiting intermediate degrees of differentiation between well and poorly differentiated forms would be expected to be derived from stem cell progeny targeted during intermediate stages of maturation. Thus, in this view, the ability of neoplasms to exhibit particular patterns of tissue specific differentiation and oncodevelopmental expression can be considered to be a function of the state of differentiation of a given target stem cell in carcinogenesis. This carcinogenic event, in turn, is believed by some to result in a block, arrest, or derangement in differentiation, which occurs during the stages of normal stem cell maturation,[90,91,97] or it may be the cause of an imbalance between cellular proliferation and differentiation.[90]

In emphasizing the importance of studies on fetal tissues, when evaluating the biochemistry of malignant neoplasia, Potter first put forth the concept of oncogeny as blocked ontogeny in 1969.[93,98] This concept, which was developed in large part from studies done on biochemically diverse transplantable hepatocellular carcinomas and preneoplastic liver of the rat, holds that adult tissue cells that undergo differentiation by a process of reontogeny following cell division may be blocked during carcinogenesis at any one of a number of intermediate stages of differentiation.[98] Phenotypic heterogeneity and patterns of oncodevelopmental expression shown by resulting neoplasms would then be dictated by combinations of blocks and by the stages at which the blockages of differentiation occurred.[98] Potter further emphasized his view that this concept should be particularly understood in terms of blocks in the ontogeny of individual proteins[6] and that, while malignant neoplastic tissues might express fetal characteristics, they are also quite distinct from fetal tissues, since they are unable to recapitulate the total program that develops during normal differentiation because this program is blocked.[6]

In 1978, Potter extended his concept of oncogeny as blocked ontogeny by formulating the concept of partially blocked ontogeny.[94] In particular, this extension was intended to account for the highly differentiated slow-growing tumors containing some cells that have left the proliferating pool to differentiate along the normal pathways, but that are blocked somewhere short of the final differentiation state. Potter labeled the products of differentiated cell as organism-serving molecules. In this context, he proposed that any neoplasm that produces an organism-serving molecule is an example of partially blocked ontogeny.

While blocked differentiation does fit with the process of neoplastic development from targeted stem cells or from adult cells undergoing reontogeny, the concept of reversion of adult cells must also be considered as a way of explaining oncodevelopmental expression by neoplastic tissues. In this regard, Uriel[95,96] suggested that retrodifferentiation may be implicated in the carcinogenic induction of neoplasms emerging from adult differentiated tissues. Retrodifferentiation refers to the sequence of nucleocytoplasmic events that are inverse to those of differentiation. Thus, it indicates a stepwise reversion during carcinogenesis of the normal adult cell state of differentiation to pre-neoplastic and neoplastic stages that then exhibit varying and progressive degrees of immaturity.

While there is evidence to support all three of these concepts, generalizations concerning the overall application and validity of each are subject to question. This is so, by virtue of (1) the existence of specific exceptions, (2) the lack of appropriate studies designed to distinguish between them,[99] and (3) doubts that have arisen concerning the making of generalizations that relate neoplasia to embryologic or fetal states of differentiation and carcinogenesis to some disturbance in the normal pattern of differentiation.[100] Thus, while the presence of stem cell populations is evident in a variety of adult organs and tissues, such as epidermis, intestinal mucosa, and hematopoietic organs, to date, no such cell population has been clearly defined for the normal parenchymal cells of liver and pancreas. Here, however, it should be pointed out that for rat liver, it has been hypothesized that the oval or bile ductular cell might be acting as a facultative stem cell during some forms of chemical hepatocarcinogenesis.[101,102] Furthermore, while it has been hypothesized that neoplasia may result from blocked ontogeny, numerous studies have characterized specific stages in the development of malignant neoplasia.[103] In addition, many of the studies done in the past have largely failed to distinguish between the various concepts detailed above because they have been concerned mostly with malignant neoplasms themselves, and not with cellular changes which occur early in carcinogenesis.[99] The role of karyotypic or genetic instability in neoplasms must also be considered as an additional feature that may further affect changes in their differentiation states. Finally, as a result of his experience with hepatocarcinogenesis, Farber[100] recently suggested that hyperplastic hepatocellular nodules, induced in rat liver by various chemical carcinogens, and from which hepatocellular carcinomas have been shown to originate, may be comprised of hepatocytes which are exhibiting a new physiologically adapted state. In this context, he argued that any direct comparisons between hepatocellular carcinomas and embryonic, fetal, neonatal, or adult liver should not be considered as being meaningful unless each is related to the "new state of differentiation in hepatocyte nodules."[100]

## 4. EXPRESSION OF DEVELOPMENTAL GENES DURING VARIOUS NON-NEOPLASTIC CONDITIONS AND IN CELL CULTURE

The elaboration of oncodevelopmental gene products is not unique to neoplastic cells but has also been demonstrated in non-neoplastic adult cells, both *in vivo* during a variety of pathologic conditions and in cell culture as a result of adaptive responses to changes or alterations in their normal homeostatic environment. For example, AFP is elevated, albeit at generally lower levels than those associated with hepatocellular carcinoma, in the sera of patients with several types of benign liver diseases, including cirrhosis and hepatitis,[65,77] as well as during other forms of non-neoplastic disease, such as tyrosinosis and ataxia telangiectasia.[77] Similarly, elevated serum levels of CEA have been demonstrated in a variety of non-neoplastic human diseases, including severe alcoholic liver disease, extrahepatic biliary obstruction, pancreatitis, colitis, chronic bronchitis, emphysema, and tuberculoses.[12,65,104,105] In addition, murine γ-fetal antigen has been shown to be expressed in spleen and in hematopoietic tissue, particularly bone marrow, of the normal adult mouse.[31]

Fetal enzymes have also been found in adult tissues during various non-neoplastic states. In rat liver, γ-glutamyl transpeptidase has been shown to be induced in periportal hepatocytes during chronic alcohol consumption, following portal caval shunting, during aging, after partial hepatectomy (in certain strains), and as a result of specific treatments with certain drugs, hormones, and hepatotoxins.[106-112] It should be noted, however, that variant forms of this enzyme have been reported to be expressed during hepatocarcinogenesis in rats and in the sera of humans with hepatocellular carcinomas.[113-116]

Fetal liver isozymes were also demonstrated in regenerating rat liver following partial hepatectomy. In this regard, Curtin and Snell[99] reported that regenerating rat liver at three days posthepatectomy possessed an enzymatic pattern similar to that of both fetal and neoplastic liver but, unlike neoplastic liver, retained the capacity to undergo redifferentiation toward a normal adult biochemical pattern. On the other hand, it was recently found by Fausto and associates[117] and by Huber et al.[118] that the overall patterns of gene expression during liver regeneration after partial hepatectomy in the rat deviates little from that of the normal adult liver.

The production of oncodevelopmental substances by both malignant neoplastic cells and by transformed cells in culture is well established.[103,119-121] However, normal untransformed adult cells have also been observed to exhibit embryonic or fetal gene expression in cell culture. This phenomenon is particularly evident in the case of normal adult rat hepatocytes maintained in relatively short-term primary cultures. Under such conditions, these cells were shown to express within a few days of culture a number of fetal liver isozymes,[122,123] γ-glutamyl transpeptidase,[123] and AFP.[122,123] Furthermore, a number of the fetal changes shown by adult rat hepatocytes in primary culture have been found to be regulated by the inclusion of specific hormones, or of ADP-ribosylation inhibitors in the culture medium.[124-126]

## 5. POSSIBLE MECHANISMS FOR DEVELOPMENTAL GENE EXPRESSION IN NEOPLASTIC AND NON-NEOPLASTIC CELLS OF THE ADULT ORGANISM

It may be inappropriate to view oncodevelopmental expression as being a function of fixed blocks in target cell differentiation. In this regard, there is increasing evidence to indicate that the development of malignant neoplasms in many tissues and organs is a multistep process involving the appearance of altered cell populations at different stages.[103,127] In addition, data are accumulating to suggest that neoplastic cells are more genetically labile than normal cells and that tumor progression, which includes such changes as an increased expression by malignant neoplastic cells of embryonic and fetal properties, may be linked to a cascade of genetic instability.[128] Nowell[128] also pointed out that there continues to be considerable debate as to whether the loss of differentiation exhibited by malignant neoplasms reflects an actual block in differentiation or simply an increased growth fraction with a higher proportion of cells remaining in an undifferentiated state. However, it is also apparent that while the expression of some oncodevelopmental substances may be associated with cell proliferation and possibly even with specific stages of the cell cycle,[10,129] that of others is not.[38]

Additional evidence against fixed blocks in differentiation comes from studies of terminal differentiation of various malignant neoplastic cell types when subjected to appropriate inducers of cell differentiation[130-133] and of redifferentiation, which has been mainly investigated in early hyperplastic hepatocellular nodules produced in the Solt–Farber selection model of rat hepatocarcinogeneses.[134] In addition, Scott and associates[135,136] recently provided data to suggest that the loss of proliferative potential associated with the terminal event in cellular differentiation in cultured preneoplastic BALB/c 3T3 T mesenchymal cells is a distinct regulatory process. These investigators have further shown that arrest at both the predifferentiation state and at the nonterminal differentiation state of these cells is a completely reversible phenomenon that does not limit their subsequent growth or differentiation potential. However, when the 3T3 T cells undergoing adipocyte differentiation were induced to dedifferentiate, they subsequently were found upon re-differentiation to undergo a metaplastic change to macrophages, suggesting that such preneoplastic cells express defects in the stringency with which the integrated control of cellular differentiation and proliferation is regulated.[136]

It is now clear that the expression of some oncodevelopmental substances, such as AFP, are regulated mainly at the transcriptional level.[137-139] Transcriptional control, in turn, is consistent with the interpretation that oncodevelopmental gene expression occurs either as a result of an activation of developmental genes in normal differentiated or partially differentiated cells during carcinogenesis or to the continued expression of such genes in undifferentiated stem cell targets.[140] On the other hand, regulation at translational steps has also been proposed to be associated with controlling differentiation during development and in neoplasia,[3] and post-translational modification of oncodevelopmental glycoproteins, such as AFP, γ-glutamyl transpeptidase, and CEA, have been linked to the emergence of variant forms exhibiting heterogeneity in their oligosaccharide chains.[38,105,141,142]*

A number of important factors have been implicated in regulating gene expression during cell differentiation and development. These include epithelial cell interactions with specific basement membrane components and stroma,[144,145] intercellular communication,[7] DNA methylation,[146] ADP ribosylation,[125,147] modulation of distinct protein kinase activities,[148] hormones,[103,149] microenvironment,[100,128] and patterns of specific cellular protooncogene or oncogene expression.[150-155] Conceivably, alterations in any one of these factors could have significant affects on cellular differentiation, although the roles played by each in controlling or modulating embryonic and fetal gene expression either during normal development, in adult cells during various non-neoplastic conditions, or in neoplastic cells remain to be fully elucidated.

On the basis of studies with adult rat hepatocytes in primary culture, Pitot and Sirica[103] proposed that oncodevelopmental gene expression may be the result of a lack of host regulating influences on the genome of carcinogen-altered cells because of an inability of such cells to come into contact with, recognize, and/or respond to hormones and other key regulatory factors normally required to maintain the fully differentiated state. If the carcinogenic or tumor-promoting stimulus is removed at some critical point, it is still possible for the altered cells to recover their ability to respond to such regulatory signals but, as the carcinogenic process progresses, emerging neoplastic cell populations would be expected to become increasingly refractory to such signals. By comparison, Pitot and Sirica suggested that normal adult rat hepatocytes in primary culture express fetal genes because of the lack of repressive signal molecules in the basal culture medium.

While there is some support for this proposal,[124-126] further studies are required to test its validity, first by identifying the specific nature of the signals acting normally to repress embryonic and fetal genes in quiescent, fully differentiated adult hepatocytes, and second, to discover the nature of the defects occurring in the target cells during hepatocarcinogenesis that make them exhibit various degrees of nonresponsiveness to the regulatory signals of differentiation. Finally, although it appears that the expression of developmental genes during carcinogenesis is clearly not in itself an obligatory feature of neoplastic transformation, the appearance of such gene products, when persistent, can serve as important phenotypic markers. These can be useful in the diagnosis or monitoring of neoplastic disease, as well as in defining altered patterns of cell differentiation expressed during carcinogenesis and tumor progression.

---

*Another recent example implying post-translational modification is illustrated by the recent findings of Muchmore *et al.*,[143] who demonstrated a developmental regulation of *O*-acetylation of sialic acids of rat and human colon and found variable, but generally lower, levels of *O*-acetylated sialic acids in human primary colonic adenocarcinomas, as well as no detectable *O*-acetylation in four established human colon tumor cell lines when compared with normal adult colon.

# REFERENCES

1. Cohnheim, J., 1877, *Vorlesungen über allgemeine Pathologie,* A. Hirschwald, Berlin.
2. Willis, R. A., 1960, *Pathology of Tumors,* 3rd ed., Butterworth, Washington, D. C.
3. Pitot, H. C., 1974, Neoplasia and differentiation as translational functions, in: *Developmental Aspects of Carcinogenesis and Immunity. The Thirty-second Symposium of the Society for Developmental Biology* (T. J. King, ed.) pp. 79–88, Academic, New York.
4. Pierce, G. B., Shikes, R., and Fink, L. M., 1978, *Cancer: A Problem of Developmental Biology,* Prentice-Hall, Englewood Cliffs, New Jersey.
5. Rubin, H., 1985, Cancer as a dynamic developmental disorder, *Cancer Res.* **45:**2935–2942.
6. Potter, V. R., 1983, The cancer cell, in: *Concepts in Cancer Medicine* (S. B. Kahn, R. R. Love, C. Sherman, and R. Chakravorty, eds.), pp. 119–125, Grune & Stratton, New York.
7. Loch-Caruso, R., and Trosko, J. E., 1986, Inhibited intercellular communication as a mechanistic link between teratogenesis and carcinogenesis, *CRC Crit. Rev. Toxicol.* **16:**157–183.
8. Fishman, W. H., 1983, Oncodevelopmental markers, in: *Oncodevelopmental Markers: Biologic, Diagnostic, and Monitoring Aspects* (W. H. Fishman, ed.), pp. 3–19, Academic, New York.
9. Abelev, G. I., 1971, Alpha-fetoprotein in ontogenesis and its association with malignant tumors, *Adv. Cancer Res.* **141:**295–358.
10. Sell, S., Becker, F. F., Leffert, H. L., and Watabe, H., 1976, Expression of an oncodevelopmental gene product (α-fetoprotein) during fetal development and adult oncogenesis, *Cancer Res.* **36:**4239–4249.
11. Gold, P., and Freedman, S. O., 1965, Demonstration of tumor-specific antigens in human colonic carcinomata by immunological tolerance and absorption techniques, *J. Exp. Med.* **121:**439–462.
12. Neville, A. M., and Cooper, E. H., 1976, Biochemical monitoring of cancer, *Ann. Clin. Biochem.* **13:**283–305.
13. Steel, G., Jr., and Zamcheck, N., 1985, The use of carcinoembryonic antigen in the clinical management of patients with colorectal cancer, *Cancer Detection Prev.* **8:**421–427.
14. Bleday, R., Song, J., Walker, E. S., Salcedo, B. F., Thomas, P., Wilson, R. E., Chen, L. B., and Steel, G., Jr., 1986, Characterization of a new monoclonal antibody to a cell surface antigen on colorectal cancer and fetal gut tissues, *Cancer* **57:**433–550.
15. Decaens, C., Bara, J., Rosa, B., Daher, N., and Burtin, P., 1983, Early oncofetal antigenic modifications during rat colonic carcinogenesis, *Cancer Res.* **43:**355–362.
16. Bara, J., Gautier, R., Daher, N., Zaghouani, H., and Decaens, C., 1986, Monoclonal antibodies against oncofetal mucin $M_1$ antigens associated with precancerous colonic mucosae, *Cancer Res.* **46:**3983–3989.
17. Shi, Z. R., McIntyre, L. J., Knowles, B. B., Solter, D., and Kim, Y. S., 1984, Expression of a carbohydrate differentiation antigen, stage-specific embryonic antigen 1, in human colonic adenocarcinoma, *Cancer Res.* **44:**1142–1147.
18. Itzkowitz, S. H., Shi, Z. R., and Kim, Y. S., 1986, Heterogeneous expression of two oncodevelopmental antigens, CEA and SSEA-1, in colorectal cancer, *Histochem. J.* **18:**155–163.
19. Higgins, P. J., Friedman, E., Lipkin, M., Hertz, R., Attiyeh, F., and Stonehill, E. H., 1983, Expression of gastric-associated antigens by human premalignant and malignant colonic epithelial cells, *Oncology* **40:**26–30.
20. Biasco, G., Lipkin, M., Minarini, A., Higgins, P., Miglioli, M., and Barbara, L., 1984, Proliferative and antigenic properties of rectal cells in patients with chronic ulcerative colitis, *Cancer Res.* **44:**5450–5454.
21. Thor, A., Ohuchi, N., Szpak, C. A., Johnston, W. W., and Schlom, J., 1986, Distribution of oncofetal antigen tumor-associated glycoprotein-72 defined by monoclonal antibody B 72.3, *Cancer Res.* **46:**3118–3124.
22. Fritsché, R., and Mach, J.-P., 1975, Identification of a new oncofoetal antigen associated with several types of human carcinomas, *Nature (Lond.)* **258:**735–737.
23. Kim, Y. S., and McIntyre, L. J., 1983, Markers of gastrointestinal cancer, in: *Oncodevelopmental Markers: Biologic Diagnostic, and Monitoring Aspects* (W. H. Fishman, ed.), pp. 299–313, Academic, New York.
24. Banwo, O., Versey, J., and Hobbs, J. R., 1974, New oncofetal antigen for human pancreas, *Lancet* **1:**643–645.
25. Nishida, K., Sugiura, M., Yoshikawa, T., and Kondo, M., 1985, Enzyme immunoassay of pancreatic oncofetal antigen (POA) as a marker of pancreatic cancer, *Gut* **26:**450–455.
26. Carré-Llopis, A., and Escribano, M. J., 1986, Isolation and characterization of two oncofetal glycoproteins from hamster pancreas using concanavalin A and preparative electrophoresis, *Biochem. Biophys. Acta* **880:**101–107.

27. Rees, W. V., Irie, R. F., and Morton, D. L., 1981, Oncofetal antigen-1:distribution in human tumors, *J. Natl. Cancer Inst.* **67:**557–562.

28. Tong, C., Stonehill, E. H., Higgins, P. J., and Bendich, A., 1978, A fetal antigen in a mouse fibrosarcoma with possible cross-reactivity with an adult mouse skin component, *Eur. J. Cancer* **14:**147–152.

29. Higgins, P. J., Tong, C., and Borenfreund, E., 1981, Presence of anti-γ-FA-reactive antigens in spontaneous and carcinogen-induced malignancies of experimental animals, *Oncology* **38:**340–345.

30. Higgins, P. J., Marcus, S., and Hawrylko, E., 1981, Progressive growth of transplanted tumors is accompanied by increasing serum concentrations of murine gamma fetal antigen, *Oncodev. Biol. Med.* **2:**77–87.

31. Higgins, P. J., Silverstone, A. E., Bueti, C., Pizzi, V. F., Melamed, M. R., Lipkin, M., and Traganos, F., 1986, Expression of murine gamma fetal antigen in adult hematopoietic tissue and during induced differentiation of Friend erythroleukemia cells, *J. Natl. Cancer Inst.* **76:**885–893.

32. Bartal, A. H., Lichtig, C., Cardo, C. C., Feit, C., Robinson, E., and Hirshaut, Y., 1986, Monoclonal antibody defining fibroblasts appearing in fetal and neoplastic tissues, *J. Natl. Cancer Inst.* **76:**415–421.

33. Kasai, M., Takashi, T., Takahashi, T., and Tokunaga, T., 1984, Two new fetal thymocyte antigens, FT-1 and FT-2, *Immunol. Rev.* **82:**105–115.

34. Drysdale, J. W., and Alpert, E., 1975, Carcinofetal human isoferritins, *Ann. NY Acad. Sci.* **259:**427–434.

35. Bernard, B. A.. Robinson, S. M., Semat, A., and Darmon, M., 1985, Reexpression of fetal characters in Simian Virus 40-transformed human keratinocytes, *Cancer Res.* **45:**1707–1716.

36. Matsuura, H., and Hakomori, S-I, 1985, The oncofetal domain of fibronectin defined by monoclonal antibody FDC-6: Its presence in fibronectins from fetal and tumor tissues and its absence in those from normal adult tissues and plasma, *Proc. Natl. Acad. Sci. USA* **82:**6517–6521.

37. Durban, E., Roll, D., Beckner, G., and Busch, H., 1981, Purification and characterization of a nuclear DNA-binding phosphoprotein in fetal and tumor tissues, *Cancer Res.* **41:**537–545.

38. Hanigan, M. H., and Pitot, H. C., 1985, Gamma-glutamyl transpeptidase—Its role in hepatocarcinogenesis, *Carcinogenesis* **6:**165–172.

39. Gerber, M. A., and Thung, S. N., 1980, Enzyme patterns in human hepatocellular carcinoma, *Am. J. Pathol.* **98:**395–400.

40. Schapira, F., Reuber, M. D., and Hatzfeld, A., 1970, Resurgence of two fetal-type of aldolases (A and C) in some fast-growing hepatomas, *Biochem. Biophys. Res. Commun.* **40:**321–327.

41. Weinhouse, S., Shatton, J. B., Criss, W. E., Farina, F. A., and Morris, H. P., 1972, Isozymes in relation to differentiation in transplantable rat hepatomas, *GANN Monog. Cancer Res.* **13:**1–37.

42. Schwartz, M. K., 1973, Enzymes in cancer, *Clin. Chem.* **19:**10–22.

43. Stefanini, M., 1985, Enzymes, isozymes, and enzyme variants in the diagnosis of cancer—A short review, *Cancer* **55:**1931–1936.

44. Walker, P. R., and Potter, V. R., 1972, Isozymes studies on adult, regenerating, precancerous and developing liver in relation to findings in hepatomas, in: *Advances in Enzyme Regulation,* Vol. 10 (G. Weber, ed.), pp. 339–364, Pergamon, Oxford.

45. Farina, F. A., Shatton, J. B., Morris, H. P., and Weinhouse, S., 1974, Enzymes of pyruvate kinase in liver and hepatomas of the rat, *Cancer Res.* **34:**1439–1446.

46. Ibsen, K. H., Basabe, J. R., and Lopez, T. P., 1975, Extraction of a factor from Ehrlich acites tumor cells that increases the activity of the fetal isozyme of pyruvate kinase in mouse liver, *Cancer Res.* **35:**180–188.

47. Goldfarb, S., and Pitot, H. C., 1976, Enzymology of highly differentiated hepatocellular carcinomas, in: *Frontiers of Gastrointestinal Research,* Vol. 2 (L. van der Reis, ed.), pp. 194–242, S. Karger AG, Basel.

48. Sato, K., Takaya, S., Imai, F., Hatayama, I., and Ito, N., 1978, Different deviation patterns of carbohydrate-metabolizing enzymes in primary rat hepatomas induced by different chemical carcinogens, *Cancer Res.* **38:**3086–3093.

49. Shatton, J. B., Morris, H. P. and Weinhouse, S., 1969, Kinetic, electrophoretic, and chromatographic studies on glucose-ATP phosphotransferases in rat hepatomas, *Cancer Res.* **29:**1161–1172.

50. Sato, S., Matsushima, T., and Sugimura, T., 1969, Hexokinase isozyme patterns of experimental hepatomas of rats, *Cancer Res.* **29:**1437–1446.

51. Ogawa, K., and Ichihara, A., 1972, Isozymes patterns of branched-chain amino acid transaminase in various rat hepatomas, *Cancer Res.* **32:**1257–1263.

52. Ichihara, A., 1975, Isozyme patterns of branched-chain amino acid transaminase during cellular differentiation and carcinogenesis, *Ann. NY Acad. Sci.* **259:**347–354.

53. Katunuma, N., Kuroda, Y., Yoshida, T., Sanada, Y., and Morris, H. P., 1972, Relationship between degree of differentiation and growth rate of minimal deviation hepatomas and kidney cortex tumors studied with glutaminase isozymes, *GANN Monog. Cancer Res.* **13:**143–151.

54. Yin, Z., Sato, K., Tsuda, H., and Ito, N., 1982, Changes in activities of uridine diphosphate-glucuronyl-transferases during chemical hepatocarcinogenesis, *Gann* **73:**239–248.

55. Sato, K., Kitahara, A., Yin, Z., Ebina, T., Satoh, K., Tsuda, H., Ito, N., and Dempo, K., 1983, Molecular forms of glutathione S-transferase and UDP-glucuronyltransferase as hepatic preneoplastic marker enzymes, *Ann. NY Acad. Sci.* **417:**213–223.

56. Kitahara, A., Satoh, K., Nishimura, K., Ishikawa, T., Ruike, K., Sato, K., Tsuda, H., and Ito, N., 1984, Changes in molecular forms of rat hepatic glutathione S-transferase during chemical hepatocarcinogenesis, *Cancer Res.* **44:**2698–2703.

57. Bull, D. L., Taylor, A. T., Austin, D. M., and Jones, O. W., 1974, Stimulation of fetal thymidine kinase in cultured human fibroblasts transformed by SV40 virus, *Virology* **57:**279–284.

58. Salser, J. S., and Balis, M. E., 1976, Foetal thymidine kinase in tumours and colonic flat mucosa of man, *Nature (Lond.)* **260:**261–262.

59. Javre, J.-L., Hannouche, N., Samperez, S., and Jouan, P., 1986, Mise en évidence de la thymidine kinase de type foetal dans les cancers du sein, *Bull. Cancer (Paris)* **73:**8–16.

60. Hall, M., Silverman, L., Wenger, A. S., and Mickey, D. D., 1985, Oncodevelopmental enzymes of the Dunning rat prostatic adenocarcinoma, *Cancer Res.* **45:**4053–4059.

61. Fishman, W. H., Inglis, N. I., Stolbach, L. L., and Krant, M. J., 1968, A serum alkaline phosphatase isoenzyme of human neoplastic cell origin, *Cancer Res.* **28:**150–154.

62. Herz, F., 1985, Alkaline phosphatase isozymes in cultured human cancer cells, *Experientia* **41:**1357–1361.

63. Sato, K., Kitahara, A., Satoh, K., Ishikawa, T., Tatematsu, M., and Ito, N., 1984, The placental form of glutathione S-transferase as a new marker protein for preneoplasia in rat chemical hepatocarcinogenesis, *Gann* **75:**199–202.

64. Kodate, C., Fukushi, A., Narita, T., Kudo, H., Soma, Y. and Sato, K., 1986, Human placental form of glutathione S-transrerase (GST-π) as a new immunohistochemical marker for human colonic carcinoma, *Jpn. J. Cancer Res. (Gann)* **77:**226–229.

65. Bates, S. E., and Logo, 1985, Tumor markers: value and limitations in the management of cancer patients, *Cancer Treatm. Rev.* **12:**163–207.

66. Braunstein, G. D., 1983, hCG expression in trophoblastic and nontrophoblastic tumors, in: *Oncodevelopmental Markers: Biologic, Diagnostic, and Monitoring Aspects* (W. H. Fishman, ed.), pp. 351–371, Academic, New York.

67. Bohn, H., 1983, Systematic identification of specific oncoplacental proteins, in: *Oncodevelopmental Markers: Biologic, Diagnostic, and Monitoring Aspects* (W. H. Fishman, ed.), pp. 69–86, Academic, New York.

68. Nakajima, T., Okazaki, N., Morinaga, S., Tsumuraya, M., Shimosato, Y., and Saiki, S., 1985, A case of alpha-fetoprotein-producing rectal carcinoma, *Jpn. J. Clin. Oncol.* **15:**679–685.

69. Zamcheck, N., 1983, Colorectal cancer markers: Clinical value of CEA, in: *Oncodevelopmental Markers: Biologic, Diagnostic, and Monitoring Aspects* (W. H. Fishman, ed.), pp. 333–349, Academic, New York.

70. Busch, H., Chan, P., Takahashi, K., Busch, R. K., Kelsey, D., Spohn, W.,H., and Son, M., 1983, Human tumor nucleolar antigens, in: *Oncodevelopmental Markers: Biologic, Diagnostic, and Monitoring Aspects* (W. H. Fishman, ed). pp. 37–67, Academic, New York.

71. Soma, G.-I., Kitahara, N., and Andoh, T., 1984, Molecular cloning and characterization of a cDNA clone for a protein specifically expressed in embryo as well as in a chemically induced pancreatic β cell tumor of rat, *Biochem. Biophys. Res. Commun.* **124:**164–171.

72. Sato, K., Kitahara, A., Yin, Z., Waragai, F., Nishimura, K., Hatayama, I., Ebina, T., Yamazaki, T., Tsuda, H., and Ito, N., 1984, Induction by butylated hydroxyanisole of specific molecular forms of glutathione S-transferase and UDP-glucuronyltransferase and inhibition of development of γ-glutamyl transpeptidase-positive foci in rat liver, *Carcinogenesis* **5:**473–477.

73. Decaens, C., Gautier, R., Bara, J., Daher, N., Le Pendu, J., and Burtin, P., 1988, A new mucin-associated oncofetal antigen, a marker of early carcinogenesis in rat colon, *Cancer Res.* **48:**1571–1577.

74. Hanausek-Walaszek, M., Walaszek, Z., Lang, R. W., and Webb, T. E., 1984, Characterization of a 60,000-dalton oncofetal protein from the plasma of tumor-bearing rats, *Cancer Invest.* **2:**433–441.

75. Hanausek-Walaszek, M., Walaszek, Z., and Webb, T. E., 1985, Chemical carcinogens as specific inducers of a 60-kilodalton oncofetal protein in rats, *Carcinogenesis* **6:**1725–1730.

76. Webb, T. E., Hanausek-Walaszek, M., and Walaszek, Z., 1986, Persistence of the hepatocarcinogen-induced 60 kd oncofetal protein in rat liver and blood plasma, *Proc. Am. Assoc. Cancer Res.* **27:**81.

77. Sell, S., and Becker, F. F., 1978, Alpha-fetoprotein, *J. Natl. Cancer Inst.* **60:**19–26.

78. Hirai, H., 1982, Alpha fetoprotein, in: *Biochemical Markers for Cancer* (T. Ming Chu, ed.), pp. 25–59, Dekker, New York.

79. Koen, H., Pugh, T. D., Nychka, D., and Goldfarb, S., 1983, Presence of α-fetoprotein-positive cells in hepatocellular foci and microcarcinomas induced by single injections of diethylnitrosamine in infant mice, *Cancer Res.* **43:**702–708.

80. Jalanko, H., and Rouslahti, E., 1979, Differential expression of α-fetoprotein and γ-glutamyl transpeptidase in chemical and spontaneous hepatocarcinogenesis, *Cancer Res.* **39:**3495–3501.

81. Sakakibara, K., and Tsukada, Y., 1980, Lack of correlation among γ-glutamyltranspeptidase activity, production of α-fetoprotein, and transplantability in rat liver epithelial-like cell cultures, *Gann* **71:**679–685.

82. Sato, K., Hatayama, I., Hoshino, K., Imai, F., Tsuchida, S., Sato, T., Nishimura, K., Tatematsu, M., and Ito, N., 1981, Enzyme deviation patterns in primary rat hepatomas induced by sequential administration of two chemically different carcinogens, *Cancer Res.* **41:**4147–4153.

83. Daimon, M., Tsutsumi, K., Sato, J., Tsutsumi, R., and Ishikawa, K., 1984, Changes of aldolase A and B messenger RNA levels in rat liver during azo-dye-induced hepatocarcinogenesis, *Biochem. Biophys. Res. Commun.* **124:**337–343.

84. Cameron, R., Kellen, J., Kolin, A., Malkin, A., and Farber, E., 1978, γ-Glutamyltransferase in putative premalignant liver cell populations during hepatocarcinogenesis, *Cancer Res.* **38:**823–829.

85. Sell, S., 1978, Distribution of α-fetoprotein- and albumin-containing cells in the livers of Fischer rats fed four cycles of N-2-fluorenylacetamide, *Cancer Res.* **38:**3107–3113.

86. Peraino, C., Richards, W. L., and Stevens, F. J., 1983, Multistage hepatocarcinogenesis, in: *Mechanisms of Tumor Promotion* Vol. 1: *Tumor Promotion in Internal Organs* (T. J. Slaga, ed.), pp. 1–53, CRC Press, Boca Raton, Florida.

87. Wirth, P. J., Benjamin, T., Schwartz, D. M., and Thorgeirsson, S. S., 1986, Sequential analysis of chemically induced hepatoma development in rats by two dimensional electrophoresis, *Cancer Res.* **46:**400–413.

88. Roomi, M. W., Ho, R. K., Sarma, D. S. R., and Farber, E., 1985, A common biochemical pattern in preneoplastic hepatocyte nodules generated in four different models in the rat, *Cancer Res.* **45:**564–571.

89. Rao, M. S., Tatematsu, M., Subbarao, V., Ito, N., and Reddy, J. K., 1986, Analysis of peroxisome proliferator-induced preneoplastic and neoplastic lesions of rat liver for placental form of glutathione S-transferase and γ-glutamyltranspeptidase, *Cancer Res.* **46:**5287–5290.

90. Pierce, G. B., 1970, Differentiation of normal and malignant cells, *Fed. Proc.* **29:**1248–1254.

91. Buick, R. N., and Pollak, M. N., 1984, Perspectives on clonogenic tumor cells, stem cells, and oncogenes, *Cancer Res.* **44:**4909–4918.

92. Katenkamp, D., and Raikhlin, N. T., 1985, Stem cell concept and heterogeneity of malignant soft tissue tumor—A challenge to reconsider diagnostics and therapy?, *Exp. Pathol.* **28:**3–11.

93. Potter, V., 1969, Recent trends in cancer biochemistry: The importance of studies on fetal tissue, *Can. Cancer Conf.* **8:**9–30.

94. Potter, V., 1978, Phenotypic diversity in experimental hepatomas: The concept of partially blocked ontogeny, *Br. J. Cancer* **38:**1–23.

95. Uriel, J., 1976, Cancer, retrodifferentiation, and the myth of Faust, *Cancer Res.* **36:**4269–4275.

96. Uriel, J., 1979, Retrodifferentiation and the fetal patterns of gene expression in cancer, *Adv. Cancer Res.* **29:**127–174.

97. Drexler, H. G., Gaedicke, G., and Minowada, J., 1985, Biochemical enzyme analysis in acute leukaemia, *J. Clin. Pathol.* **38:**117–127.

98. Walker, P. R., and Potter, V. R., 1972, Isozyme studies on adult, regenerating, precancerous and developing liver in relation to findings in hepatomas, in: *Advances in Enzyme Regulation*, Vol. 10 (G. Weber, ed.), pp. 339–364, Pergamon, Oxford.

99. Curtin, N. J., and Snell, K., 1983, Enzymic retrodifferentiation during hepatocarcinogenesis and liver regeneration in rats *in vivo*, *Br. J. Cancer* **48:**495–505.

100. Farber, E., 1984, Cellular biochemistry of the stepwise development of cancer with chemicals: G. H. A. Clowes Memorial Lecture, *Cancer Res.* **44:**5463–5474.

101. Grisham, J. W., 1980, Cell types in long-term propagable culture of rat liver, *Ann. NY Acad. Sci.* **349:**128–137.

102. Hayner, N. T., Braun, L., Yaswen, P., Brooks, M., and Fausto, N., 1984, Isozyme profiles of oval cells, parenchymal cells, and biliary cells isolated by centrifugal elutriation from normal and preneoplastic livers, *Cancer Res.* **44:**332–338.

103. Pitot, H. C., and Sirica, A. E., 1980, Hepatocarcinogenesis as a problem in developmental biology, in: *Differentiation and Neoplasia* (R. G. McKinnell, M. A. DiBerardino, M. Blumenfeld, and R. D. Bergad, eds.), pp. 241–250, Springer-Verlag, Berlin.

104. Holyoke, E. D., Evans, J. T., Mittleman, A., and Chu, T. M., 1982, Carcinoembryonic antigen as a tumor marker, in: *Biochemical Markers for Cancer* (T. Ming Chu, ed.), pp. 61–80, Dekker, New York.

105. Burtin, P., and Escribano, M. J., 1983, The carcinoembryonic antigen and its cross-reacting antigens, in: *Oncodevelopmental Markers: Biologic, Diagnostic, and Monitoring Aspects* (W. H. Fishman, ed.), pp. 315–332, Academic, New York.

106. Yamada, S., Wilson, J. S., and Lieber, C. S., 1985, The effects of ethanol and diet on hepatic and serum γ-glutamyl transpeptidase activities in rats, *J. Nutr.* **115**:1285–1290.

107. Colombo, J. P., and Gigon, P. L., 1979, γ-Glutamyltranspeptidase (GGTP) and cytochrome P-450 after portacaval shunt in the rat, *Experientia* **35**:1005–1006.

108. Ogawa, K., Onoé, T., and Takeuchi, M., 1981, Spontaneous occurrence of γ-glutamyl transpeptidase positive hepatocytic foci in 105-week-old Wistar and 72-week-old Fisher 344 Male rats, *J. Natl. Cancer Inst.* **67**:407–412.

109. Bone, S. N. III, Michalopoulos, G., and Jirtle, R. L., 1985, Ability of partial hepatectomy to induce γ-glutamyl transpeptidase in regenerated and transplanted hepatocytes of Fisher 344 and Wistar-Furth rats, *Cancer Res.* **45**:1222–1228.

110. Galteau, M. M., Siest, G., and Ratanasavanh, D., 1980, Effect of phenobarbital on the distribution of gamma-glutamyltransferase between hepatocytes and nonparenchymal cells in the rat, *Cell. Mol. Biol.* **26**:267–273.

111. Barouki, R., Chobert, M. N., Finidori, J., Billon, M. C., and Hanoune, J., 1983, The hormonal induction of gamma glutamyltransferase in rat liver and in a hepatoma cell line, *Mol. Cell. Biochem.* **53/54**:77–78.

112. Garcia, B. M., and Mourelle, M. 1984, Gamma-glutamyl transpeptidase: A sensitive marker in DDT and toxaphene exposure, *J. Appl. Toxicol.* **4**:246–248.

113. Sato, K., Tsuchida, S., Waragai, F., Yin, Z., and Ebina, T., 1983, Properties of molecular forms of γ-glutamyl transpeptidase and uridine diphosphate-glucuronyltransferase as hepatic preneoplastic marker enzymes, *Gann Monog. Cancer Res.* **29**:23–31.

114. Yamashita, K., Hitoi, A., Taniguchi, N., Yokosawa, H., Tsukada, Y., and Kobata, A., 1983, Comparative study of the sugar chains of γ-glutamyltranspeptidase purified from rat liver and rat AH-66 hepatoma cells, *Cancer Res.* **43**:5059–5063.

115. Nemesánszky, E., and Lott, J. A., 1985, Gamma-glutamyltransferase and its isoenzymes: Progress and problems, *Clin. Chem.* **31**(6):787–803.

116. Taniguchi, N., House, S., Kuzumaki, N., Yokosawa, N., Yamagiwa, S., Iizuka, S., Makita, A., and Sekiya, C., 1985, A monoclonal antibody against γ-glutamyltransferase from human primary hepatoma: Its use in enzyme-linked immunosorbent assay of sera of cancer patients, *J. Natl. Cancer Inst.* **75**:841–847.

117. Petropoulos, C. J., Lemire, J. M., Goldman, D., and Fausto, N., 1985, Homology between rat liver RNA populations during development, regeneration, and neoplasia, *Cancer Res.* **45**:5114–5121.

118. Huber, B. E., Heilman, C. A., Wirth, P. J., Miller, M. J., and Thorgeirsson, S. S., 1986, Studies of gene transcription and translation in regenerating rat liver, *Hepatology* **6**:209–219.

119. Ting, C.-C., Sandford, K. K., and Price, F. M., 1978, Expression of fetal antigens in fetal and adult cells during long-term culture, *In Vitro* **14**:207–211.

120. Ruddon, R. W., Marker expression by cultured cancer cells, in: *Oncodevelopmental Markers: Biologic, Diagnostic, and Monitoring Aspects* (W. H. Fishman, ed.), pp. 87–108, Academic, New York.

121. Chou, J. Y., and Savitz, A. J., 1986, Alpha-fetoprotein synthesis in transformed fetal rat liver cells, *Biochem. Biophys. Res. Commun.* **135**:844–851.

122. Leffert, H., Moran, T., Sell, S., Skelly, H., Ibsen, K., Mueller, M., and Arias, I., 1978, Growth state-dependent phenotypes of adult hepatocytes in primary monolayer culture, *Proc. Natl. Acad. Sci. USA* **75**:1834–1837.

123. Sirica, A. E., Richards, W., Tsukada, Y., Sattler, C. A., and Pitot, H. C., 1979, Fetal phenotypic expression by adult rat hepatocytes on collagen gel/nylon meshes, *Proc. Natl. Acad. Sci. USA* **76**:283–287.

124. Spence, J. T., and Pitot, H. C., 1980, Maintenance of glucokinase acitivty in primary hepatocyte cultures, *J. Cell. Physiol.* **103**:173–178.

125. Althaus, F. R., Lawrence, S. D., He, Y-Z., Sattler, G. L., Tsukada, Y., and Pitot, H. C., 1982, Effects of altered [ADP-ribose]$_n$ metabolism on expression of fetal functions by adult hepatocytes, *Nature (Lond.)* **300**:366–368.

126. Colbert, R. A., Amatruda, J. M., and Young, D. A., 1984, Changes in the expression of hepatocyte

protein gene-products associated with adaption of cells to primary culture, *Clin. Chem.* **30**(12):2053–2058.

127. Farber, E., 1984, The multistep nature of cancer development, *Cancer Res.* **44**:4217–4223.
128. Nowell, P. C., 1986, Mechanisms of tumor progression, *Cancer Res.* **46**:2203–2207.
129. Sasaki, K., Murakami, T., Kawasaki, S., Okita, K., Tukemoto, T., and Takahashi, M., 1985, Change of α-fetoprotein content during cell cycle of human hepatoma cells *in vitro:* Flow cytometric analysis, *Tumor Biol.* **6**:483–489.
130. Friend, C., Scher, W., Holland, J. G., and Sato, T., 1971, Hemoglobin synthesis in murine virus induced leukemic cells *in vitro:* Stimulation of erythroid differentiation by dimethyl sulfoxide, *Proc. Natl. Acad. Sci. USA* **68**:378–382.
131. Collins, S. J., Ruscetti, F. W., Gallagher, R. E., and Gallo, R. C., 1978, Terminal differentiation of human promyelocytic cells induced by dimethyl sulfoxide and other polar compounds, *Proc. Natl. Acad. Sci. USA* **75**:2458–2462.
132. Rifkind, R. A., Sheffery, M., and Marks, P. A., 1984, Induced differentiation of murine erythroleukemia cells: Cellular and molecular mechanisms, *Adv. Cancer Res.* **42**:149–166.
133. Yun, K., and Sugihara, H., 1986, Cell differentiation and cell cycle effects on human promyelocytic leukemia cells induced by 12-*O*-tetradecanoylphorbol-13-acetate, *Lab. Invest.* **54**:336–344.
134. Tatematsu, M.. Nagamine, Y., and Farber, E., 1983, Redifferentiation as a basis for remodeling of carcinogen-induced hepatocyte nodules to normal appearing liver, *Cancer Res.* **43**:5049–5058.
135. Wier, M. L., and Scott, R. E., 1986, Regulation of the terminal event in cellular differentiation: Biological mechanisms of the loss of proliferative potential, *J. Cell Biol.* **102**:1955–1964.
136. Sparks, R. L., Seibel-Ross, E. I., Wier, M. L., and Scott, R. E., 1986, Differentiation, dedifferentiation, and transdifferentiation of BALB/c 3T3 T mesenchymal stem cells: Potential significance in metaplasia and neoplasia, *Cancer Res.* **46**:5312–5319.
137. Nahon, J. L., Gal, A., Frain, M., Sell, S., and Sala-Trepat, J. M., 1982, No evidence for post-transcriptional control of albumin and α-fetoprotein gene expression in developing rat liver and neoplasia, *Nucleic Acad. Res.* **10**:1895–1911.
138. Muglia, L., and Locker, J., 1984, Developmental regulation of albumin and α-fetoprotein gene expression in the rat, *Nucleic Acid Res.* **12**:6751–6762.
139. Poliard, A. M., Bernuau, D., Tournier, I., Legrès, L. G., Schoevaert, D., Feldmann, G., and Sala-Trepat, J. M., 1986, Cellular analysis by in situ hybridization and immunoperoxidase of alpha-fetoprotein and albumin gene expression in rat liver during the perinatal period, *J. Cell Biol.* **103**:777–786.
140. Klavins, J. V., 1985, *Tumor Markers: Clinical and Laboratory Studies*, pp. 4–5, Liss, New York.
141. Bayard, B., Debray, H., Kerckaert, J.-P., and Biserte, G., 1977, Rat alpha-fetoprotein heterogeneity, *FEBS Lett.* **80**:35–40.
142. Ishiguro, T., Sakaguchi, H., Fukui, M., and Sugitachi, I., 1986, Serum alpha-fetoprotein subfractions in hepatic malignancies identified by different reactivities with concanavalin A, lentil lectin, or phytohemagglutinin-E, *Jpn. J. Surg.* **16**:16–21.
143. Muchmore, E. A., Varki, N. M., Fukuda, M., and Varki, A., 1987, Developmental regulation of sialic acid modifications in rat and human colon, *FASEB J.* **1**:229–235.
144. Kleinman, H. K., Cannon, F. B., Laurie, G. W., Hassell, J. R., Aumailley, M., Terranova, V. P., Martin, G. R., and DuBois-Dalcq, M., 1985, Biological activities of laminin, *J. Cell. Biochem.* **27**:317–325.
145. Kratochwil, K., 1986, The stroma and the control of cell growth, *J. Pathol.* **149**:23–24.
146. Jones, P. A., 1986, DNA methylation and cancer, *Cancer Res.* **46**:461–466.
147. Farzaneh, F., Zalin, R., Brill, D., and Shall, S., 1982, DNA strand breaks and ADP-ribosyl transferase activation during cell differentiation, *Nature (Lond.)* **300**:362–366.
148. Fontana, J. A., Reppucci, A., Durham, J. P., and Miranda, D., 1986, Correlation between the induction of leukemic cell differentiation by various retinoids and modulation of protein kinases, *Cancer Res.* **46**:2468–2473.
149. Greengard, O., 1970, The developmental formation of enzymes in rat liver, in: *Biochemical Actions of Hormones*, Vol. 1 (G. Litwack, ed.), pp. 53–87, Academic, New York.
150. Lachman, H. M., and Skoultchi, A. I., 1984, Expression of c-myc changes during differentiation of mouse erythroleukaemia cells, *Nature (Lond.)* **310**:592–594.
151. Kaczmarek, L., 1986, Biology of disease: Protooncogene expression during the cell cycle, *Lab. Invest.* **54**:365–376.
152. Lebovitz, R. M., 1986, Oncogenes as mediators of cell growth and differentiation, *Lab Invest.* **55**:249–251.
153. Zimmerman, K. A., Yancopoulos, G. D., Collum, R. G., Smith, R. K., Kohl, N. E., Denis, K. A., Nau,

M. M., Witte, O. N., Toran-Allerand, D., Gee, C. E., Minna, J. D., and Alt, F. W., 1986, Differential expression of myc family genes during murine development, *Nature (Lond.)* **319:**780–783.

154. Coppola, J. A., and Cole, M. D., 1986, Constitutive c-myc oncogene expression blocks mouse erythro-leukaemia cell differentiation but not commitment, *Nature (Lond.)* **320:**760–763.

155. Huber, B. E., Heilman, C. A., and Thorgeirsson, S. S., 1986, Gene expression in the progressive development of hepatocellular carcinoma (HCC) in the rat, *Proc. Annu. Meeting Am. Assoc. Cancer Res.* **27:**7.

# 22

# Expression of Differentiated Function in Neoplasms

## Robert G. McKinnell

## 1. EMBRYOS, STEM CELLS, AND CANCER CELLS

"Once a cancer cell, always a cancer cell" is classic dogma that arose quite naturally from observation of the usual intractable course of cancer in human beings.[1] Yet as difficult to manage as clinical cancer may be, the realization is emerging that some cancer cells in certain situations may give rise to cell progeny that are postmitotic and terminally differentiated.

The study of growth and differentiation of normal cells had suggested to a number of pathobiologists that an understanding of normal differentiation might lead to useful insights into the control of malignant neoplasia, often described as a disease of cells that appear to be undifferentiated, dedifferentiated, or inappropriately differentiated.[2] Some of this history is reviewed in this chapter. While the precise cell of origin of most tumors is unknown,[3,4] it now seems reasonable to view some cancers as being composed of abnormal stem cells that generally fail to give rise to mature progeny, but that, under certain circumstances, can be induced to mature into differentiated postmitotic benign cells.

### 1.1. Similarities between Normal Cells and Cancer Cells

Is a developmental approach reasonable for considering the neoplastic process? An abiding proposition has emerged during the second half of the twentieth century that holds that cancer cells are much like normal cells, a view derived from cell morphology and biochemistry. Since the late 1940s, fine structure studies with transmission electron microscopy (TEM) made it manifestly clear that the architecture of normal and neoplastic cells differed little. All the organelles of normal cells such as the nucleus, mitochondria, Golgi apparatus, and rough endoplasmic reticulum are found in neoplastic cells.[5] Similarly, as more and more tumors were scrutinized with the powerful probes of the biochemists and molecular biologists, it became clear that cancer cells could not survive and function were they not equipped with the customary array of nucleic acids, enzymes, and physiologically essential molecules.[1] Compared with normal adult cells, however, cancer cells appear incompletely or improperly differentiated.[2]

The enormous diversity of cell types in an adult mammal arises by differentiation. Associated

---

*Robert G. McKinnell* • Department of Genetics and Cell Biology, University of Minnesota, St. Paul, Minnesota 55108-1095.

with differentiation is the loss of mitotic activity. Once achieved, differentiation is remarkably stable; i.e., normal liver does not become striated muscle and keratinized skin cells do not become β-cells in the pancreas. (*Note:* The generalization made here is made with the knowledge that the differentiated state can be disrupted under certain experimental conditions[6-8].)

During embryonic development, a large proportion of cells are mitotically active, and many cells progress through a series of cell-type changes. Undifferentiated ectoderm, for example, may specialize first as neural plate, then forebrain, then cerebrum. In the case of embryonic ectoderm, at least, a bewildering array of chemical substances with no obvious relationship to each other has proven capable of inducing neural differentiation, as does chordamesoderm tissue, which is the inducer *in vivo*.

Also noteworthy when studying the characteristics of embryonic cells is their propensity to translocate along specific pathways during the course of normal development. Primordial germ cells and neural crest cells exemplify migratory behavior in the embryo.[9,10] Malignant neoplastic cells also translocate by the process of invasion and metastasis[11-13] (see Chapter 27).

Among the many kinds of tissues found in adult organisms are those that retain populations of undifferentiated stem cells which retain mitotic potential. Their proliferation provides daughter cells that differentiate and replenish cells lost due to wear or senescence. As daughter cells differentiate, their mitotic potential is lost. Only the stem cells retain their proliferative potential. Among the adult tissues that depend on resupply by an undifferentiated and proliferating stem cell population are the skin, the inner lining of the gut, and blood. If we accept the notion that cancer cells are more similar to normal cells than they are different, then we might consider the possibility that the undifferentiated appearance of some cancers is due not to dedifferentiation (an unlikely event due to the stability of the differentiated state), but rather to the overproduction of undifferentiated mitotically active stem cells, each of which resembles the normal regulated stem cell. Perhaps, if enough is learned about normal differentiation, it follows that the less than fully differentiated neoplastic cells can be induced to differentiate and become postmitotic benign cells without the usual need to kill either the neoplastic cells intentionally or normal cells inadvertently.

If only one or a very few malignant tumor types could be induced to differentiate into nonmalignant postmitotic cells, then the phenomenon would be more apt to have curiosity value only. However, a relatively large number of neoplasms have now been described, including a plant teratoma, tumors of lower vertebrates, and a number of cancers of lower mammals and humans (including cancers derived from each of the three embryonic germ layers), all of which produce differentiated postmitotic benign cell progeny. Induction of the differentiated phenotype occurs spontaneously or as a result of treatment with a vast number of apparently unrelated chemical substances. Chemical induction of differentiation in cancer cells is reminiscent of studies of the chemical nature of the amphibian organizer. Perhaps useful insight will be obtained concerning both phenomena by comparing the two.

A consideration of the differentiation of cancer cells is of theoretical importance to cell and developmental biology. It also has enormous practical significance to pathobiology because of the possibility of cancer treatment, not with conventional cytotoxic agents, but with substances that function to modulate or alter gene expression resulting in the maturation or differentiation of cancer cells.[4,14-28]

## 1.2. Historic Considerations

The idea that malignant tumors could arise by faulty differentiation had its origin in the mid-19th century. Robert Remak in 1854 proposed that faulty embryological development led to epithelial tumors discovered in bone marrow.[29] Similarly, a few years later, Cohnheim was called upon to explain the origin of striated muscle fibers in a kidney tumor of a 5-year-old girl. Cohnheim speculated that the stem cells of muscle, due to a developmental error, ended up in the kidney rudiment of the embryo where they persisted and ultimately became reactivated and the source of the striated muscle of the tumor.[30] Later, Cohnheim enunciated his ideas in a book in which he described his belief that during embryonic development more cells are produced than are needed or could be used by the embryo. The excess cells, stated Cohnheim, failed to mature and thus remained embryonic, and "owing to their embryonic character," were endowed with a marked capacity for proliferation. The reactivation of the embryonic cells resulted in cancer.[31] Another early investigator who believed he detected a relationship between development and neoplasia was Beard.[32] He suggested that some tumors could evolve from misplaced germ cells that, owing to their origin and anatomically inappropriate location, could give rise to cancer. Clearly, the early pioneers conceived of a relationship between development and malignancy. Their views led to the embryonic rest theory of the origin of cancer, which has been largely discredited. However, it is interesting to note that their ideas are remarkably compatible with contemporary views of the stem cell origin of cancer. Both invoke the need to consider the origin of cancer cells as it relates to morphology (i.e., differentiation) and proliferative potential.

An approach to achieving cancer cell differentiation experimentally was suggested by Needham.[33,34] Aware of the extensive differentiation that occurs in the limb regeneration blastema of adult tailed amphibians (*Urodeles*), and familiar with the description by Lucké[35] of a renal adenocarcinoma of the leopard frog (see Section 2.3), Needham wondered whether the "wildly growing material could be mastered" by an influence from the regeneration blastema. Rose and Wallingford[36] and Rose[37] attempted to answer that question by grafting pieces of the frog renal carcinoma into urodele limbs. After the graft grew, the limbs were amputated across the graft. Normal muscle, cartilage, and connective tissue cells of frog origin were reportedly detected in the regenerating urodele limb. Although the tumor cells appeared to have responded to the regeneration blastema environment by differentiation, the experiments could not be continued due to the unavailability of means to forestall graft rejection. Since that time, immunosuppressive agents have become available which induce long-term tolerance in amphibians[38,39] and could be used if these experiments were to be extended. It should be noted, however, that other laboratories were unable to duplicate these results with either frog renal carcinoma or other tumors.[40–44]

Moreover, when one considers the stability of cell-type specialization of most tissues of adult animals, it seems unlikely that renal adenocarcinoma is capable of differentiating as limb muscle and cartilage. If the implanted kidney cancer in the blastema gave rise to normal cells, it would probably give rise to kidney cells. In addition, the limb would be an inappropriate site for induction of kidney cell differentiation, since there appears to be specificity to the environment which induces cancer cells[45] to differentiate. Thus, teratocarcinoma cells differentiate in the blastocyst[45] (see Section 2.6), while neuroblastoma cells differentiate in a neurula[18] (see Section 2.4). Following this line of thought, an appropriate site for induction of differentiation of renal carcinoma would be the developing mesonephros of an amphibian embryo. Lamentably, renal tumor cells have thus far not been transplanted to that site. It thus seems that Needham was probably wrong in his suggested limb-blastema induced differentiation of frog renal adenocarcinoma. However, his ideas were seminal and ahead of their time; study of these ideas further aids in clarifying an understanding of the need for special environments that lead to cancer cell differentiation.

Cohnheim and Needham were not alone. Many other pioneers believed that an understanding of normal differentiation is fundamental to the study of cancer. By contrast, Lockhart-Mummery[46] enunciated the idea that gene mutation in a normal cell was the central event which led to malignancy. Haldane[47] argued that "until it can be shown that differentiation is due to gene mutation it seems reasonable to regard carcinogenesis as *anomalous differentiation* (italics added) rather than mutation." Needham[34] agreed with Haldane to the extent that he found it appropriate to discourse on cancer in a book on embryology. Others who expressed hope that from an understanding of normal differentiation there might emerge the potential for controlled differentiation of cancer cells included Waddington,[48] Berrill,[49] Pierce,[50] and Markert.[51]

When later investigators sought to modulate gene expression of tumor cells in the laboratory with the production of phenotypically normal or near normal cell progeny, they met with considerable success. That is the subject of this chapter.

## 2. DIFFERENTIATED CELL PROGENY OBTAINED FROM TUMOR CELLS

### 2.1. A Plant Tumor

A generalization exists that all multicellular organisms that undergo differentiation are vulnerable to neoplastic transformation. This applies as much to plants as it does to animals.[52–54] Dicotyledonous plants may become afflicted with a non-self-limiting neoplastic disease known as crown gall[55–58] that is initiated by the $T_i$ plasmid[59–62] transmitted to a wound on a susceptible plant by a specific bacterium, *Agrobacterium tumefaciens*[63] (see also Chapter 25). Crown galls resemble embryonic plants in that they produce auxin and cytokinin, growth-regulating substances produced at reduced levels by fully mature plants.

Normal cells and tissues from a diversity of mature plants can be cultured *in vitro*[64] and certain somatic cells and protoplasts appear totipotent by virtue of their capacity to grow and differentiate into cells of all the parts of a whole plant.[65–68] Cells from the normal tobacco plant exhibit such totipotency.[69,70] A plant tumor with a known etiology and a well-characterized mode of transfection, coupled with advanced plant cell culture technique, made the crown gall and related teratomas ideal subjects for characterization of tumor cell differentiation potential.

After transfection with the $T_i$ plasmid, tumors of the tobacco plant *Nicotiana tabacum* may grow as typical crown gall or as teratomas depending upon the plant host and other factors.[71] Teratomas grow as a chaotic assortment of tissues and organs of varying degrees of morphological development including abnormal structures resembling shoots and leaves. The abnormal shoots and leaves may be grafted serially (i.e., tumor tissue may be grafted to several hosts successively). Under these conditions, some grafts undergo normal morphogenesis into functional leaves, stems, diploid flower parts such as petals and filaments, and all other specialized tissue types.[72–75]

One could ask whether the abnormal shoots and leaves that developed on the surface of the teratomas were produced by inappropriate cell differentiation of the teratoma cells or from normal cells swept along from normal portions of the plant by the rapidly growing tumor. To answer that question, tumors were produced by cloning single teratoma cells. The clones developed as teratomas. The cloned teratomas produced the expected disorganized cells plus abnormal shoots and leaves. These cloned structures were then grafted serially to normal hosts where the grafts differentiated into normal plants that had the capacity to flower and set seed[56,58,75,76] (Fig. 1). The experiments with tobacco teratoma cells demonstrate unequivocally that the transformed condition can be reversed with tumor cells giving rise to the full gamut of normal cell types. Thus, tumorigenesis in the crown-gall teratoma is not attributable to a deletion or other irreversible alteration in the genome of the tobacco cell but is epigenetic and results from inappropriate gene activity. The inappropriate gene activity can be normalized by serial grafting which alters the tumor environment sufficiently to permit normal differentiation.

### 2.2. Fish Pigment Cell Neoplasm

Spontaneous neoplasms have been reported in many species of aquatic vertebrates.[77,78] Invasive tumors of the goldfish, *Carassius auratus*, are one example.[79] Cell lines produced from nonmelanin pigment cell tumors arising in these fish[80] may proliferate indefinitely as stem cells or differentiate in response to agents such as dimethylsulfoxide (DMSO), 12-O-tetradecanoyl-phorbol 13-acetate (TPA), or autologous serum. The tumor-derived cell lines differentiate a variety of pigments, dermal bonelike structures, scales, fin rays, teeth, neuronlike cells, and lentoid bodies.[81–84]

### 2.3. Amphibian Tumor: The Lucké Renal Adenocarcinoma

The northern leopard frog, *Rana pipiens*, may become afflicted with a herpesvirus-induced renal adenocarcinoma.[35,85–87] The tumor is spontaneously metastatic.[88–90] A number of years ago, there was disputed evidence from regeneration studies that the frog renal adenocarcinoma is pluripo-

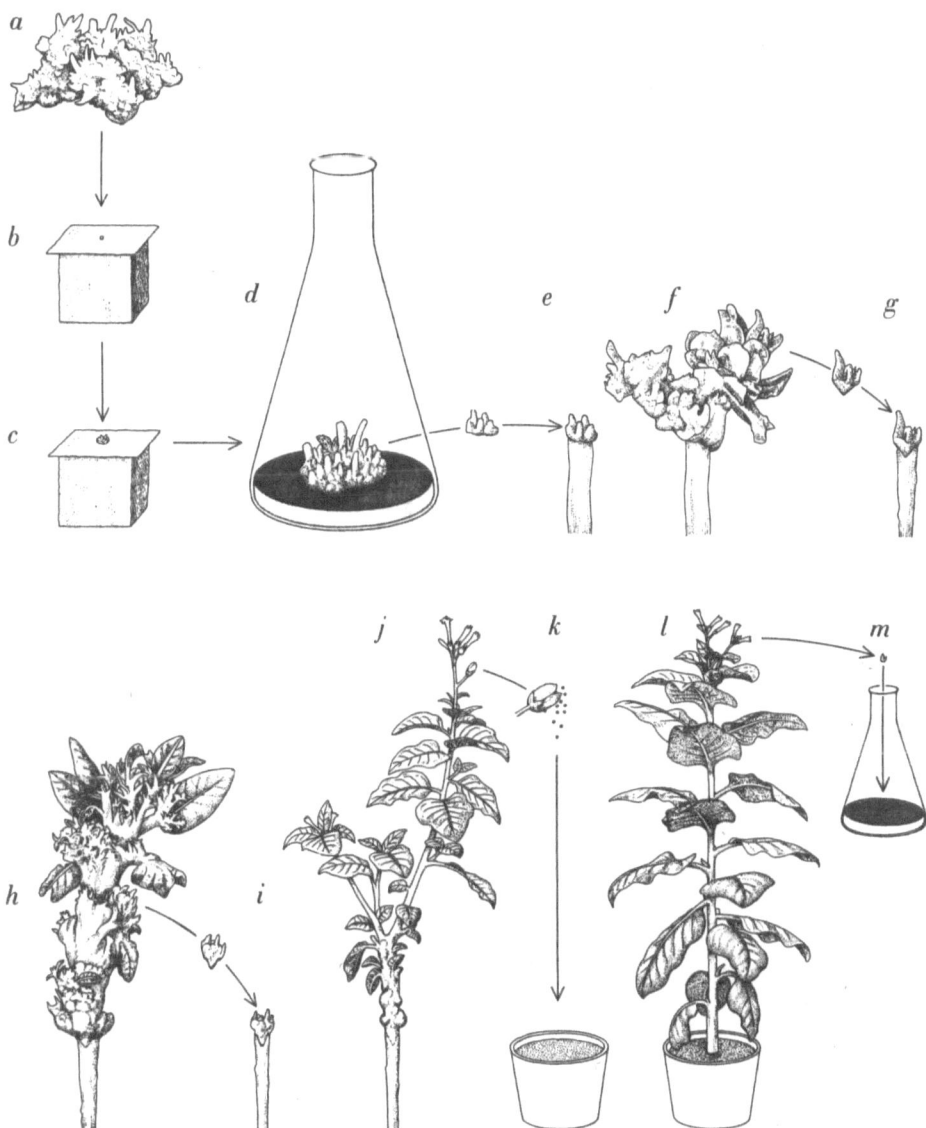

*Figure 1.* Mitotic progeny of tobacco teratoma have the capacity to differentiate all of the tissues of a normal tobacco plant. The teratoma (a) provides a single cell (b), which is isolated from its nurse tissue by a filter. The cloned cell grows into a small teratoma (c) which is further cultured in a flask with medium suitable for culture of teratoma cells (d). A leaflike bud from cultured teratoma is grafted to a normal but genetically different tobacco plant (e), where it continues to proliferate and produce buds (f) that are serially grafted (g, h, i) inducing normal tissue differentiation. The graft flowers (j) and sets seed (k). A normal tobacco plant grows from the seed (1). Cells from the normal plant, genetically identical to the teratoma and distinct from the host plant, fail to grow on culture medium (m) suitable only for tobacco teratoma cells. (From ref. 72a. Copyright © 1965, by Scientific American, Inc. All rights reserved.)

tent and has the capacity to produce normally differentiated cellular progeny (see Section 1.1). A different experimental approach and one which is extraordinarily potent in its capacity to reveal differentiation potential is nuclear transplantation. An early use of the procedure was with the tumor of *Rana pipiens.*

Nuclear transplantation was developed first in *R. pipiens* for the purpose of disclosing the developmental potential of embryonic somatic nuclei.[91-95] Transplantation of early embryonic nuclei into enucleated mature ova results in embryos that develop into frogs capable of reaching sexual maturity. Transplantation of nuclei from older embryos into enucleated ova, however, results in progressively fewer embryos that are able to reach maturity. No enucleated ovum receiving an adult nucleus has ever developed to maturity.

While current nuclear transfer technique suggests that adult nuclei are unable to program for all aspects of normal development, even terminally differentiated nuclei prove competent to program for a number of cell types when tested by nuclear transplantation. DiBerardino and colleagues demonstrated that erythrocyte nuclei, when pretreated by transfer into oocyte cytoplasm followed by retransfer into mature egg cytoplasm, are able to program for all the tissue types of swimming larvae that feed and that develop limb buds.[8,96,97] These erythrocyte nuclear transfer larvae exhibit the most advanced development obtained by the transfer of adult nuclei thus far and clearly indicate that the potential exists in the terminally differentiated postmitotic erythrocyte nucleus for differentiating many cell types. Nuclear transplantation, and the attendant procedures for enhancing nuclear potential, may thus be used to gauge the abilities of different types of nuclei to program for cell differentiation.

Several years ago, nuclear transplantation studies were started with diploid nuclei of the frog renal adenocarcinoma (Fig. 2). Renal tumor nuclei were inserted into previously enucleated mature ova.[98-101] In the best experiments, swimming tadpoles ensued (Fig. 3). No pretreatments of nuclei with oocyte cytoplasm were required to obtain this result. The tadpoles exhibited the entire range of differentiated tissues appropriate for a tadpole, including a central nervous system (CNS), notochord, skin, muscle, heart, blood vessels, and gills. The central nervous system was differentiated into white and gray matter and had a morphology appropriate for its anatomical region. Avoidance swimming, elicited by stimulation of the tadpole, demonstrated that not only were appropriately formed muscles and nerves present but their function was fully coordinated.

Because the yield of tadpoles programmed by cancer nuclei was relatively low [in one experiment, 12 of 161 (7.4%) developed past the gastrula stage[102]], it was decided to produce tumors that were chromosomally distinct from ordinary frog cells (diploid number: 26) to serve as cytogenetically labeled nuclear donors. This would provide the means to ensure that the differentiating tadpole cells were truly descended from the transplanted tumor nucleus and not from an inadvertently surviving egg nucleus. Triploid tumors (chromosome number: 39) were produced by injecting Lucké tumor herpesviruses into prefeeding triploid embryos. Some of the treated embryos became adult frogs with triploid tumors.[103] The triploid tumors then became donors for nuclear transplantation experiments. Seven tadpoles were produced in the triploid tumor study (Fig. 4). All the nuclear transplant tadpoles were triploid.[104] The triploidy of the nuclear transplant tadpoles excluded the remote possibility that the tadpoles developed by parthenogenesis and provided direct cytogenetic evidence that nuclei from the renal adenocarcinoma were reprogrammed to give rise to all tissue types of prefeeding larvae.

Once the triploid studies had established that the donor nucleus was of tumor origin, it was desirable to determine whether the donor nucleus originated from the tumor's malignant epithelium or from the connective tissue stroma. To this end, dissociated cells of tumors were studied by their fluorescence in the ultraviolet after staining with acridine orange.[105,106] Almost all (98.5%) of the dissociated cells were carcinoma,[107,108] providing supports for the view that the tadpoles previously reported could only have developed in response to the injection of a tumor nucleus into an enucleated ovum.

In addition, there is evidence from another source to indicate that nuclei from renal adenocarcinoma cells provide the genome for the reported tadpoles. That evidence was obtained by transplantation of cultured carcinoma nuclei. The cultures were epithelial in appearance, as would be

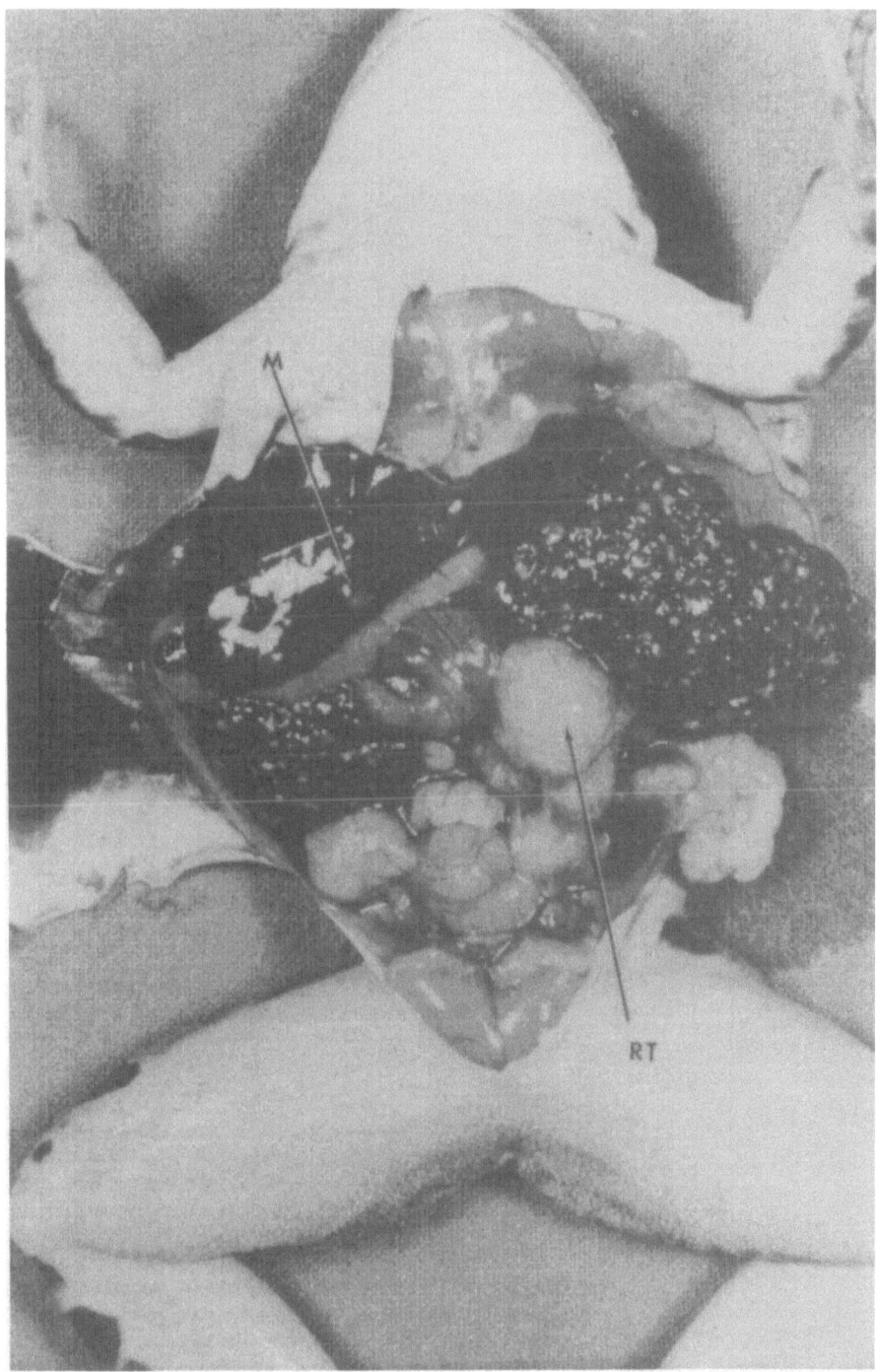

*Figure 2.* The tumor mass (RT) in the region of the mesonephros of this frog is a Lucké renal adenocarcinoma. There is a metastatic nodule (M) in the liver. (From McKinnell *et al.*[107])

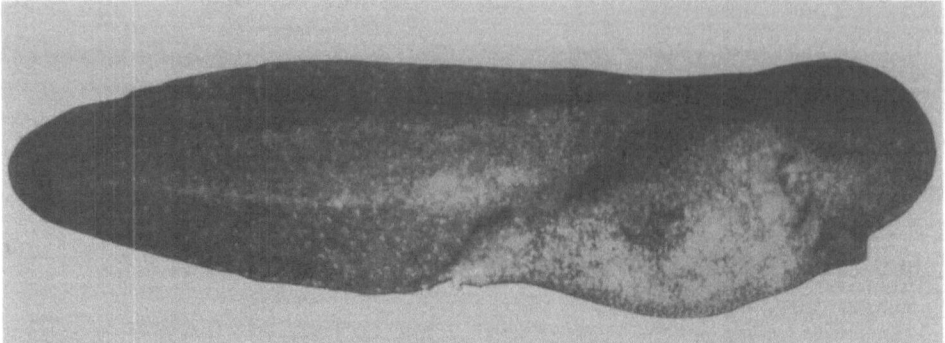

*Figure 3.* Swimming stage larva of frog produced by transplanting a Lucké renal adenocarcinoma nucleus into an enucleated frog egg. (From McKinnell.[100a])

expected from a carcinoma, and larvae were produced from transplanted nuclei from the cultured carcinoma cells, further corroborating and strengthening the earlier studies.[109] The inescapable conclusion is that mitotic descendants of Lucké renal carcinoma nuclei are able to differentiate into all larval cell types.

Differentiation has been demonstrated to occur in the frog renal adenocarcinoma as a consequence of a changed cytoplasmic environment (the egg cytoplasm). The molecular mechanisms controlling differentiation are, of course, yet to be explained. The frog renal adenocarcinoma is but one amphibian tumor. Other amphibians are also known to be afflicted with neoplasms,[87,110] at least one of which differentiates spontaneously.[111]

As is true of most tumors,[3,4,28] the cell type of origin of the Lucké renal adenocarcinoma remains unknown. However, it can be questioned as to whether the cancer occurs as a result of

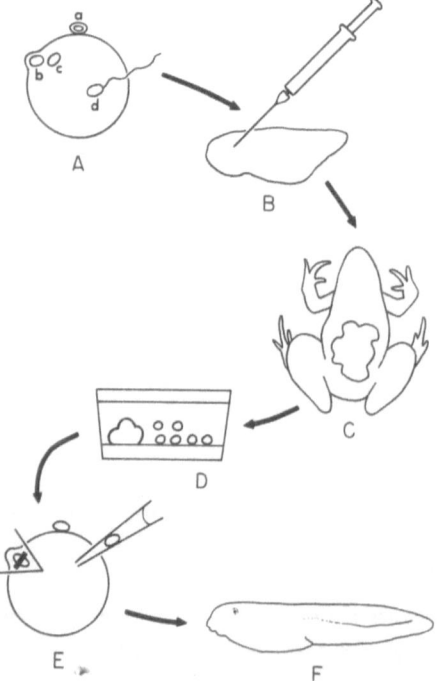

*Figure 4.* Triploidy of swimming larvae provides cytogenetic evidence that a renal adenocarcinoma nucleus programs for differentiated tissues. A triploid zygote (A) is produced by retention of the second polar body. When the triploid zygote attains a prehatching embryo stage (B), it is injected with a Lucké tumor herpesvirus preparation. A triploid frog (C) develops with a triploid renal adenocarcinoma. The latter is dissociated (D) and a triploid Lucké renal adenocarcinoma nucleus in injected into a previously enucleated egg (E). Triploidy is evidence that the donor renal adenocarcinoma nucleus provided the genome for the swimming larva (F). (From McKinnell and Ellis[104a].)

dedifferentiation of an adult cell into a mitotically active neoplastic cell, or if the cancer results from the transformation of already mitotically active, not fully differentiated, kidney stem cells during embryogenesis. While adult kidney is not an organ subject to extensive tissue renewal, it can under certain circumstances, such as nephrectomy, resume mitotic activity.[112-115]

However, two kinds of evidence argue compellingly against the transformation of fully differentiated adult cells into mitotically active neoplastic cells and favor the interpretation that the target cell for neoplastic change is a stem cell. The first of these lines of evidence relates to the developmental stages that are vulnerable to Lucké tumor herpesvirus (LTHV) transformation. Only eggs, embryos, and larvae are susceptible to the oncogenic effect of LTHV injection.[103,116] Furthermore, there is direct experimental evidence from virus injection experiments that a pronephric cell or some antecedent stem cell of the pronephros can be transformed by the virus resulting in the appearance of pronephric tumors at metamorphosis.[117] Since the pronephros exists only in immature stages, the virus injection experiments support the view that a stem cell, not a fully differentiated adult cell, is the target for LTHV transformation. Cancer induction by LTHV in immature frog stages has interesting counterparts in the experimental induction of some tumors in mammals by viruses and chemical carcinogens that seem most effective when administered to neonatal animals with their less than fully differentiated cells.[118-121]

A second kind of evidence derives from the extensive embryonic development obtained when frog renal tumor nuclei were transplanted to enucleated eggs. Normal development or extensive embryonic development in nuclear transfer embryos is characteristic only of transplanted embryonic nuclei. Specialized nuclei direct such extensive development only after pretreatment by exposure to low temperature and a polycationic amine[122] or incubation in oocyte cytoplasm.[8,94] No pretreatment of any kind is required to condition renal adenocarcinoma nuclei to participate in embryonic development after nuclear transplantation. In other words, they behave as if they were embryonic nuclei. This could possibly be, as is suggested here, because the carcinoma cells are transformed stem cells that are frozen in an immature stage of differentiation by exposure to an oncogenic virus. Thus, the frog renal adenocarcinoma may have a stem cell origin, as many other tumors are thought to have.[1,3,22,24,123]

Studies of frog renal tumors would be of limited value if they had no relevance to tumors of higher organisms. However, they do have relevance. For example, it has been reported that a human congenital nephroma, which grew *in vitro* as sheets of spindle-shaped cells totally devoid of typical renal structures, could be cocultured with fetal mouse dorsal spinal cord with the result that the nephroma differentiated fetal nephrons with Bowman's capsules, glomeruli, and proximal tubules.[124] The human nephroma thus had the capacity to differentiate when confronted with a previously described kidney tubule inducer[125,126] and in that restricted sense shares an attribute with the Lucké renal adenocarcinoma of the frog.

## 2.4. Neuroblastomas

The potentiality for induced expression of differentiated function in human neuroblastomas was reported more than 40 years ago, although the significance of the observations to the concept of cancer cell differentiation may have escaped the authors. Eight human neuroblastomas were cultured *in vitro* as a means of making a differential diagnosis among this tumor and lymphosarcomas and small cell carcinomas. The most conspicuous trait of the cultured neuroblastomas was the outgrowth of dendritic processes and axons, otherwise referred to as neurites.[127] Since those early observations, others have reported the same phenomenon, i.e., that neuroblastomas, which typically resemble masses of small lymphocytes, will in culture differentiate and mature[128,129] (Fig. 5).

Maturation is characterized by the coalescence of previously dispersed microtubules proximal to the site of neurite outgrowth.[130-133] There is an increase in Nissl substance, increase in nuclear size, and growth of one or more neurites. Maturation of murine or human neuroblastoma cells may occur spontaneously in culture[127,128] or as a result of growth in serum-free medium or treatment with various chemicals, vitamins, or chemotherapeutic agents.[129,130,134-139]

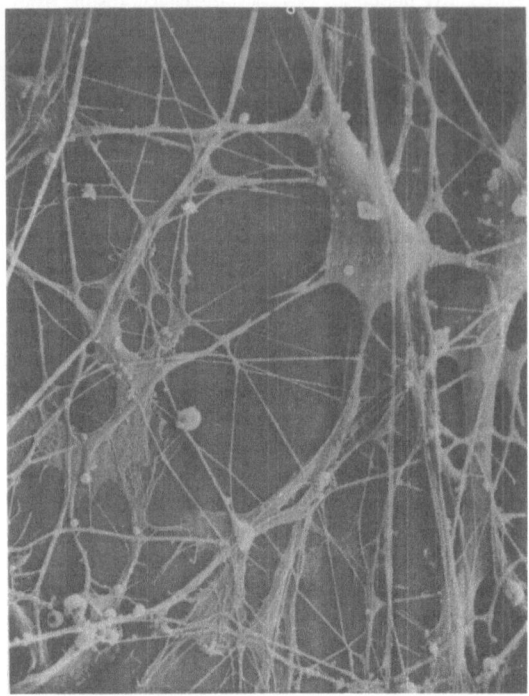

*Figure 5.* Human neuroblastoma cells differentiated after culture for 44 days in medium containing mitomycin-C. The scanning electron micrograph shows a ganglion cell and network of interlacing neurites. (From Goldstein and Plurad.[137])

Teratocarcinoma cells have been observed to differentiate in the presence of unidentified substances in the blastocyst. Is there an analogous differentiating environment that can exert biologic control on neuroblastoma cells? An answer is emerging from experiments in which neuroblastoma cells are injected into the neural crest migratory route[18]* and into the embryonic adrenal gland at the time when normal neural crest cells arrive at that organ.[140] Whatever the fate of the injected neuroblastoma cells, it is evident that tumors fail to occur in expected numbers. The observed maturation of neuroblastoma cells *in vitro* and *in vivo* lends credence to the early observation of spontaneous differentiation of a human malignant tumor to a benign ganglioneuroma.[141]

## 2.5. Rhabdomyosarcoma

Skeletal muscle tumors of humans[142] and rats[143] contain both mononucleated round or spindle-shaped cells and multinucleated striated muscle fibers. The nonstriated mononucleated cells are mitotically active, incorporate [³H]thymidine, and have quantitative Feulgen DNA values typical of proliferating cells. By contrast, the multinucleated cells are striated postmitotic differentiated cells that are not labeled with [³H]thymidine after a 2-hr exposure. However, if the cells are incubated an additional 16 hr, after unincorporated radioactive precursors have been removed, the multinucleated cells become labeled, which indicates that the origin of the differentiated myotubules is from the mononucleated cells.[144]

Mouse skeletal muscle tumor cells, in confluent culture, are similarly incompletely differenti-

---

*Tsokos *et al.*[139a] recently have provided morphologic and biochemical evidence for the potential of human neuroblastoma cell lines to undergo neuronal, melanocytic, and Schwann cell differentiation in response to treatments *in vitro* with dibutyryl cyclic adenosine monophosphate and retinoic acid. These investigators further suggested that differentiation of these malignant neoplasms actually recapitulates different stages of neural crest development.

ated. Treatment of these cells with *N-N*-dimethylformamide induces differentiation. As would be expected, fewer animals receiving injections of differentiated cells develop tumors compared with animals receiving uninduced cells.[145]

More recently, it was reported that rat rhabdomyosarcoma cells will differentiate in response to hydrocortisone, in turn inhibiting metastases to lungs and lymph nodes. Metastasis is a fundamental characteristic of malignancy. Postmitotic differentiated cells should, and apparently do, fail to metastasize.[146]

## 2.6. Teratocarcinomas

Early evidence that malignant cells could differentiate came from studies of teratocarcinomas. The tumors arise spontaneously in the gonads of certain strains of mice[147] or can be produced experimentally by grafting embryos to ectopic sites.[148–150] While experimentation relating to differentiation of teratocarcinomas is confined to mice, germ cell tumors of humans, like their murine counterparts, are known in some cases to undergo maturation.[151,152]

The highly malignant mouse teratocarcinomas are composed of varying proportions of undifferentiated embryonal carcinoma cells and a wide diversity of tissues in various stages of differentiation, including CNS tissue, cartilage, bone, stratified squamous epithelium, striated muscle fibers, respiratory and alimentary muscosae, glands, and so forth,[153–157] in an anatomic arrangement described by Needham[34] as an ''approximation to chaos.'' Sometimes in these bizarre neoplasms there appear structures with a marked resemblance to early human embryos.[158] These are called embryoid bodies.

Free-floating cell aggregates, which resemble naturally occurring embryoid bodies, can be produced in the laboratory by injecting a suspension of teratocarcinoma cells into mice. These experimentally produced structures are composed of embryonal carcinoma cells covered by a layer of visceral yolk sac. The internal cells were thought to be multipotential and were believed to give rise to various somatic cells by differentiation.[159] Experimental verification of the multipotentiality of embryoid bodies was obtained by grafting these structures to the anterior eye chamber[160] or subcutaneously in mice.[161] A diversity of differentiated tissue types formed. A direct test of the capacity of single teratocarcinoma cells to differentiate was provided by Klinesmith and Pierce.[162] They transplanted single cells into mice and obtained teratocarcinomas composed of embryonal carcinoma and up to 14 well-differentiated somatic tissues. Their results clearly demonstrate the multipotentiality of single embryonal carcinoma cells. The cells replicate not only more cells like themselves but, in addition, produce an array of differentiated nonmalignant cell types.

One could postulate that an embryonic environment could have a profound effect on gene expression in teratocarcinoma cells. It does. Teratocarcinoma cells, transferred to a mouse blastocyst, will participate in normal development. This phenomenon was first demonstrated by Brinster,[163] who illustrated his study with a random bred Swiss albino mouse displaying a stripe of agouti fur. He thus demonstrated unequivocally that the injected teratocarcinoma cells, carrying the genotype for agouti color, had differentiated into an adult tissue (agouti fur) in the presence of the normally differentiating embryonic host cells. These studies were extended by others[164–169] who injected genetically marked teratocarcinoma core cells derived from embryoid bodies, either singly or in small numbers, into mouse blastocysts. The operated blastocysts were inserted into a foster female and, upon completion of gestation, normal live mosaic mice were born. The mice contained normal differentiated tissues of teratocarcinoma origin. The tissue types included those previously seen in mouse teratomas as well as liver, thymus, and kidney. The teratocarcinoma cells were judged to be totipotent.

An intact genome is believed to be a prerequisite for totipotency. Many tumors are aneuploid or show other chromosomal alterations.[170,171] Therefore, the chromosomal composition of the totipotential teratocarcinoma cells was examined. They proved to be euploid or near euploid.[172] Some teratocarcinoma-injected blastocysts develop as chimeras with tumors.[167,168] The failure of the blastocyst environment to regulate all teratocarcinoma cells may occur even if the cells are euploid.[173]

Teratocarcinoma cells thus exhibit the capacity to differentiate into a number of mature tissues when grafted to adult hosts or to the embryonic environment of a blastocyst. Cell lines derived from teratocarcinomas have been shown to differentiate *in vitro*. When isolated single cells were cultured they divided and formed small aggregates which subsequently detached giving rise to typical embryoid bodies.[174]

Retinoic acid in concentrations as low as $10^{-9}$ M has been shown to induce phenotypic changes in teratocarcinoma-derived cell lines.[175] Morphologic changes observed in monolayer culture suggested the differentiation of endodermal cells like those that form the exterior coat of embryoid bodies. Moreover, the retinoic acid-treated cells produce plasminogen activator that is not secreted in appreciable levels by embryonal carcinoma cells but is secreted by endoderm cells differentiated from embryonal carcinoma cells. Furthermore, the retinoic acid differentiated cells produce a collagenlike protein identical to that elaborated by parietal endoderm cells.

Since these pioneering studies of retinoic acid-induced differentiation, many additional investigations have reported the efficacy of retinoic acid in promoting differentiation *in vitro*. Cultures of human teratoma, for example, contain a small fraction of cells that respond to retinoic acid treatment by differentiating as neurons.[176–178]

Depending on the concentration of retinoic acid used, different cell types are observed to differentiate. Using a subclone of P19 teratocarcinoma cells, retinoic acid at $10^{-9}$ M caused the differentiation of cardiac cells, retinoic acid at $10^{-8}$ M induced skeletal cells, and retinoic acid at $10^{-5}$–$10^{-7}$ M caused the differentiation of neurons and astroglia.[179] Recently, it has been shown that retinoic acid treatment of teratocarcinoma cells will affect DNA methylation,[180] expression of homeo-box genes,[181,182] X-chromosome inactivation,[183] and decreased poly(ADP-ribose) synthesis.[184]

There is a teratocarcinoma cell line which, after subcutaneous injection into recipient mice, has the capacity to differentiate chondroblasts and chondrocytes that subsequently form bonelike ossicles complete with marrow populated with erythrocytes, granulocytes, and megakaryocytes. The ossicles may persist for a year with little or no change. However, some recipient mice develop osteosarcomas, chondrosarcomas, and fibrosarcomas.[185] Thus, while differentiation is thought to abrogate malignancy (and usually does), there are cases (such as these bone-forming cells and *some* mice that as blastocysts received teratocarcinoma cells) in which differentiation has occurred but the potential for malignancy has persisted.

## 2.7. Squamous Cell Carcinoma

Skin tumors of rats, produced by dietary administration of the chemical carcinogen $N,N'$-2,7-fluorenylenebisacetamide, were found to be of several histological types,[186] including one that was established as a transplantable squamous cell carcinoma that exhibited islands of well-differentiated keratinizing epithelial pearls scattered throughout the neoplasm similar to those seen in human squamous cell carcinoma of the skin (Fig. 6). Rats bearing this tumor were pulse-labeled with [$^3$H]thymidine in an experiment designed to detect the origin of the epithelial pearls. Many squamous cell carcinoma nuclei were labeled after 2 hr but epithelial pearls were unlabeled. However, at 96 hr after labelling, epithelial pearls were also labeled.[187] This experiment indicated that the well-differentiated pearls were derived from the squamous cell carcinoma. The designations squamous cell carcinoma and epithelial pearl are morphologic and do not reveal the capacity of either to produce tumors. Small fragments of undifferentiated squamous cell carcinoma and dissected epithelial pearls were therefore grafted subcutaneously into rats. In this regard, only the squamous cell carcinoma, produced tumors while the epithelial pearls differentiated, became postmitotic, and lost the capacity to form tumors when grafted.[187]

## 2.8. Myeloid Leukemia

Factors that control growth, viability, and differentiation of the normal stem cells that give rise to granulocytes and macrophages have been characterized and are known as colony-stimulating

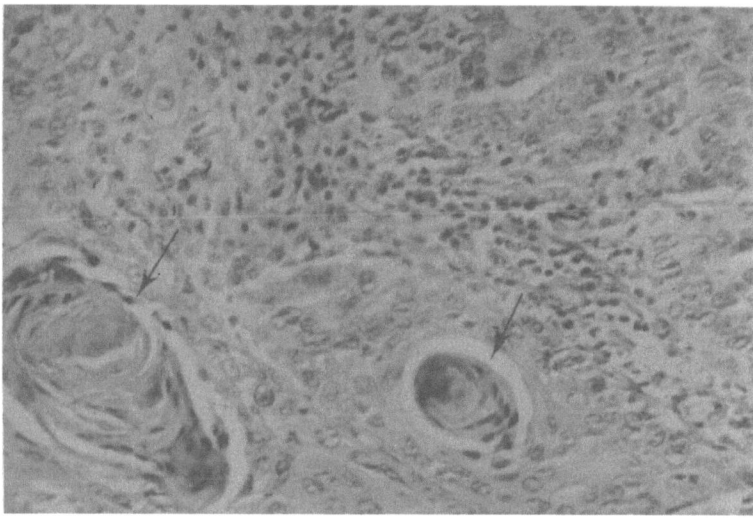

*Figure 6.* Squamous cell pearls (arrows) in a human skin squamous cell carcinoma. (Courtesy of Dr. Alphonse E. Sirica, Medical College of Virginia-VCU.) (H&E, ×320)

factors or macrophage granulocyte inducers (MGI). Thus far, four major colony-stimulating factors have been purified from the mouse, and all have been shown to be glycoproteins produced by a variety of normal tissues. These factors can induce cultured murine myeloid leukemic cells to differentiate *in vitro*.[188] Induced differentiation occurs also in human myeloid leukemic cell lines ML-1 and HL-60[189,190] (Fig. 7). Recently, a pluripotent human colony-stimulating factor similar to murine granulocyte colony-stimulating factor, with the capacity to induce terminal differentiation of certain murine and human leukemic cell lines, was produced using recombinant DNA (rDNA) procedures.[191]

As would be expected, not all myeloid leukemia cells respond in the same manner. Some myeloid cell lines have the capacity for continued growth but fail to differentiate properly. The cells seem to have escaped from the need for growth inducers that are ordinarily supplied extrinsically. It would seem that they need less growth factor for replication or that they produce their own growth factor intrinsically. Some of these cells, designated D+ for differentiation-positive, will respond to an exogenous supply of the differentiation inducer by differentiating into cells which are morphologically and physiologically indistinguishable from normal macrophages and granulocytes. The differentiation-positive cells respond not only to the natural inducer but also to a relatively long list of chemical inducers.[192] The differentiated macrophages and granulocytes are mitotically inactive.

Other kinds of leukemic cells, designated D− for differentiation-negative, fail to respond to natural differentiation inducers and perhaps represent a more advanced stage of malignancy than the D+ type cells. However, this latter type of myeloid leukemic cell may respond to other agents, or combination of agents, together with normal differentiation factor, to produce differentiated, postmitotic myeloid blood cells. The substances to which D− cells may respond include some steroid hormones, low doses of X-rays, some vitamins, insulin, lectins, some phorbol esters, and low doses of conventional chemotherapeutic agents such as cytosine arabinoside, adriamycin, and methotrexate.[22,23] Thus, both the differentiation-positive and the differentiation-negative cells have retained the genes necessary for differentiation, even though their chromosomes may vary from the normal karyotype.[193] This indicates that while there is a genetic basis for the malignant behavior of the leukemic cells, the genetic defect can be bypassed with appropriate treatment of leukemic cells *in vitro* or experimental treatment *in vivo*.[25,192,194,195]

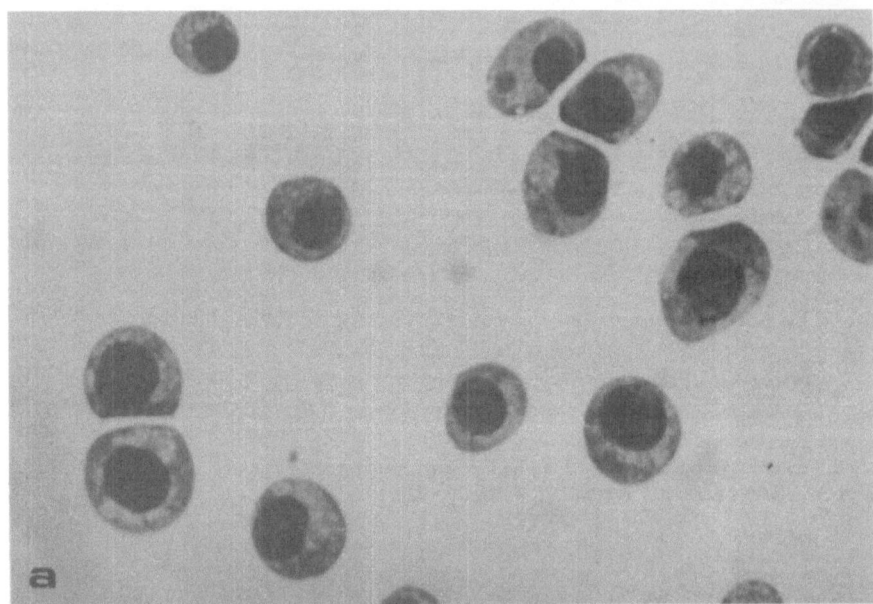

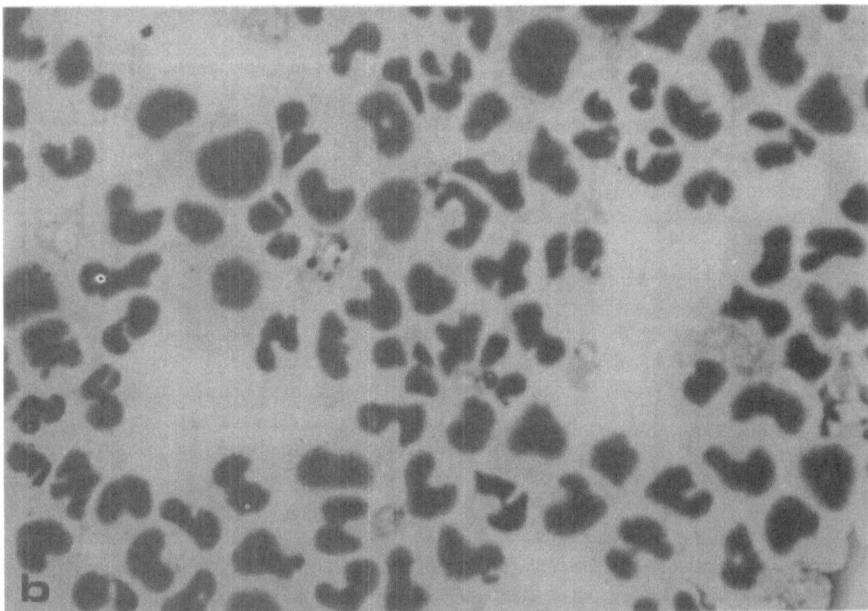

*Figure 7.* Induction of granulocyte differentiation in the human promyelocytic leukemia cell line HL-60. (a) Undifferentiated leukemic promyeloblasts. (b) Granulocyte differentiation induced by 6 days of exposure to 1.25% DMSO. (Courtesy of Dr. Eric Westin, Medical College of Virginia, VCU.) (Wright stain, ×320)

## 2.9. Murine Erythroleukemia

Murine erythroleukemia cell (MELC) lines were derived from reticulum cell sarcomas which developed from subcutaneous grafts of spleen or liver obtained from mice afflicted with Friend virus-induced leukemia.[196–198] The cell lines are malignant, as evidenced by the tumors formed when cells are injected into appropriate murine hosts. The tumors so produced are indistinguishable from those from which the cell lines were derived. MELC grows as a pleomorphic population of cells composed of undifferentiated cells and cells at various levels of erythroid differentiation. Most are primitive erythroid cells, but some become more mature and resemble normoblasts. Most MELC cell lines display a low level of spontaneous differentiation as evidenced by the benzidine reaction for hemoglobin. Erythroid differentiation is enhanced by treatment of the cells with dimethylsulfoxide (DMSO). Similarly, sodium butyrate induces erythroid differentiation in the equivalent human leukemic cell line K562 with an associated loss of proliferative capacity.[199] A number of significant changes in the MELC cells occurs with differentiation, including greatly increased levels of globin mRNA, $\alpha$- and $\beta$-globin synthesis, appearance of erythrocyte membrane antigens, synthesis of heme and hemoglobin, decreased cell volume, and a limited capacity for cell renewal.[198,200] Induced differentiation of MELC cells thus shares similarities to erythropoietin-regulated differentiation of normal cells, but the MELC themselves (and K562 cells) are unresponsive to erythropoietin, and the MELC cells do not achieve a completely normal erythroid phenotype with nuclear ejection. Virus proliferation continues even during induced maturation, indicating that the phenomena are not mutually exclusive events.

Spleen colonies of MELC form when the cells are inoculated intravenously into irradiated mice. The colonies are composed of neoplastic cells and cells that differentiate along the erythroid pathway as proerythroblasts and normoblasts.[201] Hence, erythroid differentiation occurs either *in vitro* or in spleen colonies *in vivo*. It occurs spontaneously, or it can be induced.

A diversity of chemicals induce differentiation of murine erythroleukemia. They include DMSO, as well as hexamethylene bisacetamide (HMBA), purines and purine analogues, short-chain fatty acids, hemin, cardiac glycosides, metabolic inhibitors, and so forth.[198,202–204] Recently, the antifungal antibiotic trichostatins were shown to be potent inducers of MELC differentiation[205] and thus may be added to the more than 300 inducers of MELC differentiation. As in other tumor systems, a marked decrease in oncogenicity appears to be directly related to enhanced differentiation.[202]

## 2.10. Other Tumors That Differentiate

Space precludes discussion of all tumors reported to differentiate. Some others reported to do so include breast cancer,[206,207] glioma,[208,209] melanoma,[210,211] colon cancer,[212,213] and Burkitt lymphoma.[214]

## 3. PRIMARY INDUCTION IN THE VERTEBRATE EMBRYO COMPARED WITH THE INDUCTION OF CANCER CELL DIFFERENTIATION

Embryonic induction refers to the interaction of two tissues in which one, the inducer, after coming into close proximity with the responding tissue, causes that tissue to differentiate. To be effective, this inductive influence must occur within a brief developmental period during which the responding tissue is described as being "competent" to respond to the induction. The best known and most studied example of induction is that of neural plate and embryonic axis by the underlying chordamesoderm cells of the amphibian embryo,[215–218] although induction has also been studied in the avian and mammalian embryo. Embryonic inductions are not limited to the neural plate but include a whole host of secondary and tertiary inductions, including the lens of the eye, which is induced by the optic cups,[219] as well as the induction by embryonic mammalian spinal cord of tubule development in metanephrogenic mesenchyme.[125,220]

Initially, the inductive potency of the dorsal lip of the amphibian blastopore was studied by transplantation to a heterotopic site where it induced a neural plate, embryonic axis, and, ultimately, a secondary embryo. These experiments showed that most regions of the embryonic ectoderm would respond to subjacent chordamesoderm by differentiating a neural plate and neural tube. Primary induction was also demonstrated *in vitro* in sandwiches of inducers and responding tissue.

It was not long, moreover, before it was discovered that the inducer tissue may be killed physically (e.g., crushing, freezing, or heating) or by chemical treatment (e.g., alcohol, ether, or other solvents) and still retain its efficacy in induction. The demonstration of induction by nonliving tissue strongly suggested that induction occurs as a result of a chemical, not a biologic, event.[217,221] A flurry of activity accompanied the realization that a chemical might be identified that controlled normal cell differentiation. Within a short period, many unrelated chemical substances were identified that had the capacity to induce amphibian neural tissue—including silica, calcium carbonate,[222] digitonin, cephalin, various buffers,[223] thiocyanate,[224] sulfhydryl compounds,[225] certain dyes,[226] and even a hydrocarbon carcinogen.[227] The problem was complicated when it was reported that neural differentiation would occur with no inducer at all.[228] The great variety of apparently unrelated factors that can induce embryonic ectoderm to differentiate as neural tube suggests that embryonic ectoderm, before induction, is already fully equipped to carry out neural differentiation, and is arrested by no more than a hair trigger. Many relatively unspecific influences might then propel embryonic ectoderm to its neural destiny. Yet it must be remembered that most embryonic ectoderm, in the absence of induction by the chordamesoderm, differentiates as epidermis. Despite years of study of the phenomenon, Gurdon recently commented that the "molecular basis of induction and the inductive response remain almost totally obscure."[218]

In sum, differentiation of the neural plate can occur *in vivo* after induction of the chordamesoderm. *In vitro* it can occur spontaneously, or it can be induced by proximity to natural inducers or by a wildly divergent array of chemical substances.

Differentiation of cancer cells, in general, seems to share similarities with the embryonic cell differentiation. For example, spontaneous differentiation of cancer cells occurs *in vivo*, but the phenomenon appears to be rare. When it occurs, it is sometimes referred to as spontaneous regression, but it is in fact maturation or differentiation.[151,229] Such a case was described above in the discussion of neuroblastoma[141] (see Section 2.4). Cancer cell differentiation also occurs spontaneously *in vitro;* the differential diagnostic procedure to identify the cell of origin of neuroblastomas by determining the type of growth *in vitro* is an example.[127]

Maturation of cancer cells occurs *in vitro* in response to biologic substances and to a diversity of chemical substances as bewildering as those which effect neural plate differentiation in the amphibian embryo. Exemplifying the biologic response modifiers discussed with regard to myeloid leukemia (see Section 2.8) are the macrophage granulocyte inducers (MGI), also known as granulocyte–macrophage colony-stimulation factor (GM-CSF).[23,188] Another biologic substance reported to affect both normal and tumor cells is the glia maturation factor (GMF), an acidic protein of the brain, capable of promoting differentiation of cultured astroblasts. Contact inhibition is restored and proliferation is limited when the C6 rodent and HG-1 human glioma cell lines are cultured with GMF. Differentiation to mature astrocytic cells occurs *in vivo* with inoculation of C-6 cells into nude mice treated with GMF.[209]

There are other biologic factors that can effect differentiation of cancer cells, but they remain undefined. Included in this category are factors in the cytoplasm of the amphibian egg that inhibit the expression of those genes characteristic of the frog renal carcinoma and awake from dormancy the genes associated with normal differentiation of amphibian larvae (see Section 2.3). Also included in this category is the interior of the murine blastocyst, which permits differentiation of teratocarcinoma cells (see Section 2.6).

Just as embryonic cells can be induced to differentiate *in vitro* with a diversity of chemical compounds, so too do certain cancers respond to a wide spectrum of chemicals. These include, but are not limited to, the induced differentiation of teratocarcinoma cells by retinoic acid,[230] retinal, retinol, 5-bromouracil 2′-deoxyribose (BUdR), 5-iodouracil 2′-deoxyribose (IUdR), (HMBA), dimethylacetamide (DMA), and (DMSO).[231] Promyelocytic leukemia cells (HL-60) are induced to differentiate by retinoic acid, 12-*O*-tetradecanoyl-phorbol 13-acetate (TPA), and phytohemag-glutinin-leukocyte conditioned medium,[232,233] cyclopentenyl and cyclopentyo analogues of cytidine,[234] DMSO and dimethylformamide (DMF),[235] as well as recombinant human leukocyte interferon in combination with other inducers.[236]

Waxman and colleagues[204] stated that about 300 agents have induced differentiation in the mouse erythroleukemia cell system but with varying efficacy. It is beyond the scope of this paper to either list all of the inducers or to provide an explanation of how they function. A useful summary which sorts differentiation inducers into five categories has been provided by Gabrilove.[27] She divided inducers into chemotherapeutic agents, polar compounds, phorbol esters, vitamin ana-logues, and physiologically important cytokines. A similar table of agents that induce differentiation of cancer cells can be found in Freshney's report.[28]

Rather than go into detail concerning the proposed mechanisms for induction, it is the purpose here to emphasize that many cancer cells have the latent competence to respond to stimulation by differentiation. It is as if they are primed and need only be cued to initiate terminal differentiation. Terminal differentiation abrogates malignancy, and that is the rationale for continued study of cancer cell differentiation.

ACKNOWLEDGMENTS. The author acknowledges with appreciation the valuable comments made to an early version of this paper by Dr. G. Barry Pierce and Dr. Marion Namenwirth. Barbara Hunter and Debra Kane helped with the preparation of this manuscript, which was typed by Tina Lorsung. Beverly W. Kerr and Susan McKinnell proofread the final version of the paper. Work from the author's laboratory was supported by grants RD-248 and IN-Y-8 from the American Cancer Society and by grant 84/0438 from NATO.

# REFERENCES

1. Pierce, G. B., Shikes, R., and Fink, L. M., 1978, *Cancer, A Problem of Developmental Biology*, Prentice-Hall, Englewood Cliffs, New Jersey.
2. Siminovitch, L., and Axelrad, A. A., 1963, Cell-cell interactions *in vitro:* Their relation to differentiation and carcinogenesis, *Can. Cancer Conf.* **5:**149–165.
3. Mintz, B., 1978, Gene expression in neoplasia and differentiation, *Harvey Lect.* **71:**193–246.
4. Pierce, G. B., and Speers, W. C., 1988, Tumors as caricatures of the process of tissue renewal: Prospects for therapy by directing differentiation, *Cancer Res.* **48:**1996–2004.
5. Bernhard, W., 1969, Ultrastructure of the cancer cell, in: *Handbook of Molecular Cytology* (A. Lima-de-Faria, ed.), pp. 687–715, North-Holland, Amsterdam.
6. DiBerardino, M. A., Hoffner, N. J., and Etkin, L., 1984, Activation of dormant genes in specialized cells, *Science* **224:**946–952.
7. Blau, H. M., Pavlath, G. K., Hardeman, E. C., Chiu, C-P., Silberstein, L., Webster, S. G., Miller, S. C., and Webster, C., 1985, Plasticity of the differentiated state, *Science* **230:**758–766.
8. DiBerardino, M. A., Orr, N. H., and McKinnell, R. G., 1986, Feeding tadpoles cloned from *Rana* erythrocyte nuclei, *Proc. Natl. Acad. Sci. USA* **83:**8231–8234.
9. Armstrong, P. B., 1984, Invasiveness of non-malignant cells, in: *Invasion, Experimental and Clinical Implications*, pp. 126–167, Oxford University Press, Oxford.
10. Bronner-Fraser, M., 1984, Latex beads with defined surface coats as probes of neural crest migratory pathways, in: *The Role of Extracellular Matrix in Development* (R. L. Trelstad, ed.), pp. 399–432, Liss, New York.
11. Liotta, L. A., 1986, Tumor invasion and metastasis—Role of the extracellular matrix, *Cancer Res.* **46:**1–7.
12. Mareel, M. M., and Calman, K. C., 1984, *Invasion: Experimental and Clinical Implications*, Oxford University Press, Oxford.
13. McKinnell, R. G., Bruyneel, E. A., Mareel, M. M., Tweedell, K. S., and Mekela, P., 1988, Tem-perature-dependent malignant invasion *in vitro* by frog renal carcinoma-derived PNKT-4B cells, *Clin. Exp. Metast.* **6:**49–59.

14. Pierce, G. B., 1961, Teratocarcinomas, in: *Teratocarcinomas, A Problem in Developmental Biology*, Fourth Canadian Cancer Conference, Vol. 4 (R. Begg, ed.), pp. 119–137, Academic, New York.

15. Pierce, G. B., 1974, The benign cells of malignant tumors, in: *Developmental Aspects of Carcinogenesis and Immunity* (T. J. King, ed.), pp. 3–22, Academic, New York.

16. Pierce, G. B., 1975, Teratocarcinoma: Introduction and perspectives, in: *Teratomas and Differentiation* (M. I. Sherman and D. Solter, eds.), pp. 3–12, Academic, New York.

17. Pierce, G. B., and Johnson, L. D., 1971, Differentiation and cancer, *In Vitro* 7:140–145.

18. Podesta, A. H., Mullins, J., Pierce, G. B., and Wells, R. S., 1984, The neurula-stage mouse embryo in control of neuroblastoma, *Proc. Natl. Acad. Sci. USA* 81:7608–7611.

19. Sporn, M. B., and Roberts, A. B., 1984, Role of retinoids in differentiation and carcinogenesis, *J. Natl. Cancer Inst.* 73:1381–1387.

20. Sachs, L., 1980, Activation of normal differentiation genes and the origin and development of myeloid leukemia, in: *Differentiation and Neoplasia* (R. G. McKinnell, M. A. DiBerardino, M. Blumenfeld, and R. D. Bergad, eds.), pp. 213–216, Springer-Verlag, Berlin.

21. Sachs, L., 1985, Regulators of growth, differentiation, and the reversal of malignancy: Normal hematopoiesis and leukemia, in: *Molecular Biology of Tumor Cells* (B. Wahren, G. Holm, S. Hammarström, and P. Perlmann, eds.), pp. 257–280, Raven, New York.

22. Sachs, L., 1986, Growth, differentiation and the reversal of malignancy, *Sci. Am.* 254:40–47.

23. Sachs, L., 1987, Cell differentiation and bypassing of genetic defects in the suppression of malignancy, *Cancer Res.* 47:1981–1986.

24. Paul, J., 1978, Cell differentiation and cancer—A summary, in: *Cell Differentiation and Neoplasia* (G. F. Saunders, ed.), pp. 525–532, Raven, New York.

25. Lotem, J., and Sachs, L., 1984, Control of *in vivo* differentiation of myeloid leukemic cells. IV. Inhibition of leukemia development by myeloid differentiation-inducing protein, *Int. J. Cancer* 33:147–154.

26. Marks, P. A., and Rifkind, R. A., 1984, Differentiation modifiers, *Cancer* 54 (suppl. 11):2766–2769.

27. Gabrilove, J. L., 1986, Differentiation factors, *Semin. Oncol.* 13:228–233.

28. Freshney, R. I., 1985, Induction of differentiation in neoplastic cells, *Anticancer Res.* 5:111–130.

29. Rather, L. J., 1978, *The Genesis of Cancer*, Johns Hopkins Press, Baltimore.

30. Cohnheim, J., 1875, Congenitales, quergestreiftes Muskelsarkom der Nieren, *Arch. Pathol. Anat. Physiol. Klin. Med.* 65:64–69.

31. Cohnheim, J., 1889, *Lectures on General Pathology*, The New Sydenham Society, London (translated from the German by A. B. McKee).

32. Beard, J., 1911, The enzyme treatment of cancer and its scientific basis, *Collected papers*, Chatto and Windus, London.

33. Needham, J., 1936, New advances in the chemistry and biology of organized growth, *Proc. R. Soc. Med.* 29:1577–1626.

34. Needham, J., 1942, *Biochemistry and Morphogenesis*, Cambridge University Press, Cambridge.

35. Lucké, B., 1934, A neoplastic disease of the kidney of the frog, *Rana pipiens*, *Am. J. Cancer* 20:352–379.

36. Rose, S. M., and Wallingford, H. M., 1948, Transformation of renal tumors of frogs to normal tissue in regenerating limbs of salamanders, *Science* 107:457.

37. Rose, S. M., 1949, Transformed cells, *Sci. Am.* 181(6):22–24.

38. Rollins, L. A., and McKinnell, R. G., 1980, The influence of glucocorticoids on survival and growth of allografted tumors in the anterior eye chamber of leopard frogs, *Dev. Comp. Immunol.* 4:283–294.

39. Tarin, D., McKinnell, R. G., and Nace, G. W., 1984, Artificially induced metastasis by cells from spontaneous Lucké renal adenocarcinoma, *Invasion Metast.* 4:198–208.

40. Ruben, L. N., 1955, The effects of implanting anuran cancer into nonregenerating and regenerating larval urodele limbs, *J. Exp. Zool.* 128:29–51.

41. Ruben, L. N., 1956, The effects of implanting anuran cancer into regenerating adult urodele limbs. I. Simple regenerating systems, *J. Morphol.* 98:389–403.

42. Ruben, L. N., and Balls, M., 1964, The implanting of lymphosarcoma of *Xenopus laevis* into regenerating and non-regenerating forelimbs of that species, *J. Morphol.* 115:225–238.

43. Sheremetieva, E. A., 1965, Spontaneous melanoma in regenerating tails of axolotls, *J. Exp. Zool.* 158:101–122.

44. Tsonis, P. A., 1984, Limb regeneration in newts with spontaneous skin cancer, *Can. J. Zool.* 62:2681–2685.

45. Pierce, G. B., Arechaga, J., Jones, A., Lewellyn, A., and Wells, R. S., 1987, The fate of embryonal-carcinoma cells in mouse blastocysts, *Differentiation* 33:247–253.

46. Lockhart-Mummery, J. P., 1934, *The Origin of Cancer,* Churchill, London.

47. Haldane, J. B. S., 1934, The origin of cancer, *J. Pathol.* **38:**507–508.

48. Waddington, C. H., 1935, Cancer and the theory of organizers, *Nature (Lond.)* **135:**606–608.

49. Berrill, N. J., 1943, Malignancy in relation to organization and differentiation, *Physiol. Rev.* **23:**101–123.

50. Pierce, G. B., 1967, Teratocarcinoma: Model for a developmental concept of cancer, in: *Current Topics in Developmental Biology* (A. A. Moscona and A. Monroy, eds.), pp. 223–246, Academic, New York.

51. Markert, C. L., 1968, Neoplasia: A disease of cell differentiation, *Cancer Res.* **28:**1908–1914.

52. Levin, I., and Levine, M., 1920, Malignancy of the crown-gall and its analogy to animal cancer, *J. Cancer Res.* **5:**243–260.

53. Lippincott, J. A., and Lippincott, B. B., 1981, Crown gall, a "malignant plant tumor," in: *Neoplasms Comparative Pathology of Growth in Animals, Plants, and Man* (H. E. Kaiser, ed.), pp. 833–839, Williams & Wilkins, Baltimore.

54. Kalil, M., and Hildebrandt, A. C., 1981, Pathology and distribution of plant tumors, in: *Neoplasms— Comparative Pathology of Growth in Animals, Plants, and Man* (H. E. Kaiser, ed.), pp. 813–821, Williams & Wilkins, Baltimore.

55. Braun, A. C., 1947, Thermal studies on the factors responsible for tumor initiation in crown-gall, *Am. J. Bot.* **34:**234–240.

56. Braun, A. C., 1968, The multipotential cell and the tumor problem, in: *The Stability of the Differentiated State* (H. Ursprung, ed.), pp. 128–135, Springer-Verlag, New York.

57. Braun, A. C., 1972, The usefulness of plant tumor systems for studying the basic cellular mechanisms that underlie neoplastic growth generally, in: *Cell Differentiation* (R. Harris, P. Allin, and D. Viza, eds.), pp. 115–118, Munksgaard, Copenhagen.

58. Meins, F., Jr., 1974, Mechanisms underlying tumor transformation and tumor reversal in crown-gall, a neoplastic disease of higher plants, in: *Developmental Aspects of Carcinogenesis and Immunity* (T. J. King, ed.), pp. 23–39, Academic, New York.

59. Watson, B., Currier, T. C., Gordon, M. P., Chilton, M. D., and Nester, E. W., 1975, Plasmid required for virulence of *Agrobacterium tumefaciens, J. Bacteriol.* **123:**255–264.

60. Schilperoort, R. A., Klapwijk, P. M., Hooykaas, P. J. J., Koekman, B. P., Ooms, G., Otten, L. A. B. M., Wurzer-Figurelli, E. M., Wullems, G. J., and Rörsch, A., 1978, *A. tumefaciens* plasmids as vectors for genetic transformation of plant cells, in: *Frontiers of Plant Tissue Culture 1978* (T. A. Thorpe, ed.), pp. 85–94, The International Association for Plant Tissue Culture, Calgary.

61. Ream, L. W., and Gordon, M. P., 1982, Crown gall disease and prospects for genetic manipulation in plants, *Science* **218:**854–859.

62. Thomashow, M. F., Hugly, S., Buchholz, W. G., and Thomashow, L. S., 1986, Molecular basis for auxin-independent phenotype of crown gall tumor tissues, *Science* **231:**616–618.

63. Smith, E. F., and Townsend, C. O., 1907, A plant-tumor of bacterial origin, *Science* **25:**671–673.

64. Torrey, J. G., 1985, The development of plant biotechnology, *Am. Sci.* **73:**354–363.

65. Muir, W. H., Hildebrandt, A. C., and Riker, A. J., 1958, The preparation, isolation, and growth in culture of single cells from higher plants, *Am. J. Bot.* **45:**589–597.

66. Steward, F. C., Mapes, M. O., Kent, A. E., and Holsten, R. D., 1964, Growth and development of cultured plant cells, *Science* **143:**20–27.

67. Steward, F. C., Ammirato, P. V., and Mapes, M. O., 1970, Growth and development of totipotent cells, *Ann. Bot.* **34:**761–787.

68. Earle, E. D., and Torrey, J. G., 1965, Morphogenesis in cell colonies grown from *Convolvulus* cell suspensions plated on synthetic media, *Am. J. Bot.* **52:**891–899.

69. Takebe, I., Labib, G., and Melchers, G., 1971, Regeneration of whole plants from isolated mesophyll protoplasts of tobacco, *Naturwissenschaft* **58:**318–320.

70. Vasil, V., and Hildebrandt, A. C., 1965, Differentiation of tobacco plants from single, isolated cells in microculture, *Science* **150:**889–892.

71. Braun, A. C., 1953, Bacterial and host factors concerned in determining tumor morphology in crown gall, *Bot. Gaz.* **114:**363–371.

72. Braun, A. C., 1951, Recovery of crown-gall tumor cells, *Cancer Res.* **11:**839–844.

72a. Braun, A. C., 1965, The reversal of tumor growth, *Sci Am.* **213**(5):75–83.

73. Braun, A. C., and Wood, H. N., 1976, Suppression of the neoplastic state with the acquisition of specialized functions in cells, tissues, and organs of crown gall teratomas of tobacco, *Proc. Natl. Acad. Sci. USA* **73:**496–500.

74. Turgeon, R., Wood, H. N., and Braun, A. C., 1976, Studies on the recovery of crown gall tumor cells, *Proc. Natl. Acad. Sci. USA* **73:**3562–3564.

75. Binns, A. N., Wood, H. N., and Braun, A. C., 1981, Suppression of the tumorous state in crown gall teratomas of tobacco: A clonal analysis, *Differentiation* **19**:97–102.

76. Braun, A. C., 1959, A demonstration of the recovery of the crown-gall tumor cell with the use of complex tumors of single-cell origin, *Proc. Natl. Acad. Sci. USA* **45**:932–938.

77. Schlumberger, H. G., and Lucké, B., 1948, Tumors of fishes, amphibians and reptiles, *Cancer Res.* **8**:657–754.

78. Harshbarger, J. C., Charles, A. M., and Spero, P. M., 1981, Collection and analysis of neoplasms of sub-homeothermic animals from a phyletic point of view, in: *Phyletic Approaches to Cancer* (C. J. Dawe, J. C. Harshbarger, S. Kondo, T. Sugimura, and S. Takayama, eds.), pp. 357–384, Japan Scientific Societies Press, Tokyo.

79. Ishikawa, T., Prince Masahito, Matsumoto, J., and Takayama, S., 1978, Morphologic and biological characterization of erythrophoromas in goldfish (*Carassius auratus*), *J. Natl. Cancer Inst.* **61**:1461–1470.

80. Matsumoto, J., Ishikawa, T., Prince Masahito, and Takayama, S., 1980, Permanent cell lines from erythrophoromas in goldfish (*Carassius auratus*), *J. Natl. Cancer Inst.* **64**:879–890.

81. Matsumoto, J., Ishikawa, T., Prince Masahito, Oikawa, A., and Takayama, S., 1981, Multiplicity in phenotypic expression of fish erythrophoroma and irido-melanophoroma cells *in vitro*, in: *Phyletic Approaches to Cancer* (C. J. Dawe, J. C. Harshbarger, S. Kondo, T. Sugimura, and S. Takayama, eds.), pp. 253–266, Japan Scientific Societies Press, Tokyo.

82. Matsumoto, J., Lynch, T. J., Grabowski, S., Richards, C. M., Lo, S. L., Clark, C., Kern, D., Taylor, J. D., Tchen, T. T., Ishikawa, T., Prince Masahito, and Takayama, S., 1983, Fish tumor pigment cells: Differentiation and comparison to their normal counterparts, *Am. Zool.* **23**:569–580.

83. Matsumoto, J., Akiyama, T., Taylor, J. D., and Tchen, T. T., 1985, Modification of differentiation programs of goldfish erythrophoroma cells by dual applications of different inducing agents: A problem of blast (stem) cells, in: *Pigment Cell 1985: Biological, Molecular, and Clinical Aspects of Pigmentation* (J. T. Bagnara, S. N. Klaus, E. Paul, and M. Schartl, eds.), pp. 333–340, Tokyo University Press, Tokyo.

84. Akiyama, T., Matsumoto, J., Ishikawa, T., and Eguchi, G., 1986, Production of crystallins and lens-like structures in differentiation-induced neoplastic pigment cells (goldfish erythrophoroma cells) in vitro, *Differentiation* **33**:34–44.

85. Naegele, R. F., Granoff, A., and Darlington, R. W., 1974, The presence of the Lucké herpesvirus genome in induced tadpole tumors and its oncogenicity: Koch-Henle postulates fulfilled, *Proc. Natl. Acad. Sci. USA* **71**:830–834.

86. McKinnell, R. G., 1984, Lucké tumor of frogs, in: *Diseases of Amphibians and Reptiles* (G. L. Hoff, F. L. Frye, and E. R. Jacobson, eds.), pp. 581–605, Plenum, New York.

87. Asashima, M., Oinuma, T., and Meyer-Rochow, V. B., 1987, Tumors in amphibia, *Zool. Sci.* **4**:411–425.

88. Lucké, B., and Schlumberger, H., 1949, Induction of metastasis of frog carcinoma by increase of environmental temperature, *J. Exp. Med.* **89**:269–278.

89. McKinnell, R. G., and Cunningham, W. P., 1982, Herpesviruses in metastatic Lucké renal adenocarcinoma, *Differentiation* **22**:41–46.

90. McKinnell, R. G., and Tarin, D., 1984, Temperature-dependent metastasis of the Lucké renal carcinoma and its significance for studies on mechanisms of metastasis, *Cancer Metast. Rev.* **3**:373–386.

91. Briggs, R., and King, T. J., 1952, Transplantation of living nuclei from blastula cells into enucleated frogs' eggs, *Proc. Natl. Acad. Sci. USA* **38**:455–463.

92. DiBerardino, M. A., 1980, Genetic stability and modulation of metazoan nuclei transplanted into eggs and oocytes, *Differentiation* **17**:17–30.

93. DiBerardino, M. A., and Hoffner, N. J., 1980, The current status of cloning and nuclear reprogramming in amphibian eggs, in: *Differentiation and Neoplasia* (R. G. McKinnell, M. A. DiBerardino, M. Blumenfeld, and R. D. Bergad, eds.), pp. 53–64, Springer-Verlag, Berlin.

94. McKinnell, R. G., 1978, *Cloning, Nuclear Transplantation in Amphibia*, University of Minnesota Press, Minneapolis.

95. McKinnell, R. G., 1985, *Cloning of Frogs, Mice and Other Animals*, University of Minnesota Press, Minneapolis.

96. DiBerardino, M. A., and Hoffner, N. J., 1983, Gene reactivation in erythrocytes: Nuclear transplantation in oocytes and eggs of *Rana*, *Science* **219**:862–864.

97. Orr, N. H., DiBerardino, M. A., and McKinnell, R. G., 1986, The genome of frog erythrocytes displays centuplicate replication, *Proc. Natl. Acad. Sci. USA* **83**:1369–1373.

98. King, T. J., and McKinnell, R. G., 1960, An attempt to determine the developmental potentialities of the cancer cell nucleus by means of transplantation, in: *Cell Physiology of Neoplasia*, pp. 591–617, University of Texas Press, Austin.

99. King, T. J., and DiBerardino, M. A., 1965, Transplantation of nuclei from the frog renal adenocarcinoma. I. Development of tumor nuclear-transplant embryos, *Ann. NY Acad. Sci.* **126:**115–126.

100. McKinnell, R. G., 1973, Nuclear transplantation, in: *Seventh National Cancer Conference Proceedings,* pp. 65–72, J. B. Lippincott, Philadelphia.

100a. McKinnell, R. G., 1972, Nuclear transfer in *Xenopus* and *Rana* compared, in: *Cell Differentiation* (R. Harris, P. Allin, and D. Viza, eds.), pp. 61–64, Munksgaard, Copenhagen.

101. McKinnell, R. G., 1979, The pluripotential genome of the frog renal tumor cell as revealed by nuclear transplantation, *Int. Rev. Cytol. Suppl.* **9:**179–188.

102. DiBerardino, M. A., King, T. J., and McKinnell, R. G., 1961, Embryonic development and the frog renal adenocarcinoma, in: *Frog Kidney Adenocarcinoma Conference* (W. R. Duryee and L. Warner, eds.), pp. 81–90, National Institutes of Health, Bethesda.

103. McKinnell, R. G., and Tweedell, K. S., 1970, Induction of renal tumors in triploid leopard frogs, *J. Natl. Cancer Inst.* **44:**1161–1166.

104. McKinnell, R. G., Deggins, B. A., and Labat, D. D., 1969, Transplantation of pluripotential nuclei from triploid frog tumors, *Science* **165:**394–396.

104a. McKinnell, R. G., and Ellis, V. L., 1972, Epidemiology of the frog renal tumour and the significance of tumour nuclear transplantation studies to a viral aetiology of the tumour: a review, in: *Oncogenesis and Herpesviruses* (P. M. Biggs, G. de Thé, and L. N. Payne, eds.), pp. 183–197, International Agency for Research on Cancer, Lyon.

105. Tweedell, K. S., 1965, Cytopathology of a frog renal adenocarcinoma *in vitro* with fluorescence microscopy, *Ann. NY Acad. Sci.* **126:**170–187.

106. Harrison, F. W., Zambernard, J., and Cowden, R. R., 1975, Fluorescent cytochemistry of calid and algid normal and Lucké tumor-bearing kidneys, *Acta Histochem.* **54:**295–306.

107. McKinnell, R. G., Steven, L. M., Jr., and Labat, D. D., 1976, Frog renal tumors are composed of stroma, vascular elements, and epithelial cells: What type nucleus programs for tadpoles with the cloning procedure?, in: *Progress in Differentiation Research* (N. Müller-Berat, ed.), pp. 319–330, North-Holland, Amsterdam.

108. Seppanen, E. D., McKinnell, R. G., Tarin, D., Rollins-Smith, L. A., and Hanson, W., 1984, Temperature-dependent dissociation of Lucké renal adenocarcinoma cells, *Differentiation* **26:**227–230.

109. DiBerardino, M. A., Mizell, M., Hoffner, N. J., and Friesendorf, D. G., 1983, Frog larvae cloned from nuclei of pronephric adenocarcinoma, *Differentiation* **23:**213–217.

110. Balls, M., and Clothier, R. H., 1974, Spontaneous tumors of amphibia, *Oncology* **29:**501–519.

111. Seilern-Aspang, F., and Kratochwil, K., 1962, Induction and differentiation of an epithelial tumor in the newt (*Triturus cristatus*), *J. Embryol. Exp. Morphol.* **10:**337–356.

112. Simnett, J. D., and Chopra, D. P., 1969, Organ specific inhibitor of mitoses in amphibian kidney, *Nature (Lond.)* **222:**1189–1190.

113. Chopra, D. P., and Simnett, J. D., 1970, Stimulation of cell division in pronephros of embryonic grafts following partial nephrectomy in the host (*Xenopus laevis*), *J. Embryol. Exp. Morphol.* **24:**525–533.

114. Goldin, G., and Fabian, B., 1978, The regulation of growth in the mesonephric kidney of adult *Xenopus laevis* by an endogenous inhibitor of cell proliferation, *Dev. Biol.* **66:**529–538.

115. Skraastad, O., 1987, Compensatory cell proliferation in the kidney after unilateral nephrectomy in mice, *Virchows Arch. B* **53:**97–101.

116. Tweedell, K. S., 1967, Induced oncogenesis in developing frog kidney cells, *Cancer Res.* **27:**2042–2052.

117. Tweedell, K. S., 1978, Pronephric tumor cell lines from herpesvirus transformed cells, *Int. Agency Res. Cancer, Sci. Pub. 24* (**II**):609–616.

118. Gross, L., 1951, "Spontaneous" leukemia developing in C3H mice following inoculation, in infancy, with AK-leukemic extracts, or AK-embryos, *Proc. Soc. Exp. Biol. Med.* **76:**27–32.

119. Pietra, G., Spencer, K., and Shubik, P., 1959, Response of newly born mice to a chemical carcinogen, *Nature (Lond.)* **183:**1689.

120. Dawe, C. J., and Law, L. W., 1959, Morphologic changes in salivary-gland tissue of the newborn mouse exposed to parotid-tumor agent *in vitro, J. Natl. Cancer Inst.* **23:**1157–1177.

121. Baluda, M. A., and Jamieson, P. P., 1961, *In vivo* infectivity studies with avian myeloblastosis virus, *Virology* **14:**33–45.

122. Hennen, S., 1970, Influence of spermine and reduced temperature on the ability of transplanted nuclei to promote normal development in eggs of *Rana pipiens, Proc. Natl. Acad. Sci. USA* **66:**630–637.

123. Prescott, D. M., and Flexer, A. S., 1986, *Cancer, The Misguided Cell,* 2nd ed., Sinauer Associates, Sunderland, Massachusetts.

124. Crocker, J. F. S., and Vernier, R. L., 1972, Congenital nephroma of infancy: Induction of renal structures by organ culture, *J. Pediatr.* **80:**69–73.

125. Grobstein, C., 1955, Inductive interaction in the development of the mouse metanephros, *J. Exp. Zool.* **130:**319–339.
126. Unsworth, B., and Grobstein, C., 1970, Induction of kidney tubules in mouse metanephrogenic mesenchyme by various embryonic mesenchymal tissues, *Dev. Biol.* **21:**547–556.
127. Murray, M. R., and Stout, A. P., 1947, Distinctive characteristics of the sympathicoblastoma cultivated *in vitro, Am. J. Pathol.* **23:**429–441.
128. Goldstein, M. N., Burdman, J. A., and Journey, L. J., 1964, Long-term tissue culture of neuroblastomas. II. Morphologic evidence for differentiation and maturation, *J. Natl. Cancer Inst.* **32:**165–199.
129. Prasad, K. N., 1982, Maturation of neuroblastoma, in: *Prolonged Arrest of Cancer* (B. A. Stoll, ed.), pp. 281–308, Wiley, Chichester.
130. Spiegelman, B. M., Lopata, M. A., and Kirschner, M. W., 1979, Aggregation of microtubule initiation sites preceeding neurite outgrowth of mouse neuroblastoma cells, *Cell* **16:**253–263.
131. Marchisio, P. C., Weber, K., Osborn, M., 1979, Identification of multiple microtubule initiating sites in mouse neuroblastoma cells, *Eur. J. Cell Biol.* **20:**45–50.
132. Sharp, G. A., Osborn, M., and Weber, K., 1981, Ultrastructure of multiple microtubule initiation sites in mouse neuroblastoma cells, *J. Cell Sci.* **47:**1–14.
133. Kirschner, M., 1982, Microtubules and their role in cell, tissue, and organismal polarity, in: *Developmental Order: Its Origin and Regulation* (S. Subtelny and P. B. Green, eds.), pp. 117–132, Liss, New York.
134. Schubert, D., Humphreys, S., Baroni, C., and Cohn, M., 1969, *In vitro* differentiation of a mouse neuroblastoma, *Proc. Natl. Acad. Sci. USA* **64:**316–323.
135. Schubert, D., Humphreys, S., DeVitry, F., and Jacob, F., 1971, Induced differentiation of a neuroblastoma, *Dev. Biol.* **25:**514–546.
136. Seeds, N. W., Gilman, A. G., Amano, T., and Nirenberg, M. W., 1970, Regulation of axon formation by clonal lines of a neural tumor, *Proc. Natl. Acad. Sci. USA* **66:**160–167.
137. Goldstein, M. N., and Plurad, S., 1980, Drug-induced differentiation of human neuroblastoma: Transformation into ganglion cells with mitomycin-C, in: *Differentiation and Neoplasia* (R. G. McKinnell, M. A. DiBerardino, M. Blumenfeld, and R. D. Bergad, eds.), pp. 259–264, Springer-Verlag, Berlin.
138. Sidell, N., 1981, Retinoic acid induced growth inhibition and morphologic differentiation of human neuroblastoma cells *in vitro, J. Natl. Cancer Inst.* **68:**589–596.
139. Mattsson, M. E. K., Ruusala, A. I., and Pahlman, S., 1984, Changes in inducibility of ornithine decarboxylase activity in differentiating human neuroblastoma cells, *Exp. Cell Res.* **155:**105–112.
139a. Tsokos, M., Scarpa, S., Ross, R. A., and Triche, T. J., 1987, Differentiation of human neuroblastoma recapitulates neural crest development: Study of morphology, neurotransmitter enzymes, and extracellular matrix proteins, *Am. J. Pathol.* **128:**484–496.
140. Wells, R. S., and Miotto, K. A., 1986, Widespread inhibition of neuroblastoma cells in the 12- to 17-day old mouse embryo, *Cancer Res.* **46:**1659–1662.
141. Cushing, H., and Wolbach, S. B., 1927, The transformation of a malignant paravertebral sympathicoblastoma into a benign ganglioneuroma, *Am. J. Pathol.* **3:**203–216.
142. Kroll, A. J., Kuwabara, T., and Howard, G. M., 1963, Electron microscopy of rhabdomyosarcoma of the orbit, *Invest. Ophthalmol.* **2:**523–537.
143. Corbeil, L. B., 1967, Differentiation of rhabdomyosarcoma and neonatal muscle cells *in vitro, Cancer,* **20:**572–578.
144. Nameroff, M. A., Reznik, M., Anderson, P., and Hansen, J. L., 1970, Differentiation and control of mitosis in a skeletal muscle tumor, *Cancer Res.* **30:**596–600.
145. Dexter, D. L., 1977, *N,N*-Dimethylformamide-induced morphological differentiation and reduction in tumorigenicity in cultured mouse rhabdomyosarcoma cells, *Cancer Res.* **37:**3136–3140.
146. Becker, M., Moczar, E., Korach, S., Lascaux, V., and Poupon, M. F., 1985, Relationship between *in vitro* effects and *in vivo* control of metastasis induced by hydrocortisone in a rat rhabdomyosarcoma, in: *Treatment of Metastasis: Problems and Prospects* (K. Hellmann and S. A. Eccles, eds.), pp. 183–186, Taylor and Francis, London.
147. Stevens, L. C., 1973, A new inbred subline of mice (129/terSv) with a high incidence of spontaneous testicular teratoma, *J. Natl. Cancer Inst.* **50:**235–242.
148. Stevens, L. C., 1970, Experimental production of testicular teratomas in mice of strains 129, A/He and their F, hybrids, *J. Natl. Cancer Inst.* **44:**923–929.
149. Stevens, L. C., 1970, The development of transplantable teratocarcinomas from intertesticular grafts of pre- and post-implantation mouse embryos, *Dev. Biol.* **21:**364–382.
150. Solter, D., Skreb, N., and Damjanov, I., 1970, Extrauterine growth of mouse egg-cylinder results in malignant teratoma, *Nature (Lond.)* **227:**503–504.

151. Smithers, D. W., 1969, Maturation in human tumours, *Lancet* **2:**949–952.
152. Carr, B. I., Gilchrist, K. W., and Carbone, P. P., 1981, The variable transformation in metastases from testicular germ cell tumors: The need for selective biopsy, *J. Urol.* **126:**52–54.
153. Askanazy, M., 1907, Teratome nach ihrem Bav, ihrem Verlauf, Ihrer Genese und im Vergleich zum experimentallen Teratoid, *Verhandl. Dtsch. Pathol. Gesellsch.* **11:**39–82.
154. Willis, R. A., 1962, *The Borderland of Embryology and Pathology,* 2nd ed., Butterworths, London.
155. Fekete, E., and Ferrigno, M. A., 1952, Studies on a transplantable teratoma of the mouse, *Cancer Res.* **12:**438–440.
156. Pierce, G. B., Dixon, F. J., Jr., and Verney, E., 1959, Testicular teratomas, I. Demonstration of teratogenesis by metamorphosis of multipotential cells, *Cancer* **12:**573–583.
157. Stevens, L. C., 1981, Genetic influences on the development of gonadal tumors in mice with emphasis on teratomas, in: *Neoplasms—Comparative Pathology of Growth in Animals, Plants, and Man* (H. E. Kaiser, ed.), pp. 467–474, Williams & Wilkins, Baltimore.
158. Dixon, F. J., and Moore, R. A., 1953, Testicular tumors, *Cancer* **6:**427–454.
159. Pierce, G. B., and Dixon, F. J., 1959, Testicular teratomas. I. The demonstration of teratogenesis by metamorphosis of multipotential cells, *Cancer* **12:**573–583.
160. Stevens, L. C., 1960, Embryonic potency of embryoid bodies derived from a transplantable testicular teratoma of the mouse, *Dev. Biol.* **2:**285–297.
161. Pierce, G. B., Dixon, F. J., and Verney, E. L., 1960, Teratocarcinogenic and tissue-forming potentials of the cell types comprising neoplastic embryoid bodies, *Lab. Invest.* **9:**583–602.
162. Kleinsmith, L. J., and Pierce, G. B., 1964, Multipotentiality of single embryonal carcinoma cells, *Cancer Res.* **24:**1544–1551.
163. Brinster, R. L., 1974, The effect of cells transferred into the mouse blastocyst on subsequent development, *J. Exp. Med.* **140:**1049–1056.
164. Mintz, B., and Illmensee, K., 1975, Normal genetically mosaic mice produced from malignant teratocarcinoma cells, *Proc. Natl. Acad. Sci. USA* **72:**3585–3589.
165. Illmensee, K., and Mintz, B., 1976, Totipotency and normal differentiation of single teratocarcinoma cells cloned by injection into blastocysts, *Proc. Natl. Acad. Sci. USA* **73:**549–553.
166. Dewey, M. J., Martin, D. W., Martin, G. R., and Mintz, B., 1977, Mosaic mice with teratocarcinoma-derived mutant cells deficient in hypoxanthine phosphoribosyl transferase, *Proc. Natl. Acad. Sci. USA* **74:**5564–5568.
167. Papaioannou, V. E., McBurney, M. W., Gardner, R. L., and Evans, M. J., 1975, Fate of teratocarcinoma cells injected into early mouse embryos, *Nature (Lond.)* **258:**70–73.
168. Papaioannou, V. E., Gardner, R. L., McBurney, M. W., Babinet, C., and Evans, M. J., 1978, Participation of cultured teratocarcinoma cells in mouse embryogenesis, *J. Embryol. Exp. Morphol.* **44:**81–92.
169. Stewart, T. A., and Mintz, B., 1981, Successive generations of mice produced from an established culture line of euploid teratocarcinoma cells, *Proc. Natl. Acad. Sci. USA* **78:**6314–6318.
170. Rowley, J. D., 1984, Biological implications of consistent chromosomal rearrangements in leukemia and lymphoma, *Cancer Res.* **44:**3159–3168.
171. Yunis, J. J., 1986, Chromosomal rearrangements, genes, and fragile sites in cancer: Clinical and biologic implications, in: *Important Advances in Oncology 1986* (V. T. DeVita, S. Hellman, and S. A. Rosenberg, eds.), pp. 93–128, J. B. Lippincott, Philadelphia.
172. Cronmiller, C., and Mintz, B., 1978, Karyotypic normalcy and quasinormalcy of developmentally totipotent mouse teratocarcinoma cells, *Dev. Biol.* **67:**465–477.
173. Rossant, J., and McBurney, M. W., 1982, The developmental potential of a euploid male teratocarcinoma cell line after blastocyst injection, *J. Embryol. Exp. Morphol.* **70:**99–112.
174. Martin, G. R., and Evans, M. J., 1975, Differentiation of clonal lines of teratocarcinoma cells: Formation of embryoid bodies in vitro, *Proc. Natl. Acad. Sci USA* **72:**1441–1445.
175. Strickland, S., and Mahdavi, V., 1978, The induction of differentiation in teratocarcinoma stem cells by retinoic acid, *Cell* **15:**393–403.
176. Webb, M., Graham, C., and Walsh, F., 1986, Neuronal differentiation of cloned human teratoma cells in response to retinoic acid *in vitro, J. Neuroimmunol.* **11:**67–86.
177. Levine, J. M., and Flynn, P., 1986, Cell surface changes accompanying the neural differentiation of an embryonal carcinoma cell line, *J. Neurosci.* **6:**3374–3384.
178. Wartiovaara, J., and Rechardt, L., 1985, Neural differentiation in embryonal carcinoma cells, *Prog. Clin. Biol. Res.* **171:**3–13.
179. Edwards, M. K., and McBurney, M. W., 1983, The concentration of retinoic acid determines the differentiated cell types formed by a teratocarcinoma cell line, *Dev. Biol.* **98:**187–191.

180. Razin, A., Webb, C., Szyf, M., Yisraeli, J., Rosenthal, A., Neven-Many, T., Scicky-Gallili, N., and Cedar, H., 1984, Variations in DNA methylation during mouse differentiation *in vivo* and *in vitro*, *Proc. Natl. Acad. Sci. USA* **81**:2275–2279.

181. Colberg-Poley, A. M., Voss, S. D., Chowdhury, K., and Gruss, P., 1985, Structural analysis of murine genes containing homeo box sequences and their expression in embryonal carcinoma cells, *Nature (Lond.)* **314**:713–718.

182. Hauser, C. A., Joyner, A. L., Klein, R. D., Learned, T. K., Martin, G. R., and Tjian, R., 1985, Expression of homologous homeo-box-containing genes in differentiated human teratocarcinoma cells and mouse embryos, *Cell* **43**:19–28.

183. Paterno, G. D., and McBurney, M. W., 1985, X chromosome inactivation during induced differentiation of a female mouse embryonal carcinoma cell line, *J. Cell Sci.* **75**:149–163.

184. Ohashi, Y., Ueda, K., Hayaishi, O., Ikai, K., and Niwa, O., 1984, Induction of murine teratocarcinoma cell differentiation by suppression of poly (ADP-ribose) synthesis, *Proc. Natl. Acad. Sci. USA* **81**:7132–7136.

185. Nicolas, J. F., Gaillard, J., Jakob, H., and Jacob, F., 1980, Bone-forming cell line derived from embryonal carcinoma cells, *Nature (Lond.)* **286**:716–718.

186. How, S-W., and Snell, K. C., 1967, Skin tumors induced in rats by the dietary administration of *N,N'*-2,7- fluorenylenebisacetamide, *J. Natl. Cancer Inst.* **38**:407–434.

187. Pierce, G. B., and Wallace, C., 1971, Differentiation of malignant to benign cells, *Cancer Res.* **31**:127–134.

188. Metcalf, D., 1985, The granulocyte-macrophage colony-stimulating factors, *Science* **229**:16–22.

189. Takeda, K., Minowada, J., and Bloch, A., 1982, Kinetics of appearance of differentiation associated characteristics in ML-1, a line of human myeloblastic leukemia cells, after treatment with TPA, DMSO, or Ara-C, *Cancer Res.* **42**:5152–5158.

190. Mendelsohn, N., Michl, J., Gilbert, H. S., Acs, G., and Christman, J. K., 1980, L-Ethionine as an inducer of differentiation in human promyelocytic leukemia cells (HL-60), *Cancer Res.* **40**:3206–3210.

191. Souza, L. M., Boone, T. C., Gabrilove, J., Lai, P. H., Zsebo, K. M., Murdock, D. C., Chazin, V. R., Bruszewski, J., Lu, H., Chen, K. K., Barendt, J., Platzer, E., Moore, M. A. S., Mertelsmann, R., and Welte, K., 1986, Recombinant human granulocyte colony-stimulating factor: Effects on normal and leukemic myeloid cells, *Science* **232**:61–65.

192. Sachs, L., 1978, The differentiation of myeloid leukemic cells: new possibilities for therapy, *Br. J. Haematol.* **40**:509–517.

193. Azumi, J-I., and Sachs, L., 1977, Chromosome mapping of the genes that control differentiation and malignancy in myeloid leukemic cells, *Proc. Natl. Acad. Sci. USA* **74**:253–257.

194. Lotem, J., and Sachs, L., 1978, *In vivo* induction of normal differentiation in myeloid leukemia cells, *Proc. Natl. Acad. Sci. USA* **75**:3781–3785.

195. Lotem, J., and Sachs, L., 1981, *In vivo* inhibition of the development of myeloid leukemia by injection of macrophage- and granulocyte-inducing protein, *Int. J. Cancer* **28**:375–386.

196. Friend, C., Patuleia, M. C., and de Harven, E., 1966, Erythrocytic maturation *in vitro* of murine (Friend) virus-induced leukemia cells, *Natl. Cancer Inst. Monog.* **22**:505–522.

197. Friend, C., 1978, The phenomenon of differentiation in murine erythroleukemic cells, *Harvey Lect.* **72**:253–281.

198. Friend, C., 1980, The regulation of differentiation in murine virus-induced erythroleukemic cells, in: *Differentiation and Neoplasia* (R. G. McKinnell, M. A. DiBerardino, M. Blumenfeld, and R. D. Bergad, eds.), pp. 202–212, Springer-Verlag, Berlin.

199. Anderson, L. G., Jokinen, M., and Gahmberg, C. G., 1979, Induction of erythroid differentiation in the human leukaemia cell line K562, *Nature (Lond.)* **278**:364–365.

200. Friend, C., Scher, W., Holland, J. G., and Sato, T., 1971, Hemoglobin synthesis in murine virus induced leukemia cells *in vitro* stimulation of erythroid differentiation by dimethyl sulfoxide, *Proc. Natl. Acad. Sci. USA* **68**:378–382.

201. Rossi, G. B., and Friend, C., 1967, Erythrocytic maturation of (Friend) virus-induced leukemic cells in spleen colonies, *Proc. Natl. Acad. Sci. USA* **58**:1373–1380.

202. Marks, P. A., and Rifkind, R. A., 1978, Erythroleukemic differentiation, *Annu. Rev. Biochem.* **47**:419–448.

203. Marks, P. A., Sheffery, M., and Rifkind, R. A., 1987, Induction of transformed cells to terminal differentiation and the modulation of gene expression, *Cancer Res.* **47**:659–666.

204. Waxman, S., Scher, W., and Scher, B. M., 1986, Basic principles for utilizing combination differentiation agents, *Cancer Detect. Prev.* **9**:395–407.

205. Yoshida, M., Normura, S., and Beppu, T., 1987, Effects of trichostatins on differentiation of murine erythroleukemia cells, *Cancer Res.* **47:**3688–3691.
206. DeCosse, J. J., Gossens, C. L., Kuzma, J. F., and Unsworth, B. R., 1973, Breast cancer: Induction of differentiation by embryonic tissue, *Science* **181:**1057–1058.
207. Okuyama, S., Mishina, H., and Maki, T., 1985, Redifferentiation of cancer cells: bestatin, estradiol, and prostaglandin D2, *Ann. NY Acad. Sci.* **459:**293–307.
208. Freshney, R. I., 1984, Effects of glucocorticoids on glioma cells in culture, *Exp. Cell Biol.* **52:**286–292.
209. Lim, R., Hicklin, D. J., Ryken, T. C., Han, X-M., Liu, K-N., Miller, J., and Baggenstoss, B. A., 1986, Suppression of glioma growth *in vitro* and *in vivo* by glia maturation factor, *Cancer Res.* **46:**5241–5247.
210. Siracky, J., Blasko, M., and Borovansky, J., 1985, Stimulation of differentiation in human melanoma cells by dimethylsulphoxide (DMSO), *Neoplasma* **32:**685–688.
211. Lotan, R., and Lotan, D., 1980, Stimulation of melanogenesis in a human melanoma cell line by retinoids, *Cancer Res.* **40:**3345–3350.
212. Dexter, D. L., Barbosa, J. A., and Calabresi, P., 1979, *N,N*-Dimethylformamide-induced alteration of cell culture characteristics and loss of tumorigenicity in cultured human colon carcinoma cells, *Cancer Res.* **39:**1020–1025.
213. Dexter, D. L., Spremulli, E. N., Matook, G. M., Diamond, I., and Calabresi, P., 1982, Inhibition of the growth of human colon cancer xenografts by polar solvents, *Cancer Res.* **42:**5018–5022.
214. Balana, A., Wiels, J., Tetaud, C., Mishal, Z., and Tursz, T., 1985, Induction of cell differentiation in Burkitt lymphoma lines. BLA: A glycolipid marker of B-cell differentiation, *Int. J. Cancer* **36:**453–460.
215. Spemann, H., and Mangold, H., 1924, Über Induktion von Embryonalanlagen durch Implantation artfremder Organisatoren, *Arch. Mikr. Anat. Entw. Mech.* **100:**599–638.
216. Spemann, H., 1938, *Embryonic Development and Induction*, Yale University Press, New Haven.
217. Saxen, L., and Toivonen, S., 1962, *Primary Embryonic Induction*, Prentice-Hall, Englewood Cliffs, New Jersey.
218. Gurdon, J. B., 1987, Embryonic induction—Molecular prospects, *Development* **99:**285–306.
219. Lewis, W. H., 1904, Experimental studies on the development of the eye of amphibia. I. On the origin of the lens, *Rana palustris*, *Am. J. Anat.* **3:**505–536.
220. Grobstein, C., 1956, Trans-filter induction of tubules in mouse metanephrogenic mesenchyme, *Exp. Cell Res.* **10:**424–440.
221. Bautzmann, H., Holtfreter, J., Spemann, H., and Mangold, O., 1932, Versuche zur Analyse der Induktionsmittel in der Embryonalentwicklung, *Naturwissenschaften* **20:**971–974.
222. Okada, Y. K., 1938, Neural induction by means of inorganic implantation, *Growth* **2:**49–53.
223. Barth, L. G., 1939, The chemical nature of the amphibian organizer: III. Stimulation of the presumptive epidermis of Ambystoma by means of cell extracts and chemical substances, *Physiol. Zool.* **12:**22–29.
224. Ranzi, S., and Tamini, E., 1939, Die Wirkung van NaSCN auf die Entwicklung von Froschembryonen, *Naturwissenschaften* **27:**566–567.
225. Brachet, J., and Rapkine, L., 1939, Oxydation et reduction d'explantats dorsaux et ventraux de gastrulas (Amphibiens), *C. R. Soc. Biol.* **131:**789–791.
226. Beatty, R. A., de Jong, S., and Zielinski, M. A., 1939, Experiments on the effect of dyes on induction and respiration in the amphibian gastrula, *J. Exp. Biol.* **16:**150–154.
227. Shen, S. C., 1939, A quantitative study of amphibian neural tube induction with a water-soluble hydrocarbon, *J. Exp. Biol.* **16:**143–149.
228. Barth, L. G., 1941, Neural differentiation without organizer, *J. Exp. Zool.* **87:**371–383.
229. Evans, A., Gerson, J., and Schnaufer, L., 1976, Spontaneous regression of neuroblastoma, *Conference on Spontaneous Regression of Cancer* (E. F. Lewison, ed.), *National Cancer Institute Monograph* **44:**49–54.
230. Moore, E. E., Mitra, N. S., and Moritz, E. A., 1986, Differentiation of F9 embryonal carcinoma cells. Differences in the effects of retinoic acid, 5-bromodeoxyuridine, and *N'-N'*-dimethylacetamide, *Differentiation* **31:**183–190.
231. Andrews, P. W., Gonczol, E., Plotkin, S. A., Dignazio, M., and Oosterhuis, J. W., 1986, Differentiation of TERA-2 human embryonal carcinoma cells into neurons and HCMV permissive cells. Induction by agents other than retinoic acid, *Differentiation* **31:**119–126.
232. Kaplinsky, C., Estrov, Z., Freedman, M. H., and Cohen, A., 1986, Induction of differentiation in HL-60 promyelocytic cells: A comparative study in two sublines, *Blood Cells* **11:**459–468.
233. Paukovits, J. B., Paukovits, W. R., and Laerum, O. D., 1986, Identification of a regulatory peptide distinct from normal granulocyte-derived hemoregulatory peptide produced by human promyelocytic HL-60 leukemia cells after differentiation induction with retinoic acid, *Cancer Res.* **46:**4444–4448.
234. Glazer, R. I., Cohen, M. B., Hartman, K. D., Knode, M. C., Lim, M. I., and Marquez, V. E., 1986,

Induction of differentiation in the human promyelocytic leukemia cell line HL-60 by the cyclopentanyl analogue of cytidine, *Biochem. Pharmacol.* **35:**1841–1848.

235. Mukherjee, A. B., Czirbik, R. J., Parsa, N. Z., and Testa, J. R., 1985, Induction of terminal differentiation and nuclear appendage(s) formation in a human myeloid leukaemia cell line (HL-60), *Cytobios* **44:**109–118.

236. Grant, S., Bhalla, K., Weinstein, B., Pestka, S., Mileno, M. D., and Fisher, P. B., 1985, Recombinant human interferon sensitizes resistant myeloid leukemic cells to induction of terminal differentiation, *Biochem. Biophys. Res. Commun.* **130:**379–388.

# 23

# *Ectopic Hormone Production and Neoplasia*

## *David P. Rose*

## 1. INTRODUCTION

When the term ''ectopic hormone production'' was coined by Liddle and colleagues,[1] the intent was to describe a situation in which hormones are secreted by tumors of tissues not normally responsible for their production. The classic clinical presentation was of Cushing syndrome occurring in patients with tumors which were not associated with the pituitary or adrenal glands. If effective therapy were possible, extirpation of the cancer resulted in regression of the endocrine disorder. Furthermore, cases are seen in which an endocrine tumor secretes both the hormone appropriate to its tissue of origin (eutopic production), plus others not normally produced by that endocrine gland (ectopic production). While this original definition is of value clinically, it is now recognized that the range of normal cells which secrete hormones extends far beyond those associated with the classical endocrine system.

All ectopically produced hormones are glycoproteins or polypeptides. This is consistent with the view that the mechanism for their synthesis involves gene derepression, an event that occurs frequently during the process of carcinogenesis.[2] Protein synthesis is genetically coded as a single step, so that only one derepression event is required for its initiation. By contrast, steroid hormone synthesis involves a series of enzymatically regulated reactions. In this latter case, ectopic production would require virtually impossible multiple derepressions to permit the emergence of all the enzymes involved in the steroidogenic process.

The derepression hypothesis of ectopic protein and polypeptide hormone production cannot stand alone. Random derepression of the relevant gene or genes in tumor cells is not compatible with the fact that adrenocorticotropic hormone (ACTH), for example, is ectopically produced much more frequently than are some other peptides. Also, different tumor types vary in their propensity for association with ectopic hormone production. Thus, small cell carcinoma of the lung is the tumor most often responsible for the production of ACTH, β-lipotropin, vasopressin, and, excluding trophoblastic cancers, the gonadotropins. By contrast, breast cancer, another common tumor, is a rare cause of ectopic hormone syndrome, although some do secrete the β-subunit of human chorionic gonadotropin (hCG),[3] and calcitonin.[4]

The concept of the APUD series of endocrine cells, originally developed by Pearse and colleagues[5] at the Postgraduate Medical School, London, continues to be favored in discussions of

*David P. Rose* • Division of Nutrition and Endocrinology, American Health Foundation, Valhalla, New York 10595.

the cellular basis of tumor ectopic hormone production. APUD cells, the acronym that describes the cytochemical characteristics arising from *amine precursor uptake and decarboxylation*, are considered to arise embryologically from the neural crest. Under physiologic circumstances, these cells secrete catecholamines and 5-hydroxytryptamine (5-HT), and they may continue to do so even after neoplastic transformation, as in the case of 5-HT production by a carcinoid tumor arising from enterochromaffin cells. During embryonic development, APUD cells migrate throughout the primitive gut but are especially abundant in the foregut. It is their presence in primitive entoderm-derived structures, such as the thyroid and parathyroid glands, and the pancreatic islets, which confers endocrine function to these organs. Similarly, when the stomach, duodenum, and small intestine form from the primitive entodermal canal, the presence of APUD cells provides the primary source of the gastrointestinal hormones.

If derepression of a peptide hormone gene occurs during malignant transformation involving APUD cells, the result could be, for example, the emergence of a carcinoid tumor of the bronchus producing ectopic ACTH as well as eutopic 5-HT. In this case, the endocrine APUD cell hypothesis can explain ectopic hormone production. Small cell carcinoma of the lung, the most common source of most ectopic hormones, may arise from the argentaffin, Kultschitzky-like cells of the bronchial mucosa,[6] and so, here too there is no inconsistency with the APUD hypothesis. Occasionally, squamous cell carcinomas and adenocarcinomas of the lung also produce ACTH,[7,8] but L-DOPA decarboxylase activity, a key component of APUD cells, also occurs in these tumors. Baylin *et al.*[9] found this decarboxylase enzyme to be highest in small cell carcinomas, but some adenocarcinomas also had pronounced, overlapping levels of activity. In addition, all but one of five squamous cell carcinomas had detectable activity, as did four of five large cell carcinomas. These investigators concluded that all four principal types of lung cancers are related, and have the potential for developing APUD characteristics and endocrine activity as expressed by the production of small peptides, such as ACTH and vasopressin. In a second publication from the same laboratory, it was reported that all four of these lung cancers may possess not only L-DOPA decarboxylase and histaminase activity, but also synthesize calcitonin.[10] Baylin *et al.* postulated that all these forms arise from a single cell system, but become distinguished one from another by their degree of differentiation. This, in turn, determines the nature of their ectopic hormone production. Thus, small polypeptides such as ACTH, β-lipotropin, β-endorphin, and calcitonin frequently coexist[11,12] and are usually associated with retention of L-DOPA decarboxylase activity. At the other end of the spectrum are anaplastic tumors, such as large cell carcinomas of the lung, which lack the biochemical features of APUD cells, and produce protein hormones of high molecular weight, such as hCG.[13]

Peptide hormones are synthesized in a sequence that involves initial production of a high molecular weight, biologically inert precursor, that is then cleaved to form the active hormone. Some, such as prolactin and growth hormone, occur in three or more molecular forms of differing biological activities.[14,15] The precursor of ACTH and related peptides is pro-opiomelanocortin (POMC), a 31,000-$M_r$ glycoprotein that is cleaved within the corticotropic cells to yield ACTH (4507 $M_r$); β-lipotropin, which is a 91-amino acid carboxyterminal fragment; and a 78-amino acid aminoterminal glycopeptide. Further cleavage of β-lipotropin occurs to produce β-endorphin and γ-lipotropin. The ACTH molecule contains a 13-amino acid sequence that constitutes α-melanocyte-stimulating hormone (α-MSH), while β-lipotropin contains the 18-amino acid sequence of β-MSH.

Human chorionic gonadotropin, like luteinizing hormone (LH), follicle-stimulating hormone (FSH), and thyroid-stimulating hormone (TSH), is a glycoprotein composed of two chains. The α-chains are similar in amino acid sequence for all four of these hormones, although the hCG α-chain differs from the other three by having a 2-amino acid inversion and a 3-amino acid deletion at the NH$_2$ terminal. The β-chains are different for each and confer specificity of hormone action. Neither the α- or β-chains by themselves possesses biologic activity.

These variations in structural components, the existence of high-molecular-weight precursors, the need for cleavage to produce biologically active peptides, and the occurrence of similar and dissimilar chains in the glycoprotein hormones, have profound implications for understanding ectopic hormone production. Depending upon the presence or absence of the processing enzymes necessary for the cleavage of inactive prohormone, the precursor alone may be secreted, in which case clinical manifestations will not occur. Alternatively, either the active hormone may be formed, leading to an ectopic hormone syndrome, or fragments may appear in the circulation in abnormally large amounts.

The ectopic secretion of ACTH provides an excellent example of these three possible outcomes. Gewirtz and Yalow[7] originally described lung cancer patients without clinical evidence of hyperadrenocorticism in whom immunoreactive, but biologically inactive ACTH (frequently referred to as big ACTH because of its large molecular size) was detectable in the tumor tissue. When cancers are associated with Cushing syndrome the tumor tissue contains bioactive hormone.[16] Finally, some patients have tumors that secrete β-lipotropin into the circulation, where it may provide a biologic marker of early lung cancer.[17]

A wide variety of clinical syndromes have been described in association with ectopic hormone production by tumors. These syndromes are summarized, along with the tumors most often responsible, in Table I. None of them is common; for example, Cushing syndrome occurs in only some 3–5% of patients with small cell carcinoma of the bronchus. These endocrinopathies and metabolic disorders are important because they may be the presenting feature of an otherwise occult neoplasm.

## 2. ACTH, POMC-DERIVED PEPTIDES, CRH

Cushing syndrome arising in association with nonendocrine tumors is the most frequently seen clinical manifestation of ectopic hormone production. Azzopardi and Williams[18] gathered together 133 cases from the literature, and found that small cell carcinomas of the lung were responsible for 53%, while thymomas and pancreatic cancers accounted for another 25%. Less common causes of Cushing syndrome are the neuroectodermal tumors, principally pheochromocytomas, medullary thyroid carcinomas, and bronchial carcinoid tumors.

*Table I. Clinical Syndromes and Most Frequently Associated Tumors*

| Hormone | Associated tumors | Syndrome |
|---|---|---|
| ACTH and pro-opiomelanocortin-derived peptides | Bronchial carcinoma (especially small cell); thymoma; islet cell pancreatic tumor; neuroectodermal tumors; bronchial adenoma, including carcinoid medullary thyroid carcinoma | Cushing syndrome, notably hypokalemic alkalosis, myopathy |
| Vasopressin | Small cell bronchial carcinoma; other lung cancers | Dilutional hyponatremia, psychiatric disturbance, convulsions, coma |
| Gonadotropins | Large cell bronchial carcinoma; hepatoblastoma; hepatoma | Precocious puberty gynecomastia |
| Parathormone-related and other osteolytic agents | Bronchial, usually squamous carcinoma; renal cell carcinoma; ovarian carcinoma | Hypercalcemia |
| Insulinlike hypoglycemic agents | Mesenchymal tumors; hepatoma | Hypoglycemia |
| Erythropoietin | Cerebellar hemangioblastoma; uterine and ovarian tumors | Erythrocytosis |
| Vasoactive intestinal peptide (VIP) | Bronchial carcinoma | Watery diarrhea, hypokalemic alkalosis |
| Prolactin | Renal cell and bronchial carcinoma | Galactorrhea |

Most patients with Cushing syndrome due to ectopic ACTH production by a tumor do not develop the classic physical signs, such as truncal obesity, cutaneous striae, and osteoporosis. These take several months or years to develop, whereas the changes due to a lung cancer, for example, appear rapidly and are usually accompanied by acute clinical deterioration. The most frequently seen features of the ectopic hormone-induced Cushing syndrome are hypokalemic alkalosis, muscle weakness, hypertension, carbohydrate intolerance, and hyperpigmentation. Hypokalemia is much more common in patients with ectopically produced ACTH than in nonmalignant Cushing syndrome because the circulating cortisol levels are often extremely high and produce severe renal losses of potassium. Indeed, the presence of hypokalemia in the absence of another explanation should always suggest a diagnosis of ectopic ACTH syndrome. Plasma ACTH levels often exceed 200 pg/ml, with plasma cortisol concentrations being above 40 μg/dl. Typically, they are not suppressed by dexamethasone at a dose which does affect plasma cortisol and urinary 17-hydroxycorticosteroids in patients with Cushing disease of pituitary origin.

In 1971, Upton and Amatruda[19] reported the first case of ectopic ACTH syndrome due to the production of a corticotropin-releasing factor (CRF) by tumors. However, this observation predated the identification of corticotropin-releasing hormone (CRH) by 10 years.[20,21] Further examples followed[22,23]; more recently, Carey et al.[24] used immunocytochemistry to demonstrate CRH in a metastatic prostate cancer and its coelution with authentic human and rat CRH on high-performance liquid chromatography (HPLC).

Although, perhaps 5% or less of patients with small cell lung cancer are recognized clinically as having ectopic Cushing syndrome, ACTH is frequently detectable in the plasma by radioimmunoassay (RIA). This is due to the secretion of immunoreactive, but biologically inert, big ACTH. Yalow et al.[7,25] first demonstrated the presence of big ACTH in the tumors and plasma of patients with a thymona or lung cancer. In their study of 28 bronchial carcinoma patients, none of whom had Cushing syndrome, 14 of 15 primary tumors, and all of 13 metastases contained immunoreactive ACTH, most of which was big ACTH.[7] Histologically, small cell carcinomas, adenocarcinomas, and squamous cell carcinomas were about equally represented, although, as already noted, when ectopic ACTH syndrome occurs, it is nearly always associated with the small cell form. The obvious conclusion is that of the different histological types of lung cancer, only small cell carcinomas are likely to possess the proteolytic cleavage enzyme necessary for the production of bioactive ACTH from its precursor molecule.

Gewirtz and Yalow[7] also assayed plasma ACTH in 83 lung cancer patients. Controls were either healthy persons, patients with chronic obstructive pulmonary disease, or those with other forms of lung disease. Just over one half the lung cancer patients and one third of those with obstructive lung disease had elevated plasma ACTH levels, with most of the excess being due to the presence of big ACTH. Wolfsen and Odell[8] also determined plasma ACTH by RIA in patients with chronic obstructive pulmonary disease. Twenty of 111 of these had elevated levels, five of whom were found to have developed lung cancer within a 2½-year follow-up period.

There have been several reports of MSH production in association with ectopic ACTH.[11,26,27] In fact, β-MSH per se is not secreted from the human pituitary gland, and its presence appears to be an artifact of the extraction–purification procedure. This, in turn, causes formation of the immunoreactive peptide from a precursor[28] (most likely β-lipotropin), which contains within its structure the entire amino acid sequence of β-MSH. β-Lipotropin may also be a prohormone for β-endorphin,[29] both of which have been shown to be ectopically produced by nonendocrine tumors.[12,17] Odell et al.[17] assayed 79 carcinomas arising from the lung, colon, stomach, esophagus, or breast and found all to contain β-lipotropin at concentrations greater than those in plasma. Sixty-one of the 79 malignant tumors had levels higher than those detected in the corresponding normal tissues.

Bertagna et al.[12] also obtained evidence indicating that a common precursor for ACTH, lipotropin, and β-endorphin is produced by tumors secreting ectopic ACTH when they showed the presence of a high-molecular-weight secretory product which possessed immunoreactivity to all three peptides. Subsequently, RNA which directed the synthesis of a protein with ACTH and β-endorphin immunoreactivity was extracted from an ACTH-producing thymic carcinoid.[30]

## 3. VASOPRESSIN

The original published cases of ectopic vasopressin, or antidiuretic hormone (ADH), production was not recognized as such by Schwartz *et al.*[31] They described two patients with bronchial carcinomas, hyponatremia, persistently hyperosmotic urine, and failure to conserve sodium despite their depleted state. It was concluded, however, that the tumors had stimulated inappropriate ADH secretion from the neurohypophysis. Later, Amatruda *et al.*[32] had the opportunity to observe a similar patient and demonstrated the presence of ADH-like activity in the tumor extract.

The ectopically produced peptide appears to be identical to the normally secreted arginine vasopressin. Yamaji *et al.*[33] examined ADH production by a transplantable small cell carcinoma of the lung and showed that its synthesis, as in the hypothalamus, proceeds via post-translational processing of a glycosylated 20,000-$M_r$ protein (propressophysin) that yields both vasopressin and its carrier protein, neurophysin. Propressophysin occurs in the plasma of patients with small cell carcinoma of the lung, but not that of patients with inappropriate antidiuresis due to neurologic disease, suggesting that it may provide a marker for ectopic ADH production.[34]

Over the years, most cases of ectopic ADH syndrome have continued to be associated with small cell lung cancer. In this regard, approximately 7% of patients with this tumor type have clinically manifest inappropriate ADH secretion.[35] Other tumors that have been shown to be responsible include bronchial carcinoids,[36] pancreatic adenocarcinoma,[37] and prostatic cancer.[38] Rees *et al.*[39] described a patient who presented with a small cell lung cancer and Cushing syndrome due to ectopic ACTH production. When the hypercorticoidism was suppressed with aminoglutethimide, hyponatremia was unmasked, which was due to inappropriate ADH secretion. The tumor was subsequently found to have been producing arginine vasopressin, oxytocin, neurophysin, ACTH, corticotropin-like intermediate lobe peptide, insulin, prolactin, and perhaps as an artifact, β-MSH.

Ectopic production of ADH without hyponatremia may be very common in lung cancer patients. Gilby *et al.*[40] concluded that it occurs in about 40% of small cell lung cancers. Also, Odell *et al.*,[41] employing an antiserum reactive with both arginine vasopressin and the fetal peptide arginine vasotocin, showed that elevated levels of the hormone(s) were present in 41% of 41 patients with lung cancer of various histologic types and in 37% of 30 patients with colon cancer.

## 4. HUMAN CHORIONIC GONADOTROPIN

The production of hCG is typically associated with trophoblastic tumors, when it is not ectopic in origin. However, ectopic secretion of bioactive gonadotropin does occur and has been associated with precocious puberty in young boys with hepatoblastoma,[42] as well as with gynecomastia in adult male lung cancer patients.[43] The early descriptions of ectopic gonadotropin secretion were made before the availability of assays capable of distinguishing between LH and hCG. Only later was it apparent that hCG is almost entirely responsible for the clinical syndromes.

With the development of RIAs specifically for the α and β-chains of hCG, it became possible to define the frequency with which these subunits are produced ectopically, and their potential as tumor markers. When plasma or serum was assayed, it was found that detectable levels of immunoreactive hCG occur in nonpregnant normal subjects. For example, the radioimmunoassays used by Kahn *et al.*[44] set the upper limits of normal for hCG-α, hCG-β, and hCG at 2.5, 2.0, and 3.0 ng/ml, respectively, for males and premenopausal females. For postmenopausal women, the upper limits of normal increased to 7.0, 3.0, and 7.5 ng/ml, respectively. The higher hCG-α values in postmenopausal women are presumably of pituitary origin and are a consequence of their high serum LH levels. The elevated complete hCG levels may also be due to cross-reaction of antibody with LH, as suggested by Monteiro *et al.*[45]

Braunstein *et al.*[3] evaluated a large series of patients with various types of cancer including carcinomas of the stomach, liver, pancreas, and breast, and found the serum hCG to be elevated in

7% of nontesticular tumors. Serum hCG-α is elevated in a minority of patients with lung cancers (5%) and with nonislet cell gastrointestinal (GI) tract malignancies (4%).[46]

Kahn et al.[44] studied 76 patients with islet cell tumors of the pancreas. There were 27 with functioning islet cell carcinomas, 17 (63%) of whom had elevated levels of plasma hCG, or one of its subunits. None of 43 patients with benign tumors, or six with nonfunctioning malignant islet cell tumors had increased levels of complete hCG, hCG-α, or hCG-β. Thus, when present, these proteins appear to provide a reliable indicator of malignancy in patients already known to have an islet cell tumor. The most consistent abnormality in this study was an elevation in hCG-α, the chain common to hCG, LH, and TSH. Increased plasma levels were present in 14 of the 27 patients (52%).

Naughton et al.[47] used an immunoperoxidase technique to examine a variety of cancer tissues for hCG-β. Ten of these samples were regarded as clearly positive, including two carcinomas of the breast, while another five gave equivocal results. Odell and Wolfsen[48] postulated that all cancers synthesize hCG-like material, although it frequently fails to appear in the circulation in detectable amounts. This may be because the protein never reaches the plasma, or it could be the result of its rapid enzymatic degradation. In this context, it is probably relevant that the carbohydrate component of hCG normally retards degradation, thereby maintaining bioactivity of the hormone,[49] and that ectopically produced hCG is deficient in carbohydrate.[50] Before leaving the issue of hCG in tumors, it must be pointed out that there is not universal agreement concerning the frequency with which this protein is detectable, at least by immunohistochemical techniques. Bellet et al.,[51] using a highly specific hCG-β antiserum, found only seven out of 93 tumors to be positive. Five of these were testicular cancers, while the other two were among 53 breast cancers examined. Another study[45] examined 18 breast cancers and demonstrated that 16 were negative for hCG, with two exhibiting only a minimal positive staining for this hormone.

The story of ectopic production of hCG is complicated further by reports of its presence not only in the plasma of individuals without malignant disease, but also in normal tissues.[52,53] When extracts of normal tissues were tested for hCG-β by RIA, and hCG-like protein by a radioreceptor assay, material that reacted like complete hCG, rather than just the β-chain, was found consistently in kidney, lung, stomach, colon, liver, and heart.[53] This material, like that secreted by tumors, contains little carbohydrate, and so probably exerts little bioactivity. Morrish et al.[54] further demonstrated the synthesis of hCG-like protein by normal tissues in vitro together with its secretion into the culture medium. Thus, it appears that the genome for hCG is not completely suppressed in adult nonendocrine tissues, again raising the question: "When is 'ectopic' not ectopic?"

## 5. PARATHORMONE (PTH) AND OTHER HYPERCALCEMIA-INDUCING FACTORS

Hypercalcemia is a common feature in cancer patients, but demonstrable bone metastases are not always present. Its occurrence in patients with solid tumors without evidence of osteolytic bone destruction was attributed to the ectopic production of PTH.[55,56] In one study,[57] PTH was measured by radioimmunoassay in both arterial and venous renal blood from an adenocarcinoma-bearing kidney. There was an arteriovenous gradient in PTH concentration, the venous sample containing approximately four times the level detected in the arterial blood.

Despite these positive findings, others failed to demonstrate either immunoreactive PTH in the tumor tissue or elevated levels in the serum of cancer patients with hypercalcemia but without osteolytic metastases.[58,59] These conflicting reports can be ascribed at least in part to difficulties in the RIA itself, and particularly to the heterogeneity of the PTH protein fragments used in preparing the antiserum. More recently, in order to circumvent the technical problems of the radioimmunoassay, a cloned PTH DNA was used in a DNA–RNA hybridization assay in order to detect PTH RNA in tumor tissues.[60] None of 13 human cancers, including five associated with hypercalcemia at the time of tumor excision, contained PTH RNA transcripts. Although it would be premature to reach a final verdict, these preliminary results call into question the role of PTH in the cancer-related humoral hypercalcemia.

While further studies using the hybridization technique are indicated, other possible mechanisms require serious consideration. Stewart *et al.*[59] identified a subgroup of cancer patients with hypercalcemia as having a higher urinary calcium excretion and lower plasma 1,25-dihydroxy vitamin D than that usually seen in primary hyperparathyroidism. Furthermore, excretion of nephrogenous cyclic adenosine monophosphate (cAMP) was elevated without detectable immunoreactive PTH in their serum. The conclusion that these tumors produce factors displaying PTH-like biologic activities, but distinct from the normal hormone, was later supported by the demonstration that they stimulate adenylate cyclase activity *in vitro* by binding to renal receptors.[61,62] These factors may bear sufficient structural similarity to PTH for them to be recognized by the antibodies used in some of the radioimmunoassays. Several earlier studies suggested that there are immunoreactive differences between parathyroid gland-secreted PTH and the hormone produced ectopically by tumors.[56,63]

Prostaglandins stimulate bone resorption *in vitro*, and they have been associated with the resorption induced by mouse fibrosarcoma cells.[64] Inhibitors of prostaglandin synthesis were also shown to be effective in reducing metastasis in an animal tumor model.[65] In humans, prostaglandin metabolites were demonstrated in the urine of some hypercalcemic cancer patients and inhibition of prostaglandin synthesis by aspirin or indomethacin produced a reduction in the urinary excretion of both the metabolite and calcium.[66] Nevertheless, only limited clinical success has been achieved with indomethacin therapy,[67] and it seems doubtful that prostaglandins play a major role in human cancer-related hypercalcemia.

An exciting new development is that tumor-secreted growth factors induce hypercalcemia. Transforming growth factor-$\alpha$ is biologically related to epidermal growth factor (EGF), which is known to possess bone-resorbing properties.[68] EGF-like proteins have been shown to be secreted into the medium by cultured human cancer cells[69,70] and are detectable in the urine of patients with advanced disease.[71] In addition, Ibbotson *et al.*[72] recently obtained evidence that a transforming growth factor is responsible for the mobilization of calcium from bone in a rat Leydig cell tumor model for humoral hypercalcemia.

## 6. INSULINLIKE HYPOGLYCEMIC FACTORS

Hypoglycemia has been described as a complication of various tumors other than those arising from the pancreatic islet cells. They are often large and of mesenchymal origin, including fibrosarcomas, leiomyosarcomas, and lymphosarcomas. Also, primary hepatic tumors account for about 20% of cases. In one series of 100 cases occurring in adults, all the tumors weighed between 800 and 10,000 g, with an average weight of 2000 g.[73]

Until recently, there was confusion concerning the mechanism responsible for the hypoglycemic syndrome. The size of most of the tumors involved, and the finding of a high tumor glycogen content suggested excessive glucose utilization with consequent low blood glucose in the host.[74] However, this finding was not supported by attempts to demonstrate an arteriovenous glucose gradient across the tumor.[75] Early reports that immunoreactive insulin was detectable in tumors associated with hypoglycemia were not confirmed by later studies, and Skrabanek and Powell,[76] after a detailed examination of the literature, concluded that there is no support for the occurrence of ectopic insulin production.

Insulinlike biologic activity in plasma is due to a number of factors other than insulin itself. Nonsuppressible insulinlike activity (NSILA) was identified as an acetic acid, ethanol-soluble peptide that behaved biologically like insulin both *in vivo* and *in vitro* but did not react with anti-insulin antibodies.[77] In fact, NSILA comprises a family of small proteins generally referred to as somatomedins, and include insulinlike growth factors I and II (IGF I and IGF II). Specific radioimmunoassay and radioreceptor assays are available for their detection, and recent studies have demonstrated their secretion by human cancer cells in culture.[78,79] Megyesi *et al.*[80] first employed a radioreceptor assay to show the presence of elevated NSILA levels in the plasma of five patients with hypoglycemia complicating extrapancreatic tumors, and similar observations have been made since that time.[81,82] It now seems likely that most cases of ectopically produced hypoglycemia will prove to be due to tumor production of IGF.

## 7. GROWTH HORMONE-RELEASING FACTOR

The production of growth hormone-releasing factor (GHRF) by tumors is of special interest because it provided the source of material in quantities sufficient for establishing the structure of this polypeptide.[83,84] In 1960, Southern[85] described a patient with a metastatic bronchial carcinoid, elevated serum and cerebrospinal 5-HT levels, a pituitary adenoma, and clinical features of acromegaly. Since that time, there have been a number of reports of bronchial carcinoid tumors occurring in association with acromegaly.[86-88] In two patients, operative removal of the tumors was followed by correction of the high serum growth hormone levels.[87]

Frohman and colleagues demonstrated the stimulation of growth hormone release from cultured rat anterior pituitary cells by a bronchial carcinoid tissue extract[89] and a similar effect using a pituitary perfusion system.[90] These investigators also went some way in purifying GHRF, which they found to be present in 15 of 46 tumors examined, including eight of 15 carcinoids, two of four pancreatic islet cell tumors, and three of seven small cell carcinomas of the lung. However, sequencing of the peptide was completed by the research teams led by Guillemin[83] and Vale,[84] both of whom used pancreatic islet cell tumors as their starting material. The structures described were identical (Fig. 1), except that Vale's group omitted the last four of the 44-amino acid sequence. Structure–function relationships indicated that nearly all of the biologic activity was ascribable to the 1–27-amino acid sequence.

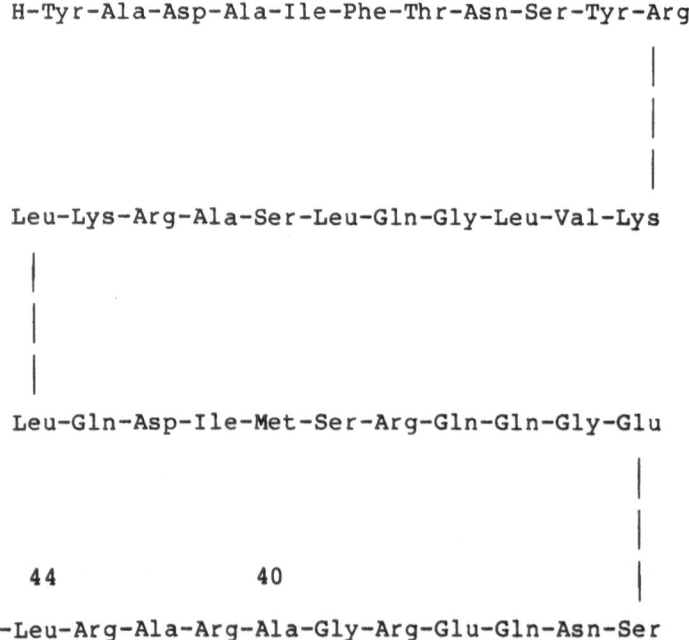

```
H-Tyr-Ala-Asp-Ala-Ile-Phe-Thr-Asn-Ser-Tyr-Arg
                                              |
                                              |
                                              |
Leu-Lys-Arg-Ala-Ser-Leu-Gln-Gly-Leu-Val-Lys
 |
 |
 |
Leu-Gln-Asp-Ile-Met-Ser-Arg-Gln-Gln-Gly-Glu
                                            |
                                            |
  44             40                         |
NH2-Leu-Arg-Ala-Arg-Ala-Gly-Arg-Glu-Gln-Asn-Ser
```

*Figure 1.* Structure of human growth hormone-releasing factor, material sequenced after isolation from an islet cell tumor of the pancreas.

## 8. OTHER ECTOPICALLY PRODUCED HORMONES

### 8.1. Calcitonin

Calcitonin is normally produced by the parafollicular C cells of the thyroid gland; thus, the increased circulating level seen in medullary thyroid carcinomas is not categorized as ectopic hormone production. The first demonstrated case of truly ectopic calcitonin production by a tumor was in a patient with a small cell carcinoma of the bronchus.[91] There was a high serum calcitonin level, which fell after chemotherapy, and a pronounced arteriovenous gradient in calcitonin concentration across the tumor vascular bed. Since that time, ectopic calcitonin production has been associated with various tumor types and demonstrated both in cell culture[4,92] and in human cancer-bearing athymic nude mice.[4]

Serum calcitonin RIA has been proposed as a cancer biomarker. Coombes *et al.*[4] reported detectable levels of calcitonin, which does not occur in healthy adults, in 23 of 28 patients with metastatic breast cancer, but only 1 of 13 with disease restricted to breast and regional lymph nodes. In another study, 84% of patients with extensive small cell carcinomas of the lung had high serum calcitonin concentrations.[93] Calcitonin production by tumors other than medullary cell carcinomas of the thyroid, where it may be responsible for flushing and diarrhea, is not usually associated with any clinical manifestations.

### 8.2. Prolactin

Turkington[94] described a woman with a renal cell carcinoma, galactorrhea, and hyperprolactinemia. Surgical resection of the tumor produced a prompt reduction in serum prolactin to normal levels, and ectopic secretion of the hormone was confirmed by its secretion in cell culture. Davis *et al.*[95] reported hyperprolactinemia in 33% of bronchogenic carcinomas, but without exclusion of prolactin response to stress, drugs, and surgery or radiation to the chest wall,[96] these cases cannot be accepted as examples of ectopic production of the hormone. Of more interest is the report by Rosen *et al.*[97] demonstrating that eight of 32 cancer cell lines examined synthesized prolactin *in vitro*, although the hormone was not secreted into the culture medium.

### 8.3. Gastrin-Releasing Peptide

This is one of several GI small peptides that have recently been shown to be produced ectopically by various tumors. Gastrin-releasing peptide is a 27-residue peptide, the carboxy-terminal amino acid sequence of which shares close structural homology with the amphibian peptide bombesin. Earlier reports in which the ectopically derived peptide was referred to as bombesin now appear to have been in error. Its structure is closer to that of normally produced GRP than it is to bombesin.[98]

The production of GRP has been associated particularly with small cell carcinomas of the lung,[99] although it occurs also in other types of lung cancer,[100] and in medullary carcinomas of the thyroid.[101]

### 8.4. Vasointestinal Peptide

Vasointestinal peptide (VIP) is a 28-amino acid peptide structurally similar to secretin and glucagon. It has a relaxant effect on gastric and gall bladder muscle, but stimulates intestinal muscle to contract. Bloom *et al.*[102] described five patients, four with pancreatic carcinomas and one with a retroperitoneal ganglioneuroblastoma, who exhibited watery diarrhea, hypokalemia, and achlorhydria. The tumor tissues all contained immunoreactive VIP, and high levels were present in the plasma. The same syndrome has also been reported in association with other tumors, including lung cancers and pheochromocytomas.[103]

## 8.5. Erythropoietin

Renal cell carcinoma is the tumor most frequently associated with erythrocytosis due to excessive erythropoietin production, but, as is also true of hepatoma, this is not of ectopic origin, since the kidney and liver are the normal sites of secretion of this hormone. Erythrocytosis is said to occur in 10–20% of patients with cerebellar hemangioblastomas,[73] but usually the demonstration of ectopic erythropoietin production has not been attempted in these cases. Wrigley *et al.*[104] described erythrocytosis that regressed after removal of a uterine fibromyoma. In this case, bioassay demonstrated erythropoietin in both tumor time extracts and in fluid from cysts that had formed within the tumor. A similar case was reported by Ossias *et al.*[105] in which erythropoietinlike activity from the fibromyoma extract was abolished by antiserum to erythropoietin. Anagnostou *et al.*[106] described a patient with a hemangioblastoma in whom bioassay for erythropoietin activity showed a high level in an extract of the tumor tissue. Plasma bioassay was used to follow disease response to surgery. Here, increased plasma erythropoietin activity predated the clinical manifestations of recurrent disease.

The available bioassays for erythropoietin are both complex and insensitive. Further understanding of erythropoietin pathophysiology and ectopic production is likely to follow the recent development of reliable RIA.[107]

## 9. CONCLUSION

The introduction of radioimmunoassay by Berson and Yalow during the 1950s was largely responsible for the accelerated recognition of the ectopic hormone syndromes, and now the new techniques of molecular biology are providing a clearer picture of the basic mechanisms involved in their production by tumor cells. But, the benefits have not all been in one direction. The study of patients with ectopic hormone syndromes has also contributed to basic research, a nice example being the determination of the structure of GHRF, for which a pancreatic islet cell tumor was used as the starting material.

Tumor cell culture and the *in vivo* growth of solid human tumors in athymic nude mice are two procedures which are now being widely used to demonstrate ectopic hormone production. These techniques have been invaluable in the study of growth factor synthesis by tumors and the autocrine and paracrine stimulation of cell proliferation. Examples include the secretion of somatomedin and EGF-like polypeptides. An exciting prospect is that these new discoveries may provide a molecular approach to cancer therapy, by the development of either synthetic antitumor growth factors or of antibodies directed against receptors on the tumor cell membrane. It seems to this reviewer that these areas are going to provide major contributions to clinical oncology over the next decade or so.

By contrast, the clinical application of circulating ectopically produced hormones as biomarkers for early cancer detection has not fulfilled its initial promise. This is because elevations in the plasma hormone levels usually occur only in cases in which the tumor burden is large, and metastasis has often already taken place. A potential exception is the finding by Wolfsen and Odell[8] that radioimmunoassayable plasma ACTH may be increased in patients with chronic obstructive pulmonary disease, in whom lung cancer subsequently develops.

## REFERENCES

1. Liddle, G. W., Island, D., and Meador, C. K., 1962, Normal and abnormal regulation of corticotropin secretion in man, *Recent Progr. Horm. Res.* **18**:125–166.
2. Shields, R., 1977, Gene derepression in tumors. *Nature (Lond.)* **209**:752–753.
3. Braunstein, G. D., Vaitukaitis, J. L., Carbone, P. P., and Ross, G. T., 1973, Ectopic production of human chorionic-gonadotropin by neoplasms, *Ann. Intern. Med.* **78**:39–45.
4. Coombes, R. C., Easty, G. C., Detre, S. I., Hillyard, C. J., Stevens, U., Girgis, S. I., Galante, L. S.,

Heywood, L., MacIntyre, I., and Neville, A. M., 1975, Secretion of immunoreactive calcitonin by human breast carcinomas, *Br. Med. J.* **4:**197–199.

5. Pearse, A. G. E., 1969, The cytochemistry and ultrastructure of polypeptide hormone-producing cells of the APUD series and the embryologic, physiologic and pathologic implications of the concept, *J. Histochem. Cytochem.* **17:**303–313.

6. Bensch, K. G., Corrin, B., Pariente, R., and Spencer, H., 1968, Oat cell carcinoma of the lung. Its origin and relationship to bronchial carcinoid, *Cancer* **22:**1163–1172.

7. Gewirtz, G., and Yalow, R. S., 1974, Ectopic ACTH production in carcinoma of the lung, *J. Clin. Invest.* **53:**1022–1032.

8. Wolfsen, A. R., and Odell, W. D., 1979, Pro ACTH: Use for early detection of lung cancer, *Am. J. Med.* **66:**765–772.

9. Baylin, S. B., Abeloff, M. D., Goodwin, G., Carney, D. N., and Gazdar, A. F., 1980, Activities of L-dopa decarboxylase and diamine oxidase (histaminase) in human lung cancers and carboxylase as a marker for small (oat) cell cancer in cell culture, *Cancer Res.* **40:** 1990–1994.

10. Berger, C. L., Goodwin, G., Mendelsohn, G., Eggleston, J. C., Abeloff, M. D., Aisner, S., and Baylin, S. B., 1981, Endocrine-related biochemistry in the spectrum of human lung carcinoma, *J. Clin. Endocrinol. Metab.* **53:**422–429.

11. Abe, K., Adachi, I., Miyakawa, S., Tanaka, M., Yamaguchi, K., Tanaka, N., Kameya, T., and Shimosato, Y., 1977, Production of calcitonin, adrenocorticotropic hormone and β-melanocyte-stimulating hormone in tumors derived from amine precursor uptake and decarboxylation cells, *Cancer Res.* **37:**4190–4194.

12. Bertagna, X. Y., Nicholson, W. E., Sorenson, G. D., Pettengill, O. S., Mount, C. D., and Orth, D. N., 1978, Corticotropin, lipotropin, and β-endorphin production by a human non-pituitary tumor in culture: Evidence for a common precursor, *Proc. Natl. Acad. Sci. USA* **75:**5160–5164.

13. Weintraub, B. D., and Rosen, S. W., 1971, Ectopic production of human chorionic somatomammotropin by nontrophoblastic cancers, *J. Clin. Endocrinol. Metab.* **32:**94–101.

14. Whitaker, M. D., Klee, G. G., Kao, P. C., Randall, R. V., and Heser, D. W., 1983, Demonstration of biological activity of prolactin molecular weight variants in human sera, *J. Clin. Endocrinol. Metab.* **58:**826–830.

15. Stolar, M. W., Amburn, K., and Baumann, G., 1984, Plasma "big" and "big big" growth hormone (GH) in man: An oligomeric series composed of structurally diverse GH monomers, *J. Clin. Endocrinol. Metab.* **59:**212–218.

16. Liddle, G. W., Nicholson, W. E., and Island, D. P., 1969, Clinical and laboratory studies of ectopic hormonal syndromes, *Recent Prog. Horm. Res.* **25:**283–314.

17. Odell, W. D., Wolfsen, A. R., Bachelot, I., and Hirose, F. M., 1979, Ectopic production of lipotropin by cancer, *Am. J. Med.* **66:**631–638.

18. Azzopardi, J. G., and Williams, E. D., 1968, Pathology of "nonendocrine" tumors associated with Cushing's syndrome, *Cancer* **22:**274–286.

19. Upton, G. V., and Amatruda, T. T. Jr., 1971, Evidence for the presence of tumor peptides with corticotropin-releasing factor-like activity in the ectopic ACTH syndrome, *N. Engl. J. Med.* **285:**419–424.

20. Vale, W., Spiess, J., Rivier, C., and Rivier, J., 1981, Characterization of a 41-residue ovine hypothalamic peptide that stimulates secretion of corticotropin and β-endorphin, *Science* **213:**1394–1397.

21. Shibahara, S., Morimoto, Y., Furutani, Y., Notake, M., Takahashi, H., Shimizu, S., Horikawa, S., and Numa, S., 1983, Isolation and sequence analysis of the human corticotropin-releasing factor precursor gene, *EMBO J.* **2:**775–779.

22. Yamamoto, H., Hirata, Y., Matsukura, S., Imura, H., Nakamura, M., and Tanaka, A., 1976, Studies on ectopic ACTH-producing tumors. IV. CRF-like activity in tumour tissue, *Acta Endocrinol. (Copenh.)* **82:**183–192.

23. Suda, T., Demura, H., Demura, R., Wakabayashi, I., Nomura, K., Odagiri, E., and Shizume, K., 1977, Corticotropin-releasing factor-like activity in ACTH producing tissues, *J. Clin. Endocrinol. Metab.* **44:**440–446.

24. Carey, R. M., Varma, S. K., Drake, C. R., Thorner, M. O., Kovacs, K., Rivier, J., and Vale, W., 1984, Ectopic secretion of corticotropin-releasing factor as a cause of Cushing's syndrome: A clinical, morphological and biochemical study, *N. Engl. J. Med.* **311:**13–20.

25. Yalow, R. S., and Berson, S. A., 1971, Size heterogeneity of immunoreactive human ACTH in plasma and in extracts of pituitary glands and ACTH-producing thymoma, *Biochem. Biophys. Res. Commun.* **44:**439–445.

26. Law, D. A., Liddle, G. W., Scott, H. W., Jr., and Tauber, S. D., 1965, Ectopic production of multiple hormones (ACTH, MSH and gastrin) by a single malignant tumor, *N. Engl. J. Med.* **273**:292–296.

27. Shapiro, M., Nicholson, W. E., Orth, D. N., Mitchell, W. M., and Liddle, G. W., 1971, Differences between ectopic MSH and pituitary MSH, *J. Clin. Endocrinol. Metab.* **33**:377–381.

28. Bachelot, I., Wolfsen, A. R., and Odell, W. D., 1977, Pituitary and plasma lipotropins: Demonstration of the artificial nature of beta MSH, *J. Clin. Endocrinol. Metab.* **44**:939–946.

29. Chretien, M., Seidah, N. G., Benjannet, S., Dragon, N., Routhier, R., Motomatsu, T., Crine, P., and Lis, M., 1977, A βLPH precursor model: Recent developments concerning morphine-like substances, *Ann. NY Acad. Sci.* **297**:84–107.

30. Tsukada, T., Nakai, Y., Jingami, H., Imura, H., Taii, S., Nakanishi, S., and Numa, S., 1981, Identification of the mRNA coding for the ACTH-beta-lipotropin precursor in a human ectopic ACTH-producing tumor, *Biochem. Biophys. Res. Commun.* **98**:535–540.

31. Schwartz, W. B., Bennett, W., Curelop, S., and Bartter, F. C., 1957, A syndrome of renal sodium loss and hyponatremia probably resulting from inappropriate secretion of antidiuretic hormone, *Am. J. Med.* **23**:529–542.

32. Amatruda, T. T., Jr., Mulrow, P. J., Gallagher, J. C., and Sawyer, W. H., 1963, Carcinoma of the lung with inappropriate antidiuresis, *N. Engl. J. Med.* **269**:544–549.

33. Yamaji, T., Ishibashi, M., Katayama, S., Itabashi, A., Ohsawa, N., Kondo, Y., Mizumoto, Y., and Kosaka, K., 1981, Neurophysin biosynthesis in vitro in oat cell carcinoma of the lung with ectopic vasopressin production, *J. Clin. Invest.* **68**:1441–1449.

34. Yamaji, T., Ishibashi, M., and Hori, T., 1984, Propressophysin in human blood: A possible marker of ectopic vasopressin production, *J. Endocrinol. Metab.* **59**:505–512.

35. Hainsworth, J. D., Workman, R., and Greco, F. A., 1983, Management of the syndrome of inappropriate antidiuretic hormone secretion in small cell lung cancer, *Cancer* **51**:161–165.

36. Hamilton, B. P. M., Upton, G. V., and Amatruda, T. T., Jr., 1972, Evidence for the presence of neurophysin in tumors producing the syndrome of inappropriate antidiuresis, *J. Clin. Endocrinol. Metab.* **35**:764–767.

37. Marks, L. J., Berde, B., Klein, L. A., Roth, J., Goonan, S. R., Blumen, D., and Nasbeth, D. C., 1968, Inappropriate vasopressin secretion and carcinoma of the pancreas, *Am. J. Med.* **45**:967–974.

38. Bartter, F. C., and Schwartz, W. B., 1967, The syndrome of inappropriate secretion of antidiuretic hormone, *Am. J. Med.* **42**:790–806.

39. Rees, L. H., Bloomfield, G. A., Rees, G. M., Corrin, B., Franks, L. M., and Ratcliffe, J. G., 1974, Multiple hormones in a bronchial tumor, *J. Clin. Endocrinol. Metab.* **38**:1090–1097.

40. Gilby, E. D., Bondy, P. K., and Fosling, M., 1976, Impaired water excretion in oat cell lung cancer, *Br. J. Cancer* **34**:323–324.

41. Odell, W., Wolfsen, A., Yoshimoto, Y., Weitzman, R., Fisher, D., and Hirose, F., 1977, Ectopic polypeptide synthesis: A university concomitant of neoplasia, *Trans. Assoc. Am. Physicians* **90**:204–227.

42. McArthur, J. W., Toll, G. D., Russfield, A. B., Reiss, A. M., Quinby, W. C., and Baker, W. H., 1973, Sexual precocity attributable to ectopic gonadotropin secretion by hepatoblastoma, *Am. J. Med.* **54**:390–403.

43. Fusco, F. D., and Rosen, S. W., 1966, Gonadotropin-producing anaplastic large-cell carcinomas of the lung, *N. Engl. J. Med.* **275**:507–515.

44. Kahn, R., Rosen, S. W., Weintraub, B. D., Fajans, S. S., and Gorden, P., 1977, Ectopic production of chorionic gonadotropin and its subunits by islet-cell tumors, *N. Engl. J. Med.* **297**:565–569.

45. Monteiro, J. C. M. P., Ferguson, K. M., McKinna, J. A., Greening, W. P., and Neville, A. M., 1984, Ectopic production of human chorionic gonadotropin-like material by breast cancer, *Cancer* **53**:957–962.

46. Kourides, I. A., and Schorr-Toshav, N. L., 1981, Alpha subunit of glycoprotein hormones: Secretion by human malignancies, *Clin. Bull.* **11**:106–109.

47. Naughton, M. A., Merrill, D. A., McManus, L., Fink, L. M., Berman, E., White, M. J., and Hernandez, A. M., 1975, Localization of the β chain of human chorionic gonadotropin on human tumor cells and placental cells, *Cancer Res.* **35**:1887–1890.

48. Odell, W. D., and Wolfsen, A. R., 1980, Hormones from tumors: Are they ubiquitous?, *Am. J. Med.* **68**:317–318.

49. Van Hall, E. V., Vaitukaitis, J. L., and Ross, G. T., 1971, Immunological and biological activity of hCG following progressive desialylation, *Endocrinology* **88**:456–464.

50. Yoshimoto, Y., Wolfsen, A. R., and Odell, W. D., 1979, Glycosylation, a variable in the production of hCG by cancers, *Am. J. Med.* **67**:414–420.

51. Bellet, D., Arrang, J. M., Contesso, G., Cailland, J. M., and Bohuon, C., 1980, Localization of the β subunit of human chorionic gonadotropin on various tumors, *Eur. J. Cancer* **16**:433–439.
52. Yoshimoto, Y., Wolfsen, A. R., and Odell, W. D., 1977, Human chorionic gonadotropin-like substance in nonendocrine tissues of normal subjects, *Science* **197**:575–577.
53. Yoshimoto, Y., Wolfson, A. R., Hirose, F., and Odell, W. D., 1979, Human chorionic gonadotropin-like material: Presence in normal human tissues, *Am. J. Obstet. Gynecol.* **134**:729–733.
54. Morrish, D. W., Wolfsen, A. R., and Odell, W. D., 1980, hCG-like substance in normal tissues: In vitro synthesis. *Clin. Res.* **28**:25A.
55. Roof, B. S., Carpenter, B., Fink, D. J., and Gordan, G. S., 1971, Some thoughts on the nature of ectopic parathyroid hormones, *Am. J. Med.* **50**:686–691.
56. Benson, R. C., Jr., Riggs, B. L., Pickard, B. M., and Arnaud, C. D., 1974, Immunoreactive forms of circulating parathyroid hormone in primary and ectopic hyperparathyroidism, *J. Clin. Invest.* **54**:175–181.
57. Buckle, R. M., McMillan, M., and Mallison, C., 1970, Ectopic secretion of parathyroid hormone by a renal adenocarcinoma in a patient with hypercalcaemia, *Br. Med. J.* **4**:724–726.
58. Powell, D., Singer, F. R., Murray, T. M., Minkin, C., and Potts, J. T., Jr., 1973, Nonparathyroid humoral hypercalcemia in patients with neoplastic diseases, *N. Engl. J. Med.* **289**:176–181.
59. Stewart, A. F., Horst, R., Deftos, L. J., Cadman, E. C., Lang, R., and Broadus, A. E., 1980, Biochemical evaluation of patients with cancer-associated hypercalcemia: Evidence for humoral and non-humoral groups, *N. Engl. J. Med.* **303**:1377–1383.
60. Simpson, E. L., Mundy, G. R., D'Souza, S. M., Ibbotson, K. J., Bockman, R., and Jacobs, J. W., 1983, Absence of parathyroid hormone messenger RNA in nonparathyroid tumors associated with hypercalcemia, *N. Engl. J. Med.* **309**:325–330.
61. Stewart, A. F., Insogna, K. L., Goltzman, D., and Broadus, A. E., 1983, Identification of adenylate cyclase-stimulating activity and cytochemical glucose-6-phosphate dehydrogenase-stimulating activity in extracts of tumors from patients with humoral hypercalcemia of malignancy, *Proc. Natl. Acad. Sci. USA* **80**:1454–1458.
62. Strewler, G. J., Williams, R. D., and Nissenson, R. A., 1983, Human renal carcinoma cells produce hypercalcemia in the nude mouse and a novel protein recognized by parathyroid hormone receptors, *J. Clin. Invest.* **71**:769–774.
63. Riggs, B. L., Arnaud, D. C., Reynolds, J. C., and Smith, L. H., 1971, Immunologic differentiation of primary hyperparathyroidism from hyperparathyroidism due to nonparathyroid cancer, *J. Clin. Invest.* **50**:2079–2083.
64. Tashjian, A. H., Jr., Voelkel, E. F., Levine, L., and Goldhaber, P., 1972, Evidence that the bone resorption stimulating factor produced by mouse fibrosarcoma cells is prostaglandin $E_2$: A new model for the hypercalcemia of cancer, *J. Exp. Med.* **136**:1329–1343.
65. Powles, T. J., Clark, S. A., Easty, D. M., Easty, G. C., and Munro, N. A., 1973, The inhibition by aspirin and indomethacin of osteolytic tumour deposits and hypercalcaemia in rats with Walker tumour, and its possible application to human breast cancer, *Br. J. Cancer* **28**:316–321.
66. Seyberth, H. W., Segre, G. V., Morgan, J. L., Sweetman, B. J., Potts, J. T., and Oates, J. A., 1975, Prostaglandins as mediators of hypercalcemia associated with certain types of cancer, *N. Engl. J. Med.* **293**:1278–1283.
67. Mundy, G. R., Wilkinson, R., and Heath, D. A., 1983, A comparative study of available medical therapy for hypercalcemia of malignancy, *Am. J. Med.* **74**:421–432.
68. Raisz, L. G., Simmons, H. A., Sandberg, A. L., and Canalis, E., 1980, Direct stimulation of bone resorption by epidermal growth factor, *Endocrinology* **107**:270–273.
69. Dickson, R. B., Bates, S. E., McManaway, M. E., and Lippman, M. E., 1986, Characterization of estrogen responsive transforming activity in human breast cancer cell lines, *Cancer Res.* **46**:1707–1713.
70. Bauknecht, T., Kiechle, M., Bauer, G., and Siebers, J. W., 1986, Characterization of growth factors in human ovarian carcinomas, *Cancer Res.* **46**:2614–2618.
71. Kimball, E. S., Bohn, W. H., Cockley, K. D., Warren, T. C., and Sherwin, S. A., 1984, Distinct high-performance liquid chromatography pattern of transforming growth factor activity in urine of cancer patients as compared with that of normal individuals, *Cancer Res.* **44**:3613–3619.
72. Ibbotson, K. J., D'Souza, S. M., Ng, K. W., Osborne, C. K., Niall, M., Martin, T. J., and Mundy, C. R., 1983, Tumor-derived growth factor increases bone resorption in a tumor associated with humoral hypercalcemia of malignancy, *Science* **221**:1292–1294.
73. Lipsett, M. B., Odell, W. D., Rosenberg, L. E., and Waldman, T. A., 1964, Humoral syndromes associated with nonendocrine tumors, *Ann. Intern. Med.* **61**:733–756.

74. McFadzean, A. J. S., and Yeung, R. T. T., 1956, Hypoglycemia in primary carcinoma of the liver, *Arch. Intern. Med.* **98:**720–731.

75. Butterfield, W. J. H., Kinder, C. H., and Mahler, R. F., 1960, Hypoglycaemia associated with sarcoma, *Lancet* **1:**703.

76. Skrabanek, P., and Powell, D., 1978, Ectopic insulin and Occam's razor: Reappraisal of the riddle of tumour hypoglycaemia, *Clin. Endocrinol.* **9:**141–154.

77. Rinderknecht, E., and Humbel, R. E., 1976, Polypeptides with nonsuppressible insulin-like and cell-growth promoting activities in human serum: Isolation, chemical characterization, and some biological properties of forms I and II, *Proc. Natl. Acad. Sci. USA* **73:**2365–2369.

78. Huff, K. K., Kaufman, D., Gabbay, K. H., Spencer, E. M., Lippman, M. E., and Dickson, R. B., 1986, Secretion of an insulin-like growth factor-I-related protein by human breast cancer cells, *Cancer Res.* **46:**4613–4619.

79. Atkison, P. R., Hayden, L. J., Bala, R. M., and Hollenberg, M. D., 1984, Production of somatomedin-like activity by human adult tumor-derived, transformed, and normal cell cultures and by cultured rat hepatocytes: Effects of culture conditions and of epidermal growth factor (urogastrone), *Can. J. Biochem. Cell Biol.* **62:**1343–1350.

80. Megyesi, K., Kahn, C. R., Roth, J., and Gorden, P., 1974, Hypoglycemia in association with extra-pancreatic tumors: Demonstration of elevated plasma NSILA-S by a new radioreceptor assay, *J. Clin. Endocrinol. Metab.* **38:**931–934.

81. Hyodo, T., Megyesi, K., Kahn, C. R., McLean, J. P., and Friesen, H. G., 1977, Adrenocortical carcinoma and hypoglycemia: Evidence for production of nonsuppressible insulinlike activity by the tumor, *J. Clin. Endocrinol. Metab.* **44:**1175–1184.

82. Plovnick, H., Ruderman, N. B., Aoki, T., Chideckel, E. W., and Poffenbarger, P. L., 1979, Non-β-cell tumor hypoglycemia associated with increased nonsuppressible insulin-like protein (NSILP), *Am. J. Med.* **66:**154–159.

83. Guillemin, R., Brazeau, P., Bohlen, P., Esch, F., Ling, N., and Wehrenberg, W. B., 1982, Growth hormone-releasing factor from a human pancreatic tumor that caused acromegaly, *Science* **218:**585–587.

84. Rivier, J., Spiess, J., Thorner, M., and Vale, W., 1982, Characterization of a growth hormone-releasing factor from a human pancreatic islet tumor, *Nature (Lond.)* **300:**276–278.

85. Southern, A. L., 1960, Functioning metastatic bronchial carcinoid with elevated levels of serum and cerebrospinal fluid serotonin and pituitary adenoma, *J. Clin. Endocrinol. Metab.* **20:**298–305.

86. Dabek, J. T., 1974, Bronchial carcinoid tumor with acromegaly in two patients, *J. Clin. Endocrinol. Metab.* **38:**329–333.

87. Sonksen, P. H., Ayres, A. B., Briambridge, M., Corrin, B., Davies, D. R., Jeremiah, G. M., Oaten, S. W., Lowy, C., and West, T. E. T., 1976, Acromegaly caused by pulmonary carcinoid tumors, *Clin. Endocrinol.* **5:**503–513.

88. Shalet, S. M., Beardwell, C. G., MacFarlane, I. A., Ellison, M. L., Norman, C. M., Rees, L. H., and Hughes, M., 1979, Acromegaly due to production of a growth hormone releasing factor by a bronchial carcinoid tumor, *Clin. Endocrinol.* **10:**61–67.

89. Zafar, M. S., Mellinger, R. C., Fine, G., Szabo, M., and Frohman, L. A., 1979, Acromegaly associated with a bronchial carcinoid tumor: Evidence for ectopic production of growth hormone-releasing activity, *J. Clin. Endocrinol. Metab.* **48:**66–71.

90. Frohman, L. A., Szabo, M., Berelowitz, M., and Stachura, M. E., 1980, Partial purification and characterization of a peptide with growth hormone-releasing activity from extrapituitary tumors in patients with acromegaly, *J. Clin. Invest.* **65:**43–54.

91. Silva, O. L., Becker, K. L., Primack, A., Doppman, J., and Snider, R. H., 1973, Ectopic production of calcitonin, *Lancet* **2:**317.

92. Ellison, M., Woodhouse, D., Hillyard, C., Dowsett, M., Coombes, R. C., Gilby, E. D., Greenberg, P. B., and Neville, A. M., 1975, Immunoreactive calcitonin production by human lung carcinoma cells in culture, *Br. J. Cancer* **32:**373–379.

93. Wallach, S. R., Royston, I., Taetle, R., Wohl, H., and Deftos, L. J., 1981, Plasma calcitonin as a marker of disease activity in patients with small cell carcinoma of the lung, *J. Clin. Endocrinol. Metab.* **53:**602–606.

94. Turkington, R. W., 1971, Ectopic production of prolactin, *N. Engl. J. Med.* **285:**1455–1458.

95. Davis, S., Proper, S., May, P. B., and Ertel, N. H., 1979, Elevated prolactin levels in bronchogenic carcinoma, *Cancer* **44:**676–679.

96. Rose, D. P., and Pruitt, B. T., 1981, Plasma prolactin levels in patients with breast cancer, *Cancer* **48:**2687–2691.

97. Rosen, S. W., Weintraub, B. D., and Aaronson, S. W., 1980, Nonrandom ectopic protein production by malignant cells: Direct evidence in vitro, *J. Clin. Endocrinol. Metab.* **50:**834–841.

98. Yamaguchi, K., Abe, K., Kameya, T., Adachi, I., Taguchi, S., Otsubo, K., and Yanaihara, N., 1983, Production and molecular size heterogeneity of immunoreactive gastrin-releasing peptide in fetal and adult lungs and primary lung tumors, *Cancer Res.* **43:**3932–3939.

99. Moody, T. W., Pert, C. B., Gazdar, A. F., Carney, D. N., and Minna, J. D., 1981, High levels of intracellular bombesin characterize human small-cell lung carcinoma, *Science* **214:**1246–1248.

100. Abe, K., Yamaguchi, K., Adachi, I., Suzuki, M., Kimura, S., Shimada, A., Maruno, K., and Yanaihara, N., 1984, Production of gastrin-releasing peptide (bombesin) by tumors, in: *Endocrinology* (F. Labrie and L. Proulx, eds.), pp. 77–80, Elsevier, Amsterdam.

101. Matsubayashi, S., Yanaihara, C., Ohkubo, M., Fukata, S., Hayashi, Y., Tamai, H., Nakagawa, T., Miyauchi, A., Kuma, K., Abe, K., Suzuki, T., and Yanaihara, N., 1984, Gastrin-releasing peptide immunoreactivity in medullary thyroid carcinoma, *Cancer* **53:**2472–2477.

102. Bloom, S. R., Polak, J. M., and Pearse, A. G. E., 1973, Vasoactive intestinal peptide and watery diarrhoea syndrome, *Lancet* **2:**14–16.

103. Said, S. I., and Faloona, G. R., 1975, Elevated plasma and tissue levels of vasoactive intestinal polypeptide in the watery-diarrhea syndrome due to pancreatic, bronchogenic and other tumors, *N. Engl. J. Med.* **293:**155–160.

104. Wrigley, P. F. M., Malpas, J. S., Turnbull, A. L., Jenkins, G. C., and McArt, A., 1971, Secondary polycythaemia due to a uterine fibromyoma producing erythropoietin, *Br. J. Haematol.* **21:**551–555.

105. Ossias, A. L., Zanjani, E. D., Zalusky, R., Estren, S., and Wasserman, L. R., 1973, Case report: Studies on the mechanism of erythrocytosis associated with a uterine fibromyoma, *Br. J. Haematol.* **25:**179–185.

106. Anagnostou, A., Chawla, M. S., Poloi, L., and Fried, W., 1979, Determination of plasma erythropoietin levels. An early marker of tumor activity, *Cancer* **44:**1014–1016.

107. Cohen, R. A., Clemons, G., and Ebbe, S., 1985, Correlation between bioassay and radioimmunoassay for erythropoietin in human serum and urine concentrates, *Proc. Soc. Exp. Biol. Med.* **179:**296–299.

# 24

# Metaplastic Transformation of Pancreatic Cells to Hepatocytes

## Dante G. Scarpelli, Janardan K. Reddy, and Sambasiva M. Rao

## 1. INTRODUCTION

The dogma that the differentiated state in non-neoplastic cells is stable and irreversible is clearly no longer tenable in the face of the numerous examples in the literature that document its plasticity under certain circumstances. The earliest examples of the transformation of one differentiated cell type to another, referred to as metaplasia, were encountered by pathologists during their histologic studies of human tissues affected by processes such as inflammation and neoplasia.[1] While relatively common, the occurrence of metaplasia in association with these conditions is extremely variable from case to case, suggesting that its development depends on a very specific set of conditions. Although metaplasia has long been known and is well documented in both epithelial and mesenchymal cells, details of its histogenesis remain controversial. This is based largely on the issue of whether one fully differentiated cell type can indeed directly undergo transformation to another, or whether as some hold, metaplastic cells must arise from undifferentiated precursor cells that persist in the adult state and under abnormal conditions undergo atypical differentiation.

There are a number of examples of experimental systems in which metaplasia can be induced which have served as models for its detailed study. The earliest, most studied, and best known of these involves both epithelial and mesenchymal cells during retinal regeneration in eyes of adult salamanders where pigment cells of the retina lose their pigment and are transformed into neural cells.[2-4] Later, again in urodeles, it was shown that pigmented cells of the iris can be induced to proliferate and differentiate into lens cells and lens fibers.[5-8] Comparable cellular transformations in ocular tissues have also been experimentally induced in embryonic chick and rat eyes, so that these striking examples of redirected differentiation are not limited to the lower vertebrates.[5] The latter model, however, may not be entirely appropriate to study metaplasia since it entails the use of embryonic tissues, which, it may be argued, are probably more multipotent than their adult counterparts. All of these tissues have a common embryologic derivation from gastrular ectoderm and the transformations they are capable of appear to be limited to a certain spectrum or "developmental family" of tissues in the eye.[5]

In the human lung, the epithelium lining bronchi is frequently the site of squamous metaplasia as the result of injury due to chronic exposure to noxious atmospheric pollutants, or repeated

Dante G. Scarpelli, Janardan K. Reddy, and Sambasiva M. Rao  •  Department of Pathology, Northwestern University Medical School, Chicago, Illinois 60611.

infections. Experiments in which tracheal epithelium was subjected to mechanical injury clearly established that squamous cells are derived directly from the transformation of preexisting columnar epithelial cells.[9] Experimental induction of metaplasia of mesenchymal cells has also been reported[10] and more recently has been employed as a model to study some of the mechanisms involved in differentiation.[11]

Another focus of tissues identified as being capable of undergoing metaplastic transformation with significant regularity involves those derived from gut endoderm, namely liver,[12] stomach,[13,14] and more recently, pancreas.[15] The earliest examples were described in the liver of adult rats during carcinogenesis studies in which neoplastic cells with the phenotype of intestinal epithelium were encountered. Intestinal epithelium and cells resembling hepatocytes have also been reported in the human stomach, especially during the development of human cancer; the precise details of these transformations remain to be established. Until recently, unequivocal evidence of metaplasia had not been documented in the pancreas despite the presence of cells in the normal organ of many species with the phenotypic characteristics of both islet and acinar cells, so-called intermediate cells.[16] It turns out that cells in the regenerating pancreas of adult rodents are susceptible to alterations of gene expression such that they undergo transformation into cells that are morphologically and functionally indistinguishable from hepatocytes.[15,17] The extent and reproducibility with which this transformation can be induced makes this a promising model to study the regulation of cell differentiation and its alteration by chemical carcinogens, and is the *raison d'être* for the inclusion of this chapter in this volume.

## 2. ANIMAL MODELS

### 2.1. Hamster

The experimental induction of hepatocytes in pancreas of rodents has been accomplished only in the hamster[15] and rat[17]; several attempts to do this in mice have thus far been negative. In the hamster, the conversion of pancreatic cells to cells with a phenotype resembling hepatocytes was first achieved by the injection of a single dose of the pancreatic carcinogen, N-nitrosobis(2-oxopropyl)amine (BOP) during pancreatic regeneration.[18] The most reproducible results were obtained when BOP was given 60 hours after the induction of regeneration by restitution of methionine to animals previously maintained on a methionine deficient diet and intoxicated with ethionine for 8 days. It turns out that at 60 hr, regeneration is at its peak as reflected by the fact that approximately 22.4% of acinar cells, the largest cell component of the pancreas, are in S phase of the cell cycle. In our first description of this model and subsequently, it was clear that hepatocytes can also be induced, though with less regularity and in smaller numbers, by BOP alone, or by pancreatic regeneration alone, including that induced by localized trauma produced by crush injury (M. S. Rao and D. G. Scarpelli, unpublished observations). More recently, we have determined that known tumor-promoting agents such as 12-O-tetradecanoyl phorbol-13-acetate (TPA) (T. Makino and D. G. Scarpelli, unpublished observations) and 2,3,7,8-tetrachlorodibenzo-p-dioxin (TCDD) (M. S. Rao and D. G. Scarpelli, unpublished observations) can also trigger the metaplastic transformation, the former when given as a single dose of 1000 μg/kg b.w. administered at the peak of regeneration, the latter as the result of repeated monthly injections of 50 μg/kg b.w. over a 5-month period.

There is considerable variation between different animals in the extent of the metaplastic response they show. This can range from numerous nests of hepatocytes seen in a segment of the pancreas to single liver cells scattered in the organ. It is worthy to note that "eosinophilic cells" morphologically identical to hepatocytes have also been identified in the pancreas of aged hamsters in two studies of large colonies.[19,20] These cells were originally interpreted as resulting from a metaplastic reaction involving fat cells. Their variable infrequency in these colonies (0.46% and 6%, respectively) and presence exclusively in old animals, coupled with the finding that they can be readily induced by even brief exposure to various carcinogens, suggests that the "spontaneous" appearance of hepatocytes in the pancreas of aged hamster may be due, in part, to their exposure to an ambient environmental mutagen or carcinogen. The foregoing studies have been corroborated by a more recent report[21] describing similar cells which have been interpreted by the authors as representing altered pancreatic islet cells encountered in mature hamsters in a long-term study of unspecified nature. The relative ease with which pancreatic cells can be transformed to hepatocytes in the hamster suggests that the stability of the regulatory gene controls in these cells may be limited, and that their instability is enhanced during cell replication.

## 2.2. Rat

In the rat the induction of pancreatic hepatocytes has been accomplished by protracted treatment with the peroxisome proliferator drugs, Wy, 14-643 ([4-chloro-6-(2,3-xylidino)-2-pyrimidinylthio]acetic acid).[17] or ciprofibrate; i.e., 2-[4(2,2-dichlorocyclopropyl)penoxy]-2-methylpropionic acid.[22] In both instances, the transformation was accomplished in the non-regenerating pancreas. The second variant model was discovered in experiments in which a single dose of the pancreatic carcinogen, 4-hydroxyaminoquinoline-1-oxide (4HAQO) was followed by pancreatic regeneration induced by restitution of dietary copper to copper deficient animals with severe acinar cell atrophy.[23] Subsequent experiments without 4HAQO have shown that copper-induced regeneration in copper deficient animals alone is sufficient to induce a metaplastic response which is quantitatively indistinguishable from that obtained when carcinogen treatment is followed by regeneration, suggesting that regeneraton may be the major stimulus.[24] Protracted dietary restriction of methyl-rich nutrients such as methionine and choline as well as factors necessary for mediating transmethylation; i.e., folate and vitamin $B_{12}$, also lead to the development of pancreatic hepatocytes in male F-344 rats.[25] In these experiments, which lasted for 1.4 and 1 years, respectively, animals also injected with the carcinogen diethyl-nitrosamine and allowed to survive longer developed such cells more readily than their counterparts receiving saline alone. The apparent synergistic effect of longevity on the formation of hepatocytes in rat pancreas suggested these findings to be in keeping with similar results previously documented in aged hamsters. The various experimental and natural circumstances in which hepatocytes have been induced or are encountered are summarized in Table I.

Eosinophilic cells resembling hepatocytes have also been reported recently[26] in rats used in the routine safety evaluation of unnamed chemicals. The slight, albeit nonsignificant, increase in

### Table I. Models of Metaplastic Transformation of Hepatocytes in Pancreas

| Species | Model | Intensity of the reaction and reproducibility | Reference |
|---------|-------|-----------------------------------------------|-----------|
| Hamster | Regeneration[a] + BOP | + + | 15,18 |
|         | Regeneration[a,b] | + | 15 |
|         | TCDD | + + | e |
|         | Regeneration[a] + TPA | ± | f |
|         | Aging | ? | 19,20 |
| Rat | Wy,14-643 ciprofibrate | ± | 17,22 |
|     | Regeneration[c] | + + | 23,24 |
|     | Methionine deficiency | ± | 25 |
| Human | Spontaneous | ?[d] | g |

[a]Induced by ethionine.
[b]Induced by crush injury.
[c]Induced by copper repletion of copper deficiency.
[d]Also observed in some patients with islet cell tumor.
[e]Unpublished observations: M.S. Rao, V. Subbarao, J.D. Prasad, and D.G. Scarpelli.
[f]Unpublished observations: T. Makino and D.G. Scarpelli.
[g]Unpublished observations: D.G. Scarpelli.

incidence of pancreatic hepatocytes encountered in the treated group suggests that the test chemical(s) may have also contributed to the metaplastic transformation. Finally, this study reports the presence of pleomorphic hepatocyte foci, which have only very rarely been seen in the pancreas of both the hamster and rat. Since the author does not specify whether the pleomorphic foci were in both the treated and control groups or only in the treated group, it is not possible to ascertain whether this cytologic alteration is truly spontaneous or the result of chemical insult.

## 2.3. Human

There is only one published report of polyhedral eosinophilic epithelial cell nests in human pancreas of patients with neoplastic and hyperplastic islet cell lesions.[30] These cells have been variously referred to in this abstract[27] as oncocytes and hepatocyte-like cells. Since immunochemical analysis was limited to staining for insulin, glucagon, pancreatic polypeptide, and neuron specific enolase, and these cells were found to be uniformly negative for these markers, their precise nature remains indeterminate. The authors suggest that the eosinophilic cells appeared to be derived from pancreatic acinar cells. We have found a single example of hepatocyte-like cells (Fig. 1) in the essentially normal pancreas obtained at the autopsy of a 58-year-old man who died in congestive heart failure and in whom no islet cell pathology was present.

# 3. CHARACTERIZATION OF THE METAPLASTIC CELLS IN PANCREAS

Detailed morphologic, cytochemical, immunochemical, biochemical, and functional studies[28,29] of hepatocyte-like cells in hamster pancreas were undertaken. By light microscopy these are round to polyhedral cells with substantial eosinophilic cytoplasm interrupted by basophilic stippling and irregular clear area, and contain a large pale central nucleus with a single prominent nucleolus. These cells vary in distribution in the pancreas from single cells to small nests localized either within or adjacent to acini (Fig. 2), adjacent to islets (Fig. 3), between fat cells in atrophic acinar tissue (Fig. 4), or in fibrous connective tissue around ductules. Nests within acini tended to retain the contour of acini and blended into surrounding pancreas. On rare occasions mitotic figures were present in the hepatocyte-like cell nests. At the level of ultrastructure these cells have all the characteristics of fully differentiated liver parenchymal cells (Fig. 5), including the three specialized cell surface membranes, namely that exposed to the perisinusoidal space, that forming the bile canaliculus, and that in contact with adjacent hepatocytes. In the nucleus, the chromatin masses are smaller, less dense, and well defined than that of adjacent smaller acinar cell nuclei. The cytoplasm contains irregular patches of parallel arrays of rough-surfaced endoplasmic reticulum cisternae, as well as those of the smooth endoplasmic reticulum consisting of anastomosing tubular structure and

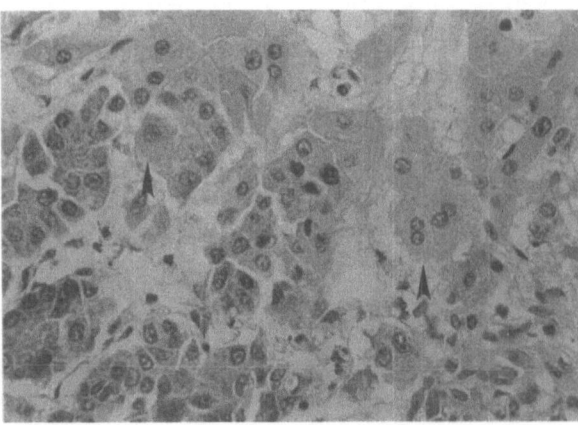

Figure 1. Human pancreas with a focus of eosinophilic cells resembling hepatocytes (arrows). (×480)

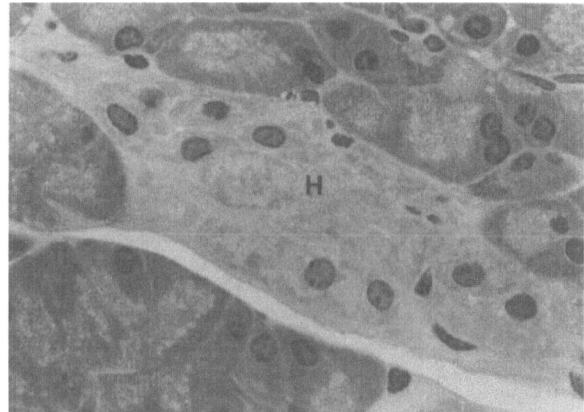

*Figure 2.* Hepatocytes (H) induced in regenerating hamster pancreas with a single injection of BOP. Note the larger nuclei and basophilic stippling of the cytoplasm of liver cells in contrast to the cytologic features of adjacent acinar cells. (×440)

vesicles. Associated with the latter, both α- and β-configurations of glycogen are almost always present, and in some cells, glycogen storage is extensive. Ovoid to short rod-shaped mitochondria with a low-density matrix and sparse cristae, as well as peroxisomes comprise the majority of free organelles. Lysosomes are sparse and largely localized in the peribiliary cytoplasm. Specializations of the plasma membrane which form the bile canaliculus with its adjacent occluding junction, the gap junctions at points of cell–cell contact, and the numerous microvilli of the cell surface facing the sinusoid are indistinguishable from those of normal hepatocytes. Kupffer cells are conspicuously absent in aggregates of pancreatic hepatocytes.

In sharp contrast to adjacent acinar cells, histochemical stains of pancreatic hepatocytes showed significant amounts of glycogen and numerous peroxisomes. These cells stained intensely for albumin (Fig. 6) and α-fetoprotein, and were negative for the acinar cell enzymes α-amylase and carboxypeptidase A. To determine further whether these cells were indeed hepatocytes, their responses to the peroxisome proliferator drug methyl clofenapate and to phenobarbital were studied. Pancreatic hepatocyte-like cells in hamsters fed a diet containing 0.2 percent methyl clofenapate for 3 weeks became hypertrophied and showed a proliferation of peroxisomes, reflected in turn by an approximately 8-fold increase in the relative cytoplasmic volume of peroxisomes and an enhanced activity of peroxisomal enzymes in pancreatic tissue that was as follows: 8.5- to 13-fold of enoyl-CoA hydratase, 1.6- to 3.4-fold of catalase, more than 2000-fold of carnitine acetyltransferase, and a 2.8- to 3.0-fold in palmitoyl CoA oxidation as compared with that in the pancreas of untreated animals. Immunochemical staining of tissue sections of pancreas containing hepatocytes with

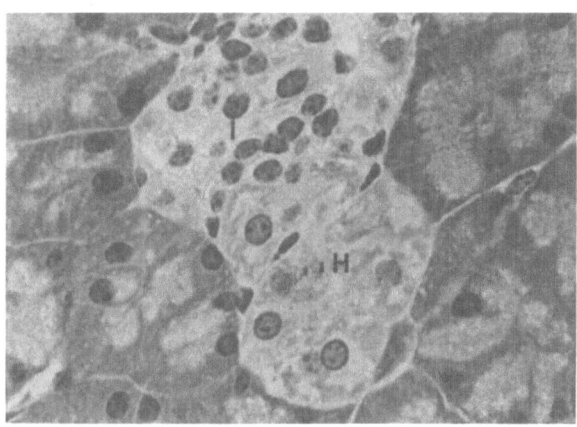

*Figure 3.* Focus of liver cells (H) adjacent to a pancreatic islet (I). (×440)

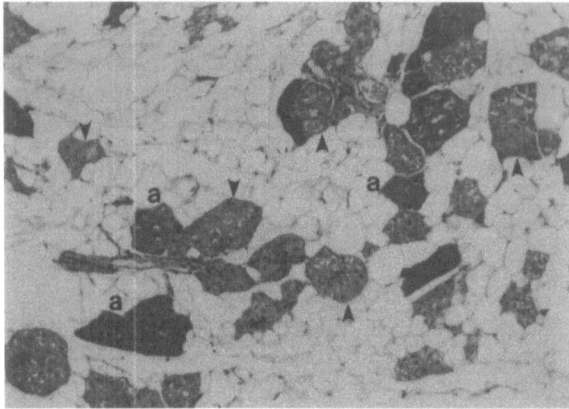

*Figure 4.* Nests of liver cells (arrows) in fat tissue in atrophic pancreas; acinar cell nests (a) are intensely basophilic. (×75)

polyclonal antibody to purified enoyl-CoA hydratase was most intense in pancreatic hepatocytes in treated animals. Pancreatic hepatocytes like their normal counterparts respond to the ingestion of 0.1% phenobarbital for 7 days by developing an increased level of arylhydrocarbon hydroxylase (AHH) such that whole pancreas containing such cells has a 31-fold higher level of AHH activity than normal pancreas in control hamsters. Surgical removal of the median and left lateral lobes of the liver of hamsters bearing pancreatic hepatocytes triggers them to enter S phase 24 hr later, followed by mitoses at 30 hr, a pattern identical to that which is seen in the partially hepatectomized liver. Pancreatic hepatocytes also accumulate iron during iron overload induced by daily subcutaneous injection of iron dextran for 8 days, a pathologic reaction also seen in normal liver cells during iron excess. In the rat,[30,31] the identity of pancreatic hepatocytes as true liver cells has also been expanded to include their expression of the hepatocyte-specific mitochondrial enzyme carbamoyl phosphate synthetase (Fig. 7). The foregoing functional characteristics of pancreatic hepatocytes summarized in Table II, although not by any means exhaustive, nonetheless indicate that in many ways pancreatic hepatocytes are identical to normal liver parenchymal cells. However, in striking contrast to the hamster, rat pancreatic hepatocytes at some stage of their development contain secretion granules resembling those found in the β-cells of islets, and zymogen granules identical to those present in normal pancreatic acinar cells. These unique morphologic features of hepatocytes induced in rat pancreas are considered in some detail in the subsequent section as part of the discussion of their cytogenesis. Moreover, it should be noted that pancreatic hepatocytes, once induced in either the rat or hamster, appear to persist even in those instances in which the protracted

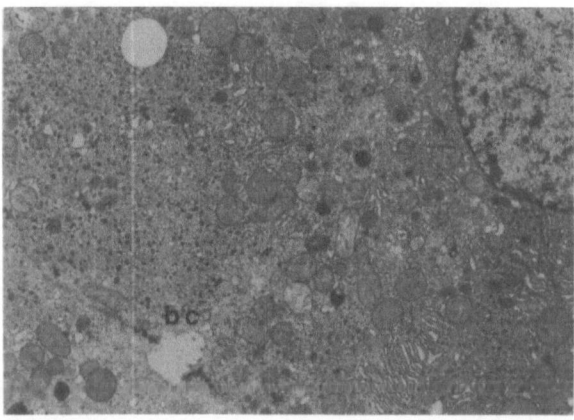

*Figure 5.* Ultrastructure of a pancreatic hepatocyte showing mitochondria, ER, microbodies, and bile canaliculus (bc) characteristic of liver cells. (×8000)

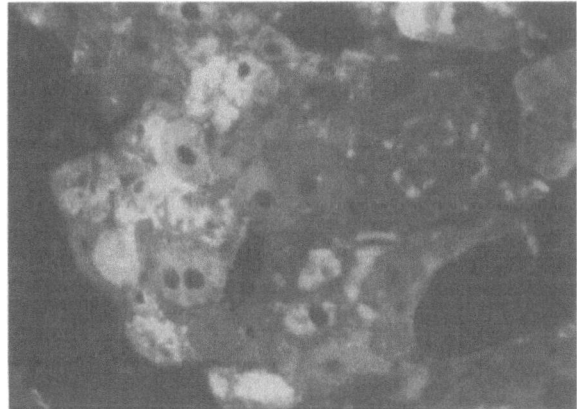

*Figure 6.* Immunochemical staining of albumin in pancreatic hepatocytes. Note the unstained centrally placed nuclei. (×350)

dietary manipulations or administration of the chemicals responsible for their appearance are discontinued. In the hamster, in which their permanence was documented,[15] they persisted for as long as 1 year after their formation, indicating that the metaplastic transformation is long-lived and stable.

## 4. CELLS OF ORIGIN

### 4.1. Hamster

In the hamster pancreas, induced hepatocytes are localized at four sites in the following decreasing order of frequency: in acinar cell lobules, adjacent to the islets of Langerhans, in fatty tissue replacing foci of atrophic pancreas, and in ductules and periductular connective tissue. Such a wide distribution of hepatocyte in the pancreas raises some interesting questions about the nature of the precursor cells from which they are derived. This is especially so in the hamster, since, unlike the rat, no one has been able to identify unequivocally any intermediate cells in this species which might be considered as a likely candidate as a cell of origin for hepatocytes. Furthermore, the pancreas in all vertebrate species is an organ which consists only of well differentiated cells, and thus far, a stem cell population or its equivalent has not been identified.[32] Regeneration of the pancreas is accomplished largely if not exclusively, by proliferation of acinar cells, which represent the largest component cell population. In none of the numerous studies of pancreatic regeneration in rodent species has any cell that might be considered a stem cell been observed.[33-35] In an effort to

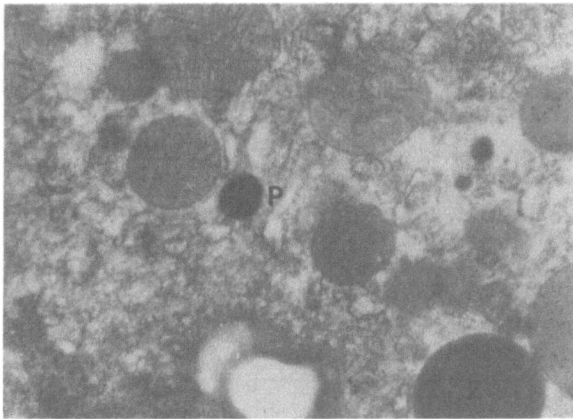

*Figure 7.* Immunogold protein-A staining of carbamoyl phosphate synthetase (fine granules) in mitochondria and a zymogen granule (z) and peroxisome (p) in a pancreatic hepatocyte in rat. (×13,800)

*Table II. Functional Characteristics of Pancreatic Hepatocytes*

Synthesis of export molecules
    Glycogen (expression of glycogen synthetase enzyme)
    Albumin
    α-Fetoprotein
Response to peroxisome proliferator compounds
    Peroxisome proliferation
    Increased activity of enzymes (catalase, carnitine acetyltransferase, β-oxidation system enzymes)
Expression of carbamoyl phosphate synthetase, a liver-specific mitochondrial enzyme
Induction of aryl hydrocarbon hydroxylase enzyme by treatment with phenobarbital
Proliferation following subtotal hepatectomy of host liver
Accumulation of iron during iron overload

test the possibility that acinar cells might be involved, advantage was taken of the anatomic organization of the hamster pancreas into distinct segments. The major duct of gastric segment was ligated with care taken not to compromise its blood supply while leaving the duodenal and splenic segments intact. Within 3 or so weeks, the ligated segment undergoes atrophy characterized by a total disappearance of acinar cells while the major ducts, some ductules, and islets remain and appear intact. When pancreatic regeneration was induced in such animals (D. G. Scarpelli and M. S. Rao, unpublished observations), during which they were experimentally manipulated as described previously, hepatocytes were induced only in the nonligated segments of the pancreas. This, coupled with the simultaneous immunochemical demonstration of α-amylase, carboxypeptidase A, and albumin in cells with the lobular distribution and cytologic characteristics of acinar cells was interpreted as presumptive evidence that acinar cells were probably involved in the metaplastic transformation. However, the foregoing results must be interpreted with some caution since we have not clearly identified cells simultaneously possessing phenotypic markers of both acinar cells and hepatocytes in hamsters as has been done in the rat. More recently in yet unpublished studies (T. Makino and D. G. Scarpelli, unpublished observations), cells with the morphologic characteristics of hepatocytes have been found lining ductules (Fig. 8), and ductlike structures have been identified (Fig. 9) in some nests of pancreatic hepatocytes. In addition, cells morphologically intermediate between hepatocytes and ductular cells at the level of ultrastructure have also been identified. Such cells are most readily apparent within one to several days after the administration of carcinogen at the height of S phase during regeneration. The accumulation of lipid droplets and glycogen, and the appearance of small patches of rough surfaced endoplasmic reticulum appear to be among the earliest functional and morphologic markers presaging the development of fully differentiated hepatocytes, antedating the appearance of plump eosinophilic cells containing a large pale centrally placed nucleus identical to hepatocytes. The identification in the hamster pancreas of hepatocytes in the cells lining ductules is consonant with the observation made more than 85 years ago[36] and amply supported since then by numerous developmental studies, i.e., that ductules are the earliest recognizable structure in the embryonic pancreas and form a developmental continuum with islet and acinar cells. Since ductules appear to be involved in the histogenesis of hepatocytes in the intact hamster pancreas, the failure to induce them in the atrophic segment following duct ligation, wherein acinar cells are absent, while ductules, ducts, and islets remain suggests that perhaps cell–cell interaction between the acinar cell or another cell type and ductular cells is necessary for the metaplastic transformation. While the identity of the pancreatic cell(s) from which hepatocytes develop in the hamster remains to be unequivocally established, sufficient data exist to suggest that either acinar or ductular cells or both may be involved in the transformation. Such would be in keeping with the known multipotent potential of the adult pancreas and other tissues of endodermal derivation.

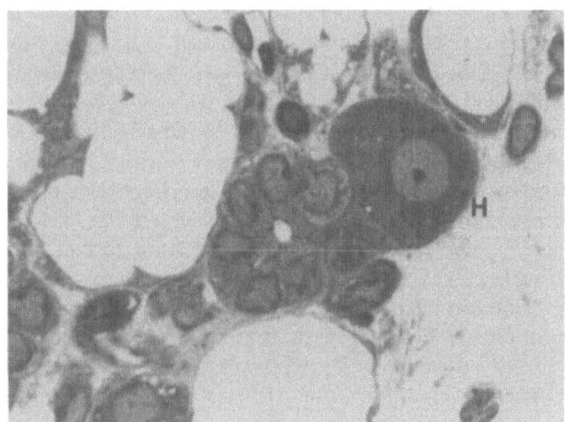

*Figure 8.* Pancreatic hepatocyte (H) appearing to arise from a cell lining a pancreatic ductule in hamster. (×900)

## 4.2. Rat

In the rat,[17,22–24] the histogenesis of pancreatic hepatocytes appears to be less complex, and the nature of the pancreatic cells from which hepatocytes are induced is somewhat clearer than in the hamster, though it is by no means completely understood. The rat is among those species in which cells in the pancreas with structural features of both exocrine and endocrine cell types (referred to as intermediate cells) have been well documented. Morphologic features suggesting the presence of such hybrid cells were first described in human pancreas at the beginning of this century.[37,38] Subsequent studies[39–41] using electron microscopy have confirmed their existence and extended their presence to many other species including lower vertebrates, such as the toad (*Bufo vulgaris formosus*), frog (*Rana esculenta*), and lizard (*Amphisbaena*), as well as some birds, rodents, the guinea pig, cat, goat, and *Saimiri* and *Rhesus* monkeys. The frequency of hybrid acinar-β cells is highest in the lower vertebrates, in which the exocrine and endocrine cells of the pancreas are normally intermingled, and rarer in higher vertebrates, in which these cellular elements are segregated. The hamster is a species in which such pancreatic cells are either extremely rare or do not exist. Repeated attempts by us to identify them by electron microscopy have been unsuccessful. In this regard, it should be noted that early reports of hybrid cells in the hamster pancreas were based solely on the study of hematoxylin–eosin (H & E) stained tissue sections, and their presence in this species has not been corroborated by ultrastructural, histochemical, or immunochemical studies.

A study of the histogenesis of the induction of pancreatic hepatocytes in both the ciprofibrate[22]

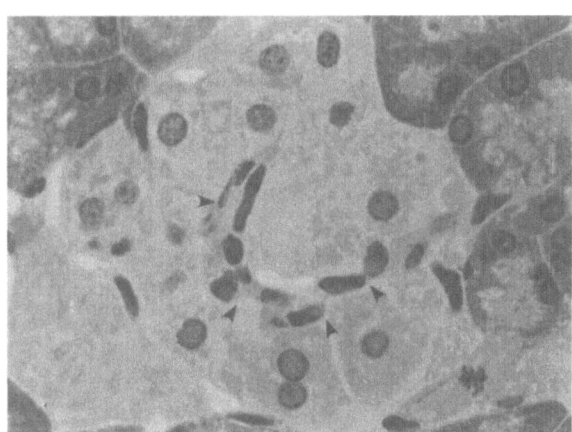

*Figure 9.* Focus of pancreatic hepatocytes showing a ductlike profile in its center (arrows). (×440)

and copper depletion–repletion rat models[23,24,31] clearly identified a hitherto undescribed hybrid pancreatic cell, one with the simultaneous expression of morphologic markers of islet, acinar, and hepatic cells, i.e., β-granules, zymogen granules, and peroxisomes. In these studies, a refinement in the selection of hepatocyte-specific markers, namely the morphologic appearance of peroxisomes containing uricase crystalloids, and the immunochemical localization of the mitochondrial enzyme carbamoyl-phosphate synthetase further corroborated earlier findings that the cells induced in the pancreas were truly hepatocytes. In the ciprofibrate model, pancreatic hepatocytes were usually localized adjacent to islets with extension into the surrounding acinar tissue. In addition to perinsular hepatocytes, in the copper depletion–repletion model, where there is pancreatic atrophy characterized by a marked loss of acinar tissue and fatty infiltration, hepatocytes either singly or in nests are also present in fat tissue. In contrast to the situation in the hamster, ductules have not been implicated in the histogenesis of hepatocytes in the rat.

The fact that pancreatic cells can, under the proper conditions, be induced to transform into apparently well-differentiated and stable hepatocytes was unexpected, since it has long been held that the adult pancreas consists exclusively of well-differentiated component cells and is a slow-growing organ that lacks stem cells.[32] The identity of the cell of origin in the hepatocyte transformation in the pancreas is obscured by the conflicting evidence in hamster as compared to that obtained in the rat. While it is quite possible that a stem cell may be involved in the genesis of hepatocytes, various efforts to identify that such a cell population indeed exists in the pancreas have been unsuccessful thus far. It would have to be a cell other than those identified as the component cells of the pancreas, which is normally quiescent ($G_o$) and which is triggered to enter $G_1$ and replicate when an appropriate stress is applied which necessitates cell replacement. Although it has been suggested that intermediate cells might be derived from stem cells, the current view is that they probably exist as hybrid cells from the beginning. From the foregoing two sections, it is quite evident that although the plasticity of pancreatic cells has been known from some time, its span appears to be somewhat greater than previously appreciated.

## 5. OTHER EXAMPLES OF METAPLASIA IN GUT ENDODERM-DERIVED TISSUES

As the metaplastic conversion of pancreatic cells to liver in rodents flows against the usual direction of embryonic differentiation of gut endoderm, and occurs with relative ease, requiring only regeneration in both the hamster and rat, one could ask whether the reverse program of metaplasia exists, i.e., the transformation of hepatocytes to pancreas. It turns out that there are not only examples of this in the rat, but surprisingly in a lower vertebrate, the rainbow trout, as well (see Section 5.2).

### 5.1. Rat

The conversion of cells in rat liver to fully differentiated acinar cells which were interpreted to be of pancreatic type was reported following exposures to hepatoxic polychlorinated biphenyls which induced extensive cholangiofibrosis.[42] Most recently,[43] these paraffin-embedded tissues were reprocessed for electron microscopy and studied immunochemically at the level of ultrastructure. It was found by both light and electron microscopy that these were indeed morphologically identical to pancreatic acinar cells (Fig. 10) and that the zymogen granules contained the pancreatic specific enzyme markers α-amylase and carboxypeptidase A. No examples of cells with morphologic features of both hepatocytes and acinar cells were found, and the cell in liver from which pancreatic cells are derived remains unknown. In addition to the metaplastic transformation just described, cells in rat liver are also capable of undergoing conversion to other epithelial cell types in the gut, such as those lining the small intestine and bile ductules. Intestinal metaplasia in liver, first described about 9 years ago, in hepatocarcinomas induced by the carcinogen 3-methyl-4-dimethylaminoazobenzene[12] is also a metaplastic transformation that is not well understood. The

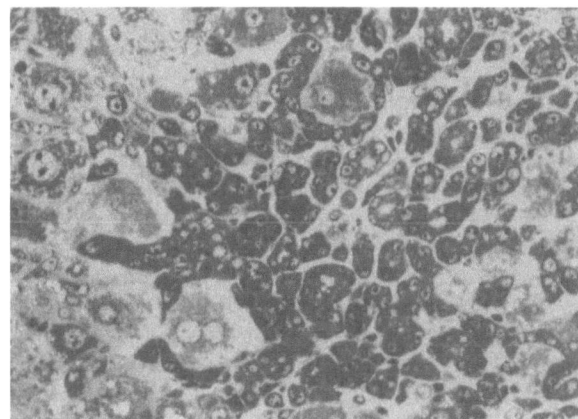

*Figure 10.* Group of intensely basophilic pancreatic acinar cells in rat liver induced by protracted treatment with polychlorinated biphenyls. (×250)

current state of knowledge suggests that such cells may be derived from "oval" cells[44,45] which presumably arise from biliary ductules. Some believe oval cells to be hepatic stem cells based on their formation of transitional cells intermediate between biliary ductular cells and hepatocytes, coupled with their expression of hepatocyte-specific protein markers such as $\alpha$-fetoprotein (AFP), albumin, and fetal liver aldolases.[46,47] A more recent study[48] in which small intestinal epithelial cells were induced in rat liver by feeding the hepatocarcinogen 2-acetylaminofluorene has shown that these cells arise from oval cells during a complex program of differentiation in which they subsequently undergo transformation to biliary ductular cells without clear evidence of the involvement of hepatocytes. This interpretation of events is supported by the retention of [³H]thymidine label by oval cells, their acquisition of leucine aminopeptidase and $\gamma$-glutamyltranspeptidase enzyme activities, and more importantly, the ultrastructural features of intestinal cells during the conversion. Despite these complexities regarding the cell of origin, the preceding example further documents the surprising plasticity of gut endoderm-derived tissues, which persists into adult life.

## 5.2. Rainbow Trout

Pancreatic acinar cells have also been found in the livers of rainbow trout as a consequence of treatment with aflatoxin $B_1$ or of prolonged feeding of cyclopropenoid fatty acids (CPFA), both of which are hepatotoxic and hepatocarcinogens. CPFA are also potent promoters of aflatoxin $B_1$-induced carcinogenesis for trout liver.[49] These fatty acids are components of the residual oil in cottonseed meal and are also mitogenic for liver cells.[50] The kinetics of the transformation and the cellular derivation of acinar cells in this cell system remains to be elucidated.

## 5.3. Human

The susceptibility of tissues derived from gut endoderm in humans to metaplastic transformation has been well documented for some time. The earliest identified and probably the most commonly encountered[51,52] examples involved the transformation of epithelium of the stomach to that normally found in the small intestine, which has special significance because it presages the subsequent development of adenocarcinoma of the gastric mucosa and is considered to be a precancerous lesion.[53] It is not uncommon to find gastric cancer arising in foci of intestinal metaplasia. The metaplastic change converts gastric mucosa from a complex epithelium of surface glands lined by tall columnar cells beneath which lie acid-producing glands consisting of oxyntic cells intermixed with a layer of zymogen glands which produce pepsin, to a simpler epithelium lined by tall columnar and mucin-secreting goblet cells beneath which lies a thin layer of atrophic gastric glands. These morphologic changes are accompanied by functional ones, which include a greatly reduced production of gastric acid and the enzyme pepsin coupled with the appearance of leucine aminopeptidase[54] and disaccharidase enzymes[55] characteristic of small intestinal epithelium. Intestinal metaplasia has also been described, although more rarely, in the gallbladder, where it may be associated with adenocarcinoma.[56] Our present state of knowledge of this lesion is insufficient to determine whether, like that in the stomach, it truly is a preneoplastic lesion. These are only two of a number of examples in human pathology in which the neoplastic transformation appears to be preceded or accompanied by the expression of an inappropriate program of non-neoplastic differentiation.

In some cases of gastric cancer, an even more impressive metaplastic reaction has been described with the identification of cells with morphologic and some functional features resembling those of malignant hepatocytes,[57–59] so-called hepatoid adenocarcinoma. The liver-specific protein markers AFP, $\alpha_1$-antitrypsin, transferrin, and albumin have been localized in these tumor cells,[58] and in one case an extremely elevated serum level (12,000 ng/ml) of AFP was present.[59]

The large pancreatic ducts in patients with gall stones and chronic inflammation of the gallbladder are the frequent focus of a metaplastic transformation of epithelium resembling that normally present in the pylorus of the stomach,[60,61] that portion which is immediately adjacent to the small intestine. Histochemical studies have documented that these cells produce a neutral mucin characteristic of pyloric epithelial cells as contrasted with the sulfated variety present in normal pancreatic duct epithelium.[61] In addition to the foregoing, there are other sites in the gastrointestinal tract that are involved by metaplasia in various disease states. However, these are somewhat less common than those just described.

## 6. POSSIBLE GENETIC AND DEVELOPMENTAL MECHANISMS INVOLVED IN METAPLASIA

The number of different animal species whose gut endoderm-derived tissues are susceptible to metaplastic transformation, the apparent ease and regularity with which some of these can be induced, and the highly differentiated cells formed raises some interesting questions about determination and the range of cell differentiation in metaplasia. At certain times during development, each region of the embryo loses its multipotent capabilities and becomes committed to a specific and more limited program of structural and functional differentiation. In the case of gut endoderm, the program appears to retain multiple options which persist into adult life and under the proper conditions, allows well differentiated cells to undergo transformation to other cells of equally highly differentiated types.[62] From the foregoing, one can conclude determination when it occurs does not necessarily limit a germ layer to a rigidly fixed developmental program and even more unexpected, that highly differentiated cells derived from it retain a spectrum of options that allow them to develop along one of several different and sometimes divergent lines, e.g., pancreatic cells into hepatocytes, intrahepatic bile ductular cells into small intestinal cells, and unidentified cells in liver into pancreatic acinar cells. These transformations may be the first documented examples of conversions of one well-differentiated cell type to another equally well-differentiated one; transformations that most students of metaplasia did not believe could occur among essentially normal non-neoplastic cells.[5] Although these generalizations are certainly worthy of consideration, they do not shed light on the possible mechanisms involved in the stable transformations of one cell type to another. While pancreatic hepatocytes are long-lived and the change appears to be heritable, since their replication gives rise to hepatocytes, triggering this metaplastic transformation by simply inducing pancreatic regeneration suggests that it may not involve a stable genetic mutation. On the other hand, it should be pointed out that in the hamster, regeneration requires protracted treatment with the hepatocarcinogen ethionine, which binds to DNA to the very limited extent of $10^{-10}$ mole per nucleotide residue, but binds nonetheless, and in the rat a significant level of copper deficiency is required prior to the metaplastic transformation induced by pancreatic regeneration. Thus, both of these models involve experimental conditions that might well alter gene structure and function.

## 6.1. Gene Regulation of Determination

Any discussion of the control of embryogenesis that serves to determine the ultimate adult structures of an organism must draw heavily upon studies involving the detailed developmental analysis of the fruit fly *Drosophila melanogaster* and the nematode *Caenorhabditis elegans*. Although, at first glance it might seem highly unlikely that invertebrate systems could serve to contribute to our understanding of the genetic control of mammalian development and its aberrations, an emerging body of knowledge would suggest otherwise. In *Drosophila*, some important clues concerning the regulation of development have come from the study of the evolution of larvae through molting and pupation into adult flies. Major adult body structures, such as eyes, antennae, legs, and wings, develop from multiple distinct cellular aggregates called imaginal discs which are distributed axially at specific sites along the length of the larvae. The embryonic determination of imaginal discs has been clearly established by the finding that a transplanted disc in the larva develops into the same body structure it would have, had it been allowed to remain at its original site. In other words, its developmental fate had already been determined in the embryonic stage.

In certain strains of *Drosophila* that bear a mutation in the genes that control the development of each body segment, and direct each committed imaginal disc to form its appropriate adult structure, extreme and inappropriate displacement of body parts develop such as a wing in the thorax in place of a haltere, legs on the head instead of antennae, legs where the proboscis or feeding tube should be, or wings in place of eyes, a phenomenon referred to as transdetermination. Such mutations are termed as homeotic, meaning that they lead to the transformation of one body part into another that is normally found in a different segment of the fly. The homeotic gene families responsible for directing normal anterior and posterior body development are quite large and complex. These genes have been isolated and subjected to molecular analysis, which has identified common DNA sequences designated as the homeobox[63] consisting of stretches of about 180 base pairs in length coding for proteins containing 60 amino acids.[64] If, as the foregoing suggests, homeotic genes function as master controllers of development by their capacity to turn genes on or off, the proteins they encode for should readily interact with DNA. Although their functions remain to be experimentally established, the proteins of homeotic genes all have domains rich in the basic amino acids lysine and arginine, which suggests that they are indeed capable of such interactions with DNA.

Using cDNA complementary to mRNA of homeotic genes as probes for DNA of other species, the homeobox sequences have been identified in the genomes not only of other insects that produce homeotic mutants, but surprisingly also in all the invertebrate and vertebrate species thus far studied, including humans.[65-68] The vertebrate species sequences and those of *Drosophila* exhibit from 70% to more than 90% sequence conservation. Although homology of DNA sequences must be interpreted carefully, the extent of genetic conservation in evolution represented by the homeobox sequences is quite impressive. It suggests that the homeobox sequences encode for proteins which are of central importance in cell differentiation in organisms at many different levels of organization and complexity. The reader has by now no doubt appreciated the biological parallels that appear to exist between the inappropriate differentiations expressed in homeotic mutants of *Drosophila* and metaplasia or transdifferentiations encountered in the tissues of higher animals such as human beings. Both involve the unexpected and incongruous transformation of one cell type to another, and both appear to be permanent. While both models clearly involve alterations in the program of differentiation in cells that have been presumably previously determined to a different line of development, the situation in *Drosophila* may include genetic control at a higher and more fundamental level of hierarchical control than those operative in metaplasia.

## 6.2. Role of Gene Switching in Cell Specialization

Since all cells in a multicellular organism contain the same DNA, the development of diverse cell types necessitates special strategies to accomplish the development of primitive cells into more specialized ones. The current notion of how this might be accomplished is based on principles learned from studies of gene regulation in *Escherichia coli*,[69] which involves various repressor proteins that interact with DNA to inhibit the transcription of certain genes. For example, the best studied of these is the lactose repressor protein, which binds to the DNA of genes that code for the three proteins involved in the metabolic breakdown of lactose and thus represses their expression. The repressor is regulated in turn by the presence of lactose in the cells, loosening its binding to DNA and permitting gene expression and the subsequent synthesis of the relevant proteins. In this primitive cell system, regulation is afforded by simple on and off switching of genes.

In more complex cells such functions are regulated by a different and somewhat more flexible mechanism in which the negative regulation just described has evolved into one of positive regulation where binding proteins activate genes rather than repress them by binding to DNA at the edge of the RNA polymerase site rather than occupying it as do repressor proteins.[69] Thus, more transcription occurs in the presence of gene regulatory proteins than in their absence. Since these proteins bind to specific sites which can increase or decrease their affinity for DNA, they are capable of turning on or off. The complexity and need for fine tuning of gene function in eukaryotic cells even requires still more flexibility than that afforded by the relatively simple regulatory system just described.

Our abysmal state of ignorance about the molecular mechanisms that switch banks of many genes on or off in an orderly fashion in such cells does not allow for a substantive discussion about how this is accomplished. However, in the absence of firm understanding, once again some clues have been gleaned from studies of gene control in primitive life forms, in this case, the bacterial virus λ bacteriophage.[70] This system of gene regulation involves two regulatory proteins, λ repressor protein and cro protein, which serve to determine whether the virus will integrate into the host cell DNA and be passed on to subsequent generations, or whether it will replicate in the cytoplasm and ultimately kill the cell. In the lysogenic state, large amounts of λ repressor protein is synthesized which in turn shuts off the synthesis of cro protein and allows viral DNA to become integrated into the bacterial cell's DNA; in the lysis state, on the other hand, large amounts of cro protein is synthesized which then turns off the synthesis of lambda repressor protein and permits the rapid replication of viral DNA that eventually leads to killing of the cell. This pattern of regulation consists of two interacting regulatory proteins that bind to the operator site of the genes responsible for each other's synthesis, turning one set of genes on and the other off, or vice versa.

In eukaryotic cells it is hypothesized that a somewhat analogous, although expanded, strategy is employed involving different sets of regulatory proteins that act on multiple genes simultaneously in various combinations to generate many diverse cell types from a precursor cell, so-called combinatorial gene regulation.[71] The hypothetical scheme that is now described encompasses not only the generation of different types of cells from a single precursor cell by different combinations of regulatory proteins, but also takes into account the fact that the relative position (e.g., right and left) that the cells occupy in an embryonic field may affect their differentiation. This model also emphasizes the importance of cell replication in differentiation, i.e., that heritable changes in cell state occur only in association with mitosis.[72] The activation of a master gene or genes in the embryonic progenitor cell results in the induction of a regulatory protein designated protein 1 in the daughter cell in the right hand side of the field, and none in the daughter cell on the left following their division. This is repeated after the second division where proteins 2 or 3 are induced such that the two daughter cells in the right field contain proteins 1 and 2, and 1 and 3, respectively, while in cells on the left only the single protein 2 or 3 is induced. Following the third round of mitoses, proteins 4 or 5 are induced and the distribution of the various triplet combinations of regulatory proteins in the 4 cells on the right would be 1,2,4; 1,2,5; 1,3,4; and 1,3,5, respectively, each giving rise to a different cell type. While on the left where the following doublet combinations exist, 2,4; 2,5; 3,4; and 3,5, cells differing from those on the right would be formed. Several different gene regulatory proteins probably act in concert to turn on a single gene.[73] Thus, a relatively few master regulatory genes could induce the formation of many different cell types.

In addition to the foregoing gene regulatory mechanisms which exist in prokaryotes and could also operate in eukaryotes, there are two additional ones that bear mention that are found only in eukaryotes. The first consists of a loosening or decondensation of chromatin structure along a stretch of a gene that is activated,[74] as demonstrated by susceptibility of its sequences of DNA to degradation by DNase 1. Although the bases for these changes are not entirely clear, they may be related to the decrease binding of histone H1, as well as its acetylation in transcriptionally active DNA. A second mechanism involves the binding of regulatory proteins to specific sites in the loci of decondensed chromatin, which then induces binding and activation of RNA polymerase and synthesis of RNA.

Using the foregoing schemes as a model, it is possible to further hypothesize at least two levels of gene control that might be disturbed in the metaplastic transformation. The first would be at the level of the master gene or genes proximal to the precursor cell, which would be consonant with the view that stem cells are involved. In this scenario, relatively undifferentiated although committed (determined) cells would be programmed to synthesize an inappropriate combination of regulatory proteins, which in turn, would lead to the development of an unexpected cell type. A second equally plausible possibility involves altered gene function in daughter cells more distal from their progenitor, where again inappropriate combinations of regulatory proteins would be induced and transdifferentiation would result. If the latter is the case, according to this scheme, a pancreatic cell may differ from a liver cell because of the difference of perhaps only 1, 2, or 3 gene regulatory proteins, since as one proceeds more distally, minor changes in the combinations of regulatory proteins could result in the formation of a different cell type.

Before concluding this section, which deals with the role of the nucleus in differentiation, mention should be made of the provocative experiments[75] that use muscle/nonmuscle cell heterokaryons to analyze how tissue-specific phenotypes arise and are maintained. Differences in the kinetics, frequency, and gene dosage requirements for gene expression among the different nonmuscle cell/muscle cell heterokaryons suggest the presence of cytoplasmic factors. These results also indicate that gene expression in the nuclei of differentiated cells is highly plastic, involves multiple chromosomes, and appears to be modulated by diffusable transacting molecules in the cytoplasm. Detailed molecular analysis of metaplasia will no doubt add important new insights to our understanding of gene regulation and the control of differentiation.

## 6.3. DNA Methylation and Gene Expression

Since several of the experimental protocols which lead to the induction of pancreatic hepatocytes are also known to impair methylation, it seems reasonable to consider how hypomethylation of DNA is thought to be involved in gene expression. The modification of DNA following synthesis by enzymatic methylation of cytosine residues has been shown to occur in most living systems, including higher organisms. In mammalian DNA, for example, as much as 7% of the total cytosine may be converted to the 5-methyl derivative. Although the precise biologic role of 5-methyl cytosine in DNA is not entirely clear, its apparent conservation throughout evolution, coupled with the fact that it constitutes a significant proportion of the total bases in DNA, suggests that it probably serves an important function.[76] Since it has been shown that active gene sequences in many cell systems are undermethylated, it has been suggested that methylation of CG sequences of DNA may be involved in gene expression.[77] In this regard, it is important to mention that different classes of carcinogens, including ethionine, inhibit DNA methylation in a variety of normal and neoplastic cells presumably due to interference with the activity of DNA transmethylase. In the hamster and rat pancreas, induction of the metaplastic transformation of pancreatic cells to hepatocytes by chemical carcinogens, and in the rat that produced by prolonged maintenance on a methyl-deficient diet suggest that hypomethylation of DNA may be involved. In addition to its role in gene expression, it turns out that because hypomethylation patterns resist further methylation, they are heritable, especially when they have been induced by carcinogens. Although the mechanism(s) responsible for heritability is not clear, it is postulated that carcinogen binding and adduct formation involving guanine residues adjacent and opposite cytosine in DNA may alter its recognition by methyltransferase, inhibit its methylation, and the hypomethylated sequences are replicated during subsequent DNA synthesis.[78] If hypomethylation is indeed involved in the conversion of pancreatic cells to hepatocytes, the foregoing could serve to explain its stability and heritability.

## 7. SUMMARY

The transformation of one differentiated cell type to another, also referred to as metaplasia or transdifferentiation, is a general phenomenon which occurs in numerous living systems ranging from the fruit fly to humans, and involves cells at various levels of development and differentiation. The development of hepatocytes in pancreas is noteworthy because it appears to involve the conversion of one highly specialized cell to another equally developmentally complex one; the change is irreversible and can be readily induced experimentally in adult animals. Furthermore, the transformation in rodents can be induced by a number of manipulations, including pancreatic regeneration, methyl deficiency, and exposure to chemical carcinogens, and some tumor promoters.

While the question of the cell of origin remains open, evidence in the hamster suggests that it involves a differentiated pancreatic cell, a view that is strengthened by the failure thus far by investigators to identify a stem cell in pancreas. This pancreatic conversion is but one of a number of metaplastic transformations that have been documented in adult tissues derived from gut endoderm in rodents, rainbow trout, and humans. The molecular mechanisms by which dormant or repressed genes can be activated include DNA protein interactions, alterations of chromatin structure, methylation of DNA, and perhaps gene rearrangements.

## REFERENCES

1. Willis, R. A., 1960, *Pathology of Tumors,* 3rd ed., Butterworths, Washington, D.C.
2. Stone, L. S., 1950, The role of retinal pigment cells in regenerating neural retinae of adult salamander eyes, *J. Exp. Zool.* **113:**9–31.
3. Stone, L. S., 1950, Neural retina degeneration followed by regeneration from surviving retinal pigment cells in grafted adult salamander eyes, *Anat. Rec.* **106:**89–109.
4. Stone, L. S., Regeneration of the iris and lens from retina pigment cells in adult newt eyes, *J. Exp. Zool.* **129:**505–533.
5. Grobstein, C., 1959, Differentiation of vertebrate cells, in: *The Cell,* Vol. 1 (J. Brachet and A. E. Mirsky, eds.), pp. 437–496, Academic, New York.
6. Okada, T. S., 1980, Cellular metaplasia or transdifferentiation as a model for retinal cell differentiation, *Current Top. Dev. Biol.* **16:**349–390.
7. Eguchi, G., Masuda, A., Karasawa, Y., Kodama, R., and Itoh, Y., 1981, Microenvironments controlling the transdifferentiation of vertebrate pigmented epithelial cells in *in vitro* culture, *Adv. Exp. Med. Biol.* **158:**209–221.
8. Yamada, T., 1982, Transdifferentiation of lens cells and its regulation, in: *Cell Biology of the Eye* (D. S. McDevitt, ed.), pp. 193–242, Academic, New York.
9. McDowell, E., Becci, P., Schürch, W., and Trump, B., 1979, The respiratory epithelium. VII. Epidermoid metaplasia of hamster tracheal epithelium during regeneration following mechanical injury, *J. Natl. Cancer Inst.* **62:**995–1008.
10. Reddi, A. H., and Huggins, C. B., 1975, Formation of bone marrow in fibroblast-transformation ossicles. *Proc. Natl. Acad. Sci. USA* **72:**2212–2216.
11. Taylor, S. M., and Jones, P. A., 1979, Multiple new phenotypes induced in 10T1/2 and 3T3 cells treated with 5-azacytidine, *Cell* **17:**771–779.
12. Yoshida, Y., Kaneko, A., Chisaka, N., and Onoe, T., 1978, Appearance of intestinal type of tumor cells in hepatoma tissue induced by 3′-methyl-4-dimethylaminoazobenzene, *Cancer Res.* **38:**2753–2758.
13. Matsukara, N., Suzuki, K., Kawochi, T., Aoyagi, M., Sugimura, T., Kitaoka, H., Numajiri, H., Shirota, A., Itaboshi, M., and Hirota, T., 1980, Distribution of marker enzyme and mucin in intestinal metaplasia in human stomach and relation of complete and incomplete types of metaplasia to minute gastric carcinomas, *J. Natl. Cancer Inst.* **65:**231–240.
14. Wattenberg, L. W., 1959, Histochemical study of aminopeptidase in metaplasia and carcinoma of the stomach, *Arch. Pathol. Lab. Med.* **67:**281–286.

15. Scarpelli, D. G., and Rao, M. S., 1981, Differentiation of regenerating pancreatic cells into hepatocyte-like cells, *Proc. Natl. Acad. Sci. USA* **78**:2577–2581.

16. Melmed, R. N., Benitez, C. J., and Holt, S. J., 1972, Intermediate cells of the pancreas. I. Ultrastructural characterization, *J. Cell Sci.* **11**:449–475.

17. Lalwani, N. D., Reddy, M. K., Qureshi, S. A., and Reddy, J. K., 1981, Development of hepatocellular carcinomas and increased peroxisomal fatty acid β-oxidation in rats fed [4-chloro-6-(2,3-xylidino)-2-pyrimidinylthio]acetic acid (Wy-14,643) in the semipurified diet, *Carcinogenesis* **7**:645–650.

18. Scarpelli, D. G., and Rao, M. S., 1981, Early changes in regenerating hamster pancreas following a single dose of *N*-nitrosobis(2-oxopropyl)amine (NBOP) administered at the peak of DNA synthesis, *Cancer* **47**:1552–1561.

19. Pour, P., Mohr, U., Althoff, J., Cardesa, A., and Kmoch, N., 1976, Spontaneous tumors and common diseases in two colonies of Syrian hamsters. III. Urogenital system and endocrine glands, *J. Natl. Cancer Inst.* **56**:949–961.

20. Takahashi, M., and Pour, P., 1978, Spontaneous alterations in the pancreas of the aging Syrian hamster, *J. Natl. Cancer Inst.* **60**:355–364.

21. Murgatroyd, L. B., and Tucker, M. J., 1981, Pancreatic islet cell hypertrophy in the Syrian hamster, *J. Comp. Pathol.* **91**:455–459.

22. Reddy, J. K., Rao, M. S., Qureshi, S. A., Reddy, M. K., Scarpelli, D. G., and Lalwani, N. D., 1984, Induction and origin of hepatocytes in rat pancreas, *J. Cell Biol.* **98**:2082–2090.

23. Rao, M. S., Subbarao, V., Scarpelli, D. G., and Reddy, J. K., 1985, Pancreatic hepatocytes in rats, *Toxicologist* **5**:160a.

24. Rao, M. S., Subbarao, V., and Reddy, J. K., 1986, Induction of hepatocytes in the pancreas of copper depleted rats following copper repletion, *Cell Diff.* **18**:109–117.

25. Hoover, K. L., and Poirer, L. L., 1986, Hepatocyte-like cells within the pancreas of rats fed methyl-deficient diets, *J. Nutr.* **116**:1569–1575.

26. Chiu, T., 1987, Focal eosinophilic hypertrophic cells of the rat pancreas, *Toxicol. Pathol.* **15**:1–6.

27. O'Leary, T. J., Costa, J., and Roth, J., 1982, Oncocytic nodules of the pancreas, *Lab. Invest.* **46**:63a.

28. Rao, M. S., Reddy, M. K., Reddy, J. K., and Scarpelli, D. G., 1982, Response of chemically induced hepatocyte-like cells in hamster pancreas to methyl clofenapate, a peroxisome proliferator, *J. Cell Biol.* **95**:50–56.

29. Rao, M. S., Subbarao, V., Luetteke, N., and Scarpelli, D. G., 1983, Further characterization of carcinogen-induced hepatocyte-like cells in hamster pancreas, *Am. J. Pathol.* **110**:89–94.

30. Rao, M. S., Bendayan, M., and Reddy, J. K., 1985, Localization of carbamyl phosphate synthetase (ammonia) (CPS) in pancreatic hepatocytes of rat, *Fed. Proc.* **44**:740a.

31. Rao, M. S., Scarpelli, D. G., and Reddy, J. K., 1986, Transdifferentiated hepatocytes in rat pancreas, *Current Top. Dev. Biol.* **20**:63–77.

32. Leblond, C. P., 1964, Classification of cell populations on the basis of their proliferative behavior, *Natl. Cancer Inst. Monog.* **14**:119–150.

33. Fitzgerald, P. J., 1960, The problem of the precursor cell of regenerating pancreatic acinar epithelium, *Lab. Invest.* **9**:67–84.

34. Fitzgerald, P. J., Herman, L., Carol, B., Roque, A., Marsh, W. H., Rosenstock, L., Richardson, C., and Perl, D., 1968, *Am. J. Pathol.* **52**:983–1011.

35. Scarpelli, D. G., Rao, M. S., Subbarao, V., and Beversluis, M., 1981, Regeneration of Syrian golden hamster pancreas and covalent binding of *N*-nitroso-2,6-[³H]dimethylmorpholine, *Cancer Res.* **41**:1051–1057.

36. Laguesse, E., 1895, Recherches sur l'histogénie due pancreas chez le mouton, *J. Anat. Physiol. (Paris)* **31**:475–504.

37. Mankowski, A., 1902, Ueber die mikroskopischen Veränderungen des Pankreas nach Unterbindung einzelner Theile und über einige mickrochemische Besonderheiten der Langerhan 'schen inseln, *Arch. Mikrosk, Anat. Entwicklungsmech.* **59**:286–294.

38. Laguesse, M. E., 1905, Ilots endocrines et formes de transition dans le lobule pancréatique (homme), *C. R. Soc. Biol. (Paris)* **58**:542–544.

39. Herman, L., Sato, T., and Fitzgerald, P. J., 1963, Electron microscopy of acinar-islet cells in the rat pancreas, *Fed. Proc.* **22**:603.

40. Melmed, R. N., Benitz, C. J., and Holt, S. J., 1972, Intermediate cells of the pancreas. I. Ultrastructural characterization, *J. Cell Sci.* **11**:449–475.

41. Melmed, R. N., 1979, Intermediate cells of the pancreas. An appraisal, *Gastroenterology* **76**:196–201.

42. Kimbrough, R., 1973, Brief communication: Pancreatic-type tissue in livers of rats fed polychlorinated biphenyls, *J. Natl. Cancer Inst.* **51**:679–681.

43. Rao, M. S., Bendayan, R. D., Kimbrough, R. D., and Reddy, J. K., 1986, Characterization of pancreatic-type tissue in the liver of rat induced by polychlorinated biphenyls, *J. Histochem. Cytochem.* **34:**197–201.

44. Sasaki, T., and Yoshida, T., 1935, Experimentelle Erzeugung des Lebercarcima durch Futterung mit *O*-Amidoazotoluol, *Virchows Arch. (Pathol. Anat. Physiol. Klin. Med.)* **295:**175–200.

45. Edwards, J. E., and White, J., 1941, Pathologic changes with special reference to pigmentation and classification of hepatic tumors in rats fed *p*-dimethylaminoazobenzene (butter yellow), *J. Natl. Cancer Inst.* **2:**157–183.

46. Yaswen, P., Hayner, N. T., and Fausto, N., 1984, Isolation of oval cells by centrifugal elutriation and comparison with other cell types purified from normal and neoplastic livers, *Cancer Res.* **44:**324–331.

47. Hayner, N. T., Braun, L., Yaswen, P., Brooks, M., and Fausto, N., 1984, Isozyme profiles of oval cells, parenchymal cells and biliary cells isolated by centrifugal elutriation from normal and preneoplastic livers, *Cancer Res.* **44:**332–338.

48. Tatematsu, M., Kaku, T., Medline, A., and Farber, E., 1985, Intestinal metaplasia as a common option of oval cells in relation to cholangiofibrosis in liver of rats exposed to 2-acetylaminofluorene, *Lab. Invest.* **52:**354–362.

49. Hendricks, T. R., Meyers, T. R., and Shelton, D. W., 1984, Histologic progression of hepatic neoplasia in rainbow trout (*Salmo gairdneri*), in: *Use of Small Fish Species in Carcinogenicity Testing*, Journal of the National Cancer Institute Monographs, Vol. 65 (K. L. Hoover, ed.), pp. 321–336, National Cancer Institute, Bethesda.

50. Scarpelli, D. G., 1974, Mitogenic activity of sterculic acid, a cyclopropenoid fatty acid, *Science* **185:**958–960.

51. Magnus, H. A., 1937, Observations on the presence of intestinal epithelium in the gastric mucosa, *J. Pathol.* **44:**389–398.

52. Warren, S., and Meissner, W. A., 1944, Chronic gastritis and carcinoma of the stomach, *Gastroenterology* **3:**251–256.

53. Morson, B. C., 1956, Intestinal metaplasia of the gastric mucosa, *Gastroenterologia (Basel)* **86:**353–355.

54. Wattenberg, L. W., 1959, Histochemical study of aminopeptidase in metaplasia and carcinoma of the stomach, *AMA Arch. Pathol.* **67:**281–286.

55. Matsukura, N., Suzuki, K., Kawachi, T., Aoyagi, M., Sugimura, T., Kitaoka, H., Numajiri, H., Shirota, A., Itaboshi, M., and Hirota, T., 1980, Distribution of marker enzymes and mucin in intestinal metaplasia in human stomach and relation of complete and incomplete types of intestinal metaplasia to minute gastric carcinomas, *J. Natl. Cancer Inst.* **65:**231–240.

56. Albores-Saavedra, J., Nadji, M., and Henson, D. E., 1986, Intestinal-type adenocarcinoma of the gallbladder. A clinicopathologic and immunocytochemical study of seven cases, *Am. J. Surg. Pathol.* **10:**19–25.

57. Okita, K., Noda, K., and Kodama, T., 1977, Carcino-fetal proteins and gastric cancer: the site of alpha-fetoprotein synthesis in gastric cancer, *Gastroenterol. Jpn.* **12:**400–406.

58. Kodama, T., Kameya, T., and Hirota, T., 1981, Production of alpha-fetoprotein, normal serum proteins, and human chorionic gonadotropin in stomach cancer: Histologic and immunohistochemical analyses of 35 cases, *Cancer* **48:**1647–1655.

59. Ishikura, H., Fukasawa, Y., Ogasawara, K., Natori, T., Tsukada, Y., and Aizawa, M., 1985, An AFP-producing gastric carcinoma with features of hepatic carcinoma, *Cancer* **56:**840–848.

60. Walters, M. N-I., 1965, Goblet-cell metaplasia in ductules and acini of the exocrine pancreas, *J. Pathol.* **89:**569–572.

61. Roberts, P. F., 1974, Pyloric gland metaplasia of the human pancreas. A comparative histochemical study, *Arch. Pathol. Lab. Med.* **97:**92–95.

62. Scarpelli, D. G., 1985, Multipotent developmental capacity of cells in the adult animal, *Lab. Invest.* **52:**331–333.

63. McGinnis, W., Levine, M. S., Hafen, E., Kuroiwa, A., and Gehring, W. J., 1984, A conserved DNA sequence in homeotic genes of the *Drosophila antennapedia* and bithorax complexes, *Nature (Lond.)* **308:**428–433.

64. Fjose, A., McGinnis, W. J., and Gehring, W. J., 1985, Isolation of a homeobox-containing gene from the engrailed region of Drosophila and the spatial distribution of its transcripts, *Nature (Lond.)* **313:**284–289.

65. Shepard, J. C. W., McGinnis, W., Carrasco, A. J., De Robertis, E. M., and Gehring, W. J., 1984, Fly and frog homeo domains show homologies with yeast mating type regulatory proteins, *Nature (Lond.)* **310:**70–71.

66. McGinnis, W., Garber, R. L., Wirz, J., Kuroiwa, A., and Gehring, W. J., 1984, A homologous protein-coding sequence in drosophila homeotic genes and its conservation in other metazoans, *Cell* **37:**403–408.

67. Manley, J. L., and Levine, M. S., 1985, The homeo box and mammalian development, *Cell* **43:**1–2.

68. Gehring, W. J., 1987, Homeoboxes in the study of development, *Science* **236**:1245–1252.
69. Miller, J. H., and Reznikoff, W. S. (eds.), 1978, *The Operon*, Cold Spring Harbor Laboratory, Cold Spring Harbor, New York.
70. Ptashne, M., 1980, How the lambda repressor and cro work, *Cell* **19**:1–11.
71. Gierer, A., 1974, Molecular models and combinatorial principles in cell differentiation and morphogenesis, *Cold Spring Harbor Symp. Quant. Biol.* **38**:951–961.
72. Holtzer, H., Weintraub, H., Mayne, R., and Mochen, R., 1972, The cell cycle, cell lineages, and cell differentiation, *Curr. Top. Dev. Biol.* **7**:229–256.
73. Ogden, S., Haggerty, D., Stoner, C. M., Kolodrubetz, D., and Schleif, R., 1980, The *E. coli* L-arabinose operon binding sites of the regulatory proteins and a mechanism of positive and negative regulation, *Proc. Natl. Acad. Sci. USA* **77**:3346–3550.
74. Weintraub, H., and Groudine, M., 1976, Chromosomal subunits in active genes have an altered conformation, *Science* **193**:848–856.
75. Blau, H. M., Plavath, G. K., Hardeman, E. C., Chiu, C-P., Silberstein, L., Webster, S. G., Miller, S. C., and Webster, C., 1985, Plasticity of the differentiated state, *Science* **230**:758–766.
76. Razin, A., and Riggs, A. D., 1980, DNA methylation and gene function, *Science* **210**:604–610.
77. Navath-Many, T., and Cedar, H., 1981, Active gene sequences are undermethylated, *Proc. Natl. Acad. Sci. USA* **78**:4246–4250.
78. Riggs, A. D., and Jones, P. A., 1983, 5-Methylcytosine, gene regulation, and cancer, *Adv. Cancer Res.* **40**:1–29.

# 25

# *Crown Gall Neoplasms*

## *Joseph V. Formica*

## 1. INTRODUCTION

Crown gall, a neoplastic disease of worldwide distribution, affects woody and herbaceous plants. Although this neoplasm occurs primarily in dicotyledons, it has also been found in gymnosperms and monocotyledons.[1] Crown gall is characterized by the formation of tumors or galls of varying size and form which may occur on stems, roots, and leaves of plants. Plants with the disease become stunted, produce small chlorotic leaves and exhibit increased susceptibility to adverse environmental conditions, especially winter injury and suprainfection.[2]

Historically, Smith and Townsend[3] are credited with publishing the first account of crown gall disease in which the proximate cause was characterized experimentally. The pioneer investigations of Armin Braun established *Agrobacterium tumefaciens* as the causative agent. In addition, he demonstrated that crown gall tissue was permanently transformed after exposure to the bacterial pathogen.[4] Furthermore, he demonstrated that this tissue could be grown axenically (in the absence of bacteria) in a phytohormone-free medium.[5] These early investigations implicated a tumor-inducing principle (TIP) transmitted by the bacteria which resulted in the transformed state. Later, as a result of the significant work of Zaenen *et al.*,[6] Chilton *et al.*,[7] and van Larebeke *et al.*,[8,9] the transforming principle was demonstrated to be plasmid DNA. These latter investigators established that tumorigenic strains contain large tumor-inducing (Ti) plasmids, sequences from which are transferred (referred to as T-DNA) to the host plant cell.[10]

As currently envisioned, the organism multiplies in an extracellular environment, and after a critical mass has been achieved, bacterial DNA sequences are transferred to the host cells. The microorganism itself does not persist intracellularly. The transferred DNA then becomes integrated into the plant chromosomal DNA and subsequently replicates with host DNA. Expression of this integrated DNA results in alterations in phytohormone (auxins and cytokinins) levels, resulting in unregulated growth and the subsequent formation of crown gall tumors, teratomas, and abnormal proliferation of roots.[11] In addition, the integrated DNA directs the synthesis of unusual amino acid compounds, termed opines (e.g., octopine, nopaline, agropine), which are used by the inciting bacteria as a source of carbon and nitrogen.[12] In this manner, the microorganism creates a unique ecological niche in which the inoculum is perpetuated.[13]

Crown gall is unique because it is the only known instance in which the etiologic agent associated with neoplastic transformation involves a bacterial vector. Also, because transformation involves intrakingdom conjugative transfer resulting in the natural insertion and covalent linkage of procaryotic with eucaryotic DNA. Furthermore, crown gall represents an interesting model for investigating the reversal of the tumorous state.

*Joseph V. Formica* • Department of Microbiology and Immunology, School of Basic Health Sciences, Virginia Commonwealth University, Richmond, Virginia 23298.

## 2. PATHOLOGY

### 2.1. Symptoms

Crown gall tumors first appear as small overgrowths on stems or roots located near the soil line. Early tumors are spherical, white to flesh colored, and soft. At first, the tumor resembles a callus or plant scar tissue. As the tumor enlarges, however, it becomes less convoluted and its color changes to a dark brown or black. This change in color has been shown to be the result of necrosis of peripheral cells.[2]

The tumor on the surface of host plant is connected to the host by a narrow neck of tissue. A particular tumor may decay but new tumors can also appear in other parts of the host plant during the same growing season or during a subsequent growing season.[2] When these secondary tumors develop at points distant from the primary tumor, they are found to be free of bacteria.[14]

### 2.2. Pathogen

The genus *Agrobacterium* is a member of the family *Rhizobiaceae*. Four species are recognized within this genus: *A. rhizogenes*, the causative agent of the disease hairy root; *A. rubi*, the causative agent of aerial galls or spherical growths on black and purple cane raspberries; *A. tumefaciens*, the causative agent of crown gall disease; and *A. radiobacter*, the only nonpathogenic member of this genus.[15]

The agrobacteria are gram-negative rods measuring 0.6–1.0 $\mu$m in length. They are motile by means of polar or peritrichous flagellation. The agrobacteria grow optimally at 29–30°C, can use L-ornithine and L-asparagine, are able to reduce nitrite, and can produce $H_2S$ from cysteine. In addition, this genus is catalase positive and has been shown to be sensitive to the tetracyclines, gentamycin, neomycin, and novobiocin.[16]

Three biotypes are differentiated within the species *A. tumefaciens* by their ability to reduce lactose to its keto-derivative.[17] Biotype 1 is ketolactose positive and forms beige-colored mucous colonies; biotype 2 is ketolactose negative and forms white mucous colonies; and biotype 3, which is also ketolactose negative, forms pearly-white translucent moist colonies.[16] It is distinguished from biotype 2 by its inability to utilize erythritol, or grow on New and Kerr[18] selective media. Biotypes 1 and 2 generally affect fruit trees and are considered to have a broad host range, while biotype 3 appears to be restricted to grapevines, hence exhibiting a very limited host range.[19]

All pathogenic strains of agrobacteria isolated from nature possess Ti-plasmids.[7,8] Classification of these plasmids is based on their ability to code for the metabolism of specific opines such as octopine, nopaline, and agropine.[20] Furthermore, the Ti-plasmids are transferable not only among *Agrobacterium* strains, but also to some *Rhizobium* strains[21]; consequently, physiologic properties coded by them are not as reliable for taxonomy of the bacteria as the more stable chromosomally determined characteristics described above.[16]

### 2.3. Development of Disease

*Agrobacterium tumefaciens* enters roots or stems near the soil line through recent wounds. Wounds result from agricultural practices, grafting, winter damage, or insects. Once the bacterium invades, it multiplies in the extracellular space. Following transformation, whorls of proliferating neoplastic cells appear in the cortex or in the cambial layer of the plant, depending on the depth of the wound. These neoplastic plant cells, which may be multinucleated, divide rapidly and exhibit the features of anaplasia. In general, a tumor or gall becomes grossly visible by 10–14 days after inoculation of the wound.[2]

As the tumor continues its growth, its center may be free of bacteria. However, *A. tumefaciens* can be found in its periphery. Although tracheids or vessels develop to some extent within the tumor, there is little orientation or connection between these and the vascular system of the host plant. Growth of the tumor eventually exerts pressure on normal tissue and can crush xylem vessels, thus compromising flow of water to the upper parts of the plant.[2]

The early tumor is not covered with a protective epidermis. Consequently, the lack of hardened surface tissue makes this area susceptible to secondary invaders such as insects and saprophytic or pathogenic microorganisms. This results in decay and discoloration of the tumor, causing the peripheral surface to turn brown or black. Subsequently, the tumor breaks down, releasing *A. tumefaciens* to the soil where, if given the opportunity, it may invade another host. If the tumor does not succumb to secondary effects, it will mature.[2]

The mature tumor can become woody and hard, consisting of lignified vascular bundles and woody fibers mingled with parenchymal tissue. Compression of the surrounding normal plant tissue by the expanding tumor results in a decrease in its supply of water and nutrients. The vascular bundles in the tumor are ineffective because they are incomplete and disarranged. Thus, as the tumor becomes starved of nutrients, further growth is stopped and it begins to decay with a sloughing of necrotic tissue. Regression may occur, but more often than not, the tumor will remain viable and form additional tumors in the same or subsequent seasons. Secondary tumors usually arise above the primary tumor on unwounded parts of the stem. The starting point of the secondary tumor appears to be associated with the xylem or the vascular bundles of the primary tumor and the two are connected by tumor strands made up of dividing cells. Secondary tumors are free of bacteria. If they are grafted onto healthy plants, they enlarge and develop like the primary tumor from which they were derived.[2]

## 2.4. Genetic Organization

All tumorigenic strains of *A. tumefaciens* contain a Ti-plasmid, which can vary in size from 200 to 400 kilobases.[6,22,23] In addition, these plasmids vary in DNA homology. For instance, there is only a 74% homology between plasmid DNAs obtained from various octopine strains of *A. tumefaciens* and from 28 to 95% homology between plasmid DNAs of various nopaline strains.[24] Also, there is only a 6–36% homology between the plasmid DNA derived from octopine strains and the plasmid DNA derived from nopaline strains of *A. tumefaciens*.[25] However, T-DNA, the common sequence in the Ti-plasmids that becomes incorporated into plant cell DNA, is highly conserved and is essential for oncogenicity.[7,25] This common sequence is homologous in all Ti-plasmids investigated from wide host range strains of *A. tumefaciens*. By contrast, the limited host range agrobacteria contain Ti-plasmids that have little homology to this common sequence. On the other hand, the virulence region or the region related to host range of susceptable plants, demonstrated homology between octopine and nopaline plasmids.[25]

Octopine and nopaline Ti-plasmids were found to be incompatible since they were unable to coexist in the same bacterial cell. They, along with the limited host range Ti-plasmids, belong to the incompatibility group *inc* Rh-1. The agropine Ti-plasmid belongs to incompatability group *inc* Rh-2, and Ri-plasmids belong to *inc* RH-3. Plasmids from different incompatibility groups, however, may be stably maintained within one cell.[26]

The following plasmid-borne traits have been identified on Ti-plasmids of agrobacteria: oncogenicity, tumor morphology, opine synthesis, opine utilization, conjugative plasmid transfer, agrocin sensitivity, binding to plant cells, host range, exclusion of the bacteriophage AP-1, incompatibility, T-DNA region, and phytohormone synthesis[20] (Fig. 1).

There are two regions on the Ti-plasmid essential for tumor induction: the T-DNA region that is transferred and incorporated into host plant DNA,[7,10] and the virulence (*vir*) region, which is outside the T-region and is expressed inside the bacterium.[27,28] The virulence region, although essential for tumorigenesis, is not integrated or maintained in the transformed plant cells.

The T-region from octopine strains consists of a left ($T_L$) and right ($T_R$) segment separated by a 16- to 19-kilobase pair segment of DNA.[29] $T_L$ is responsible for tumor maintenance (phytohormone synthesis) and for octopine synthesis,[30] whereas $T_R$ is responsible for the synthesis of secondary opines (i.e., agropine).[28,29,31] By contrast, in nopaline strains, the T-DNA is one continuous piece, coding for both tumor maintenance and opine synthesis.[32,33]

The T-DNA is flanked by 25 base pair imperfect direct repeat sequences (border sequences) that are apparently involved in the excision and transfer of the T-DNA to the host plant cell.[34–42]

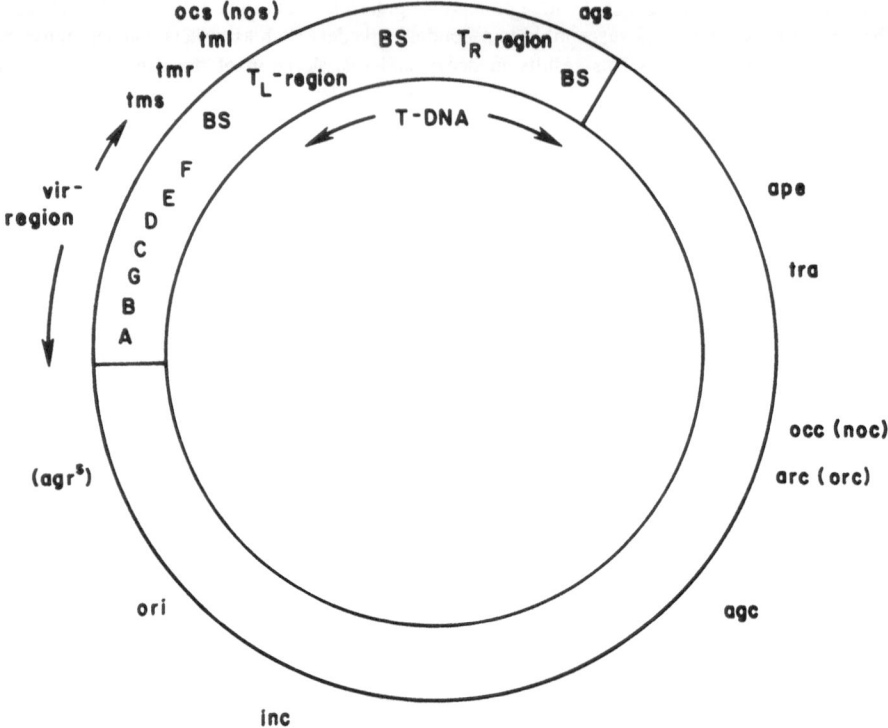

*Figure 1.* Composite Ti-plasmid showing the location of genetic determinants: tms, tumor morphology (shoot); tmr, tumor morphology (root); tml, tumor morphology (large); ocs, octopine synthesis (or, nos, nopaline synthesis); ags, agropine synthesis; ape, phage AP-1 exclusion; tra, conjugative transfer; occ, octopine catabolism (or, noc, nopaline catabolism); arc, arginine catabolism (or, orc, ornithine catabolism); agc, agropine catabolism; inc, incompatibility; ori, origin of replication; (agr$^s$), Agrocin 84 sensitivity. Other physical regions include BS, border sequences; T-DNA, transfer DNA; $T_L$, left region; $T_R$, right region; vir, virulence region.

## 3. THE INFECTIOUS PROCESS

The model proposed for the initiation of infection involves specific receptors both on the bacterial surface and on the plant surface. After the bacteria are bound, the pathogen produces cellulose fibrils that anchor the bacteria in place and simultaneously entrap daughter and/or additional bacterial cells, forming an aggregate or bacterial colony enmeshed in cellulose fibers at the wound site. This bacterial colony may secrete substances such as pectinase or cellulase, leading to the digestion of plant cell wall material, and hence, provides a possible mechanism whereby contact can occur between the bacterial and plant cell membranes. This intimate contact facilitates transfer of the Ti-plasmid by an as yet unknown mechanism.

### 3.1. Recognition and Attachment

Initial investigations by Braun[4] demonstrated a temporal relationship between inoculation and tumor formation. In this respect, the infected plant cells were observed to become increasingly autonomous by 32 hr after inoculation; by 48 hr they were in a full autonomous state. Maintaining the plant at 34°C within the first 32 hr, however, prevented tumor formation.

This protocol was refined using cellulose negative stains.[43] It was easier to control contact time with these strains because, lacking cellulose fibrils for anchorage, they could be easily washed off the plant. When washed off within 2 hr, no tumors were formed. However, if left on for 8 hr, tumors formed at the wound site. The time factor requirement may be needed to permit multiple transfers of DNA to occur into the same host plant cell or perhaps for the integration of T-DNA into a site where it could be maximally expressed or amplified.

Recognition and attachment as necessary requirements for pathogenicity have been demonstrated by showing that tumor formation can be prevented by co-infection or prior infection with nonpathogenic agrobacteria.[44] Furthermore, prior application of cell wall material from pathogenic agrobacteria[45] or with cell wall material prepared from dicotyledons also prevented tumor formation.[46] In addition, a study with insertional mutants revealed that if the A. tumefaciens lost its ability to bind, it also lost pathogenicity. Revertants of this group simultaneously gained binding capacity and tumorigenicity.[47,48] The mechanisms involved in recognition, attachment, and binding, however, are still unclear.

The chemical nature of the binding sites on the plant cells was investigated by applying various compounds to the system or by employing various enzymatic treatments.[49] Factors found to diminish binding of A. tumefaciens was protease treatment of plant material, the addition of poly-L-lysine to the medium, or the addition of pectin to the host plant cells. However, pectin treated with pectin methyltransferase reduced its inhibitory effect, but inhibition could be restored with pectin esterase treatment. Furthermore, protease-treated plant cells regained binding ability after incubation in complete media. Binding ability was not regained in the presence of cycloheximide. These observations suggested that the attachment site is a protein–pectin complex in which the pectin is not fully methylated.[50,51]

The role of the bacterium in attachment is a more active one. For instance, only living bacteria can bind and attach either to live or dead plant cells. In addition, A. tumefaciens binds even in the presence of tetracycline or chloramphenicol,[48] indicating that the binding site is constitutively produced rather than induced. The formation of cellulose fibrils (attachment), however, would be affected by these antibiotics.[50]

A lipopolysaccharide (LPS) fraction prepared from virulent agrobacteria prevented tumor formation if placed in the wound prior to the application of the pathogenic bacterium.[45] Similar types of experiments using LPS from nonpathogenic strains did not prevent tumor formation, suggesting that the bacterial binding site is associated only with the LPS fraction of pathogenic strains. Furthermore, it was demonstrated that the polysaccharide portion of LPS, and not the lipid A component, was responsible for interference with tumorigenesis.[51]

The Ti-plasmid was also implicated in directing the synthesis of binding sites in the LPS. Although prior or co-infection with non-pathogenic (Ti-plasmidless) agrobacteria can prevent tumor formation, they bind poorly or not at all to plant cells.[44,52] However, if a Ti-plasmid is transferred to a nonpathogenic strain by conjugation, not only can the recipient bind to plant cells, but it becomes pathogenic and causes tumor formation. The converted bacteria can now produce an LPS that inhibits tumor formation when applied to wounds prior to the application of pathogenic agrobacteria.

Douglas et al.[47,53] demonstrated, using Tn5 insertional mutations, that attachment involved the activation of bacterial chromosomal chv genes. Subsequently, Stachel et al.[54] identified acetosyringone and α-hydroxyacetosyringone as the molecules that trigger recognition and attachment. Wounding of the plant apparently was necessary for the production of these phenolic compounds, which were found in the exudate. These signal molecules were further shown to activate chvA and chvB, which have been implicated in the production of (1-2)-β-glucan[55] as well as in the induction of the virulence (vir) region on the Ti-plasmid.[56] Furthermore, it was speculated that the true nature of acetosyringone and α-hydroxyacetosyringone production may be related to lignin repair of wounds since sinapinic acid, a precursor of lignin, also displays acetosyringone-like activity.[54]

Once the bacteria attached to the binding site, cellulose synthesis commenced resulting in the aggregation of bacteria.[50,51] Binding with cellulose fibrils has been shown to be a necessary condition for the induction of tumors.[43]

## 3.2. DNA Transfer

After attachment and aggregate formation, DNA is passed into and transforms the host plant cell. The mechanism by which this transfer occurs is becoming better understood.

Only the T-DNA of the Ti-plasmid becomes integrated into plant cell chromosomal DNA.[7] The *vir* region, located outside the T-DNA region, and the border sequences that flank the T-DNA, are both involved in tumorigenesis, presumably by mobilizing and transferring genomic material in a manner similar to that of bacterial conjugation.[40,57]

Conjugation requires cell to cell contact implicating the formation of an unidentified channel between juxtaposed plant and bacterial cells. The mechanism of transfer envisioned is as follows: Phenolic compounds induce the *vir*-region to produce a gene product which generates "nicks" in the borders flanking the T-DNA,[57,58] which in turn results in the circularization of the T-DNA.[59] A single strand, the T-strand, is excised from the circularized form by unwinding in a 5′ to 3′ direction and is subsequently transferred to the recipient cell, presumably as a DNA–protein complex.[60] The transfer is associated with conjugal synthesis of the replacement strand in the donor and synthesis of the complimentary strand in the recipient.[57] It has also been shown to be associated with RNA-primed conjugal DNA synthesis.[57,58] However, the mechanisms governing the excision, transfer, and integration of T-DNA into plant cell chromosomal DNA are still not known.

## 4. DIFFERENTIATION OF CROWN GALL CELLS

The phenotypic traits expressed by the transformed plant cell resulting from the integration of T-DNA include phytohormone autotrophy, opine synthesis, and the formation of galls, abnormal roots, or teratomas. In the reversal of transformation, these traits are either suppressed or the genetic material encoding for these responses are eliminated. Either way, a normal fertile plant can be regenerated.

### 4.1. Phytohormone Synthesis and Differentiation

Phytohormone autotrophy was first demonstrated by Braun, who showed that crown gall cells free of bacteria could grow in cell culture without the addition of auxin or cytokinin. By contrast, normal cells in culture require the addition of these hormones for growth and maintenance.[5,14] Moreover, autotrophic tumor callus cell lines revealed twice or greater levels of auxin (indole-3-acetic acid) as well as higher levels of cytokinin, than did normal cells.[61–64] In addition, tumor morphology was found to be a consequence of imbalances in phytohormone levels.[11,64–66] For example, friable tumors were found to contain 10–30 times more indole-3-acetic acid than either teratomas or compact tumors.[64]

Ooms *et al.*[65] demonstrated this relationship using insertional mutations. Transposon insertions in the left portion of T-DNA in a pathogenic strain of *A. tumefaciens* resulted in the shooter mutants, designated LBA 1501 and LBA 4060. When used to infect *Kalanchoe* or tobacco, tumors formed in which shoots appeared from auxiliary bud sites. This was considered to be a cytokininlike effect, since Skoog and Miller[67] had previously demonstrated that tobacco callus developed shoots if the level of cytokinin in the medium was high compared with that of auxin. Conversely, it was demonstrated that if the level of auxin was high compared with cytokinin, tobacco calli developed roots and, when neither hormone dominated, the calli remained amorphous. Similarly, Ooms *et al.*[65] showed this auxinlike effect with plants infected with the "rooter" mutant, LBA 4210, which had a transposon inserted into the right portion of the $T_L$ region. Simultaneous infection with both "shooter" and "rooter" mutants resulted in tumors identical to the wild type. Tumors incited by the shooter mutants were found to contain relatively high cytokinin levels compared with the wild-type tumor, while those incited by the rooter mutant had relatively low cytokinin levels. By contrast, the auxin levels in the "shooter," "rooter," and wildtype tumors were about the same.[11,65]

The auxin and cytokinin loci in the Ti-plasmid were located more accurately by Garfinkel *et* al.[68] and Leemans et al.[28] By introducing transposons in the left portion of T-DNA ($T_L$ segment) of an octopine plasmid, the site of tumor induction and shoot development was identified. Transposons in the middle of $T_L$ showed the presence of root production site. Tumors incited by rooter mutants were made into wild-type tumors by the addition of cytokinin to the callus, while tumors incited by shooter mutants were made into wild-type tumors by the addition of auxin.[65] These transposon insertions in the T region resulted in the mapping of four loci in $T_L$: (1) tmr locus, responsible for the synthesis of cytokinin,[66,68] a mutation at this site results in auxin dominance, hence root growth[69]; (2) tms locus, responsible for auxin synthesis,[70–73] a mutation at this site results in cytokinin dominance, hence shoot growth[11,73]; (3) tml locus, responsible for the production of large tumors; and (4) ocs, the locus responsible for octopine synthesis. The loci tmr, tms, and tml are highly conserved, showing homology in both octopine and nopaline plasmids; however, the ocs locus did not share homology in the nopaline region. Interestingly, tmr, ocs, and nos were found to contain eucaryotic regulatory sequences.

The correlation between pathogenicity and the amount of indole-3-acetic acid produced was reported by Liu and Kado,[71] who demonstrated that even non-pathogenic or plasmidless A. tumefaciens strains produced indole-3-acetic acid, albeit in smaller amounts compared to pathogenic strains. This finding suggested that the tms site was not the only genetic site involved in auxin production. If the Ti-plasmid was reintroduced, indole-3-acetic acid synthesis was restored, particularly if the bacteria were grown in medium containing tryptophan.

Liu et al.[72] further showed that the tryptophan transminase gene was coded for by the bacterial chromosome (iaaC) and that the Ti-plasmid also contained genes in the vir region necessary for indole-3-acetic acid production (iaaP). A plasmid-free mutant, defective in the chromosomal iaaC gene, could be restored to pathogenicity and full indole-3-acetic acid production by transformation with either nopaline or octopine plasmid DNA, suggesting that Ti-plasmid DNA contained genetic determinants that encoded for indole-3-acetic acid production. However, when the plasmid of a mutant defective in the iaaP site was introduced into the iaaC mutant strain, no increase in indole-3-acetic acid production or restoration of pathogenicity was observed. Apparently the defective plasmid could not compensate for the defect in the bacterial chromosome, suggesting that both code for a similar gene product.

What has not been resolved is how indole-3-acetic acid is produced in the transformed plant cell, which only contains the tms gene. The iaaP gene in the vir-region is presumably not integrated into host nuclear DNA, since it is outside the T-DNA region. Nor is chromosomal DNA integrated. It has been speculated that high levels of indole-3-acetic-acid produced by A. tumefaciens induce the expression of indole-3-acetic acid production genes in the plant that are normally repressed. When the plant genes are switched on production is stably maintained.[75]

## 4.2. Opine Synthesis and Utilization

The genes for opine synthesis (ocs, nos, ags) are part of T-DNA, while opine catabolism (occ, noc, agc) genes reside on the Ti-plasmid distal to the vir region. In the bacterium, the opine synthesis genes are silent but, once the plant cell is transformed by A. tumefaciens, the host cell directs the synthesis of these unusual nitrogenous compounds encoded by the inciting Ti-plasmid.[9,12] Some Ti-plasmids encode for the synthesis of octopine and agropine,[76] while others encode only for nopaline synthesis[77] and still others have been shown to encode for neither octopine or nopaline but they may encode for the synthesis of agropine[78] or other similar compounds.[79] The enzymes responsible for the synthesis of octopine and nopaline have been purified and characterized.[20]

Octopine strains of A. tumefaciens generally incite unorganized tumors that have a rough surface and are surrounded by adventitious roots (Fig. 2). The tms and tmr sites, rather than the ocs site, contribute to this phenotype, which results from auxin dominance.[65] Nopaline tumors, on the other hand, can be unorganized, or they may produce teratomas (with high cytokinin levels) and have a smooth surface with roots at the bottom of the tumor[64] (Fig. 3). They may also exhibit

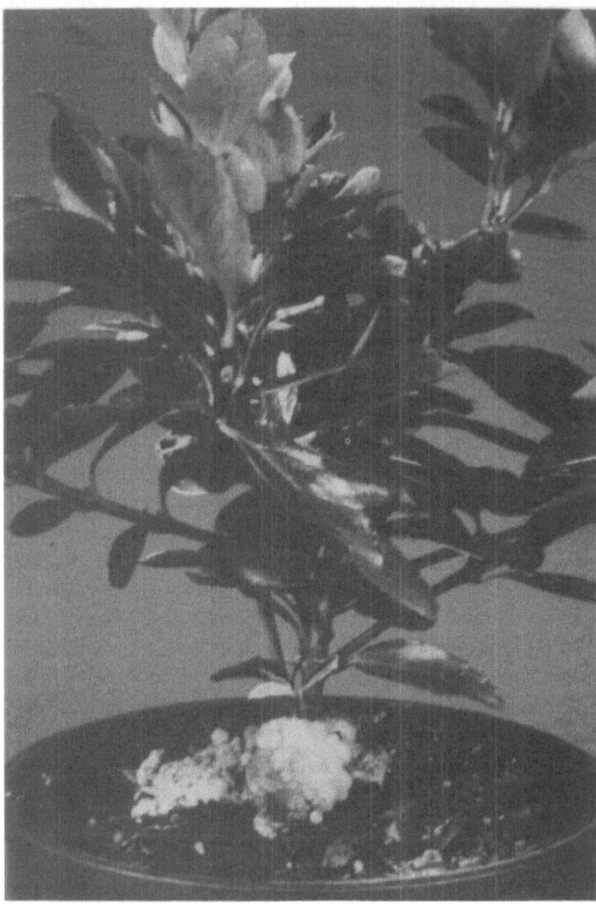

*Figure 2.* Gross pathology of a rough octopine-type gall on euonymus (*Euonymus japonicus* L.)

leaflike structures. By contrast, agropine tumors have a rough surface with few or no roots at the bottom of the tumor.[80]

Utilization of the opines by agrobacteria is directed by catabolism (*occ, noc*) genes present in the Ti-plasmid. If *A. tumefaciens* is freed of its octopine Ti-plasmid, it no longer is able to use octopine as a source of carbon and nitrogen, nor is it able to incite tumor formation. If the Ti-plasmid is reintroduced, the *A. tumefaciens* regains not only tumorigenicity but also the ability to use octopine.

When nopaline agrobacterial strains were freed of this plasmid, and the octopine Ti-plasmid introduced instead, the bacterium could then catabolize octopine, as well as incite the formation of octopine-producing tumors. Using this approach Bomhoff *et al.*[81] and Kerr *et al.*[82] demonstrated that the Ti-plasmid determined the type of opine synthesized by the transformed plant cell, and the type of opine catabolized by the inciting bacteria. However, opine catabolism genes apparently were not required for pathogenicity, since Ti mutants unable to catabolize octopine were still able to incite the formation of octopine-producing tumors.[83]

The specific tumor phenotypes found in nature led to the formulation of the opine concept,[79,81,84] which states that overgrowths elicited by pathogenic strains of agrobacteria are actually ecologic niches in which a favorable environment is created for the propagation of the pathogen. The opine elicited by the transformed plant cell assists in propagating the inoculum. The opines are also conjugal inducers that trigger conjugal activity of the Ti-plasmid, resulting in its transfer to a nonpathogenic *Agrobacterium* strain.[8,9] The nonpathogenic strain is thus converted to a pathogen.

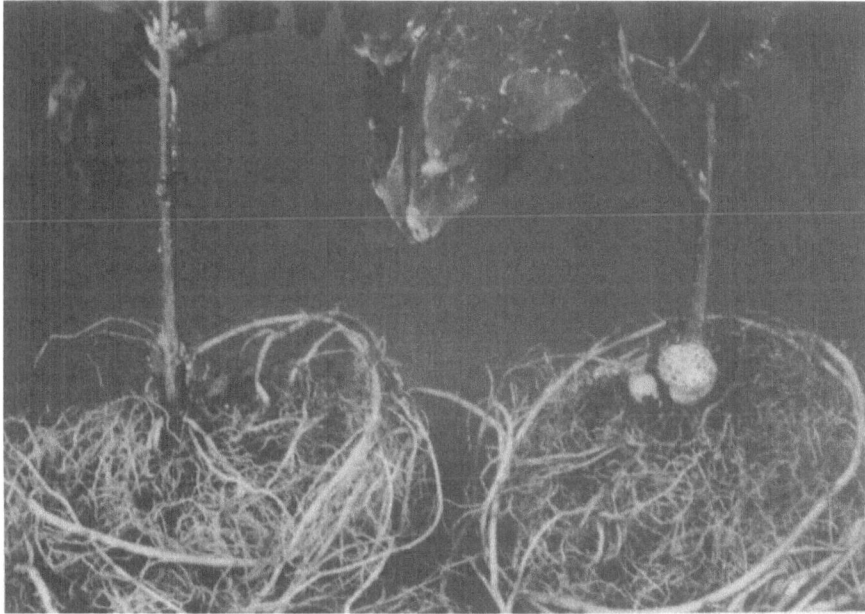

*Figure 3.* Gross pathology of a smooth nopaline-type tumor on forsythia [*Forsythia suspensa* (Thunb.) Vahl].

The expression of opine related functions provides the selective pressure required for their maintenance.

## 4.3. Reversal of the Tumorous State in Crown Gall

Reversal of the tumorous state in plants has been studied in habituated cell cultures,[85,86] in the Kostoff tumor system,[87] and in the crown gall tumor system. In this chapter only crown gall will be considered and the reader is referred to the references listed for the other systems.

Most investigations of differentiation or reversal of the tumorous state in plants have been conducted with the crown gall system. Crown gall tumors have been characterized as having the properties of rapid proliferation but a limited ability to differentiate. By contrast, normal plant cells also proliferate rapidly, but their subsequent elongation results in the differentiation of meristematic cells into organized structures, particularly at the extreme apex of the shoot or root. The apices have properties characteristic of embryonic tissue in that auxin acts synergistically with cytokinins to regulate growth and cell division. Duplication of this phenomenon *in vitro* requires the exogenous addition of phytohormones to callus cell cultures.[87]

Crown gall cells maintained in conventional media do not organize into roots or stems, but under similar conditions, normal cells can regenerate into whole plants. This phenomenon can occur because a culture of normal cells contain a population of totipotential cells. If totipotential cells are transformed *in planta* by A. *tumefaciens*, the transformed cell develops into a teratoma.[88]

A teratoma (Fig. 4) is composed of a chaotic assembly of tissues and organs showing varying grades of morphological development. In many ways it is a caricature or a monster plant. Tissue excised from a teratoma can grow indefinitely in cell culture on a minimal medium without the addition of phytohormones. The same situation is obtained with unorganized tissue from crown gall tumors. Unlike crown galls, however, teratoma-derived cells retain the capacity to organize into buds and shoots. Reversal of the tumorous state has been shown to occur by effecting the elimination of T-DNA or by suppressing the expression of T-DNA. Braun et al.[89,90] demonstrated suppression by showing that shoots derived from teratomas can be tip-grafted to healthy plant stock, and

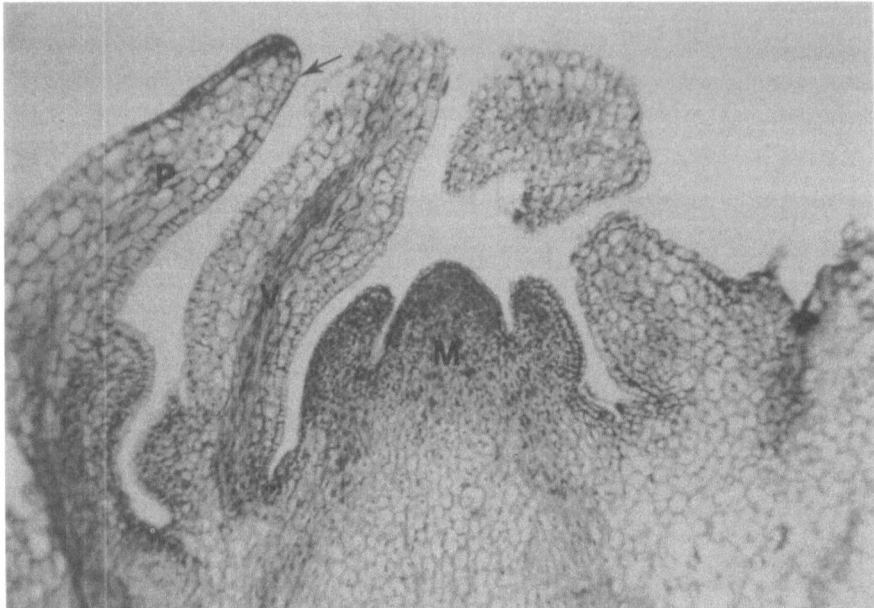

*Figure 4.* Histopathology of a spontaneous nopaline-type teratoma on Japanese holly (*Ilex crenata* Thunb.) showing differentiating apical meristem (M), leaf primordia (P), vascular tissue (V), and epidermal cells ( ↑ ). (×80)

after serial grafting, they gradually recovered from the tumorous state. These shoots developed into plants that flowered and set fertile seed. This apparent differentiation to the normal state appeared to represent a suppression of the tumorous state because the grafted shoot developed stems and leaves that looked normal. But, when these leaves were transferred to cell culture, they assumed neoplastic properties like phytohormone independence, opine synthesis, and morphology of the original teratoma. All in all, this reversal suggested persistance of T-DNA.[90–94]

Sacristan and Melchers[95] presented evidence for the elimination of genetic material. The cells from a tumor incited on a tobacco plant were cloned and grown axenically until a callus formed. Out of 253 clones examined only three were phytohormone independent and could also differentiate into whole plants. Leaves taken from the regenerated plant, when placed in cell culture, required phytohormone supplementation, suggesting that differentiation of the tumor resulted from the loss or removal of T-DNA.

Loss of T-DNA in the $F_1$ generation was also suspected because the seed that developed when the grafted shoot matured provided an apparently normal $F_1$ generation. Tissue from the $F_1$ generation when grown in callus cell culture required phytohormones and did not produce nopaline, suggesting T-DNA was lost during meiosis.[94,95] Yang *et al.*[95] found that the common sequences of T-DNA were indeed missing, but that the border sequences of T-DNA persisted in plant chromosomal DNA. These sequences were carried over apparently from the parental teratoma indicating that at least part of the T-DNA can survive meiosis. In addition, the retained border sequences were transmitted in a mendelian fashion.[96–98] Other investigations revealed that the absence of intact auxin and cytokinin loci resulted in complete suppression of the tumorous state and regeneration of a normal plant.[99,100]

Reversion appears to occur in two stages. In the initial stage, the tumorous traits are suppressed, since apparently normal shoots continued to produce nopaline and did not require phytohormone supplementation.[90–94] In the second stage, following meiosis, there is a complete loss of tumor traits. $F_1$ cells in culture no longer produce nopaline and require phytohormone supplementation, suggesting T-DNA may not survive meiosis; however Yang *et al.*[96] and others[97,98] demonstrated that at least the border sequence can survive meiosis.

Still another mechanism of suppression was demonstrated by Amasino *et al.*[80] They were able to obtain fertile plants from calli that contained intact *tms* and *tmr* regions of the T-DNA but in which the T-DNA was not transcribed. In culture, this cell line required the exogenous addition of phytohormones even though it had the genetic information to make its own phytohormones. But, if the culture was treated with 5-azacytidine, it became autotrophic for phytohormones and displayed autonomous growth. Apparently the azacytidine treatment, which presumably blocked DNA methylation, allowed the T-DNA to be transcribed, resulting in phytohormone autotrophy. What prevented transcription in the first place was not shown.

Additional evidence of the effect of hormone imbalance on tumor morphology and differentiation comes from the work of Barton *et al.*[101] They used an *A. tumefaciens* nopaline strain with a mutation in the *tmr* locus (cytokinin deficient) to produce teratoma from which a fertile plant was generated. The T-DNA in the subsequent $F_1$ generation was shown to survive meiosis. This type of mutation implies auxin dominance, but in the nopaline plasmid the *tms* locus does not support a high enough auxin level to suppress differentiation. This may explain why nopaline strains produce teratomas, tumors in which differentiation is not completely suppressed. In Barton's strain, with the mutation in the *tmr* locus, and in the presence of a weak *tms* locus with its inherent deficiency in auxin production, the teratoma could be easily reversed or differentiated. This probably could not occur with octopine strains, which generally incite unorganized tumors.

## 5. SUMMARY AND CONCLUSIONS

Crown gall disease is a unique biological system. The transfer of plasmid DNA to the plant cell resembles bacterial conjugation, but in this case it is occurring between a prokaryotic and eukaryotic cell. Similarly, the covalent linking of procaryotic DNA sequences with plant chromosomal DNA is in itself unusual.

Once the plasmid DNA is integrated, the plant pathogen has essentially diverted the plant's differentiation machinery to create tumors with unique phenotypes. The incorporated DNA sequences encode for the maintenance of the tumorous state by exercising an ability to synthesize and induce the production of phytohormones. The imbalances in phytohormone level that this creates are responsible for the tumor phenotype, as well as for maintenance of the tumorous state. By the same token reversal of the tumorous state can be made to occur by readjusting the hormonal environment. Furthermore, the ability to incorporate disarmed T-DNA (lacking *tms* and *tmr* loci) into plant nuclear DNA, and have it survive meiosis, provides a mechanism for the modification of the capability of plants.

In addition to phytohormones, the integrated DNA encodes for the synthesis of unusual amino acids known collectively as the opines. These opines are chemical mediators of parasitism because they act as inducers of conjugation, which allows the Ti-plasmid to be passed to a competent saprophyte and thus convert it to a pathogenic organism. In addition, opines serve as a metabolic source of carbon and nitrogen for the inciting microorganism, thus creating a unique ecological niche for self-perpetuation. It is this self-perpetuating mode that makes control of this disease difficult. However, during the early 1970s, Allen Kerr[102] demonstrated field control of crown gall disease by dipping stone-fruit seedlings in a suspension of *Agrobacterium radiobacter* strain K84 prior to planting. It was soon learned that this strain contained a plasmid, now called pAgK84, which encoded for the synthesis of an antibiotic referred to as Agrocin 84.[103,104] This antibiotic is described chemically as a fradulent nucleotide with a 9-(3'-deoxy-β-D-threopentofuranosyl)adenine nucleoside core.[105]

Sensitivity to the killing effects of this antibiotic correlated with tumorigenicity,[8] but only in those biotype 1 and 2 strains of *A. tumefaciens* that carried nopaline plasmids.[106] Because of this restrictive inhibitory specificity, this substance may actually be a bacteriocin. If so, it may be the first example of a nucleotide bacteriocin. Most other bacteriocins are polypeptides. Other strains of agrobacteria have been isolated that have properties similar to strain K84 and thus may be of use in designing additional controls for this disease.

ACKNOWLEDGMENT. I am indebted to Dr. George H. Lacy of Virginia Polytechnic Institute and State University, Blacksburg, Virginia for his careful criticism of this manuscript and to his colleagues, Dr. Robert C. Lambe and Dr. Robert Wick for providing the photographs for Figs. 2–4.

## REFERENCES

1. DeCleene, M., and DeLey, J., 1976, A survey of host plants for *Agrobacterium tumefaciens, Bot. Rev.* **42:**389–466.
2. Agrios, G. N., 1978, *Plant Pathology,* pp. 483–488, Academic, New York.
3. Smith, E. F., and Townsend, C. O., 1907, A plant-tumor of bacterial origin, *Science* **25:**671–673.
4. Braun, A. E., 1943, Studies on tumor inception in crown gall disease, *Am. J. Bot.* **30:**674–677.
5. Braun, A. C., 1956, The activation of two growth substance systems accompanying the conversion of normal to tumor cells in crown gall, *Cancer Res.* **16:**53–56.
6. Zaenen, I., van Larebeke, N., Teuchy, H., van Montagu, M., and Schell, J., 1974, Supercoiled circular DNA in crown-gall inducing *Agrobacterium* strains, *J. Mol. Biol.* **86:**109–127.
7. Chilton, M-D., Drummond, M. H., Merlo, D. J., Sciaky, D., Montoya, A. L., Gordon, M. P., and Nester, E. W., 1977, Stable incorporation of plasmid DNA into higher plants: The molecular basis of crown gall tumorigenesis, *Cell* **11:**263–271.
8. van Larebeke, N., Genetello, C., Schell, J., Schilperoort, R. A., Hermans, A. K., Hernalsteens, J. P., and van Montagu, M., 1975, Acquisition of tumor-inducing ability of non-oncogenic agrobacteria as a result of plasmid transfer, *Nature (Lond.)* **255:**742–743.
9. van Larebeke, N., Genetello, C., Hernalsteens, J. P., DePicker, A., Zaenen, I., Messens, E., van Montaju, M., and J. Schell, J., 1977, Transfer of Ti plasmids between *Agrobacterium* strains by mobilization with the conjugative plasmid RP4, *Mol. Gen. Genet.* **152:**119–124.
10. Chilton, M-D., Saiki, R. K., Yadav, N., Gordon, M. P., Quetier, F., 1980, T-DNA from *Agrobacterium* Ti plasmid is in the nuclear fraction of crown gall tumor cells, *Proc. Natl. Acad. Sci. USA* **77:**4060–4064.
11. Akiyoshi, D. E., Morris, R. O., Hinz, R., Mishke, B. S., Kosuge, T., Garfinkel, D. J., Gordon, M. P., and Nester, E. W., 1983, Cytokinin-auxin balance in crown gall tumors is regulated by specific loci in the T-DNA, *Proc. Natl. Acad. Sci. USA* **80:**407–411.
12. Petit, A., Delhaye, S., Tempe, J., Morel, G., 1970, Recherches sur les guanidines des tissus de crown gall. Mise en evidence d'une rélation biochemique spécifique entre les souches d'*Agrobacterium tumefaciens* et les tumeurs quielles induisent, *Physiol. Veg.* **8:**205–213.
13. Petit, A., David, C., Dabb, G., Ellis, J. G., Casse-Delboart, F., and Tempe, J., 1983, Further extension of the opine concept: Plasmids in *Agrobacterium. rhizogenes* cooperate for opine degradation, *Mol. Gen. Genet.* **190:**204–214.
14. White, P. R., and Braun, A. C., 1942, A cancerous neoplasm of plants: Autonomous bacteria-free crown gall tissue, *Cancer Res.* **2:**597–617.
15. Buchanan, R. E., and Gibbons, N. E. (eds.), 1974, *Bergey's Mannual of Determinative Bacteriology,* 8th ed., Williams & Wilkins, Baltimore.
16. Kersters, K., DeLay, J., Sneath, P. H. A., and Sackin, M., 1973, Numerical taxonomic analysis of *Agrobacterium, J. Gen. Microbiol.* **78:**227–239.
17. Kerr, A., and Panagopoulos, C. G., 1977, Biotypes of *Agrobacterium radiobacter* var. *tumefaciens* and their biological control, *Phytopathol. Z.* **90:**172–179.
18. New, P. B., and Kerr, A., 1971, A selective medium for *Agrobacterium radiobacter* biotype 2, *J. Appl. Bacteriol.* **34:**233–236.
19. Perry, K. L., and Kado, C. I., 1982, Characteristics of Ti plasmids from broad-host range and ecologically specific biotype 2 and 3 strains of *Agrobacterium tumefaciens, J. Bacteriol.* **151:**343–350.
20. Nester, E. W., and Kosuge, T., 1981, Plasmids specifying plant hyperplasia, *Annu. Rev. Microbiol.* **35:**531–565.
21. Hooykaas, P. J. J., Klapwijk, P. M., Nuti, M. P., Schilperoort, R. A., and Rorsch, A., 1977, Transfer of the *Agrobacterium tumefaciens* Ti-plasmid to avirulent *Agrobacteria* and to *Rhizobia ex planta. J. Gen. Microbiol.* **98:**477–484.
22. Van Zarebeke, N., Engler, G., Holster, M., van den Elsacker, S., Zaenen, I., Schilperoort, R. A., and

Schell, J., 1974, Large plasmid in *Agrobacterium tumefaciens* essential for crown gall-inducing activity, *Nature (Lond.)* **252:**169–170.

23. Watson, B., Currier, T. C., Gordon, M. P., Chilton, M-D., and Nester, E. W., 1975, Plasmid required for virulence of *Agrobacterium tumefaciens*, *J. Bacteriol.* **123:**255–264.

24. Currier, T. C., and Nester, E. W., 1976, Evidence for diverse types of large plasmids in tumor-inducing strains of *Agrobacterium*, *J. Bacteriol.* **126:**157–165.

25. Drummond, M. H., and Chilton, M-D., 1978, Tumor-inducing (Ti) plasmids of *Agrobacterium* share extensive regions of DNA homology, *J. Bacteriol.* **136:**1178–1183.

26. Hille, J., Hoekema, A., Hooykaas, P., and Shilperoort, R. A., 1984, Gene organization of the Ti-plasmid, in: *Plant Gene Research: Genes Involved in Microbe–Plant Interactions* (D. P. S. Verma and T. Holn, eds.), pp. 287–309, Springer-Verlag, New York.

27. Willmitzer, L., Simons, G., and Schell, J., 1982, The $t_1$-DNA in octopine crown gall tumors codes for seven well defined polyadenylated transcripts, *EMBO J.* **1:**139–146.

28. Leemans, J., Deblaere, R., Willmitzer, L., DeGreve, H., Hernalsteens, J. P., Van Montagu, M., and Schell, J., 1982, Genetic identification of functions of $t_1$-DNA transcripts in octopine crown galls, *EMBO. J.* **1:**147–152.

29. Hood, E. E., Chilton, W. S., Chilton, M-D., and Fraley, R. T., 1986, T-DNA and opine synthetic loci in tumors incited by *Agrobacterium tumefaciens* A281 on soybean and alfalfa plants, *J. Bacteriol.* **168:**1283–1290.

30. DeGreve, H., Dhaese, P., Seruinck, J. Lemmers, M., Van Montagu, M., and Schell, J., 1983, Nucleotide sequence and transcript map of the *Agrobacterium tumefaciens* Ti plasmid-encoded octopine synthase gene, *J. Mol. Appl. Genet.* **1:**499–511.

31. Komro, C. T., Dirita, V. G., Gelvin, S. B., and Kemp, J. D., 1985, Site-specific mutagenesis in the Tr-DNA region of octopine-type Ti-plasmids, *Plant Mol. Biol.* **4:**253–263.

32. Lemmers, M., Debeuckeleer, M., Holsters, M., Zambryski, P., Depicker, A., Hernalsteens, J. P., Van Montagu, M., and Schell, J., 1980, Internal organization, boundaries and integration of Ti plasmid DNA in nopaline crown gall tumors, *J. Mol. Biol.* **144:**353–376.

33. Depicker, A., Stachel, S., Dhaese, P., Zambryski, P., and Goodman, H. M., 1982, Nopaline synthase: Transcript mapping and DNA sequence, *J. Mol. Appl. Genet.* **1:**561–573.

34. Zambryski, P., Depicker, A., Kruger, K., and Goodman, H., 1982, Tumor induction by *Agrobacterium tumefaciens:* Analysis of the boundaries of T-DNA, *J. Mol. Appl. Genet.* **1:**361–370.

35. Yadav, N. S., Vanderleyden, J., Bennet, D. R., Barnes, W. M., and Chilton, M-D., 1982, Short direct repeats flank the T-DNA on a nopaline Ti plasmid, *Proc. Natl. Acad. Sci. USA* **79:**6322–6326.

36. Simpson, R. B., O'Hara, P. J., Kwok, W., Montaya, A. L., Lickenstein, C., Gordon, M. P., and Nester, E. W., 1982, DNA from the A6S/2 crown gall tumor contains scrambled Ti-plasmid sequences near its junctions with plant DNA, *Cell* **29:**1005–1014.

37. Holsters, M., Villarroel, R., Gielen, J., Seruenck, J., DeGreve, H., Van Montagu, M., and Schell, J., 1983, An analysis of the boundaries of the octopine TL-DNA in tumors induced by *Agrobacterium tumefaciens*, *Mol. Gen. Genet.* **190:**35–41.

38. Joos, H., Inze, D., Caplan, A., Sormann, M., Van Montagu, M., and Schell, J., 1983, Genetic analysis of T-DNA transcripts in nopaline crown galls, *Cell* **32:**1057–1067.

39. Shaw, C. H., Watson, M-D., Carter, G. H., and Shaw, C. H., 1984, The right hand copy of the nopaline Ti-plasmid 25 bp repeat is required for tumor formation, *Nucleic Acid Res.* **12:**6031–6041.

40. Wang, K., Herrera-Estella, L., Van Montagu, M., and Zambryski, P., 1984, Right 25 bp terminus sequences of the opaline T-DNA is essential for and determines direction for DNA transfer from *Agrobacterium* to the plant cell, *Cell* **38:**455–462.

41. Peralta, E. G., and Ream, L. W., 1985, T-DNA border sequences required for crown gall tumorigenesis, *Proc. Natl. Acad. Sci. USA* **82:**5112–5116.

42. Gardner, R. C., and Knauf, V. C., 1986, Transfer of *Agrobacterium* DNA to plants requires a T-DNA border but not the *vir* E locus, *Science* **231:**725–727.

43. Matthyses, A. G., 1983, The role of bacterial cellulose fibrils in infections by *Agrobacterium tumefaciens*, *J. Bacteriol.* **154:**906–915.

44. Lippincott, B. B., and Lippincott, J. A., 1969, Bacterial attachment to a specific wound site as an essential stage in tumor initiation by *Agrobacterium tumefaciens*, *J. Bacteriol.* **97:**620–628.

45. Whatley, M. H., Boudin, J. S., Lippincott, B. B., and Lippincott, J. A., 1976, Role for *Agrobacterium* cell envelope lipopolysaccharide in infection site attachment, *Infect. Immun.* **13:**1080–1083.

46. Lippincott, J. A., and Lippincott, B. B., 1978, Cell walls of crown-gall tumors and embryonic plant tissues lack *Agrobacterium* adherence sites, *Science* **199:**1075–1078.

47. Douglas, C. J., Halperin, W., and Nester, E. W., 1982, *Agrobacterium tumefaciens* mutants affected in attachment to plant cells, *J. Bacteriol.* **152:**1265–1275.

48. Matthysse, A. G., 1987, Characterization of nonattaching mutants of *Agrobacterium tumefaciens, J. Bacteriol.* **169:**313–323.

49. Matthysse, A. G., 1986, Initial interactions of *Agrobacterium tumefaciens* with plant host cells, *CRC Crit. Rev. Microbiol.* **13:**281–307.

50. Matthysse, A. G., Holmes, K. V., and Gurlitz, R. H. G., 1981, Elaboration of cellulose fibrils by *Agrobacterium tumefaciens* during attachment to carrot cells, *J. Bacteriol.* **145:**583–589.

51. Lippincott, J. A., and Lippincott, B. B., 1976, Nature and specificity of the bacterium-host attachment in *Agrobacterium* infection, in: *Cell Wall Biochemistry Related to Specificity in Host–Plant Pathogens Interactions* (B. Solkeim and J. Raa, eds.), pp. 439–451, Universitets-Forlaget, Tromso, Norway.

52. Matthysse, A. G., Wyman, P. M., and Holmes, K. V., 1978, Plasmid dependent attachment of *Agrobacterium tumefaciens* to plant tissue culture cells, *Infect. Immun.* **22:**516–522.

53. Douglas, C. J., Staneloni, R. J., Rubin, R. A., and Nester, E. W., 1985, *A. tumefaciens* chromosomal virulence region. *J. Bacteriol.* **161:**850–860.

54. Stachel, S. E., Messens, E., Van Montagu, M., and Zambryski, P., 1985, Identification of the signal molecules produced by wounded plant cells that activate T-DNA transfer in *Agrobacterium tumefaciens, Nature (Lond.)* **318:**624–629.

55. Dylan, T., Ielpi, L., Stanfield, S., Kashyap, L., Douglas, C., Yanofsky, M., Nester, E., Helinski, D. R., and Ditta, G., 1986, *Rhizobium meliloti* genes required for nodule development are related to chromosomal virulence genes in *Agrobacterium tumefaciens, Proc. Natl. Acad. Sci. USA* **83:**4403–4407.

56. Engstrom, P., Zambryski, P., Vannontagu, M., and Stachel, S. E., 1987, Characterization of *Agrobacterium tumefaciens* virulence proteins induced by the plant factor acetosyringone, *J. Molec. Biol.* **197:**635–646.

57. Jayaswal, R. K., Veluthambi, K., Gelvin, S. B., and Slightom, J. L., 1987, Double-stained cleavage of T-DNA and generation of single-stranded T-DNA molecules in *Escherichia coli* by a vir D-encoded border-specific endonuclease from *Agrobacterium tumefaciens, J. Bacteriol.* **169:**5035–5045.

58. Wang, K., Stachel, S. E., Timmerman, B., Van Montagu, M., and Zambryski, P. C., 1987, Site-specific nick in the T-DNA border sequence as a result of *Agrobacterium vir* gene expression, *Science* **235:**587–591.

59. Yamamoto, A., Iwahashi, M., Yanofsky, M. F., Nester, E. W., Takebe, I., and Machida, Y., 1987, The promoter proximal region in the *virD* locus of *Agrobacterium tumefaciens* is necessary for the plant-inducible circularization of T-DNA, *Mol. Gen. Genet.* **206:**174–177.

60. Gietl, C., Koukolikova-Nicola, Z., and Han, B., 1987, Mobilization of T-DNA from *Agrobacterium* to plant cells involves a protein that binds single-stranded DNA, *Proc. Natl. Acad. Sci. USA* **84:**9006–9010.

61. Beaty, J. S., Powell, G. K., Lica, L., Regier, D. A., MacDonald, E. M. S., Hommes, N. G., and Morris, R. O., 1986, Tzs, a nopaline Ti plasmid gene from *Agrobacterium tumefaciens* associated with trans-zeatin biosynthesis, *Mol. Gen. Genet.* **203:**274–280.

62. Miller, C. O., 1974, Ribosyl-trans-zeatin, a major cytokinin produced by crown gall tumor tissue, *Proc. Natl. Acad. Sci. USA* **71:**334–338.

63. Scott, I. M., Browning, G., and Eagles, J., 1980, Ribosylzeatin and zeatin in tobacco crown gall tumor tissue, *Planta* **147:**269–273.

64. Weiler, E. W., and Spanier, K., 1981, Phytohormones in the formation of crown gall tumor, *Planta* **153:**326–337.

65. Ooms, G., Hooykaas, P. J. J., Moolenaar, G., and Schilperoort, R. A., 1981, Crown gall plant tumors of abnormal morphology induced by *Agrobacterium tumefaciens* carrying mutated octopine Ti plasmids: Analysis of T-DNA functions, *Gene* **14:**33–50.

66. Barry, G. F., Rogers, S. G., Fraley, R. T., and Brand, L., 1984, Identification of a cloned cytokinin biosynthetic gene, *Proc. Natl. Acad. Sci. USA* **81:**4776–4780.

67. Skoog, F., and Miller, C. O., 1957, Chemical regulation of growth and organ formation in plant tissues cultured *in vitro, Symp. Soc. Exp. Biol.* **11:**118–131.

68. Garfinkel, D. J., Simpson, R. B., Ream, L. W., White, F. F., Gordon, M. P., and Nester, E. W., 1981, Genetic analysis of crown gall: Fine structure map of the T-DNA by site-directed mutagenesis, *Cell* **27:**143–153.

69. Willmitzer, L., Sanchez-Serrano, J., Buschfeld, E., and Schell, J., 1982, DNA from *Agrobacterium rhizogenes* is transferred to and expressed in axenic hairy root plant tissue, *Mol. Gen. Genet.* **186:**16–32.

70. Goutheret, R. J., 1947, Action de l'acide indole-acétique sur le dévelopement des tissus normaux et de tissus de crown gall de topinambour cultives *in vitro, C. R. Acad. Sci.* **224:**1728–1730.

71. Liu, S. T., and Kado, C. I., 1979, Indole acetic acid production: A plasmid function of *Agrobacterium tumefaciens*, *Biochem. Biophys. Res. Commun.* **90:**171–178.

72. Liu, S. T., Perry, K. L., Shcardl, C. L., and Kado, C. I., 1982, *Agrobacterium* Ti plasmid indole acetic acid gene is required for crown gall oncogenesis, *Proc. Natl. Acad. Sci. USA* **79:**2812–2816.

73. Inze, D., Follin, A., Van Lijsebettens, M., Simoens, C., Genetello, C., Van Montagu, M., and Schell, J., 1983, Genetic analysis of the individual T-DNA genes of *Agrobacterium tumefaciens:* Further evidence that two genes are involved in indole-3-acetic acid synthesis, *Mol. Gen. Genet.* **194:**265–274.

74. Akiyoski, D. E., Klee, H., Amasino, R. M., Nester, E. W., and Gordon, M. P., 1984, T-DNA of *Agrobacterium tumefaciens* encodes an enzyme of cytokinin biosynthesis, *Proc. Natl. Acad. Sci. USA* **81:**5994–5998.

75. Kado, C. I., 1984, Phytohormone-mediated tumorigenesis by plant pathogenic bacteria, in: *Plant Gene Research. Genes Involved in Microbe–Plant Interactions* (D. P. S. Verna and T. Holn, eds.), pp. 311–336, Springer-Verlag, New York.

76. Ménagé, A., and Morel, M. G., 1964, Sur la presence d'octopine dans les tissus de crown gall, *C.R. Acad. Sci.* **259:**4795–4796.

77. Goldman, A., Thomas, D. W., and Morel, G., 1969, Sur la structure de la nopaline, metabolite anormal de certaines tumeurs de crown gall, *C.R. Acad. Sci.* **268:**852–854.

78. Firmin, J. L., and Fenwick, G. R., 1978, Agropine. A major new plasmid determined metabolite in crown gall tumors, *Nature (Lond.)* **276:**842–844.

79. Kemp, J. D., 1982, Plant pathogens that engineer their hosts, in: *Phytopathogenic Prokaryotes,* Vol. 1 (M. S. Mount and G. H. Lacy, eds.), pp. 443–457, Academic, Orlando, Florida.

80. Amasino, R. M., and Miller, C. O., 1982, Hormonal control of tobacco tumor morphology, *Plant Physiol.* **69:**389–392.

81. Bomhoff, G. H., Klapwijk, P. M., Kester, H. C. M., Schilperoort, R. A., Hernalsteens, J. P., and Schell, J., 1976, Octopine and nopaline synthesis and breakdown genetically controlled by a plasmid of *Agrobacterium tumefaciens*, *Mol. Gen. Genet.* **145:**177–181.

82. Kerr, A., Manigault, P., Tempé, J., 1977, Transfer of virulence *in vivo* and *in vitro* in *Agrobacterium*, *Nature (Lond.)* **265:**560–561.

83. Montoya, A. J., Chilton, M-D., Gordon, M. P., Sciaky, D., and Nester, E. W., 1977, Octopine and nopaline metabolism in *Agrobacterium tumefaciens* and crown gall tumor cells: Role of plasmid genes, *J. Bacteriol.* **129:**101–107.

84. Guyon, P., Chilton, M-D., Petit, A., and Tempé, J., 1980, Agropine in "null type" crown gall tumors: Evidence for the generality of the opine concept, *Proc. Natl. Acad. Sci. USA* **77:**2693–2697.

85. Limasset, P., and Gautheret, R., 1950, Sur le caractère tumoral des tissus de tabac ayant subi le phénomène d'accoutumance aux hétero-auxines, *C.R. Acad. Sci. Paris* **230:**2043–2045.

86. Binns, A., and Meins, F., Jr., 1973, Habituation of tobacco pith cells for factors promoting cell division is heritable and potentially reversible, *Proc. Natl. Acad. Sci. USA* **70:**2660–2662.

87. Braun, A. C., 1974, Epigenetic changes, in: *The Biology of Cancer,* pp. 105–109, Addison-Wesley, Reading, Massachusetts.

88. Braun, A. C., 1953, Bacterial and host factors concerned in determining tumor morphology in crown gall, *Botan. Gaz.* **114:**363–371.

89. Braun, A. C., 1959, A demonstration of the recovery of the crown-gall tumor cell with the use of complex tumors of single-cell origin, *Proc. Natl. Acad. Sci. USA* **45:**932–938.

90. Braun, A. C., and Wood, H., 1976, Suppression of the neoplastic state with the acquisition of specialized functions in cells, tissues and organs of crown gall teratomas of tobacco, *Proc. Natl. Acad. Sci. USA* **73:**496–500.

91. Turgeon, R., Wood, H. N., and Braun, A. C., 1976, Studies on the recovery of crown gall tumor cells, *Proc. Natl. Acad. Sci. USA* **73:**3562–3564.

92. Binns, A., Wood, H. N., and Braun, A. C., 1981, Suppression of the tumorous state in crown gall teratomas of tobacco: A clonal analysis, *Differentiation* **19:**97–102.

93. Wood, H. N., Binns, A. N., and Braun, A. C., 1978, Differential expression of oncogenicity and nopaline synthesis in intact leaves derived from crown gall teratoma of tobacco, *Differentiation* **11:**175–180.

94. Williams, G. J., Molendijk, L., Ooms, G., and Schelperoort, R., 1981, Differential expression of crown gall tumor markers in transformants obtained after *in vitro Agrobacterium tumefaciens* induced transformation of cell wall regenerating protoplasts derived from *Nicotiana tabacum*, *Proc. Natl. Acad. Sci. USA* **78:**4344–4348.

95. Sacristan, M. D., and Melchers, G., 1977, Regeneration of plants from "habituated" and *Agrobacterium* transformed single-cell clones of tobacco, *Mol. Gen. Genet.* **152:**111–117.

96. Yang, F-M., and Simpson, R. B., 1981, Revertant seedlings from crown gall tumors retain a portion of the bacterial Ti plasmid sequences, *Proc. Natl. Acad. Sci. USA* **78:**4151–4155.

97. Williams, G. J., Molndijk, L., Ooms, G., and Schelperoort, R. A., 1981, Retention of tumor markers in F-1 progeny plants from *in vitro* induced octopine and nopaline tumor tissue, *Cell* **24:**719–727.

98. Wostemeyer, A., Otten, L., DeGreve, H., Hernalsteens, J. P., and Leemans, J., 1982, Regeneration of plants from crown gall cells, in: *Genetic Engineering in Eucaryotes* (P. F. Lurquin and A. Kleinhofs, eds.), pp. 137–151, Plenum, New York.

99. Yang, F-M, Montoya, A. L., Merlo, D. J., Drummond, M. H., and Chilton, M-D, 1980, Foreign DNA sequences in crown gall teratomas and their fate during the loss of the tumorous traits, *Mol. Gen. Genet.* **177:**704–714.

100. DeGreve, H., Leemans, J., Hernalsteens, J. P., Thia-Toong, L., and DeBeuckeleer, M., 1982, Regeneration of normal and fertile plants that express octopine synthase from tobacco crown galls after deletion of tumor-controlling functions, *Nature (Lond.)* **300:**752–754.

101. Barton, K. A., Binns, A. N., Matzke, A. J. M., and Chilton, M-D., 1983, Regeneration of intact tobacco plants containing full length copies of genetically engineered T-DNA and transmission of T-DNA to R1 progeny, *Cell* **32:**1033–1043.

102. Kerr, A., and Htay, K., 1974, Biological control of crown gall through bacteriocin production, *Physiol. Plant Pathol.* **4:**37–44.

103. Ellis, J. G., Kerr, A., Van Montagu, M., and Schell, J., 1979, *Agrobacterium:* Genetic studies in Agrocin 84 production and the biological control of crown gall, *Physiol. Plant Pathol.* **15:**311–319.

104. Slota, J. E., and Farrand, S. K., 1982, Genetic isolation and physical characterization of pAgK84, the plasmid responsible for Agrocin 84 production, *Plasmid* **8:**175–186.

105. Roberts, W. P., Tate, M. E., and Kerr, A., 1977, Agrocin 84 is a 6-*N*-phosphoramidate of an adenine nucleotide analogue, *Nature (Lond.)* **265:**379–381.

106. Engler, G., Holsters, M., Van Montagu, M., Schell, J., Hernalsteens, J. P., and Schelperoort, R., 1975, Agrocin 84 sensitivity: A plasmid determined property in *Agrobacterium tumefaciens, Mol. Gen. Genet.* **138:**345–349.

# 26

# Angiogenesis
## Factors and Mechanisms

## Patricia A. D'Amore and Michael Klagsbrun

## 1. TUMOR VASCULATURE

### 1.1. Background

Blood vessel proliferation is essential for the normal growth and development of tissue. In the adult, angiogenesis occurs infrequently. Exceptions are found in the female reproductive system, where angiogenesis occurs in the follicle during its development, in the corpus luteum during ovulation, and in the placenta during pregnancy. These periods of angiogenesis are relatively brief and tightly regulated. Normal angiogenesis also occurs as part of the body's repair processes, such as in the healing of wounds and fractures. On the other hand, uncontrolled angiogenesis contributes to a wide variety of serious diseases. As examples, the growth of solid tumors is dependent on vascularization, and in diabetic retinopathy vascularization of the retina often leads to blindness.

New capillaries arise as offshoots or sprouts from established vessels, mostly venules or other capillaries. This phenomenon of capillary sprouting is accomplished by a series of sequential steps[1] (Fig. 1). During the initial phase of capillary sprouting, the basement membrane of endothelial cells (EC) in the parent blood vessel is degraded. Degradation of basement membrane is thought to be accomplished by the action of proteolytic enzymes, most notably plasminogen activator and collagenase, liberated by EC in response to tumor angiogenesis factors.[2] It is also likely that tumors act directly to degrade basement membrane, via tumor-derived endoglycosidases that degrade heparan sulfate, the major glycosaminoglycan (GAG) constituent of basement membrane.[3] Once the basement membrane is degraded, EC bud out from the pre-existing vessel and migrate directionally into the perivascular space and proliferate, elongating the budding sprout. Subsequently, the EC form lumens by mechanisms that are largely unknown.[4] In the final steps, pericytes arrive at the new capillary, new basement membrane is synthesized (presumably by both cells), and a mature new capillary is established.[5]

### 1.2. Differences between Normal and Tumor Vessels

Tumors have long been noted for their rich blood supply.[6] Goldman has described the peculiarities of tumor vessel growth, calling attention to their (1) dilation, (2) accelerated proliferation,

*Patricia A. D'Amore* • Laboratory of Surgical Research and Department of Pathology, Children's Hospital and Harvard Medical School, Boston, Massachusetts 02115. *Michael Klagsbrun* • Laboratory of Surgical Research and Department of Biological Chemistry, Children's Hospital and Harvard Medical School, Boston, Massachusetts 02115.

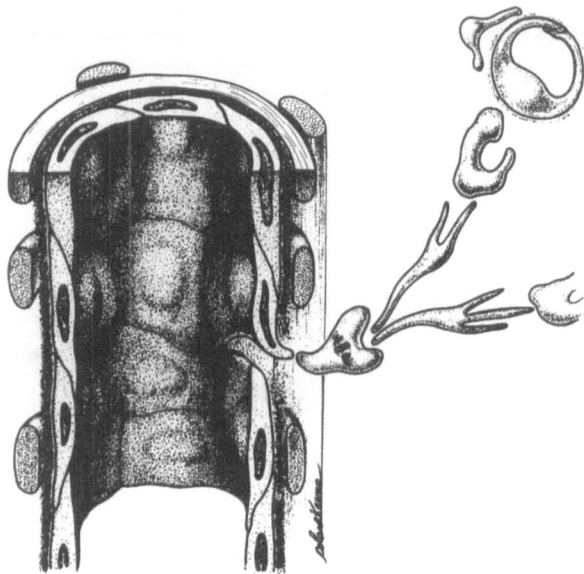

*Figure 1.* Schematic of the events involved in new capillary growth. (Adapted from the work of Ausprunk and Folkman.[1])

and (3) irregular arrangement.[7] These early observations together with subsequent studies on the vascularization of malignant tumors by Ide *et al.*[8] and Algire and Chalkley[9] have led to a complete description of tumor vessel development. This was clearly summarized in a paper by Urbach,[10] in which he made the following distinctions between the vascularization of normal homologous tissue and the vascularization of an immunolologically compatible tumor:

1. Proliferation of vessels into the tumor begins much earlier and is much greater in the case of the tumor implant than in the control implants of normal tissue.
2. During the course of vascularization of normal tissue, there is a gradual differentiation into arterioles, pre-arterioles, capillaries, venules, and veins. By contrast, most of the tumor vessels "consist of endothelial channels with wide diameter, with little or no differentiation into arterioles or venules."
3. Unlike the vasculature of normal transplanted tissue, most of the tumor vessels collapse instantly upon the death of the animal or mild reduction of arterial blood pressure.

A number of differences have also been demonstrated between the function of vessels in tumors and normal tissues. Hypotension induced by pharmacologic agents leads to the collapse of tumor vessels, presumably due to the lack of basement membrane along the undifferentiated capillaries and pressure of the tissue mass.[11] This same explanation is likely to account for the elevated permeability known to be associated with tumor vessels.[12]

Denekamp and Hobson[13] showed a 30- to 40-fold greater proliferation rate in the vascular endothelium of tumors than in normal vessels. They found the labeling rate in most tumors to be high (a mean of 9.0% and 10–20% range), regardless of the growth rate of the tumor. This is in dramatic contrast to the low rates of labeling (0.01%) that have been reported for both large[14] and microvessel[15] EC in normal tissues. The correlation between EC doubling time and tumor doubling time is not absolute, however, it has been shown that the proportion of effective vasculature decreases with increasing tumor size.[16]

## 1.3. Relationship between Vascularization and Tumor Growth

Algire[17] noted that the ability of transplanted sarcomas to grow was directly related to their capacity to elicit continued proliferation of the endothelium. This was directly demonstrated by

Gimbrone and co-workers,[18] who observed that tumors implanted into isolated perfused organs grew to a limit of 2–3 mm in diameter, whereas the same tumors reimplanted into animals grew exponentially upon vascularization. Earlier, Greene[19] had reported that tumors transplanted into guinea pig eyes did not vascularize and did not grow over a 2-3 year time period. However, they resumed growth when they were transplanted back into their original host. These experimental observations provided compelling evidence for a direct relationship between tumor vascularization and subsequent growth.

## 1.4. Role for Growth Factors

There is a clear cause-and-effect relationship between tumor vascularization and the ability of the tumor to expand. Speculation concerning the signal for vascular ingrowth dates back to Ide and co-workers,[8] who observed that tumor growth did not commence until several days after the vascularization of the explant, suggesting the production of a "blood vessel growth-stimulating substance" produced by the tumor. The first demonstration of the nature of the angiogenic signal was provided by the work of Greenblatt and Shubik.[20] Tumors implanted into the rabbit ear in chambers consisting of porous membranes were capable of inducing new vessel growth, suggesting the action of a diffusible factor(s). Additional evidence for a role for a "tumor angiogenesis factor" came from the studies of Folkman and Cavallo and co-workers,[21] in which a tumor extract was demonstrated to elicit neovascularization in the rat dorsal air sac, an *in vivo* model for angiogenesis.

Subsequently, a number of tumor-derived angiogenesis factors were identified and isolated.[22–25] However, attempts to purify these factors were unsuccessful. The difficulties encountered in obtaining a purified molecule could be ascribed to the relatively low tissue levels of the highly potent angiogenesis factors as well as to the lack of suitable and reproducible bioassays. Over the past 2 years, however, these obstacles have been largely overcome. As a result, a number of angiogenesis factors have been purified from both tumors and normal tissues, their primary amino acid sequences determined and their genes cloned.

## 2. ANGIOGENESIS FACTORS

## 2.1. Introduction

Over the years, a number of factors have been shown to be angiogenic.[26,27] Angiogenesis factors are assayed both *in vivo* and *in vitro*. The latter assay systems are based on steps in capillary development that can be recapitulated *in vitro*. (These steps are described in detail in Section 1.1 and depicted schematically in Fig. 1.) The events include: (1) degradation of basement membrane, (2) increased EC motility, and (3) accelerated EC proliferation. The development of *in vitro* assays was dependent on the availability of cultured capillary EC.

Assays measuring the ability to degrade basement membranes have involved the quantification of the release of proteases such as plasminogen activator and/or latent collagenase by EC.[2] EC migration has been assayed by measuring random motility (chemokinesis) using the phagokinetic track assay[28,29] or by measuring directional EC migration (chemotaxis) in response to a concentration gradient using a Boyden migration chamber.[30] Proliferation of EC is assayed by quantifying [³H]thymidine incorporation or by determining increases in cell number.

Although these *in vitro* assays have proved useful (even essential) in screening biologic activity during purification, it must be remembered that none of these individual steps, protease production, motility, or proliferation, is synonymous with the process of angiogenesis. Each putative angiogenic factor must be assayed for its angiogenic potential in an *in vivo* system. The most commonly used bioassays for measuring angiogenesis are (1) the developing chick chorioallantoic membrane (CAM) and (2) the corneal pocket assay.

The CAM bioassay is carried out in fertilized chick eggs in which a window is prepared by removal of a section of egg shell or in which the shell is totally removed and the egg cultured in a petri dish.[31,32] Test substances are applied to filters or plastic coverslips, or are incorporated into methylcellulose and placed onto the CAM of 8- to 10-day-old fertilized chick egg. Neovascularization at the site of implantation is monitored visually for 1–2 days after implantation and the membranes are fixed and evaluated histologically. Since the CAM is undergoing rapid intrinsic neovascularization and is also highly sensitive to nonspecific inflammatory substances such as eggshell fragments, critical evaluation and proper controls must be used in evaluating CAM results.

The most reliable bioassay for angiogenesis uses the avascular cornea of either the rabbit or rat eye.[33,34] Test substances are incorporated into sustained release polymer pellets (ethylene vinyl acetate copolymer, ELVAX), which are implanted into a pocket that is surgically prepared in the cornea. In a positive response, there is directional growth of new capillaries from the limbal blood vessels toward the implant after 5–6 days, whereas in controls, the cornea remains avascular. The bioassay can be quantified by measuring the rate of vessel growth, the length, and the density of the new blood vessels. The major disadvantages of the cornea bioassay are the limitation on the number of samples that can be assayed, the expense involved, and the inability to easily quantify the results.

## 2.2. Non-Heparin-Binding Factors: Low-Molecular-Weight Factors

### 2.2.1. Chemotactic Factors

An angiogenesis factor that stimulates the migration but not the proliferation of EC has been isolated from wound fluid.[35] The factor appears to be a polypeptide with a molecular weight of 2000–14,000. The material induces angiogenesis in the corneal pocket assay at a dose of 150 ng. It stimulates the migration of capillary EC in a Boyden chamber assay but does not stimulate the proliferation of these cells. Similar chemotactic activity has been shown to be released by macrophages in response to hypoxia[36] and lactate but not pyruvate.[37] It is strongly suspected that the macrophages are the source of the biologic activity found in wound fluid.

### 2.2.2. Lipids

Several angiogenesis factors have been described that are lipid rather than peptide in nature. 3T3 cells that have undergone differentiation into adipocytes *in vitro* secrete factors that stimulate angiogenesis in the CAM.[38] These factors stimulate the motility of aortic and capillary EC in a Boyden chamber assay, but they are not mitogenic for these cells. Characterization of the angiogenesis/chemotactic factors, including chemical analysis and the use of inhibitors of prostaglandin synthesis, suggests that the major angiogenic activity may be a mixture of prostaglandins $E_1$ and $E_2$ ($PGE_1$ and $PGE_2$) and as yet uncharacterized polar lipids.[39] Distinct factors that stimulate EC proliferation but not motility are also produced by these differentiated 3T3 cells (J. J. Castellot, Jr., personal communication).[39,40] These EC mitogens apparently are not lipids, but their identity has not yet been determined.

Prostaglandins, in particular $PGE_1$ and $PGE_2$, have been shown to induce new vessel growth.[41–43] $PGE_1$ at 1 μg stimulates angiogenesis in the corneal pocket assay and $PEG_2$ at 0.2–20 ng has been shown to stimulate neovascularization in the CAM. Other prostaglandins, including the A or F series, are not angiogenic. Prostaglandin levels are elevated in tumors, activated macrophages, wounds, and inflammatory exudates.[43] Since these cells and fluids are associated with neovascularization, it may well be that certain prostaglandins play a role in angiogenesis.

A lipid factor extractable in chloroform–methanol has been identified from omentum[44] that, when assayed in the corneal pocket assay, induces intense vascularization. The omentum-derived angiogenesis factor has not yet been purified.

### 2.2.3. Tumor-Derived Angiogenesis Factors

Low-molecular-weight compounds ranging from 200 to 1000 $M_r$ that stimulate EC proliferation and angiogenesis in the CAM and cornea have been isolated from Walker 256 tumors.[23–25]

Similar factors have been found in synovial fluid.[45] These factors appear to be neither peptide, protein, nucleic acid, nor prostaglandin.

Recently, two small molecular weight molecules isolated from Walker 256 carcinoma by ethanol extraction were characterized.[46] One was definitively identified by desorption–electron-impact spectrometry, nuclear magnetic resonance (NMR) spectroscopy, and gas chromatography-mass spectrometry (GC–MS) as nicotinamide; the second active fraction contained a larger complex of which nicotinamide was a part. The material isolated from the tumor induces new vessel growth in the cornea and CAM.

## 2.3. Non-Heparin-Binding Factors: Polypeptide Factors

### 2.3.1. Angiogenin

Angiogenin was first purified from the conditioned medium of a human adenocarcinoma cell line by a combination of cation exchange and reverse phase high-performance liquid chromatography (HPLC).[47–49] This purification procedure yielded 0.5 µg angiogenin per liter conditioned medium. Angiogenin is a single-chain polypeptide of 123 amino acids with a molecular weight of 14,400 and an isoelectric point (pI) of 9.5. It has a 35% absolute sequence homology to a family of pancreatic ribonucleases. The major active site residues of ribonuclease are conserved in angiogenin as are three of the four disulfide bonds. Angiogenin is inactive toward the more conventional substrates of ribonuclease such as wheat germ RNA, poly(C), poly(U), and RNA–DNA hybrids. However, angiogenin does cleave both 28S and 18S ribosomal RNA to relatively large products 100–500 nucleotides in length.[50] Whether this relatively specific hydrolytic activity has physiologic significance is not known.

Human complementary DNA (cDNA) coding for angiogenin was isolated from a human liver cDNA library.[49] The nucleotide sequence of the angiogenin gene was determined and the predicted amino acid sequence was in agreement with that determined by amino acid sequence analysis. Angiogenin has been shown to stimulate angiogenesis in the chick CAM in the range of 0.5–290 ng/egg and at 50 ng/eye in the rabbit cornea assay.[47]

Angiogenin differs both structurally and biologically from another major class of angiogenic agents, the heparin-binding growth factors, in that (1) it lacks sequence homology to either acidic or basic fibroblast growth factor (FGF); (2) it has no affinity for heparin; (3) it has a gene sequence coding for a signal peptide of 22–24 amino acids, unlike both acidic and basic FGF, which apparently have no signal peptide domains[51,52] [this latter structural difference is consistent with the observation that angiogenin is secreted by cells in culture,[47] whereas basic FGF (bFGF) is not[53]]; and (4) angiogenin does not appear to be a growth factor for EC. In all, these results suggest that angiogenin and the family of heparin-binding EC growth factors stimulate angiogenesis via different mechanisms that have yet to be elucidated.

Recent studies by Weiner et al.[54] have used cDNA probe for human angiogenin to investigate the distribution of angiogenin messenger RNA (mRNA) in various adult and developing tissues in the rat. These investigators found that pattern of angiogenin mRNA is unrelated to vascular development but that angiogenin is expressed predominantly in the adult liver. Furthermore, transformed liver cells do not contain more angiogenin message than does normal liver. The possibility remains that the expression of angiogenin activity is controlled at the translational level. The authors suggest that if regulation is at the transcriptional level as their results indicate, then the primary function of angiogenin may not be as an angiogenic agent.

### 2.3.2. Transforming Growth Factors

Transforming growth factors (TGF) are polypeptides that were first identified on the basis of their ability to alter the phenotype of normal cells to that of transformed cells.[55] TGF-α is a 50-amino acid polypeptide synthesized by various transformed cells.[56,57] It binds to the EGF receptor and has a 35% homology with EGF. Both TGF-α and EGF stimulate microvascular EC proliferation at 1–5 ng/ml.[58] When these polypeptides are injected subcutaneously into the hamster cheek pouch, they stimulate both capillary proliferation and [3H]thymidine incorporation. However, TGF-α is a more potent angiogenic factor (active at 0.3–1 μg) than EGF, which is angiogenic only at a dose of 10 μg.[58]

TGF-β is a 25,000-$M_r$ homodimer found in tumors and normal tissue cells such as placenta, kidney, and platelets.[59–61] When injected (at a dose of 1 μg) subcutaneously into newborn mice, TGF-β induces new vessel formation and collagen production by fibroblasts to form a highly vascular granulation tissue at the site of injection in 2–3 days.[62] Neither EGF nor PDGF had the same effect in the same bioassay. On the other hand, TGF-β has been found to inhibit both baseline and FGF-stimulated proliferation of aortic EC *in vitro*.[63,64] This apparent paradox has been resolved by the demonstration that TGF-β is a potent chemotactic factor for monocytes.[65] Thus, it is suspected that the angiogenic effects of TGF-β are due to its ability to recruit monocytes, which in turn release angiogenic stimuli.

## 2.4. Heparin-Binding Growth Factors

### 2.4.1. Background

Migration and proliferation of EC are rate-limiting events in the development of new capillaries.[1] Thus, a strategy in the purification of angiogenesis factors has been to isolate growth factors that stimulate these two events *in vitro*. Among the first factors to be identified were FGF isolated from brain[65] and EC growth factor (ECGF) isolated from hypothalamus.[66] Basic FGF was initially reported to be a cationic 13,000-$M_r$ polypeptide[67] that supported the proliferation of clonally seeded EC *in vitro*[68] and elicited new blood vessels in the rabbit corneal pocket.[69] The claims that FGF had been purified to homogeneity and was structurally related to myelin basic protein were subsequently found to be erroneous.[70] ECGF was reported to be an anionic factor existing in two molecular-weight forms of 70,000 and 17,000–25,000 that stimulated the proliferation of human umbilical vein EC.[71] Other sources of EC mitogens were the retina[72] (anionic, ~50,000 $M_r$), the eye[73] (anionic, 17,500 $M_r$), and cartilage[74] (cationic, 16,400 $M_r$). Despite much effort, these EC growth factors could not be readily purified.

### 2.4.2. Heparin Affinity

A major advance in the purification of EC growth factors came as a result of the observation that an EC mitogen derived from rat chondrosarcoma adhered tightly to a column of immobilized heparin.[75] About 1.5 M NaCl was required to elute the growth factor activity from the column (Fig. 2). In the case of tissues such as hypothalamus (Fig. 3) and brain, two peaks of heparin-binding activity were found, an acidic one eluting at 1 M NaCl and a basic one eluting at 1.5 M NaCl. After extensive analysis it now appears that most, if not all, EC mitogens have a marked affinity for heparin. There are several lines of evidence that the binding of EC growth factors for heparin represents a true affinity: (1) The various EC growth factors bind to heparin so tightly that 1–1.5 M

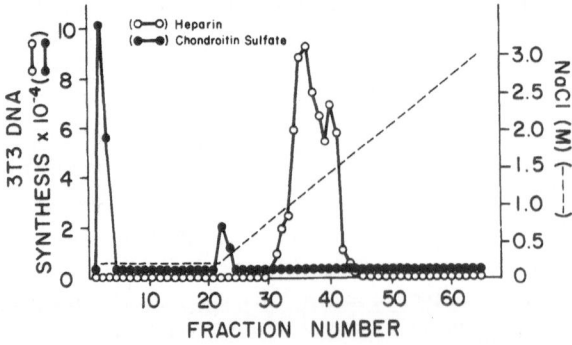

*Figure 2.* Heparin affinity chromatography of chondrosarcoma-derived bFGF. Extracts of rat chondrosarcoma were applied to columns of immobilized heparin (○) or immobilized chondroitin sulfate (●). The columns were washed with 0.1 M NaCl and growth factor was eluted with a gradient of 0.1–3M NaCl. Fractions were collected and tested for the ability to stimulate DNA synthesis in 3T3 cells.

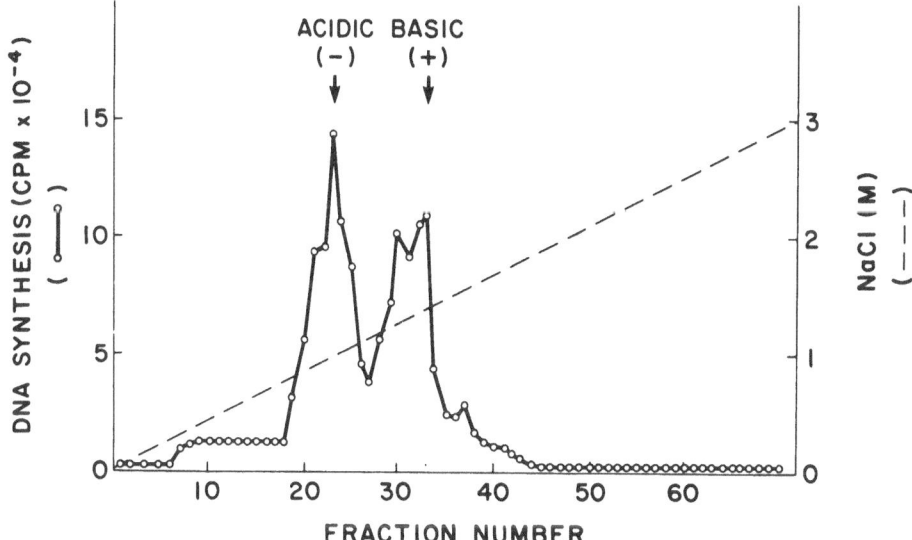

*Figure 3.* Heparin affinity chromatography of brain extracts. Extracts of brain were applied to a column of heparin–Sepharose. Growth factor activity was eluted with a gradient of 0.1 M–3M NaCl. Fractions were collected and tested for the ability to stimulate DNA synthesis in 3T3 cells. The first peak (acidic) of growth had an isoelectric point of about 5; the second (basic), an isoelectric point of about 10.

NaCl is required for their elution from heparin–Sepharose (these salt concentrations are comparable to those required to elute well known heparin-binding proteins such as antithrombin III)[76]; (2) the binding of the EC growth factors for heparin is highly specific [they do not adhere to other GAG, such as chondroitin sulfate (Fig. 2) and hyaluronic acid][77]; and (3) their binding to heparin is independent of the isoelectric point; (anionic EC growth factors isolated from hypothalamus and retina with isoelectric points of approximately 5 adhere to heparin, a polyanionic molecule).[78] In fact, the anionic EC growth factor adheres much more tightly to heparin than does PDGF, a polypeptide with an isoelectric point of 10 that is not an EC mitogen.[76–78] The comparison of the elution profiles of a number of growth factors from columns of heparin-Sepharose is summarized in Fig. 4.

## 2.4.3. Purification

The first purification of an EC growth factor to homogeneity was that of a chondrosarcoma-derived growth factor (ChDGF).[75] ChDGF, which elutes from heparin–Sepharose at 1.5 M NaCl, was purified in a two-step procedure combining cation exchange chromatography and heparin–Sepharose chromatography. ChDGF is a cationic 18,000-$M_r$ polypeptide that stimulates the proliferation of capillary EC at about 1 ng/ml.[75] Heparin–Sepharose chromatography has also been used to purify many other EC mitogens, including those found in brain,[79–82] hypothalamus,[80] eye,[78,83,84] and cartilage.[77] The brain-derived EC growth factors eluting from heparin–Sepharose at 1 M NaCl and 1.5 M NaCl have molecular weights of about 16,500 and 18,000, respectively (Fig. 5).

## 2.4.4. Classification and Distribution

Many of the EC growth factors first described during the 1970s, such as basic FGF, acidic FGF, ECGF, retina-derived growth factor, eye-derived growth factor, and cartilage-derived growth factor, have been shown to be heparin-binding growth factors. Successful purification of these heparin-binding factors has permitted comparative structural analysis that has greatly clarified the relationship of these polypeptides to one another.[85,86] The first reported primary amino acid se-

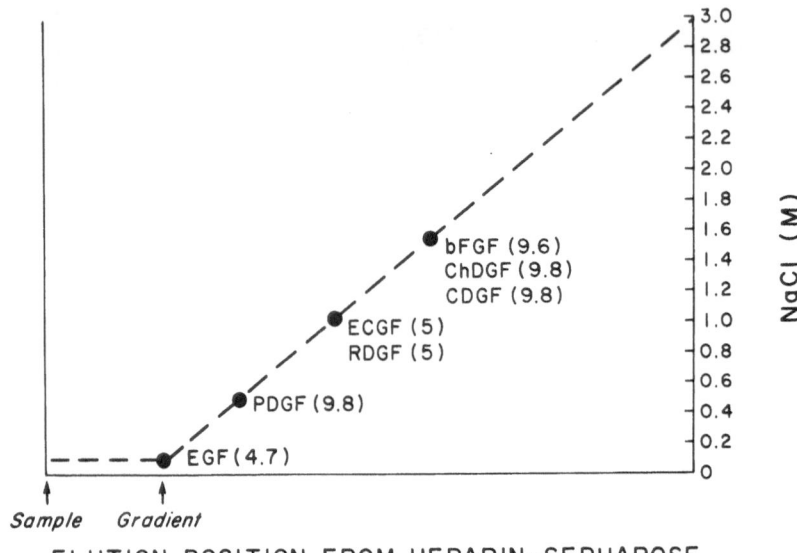

ELUTION POSITION FROM HEPARIN-SEPHAROSE

*Figure 4.* Elution position of growth factors from columns of heparin–Sepharose. A variety of growth factors were applied to heparin–Sepharose columns and eluted with a gradient of 0.1–3M NaCl. EGF, epidermal growth factor; PDGF, platelet-derived growth factor; ECGF, endothelial cell growth factor; RDGF, retina-derived growth factor; bFGF, basic fibroblast growth factor; ChDGF, chondrosarcoma-derived growth factor; CDGF, cartilage-derived growth factor. Isoelectric points are given in parentheses.

quences for heparin-binding growth factors were those of bovine pituitary bFGF, a polypeptide of 146 amino acids,[87] and of bovine brain acidic FGF (aFGF), a polypeptide of 140 amino acids.[88,89] Basic and acidic FGF were found to be structurally related, having a 53% absolute sequence homology.[89] Subsequent structural analysis of other heparin-binding EC growth factors has indicated that they can be categorized into two classes, containing growth factors structurally related to acidic and basic FGF, respectively. The growth factors within a given class are either identical or represent multiple molecular weight forms of the same polypeptide (Table I).

The class of aFGF containing anionic polypeptides that elute from heparin–Sepharose with approximately 1.0 M NaCl have isoelectric points of about 5 and molecular weights of 15,000–20,000. These heparin-binding growth factors have been found mainly in neural tissue and include brain-derived aFGF,[80,82,90] ECGF,[91] eye-derived growth factor II,[84] acidic retina-derived growth factor,[78] astroglial growth factor-1,[92] and bone-derived growth factor-1.1.[93]

The other class of heparin-binding EC mitogens consists of cationic polypeptides that elute from heparin–Sepharose with around 1.5 M NaCl, have isoelectric points of 8–10, molecular weights of 16,000–19,000, and appear to be identical to, or are multiple molecular weight forms of, bFGF. The cationic class of heparin-binding growth factors appears to be far more ubiquitous than the anionic class. Polypeptides of this class have been isolated from such sources as pituitary,[87,94] brain,[80,89] hypothalamus,[76,80] eye,[84] cartilage,[77] bone,[93] corpus luteum,[95] adrenal cortex,[96] kidney,[97] placenta,[98] macrophages,[99] chondrosarcoma,[75] hepatoma cells,[100] EC,[53,101] astroglial cells,[92] and developing brain.[102] The distribution of heparin-binding growth factors is summarized in Table II.

It appears that the various molecular-weight forms of the heparin-binding growth factors are a result of protease-mediated truncations, mostly at the amino-terminal.[103] Acidic FGF has been found in three molecular-weight forms. ECGF-β is a higher-molecular weight form (154 amino acids) of aFGF (140 amino acids) extended at the amino-terminal by 14 amino acids and blocked at its amino-terminal.[104] ECGF-β is the intact precursor form of aFGF. ECGF-α (134 amino acids) is a truncated form of aFGF, missing the 20 N-terminal amino acids of ECGF-β.

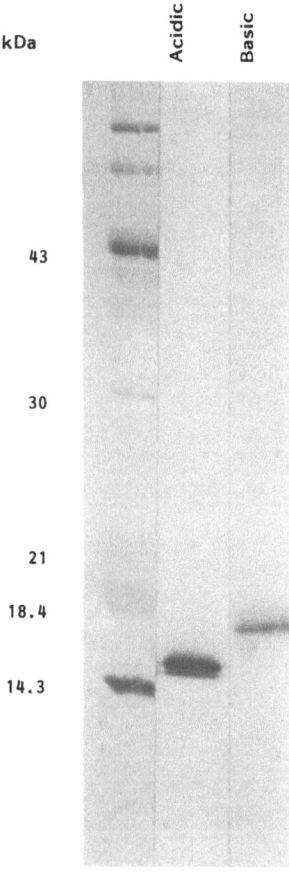

**Figure 5.** Sodium dodecyl sulfate–polyacrylamide gel electrophoresis (SDS–PAGE) of acidic and basic FGF. Brain-derived acidic and basic FGF were purified by heparin-affinity chromatography and analyzed by SDS–PAGE 0. Lane 1, molecular-weight markers; lane 2, acidic FGF; lane 3, basic FGF.

A 154-amino acid molecular-weight form of bFGF blocked at the amino-terminal has been recently described[105] and appears to be the intact form of the growth factor. Truncated forms of bFGF with 146 amino acids have been isolated from brain and with 131 amino acids have been isolated from corpus luteum, adrenal cortex, and kidney.[95–97] Truncation of bFGF to lower-molecular-weight forms is due in part to the action of acid proteinase cleavages at the amino-terminal.[103]

## 2.4.5. Gene Cloning

The availability of the primary amino acid sequences of acidic and basic FGF permitted the cloning of acidic and basic FGF genes. A human cDNA clone encoding ECGF was isolated from a human brain stem cDNA library and its nucleotide sequence determined.[51] Southern blot analysis has suggested that there is a single ECGF gene that maps to human chromosome 5. The size of the human brain stem ECGF mRNA transcript is 4.8 kilobases (kb). The predicted amino acid sequence of the open reading frame after the initiating methionine[52] is the same as the primary amino acid sequence of ECGF-β, the 154-amino acid precursor form of aFGF.[104]

A bovine cDNA clone encoding bFGF was isolated from a bovine pituitary cDNA library and the nucleotide sequence determined.[52] Basic FGF mRNA transcripts of 5 kb were found in hypothalamus and hepatoma cells[52] and EC.[101] The predicted amino acid sequence of the open reading frame corresponded to that of bFGF but appeared to have a 9-amino acid extension on the amino-terminal side. Thus, bFGF without the initiating methionine is predicted to be a 154-amino acid

*Table I. Classification of Heparin-Binding Growth Factors*

| Heparin-binding growth factor | References |
|---|---|
| Acidic FGF | |
| (pI values of 5–7, elution at 1 M NaCl) | |
| Brain-derived aFGF | 80,82,90 |
| Endothelial cell growth factor (ECGF) | 81,91 |
| Eye-derived growth factor-2 | 84 |
| Retina-derived growth factor | 78 |
| Astroglial growth factor-1 | 92 |
| Hypothalamus growth factor-α | 76 |
| Heparin-binding growth factor-α | 80 |
| Basic FGF | |
| (pI values of 8–10, elution at 1.5 M NaCl) | |
| Brain-derived bFGF | 80,89,94 |
| Eye-derived growth factor-1 | 84 |
| Astroglial growth factor-2 | 86 |
| Hypothalamus growth factor-β | 76 |
| Heparin-binding growth factor-β | 80 |
| Cartilage-derived growth factor | 77 |
| Chondrosarcoma-derived growth factor | 75 |
| Hepatoma-derived growth factor | 100 |

polypeptide[52] in agreement with structural analysis.[105] Gene and protein structural analysis suggest that both ECGF (aFGF) and bFGF are 154 amino acid polypeptides with a high degree (53%) of homology.

## 2.4.6. Receptors

Covalent crosslinking of purified [$^{125}$I]-ECGF (aFGF) and [$^{125}$I]-bFGF have resulted in the identification of FGF receptors on the surface of several different cell types. A 150,000-$M_r$ receptor for ECGF has been identified on murine lung capillary EC.[106] Two receptors for bFGF, with molecular weights of 145,000 and 125,000, have been identified on the surface of BHK-21 cells[107]; the BHK-21 cells have 120,000 binding sites per cell. Receptors (20,000 per cell) with a molecular weight of 130,000 for eye-derived growth factor 1 (EDGF-I), the retinal form of bFGF, have been identified on the surface of bovine epithelial lens cells.[108] A single receptor for both acidic and basic FGF with a molecular weight of 165,000 has been identified on the surface of Swiss 3T3 cells and myoblasts.[109] There are 60,000 binding sites on the 3T3 cells. Tyrosine phosphorylation has been demonstrated for aFGF[110] but not for bFGF.[107]

A more recent study has reported two populations of binding sites on BHK cells: a high-affinity site with a $K_d$ of 20 PM at 80,000 sites per cell and a low-affinity site with a $K_d$ of 2 nm at 600,000 sites per cell.[111] The binding to the low-affinity site could be completed by heparin and heparan sulfate but not by a variety of other GAG. Similar binding characteristics have been demonstrated for bovine capillary EC.[111] The biologic significance of the low-affinity binding site is unclear.

The data concerning FGF receptors are relatively sparse. It remains unclear whether there are distinct receptors for acidic and basic FGF or whether they share common receptors. Clarification of this issue will await the isolation and cloning of these receptor populations.

## 2.4.7. Biologic Activity *in Vitro*

Heparin binding growth factors are potent mitogens and chemoattractants for EC *in vitro* and are therefore good candidates for angiogenesis factors *in vivo*. Basic FGF induces capillary EC to

*Table II. Distribution of Acidic*
*and Basic FGF*

Acidic FGF
    Eye
    Brain
    Hypothalamus
    Bone
    Myocardium

Basic FGF
    Eye
    Brain
    Hypothalamus
    Bone
    Tumors and tumor cells
    Pituitary
    Cartilage
    Corpus luteum
    Adrenal gland
    Kidney
    Placenta
    Macrophages

migrate into three-dimensional collagen matrices *in vitro* to form capillarylike tubes,[112] mimicking events that occur during neovascularization *in vivo*.

Heparin-binding growth factors are mitogenic and chemotactic not only for EC[113] but also for fibroblasts and astroglial cells,[114] melanocytes,[115] chondrocytes,[95,116] and smooth muscle cells.[95] Thus, these polypeptides appear to be general mitogens for mesenchymal-derived cells. In addition, there is a single report that in rhabdomyosarcoma cells, bFGF is a growth factor for the tumor cells themselves.[117]

Furthermore, in some cell systems the FGF appears to function as a regulator of differentiation. FGF has been shown to stimulate the differentiation of a variety of neural cells *in vitro*, including neurite outgrowth in PC12 cells[118,119] and retinal ganglion cells,[120] the survival of cerebrocortical neurons,[121] and both survival and neurite extension of hippocampal neurons.[122] In contrast, bFGF prevents differentiation in a muscle cell line (as measured by switches in actin isoform synthesis).[123]

## 2.4.8. Biologic Activity *in Vivo*

Both basic and acidic FGF are angiogenic *in vivo* in CAM,[32,124] cornea,[124] and wound-healing models.[125,126] As little as 60 ng chondrosarcoma-derived basic FGF induces angiogenesis in the chick CAM in an 18-hr period.[32] Blood vessel growth is directional toward the site of implantation. A marked hyperplasia of connective tissue cells at the site of implantation is also found. Brain aFGF at 160 ng/egg[124] has been shown to be angiogenic in the CAM. As little as 10 ng of chondrosarcoma-derived bFGF and 80 ng brain aFGF induce new vessels in the cornea in a 6-day period.[32,124] In neither the CAM nor the cornea bioassay is there evidence of inflammation.

Cartilage-derived bFGF is active in a wound-healing model at a dose of 500 ng.[125] In this model system, polyvinyl sponges implanted into rats are injected with bFGF. After 3 days, histologic examination of the sponges reveals that bFGF induces the formation of granulation tissue that is highly vascularized with dilated blood vessels.

Lens regeneration has been shown to occur from the iris of the newt in response to acidic but not basic FGF.[127] The authors suggest that this growth factor may be the natural signal for lens regeneration produced by the retina in the newt. A recent report indicates that the role of FGF in differentiation may be even more generalized. Basic FGF has been shown to induce mesoderm formation in *Xenopus*,[128] mimicking the effect of the ventrovegetal signal. The ability of this effect to be blocked by heparin and the inability of PDGF, insulin, chorionic gonadotropin, interleukin-1, interferons, transforming growth factor-type β, or colony-stimulating factors to induce the same changes indicates a high level of specificity.

## 3. REGULATION OF ANGIOGENESIS

### 3.1. Actions of Angiogenesis Factors

It appears that a number of different factors are capable of stimulating angiogenesis *in vivo* (Table III). Some of these, such as acidic and basic FGF, angiogenin, TGF-α, and TGF-β are well characterized: they have been purified and sequenced and their genes cloned. Others have yet to be fully purified. Although all these factors are angiogenic in experimental *in vivo* assays, their effects on EC *in vitro* vary. For example, whereas acidic and basic FGF are mitogenic for EC, angiogenin appears not influence EC proliferation and TGF-β is an inhibitor of EC proliferation. Some angiogenic factors such as acidic and basic FGF stimulate both EC motility and proliferation. However, others such as the wound-derived angiogenesis factor and the 3T3 adipocyte-derived factors are only chemotactic.

These results suggest that different angiogenesis factors might act via different mechanisms. Some angiogenesis factors might act by directly stimulating EC motility and proliferation. Other factors might stimulate EC motility *in vitro* and are capable of inducing angiogenesis by positioning EC so they can be stimulated to proliferate by mitogenic factors. Yet other factors might not affect EC directly, but rather act indirectly by mobilizing secondary cells to stimulate angiogenesis. For instance, such factors might activate macrophages to produce bFGF and/or other angiogenesis factors or liberate angiogenesis factors that are stored in tissues.

### 3.2. Control of the Availability of Angiogenic Factors

The ubiquity of angiogenesis factors such as bFGF and TGF-β suggests that their availability must be tightly regulated under normal conditions. For example, considerable quantities of acidic and basic FGF are found in normal tissues such as brain, yet the vascular EC turnover time in most normal tissue is measured in years. Certain conditions, such as corpus luteum formation and wound healing, are characterized by brief angiogenesis but then return to the quiescent state. In contrast, the proliferation of tumor capillary EC is dramatically accelerated.

In light of the variety of the form and function of the microvasculature in various tissues and organs, it seems likely that there may be many forms and levels of regulators for angiogenesis. At

### Table III.  Biologic Activities of Angiogenic Factors

| Factor | Angiogenesis | EC proliferation | EC motility |
|---|---|---|---|
| Acidic FGF | Yes | Yes | Yes |
| Basic FGF | Yes | Yes | Yes |
| Angiogenin | Yes | No | N.D.[a] |
| TGF-α | Yes | Yes | N.D. |
| TGF-β | Yes | Inhibition | N.D. |
| Wound fluid | Yes | No | Yes |
| Adipocyte lipids | Yes | No | Yes |
| Prostaglandins | Yes | No | N.D. |

[a]N.D., not determined.

the molecular level, the regulation may be via: (1) controlled expression of genes for angiogenesis factors, or (2) processing and post-translational modification of the factors; (3) at the cellular level, the angiogenic factors might be sequestered to limit their availability; (4) their release could be regulated or (5) the responsiveness of the EC could be modulated; and (6) finally, the action of the factors at the tissue level could be limited via the interaction of angiogenesis stimulators with specific angiogenesis inhibitors. Thus, abnormal angiogenesis, such as occurs in tumors and diabetic retinopathy, might be the result of the breakdown of some of these postulated regulatory mechanisms.

### 3.3. Role of Ischemia in Angiogenesis

It is well documented that ischemia is a common denominator of nearly every condition in which neovascularization is observed. Basic FGF appears to remain associated with the cells that synthesize it (e.g., EC and hepatoma cells), unlike PDGF, which is secreted.[53] This result might explain an apparent paradox, that is, the finding that there are high levels of both acidic and basic FGF in tissues, such as the brain, where angiogenesis is infrequent. However, such a model poses the problem of how these factors, if not secreted, are released to stimulate new vessel growth *in vivo*. We postulate that ischemic injury or cell death permits the release of cell-associated angiogenic factors. Depending on the situation, accessory cells that are attracted by the ischemic event such as macrophages, which are known to contain angiogenic factors (bFGF, TGF-β, TNF-α), could be responsible for or augment the stimulation. In support of this, media conditioned by whole tumor suspensions or tumor-associated macrophages stimulated neovascularization in the rabbit cornea more often and more rapidly than media conditioned by tumor cells suspensions that were depleted of macrophages.[129]

### 3.4. Storage of FGF

At another level of control, bFGF has been shown to be localized in basement membranes produced by EC *in vitro*[130] and in basement membranes *in vivo*.[131] The basement membrane-associated activity can be removed by incubation with heparin or heparan sulfate but not other GAG. Furthermore, pretreatment of the extracellular matrices with heparinase or heparitinase prevents subsequent binding of the growth factor,[131] providing further evidence for an interaction between FGF and heparin in the extracellular matrix. In each of these reports, the investigators postulate a role for heparinaselike enzymes that would act to mobilize FGF from its storage site in the basement membrane. This is a particularly attractive hypothesis in light of the fact that metastasizing tumor cells are known to produce heparinases in the process of migrating through the basement membrane.[3]

### 4. SUMMARY

The rapid progress made during the past 2 years, in purifying angiogenesis factors, cloning their genes, and investigating their mechanisms of actions, promises to lead angiogenesis research into exciting new directions. Important issues that remain to be addressed include (1) identification of which cells produce and respond to the angiogenesis factors; (2) purification of angiogenesis factor receptors; (3) elucidation of the mechanisms by which angiogenesis factors act; (4) determination if and how angiogenesis activity may be modulated *in vivo;* (5) investigation of the administration of angiogenesis factors to repair damaged tissue *in vivo* such as in myocardial infarctions, wounds, and bone fractures; and (6) learning how to suppress pathologic angiogenesis such as that which occurs in tumor vascularization, proliferative diabetic retinopathy, and rheumatoid arthritis.

## REFERENCES

1. Ausprunk, D. H., and Folkman, J., 1977, Migration and proliferation of endothelial cells in preformed and newly formed blood vessels during tumor angiogenesis, *Microvasc. Res.* **14**:53–65.
2. Gross, J. L., Moscatelli, D., and Rifkin, D. B., 1983, Increased capillary endothelial cell protease activity in response to angiogenic stimuli in vitro, *Proc. Natl. Acad. Sci. USA* **80**:2623–2627.
3. Vlodavsky, I., Fuks, Z., Bar-Ner, M., Ariav, Y., and Schirrmacher, V., 1983, Lymphoma-cell mediated degradation of sulfated proteoglycans in the subendothelial cell extracellular matrix: Relationship to tumor metastasis, *Cancer Res.* **43**:2704–2711.
4. Folkman, J., and Haudenschild, C., 1980, Angiogenesis in vitro, *Nature (Lond.)* **288**:551–556.
5. Crocker, D. J., Murad, T. M., and Geer, J. C., 1970, Role of the pericyte in wound healing. An ultrastructural study, *Exp. Mol. Pathol.* **13**:51–65.
6. Virchow, R., 1863, *Die Krankhaften Geschwulste*, August Hirschwald, Berlin.
7. Goldman, E., 1907, The growth of malignant disease in man and the lower animals with special reference to the vascular system, *Lancet* **2**:1236–1237.
8. Ide, A. G., Baker, N. H., and Warren, S. L., 1939, Vascularization of the Brown-Pearce rabbit epithelioma transplant as seen in the transparent ear chamber, *AJR* **42**:891–899.
9. Algire, G. H., and Chalkley, H. W., 1945, Vascular reactions of normal and malignant tissue in vivo. I. Vascular reactions of mice to wounds and or normal and neoplastic transplants, *J. Natl. Cancer Inst.* **6**:73–85.
10. Urbach, F., The blood supply of tumors, in: *Advances in Biology of the Skin* (W. Montagna and R. A. Ellis, eds.), pp. 123–149, Pergamon, New York.
11. Algire, G. H., Legallais, F. Y., and Anderson, B. F., 1954, Vascular reactions of normal and malignant tissue in vivo. VI. The role of hypotension in the action of components of podophyllin on transplanted sarcomas, *J. Natl. Cancer Inst.* **14**:879–887.
12. Denekamp, J., 1984, Vascular endothelium as the vulnerable element in tumours, *Acta Radiol. [Oncol]* **23**:217–225.
13. Denekamp, J., and Hobson, B., 1982, Endothelial-cell proliferation in experimental tumors, *Br. J. Cancer* **46**:711–720.
14. Schwartz, S. M., and Benditt, E. P., 1977, Aortic endothelial cell replication I. Effects of age and hypertension in the rat, *Circ. Res.* **41**:248–255.
15. Hobson, B., and Dekamp, J., 1984, Endothelial proliferation in tumours and normal tissues: Continuous labelling studies, *Br. J. Cancer* **49**:405–413.
16. Tannock, I. F., 1968, The relation between cell proliferation and the vascular system in a transplanted mouse mammary tumour, *Br. J. Cancer* **22**:258–273.
17. Algire, G. H., 1947, Growth and vascularization of transplanted mouse melanomas, in: *The Biology of Melanomas*, Vol. 4, pp. 159–175, New York Academy of Science,
18. Gimbrone, M. A., Leapman, S. B., Cotran, R. S., and Folkman, J., 1972, Tumor dormancy in vivo by prevention of neovascularization, *J. Exp. Med.* **136**:261–276.
19. Greene, H. S. N., 1941, Heterologous transplantation of mammalian tumors, *J. Exp. Med.* **73**:461–473.
20. Greenblatt, M., and Shubik, P., 1968, Tumor angiogenesis: transfilter diffusion studies in the hamster by transparent chamber techniques, *J. Natl. Cancer Inst.* **41**:111–124.
21. Cavallo, T., Sade, R., Folkman, J., and Cotran, R. S., 1972, Tumor angiogenesis: Rapid induction of endothelial mitosis demonstrated by autoradiography, *J. Cell Biol.* **54**:408–420.
22. Tuan, D., Smith, S., Folkman, J., and Merler, E., 1973, Isolation of the non-histone proteins of rat Walker carcinoma 256: Their association with tumor angiogenesis, *Biochem.* **12**:3159–3165.
23. Phillips, P., Steward, J. K., and Kumar, S., 1976, Tumour angiogenesis factor (TAF) in human and animal tumours, *Int. J. Cancer* **17**:549–558.
24. McAuslan, B. R., and Hoffman, H., 1979, Endothelium stimulating factor from Walker carcinoma cells, *Exp. Cell Res.* **119**:181–190.
25. Fenselau, A., Watt, S., and Mello, R. J., 1981, Tumor angiogenic factor: Purification from the Walker 256 rat tumor, *J. Biol. Chem.* **256**:9605–9611.
26. Folkman, J., and Klagsbrun, M., 1987, Angiogenic factors, *Science* **235**:442–447.
27. D'Amore, P. A., and Braunhut, S., 1988, The role of growth factors in endothelial cell growth control, in: *Endothelial Cells* (U. Ryan, ed.), pp. 13–36, CRC Press, Boca Raton, Florida.
28. Zetter, B. R., 1980, Migration of capillary endothelial cells is stimulated by tumour-derived factors, *Nature (Lond.)* **285**:41–43.
29. Azizkhan, J., Sullivan, R., Azizkhan, R., Zetter, B., and Klagsbrun, M., 1983, Stimulation of increased

capillary endothelial cell motility by chondrosarcoma-cell-derived growth factors, *Cancer Res.* **43:**3281–3286.

30. Glaser, B. M., D'Amore, P. A., Seppa, H., Seppa, S., and Schiffman, E., 1980, Adult tissues contain chemoattractants for vascular endothelial cells, *Nature (Lond.)* **288:**483–484.

31. Ausprunk, D. H., Knighton, D. R., and Folkman, J., 1974, Differentiation of vascular endothelium in the chick chorioallantois: A structural and autoradiographic study, *Dev. Biol.* **38:**237–248.

32. Shing, Y., Folkman, J., Haudenschild, C., Lund, D., Crum, R., and Klagsbrun, M., 1985, Angiogenesis is stimulated by a tumor-derived endothelial cell growth factor, *J. Cell. Biochem.* **29:**275–287.

33. Gimbrone, M. A., Jr., Cotran, R. S., Leapman, S. B., and Folkman, J., 1974, Tumor growth and neovascularization: An experimental model using the rabbit cornea, *J. Natl. Cancer Inst.* **52:**413–427.

34. Fournier, G. A., Lutty, G. A., Watt, S., Fenselau, A., and Patz, A., 1981, A corneal micropocket assay for angiogenesis in the rat eye, *Invest. Ophthalmol. Vis. Sci.* **21:**351–354.

35. Banda, M. J., Knighton, D. R., Hunt, T. K., and Werb, Z., 1982, Isolation of a nonmitogenic angiogenesis factor from wound fluid, *Proc. Natl. Acad. Sci. USA* **79:**7773–7777.

36. Knighton, D. R., Hunt, T. K., Scheuenstuhl, H., Halliday, B. J., Werb, Z., and Banda, M. J., 1983, Oxygen tension regulates the expression of angiogenesis factor by macrophages, *Science* **221:**1283–1285.

37. Jensen, J. A., Hunt, T. K., Scheuenstuhl, H., and Banda, M., 1986, Effect of lactate, pyruvate, and PH on secretion of angiogenesis and mitogenesis factors by macrophages, *Lab. Invest.* **54:**574–578.

38. Castellot, J. J., Jr., Karnovsky, M. J., and Spiegelman, B. M., 1982, Differentiation-dependent stimulation of neovascularization and endothelial cell chemotaxis by 3T3 adipocytes, *Proc. Natl. Acad. Aci. USA* **79:**5597–5601.

39. Dobson, D. E., Castellot, J. J., and Spiegelman, B. M., 1985, Angiogenesis stimulated by 3T3-adipocytes is mediated by prostanoid lipids, *J. Cell Biol.* **101:**109a.

40. Castellot, J. J., Jr., Karnovsky, M. J., and Spiegelman, B. M., 1980, Potent stimulation of vascular endothelial cell growth by differentiated 3T3 adipocytes, *Proc. Natl. Acad. Sci. USA* **77:**6007–6011.

41. Ben Ezra, D., 1978, Neovasculogenic ability of prostaglandins, growth factors and synthetic chemoattractants, *Am. J. Ophthalmol.* **86:**455–461.

42. Ziche, M., Jones, J., and Gullino, P., 1982, Role of prostaglandin E1 and copper in angiogenesis, *J. Natl. Cancer Inst.* **69:**475–482.

43. Form, D. M., and Auerbach, R., 1983, $PGE_2$ and angiogenesis, *Proc. Soc. Exptl. Biol. Med.* **172:**214–218.

44. Goldsmith, H. S., Griffith, A. L., Kupferman, A., and Catsimpoolas, N., 1984, Lipid angiogenic factor from omentum, *JAMA* **252:**2034–2036.

45. Brown, R. A., Weiss, J. B., Tomlinson, I. W., Phillips, P., and Kumar, S., 1980, Angiogenic factor from synovial fluid resembling that from tumours, *Lancet* **29:**682–685.

46. Kull, F. C., Jr., Brent, D. A., Parikh, I., and Cuatrecasas, P., 1987, Chemical identification of a tumor-derived angiogenic factor, *Science* **236:**843–845.

47. Fett, J. W., Strydom, D. J., Lobb, R. R., Alderman, E. M., Bethune, J. L., Riordan, J. F., and Vallee, B. L., 1985, Isolation and characterization of angiogenin, an angiogenic protein from human carcinoma cells, *Biochemistry* **24:**5480–5486.

48. Strydom, D. J., Fett, J. W., Lobb, R. R., Alderman, E. M., Bethune, J. L., Riordan, J. F., and Vallee, B. L., 1985, Amino acid sequence of human tumor derived angiogenin, *Biochemistry* **24:**5486–5494.

49. Kurachi, K., Davie, E. W., Strydom, D. J., Riordan, J. F., and Vallee, B. L., 1985, Sequence of the cDNA and gene for angiogenin, a human angiogenesis factor, *Biochemistry* **24:**5494–5499.

50. Shapiro, R., Riordan, J. F., and Vallee, B. L., 1986, Characteristic ribonucleolytic activity of human angiogenin, *Biochemistry* **25:**3527–3532.

51. Jaye, M., Howk, R., Burgess, W., Ricca, G. A., Chiu, I.-M., Ravera, M. W., O'Brien, S. J., Modi, W. S., Maciag, T., and Drohan, W. N., 1986, Human endothelial cell growth factor: Cloning, nucleotide sequence, and chromosome localization, *Science* **233:**541–545.

52. Abraham, J. A., Mergia, A., Whang, J. L., Tumolo, A., Friedman, J., Hjerrild, K. A., Gospodarowicz, D., and Fiddes, J. C., 1986, Nucleotide sequence of a bovine clone encoding the angiogenic protein, basic fibroblast growth factor, *Science* **233:**545–548.

53. Vlodavsky, I., Fridman, R., Sullivan, R., Sasse, J., and Klagsbrun, M., 1987, Aortic endothelial cells synthesize basic fibroblast growth factor which remains cell associated and platelet-derived growth factor-like protein which is secreted, *J. Cell. Physiol.* **131:**402–408.

54. Weiner, H. L., Weiner, L. H., and Swain, J., 1987, The tissue distribution and developmental expression of the messenger RNA encoding angiogenin, *Science* **237:**280–282.

55. DeLarco, J. E., and Todaro, G. J., 1980, Sarcoma growth factor (SGF): Specific binding to epidermal growth factor (EGF) membrane receptors. *J. Cell. Physiol.* **102:**267–277.

56. Marquadt, H., Hunkapiller, M. W., Hood, L. E., and Todaro, G. J., 1984, Rat transforming growth factor type I: Structure and relationship to epidermal growth factor, *Science* **223**:1079–1082.

57. Derynck, R., Roberts, A. B., Eaton, D. H., Winkler, M. E., and Geodel, D. V., 1985, Human transforming growth factor-alpha: Precursor sequence, gene structure and heterologous expression, in: *Cancer Cells.* Vol. 3: *Growth Factors and Transformation* (J. Feramisco, B. Ozanne, and C. Stiles, eds.), pp. 79–86, Cold Spring Harbor Laboratory, New York.

58. Schreiber, A. B., Winkler, M. E., and Dernyck, R., 1986, Transforming growth factor-alpha: A more potent angiogenic mediator than epidermal growth factor, *Science* **232**:1250–1253.

59. Derynck, R., Jarrett, J. A., Chen, E. Y., Eaton, D. H., Bell, J. R., Assoian, R. K., Roberts, A. B., Sporn, M. B., and Goeddel, D., 1985, Human transforming growth factor-beta cDNA sequence and expression in normal and transfected cells, *Nature (Lond.)* **316**:701–705.

60. Childs, C. B., Proper, J. A., Tucker, R. F., and Moses, H. L., 1982, Serum contains a platelet-derived transforming growth factor, *Proc. Natl. Acad. Sci. USA* **79**:5312–5316.

61. Assoian, R. K., Komoriya, A., Meyers, C. A., Miller, D. M., and Sporn, M. B., 1983, Transforming growth factor-beta in human platelets. Identification of a major storage site, purification, and characterization, *J. Biol. Chem.* **258**:7155–7160.

62. Roberts, A. B., Sporn, M. B., Assoian, R. K., Smith, J. M., Roche, N. S., Wakefield, L. M., Heine, U. I., Liotta, L. A., Falanga, V., Kehrl, J. H., and Fauci, A. S., 1986, Transforming growth factor type beta: Rapid induction of fibrosis and angiogenesis in vivo and stimulation of collagen formation in vitro, *Proc. Natl. Acad. Sci. USA* **83**:4167–4171.

63. Baird, A., and Durkin, T., 1986, Inhibition of endothelial cell proliferation by type beta-transforming growth factor: Interactions with acidic and basic fibroblast growth factors, *Biochem. Biophys. Res. Commun.* **138**:476–481.

64. Heimark, R. L., Twardzik, D. R., and Schwartz, S. M., 1986, Inhibition of endothelial regeneration by type-beta transforming growth factor from platelets, *Science* **233**:1078–1080.

65. Gospodarowicz, D., Bialecki, H., and Greenburg, G., 1978, Purification of the fibroblast growth factor activity from bovine brain, *J. Biol. Chem.* **253**:3736–3743.

66. Maciag, T., Cerundolo, J., Ilsey, S., Kelley, P. R., and Forand, R., 1979, An endothelial cell growth factor from bovine hypothalamus: Identification and partial characterization, *Proc. Natl. Acad. Sci. USA* **76**:5674–5678.

67. Gospodarowicz, D., 1975, Purification of a fibroblast growth factor from bovine pituitary, *J. Biol. Chem.* **250**:2515–2520.

68. Gospodarowicz, D., Mescher, A. L., and Birdwell, C., 1977, Stimulation of corneal endothelial cell proliferation in vitro by fibroblast and epidermal growth factors, *Exp. Eye Res.* **25**:75–89.

69. Gospodarowicz, D., Bialecki, H., and Thakral, T. K., 1979, The angiogenic activity of the fibroblast and epidermal growth factor, *Exp. Eye Res.* **28**:501–514.

70. Lemmon, S. K., Riley, M. C., Thomas, K. A., Hoover, G. A., Maciag, T., and Bradshaw, R. A., 1982, Bovine fibroblast growth factor: Comparison of brain and pituitary preparations. *J. Cell Biol.* **95**:162–169.

71. Maciag, T., Hoover, G. A., and Weinstein, R., 1982, High and low molecular weight forms of endothelial cell growth factor, *J. Biol. Chem.* **257**:5333–5336.

72. D'Amore, P. A., Glaser, B. M., Brunson, S. K., and Fenselau, A. H., 1981, Angiogenic activity from bovine retina: Partial purification and characterization, *Proc. Natl. Acad. Sci. USA* **78**:3068–3072.

73. Barritault, D., Arruti, C., and Courtois, Y., 1981, Is there a ubiquitous growth factor in the eye?, *Differentiation* **18**:29–42.

74. Klagsbrun, M., and Smith, S., 1980, Purification of a cartilage-derived growth factor, *J. Biol. Chem.* **255**:10859–10866.

75. Shing, Y., Folkman, J., Sullivan, R., Butterfield, C., Murray, J., and Klagsbrun, M., 1984, Heparin affinity: Purification of a tumor-derived capillary endothelial cell growth factor, *Science* **223**:1296–1298.

76. Klagsbrun, M., and Shing, Y., 1985, Heparin affinity of anionic and cationic capillary endothelial cell growth factors: Analysis of hypothalamus-derived growth factors and fibroblast growth factors, *Proc. Natl. Acad. Sci. USA* **82**:805–809.

77. Sullivan, R., and Klagsbrun, M., 1985, Purification of cartilage-derived growth factor by heparin affinity chromatography, *J. Biol. Chem.* **260**:2399–2403.

78. D'Amore, P. A., and Klagsbrun, M., 1984, Endothelial cell mitogens derived from retina and hypothalamus: Biochemical and biological similarities, *J. Cell Biol.* **99**:1545–1549.

79. Gospodarowicz, D., Cheng, J., Liu, G.-M., Baird, A., and Bohlen, P., 1984, Isolation of brain fibroblast growth factor by heparin-Sepharose affinity chromatography: Identity with pituitary fibroblast growth factor, *Proc. Natl. Acad. Sci. USA* **81**:6963–6967.

80. Lobb, R. R., and Fett, J. W., 1984, Purification of two distinct growth factors from bovine neural tissue by heparin affinity chromatography, *Biochemistry* **23:**6295–6299.
81. Maciag, T., Mehlman, T., Friesel, R., and Schrieber, A., 1984, Heparin binds endothelial cell growth factor, the principal mitogen in the bovine brain, *Science* **225:**932–935.
82. Conn, G., and Hatcher, V. B., 1984, The isolation and purification of two anionic endothelial cell growth factors from human brain, *Biochem. Biophys. Res. Commun.* **124:**262–268.
83. Baird, A., Esch, F., Gospodarowicz, D., and Guillemin, R., 1986, Retina and eye derived endothelial cell growth factors: Partial molecular characterization and identity with acidic and basic fibroblast growth factors, *Biochemistry* **24:**7855–7860.
84. Courty, J., Loret, C., Moenner, M., Chevallier, B., Lagente, Y., Courtois, Y., and Barritault, D., 1985, Bovine retina contains three growth factor activities with different affinity to heparin: Eye derived growth factor I, II, III, *Biochim.* **67:**265–269.
85. Lobb, R., Sasse, J., Sullivan, R., Shing, Y., D'Amore, P., Jacobs, J., and Klagsbrun, M., 1986, Purification and characterization of heparin-binding endothelial cell growth factors, *J. Biol. Chem.* **261:**1924–1928.
86. Schreiber, A. B., Kenney, J., Kowalski, J., Thomas, K. A., Gimenez-Gallego, G., Rios-Candelore, M., DiSalvo, J., Barritault, D., Courty, J., Courtois, Y., Moenner, M., Loret, C., Burgess, W. H., Mehlman, T., Friesel, R., Johnson, W., and Maciag, T., 1985, A unique family of endothelial cell polypeptide mitogens: The antigenic and receptor cross-reactivity of bovine endothelial cell growth factor, brain-derived acidic fibroblast growth factor, and eye-derived growth factor II, *J. Cell Biol.* **101:**1623–1626.
87. Esch, F., Baird, A., Ling, N., Ueno, N., Hill, F., Denoroy, L., Klepper, R., Gospodarowicz, D., Bohlen, P., and Guillemin, R., 1985, Primary structure of bovine pituitary basic fibroblast growth factor (FGF) and comparison with the amino-terminal sequence of bovine brain acidic FGF, *Proc. Natl. Acad. Sci. USA* **82:**6507–6511.
88. Gimenez-Gallego, G., Rodkey, J., Bennett, C., Rios-Candelore, M., DiSalvo, J., and Thomas, K., 1985, Brain-derived acidic fibroblast growth factor: Complete amino acid sequence and homologies, *Science* **230:**1385–1388.
89. Esch, F., Ueno, N., Baird, A., Hill, F., Denroy, L., Ling, N., Gospodarowicz, D., and Guillemin, R., 1985, Primary structure of bovine brain acidic fibroblast growth factor, *Biochem. Biophys. Res. Commun.* **133:**554–562.
90. Thomas, K. A., Rios-Candelore, M., Gimenez-Gallego, G., DiSalvo, J., Bennett, C., Rodkey, J., and Fitzpatrick, S., 1985, Pure brain-derived acidic growth factor is a potent angiogenic vascular endothelial cell mitogen with sequence homology to interleukin I, *Proc. Natl. Acad. Sci. USA* **82:**6409–6413.
91. Burgess, W. H., Mehlman, T., Freisel, R., Johnson, W. V., and Maciag, T., 1985, Multiple forms of endothelial cell growth factor, *J. Biol. Chem.* **260:**11389–11392.
92. Pettmann, B., Weibel, M., Sensenbrenner, M., and Labourdette, G., 1985, Purification of two astroglial growth factors from bovine brain, *FEBS Lett.* **189:**102–108.
93. Hauschka, P., Mavarakos, A. E., Iafrati, M. D., Doleman, S. E., and Klagsbrun, M., 1986, Growth factors in bone matrix, *J. Biol. Chem.* **261:**12665–12674.
94. Bohlen, P., Baird, A., Esch, F., Ling, N., and Gospodarowicz, D., 1984, Isolation and partial molecular characterization of pituitary fibroblast growth factor, *Proc. Natl. Acad. Sci. USA* **81:**5364–5368.
95. Gospodarowicz, D., Cheng, J., Lui, G. M., Esch, F., and Bohlen, P., 1985, Corpus luteum angiogenic factor is related to fibroblast growth factor, *Endocrinology* **117:**2382–2391.
96. Gospodarowicz, D., Baird, A., Cheng, J., Lui, F., Esch, F., and Bohlen, P., 1986, Isolation of fibroblast growth factor from bovine adrenal gland: Physicochemical and biological characterization, *Endocrinology* **118:**82–90.
97. Baird, A., Esch, F., Bohlen, P., Ling, N., and Gospodarowicz, D., 1985, Isolation and partial characterization of an endothelial cell growth factor from the bovine kidney: Homology with basic fibroblast growth factor, *Regul. Peptides* **12:**201–213.
98. Moscatelli, D., Presta, M., and Rifkin, D. B., 1986, Purification of a factor from human placenta that stimulates capillary endothelial cell protease production, DNA synthesis, and migration, *Proc. Natl. Acad. Sci. USA* **83:**2091–2095.
99. Baird, A., Mormede, P., and Bohlen, P., 1985, Immunoreactive fibroblast growth factor in cells of peritoneal exudate suggests its identity with macrophage-derived growth factor, *Biochem. Biophys. Res. Commun.* **126:**358–364.
100. Klagsbrun, M., Sasse, J., Sullivan, R., and Smith, J. A., 1986, Human tumor cells synthesize an endothelial cell growth factor that is structurally related to basic fibroblast growth factor, *Proc. Natl. Acad. Sci. USA* **83:**2448–2452.

101. Schweigerer, L., Neufeld, G., Friedman, J., Abraham, J. A., Fiddes, J. C., and Gospodarowicz, D., 1987, Capillary endothelial cells express basic fibroblast growth factor, a mitogen that promotes their own growth, *Nature (Lond.)* **325:**257–259.

102. Risau, W., 1986, Developing brain produces an angiogenesis factor, *Proc. Natl. Acad. Sci. USA* **83:**3855–3859.

103. Klagsbrun, M., Sasse, J., Smith, S., and Sullivan, R., 1987, Processing of brain and tumor-derived fibroblast growth factors by acid-activated proteases, *Proc. Natl. Acad. Sci. USA* **84:**1839–1843.

104. Burgess, W. H., Mehlman, T., Marshak, D. R., Fraser, B. A., and Maciag, T., 1986, Structural evidence that endothelial cell growth factor-beta is the precursor of both endothelial cell growth factor-alpha and acidic fibroblast growth factor, *Proc. Natl. Acad. Sci. USA* **83:**7216–7220.

105. Ueno, N., Baird, A., Esch, F., Ling, N., and Guillemin, R., 1986, Isolation of an amino terminal extended form of basic fibroblast growth factor, *Biochem. Biophys. Res. Commun.* **138:**580–588.

106. Friesel, R., Burgess, W. H., Mehlman, T., and Maciag, T., 1986, The characterization of the receptor for endothelial cell growth factor by covalent ligand attachment, *J. Biol. Chem.* **261:**7581–7584.

107. Neufeld, G., and Gospodarowicz, D., 1985, The identification and partial characterization of the fibroblast growth factor receptor of baby hamster kidney cells, *J. Biol. Chem.* **260:**13860–13868.

108. Moenner, M., Chevallier, B., Badet, J., and Barritault, D., 1986, Evidence and characterization of the receptor to eye-derived growth factor I, the retinal form of basic fibroblast growth factor, on bovine epithelial lens cells, *Proc. Natl. Acad. Sci. USA* **83:**5024–5028.

109. Olwin, B. B., and Hauschka, S. D., 1986, Identification of the fibroblast growth factor receptor of Swiss 3T3 cells and mouse skeletal muscle myoblasts, *Biochemistry* **25:**3487–3492.

110. Huang, S. S., and Huang, J. S., 1986, Association of bovine brain-derived growth factor receptor with protein kinase activity, *J. Biol. Chem.* **261:**9568–9571.

111. Moscatelli, D., 1987, High and low affinity binding sites for basic fibroblast growth factor on cultured cells: Absence of a role for low affinity binding in the stimulation of plasminogen activator production by bovine capillary endothelial cells, *J. Cell. Physiol.* **131:**123–130.

112. Montesano, R., Vassalli, J-D., Baird, A., Guillemin, R., and Orci, L., 1986, Basic fibroblast growth factor induces angiogenesis in vitro, *Proc. Natl. Acad. Sci. USA* **83:**7297–7301.

113. Herman, I. M., and D'Amore, P. A., 1984, Capillary endothelial cell migration: Loss of stress fibres in response to retina-derived growth factor, *J. Muscle. Res. Cell. Motil.* **5:**697–709.

114. Senior, R. M., Huang, S. S., Griffin, G. L., and Huang, J. S., 1986, Brain-derived growth factor is a chemoattractant for fibroblasts and astroglial cells, *Biochem. Biophys. Res. Commun.* **141:**67–72.

115. Halaban, R., and Baird, A., 1987, bFGF is the putative natural growth factor for human melanocytes, *In Vitro Cell Dev. Biol.* **23:**47–52.

116. Phadke, K., 1987, Fibroblast growth factor enhances the interleukin-1-mediated chondrocytic protease release, *Biochem. Biophys. Res. Commun.* **142:**448–453.

117. Schweigerer, L., Neufeld, G., Mergia, A., Abraham, J. A., Fiddes, J. C., and Gospodarowicz, D., 1987, Basic fibroblast growth factor in human rhabdomyosarcoma cells: Implications for the proliferation and neovascularization of myoblast-derived tumors, *Proc. Natl. Acad. Sci. USA* **84:**842–846.

118. Wagner, J. A., and D'Amore, P. A., 1986, Neurite outgrowth induced by an endothelial cell mitogen isolated from retina, *J. Cell Biol.* **103:**1363–1367.

119. Togari, A., Dickens, G., Kuzuya, H., and Guroff, G., 1985, The effect of fibroblast growth factor on PC12 cells, *J. Neurosci.* **5:**307–316.

120. Lipton, S. A., Wanger, J. A., Madison, R. D., and D'Amore, P. A., 1988, Acidic fibroblast growth factor enhances regeneration of processes by postnatal mammalian retinal ganglion cells in culture, *Proc. Natl. Acad. Sci. USA* **85:**2388–2392.

121. Morrison, R. S., Sharma, A., de Vellis, J., and Bradshaw, J., 1986, Basic fibroblast growth factor supports the survival of cerebral cortical neurons in primary culture, *Proc. Natl. Acad. Sci. USA* **83:**7537–7541.

122. Walicke, P., Cowan, W. M., Ueno, N., Baird, A., and Guillemin, R., 1986, Fibroblast growth factor promotes survival of dissociated hippocampal neurons and enhances neurite extension, *Proc. Natl. Acad. Sci. USA* **83:**3012–3016.

123. Wice, B., Milbrandt, J., and Glaser, L., 1987, Control of muscle differentiation in BC3H1 cells by fibroblast growth factor and vanadate, *J. Biol. Chem.* **262:**1810–1817.

124. Lobb, R. R., Alderman, E. M., and Fett, J. W., 1985, Induction of angiogenesis by bovine brain derived class 1 heparin-binding growth factor, *Biochemistry* **24:**4869–4873.

125. Davidson, J. M., Klagsbrun, M., Hill, K. E., Buckley, A., Sullivan, R., Brewer, P. S., and Woodward,

S. C., 1985, Accelerated wound repair, cell proliferation, and collagen accumulation are produced by a cartilage-derived growth factor, *J. Cell Biol.* **100:**1219–1227.

126. Buntrock, P., Buntrock, M., Marx, I., Kranz, D., Jentzch, K. D., and Heder, G., 1984, Stimulation of wound healing, using brain extract with fibroblast growth factor (FGF) activity, *Exp. Pathol.* **26:**247–254.

127. Cuny, R., Jeanny, J-C., and Courtous, Y., 1986, Lens regeneration from cultured newt irises stimulated by retina-derived growth factors (EDGF's), *Differentiation* **32:**221–229.

128. Slack, J. M. W., Darlington, B. G., Heath, J. K., and Godsave, S. F., 1987, Mesoderm induction in early Xenopus embryos by heparin-binding growth factors, *Nature (Lond.)* **326:**197–200.

129. Polverini, P. J., and Leibovich, S. J., 1985, Induction of neovascularization and nonlymphoid mesenchymal cell proliferation by macrophage cell lines, *J. Leukocyte. Biol.* **37:**279–288.

130. Vlodavsky, I., Folkman, J., Sullivan, R., Fridman, R., Ishai-Michaeli, R., Sasse, J., and Klagsbrun, M., 1987, Endothelial cell-derived basic fibroblast growth factor: Synthesis and deposition in subendothelial extracellular matrix, *Proc. Natl. Acad. Sci. USA* **84:**2292–2296.

131. Folkman, J., Klagsbrun, M., Sasse, J., Wadzinski, M., Ingber, D., and Vlodavsky, I., 1988, A heparin-binding angiogenic protein—basic fibroblast growth factor—is stored within basement membrane, *Am. J. Pathol.* **130:**393–400.

# 27

# Tumor Invasion and Metastases
## Biochemical Mechanisms

## Lance A. Liotta, Mary L. Stracke, Ulla M. Wewer, and Elliott Schiffmann

### 1. MULTISTEP CASCADE OF METASTASES

A metastatic colony is the end result of a complicated series of tumor–host interactions.[1,2] Potential mechanisms underlying this complex process are outlined in Table I. In this regard, primary tumor initiation and promotion are followed by the transition from *in situ* to locally invasive cancer and angiogenesis.[3–6] Newly formed tumor vessels are often defective and easily invaded by tumor cells within the primary mass. At the invasion front, tumor cells also invade pre-established host blood vessels. Tumor cells are discharged into the venous drainage in single cell form and in clumps. For rapidly growing tumors 1 cm in size, millions of tumor cells can be shed into the circulation every day. Fortunately for the patient, only a very small percentage (< .01%) of circulating tumor cells initiate metastatic colonies. Tumors generally lack a well-formed lymphatic network. Therefore, communication of tumor cells with lymphatic channels occurs only at the tumor periphery and not within the tumor mass. Tumor cells entering the lymphatic drainage are carried to regional lymph nodes where they arrest in the subcapsular sinus. Within 10–60 min after initial arrest in the lymph node, a significant fraction of the tumor cells detach and enter the efferent lymphatics. These tumor cells eventually end up in the regional or systemic venous drainage due to the existence of numerous lymphatic–hematogenous communications. Thus, the regional lymph node does not function as a true mechanical barrier to tumor dissemination. Lymphatic and hematogenous dissemination occurs in parallel (see also Chapter 28).

Circulating tumor cells use a variety of means to arrest in the vessels of the target organ, where they will initiate metastatic colonies (Fig. 1). Approximately 80% of the circulating tumor cells are in single cell form and directly attach to the intact endothelial surface, or to pre-existing regions of exposed subendothelial basement membrane. Clumps of circulating tumor cells or tumor cells aggregated with host leukocytes, fibrin, or platelets can embolize directly in the precapillary venules by mechanical impaction. Tumor cells in single cell or clump form adhere to the endothelial luminal surface of arterioles. The fate and time course of the arrested tumor cells differs depending on the mechanism and location of lodgement. Tumor cells adherent to the surface of venule or capillary endothelium rapidly induce (within 1–4 hr) the active retraction of the endothelial cells. The tumor

*Lance A. Liotta, Mary L. Stracke, Ulla M. Wewer, and Elliott Schiffmann* • Laboratory of Pathology, National Cancer Institute, National Institutes of Health, Bethesda, Maryland 20892. *Present address for U.M.W.:* University Institute of Pathologic Anatomy, 2100 Copenhagen, Denmark.

Table I. Events and Potential Mechanisms
Associated with the Metastatic Cascade

| Metastatic cascade event | Potential mechanisms |
| --- | --- |
| Tumor initiation | Carcinogenic insult, oncogene activation or derepression, chromosomal rearrangement |
| Promotion and progression | Karyotypic, genetic, and epigenetic instability, gene amplification; promotion-associated genes and hormones |
| Uncontrolled proliferation | Autocrine growth factors or their receptors, receptors for host hormones such as estrogen |
| Angiogenesis | Multiple angiogenesis factors, including known growth factors |
| Invasion of local tissues and vascular walls of blood and lymphatic vessels, and intravasation | Serum chemoattractants, autocrine motility factors, attachment receptors, degradative enzymes |
| Circulating tumor cell arrest and extravasation | Tumor cell homotypic or heterotypic aggregation |
| Adherence to endothelium | Tumor cell interaction with fibrin, platelets, and clotting factors, adhesion to RGD-type receptors |
| Retraction of endothelium | Platelet factors, tumor cell factors |
| Adhesion to basement membrane | Laminin receptor, thrombospondin receptor |
| Dissolution of basement membrane | Degradative proteases, type IV collagenase, heparanase, cathepsins |
| Locomotion | Autocrine motility factors, chemotaxis factors |
| Colony formation at secondary site | Receptors for local tissue growth factors, angiogenesis factors |
| Evasion and host defenses and resistance to therapy | Resistance to killing by host macrophages, natural killer cells and activated T cells, failure to express, or blocking of, tumor-specific antigens, amplification of drug-resistant genes |

cell then attaches avidly to the exposed basement membrane. Once the tumor cells have attached, the adjacent endothelial cells extend over the tumor cell and separate it from the bloodstream. Tumor cells located between the endothelium and the basement membrane are held up in this location for 8–24 hr. Local dissolution of the basement membrane is then observed in association with a tumor cell pseudopodia traversing the basement membrane. This step is soon followed by complete extravasation of the tumor cell and quite often re-establishment of blood flow in the breached vessel. Tumor cells arrested in the arterial tree can remain in this location for two or three weeks. Endothelial retraction does not occur following arterial arrest. Intra-arterial tumor cells can actually proliferate and expand as colonies. As the tumor colonies enlarge, they become covered by a host endothelial surface that lacks a basement membrane. Once the tumor colony fills the arteriole, mechanical damage to the endothelium occurs, and this exposes the basement membrane. Tumor cells at the periphery of the interarterial colony then invade through the basement membrane and the elastic lamina of the arteriole wall to gain an extravascular position.

At all stages of the metastatic cascade, tumor cells must overcome host defenses.[3–5] Although tumor-specific antigens have been identified in animal models, it still remains unclear whether

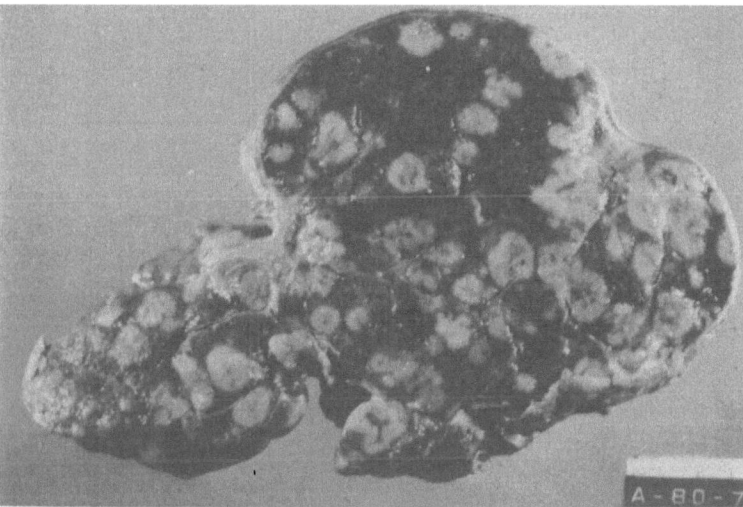

*Figure 1.* Multiple metastatic colonies in the liver of a patient who presented with an adenocarcinoma of the breast.

similar antigens play a role in human tumors, and whether the recognition of these antigens can be boosted by adjuvant immunotherapy (see Chapter 28). Limited effectiveness of adjuvent immunotherapy of metastases may be due to tumor antigen heterogeneity, tumor antigen shedding, or absence of tumor cell immunogenicity. Nonspecific host defenses such as macrophages and natural killer (NK) cells may be more effective against heterogeneous tumor cell populations. In animal models, these effector cells play an important role in the elimination of circulating tumor cells, and destruction of micrometastases.

Extravasated tumor cells proliferate as colonies but require a new vascular supply to grow larger than 0.5 mm. Thus, angiogenesis is necessary at the beginning and the end of the metastatic cascade. Metastases can themselves metastasize, further amplifying the level of disease progression. Numerous clinical reports provide circumstantial evidence for the existence of dormant metastases.[7] Up to one third of the mortality from breast cancer, for instance, occurs more than 5 years after removal of the primary tumor. Three potential mechanisms of tumor dormancy have been distinguished in animal models: (1) immunologic restraint such that the tumor population death rate equals its growth rate, (2) constitutive dependency of tumor cells on host growth factors, and (3) avascularity causing the metastasis to be limited in size due to deficiency in nutrient diffusion.

## 2. ORGAN TROPISM FOR METASTASES

The distribution of metastases varies widely depending on the histologic type and anatomic location of the primary tumor (Table II). The most frequent organ location of distant metastasis in many types of cancer appears to be the first capillary bed encountered by the circulating cells. Major pathways of metastases determined directly by anatomic considerations are listed as follows:

1. Sarcomas arising in the extremities metastasize primarily to the lungs. Sarcoma cells entering the tumor venous drainage are carried into the inferior vena cava, enter the right heart, and are carried via the pulmonary artery to the lungs.
2. Lung cancer disseminates widely to multiple organs including brain. Lung cancer is the only tumor that has direct access to the general arterial circulation via the pulmonary vein through the left heart ventricle.[3]

Table II. Autopsy Incidence of Metastases
in Humans[a]

| Organ of metastases | Primary tumor (%) | | | |
|---|---|---|---|---|
| | Lung | Colon | Breast | Melanoma |
| Liver | 30–50 | 50–60 | 40–60 | 58–70 |
| Lung | 20–40 | 25–40 | 60–80 | 66–80 |
| Bone | 30–45 | 5–10 | 50–90 | 30–48 |
| Brain | 15–43 | 0–1 | 15–30 | 40–55 |
| Adrenal | 17–38 | 14 | 38–54 | 40–47 |
| Pituitary | 0–2 | 0–1 | 20 | 18 |
| Ovary | 0–2 | 14 | 15–30 | 10–15 |
| Kidney | 16–23 | 8 | 13 | 31–35 |
| Spleen | 9 | 5 | 17 | 31 |

[a]Data adapted from reference 7 and incorporating the body of experience at the Laboratory of Pathology, NCI, NIH.

3. Colorectal carcinomas tend to metastasize to the liver. Colorectal carcinoma cells enter the mesenteric lymphatics and portal venous system and are carried to the liver.[3,7]
4. Tumors of the testicle metastasize via the lymphatics to lymph nodes of the periaortic area and then enter the subclavian veins by lymphatic–hematogenous communications. Tumor cells entering the subclavian veins go to the right heart and then to the lungs.[3,7,8]
5. Prostate cancer metastasizes primarily (90%) to vertebral bone. The anatomic route is via Batson's plexus of paravertebral veins.[8] Tumor cells entering the prostatic plexus of veins are carried to the veins about the sacrum, ilium, and the lumbar spine.
6. Patterns of head and neck cancer metastases correspond primarily to the regions of local lymphatic drainage.[7]
7. Ovarian cancer remains confined for long periods of time in the abdominal cavity. Local spread occurs to the peritoneal surfaces, the posterior paracolic gutters, and the diaphragm. These tumors invade the liver in only a small percentage of cases at a very late stage. Liver invasion is usually by direct invasion from omental disease or by mesenteric venous emboli derived from omental implants.[7]
8. Breast cancer metastases are frequently found in vertebral bone. Based on dye injection studies, it has been demonstrated that the mammary venous drainage can communicate with Batson's plexus of paravertebral veins.[8] When dye was injected into a small mammary vein, the dye was found in the clavicles, intercostal veins, head of the humerus, cervical vertebrae, and transverse cranial sinuses.

However, there are many metastatic sites which cannot be predicted based on anatomic considerations alone, and can be considered examples of organ tropism. For example, in the human, clear cell carcinoma of the kidney often metastasizes to bone and thyroid, bronchogenic carcinoma metastasizes to the adrenal, and ocular melanoma frequently metastasizes to the liver. Theoretical mechanisms for organ tropism include the following[3,5]: (1) tumor cells disseminate equally in all organs, but preferentially grow only in specific organs (preferential growth may be induced by local growth factors or hormones present in the target organ for metastases) (2) circulating tumor cells may adhere preferentially to the endothelial luminal surface only in the target organ for metastases. This hypothesis predicts organ-specific endothelial determinants and (3) circulating tumor cells may respond to soluble factors diffusing locally out of the target organ. Such factors could act in a chemotactic fashion to attract the tumor cells to extravasate. They could also cause the circulating tumor cells to aggregate and therefore embolize in the target organ. Research with animal models indicates that all of these mechanisms play a role to various degrees, depending on the tumor model system.[3,5]

## 3. TUMOR CELL INTERACTION WITH THE EXTRACELLULAR MATRIX

The mammalian organism is composed of a series of tissue compartments separated from each other by two types of extracellular matrix: basement membranes and interstitial stroma.[4] The matrix determines tissue architecture, has important biologic functions, and exists as a mechanical barrier to invasion. During the transition from *in situ* to invasive carcinoma, tumor cells penetrate the epithelial basement membrane and enter the underlying interstitial stroma. Once the tumor cells enter the stroma, they gain access to lymphatics and blood vessels for further dissemination. Fibrosarcomas and angiosarcomas, developing from stromal cells, invade surrounding muscle basement membrane and destroy myocytes. Tumor cells must cross basement membranes to invade nerve and most types of organ parenchyma. During intravasation or extravasation, the tumor cells of any histologic origin must penetrate the subendothelial basement membrane. In the distant organ where metastases colonies are initiated, extravasated tumor cells must migrate through the perivascular interstitial stroma before tumor colony growth occurs in the organ parenchyma. Therefore, tumor cell interaction with the extracellular matrix occurs at multiple stages in the metastatic cascade.

General and widespread changes occur in the organization, distribution, and quantity of the epithelial basement membrane during the transition from benign to invasive carcinoma. The human breast serves as a particularly good example for demonstrating these changes. Benign proliferative disorders of the breast such as fibrocystic disease, sclerosing adenosis, intraductal hyperplasia, fibroadenoma, and intraductal papilloma are all characterized by disorganization of the normal epithelial stromal architecture. Extreme forms can mimic the appearance of invasive carcinoma. However, no matter how extensive the architectural disorganization, these benign disorders are always characterized by a continuous basement membrane separating the epithelium from the stroma. In contrast, invasive ductual carcinoma, invasive lobular carcinoma, and tubular carcinoma all consistently possess a defective extracellular basement membrane with zones of basement membrane loss around the invading tumor cells in the stroma. The basement membrane is also markedly defective adjacent to tumor cells in lymph node and organ metastases. In some focal regions of well-differentiated carcinoma, partial basement membrane formation by differentiated structures can be identified. These findings are of direct application to diagnostic problems in surgical pathology, such as the differentiation of tangential sections of *in situ* lesions from true invasion, or differentiating severe adenosis from invasive carcinoma. Loss of basement membranes in human carcinomas significantly correlates with increased incidence of metastases and poor 5-year survival.

## 4. THREE-STEP THEORY OF INVASION

A three-step hypothesis has been proposed to describing the sequence of biochemical events during tumor cell invasion of extracellular matrix.[2,4] The first step is tumor cell attachment to the matrix. Attachment may be mediated through specific glycoproteins such as laminin and fibronectin through tumor cell plasma membrane receptors. Following attachment, the tumor cell secretes hydrolytic enzymes (or induces host cells to secrete enzymes) which can locally degrade the matrix, including degradation of the attachment glycoproteins. Matrix lysis most likely takes place in a highly localized region close to the tumor cell surface, where the amount of active enzyme outbalances the natural protease inhibitors present in the serum and in the matrix itself. In contrast to an invasive tumor cell, when a normal cell or benign tumor cell attaches to the matrix, the cell may respond by shifting into a resting or differentiated state. The third step is tumor cell locomotion into the region of the matrix modified by proteolysis. The direction of the locomotion may be influenced by chemotactic factors and autocrine motility factors. Autocrine motility factors (AMF) are a newly described class of proteins (see section below) which bind to a cell surface receptor and profoundly stimulate motility.[4] They are distinct from known growth factors, and their mechanism of action involves the membrane G protein pathway, which is inhibited by pertussis toxin. The chemotactic factors derived from serum, organ parenchyma, or the matrix itself[3,6] may influence the organ specificity of metastases. Continued invasion of the matrix may take place by cyclic repetition of these three steps.

## 5. TUMOR CELL MOTILITY FACTORS

Cell motility is necessary for tumor cells to traverse many stages in the complex cascade of invasion. Such stages could include the detachment and subsequent infiltration of cells from the primary tumor into adjacent tissue, the migration of the cells through the vascular wall into the circulation (intravasation), and the extravasation of the cells to a secondary site. The movement of cells through biologic barriers such as the endothelial basement membranes of the vasculature may well occur by means of chemotactic mechanisms. Indeed, studies on *in vitro* chemotaxis of some tumor cells indicate that a variety of compounds such as complement-derived materials, collagen peptides, formyl peptides, and certain connective tissue components can act as chemoattractants.[9,10] While these agents may well contribute to the directional aspects of a motile response, they are not sufficient to initiate the intrinsic locomotion of tumor cells. The availability of soluble attractants to the tumor cell is greatly dependent upon the host, even in those cases in which the production of attractants is the result of tumor cell-host tissue interaction. At best, it seems that the cell would have access to such motility stimuli at sporadic and irregular intervals. Such conditions are unfavorable to a sustained migration of highly invasive cells. With these considerations in mind and stimulated by the studies of Todaro and Sporn and co-workers,[11] in which they demonstrated autocrine growth factors for transformed cells, we investigated the possibility that such cells could elaborate autocrine motility factors. The action of these substances might, in part, explain both the markedly invasive character and the metastatic property of malignant neoplastic cells. Thus, under the influence of such an autocrine material, a tumor cell might move out into the surrounding host tissue and also exert a "recruiting" effect on adjacent tumor cells in the presence of a gradient of attractant (Fig. 2). Conceivably, such factors might also attract fibroblastic cells of the host, resulting in the phenomenon of desmoplasia, characteristic of invasive tumors.

We have found that the human melanoma cell line A2058 and human breast carcinoma cells produce in culture a material that markedly stimulates their own motility.[12] These cells respond in a dose-dependent manner to various concentrations of conditioned medium obtained by incubating confluent cells in serum-free medium, an indication that the motility factor is derived from the cell. Motility was measured by the modified Boyden chamber procedure. Using this assay and the checkerboard analysis,[13] we have also found that the conditioned medium factor has both chemotactic (directional) and chemokinetic (randomly motile) properties.

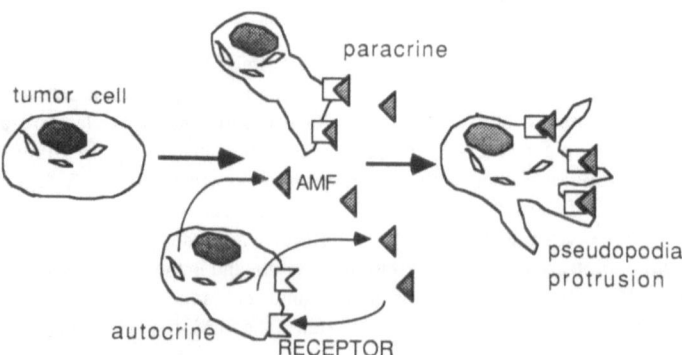

*Figure 2.* AMF hypothesis. Invasive malignant neoplastic cells produce a protein factor (AMF) that binds to specific cell-surface receptors resulting in the triggering of an intrinsic motile response. The factor(s) can also recruit neighboring cells via a paracrine mechanism.

## 6. ISOLATION AND CHARACTERIZATION OF A HUMAN MELANOMA AUTOCRINE MOTILITY FACTOR

Conditioned protein-free medium from A2058 melanoma cultures, which elicited both large (10–15% of the cells migrated) dose-dependent chemotactic and randomly motile responses (checkerboard analysis) was used to isolate AMF. The conditioned medium, after concentration by Amicon filtration, was subjected to molecular sieve chromatography. AMF emerged as a broad major peak at 40,000–65,000 $M_r$ (data not shown). The AMF was further isolated by fast-performance liquid chromatography.

The AMF activity was iodinated and found to be composed of a single major component by sodium dodecyl sulfated polyacrylamide gel electrophoresis (SDS–PAGE) of ~55,000 $M_r$ without reduction of disulfide bonds. Upon reduction with 5 mM dithiothreitol, the migration of this component on the gel became slower, indicating the existence of interchain disulfide bonds. A maximal chemotactic response to the purified AMF was elicited at a concentration of 10 nM. Amino acid analysis of AMF revealed a high content of hydrophobic residues. Both tyrosine and cysteine are present, the latter concordant with the existence of interchain disulfide bonds as indicated by the altered electrophoretic mobility of AMF before and after treatment with dithiothreitol. The amino terminal region of AMF was sequenced and found to constitute a unique protein.

## 7. TRANSDUCTION OF THE CHEMICAL SIGNAL IN THE MOTILE RESPONSE OF TUMOR CELLS

Because some cells require ongoing protein synthesis to develop a motile response, we determined if inhibition of protein synthesis affected the response of the A2058 melanoma cells to its autocrine factor. We found that concentrations of cycloheximide that eliminated *de novo* protein synthesis had no effect on stimulated cell motility. Therefore, the cell protein components required for developing a motile response appear to be stable for the duration of migration (4 hr).

Studies with leukocytes[14,15] have implicated a guanine nucleotide protein (G protein) in the receptor-mediated initiation of a motile response in these cells. The evidence is convincing that the locomotion of certain tumor cells also directly involves a G-protein.[16] Pertussis toxin, known to inhibit action of the Gi protein of the adenylate cyclase pathway,[17] profoundly and rapidly inhibited the AMF-stimulated migration *in vitro* of A2058 melanoma cells[4] and two breast cancer cell lines.[18] In the melanoma cell line, 0.5 µg/ml of pertussis toxin completely blocked motility without affecting growth in culture.[19] However, the adenylate cyclase pathway does not appear to be directly involved in the motility response, since agents that selectively modulate or have a role in this pathway (e.g., cholera toxin, forskolin, the cAMP analogue 8-bromoadenosine 3':5'-cyclic monophosphate, and the cyclase inhibitor 2',5'-dideoxyadenosine) all had minor effects on cell migration. It is likely, then, that effector systems other than that of adenylate cyclase are mediated by a G protein in producing tumor cell motility.

G proteins have been shown to act in a variety of second messenger pathways including phospholipase A2,[20] phospholipase C,[21] and activation of calcium channels.[22] Specifically, in the neutrophil, pertussis toxin inhibits both lipase enzymes as well as cell motility.[23,24] Evidence that suggests a role for phospholipase A2 in tumor cell locomotion has been obtained with the melanoma cell. Quinacrine, an agent that inhibits phospholipase A2, markedly reduced AMF-stimulated migration. In addition, deaza-adenosine, an inhibitor of biological methylation,[25] was found to markedly reduce both membrane phospholipid methylation and AMF-stimulated motility, whereas AMF itself caused a sustained increase in the incorporation of labeled methyl groups in phosphatidyl choline (Ptd Cho) in melanoma cells. Since Ptd Cho is the major substrate for phospholipase A2, these findings are consistent with a role for this enzyme in tumor cell motility.

Studies with a Walker murine carcinoma (W256) suggest that metabolism of arachidonic acid, a product of the lipase reaction, may play a role in tumor cell motility.[26] Lipoxygenase inhibitors such as quercetin, nordihydroguaretic acid, and nafazatrom significantly reduced stimulated motility, but indomethacin, a cyclo-oxygenase blocking agent, had no effect. Calmidazolium also substantially inhibited motility. Collectively, these results are in accord with both the lipoxygenase pathway for arachidonate metabolism and a calmodulin-mediated mobilization of calcium participating in migration of certain tumor cells. However, a role for the cyclo-oxygenase pathway cannot be ruled out. It has been reported that both phorbol myristate acetate- and laminin-stimulated motility in murine fibrosarcoma cells are inhibited by prostaglandins of the E series.[27] Preliminary studies (M. Stracke, unpublished material) with human melanoma cells indicate that calcium channel blocking agents inhibit AMF-stimulated motility. On the other hand, calcium ionophores were found to stimulate motility. These results are consistent with the participation of phospholipase C and the generation of inositol 1,4,5-triphosphate ($IP_3$) in initiating motility. Preliminary experiments clearly demonstrate that lithium, an inhibitor of the $IP_3$ pathway, significantly reduces AMF-induced motility (Kohn *et al.*, submitted).

From these considerations, it is likely that the generation of a motile response in tumor cells initially involves a direct role for a G-protein that interacts with an activated receptor and then transduces the signal to an effector system such as the phosphodiesterase $IP_3$ pathway and phospholipase A2 (Fig. 3). The subsequent production of arachidonate and its metabolism via lipoxygenase may contribute to the mobilization of calcium by $IP_3$ and production of diacylglycerol (DAG), which could also be required for changes in the cytoskeleton that are essential for locomo-

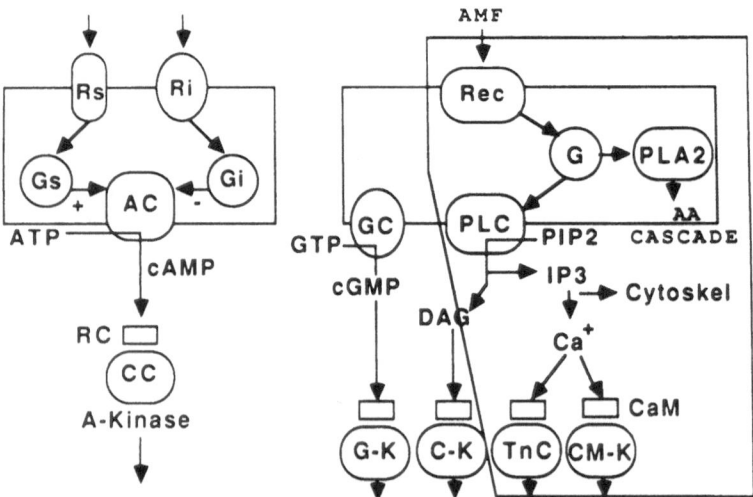

## CELLULAR RESPONSE

*Figure 3.* Signal transducer pathways potentially involved in tumor locomotion. Three major classes of second messenger pathways are depicted: the cyclic nucleotide pathway includes cyclic adenosine monophosphate (cAMP) and cyclic guanosine monophosphate (cGMP) generated adenylcyclase (AC) and guanylcyclase (GC), respectively. G proteins can regulate the production for both nucleotides through a stimulatory (Gs) and inhibitory (Gi) arms. A separate series of effector pathways involving stimulation of phospholipase $A_2$ (PLA2) and phospholipase C (phosphodiesterase PDE) are also regulated by G proteins ($G_o$). PDE results in the activation of the calcium mobilizing factor $IP_3$ (inositol triphosphate) and diacyclglycerol (DAG). All the experiments to date indicate that the cAMP and the cGMP pathway is not centrally involved in the generation of a motile response in tumor cells. The pertussis toxin-sensitive $G_o$ pathway plays a necessary role in the motile response. This pathway may mediate changes in membrane fluidity through phospholipase $A_2$ ($PLA_2$) and changes in cytoskeleton organization through PDE and the $IP_3$ pathway, which is known to alter actin-binding calcium-regulated events, such as gelsolin action. AC, adenylcyclase; CC, catalytic component; G-K, G-kinase; C-K, C-kinase; TnC, troponin C; CaM, calmodulin; CM-K, calmodulin-activated protein kinase.

tion. With respect to a role' for cathepsin B, it is conceivable that AMF may stimulate its activity within the membrane to cause a specific cleavage of a pro-enzyme whose active form (e.g., protein kinase C[26]) is required for the motile response.

Early events in migration may involve pseudopodia protrusion. During the course of invasion, the same tumor cell must interact with a variety of extracellular matrix proteins as it traverses each tissue barrier. For example, the tumor cell encounters laminin and type IV collagen when it penetrates the basement membrane, and type I collagen and fibronectin when it crosses the interstitial stroma. It has recently been shown that cells express specific cell surface receptors which recognize extracellular matrix proteins. The first example of such a receptor is the laminin receptor which binds to laminin with a nanomolar affinity. Laminin receptors have been shown to be augmented in actively invading tumor cells, and may play an important role in tumor cell interaction with the basement membrane. Arg-Gly-Asp (RGD) recognition receptors are another class of cell surface proteins which bind extracellular matrix proteins which in turn contain the protein sequence arg-gly-asp.[10] Such proteins include fibronectin, collagen type I, and vitronectin. The process of cell migration undoubtedly requires a series of adhesion and detachment steps resulting in traction and propulsion. Studies using the AMF-stimulated motility as model system have revealed an important function of pseudopodia protrusion in this process. AMF stimulates motility on a variety of different substrata. Therefore, its action is independent of the mechanism of attachment. Furthermore, AMF induces the rapid protrusion of pseudopodia in both a time- and dose-dependent manner.[28] Isolation of the induced pseudopodia reveals that they are highly enriched in their content of laminin and fibronectin matrix receptors. Since cell pseudopodia formation is known to be a prominent feature of actively motile cells, we can now set forth a working hypothesis to explain the early events in cell motility. Cytokines such as AMF which stimulate intrinsic motility may induce exploratory pseudopodia prior to cell translocation. Such pseudopodia may express augmented levels of matrix receptors (and possibly proteinases). The protruding pseudopodia may serve multiple functions including (1) acting as sense organs to interact with the extracellular matrix proteins and thereby locate directional cues, (2) providing propulsive traction for locomotion, and (3) even inducing local matrix proteolysis to assist in the penetration of the matrix.

## 8. LAMININ RECEPTORS

Cell-surface receptors for the basement membrane glycoprotein laminin mediate adhesion of tumor cells to the basement membrane prior to invasion.[4,29] Laminin as visualized by rotary shadowing electron microscopy has a distinctive cruciform shape with three short arms (35 nm) and one long arm (75 nm). All arms have globular end regions. The specialized structure of the laminin molecule may contribute to its multiple biologic functions. Laminin plays a role in cell attachment, cell spreading, mitogenesis, neurite outgrowth, morphogenesis, and cell movement. Many types of neoplastic cells contain high-affinity (nM kd) cell-surface binding sites (laminin receptors) for laminin. The molecular weight of the isolated receptor is $65,000\ M_r$.[29] The laminin receptor binds to the "B" chain (short arm) region of the laminin molecule. Laminin receptors may be altered in number or degree of occupancy in human carcinomas. This may be the indirect result of defective basement membrane organization in the carcinomas. Breast carcinoma and colon carcinoma tissue contains a higher number of exposed (unoccupied) receptors compared to benign lesions. The laminin receptors of normal epithelium may be polarized at the basal surface and occupied with laminin in the basement membrane. In contrast, the laminin receptors on invading carcinoma cells are amplified and may be distributed over the entire surface of the cell. The laminin receptor can be shown experimentally to play a role in hematogenous metastases. Treating tumor cells with the receptor-binding fragment of laminin at very low concentrations markedly inhibits or abolishes lung metastases from hematogenously introduced tumor cells. The specific mechanism of action involves adhesion of circulating tumor cells to the subendothelial basement membrane.

## 9. EFFECT OF ANTI-LAMININ RECEPTOR ANTISERA ON LAMININ-MEDIATED HAPTOTAXIS

A2058 human melanoma cells migrate in response to a gradient of laminin as assayed in a modified Boyden chamber with laminin-coated nucleopore filters. In this system, the tumor cells are placed on one side of a nucleopore (8-$\mu$m pore size) filter and the opposite face of the filter is coated with laminin (10 $\mu$g/ml). The tumor cells were allowed to attach to the filter in the lower part of the chamber. In this manner, the laminin receptor function associated with migration on laminin substrata could be separated from its effect on primary attachment. The polyclonal antiserum against the natural laminin receptor, and the polyclonal antisera against the synthetic peptides derived from the receptor cDNA clone, all inhibited the laminin haptotaxis of A2058 cells in a dose-dependent manner compared to preimmune controls. The A2058 cells also exhibited a significant haptotactic response to a gradient of fibronectin. Anti-laminin antiserum abrogated haptotactic response to laminin but not to fibronectin. In contrast, 50 $\mu$g/ml of the synthetic peptide Gly-Arg-Asp-Ser (GRGDS) significantly inhibited haptotaxis on fibronectin. The control peptide Gly-Arg-Gly-Glu-Ser (GRGES), which is not an active binding sequence of fibronectin, did not have an inhibitory effect on fibronectin haptotaxis. There was no inhibition of laminin haptotaxis with these fibronectin peptides. Furthermore, the anti-laminin receptor antisera did not significantly inhibit fibronectin haptotaxis compared to controls. These results support the concept that different receptors are involved in laminin versus fibronectin haptotaxis.

## 10. IN VIVO EXPRESSION OF LAMININ RECEPTOR IN HUMAN TUMORS CORRELATES WITH THEIR INVASIVE AND MIGRATORY CAPACITIES

Bearing in mind the *in vitro* results, we next investigated the possibility that the laminin receptor might also be preferentially associated with cells involved in *in vivo* invasion and migration. Invading trophoblasts of decidua basalis in early human pregnancy, which are characterized by invasive and migratory properties, exhibited a prominent cytoplasmic laminin receptor immunoreactivity. In the malignant human tumors investigated, the tumor cells aggressively invading the extracellular matrix also exhibited intense cytoplasmic staining with the polyclonal antilaminin receptor antisera. An identical topographic distribution pattern was found using either antiserum to the natural laminin receptor or with synthetic peptide antisera. Surrounding normal tissues showed only minimal immunoreactivity, except for some proliferating blood vessels. Metastatic carcinoma cells in liver were strongly immunoreactive, whereas the surrounding parenchyma was essentially nonreactive with these antisera (data not shown). There appeared to be a correlation between the degree of differentiation and the level of laminin receptor-positive cytoplasmic immunostaining. In 48 cases studied, the moderately or poorly differentiated carcinomas (33 cases out of 48) had more abundant and intense laminin immunoreactivity compared to the well-differentiated carcinomas (15 cases out of 48). The observation that the laminin receptor expression *in vivo* might be augmented in highly malignant tumor cells which are involved in invasion and migration is also supported by our finding that metastatic tumor tissue is a successful source for biochemical purification of the laminin receptor.[29]

## 11. RGD RECOGNITION RECEPTORS

A family of cell surface glycoproteins termed ''integrins'' has been identified which bind with low affinity ($\mu$M kd) to a variety of adhesion proteins including fibronectin, von Willebrand factor, fibrin, vitronectin, type I collagen, and thrombospondin.[30] The integrins are a complex of $\alpha$- (140,000 $M_r$) and $\beta$- (95,000 $M_r$) subunit proteins. The functions of several of the integrins are inhibited by peptides related to the Arg-Gly-Asp (RGD) sequence of fibronectin. RGD sequences present on a wide variety of proteins may serve as the recognition site for binding of the integrins. It is likely that specific ligand sequences adjacent to the RGD site may confer preferential recognition of one type of adhesion protein by certain members of the integrin family. Integrin proteins are thought to align adhesion proteins such as fibronectin on the cell surface with cytoskeletal components such as talin and actin, thus altering cell shape. Integrin type proteins may play an adhesive role in platelet–tumor cell interactions, binding of lymphoid cells to endothelium, and the interaction of circulating tumor cells with endothelial surfaces, fibrin, von Willibrand factor, or thrombospondin. In keeping with this concept, it has been reported that co-injection of tumor cells with large quantities of RGD peptides will inhibit metastases formation in animal models. The RGD peptides may interfere with the adhesion of tumor cells to the endothelial surface which may directly or indirectly be mediated through integrin proteins.

## 12. TUMOR CELL PROTEINASES

*In vitro* studies of tumor cell invasion of the extracellular matrix have shown that cell proliferation is not absolutely required. Invasion of the matrix is not merely due to passive growth pressure but requires active biochemical mechanisms. Inhibitors of protein synthesis or inhibitors of proteinases block invasion of the matrix.[4] Many research groups have proposed that invasive tumor cells secrete matrix-degrading proteinases. Collagen is an important substrate because it constitutes the structural scaffolding upon which the other components of the matrix are assembled. Tumor-derived collagenases that degrade interstitial collagen types I, II, and III have been characterized by a number of investigators. They are metal ion- (calcium and zinc) dependent enzymes that function at neutral pH. Classic collagenase produces a single cleavage in the collagen molecule (interstitial collagen types I, II, and III) producing 3/4- and 1/4-size fragments (75% of the distance from the N terminus). Tumor cells can degrade both collagenous and noncollagenous components of the basement membrane.[4,5,31] Basement membrane specific collagen types IV and V are *not* susceptible to classic collagenase, which degrades collagen types I, II, and III. A separate family of collagenolytic enzymes (type IV collagenase)[4,31] cleave the type IV collagen chain 1/4 of the distance from the amino terminus. Type IV collagenases are augmented in highly metastatic tumor cells and in endothelial cells during angiogenesis. Antibodies prepared against type IV collagenase react with invading breast carcinoma cells and breast carcinoma lymph node metastases by immunohistology. Amplification of type IV collagenase production is biochemically linked to the genetic induction of metastases in experimental models.[31,32]

## 13. MOLECULAR GENETICS OF METASTASES

It is apparent that interactions in the complicated metastatic process involve multiple gene products. A cascade or coordinated group of gene products expressed above a certain threshold level may be required for a tumor cell to traverse the successive steps successfully in the metastatic process. The crucial gene products may regulate host immune recognition of the tumor cells, cell growth, attachment, proteolysis, locomotion, and differentiation. The specific family of gene products necessary for metastases may be different for each histologic type of tumor.

The evidence linking oncogenes to the induction or maintenance of human malignancies has become increasingly compelling. In the past, oncogenes have been linked to unrestrained tumor growth. Recently, two different types of experimental approaches[5,32,33] have indicated that certain classes or combinations of oncogenes may play a role in the metastatic behavior of tumors. In the first type of experimental approach, human tumor DNA samples are surveyed for the level of oncogene expression and this is correlated with disease stage. In the second type of approach, tumor DNA or isolated oncogenes are transfected into recipient cells. The transfected cells are then studied for their metastatic propensity. Notable examples of these two approaches are work with the HER-2/neu oncogene in human breast cancer[33] and transfection of the ras oncogene in rodent systems.[31,32,34]

The HER-2/neu (neu) oncogene (also termed c-erbB-2 and HER-2) encodes a protein which is a member of the tyrosine kinase family, and is related to, but distinct from, the EGF receptor gene. At the time of this writing, the ligand for the neu oncogene encoded receptor protein had not yet been identified. A significant increase in the incidence of neu gene amplification is noted in breast cancer patients with >3 axillary lymph nodes positive for metastases.[33] Amplification of neu was also highly correlated with disease relapse (actuarial survival) as well as tumor size. Thus, even though the function of neu is unknown, its level of expression may provide important prognostic information for breast cancer (see also Chapter 10).

Transfection of members of the ras oncogene family into suitable rodent recipient cells, including diploid rat embryo fibroblasts, can induce these cells to rapidly progress to express the complete metastatic phenotype.[5,31] Other oncogenes, including myc, sarc, and fos, failed to induce metastases in rodent cells. Furthermore, when ras was transfected in combination with the adenovirus type 2 E1A oncogene, the recipient cells became very tumorigenic but totally non-metastatic.[31] Thus, some genes can suppress the action of ras to induce metastases. The current working hypothesis is that induction of the metastatic phenotype requires at least two (and possibly more) complementary genes or gene products. In the correct rodent cells, one of these genes may be the activated form of the ras oncogene. When these genes interact in the correct fashion, a cascade of specific gene products are elaborated which confer the metastatic phenotype.

## 14. CONCLUSIONS

A metastatic colony is the end result of a complicated series of steps including tumor initiation, promotion and progression, angiogenesis, invasion of local tissues and vascular channels, dissemination of circulating tumor cells, extravasation, and colony initiation and growth at the secondary site. It is assumed that in order for metastatic tumor cells to successfully traverse all of these steps, they must express the right combination of gene products. Identification of such gene products is a major goal of the investigators studying this aspect of cancer, which is the major cause of treatment failure. Identification of proteins and their associated genes, which are causally related to metastases or correlate with the level of metastatic aggressiveness should provide a number of clinical strategies for diagnosis, prognosis, and therapy. Blocking the action of proteins essential for invasion and metastases could serve as a means to prevent invasion in patients with carcinoma *in situ*, and following surgical treatment of the primary tumor. Measurement of the level of a given protein or gene product in a tumor sample or body fluid could provide a means to predict the metastatic propensity of a patient's individual tumor. Antibodies recognizing antigens associated with metastatic cells could be used to identify clinically occult metastases in the patient, and may also be used to target toxic agents to the established metastases.

Gene products associated with metastases have been identified using three major approaches as reviewed in this chapter. The first approach is to reduce metastases into defined steps and study the biochemical mechanisms involved in each step. Using this approach, a number of new proteins have been identified that facilitate tumor cell attachment, degradation, and migration through the extracellular matrix. The second approach is to transfect genes into nonmetastatic cells resulting in the expression of the metastatic phenotype. Transfection of the *ras* oncogene has been an exciting new model in this regard. Transfection of *ras* into appropriate recipient cells (including diploid fibroblasts) will cause these cells to become totally metastatic by nonimmunologic mechanisms. The *ras*-induced metastatic phenotype is accompanied by increased levels of collagenases and motility factors. Furthermore, the *ras* induction of metastases can be blocked by transfection with the adenovirus 2 E1A gene. The third approach is to compare the level of expression or amplification of genes in metastatic versus nonmetastatic human or rodent tumors. An example is the work of Slamon *et al.*,[33] who demonstrated a correlation of human breast cancer metastases and poor survival with increased amplification of the HER-2/neu oncogene. Although the function of this gene is unknown, it can be used as a tool for prognostication.

In the future, it is expected that existing research discoveries will be applied to routine use in the clinic. Undoubtedly, new metastases-associated gene products will be discovered, and their mechanisms of action delineated. This should lead to a direct clinical benefit for the high percentage of cancer patients who succumb to the direct effects of invasion or metastases.

# REFERENCES

1. Nicolson, G. L., and Milas, L. (eds.), 1984, *Cancer Invasion and Metastasis: Biological and Therapeutic Aspects,* Raven Press, New York.
2. Liotta, L. A., 1984, Tumor invasion and metastasis: Role of the basement membrane—Warner–Lambert Parke–Davis Award Lecture, *Am. J. Pathol.* **117:**339–348.
3. Schirrmacher, V., 1985, Cancer metastasis: Experimental approaches, theoretical concepts, and impacts for treatment strategies, *Adv. Cancer Res.* **43:**1–73.
4. Liotta, L. A., 1986, Tumor invasion and metastases—Role of the extracellular matrix: Rhoads Memorial Award Lecture, *Cancer Res.* **46:**1–7.
5. Nicolson, G. L., 1987, Tumor cell instability, diversification, and progression to the metastatic phenotype: From oncogene to oncofetal expression, *Cancer Res.* **47:**1473–1486.
6. Furcht, L. T., 1986, Editorial: Critical factors controlling angiogenesis: Cell products, cell matrix, and growth factors, *Lab. Invest.* **55:**505–506.
7. Sugarbaker, E. V., 1981, Patterns of metastasis in human malignancies, *Cancer Biol. Rev.* **2:**235–245.
8. Weiss, L., and Gilbert, H. A., 1981, *Bone Metastases,* GK Hall, Boston.
9. Lam, W. C., Delikatny, J. E., Orr, F. W., Wass, J., Varani, J., and Ward, P. A., 1981, The chemotactic response of tumor cells: A model for cancer metastasis, *Am. J. Pathol.* **104:**69–76.
10. McCarthy, J. B., Basara, M. L., Palm, S. L., Sas, D. F., Furcht, L. T., 1985, Stimulation of haptotaxis and migration of tumor cells by serum spreading factor, *Cancer Metast. Rev.* **4:**125–152.
11. Anzano, M. A., Roberts, A. B., Smith, J. M., Sporn, M. B., and De Larco, J. E., 1983, Sarcoma growth factors from conditioned media of virally transformed cells composed of both type α and type β growth factors, *Proc. Natl. Acad. Sci. &SA* **80:**6264–6268.
12. Liotta, L. A., Mandler, R., Murano, G., Katz, D. A., Gordon, R. K., Chiang, P. K., and Schiffmann, E., 1986, Tumor cell autocrine motility factor, *Proc. Natl. Acad. Sci. USA* **83:**3302–3306.
13. Zigmond, S. H., and Hirsch, J. G., 1973, Leukocyte locomotion and chemotaxis. New methods for evaluation and demonstration of cell-derived chemotactic factor, *J. Exp. Med.* **137:**387–410.
14. Bokoch, G. M., and Gilman, A. G., 1984, Inhibition of receptor-mediated release of arachidonic acid by pertussis toxin, *Cell* **39:**301–308.
15. Smith, C. D., Cox, C. C., and Snyderman, R., 1986, Receptor-coupled activation of phosphoinositide-specific phospholipase C by an N protein, *Science* **232:**97–100.
16. Stracke, M. L., Guirguis, R., Liotta, L. A., and Schiffmann, E., 1987, Pertussis toxin inhibits stimulated motility independently of the adenylate cyclase pathway in human melanoma cells, *Biochem. Biophys. Res. Commun.* **146:**339–345.
17. Katada, T., and Ui, M., 1982, Direct modification of the membrane adenylate cyclase system by islet-activating protein due to ADP-ribosylation of a membrane protein, *Proc. Natl. Acad. Sci. USA* **79:**3129–3133.
18. Guirguis, R., Margolies, I., Taraboletti, G., Schiffmann, E., and Liotta, L., 1987, Cytokine-induced pseudopodial protrusion is coupled to tumor cell migration, *Nature* **329:**261–263.
19. Stracke, M. L., Guirguis, R., Liotta, L., and Schiffmann, E., 1987, Pertussis toxin inhibits stimulated motility independently of the adenylate cyclase pathway in human melanoma cells, *Biochem. Biophys. Res. Commun.* **146:**339–345.
20. Okajima, F., and Ui, M., 1984, ADP-ribosylation of the specific membrane protein by islet-activating protein, pertussis toxin, associated with inhibition of a chemotactic peptide-induced arachidonate release in neutrophils. A possible role of the toxin substrate in $Ca^{2+}$-mobilizing biosignaling, *J. Biol. Chem.* **259:**13863–13871.
21. Kikuchi, A., Kozawa, O., Kaibuchi, K., Katada, T., Ui, M., and Takai, Y., 1986, Direct evidence for involvement of a guanine nucleotide-binding protein in chemotactic peptide-stimulated formation of inositol bisphosphate and trisphosphate in differentiated human leukemia (HL-60) cells. Reconstitution with Gi or Go of the plasma membranes ADP-ribosylated by pertussis toxin, *J. Biol. Chem.* **261:**11558–11562.
22. Hescheler, J., Rosenthal, W., Trautwein, W., and Schultz, G., 1987, The GTP-binding protein, Go, regulates neuronal calcium channels, *Nature (Lond.)* **325:**445–447.
23. Molski, T. F., Naccache, P. H., Marsh, M. L., Kermode, J., Becker, E. L., and Sha'afi, R. I., 1984,

Pertussis toxin inhibits the rise in the intracellular concentration of free calcium that is induced by chemotactic factors in rabbit neutrophils: possible role of the "G proteins" in calcium mobilization, *Biochem.
Biophys. Res. Commun.* **124:**644–650.

24. Lad, P. M., Olson, C. V., Grewal, I. S., and Scott, S. J., 1985, A pertussis toxin-sensitive GTP-binding
protein in the human neutrophil regulates multiple receptors, calcium mobilization, and lectin-induced
capping, *Proc. Natl. Acad. Sci. USA* **82:**8643–8647.

25. Guranowski, A., Montgomery, J. A., Cantoni, G. L., and Chiang, P. K., 1981, Adenosine analogues as
substrates and inhibitors of S-adenosylhomocysteine hydrolase, *Biochemistry* **20:**110–115.

26. Boike, G. M., Sloane, B. F., Deppe, G., Stracke, M., Schiffmann, E., Liotta, L. A., and Honn, K. V.,
1987, The role of calcium and arachidonic acid metabolism in the chemotaxis of a new murine tumor line,
*Proc. Am. Assoc. Cancer Res.* **28:**82.

27. He, X. M., Fligiel, S. E., and Varani, J., 1986, Modulation of tumor cell motility by prostaglandins and
inhibitors of prostaglandin synthesis, *Exp. Cell Biol.* **54:**128–137.

28. Guirguis, R., Margulies, I. M. K., Taraboletti, G., Schiffmann, E., and Liotta, L. A., 1987, Cytokine-
induced pseudopodial protrusion is coupled to tumour cell migration, *Nature (Lond.)* **329:**261–263.

29. Wewer, U. M., Liotta, L. A., Jaye, M., Ricca, G. A., Drohan, W. N., Claysmith, A. P., Rao, C. N.,
Wirth, P., Coligan, J. E., Albrechtsen, R., Mudryj, M., and Sobel, M. E., 1986, Altered levels of laminin
receptor mRNA in various human carcinoma cells that have different abilities to bind laminin, *Proc. Natl.
Acad. Sci. USA* **83:**7137–7141.

30. Hynes, R. O., 1987, Integrins: A family of cell surface receptors, *Cell* **48:**549–552.

31. Garbisa, S., Pozzatti, R., Muschel, R. J., Saffiotti, U., Ballin, M., Goldfarb, R. H., Khoury, G., and
Liotta, L. A., 1987, Secretion of type IV collagenolytic protease and metastatic phenotype: Induction by
transfection with c-Ha-*ras* but not c-Ha-*ras* plus Ad2-Ela, *Cancer Res* **47:**1523–1528.

32. Thorgeirsson, U. P., Turpeenniemi-Hujanen, T., Williams, J. E., Westin, E. H., Heilman, C. A., Talmadge, J. E., and Liotta, L. A., 1985, NIH/3T3 cells transfected with human tumor DNA containing
activated *ras* oncogenes express the metastatic phenotype in nude mice, *Mol. Cell. Biol.* **5:**259–262.

33. Slamon, D. J., Clark, G. M., Wong, S. G. et al., 1987, Human breast cancer: Correlation of relapse and
survival with amplification of the HER-2/*neu* oncogene, *Science* **235:**177–180.

34. Pozzatti, R. P., Muschel, R. J., Williams, J. R., Howard, B., Liotta, L. A., and Khoury, G., 1986,
Primary rat embryo cells transformed by one or two oncogenes show different metastatic potentials, *Science*
**232:**223–227.

# 28

# Phenotypic Heterogeneity and Metastasis

## James E. Talmadge and I. J. Fidler

## 1. INTRODUCTION

The movement of tumor cells from a primary neoplasm to distant organs and the subsequent outgrowth of metastases is the most devastating aspect of cancer. Metastasis is defined as "the transfer of disease from one organ, or part, to another not directly connected to it. It may be due either to the transfer of pathogenic organisms, or to transfer of cells as in malignant tumors."[1] Metastasis involves the release of cells from the primary tumor, dissemination to distant sites, arrest in the microcirculation of organs, extravasation and infiltration into the stroma of those organs, and the survival and growth, with concomitant neovascularization, into new tumor foci (Fig. 1). The outcome of this process is dependent on both host factors and tumor cell properties, and the balance and individual phenotypes of these interactions vary among tumor systems. The precise mechanisms involved in each of the steps are still not clear; however, recent work has clarified some aspects of the processes involved. Although our understanding of the pathogenesis of metastasis has evolved, a concomitant improvement in the treatment of metastatic disease from the major solid tumors of man has not occurred. Despite major advances in general patient care, in surgical techniques, and in adjuvant therapies, most deaths from cancer are caused by the growth of metastases that are resistant to therapy. In most patients, by the time of diagnosis of primary malignant neoplasms (excluding skin cancers), metastasis may well have occurred.[2-5] Metastasis can be located in different organs and in different anatomic locations within the same organ. These aspects exert a significant influence on the response of tumor cells to therapy and the efficiency of delivery of anticancer drugs to tumor foci in amounts sufficient to destroy tumor cells without concomitant host toxicity.[3] The biggest obstacle to the effective treatment of metastases is, however, the nonuniformity of cells populating both primary and metastatic neoplasms. By the time of diagnosis, and certainly in clinically advanced disease, malignant neoplasms contain heterogeneous cell populations exhibiting a wide range of biologic phenotypes such as cell-surface properties, antigenicity, immunogenicity,

*James E. Talmadge* • Smith Kline & French Laboratories, Research and Development Division, Immunology and Antiinfectives Therapy, King of Prussia, Pennsylvania 19406-0939.   *I. J. Fidler* • Department of Cell Biology, M. D. Anderson Hospital and Tumor Institute, University of Texas System Cancer Center, Houston, Texas 77030.

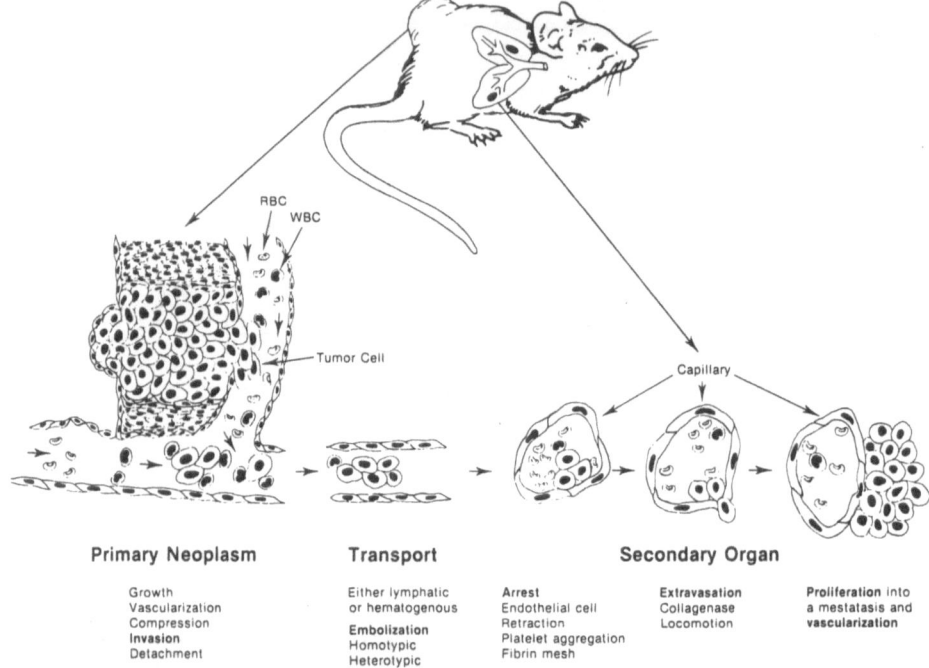

| Primary Neoplasm | Transport | Secondary Organ | | |
|---|---|---|---|---|
| Growth<br>Vascularization<br>Compression<br>Invasion<br>Detachment | Either lymphatic<br>or hematogenous<br><br>Embolization<br>Homotypic<br>Heterotypic | Arrest<br>Endothelial cell<br>Retraction<br>Platelet aggregation<br>Fibrin mesh | Extravasation<br>Collagenase<br>Locomotion | Proliferation into<br>a mestatasis and<br>vascularization |

*Figure 1.* Overview of the process of a tumor metastasis. The metastatic process is sequential and requires that cells populating metastases survive a series of highly selective events.

growth rate, karyotype, sensitivity to various cytotoxic drugs, and the ability to invade and metastasize[6-13] (see also Chapter 10). Biologic heterogeneity is equally prominent among the cells populating metastases from the same host.[6-12] Indeed, multiple metastases proliferating in different organs or even within the same organ of cancer patients can exhibit diversity in characteristics such as hormone receptors, antigenicity-immunogenicity, and sensitivity to various chemotherapeutic drugs.[3,8]

Clearly, the major goal of oncologists remains as the prevention or eradication of cancer metastasis. This chapter discusses data describing the mechanisms of tumor progression, biologic diversification, and metastasis. Those findings that have implications for the therapy of disseminated cancer are emphasized.

## 2. PATHOGENESIS OF METASTASIS (MECHANISMS)

### 2.1. Invasion

Tumor cell dissemination can occur by direct spread or migration through body coelomic cavities.[14] Such routes of dissemination, however, are involved only in a limited number of tumor histiotypes, and then only secondary to hematogenous or lymphatic spread. Invasion and infiltration into host tissues surrounding the primary tumor lead to penetration of blood, lymph vessels, or both, and provide the opportunity for widespread dispersion. Recent data have begun to reveal the mechanisms responsible for invasion of local host tissues and are discussed more extensively in Chapter 27. The production of pressure atrophy can take place regardless of rapidity of tumor proliferation. Not all invasive tumors are rapidly growing; in fact, many highly invasive tumors have very slow growth rates.[5,15] Moreover, at least *in vitro,* tumor cells added to the surface of organ explants are capable of infiltrating these tissues without any pressure factors.[16-18] Individual cell motility may play a role in tumor cell invasion, although the evidence for such a mechanism is at best circumstantial.[18-23] The investigation of variant murine tumor lines of differing invasive behavior has failed to reveal a correlation between *in vitro* motility and malignant capacity *in vivo.*[24] Interpretation of these results is difficult, since movement of cells on a two-dimensional, serum-coated plastic petri dish may not be analogous with behavior within host tissue.[24-26] However, there is little correlation between the contact inhibition of tumor cells growing as monolayer cultures and their invasive behavior when implanted in a three-dimensional developing chicken wing bud.[27] Certainly, tumor cells possess the organelles necessary for active locomotion and can form cellular cytoplasmic processes, indicative of motility, during the invasive process.[28-34] Yet the inhibition of cell motility can prevent invasion in some, but not all, *in vitro* systems.[16,18,35] Invasion by leukemic cells, without individual cell motility, is unlikely, and the situation with regard to solid tumors is less clear.[36] For all these reasons, the role of cell motility as a single factor in tumor invasion needs further investigation.

The involvement of specific tissue-destructive enzymes in tumor invasion, such as lysosomal hydrolyses and collagenases, are well defined. Destruction of host tissue by these enzymes, aided by pressure atrophy and the occlusion of blood and lymph vessels by an expanding tumor mass, appears to facilitate malignant cell infiltration. The evidence for this mechanism of invasion can be summarized as follows: Histologic examination of tissues obtained from sites of tumor invasion reveals considerable variation in the degree of tissue damage.[15,32] Many human and animal malignant neoplasms express higher levels of lytic enzymes than do benign tumors or corresponding normal tissues.[22,33-45] Although direct sampling may cause tissue damage itself and an elevation of enzyme activity, evidence for the involvement of tissue-degradative enzymes in neoplastic invasion is quite convincing.[40] Lysosomal catheptic enzymes have shown elevated levels of activity within some tumor tiuues,[40,46-48] and an increased production of cathepsin B in breast carcinomas compared with that of normal or benign tissue has been demonstrated,[47-49] suggesting a role for this enzyme in the expression of the aggressive malignant phenotype.

Enhanced production and secretion of the tissue serine protease plasminogen activator (TPA) has been associated with the neoplastic transformation of a variety of cell types.[50,51] Considerable interest has centered on the possible role of TPA in invasion and metastasis.[52] However, many normal cells produce high levels of TPA, and examination of variant murine melanoma cell lines with different invasive capacities has failed to demonstrate a consistent correlation between malignant behavior *in vivo* and TPA production or secretion.[24,42,43] Clearly, the relative importance of different enzymes and cell-adhesion molecules will vary from one tumor system to another, and within the same tumor system, from one anatomic site to another, so that one enzyme may not be critical to all types of tumor invasion.[24-26,29-31,36-53]

The penetration of blood vessels, during invasion and extravasation, is of pivotal importance in hematogenous metastasis. Therefore, it is of interest that a strong correlation has been demonstrated between the ability of murine tumor cells to produce spontaneous metastases and their production of high levels of type IV collagenase.[43,54-57] Tumor cells that invade blood vessels or leave capillaries of distant organs in which they have been arrested must penetrate the basement membrane. Dissolution of the basement membrane, suggestive of enzymatic action, has been observed in areas adjacent to arrested tumor cells.[54] Type IV collagen is a major structural protein of the basement membranes between parenchymal cells and the connective tissue on which such cells rest. Collagen IV is chemically and genetically distinct from cartilage collagen type II and stromal collagen types I and III. The collagenase prepared from metastatic murine tumor cells preferentially digests this basement membrane collagen.[55] Cells recovered from the venous effluent of a murine fibrosarcoma, potentially the invasive population, solubilized basement membrane collagen to a significantly greater extent than cells from the parent population.[56] In addition, it appears that metastatic tumor cells exhibit a preferential attachment to type IV collagen substrate.[57] Since tumor cells can arrest selectively in areas of endothelial damage, the possession of high levels of type IV collagenase could be of fundamental importance to invasion and metastasis.[43]

## 2.2. Lymphatic–Hematogenous Spread

Clinical observations suggest that carcinomas spread by the lymphatic route and mesenchymal tumors spread by means of the bloodstream.[58] This impression is erroneous; lymphatic and vascular systems have numerous connections.[59] Experimentally, it has been shown that disseminating tumor cells may pass from one system to another.[60] Therefore, the two systems are inseparable, and the division into lymphatic spread and hematogenous spread is an arbitrary one used only for the sake of clarity.

### 2.2.1. Lymphatic Spread

During tumor cell invasion, the process of infiltration and expansion into host tissues results in the penetration of small lymphatic vessels. The release of tumor cell emboli into these vessels is one mechanism for lymphatic metastases. Tumor emboli may be trapped in the first lymph node encountered on their route; alternatively, they may traverse lymph nodes or even bypass them to form distant nodal metastases (the "skip" metastasis).[61] Although this phenomenon was recognized during the late 1800s,[62] its implications for treatment were frequently ignored in the development of surgical approaches.[5,63,64]

The view that lymphatics are the primary route for the spread of carcinomas is an oversimplification of the process. What appears to be of primary importance is the role that the lymphatic system, in general, and lymph nodes, in particular, may play in the control or regulation of metastatic spread. Lymph nodes in the area of a primary neoplasm may be enlarged and clinically palpable. The enlargement could be due to either follicular hyperplasia accompanied by proliferation of reticulum cells and sinus endothelium or to growth of tumor cells. Although the use of morphologic criteria for assessing prognoses based on lymph node appearance is debatable, it has been generally accepted that inactive lymphocyte-depleted lymph nodes are indicative of a less favorable prognosis than those demonstrating reactive patterns,[65,66] and a hyperplastic response could indicate reactivity to autochthonous tumors, which may be of benefit to the host.[67]

### 2.2.2. The Barrier Function of Lymph Nodes

Whether lymph nodes can serve as a temporary "filter" for metastatic tumor cells is not clear.[5] The lymph nodes (of normal animals) can be an effective, although temporary, barrier to tumor spread. Zeidman and Buss[61] injected the Brown–Pearce variant of VX2 carcinoma cells into the afferent popliteal lymphatics of rabbits and removed the lymph nodes 1–42 days after injection. Only 2 of 30 animals developed distant metastases. This result was taken as evidence for the effectiveness of the lymph node as a temporary barrier to tumor spread. However, another experimental study with radiolabeled tumor cells from rats demonstrated that most cells that reached the lymph node rapidly entered the efferent lymphatics and then the bloodstream.[60] If, indeed, tumor cells can transfer from lymphatics to blood vessels and back with great ease, the issue may not be of clinical importance. However, it is important to note that in most experimental animal systems used to investigate this question, normal nonreactive lymph nodes have been subjected to a sudden influx of a large number of tumor cells; the situation may not be at all analogous to the regional lymph node (RLN) in the early stages of the spread of cancer.

The role of the RLN in neoplasia, in general, and in metastasis, in particular, is as controversial as it is important. Unquestionably, the RLN may be involved immunologically in the host response to neoplasms. The importance of the RLN to the initiation of systemic immunity has been established in various systems. Mitchinson[68] first reported adoptive transfer of tumor allograft immunity by the intraperitoneal administration of RLN cells of tumor-bearing animals to normal animals. Billingham *et al.*[69] showed that skin allografts lacking a lymphatic system were retained. Construction of skin pedicles in guinea pigs lacking afferent lymphatics led to indefinite retention of skin allografts.[70] By contrast, Futrell and Myers,[71] using a similar system, found that tumor allografts were rejected, although skin allografts remained viable.

Twenty years ago, Crile[72,73] challenged the classic concept of en bloc resection of primary tumors of the breast and their RLN. He advocated simple mastectomy, or lumpectomy and preservation of the RLN. The retention of the RLN free of metastatic cells was hypothesized to be important in maintaining a high level of systemic tumor immunity, which theoretically could aid in preventing growth of disseminated micrometastases. Subsequent clinical trials by Fisher and co-workers[74–76] comparing simple and radical mastectomy showed no improvement in survival rate of patients who underwent simple mastectomy.[76]

However, animal experiments complicated the interpretation of the role of the RLN in controlling tumor spread. It appears from the work of Fisher and Fisher and co-workers[77,78] that the RLN could be important for the initiation of immunity against a transplantable syngeneic tumor in mice. The effect, however, is dependent on the antigenicity of the tumor; when the tumor was weakly antigenic, the RLN were important in the initiation of systemic immunity, but this was not the case when the tumors were strongly antigenic.[77,78]

The contradictory findings on the role of the RLN in controlling cancer metastasis are not surprising. Different tumor systems, and especially different experimental conditions, would be expected to influence the relative biologic behavior of tumor cells. In many animal tumor systems, notably melanoma, tumor cells implanted intradermally will reach a draining lymph node first to then produce metastasis in visceral organs.[11] This pattern of metastasis is dependent on the nature of the tumor cells and their site of implantation. In fact, mouse melanoma cells injected intramuscularly (quadriceps femoris) will produce metastases in visceral organs without necessarily involving draining lymph nodes. Here again, one must question the biologic relevance and accuracy of such an animal model for human cutaneous melanoma. By contrast, human ocular melanoma or mucosal melanoma show early metastasis to visceral organs, and not lymph node metastases. Clearly, then, different animal tumor models (for melanoma) may or may not be applicable to one or another subtype of human melanoma. Moreover, an animal model using lymphosarcoma or leukemia cells may have little relevance to a human clinical cancer metastasis of solid tumors. The precise role of the lymph nodes draining a primary tumor in the control of metastatic spread remains uncertain. Determining this role is important, since the decision to surgically excise the RLNs must be based on the estimated risk of lymph node metastasis.

## 2.2.3. Hematogenous Spread

The widespread tumor cell dissemination is a consequence of the penetration of blood vessels or lymphatics, or both. Cells of malignant neoplasms frequently penetrate thin-walled capillaries but rarely invade artery or arteriole walls, which are rich in elastin fibers.[20] This resistance to invasion is not necessarily mediated by mechanical strength alone. Connective tissues have been shown to possess protease inhibitors, and these may block the enzyme-dependent process of invasion.[79,80] Malignant tumors do not produce their own blood vessels, but induce the growth of new capillaries from host tissue by releasing tumor angiogenesis factor[81,82] (see Chapter 26). The penetration of these vascular channels can be aided by defective or denuded endothelium and increased permeability of such vessels.

Once tumor cells have penetrated blood vessels, they can be transported or grow at the site of penetration and only subsequently release tumor emboli into the circulation. The appearance of tumor emboli correlates with the development of tumor vascularization.[83] In this regard, the rate of tumor cell release from an implanted murine fibrosarcoma was related to the development of pulmonary metastases.[84] However, the mere presence of tumor cells in the circulation does not in itself constitute metastasis,[85,86] since most cells released into the bloodstream are eliminated rapidly.[86–88] Although most tumor cells are destroyed within the bloodstream, it appears that the greater the number of cells released by a primary tumor, the greater the probability that some cells will survive to form metastases.[86] The number of tumor emboli in the circulation appears to correlate well with the size and clinical duration of the primary tumor.[5] The development of necrotic and hemorrhagic areas within large tumors facilitates this process by providing tumor cells easy access to the circulation.[19]

The rapid death of most circulating tumor cells is probably due to the traumatic nature of blood turbulence, as well as the interaction with a variety of blood components (NK cells) which is facilitated by the isolated nature of the emboli. Tumor cells can aggregate with each other (homotypic aggregation) or with host cells (heterotypic aggregation), such as platelets[88] and lymphocytes.[89,90] Formation of such multicellular emboli assists the survival of tumor cells in the circulation, and in experimental systems, the number of pulmonary metastases formed after intravenous injection of tumor cells has been related to the size of tumor emboli.[90-92] Although such an effect is presumably related to an enhanced trapping of larger emboli in the microcirculation, it can also be due to the protective effect of an outer layer of cells.[93] Metastases can result from undamaged "central" cells protected from the hostile circulatory environment, or host effector mechanisms by peripheral tumor or host cells in the embolus (Fig. 2).

Tumor cell entrapment in the capillary bed of distant organs is necessary for secondary tumor growth during hematogenous metastasis. Although the morphologic aspects of tumor cell arrest have been studied extensively, relatively little is known about the dynamics of the process.[94] Exposure of the capillary basement membrane is a result of the normal and continuous physiologic process of endothelial cell shedding and may permit adhesion of tumor emboli.[94] Platelet adherence to damaged areas (naked basement membrane) followed by degranulation can cause further retraction of endothelial cells and subsequent attachment of tumor emboli or platelet–tumor cell emboli.[89,94,95-98] Fibrin deposits around an arrested tumor embolus have frequently, but not invariably, been observed.[99-101] The role of fibrin in tumor cell arrest and metastasis is uncertain. Theoretically, a protective coat of fibrin around the tumor embolus can shield the neoplastic cells from the host immune response or blood turbulence.[101] Increased coagulability is commonly observed in

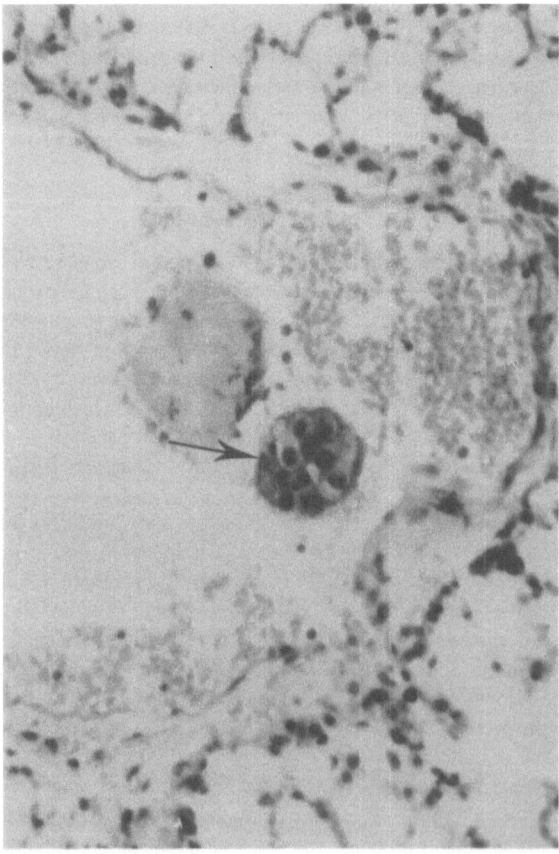

*Figure 2.* Multicellular embolus. A multicellular embolus from a B16–BL6 mouse melanoma (arrow) facilitates the arrest of the tumor cells and may assure the survival of some cells, especially those tumor cells within the clump. (HLE, ×200)

patients with cancer and could be related to the high levels of thromboplastin found in certain tumors.[102,103] Recently, it has been demonstrated that some neoplasms have the capability of producing high levels of procoagulant A activity, which can directly activate factor X in the clotting process.[102–105] A reduced rate of blood flow could lead to increased trapping of circulating tumor cells and the increased survival of already trapped cells.[3,10] The use of anticoagulants in the treatment or prevention of metastasis is based on the consideration of such factors.[106] A major limitation of this approach, however, is the increased risk of bleeding and hematoma formation in anticoagulated patients undergoing major surgery. No doubt, this has prevented expansion of the initial studies. Furthermore, such a therapeutic mechanism is predicated on a prophylaxis approach and is not therapeutically relevant, except for showers of tumor cells during surgery or metastases from metastases. Thus, the risk–potential benefit ratio appears minimal.

Extravasation of arrested tumor cells is thought to occur by mechanisms comparable to those that control invasion.[10,43] Tumor cells can grow and destroy the arresting vessel as a prelude to attaining an extravascular position, or can migrate behind white blood cells.[107] To grow in the organ parenchyma, the metastases must develop a vascular network and evade the host immune system. When the metastases have attained a certain size, they may give rise to additional metastases, the so-called "metastasis of metastases."[3,10,11] Thus, in a short time, a small primary tumor can produce a multitude of metastases.

## 3. BIOLOGIC HETEROGENEITY OF A METASTATIC TUMOR

To produce a clinically relevant metastasis, malignant tumor cells must survive a sequence of potentially lethal interactions with host homeostatic mechanisms, which include avoidance of recognition and destruction by host defenses. Failure to complete any step in the metastatic cascade leads to the elimination of the disseminating tumor cell. The complexity of the pathogenesis of metastasis explains, in part, why the process is deemed to be inefficient.[87,108] For example, the presence of tumor cells in the circulation does not predict that metastasis will occur, because most tumor cells that enter the blood stream are rapidly eliminated.[86–88] Using radiolabeled tumor cells, we have observed that by 24 hr after entry into the circulation, <1% of the cells are still viable, and <0.1% of tumor cells placed into the circulation survived to produce metastases.[86] Observations such as this prompted us to question whether the 0.1% of the circulating cells responsible for the development of metastases survived at random, or whether the cells represented the selective survival and growth of preexistent subpopulations of cells endowed with specific properties. Thus, can all cells growing in a primary neoplasm produce metastases, or can only specific and unique cells produce metastases by possessing properties that enable them to survive the potentially destructive travel from the primary tumor to the sites of metastases?

At the time of diagnosis, many human and animal neoplasms are composed of numerous subpopulations of cells with different phenotypes. Cells isolated from individual neoplasms have been shown to differ with respect to their morphology, karyotype, growth rate, antigenicity–immunogenicity, cell-surface receptors for lectins, hormone receptors, response to therapies, and potential for invasion and metastasis.[3,6–13,108] Indeed, during the last decade, the concept that neoplasms are heterogeneous and contain multiple subpopulations of cells with different biologic properties has gained wide acceptance.[6] This concept is not new. Almost a century ago, Paget[62] analyzed autopsies of a large number of patients with breast cancer and concluded that the nonrandom pattern of metastasis was not due to chance; rather, some tumor cells (seeds) traveling by vascular routes had affinity for growth in the environment provided by certain organs (soil). The development of metastases occurred only when the seed and soil were matched. Recent experiments have shown that site-specific metastasis occurs with many transplantable experimental tumors[3,10,109–112] and has been reported recently in autochthonous human tumors in patients with peritoneo-venous shunts.[113,115] A present definition of the seed and soil hypothesis could consist of three important principles. First, the process of metastasis is not random. Second, neoplasms are not uniform entities but contain cells exhibiting heterogeneous metastatic capabilities. Third, the outcome of metastasis depends on the properties of both tumor cells and host factors; the balance of these contributions varies among tumors arising in different tissues, and even among tumors of similar histologic origin in different patients.

## 3.1. Metastatic Heterogeneity of Tumor Cells in Primary Neoplasms

Cells with different metastatic properties have been isolated from parent, or primary, tumors, supporting the hypothesis that not all the cells in a primary tumor can successfully disseminate. Two general approaches have been used to isolate populations of cells that differ from the parent neoplasm in metastatic capacity. In the first, tumor cells are selected *in vivo*. These cells are either implanted subcutaneously or intramuscularly or are injected intravenously and metastasis is then allowed to occur. The metastatic lesions are harvested, and the cells that are recovered are either expanded in culture or are used immediately to repeat the process. This cycle is then repeated several times. The behavior of the cycled cells is compared with that of the cells of the parent tumor to determine whether the selection process enriched for cells of enhanced metastatic capacity.[116] The increase in metastatic capacity of the recovered cells does not result from the adaptation of tumor cells to preferential growth in a particular organ.[3,10,92,112,116-124] This procedure was originally used to obtain the B16-F10 line from the unselected B16 melanoma.[117] It has also been successfully used to produce tumor cell lines with increased metastatic capacity from many of the experimental tumors tested.

In a second approach used to support the concept of metastatic heterogeneity, cells are selected for the enhanced expression of a phenotype believed to be important in a step of the metastatic sequence, and then they are tested in the appropriate host to determine whether concomitant metastatic potential has been increased or decreased. This method has been used to examine whether properties as diverse as resistance to T lymphocytes,[124,125] adhesive characteristics,[126] invasive capacity,[127,128] lectin resistance,[129-131] resistance to natural killer cells,[132] and antibody-complement-dependent cytotoxicity[133] are important during the metastatic process.

One criticism of these studies is that the isolated tumor line may have arisen as a result of adaptive rather than selective processes. The first experimental proof for metastatic heterogeneity in neoplasms was provided by Fidler and Kripke in 1977 using the murine B16 melanoma.[133] Based on the modified fluctuation assay of Luria and Delbruck, they showed that different tumor cell clones, each derived from individual cells isolated from the parent tumor, varied dramatically in their ability to form pulmonary nodules following intravenous inoculation into syngeneic mice.[134,135] Control subcloning procedures demonstrated that the observed diversity was not a consequence of the cloning procedure.[133,134,136]

To exclude the possibility that the metastatic heterogeneity found in the B16 melanoma might have been introduced as a result of the lengthy in vivo and in vivo cultivation, the same experiment was performed with two newly induced mouse tumors. The metastatic potential of cells isolated from a UV-induced fibrosarcoma and a C3H melanoma after only five passages *in vitro* was examined.[134,136,137] The results obtained with these tumors were strikingly similar to those obtained with the B16 melanoma. Moreover, the cloned cell lines isolated from these tumors varied greatly in their ability to grow at subcutaneous sites and to produce spontaneous metastases in distant organs. In these tumor systems, the ability of cells originating from a sc tumor to produce spontaneous metastases strongly correlated with the production of artificial metastases following introduction into the venous circulation.

The finding that pre-existing tumor cell subpopulations growing in the same tumor exhibit heterogeneous metastatic potential has since been confirmed in numerous laboratories using a wide range of experimental animal tumors of different histories and histologic origins.[3] Moreover, by using young nude mice, in which natural killer cells are not yet mature, as models for metastasis of human neoplasms, it has been demonstrated that human tumor cell lines also contain subpopulations of cells with widely differing metastatic properties.[138-142]

The data demonstrating metastatic heterogeneity in neoplasms ("seed") and those showing that the outcome of metastasis is also dependent on host factors ("soil") support the concept that metastasis is selective and not a random process. Notwithstanding its short-term implications for the current therapeutic strategies, the fact that specific subpopulations of tumor cells are responsible for producing metastases offers a rational strategy for combating metastatic disease. Metastasis is a selective biologic process the outcome of which is regulated by the interaction of tumor cells with the host. As such, the process must be governed by mechanisms that can be studied and ultimately understood in sufficient detail to allow rational therapeutic interaction.

## 3.2. Origin of Cellular Diversity in Malignant Neoplasms

The issue of whether neoplasms are heterogeneous and contain subpopulations of tumor cells with different metastatic propensities is no longer controversial. The important issue is to understand how this extensive cellular heterogeneity originates and is maintained and controlled. For example, when do metastatic variants arise in a primary tumor? Do they arise early or late in the development of a malignant neoplasm? Once metastatic cells develop in a neoplasm, do they have a growth advantage over nonmetastatic cells so that with the passage of time metastatic cells constitute the majority of cells in a neoplasm? How is the proportion of metastatic cells to nonmetastatic cells regulated? Answers to some of these questions are now emerging and may help oncologists in making decisions critical to the timing and sequence of multimodality treatment for primary tumors and metastases.

Whether or not neoplasms are unicellular or multicellular in origin, most are heterogeneous with subpopulations of cells of differing biologic behavior by the time of diagnosis. Tumors can arise as the result of a rare event such as a somatic mutation, in which case their origin can be expected to be unicellular. Indeed, there is strong evidence that many forms of neoplasm are monoclonal in origin, although some are also polyclonal in origin[143–14](see Chapter 10). It is easy to understand the source of cellular diversity in neoplasms that are multicellular in their origin. Such tumors are probably populated by the progenies of several transformed cells. Thus, cells obtained from different parts of chemically induced tumors, some of which are known to be multicellular in origin, differed in their growth rate, susceptibility to cytotoxic drugs, and antigenicity.[3,5,92,148–150] However, it is more difficult to perceive the source of heterogeneity in neoplasms that are unicellular in origin.

Clinical and histologic observations of neoplasms suggested to Foulds that tumors undergo a series of changes during the course of the disease. For example, a tumor that was initially diagnosed as benign can, over a period of many months or even years, evolve into a malignant tumor.[151–152] Nowell[154] suggested that this process of tumor evolution and progression was due to acquired genetic variability within developing clones of tumors, coupled with host selection pressures, resulting in the emergence of new clonal sublines of increased growth autonomy or malignancy.

Nowell's hypothesis predicts that increasing evolution and progression toward malignancy will be accompanied by increasing genetic instability of the malignant cells. This hypothesis was examined by studying the metastatic stability and the rates of mutation to ouabain resistance and/or 6-thioguanine resistance of paired metastatic and nonmetastatic cloned lines isolated from four different mouse neoplasms.[155] In the four different tumor systems examined, highly metastatic cells were less phenotypically stable than were their nonmetastatic counterparts isolated from the same single neoplasm. This rapid generation of diversity may have been caused in part by increased genetic instability. The highly metastatic clones exhibited a rate of spontaneous mutation to ouabain and 6-thioguanine resistance severalfold higher than that found in the poorly metastatic clones.[155] These results are in accord with the hypothesis that tumor progression occurs as a result of acquired genetic alterations. Similar data have now been published by other investigators.[156–161] Additional evidence that genetic mechanisms can be responsible for tumor progression comes from mutagenesis experiments using chemical mutagens[162–164] or ultraviolet radiation.[165] Treatment of tumor cell populations resulted in the emergence of new tumor cell variants, some of which exhibited increased tumorigenicity and metastatic capacities, whereas others had decreased tumorigenic potential.[162–164] This suggests that the more metastatic a tumor cell population is, the greater the likelihood that the constituent cells will undergo spontaneous mutations, resulting in rapid phenotypic diversification and increased opportunities for escape from various therapeutic modalities.[165] This process may, in turn, be further exaggerated by the mutagenic action of many of the cytotoxic antineoplastic drugs used in current treatment regimens.

## 3.3. Instability of Heterogeneous Tumor Populations

The observation that malignant cells have higher mutation rates than benign cells is consistent with the increased metastatic capacity of cell populating metastases compared with the cells of primary tumors. Given the existence of tumor progression and lack of genetic stability, we may ask how degrees of difference can be maintained between various tumor populations. Furthermore, what has prevented these differences from being obliterated by the bidirectional emergence of new variants?

It may be that subpopulations of tumor cells within the tumor mass are not autonomous but are regulated by the proximity of other neoplastic cells. Different subpopulations of mammary tumor cells have been shown to affect the growth patterns[167–169] and chemosensitivity of other groups of cells.[168] Similar regulatory control may exist for the metastatic phenotype of different cells within a mixed tumor.[170] To test for this regulatory control, two poorly metastatic clones and two highly metastatic clones were isolated from the B16–F10 melanoma line. These clones were cultured *in vitro* or *in vivo* for 5, 10, or 20 weeks, and then subclones derived at each of these intervals were reassessed for their metastatic ability. After only 10 *in vitro* passages, many subclones that differed significantly from the parent clone were isolated. Continued cultivation introduced more variability such that by 20 and 40 passages, most clones tested differed significantly from their parent clones. In marked contrast, the metastatic phenotype of the uncloned B16 melanoma lines B16–F1 and B16–F10 remained remarkably stable over 30 *in vivo* passages or 60 *in vitro* passages. Similar stability was observed when different clones were mixed together and co-cultivated as polyclonal populations; however, the subsequent removal of all but one clone led to the rapid generation of biologic diversity in the remaining clone.[170]

The instability of metastatic properties in clones deprived of polyclonal interactions is not limited to cell lines that have been serially passaged *in vitro* or *in vivo* for considerable periods. The same phenomenon has also been identified in clones isolated from newly induced tumors and subjected to a minimum period of cultivation before assay of their metastatic properties.[171,172] Clones isolated from several UV-induced fibrosarcomas and methylcholanthrene-induced tumors that were excised within 3 months of their initial detection each contained a small, but evolving fraction of clones with varying phenotype, which increased during further passage in culture and following serial transplantation in syngeneic mice. Of more interest, however, is the finding that the proportion of unstable clones is significantly higher in cell populations before excision.[172] This indicates that unstable clones evolve *in situ* and that the proportion of such clones increases with tumor progression.

These data suggest that multiple subpopulations of tumor cells stabilize their relative proportions and thereby impose an equilibrium on the combined population. Removal of the stabilizing effect, by isolating clones or by applying a strong selection pressure such as chemotherapy, leads to rapid diversification in the resurgent populations. Although the nature of these stabilizing influences and their mode of action are not yet understood, their very existence argues against randomness in tumor development. Rather, the society of tumor cells imposes regulatory constraints on its individual members to maintain cellular diversity and its concomitant benefits for tumor survival. Certainly, this phenomenon, irrespective of its underlying mechanisms, further complicates attempts to understand the process of tumor progression toward malignancy.

## 3.4. Origin of Biologic Heterogeneity in Metastases

Biologic diversity is not restricted to primary neoplasms, since multiple metastases proliferating within the same host can also exhibit heterogeneity with regard to many characteristics such as metastatic capacity, hormone receptors, marker enzymes, growth rate, antigenicity, and response to various chemotherapeutic agents.[3,173] This diversity could result from either the process of tumor evolution or the nature of tumor cell spread, or both.

Pathologists have long recognized that primary tumors are made up of zones of morphologically distinct cells. Experimental studies have demonstrated that these zonal differences are not restricted to morphology, but include many other characteristics.[174–178] Repeated passage of small tumor fragments can rapidly impose a uniformity on tumor cell populations that is absent when larger, more representative populations are used.[178] It is conceivable that embolic aggregates may arise from a single one of these zones and thus exhibit a degree of uniformity for specific characteristics. Then, irrespective of whether only the central cell or all the cells of the clump survive, the resulting metastatic growth will be analogous to a primary tumor of unicellular origin with regard to the subsequent development of heterogeneity. The same situation could arise when the embolus is derived from an area of zonal junctions so that, although the embolus contains populations with varying phenotypes, selective cell death leads to the survival of only one cell. Alternatively, many or all of the cells forming such a mixed embolus may survive to act as the progenitor of metastatic tumors so that the generation of diversity, as in some primary tumors, is then a consequence of the multicellular origin of the neoplasm.

Metastases, like primary tumors, may have a unicellular or a multicellular origin (Fig. 3). To determine whether individual metastases are clonal and whether different metastases can be produced by different progenitor cells, a series of experiments were carried out using X-irradiated tumor cells to induce random chromosome breaks and rearrangements.[179] Metastases were examined that arose from subcutaneous tumors produced by K-1735 mouse melanoma cells that had been irradiated to induce chromosomal damage. If a metastasis were derived from a single cell, all the chromosome spreads examined within an individual metastasis would exhibit the same karyotype.

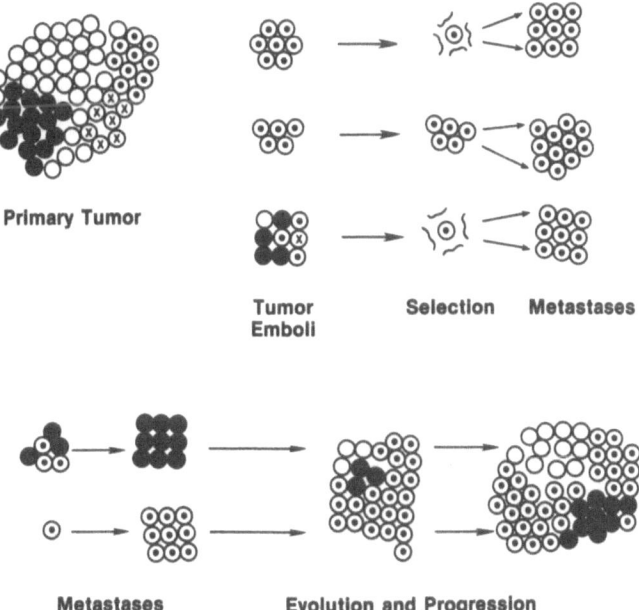

*Figure 3.* Monoclonal origin of metastases. Primary tumors generally arise from a single abnormal cell, but during tumor progression they become heterogeneous. Likewise, metastatic lesions also appear in many cases to be monoclonal in their origin. The monoclonal nature of the metastatic process could be due to the arrest of a single-cell embolus, a clonal embolus, or of a heterotypic embolus from which only one clone survives to form a metastatic lesion. Even during monoclonal metastatic formation, tumor progression continues, resulting again in a heterogeneous tumor foci.

By contrast, if a metastasis had been formed from more than one progenitor cell, its constituent cells could exhibit different chromosomal arrangements, assuming that the different cells involved carried distinguishable karyotypic markers. The cellular composition of 21 individual metastases was analyzed after cultivation of cells from individual lesions. In 10 metastases, all the chromosomes were normal, so it was impossible to establish whether they were of uni- or multicellular origin. In the other 11 lesions, unique karyotypic patterns of abnormal marker chromosomes were found, suggesting that each metastasis originated from a single progenitor cell. However, this experiment cannot resolve whether metastases arose as a consequence of individual cells surviving in the bloodstream or whether homogeneous clumps (i.e., a multicellular embolus of cells with the same chromosome marker) survived in the circulation, but it does establish that many metastases do originate from single cells. Moreover, the finding that different, individual metastases are populated by cells with various chromosome markers indicates that metastases from the same host can originate from different progenitor cells.[179]

Similar results have been obtained in experiments using B16 melanoma cell clones bearing identifiable biochemical markers.[180] This study not only revealed that the majority of metastases are of clonal origin, but also that variant clones with diverse phenotypes are formed rapidly to generate significant cellular diversity within individual metastases.[113,173,180,181] Recently, the clonality of the metastatic process was confirmed by restriction fragment length polymorphism (RFLP) following the transfection of Neo-2 plasmids as a marker of clonality. Studies based on these stably expressed markers, which are easily monitored by Southern blotting, confirmed the clonal origin of metastases.[182]

Collectively, these observations indicate that different metastases arise from different progenitor cells and account for the well-documented differences in the behavior of individual metastases in the same host, including differences in response to therapy (i.e., intralesional heterogeneity). However, within individual metastases of proven clonal origin, heterogeneity can also rapidly develop to create significant intralesional heterogeneity.

## 3.5. Development of Intralesional Heterogeneity within Metastases

The demonstration that metastatic cells exhibit higher mutation rates than nonmetastatic cells[155-158] and that heterogeneity develops more rapidly in tumors containing few subpopulations of cells[170,172] suggests that accelerated tumor evolution and progression will result in the rapid development of biologic diversity in solitary metastases, especially when such lesions are of clonal origin.[179,181,182] This question was addressed using a highly metastatic clonal line of the K-1735 melanoma that expresses a stable unique marker chromosome. Immediately after establishment *in vitro*, this *in vivo* selected line was cloned *in vitro*. The cells were also injected subcutaneously, and the local tumor and spontaneous lung metastases recovered 60–90 days later. The experimental metastatic ability was determined for each of these lines. Six of the 10 *in-vitro*-derived clones, and six of seven lines established from spontaneous metastases, differed significantly in their metastatic ability from the parental cell line. The relative sensitivities to four chemotherapeutic agents (amsacrine, vincristine, bleomycin, and doxorubicin) were also tested. Sensitivity to the drugs varied greatly among and within different metastases in clones isolated from these lesions and growth *in vitro* and in the original parent tumor cell line. These findings indicate that even within metastases of clonal origin, heterogeneity for metastasis and sensitivity to chemotherapy can develop rapidly,[181] documenting yet another mechanism for the clinical phenomenon of resistance to chemotherapy.

Isolation of multiple clones from individual lung metastases produced by the B16 melanoma has revealed that clones isolated from "early" metastases excised after 6–25 days show indistinguishable metastatic properties (i.e., intralesional clonal homogeneity).[172] This situation was found in approximately 80% of the early metastases tested, though the metastatic phenotypes of clones isolated from different metastases in the same animal do differ significantly (i.e., intralesional clonal heterogeneity). By contrast, in "late" metastases excised after 40–45 days, intralesional clonal homogeneity was found in only 25% of metastases, indicating the development of intralesional heterogeneity by diversification of the original clone that established the metastasis.

These data suggest that in the B16 melanoma, individual lung metastases are populated initially by cells with a uniform metastatic phenotype. This is in agreement with the data discussed earlier showing that most experimental metastases result from the arrest and proliferation of a single tumor cell.[179] This *in vivo* situation is therefore analogous to the *in vitro* experiments described above in which individual B16 clones grown in isolation from other clones quickly generated variant subclones with altered metastatic properties.[172]

## 4. THE CHALLENGE OF BIOLOGIC HETEROGENEITY OF NEOPLASMS

The most formidable obstacle to the successful treatment of established metastases may well be the heterogeneity of cells within neoplasms. This biologic heterogeneity, which results from the continuing evolution of tumors, is demonstrated by the emergence of variants from the primary tumor and is responsible for differences in response to treatment within cells populating a primary tumor, between the primary tumor and its metastases, and even among different metastatic lesions. The biologic diversity of neoplasms implies that the successful treatment of the disease will require the total destruction of all tumor cells. By the time primary tumors (or metastases) are diagnosed, the lesions are approximately 1 $cm^3$ in size, i.e., the resolution of X-rays and computed tomography (CT) scans and contain about $10^9$ cells. The destruction of 99.9% of the cells, a remarkable achievement indeed, still leaves $10^6$ cells to proliferate and provide a basis for the additional generation of biologic diversity, including treatment-resistant variants. Understanding the mechanisms responsible for the development of biologic heterogeneity in neoplasms and how metastatic cells spread from primary tumors to produce secondary lesions is therefore an important goal of cancer research.

The three main areas in which the biologic heterogeneity of neoplasms is likely to prove of practical importance, beyond clinical therapy, are in the detection of tumor deposits using monoclonal antibodies or tumor cell markers, in the design of screening procedures for these diagnostic techniques, and finally, in applying therapeutic regimes other than surgical resection.

Many clinical observations have demonstrated the impact of tumor cell heterogeneity on attempts to detect primary or metastatic tumor foci. For example, small cell carcinoma of the lung, medullary carcinoma of the thyroid, and carcinoid tumor can often be detected by an elevation in the serum levels of various markers, such as calcitonin, histaminase, and L-DOPA decarboxylase. When Baylin and co-workers[183,184] simultaneously sampled both primary tumors and metastases for these markers, they found a variable pattern of expression. All primary tumors produced detectable levels of each marker, whereas many of the metastases produced either low or undetectable levels. Immunohistochemical studies revealed that cells in the primary tumor varied widely in histaminase production.[183] Similarly, serial determinations of serum acid phosphatase have proved to be clinically useful for the diagnosis of advanced carcinoma of the prostate. Furthermore, a decrease in serum enzyme levels often correlates with clinical response to antiandrogen therapy. However, in 20–25% of patients with stage D (advanced) disease, the levels of this enzymatic tumor marker are normal.[185] Heterogeneity in expression and release of tumor cell markers is well documented for other neoplasms as well.[186–189] Findings such as these suggest that it may not be feasible to use a product of tumor cells for the determination of disseminated disease. Of greater importance than the implications for cancer detection are the implications of tumor cell heterogeneity for the treatment of metastatic disease. The genesis of cellular diversity within tumors via the generation and expansion of phenotypically different tumor cell clones during tumor progression provides a powerful mechanism for increasing the ability of a tumor to survive a diverse array of destructive selection pressures.

### 4.1. Effect of Tumor Cell Heterogeneity on Chemotherapy

There are numerous reports of differences in drug sensitivity among tumor cell populations growing in a parent neoplasm. Various animal or human neoplasms, such as melanoma, stomach and colon adenocarcinomas, hepatoma, breast carcinoma, ovarian carcinoma, lymphoma, glioma, and lung cancer have all been shown to contain different subpopulations of cells with different drug sensitivities.[190-196] Differences in drug response between cells that populate metastases and those isolated from the localized primary neoplasm have also been reported.[193-204] Like the drug response of cells populating primary tumors and their metastases, radiation sensitivity of cell populations of animal and human tumors is also heterogeneous.[205-207]

Tsuruo and Fidler[204] examined the *in vitro* sensitivity to various chemotherapeutic agents of tumor cells from parent tumors, their *in vitro* cloned populations, and their spontaneous metastases. Both murine tumors and a human melanoma line were evaluated. Differences in drug responsiveness were found among cells populating a parent tumor (*in vitro* clones), between the parent line and its metastatic subpopulations (*in vivo* selected lines), and among the various spontaneous metastases. These extensive differences in drug sensitivity could have profound implications for the treatment of metastases with cytotoxic drugs.

Although the growth inhibition of tumor cells *in vitro* by a drug does not always correlate with its sensitivity *in vivo*, the development of *in vitro* assays of tumor cell response to cytotoxic agents for the purpose of predicting the outcome of cancer therapy in individual patients has been pursued by many researchers. If such assays are to be meaningful, they must use a sample representative of all cells populating the tumor. The introduction of the human stem cell assay is based on the rationale that freshly isolated human tumor cells might more accurately predict the clinical response to antineoplastic agents of human tumors of similar histologic origins than cells from rodent tumors subjected to unknown selection pressures during serial passage over several months or years. However, isolation of cells from only one region of a solid tumor, which could well contain zonal heterogeneity,[178] coupled with the low cloning efficacy of most human tumor cells, may introduce severe limitations.[208,209] Additional complication are the clonal interactions between various subpopulations of cells that can influence the drug sensitivities of these subpopulations.[175]

The existence of specialized subpopulations of cells with high metastatic potential has farreaching consequences for the testing of potential agents for the treatment of metastatic disease. As recently pointed out by Schabel et al.,[210] many of the methods presently used to define the drug sensitivity of experimental animal tumors might be misleading, since tumors are not uniform entities. Partial regression of the primary tumor is an inadequate assay for screening agents for their antimetastatic activity. Assays in which a drug or combination of drugs is found to limit growth of a tumor (injected at a primary site, i.e., subcutaneously or intramuscularly) may merely reveal the presence of a subpopulation of drug-sensitive cells. It does not necessarily offer insight into the pharmacologic susceptibility of the tumor cell subpopulations that will give rise to metastases. Efforts to identify potential agents in which therapeutic agents are screened for their activity against tumor cell subpopulations with defined metastatic capabilities may be more appropriate. Stimulation of the rate of formation of tumor cell variants by restriction of subpopulation diversity may also provide an explanation for the rapid evolution of cellular diversity within individual metastases mentioned above.[171,172,180,181]

Diversification of the cellular phenotypes present in a metastasis formed by the arrest and proliferation of a single tumor cell (which may be the sole survivor from within a multicellular heterogeneous embolus) could occur by two mechanisms. The first would involve an intrinsically unstable cell that had been generating new variants at a high frequency, even while in the primary tumor. The alternative possibility is that transport of a single tumor cell from a heterogeneous primary tumor to a distant organ where, in isolation from other clonal subpopulations, its phenotypic regulation could be destabilized. In the primary tumor, interactions between the heterogeneous constituent subpopulations act to impose relative phenotypic stability and restrict the rate of formation of variants. However, for a single cell in a newly established metastasis, these interactions would be absent. The rate of formation of new tumor cell variants would thus be stimulated, quickly converting the initially clonally homogeneous metastasis to a clonally heterogeneous lesion.

The most challenging issue concerns the potential effect of therapy on the dynamics of tumor cell subpopulations. If a particular therapy were to kill the majority of cellular subpopulations in a heterogeneous tumor (as is typically the case), the surviving subpopulations might be rendered phenotypically unstable because of loss of the regulatory interaction between constituent subpopulations. By narrowing subpopulation diversity in a tumor cell population that would otherwise contain sufficient diversity to slow the formation of new clonal variants (see above), therapy could stimulate the formation of new tumor cell variants from the surviving subpopulations, i.e., iatrogenic heterogeneity.

The heterogeneous nature of the response of malignant tumor cell subpopulations to cytotoxic drugs and other therapeutic modalities makes it unlikely that a single treatment regimen will be able to kill all the cells in a tumor, even if several agents are used simultaneously. In most clinical situations, following completion of a treatment protocol that eliminates clinically detectable tumor burden, new regimens are implemented only when a patient presents at some time later with clinical evidence of recurrent disease. In this regard, the recurrent tumor cells involved could be phenotypically different from those in the original tumor; variant subpopulations would have been induced by the restriction in subpopulation diversity following or caused by the first treatment regimen. Thus, the subpopulations in the recurrent lesions could well be resistant to the therapeutic agents used in the first treatment protocol, as well as to other agents.

## 4.2. Antigenic and Immunogenic Heterogeneity

Over the years, numerous investigators have suggested that host immune mechanisms could be augmented to control cancer metastases. Several approaches utilizing both specific and nonspecific immunologic manipulation have been employed to tilt the tumor/host interaction in favor of the host. There are several major components that may inhibit the successful application of immunotherapy to the control of cancer metastasis. These components, identified by experimental studies, are (1) the heterogeneous nature of malignant neoplasms; (2) the intrinsic antigenicity of metastatic tumor cells; (3) the ability of the primary host to recognize and destroy susceptible tumor cells; (4) the inability of immunotherapy to be effective for even moderate tumor burdens; and (5) immunosuppression by prior chemoradiotherapy. Several approaches for immunologic intervention currently being studied either experimentally or clinically are increasing tumor cell antigenicity, interference with immunoregulation (by elimination of suppressor cells), specific or nonspecific immune stimulation, adoptive cell transfer (NK cells, lymphokine-activated killer cells,[211] T cells), myeloid reconstitution, or the inhibition of tumor growth or metastasis by monoclonal antibodies and immunoconjugates.

The heterogeneous nature of animal and human neoplasms with regard to antigenicity, immunogenicity, and susceptibility to lymphocyte-mediated lysis is now well recognized.[211–220] In addition, studies have shown that the antigenicity of primary tumors and their metastases and antigenicity among different metastatic lesions can also differ. Such variations may greatly influence the likelihood of success of specific immunotherapeutic modalities. For example, Olsson and Ebbesen,[221] using a number of AKR mouse lymphomas, have shown that vaccination procedures against polyclonal tumors failed because only the dominant subclone was restricted in growth. The major subpopulations, which did not constitute a sufficient mass in the vaccine to stimulate the immune response, proceeded to proliferate after the vaccination and one eventually became the dominant population.

Although there is good evidence that carcinogen-induced tumors are highly antigenic,[222] less certainty can be generated for the antigenic–immunogenic nature of autochthonous human neoplasms. This concern (are human tumors antigenic?) has evolved from the work of Hewitt *et al.*,[223] who have been unable to detect tumor-specific antigens in spontaneously arising animal tumors and thus have been unable to immunologically protect against such tumors. In any event, a promising approach for augmenting the antigenic properties of tumors, at least in animal models, has been to treat poorly immunogenic tumor cell lines with chemicals or viruses and selecting immunogenic cell variants.[162–164] Often, these variants are able to generate potent cytotoxic T cell (CTL) responses and can protect syngeneic animals against challenge with the potential tumor.[162–164,224–227]

Another issue to consider is whether the relative antigenicity of malignant cells influences their metastatic potential. A systemic study of the role of tumor cell immunogenicity and host immune status in the formation of experimental and spontaneous metastases has been reported.[215,227] Three C3H mouse fibrosarcomas with different degrees of immunogenicity were tested for growth and metastasis in normal, sham-suppressed, immunosuppressed, and immunosuppressed and immunologically reconstituted syngeneic mice. Immunosuppression affected growth and experimental metastasis of the three tumors in different ways. The highly immunogenic fibrosarcoma formed more experimental metastases in immunosuppressed mice than in normal, sham-suppressed, or immunosuppressed and immunologically reconstituted syngeneic mice. A fibrosarcoma of intermediate immunogenicity also formed more pulmonary metastases in immunosuppressed recipients, but this increase could not be reversed by reconstitution with syngeneic lymphocytes. By contrast, the least immunogenic tumor formed fewer lung metastases in immunosuppressed mice than in normal, sham-suppressed, or reconstituted mice.[215] It was concluded that the role of the immune system in experimental metastasis varies for different tumors and that no generalizations regarding the role of host immunity can be made from a single tumor system that will predict the outcome of metastasis in another tumor system.[227] Nonetheless, we can infer that the immunogenic properties of the tumor will determine, to some extent, the nature and degree of the influence of the immune system on the metastatic process.[228]

Metastatic cells can successfully evade host immune surveillance mechanisms when host immunity is suppressed. This is best exemplified in the UV light-induced skin tumors. These tumors, which are mainly squamous cell carcinomas or fibrosarcomas, are highly antigenic, and many are immunologically rejected upon transplantation to syngeneic hosts. However, these same tumors grow progressively upon transplantation to immunologically deficient recipients.[229–231] In addition, these highly antigenic UV-induced neoplasms grow progressively in syngeneic mice that have been treated for a short period of time with intermittent doses of UV radiation.[232] Studies on the mechanisms of this phenomenon revealed that the inability of precancerous UV-irradiated mice to reject challenges with syngeneic UV-induced fibrosarcomas is due to the presence of suppressor T lymphocytes on their lymphoid organs.[232–234] The reactivity of the UV-induced T suppressor cells is restricted in that these cells do not suppress the rejection of either allogeneic UV-induced fibrosarcomas or syngeneic chemically induced fibrosarcomas.[232,234] Furthermore, the immune responses of UV-irradiated mice to a variety of exogenous antigens is normal,[229–234] again suggesting that the suppressor T cells show selectivity for antigens expressed against autochthonous and syngeneic UV-induced tumors. Recent studies have suggested that in both the UV-induced tumor system and in a transplantation antigen system, the gene locus responsible for antigenicity can be lost presumably due to immunoselection.[235,236] In the transplantation antigen system,[235] the poorly antigenic B16–BL6 melanoma cell line was rendered highly antigenic by the transfection of the alloantigen H-2 $D^d$. Following transplantation to normal syngeneic hosts, the time to development of a palpable tumor was significantly increased compared to control B16–BL6 cells. However, when these animals became moribund, due to tumor burden, they had a similar amount of metastasis as those receiving control cells. Southern blot analysis showed that the metastatic cells did not express the H-2 $D^d$; indeed, they no longer had the gene. Thus, the immune response selected the rare variant that did not express the antigenic epitope. However, in the absence of a specific immune response (nude mice), the tumor growth rate and metastatic frequency was not disturbed by the presence of the alloantigen. This series of studies demonstrates that while the host specific immune system may play an important role in tumor progression and therapy, it also is a selective presence. Thus, if a tumor cell contains all the genotypes necessary for metastasis, it may be selected for, while cells with a single negative attribute are selected against, resulting subsequently in the growth of metastatic foci.

Active-specific immunotherapy, currently more in vogue than classical nonspecific immunotherapy, also has had problems. Adoptive immunization of tumor-bearing animals using T lymphocytes sensitized to tumor cells has only been partially successful in the past.[237,238] One reason is the co-transfer of suppressor T lymphocytes into the tumor-bearing host or the direct generation of these suppressor T lymphocytes by the tumor. Protocols to eradicate suppressor T lymphocytes generated in the host (irradiation or low-dose cyclophosphamide) may help, but there is still another potential problem to be resolved; the high probability of selecting for antigen-loss tumor cell variants, which could escape immune destruction.[224] Given the overwhelming data on the instability of tumor cells, the generation of such antiloss variants may be a major obstacle to specific immunotherapy. An additional possibility for further improvement of active specific immunotherapy is the use of cultured long-term lymphocyte lines expanded with interleukin-2,[210,237,239] although this approach is both labor intensive, expensive, and, to date, toxic.

Other areas of active research for the immune therapy of metastases are the use of monoclonal antibodies or immunoconjugates. Monoclonal antibodies alone may be useful to specifically block steps in the pathogenesis of metastasis.[240,241] Immunoconjugates are being used in hope that the monoclonal antibody can target these immunoconjugates to the sites of metastatic foci, allowing the toxic agent linked to these antibodies to kill those cells in the area of localization, thereby preventing their systemic deposition. It again must be realized that although promising, this therapy relies on cells in every metastatic deposit to display the specific antigen to which the monoclonal antibody is raised. As discussed previously, biochemical markers are heterogeneously expressed by both experimental and human tumor cells.[186–189] One route designed to circumvent the problem of heterogeneity with monoclonal antibody therapy is to use different combinations of monoclonal antibodies targeted to different antigens.

On the basis of many new biologic response modifiers (BRM), novel immunotherapy protocols are being devised, including interferons and their inducers, lymphokines, growth factors, antibodies, and maturation/differentiation factors.[242–244] The interferons, interleukins, and tumor necrosis factor are now in clinical trials. However, as with the chemotherapeutic agents in use, cell lines either partially or completely resistant to BRM have been observed in experimental systems, although this may not be limiting, since many of these agents are thought to be active due to immunoaugmentation of effector cell activity.

## 5. SUMMARY

Metastasis is a complex multifaceted process that is dependant on both host and tumor cell attributes. Because of tumor progression, clonal selection (associated with the metastatic process and cytoreductive therapy), and the mutagenic nature of chemo- and radiotherapy, a rapid induction of cellular heterogeneity occurs. This phenotypic and genotypic heterogeneity has tremendous implications for the successful treatment of metastasis. Heterogeneity is responsible for the failure of most therapeutic protocols. However, our understanding of the metastatic process also suggests that it may be possible to take advantage of the selective nature of the process by developing modalities directed against individual steps of the metastatic cascade. Likewise, therapies may be developed that inhibit the rapid development of genetic or epigenetic heterogeneity. Furthermore, because the metastatic process is now understood to be a selective biologic process with specific subpopulations of tumor cells responsible for producing metastasis, this now offers the potential for the development of novel and rational strategies for treating metastatic disease.

ACKNOWLEDGMENT. This research was supported by the National Cancer Institute, DHHS, under contract N01-23910 with Program Resources, Inc.

## REFERENCES

1. Dorland, W. A., 1965, *Dorland's Illustrated Medical Dictionary*, 24th ed., W. B. Saunders, Philadelphia.
2. Schabel, F. M., 1975, Concepts for systemic treatment of micrometastasis, *Cancer* **35:**15–24.
3. Fidler, I. J., 1984, The evolution of biological heterogeneity in metastatic neoplasms, in: *Cancer Invasion and Metastasis: Biologic and Therapeutic Aspects* (G. L. Nicolson and L. Milas, eds.), pp. 5–26, Raven, New York.
4. Sugarbaker, E. V., and Ketcham, A. S., 1977, Mechanisms and prevention of cancer dissemination. An overview, *Semin. Oncol.* **4:**19–32.

5. Sugarbaker, E. V., 1979, Cancer metastasis: A product of tumor–host interactions, *Curr. Probl. Cancer* **3**:1–59.

6. Hart, I. R., and Fidler, I. J., 1981, The implications of tumor heterogeneity for studies on the biology and therapy of cancer metastasis, *Biochim. Biophys. Acta* **651**:37–50.

7. Fidler, I. J., and Poste, G., 1985, The cellular heterogeneity of malignant neoplasms: Implications for adjuvant chemotherapy, *Semin. Oncol.* **12**:207–221.

8. Fidler, I. J., and Hart, I. R., 1982, Biological diversity in metastatic neoplasms: Origins and implications, *Science* **217**:998–1003.

9. Heppner, G., 1984, Tumor heterogeneity, *Cancer Res.* **44**:2259–2265.

10. Poste, G., and Fidler, I. J., 1979, The pathogenesis of cancer metastasis, *Nature (Lond.)* **283**:139–146.

11. Fidler, I. J., Gersten, D. M., and Hart, I. R., 1978, The biology of cancer invasion and metastasis, *Adv. Cancer Res.* **28**:149–250.

12. Nicolson, G. L., and Poste, G., 1982, Tumor cell diversity and host responses in cancer metastasis, *Curr. Probl. Cancer* **7**:4–83.

13. Dexter, D. L., and Calabresi, P., 1982, Intraneoplastic diversity, *Biochim. Biophys. Acta* **695**:97–112.

14. Willis, R. A., 1972, *The Spread of Tumors in the Human Body,* Butterworth, London.

15. Laerum, O. D., Bjerkvig, R., Steinsvag, S. K., and de Ridder, L., 1984, Invasiveness of primary brain tumors, *Cancer Metast. Rev.* **3**:223–236.

16. Gabbert, H., 1985, Mechanisms of tumor invasion: Evidence from *in vivo* observations, *Cancer Metast. Rev.* **4**:293–309.

17. Noguchi, P. D., Johnson, J. B., O'Donnell, R., and Petricciani, J. C., 1978, Chick embryonic skin as a rapid organ culture assay for cellular neoplasia, *Science* **199**:980–983.

18. Mareel, M. M., 1983, Invasion *in vitro:* Methods of analysis, *Cancer Metast. Rev.* **2**:201–218.

19. Weiss, L., and Ward, P. M., 1983, Cell detachment and metastasis, *Cancer Metast. Rev.* **2**:111–127.

20. Carr, I., 1983, Lymphatic metastasis, *Cancer Metast. Rev.* **22**:307–317.

21. Gail, M. H., and Boone, C. W., 1971, Density inhibition of motility in 3T3 fibroblasts and their SV40 transformation, *Exp. Cell Res.* **64**:156–162.

22. Strauli, P., and Haemmerli, O., 1984, The role of cancer cell motility in invasion, *Cancer Metast. Rev.* **3**:127–141.

23. Gershman, H., Katzin, W., and Cook, R. T., 1978, Mobility of cells from solid tumors, *Int. J. Cancer* **21**:309–316.

24. Hart, I. R., 1979, Selection and characterization of an invasive variant of the B16 melanoma, *Am. J. Pathol.* **97**:587–600.

25. Varani, J., Orr, W., and Ward, P. A., 1979, Comparison of subpopulations of tumor cells with altered migratory activity, attachment characteristics, enzyme levels and *in vivo* behavior, *Eur. J. Cancer* **15**:585–592.

26. Varani, J., Orr, W., and Ward, P. A., 1979, Hydrolytic enzyme activities, migratory activity and *in vivo* growth and metastatic potential of recent isolates, *Cancer Res.* **39**:2376–2380.

27. Tickle, C., Crawley, A., and Goodman, M., 1978, Cell movement and the mechanism of invasiveness: A survey of the behavior of some normal and malignant cells implanted into the developing chick wing bud, *J. Cell Sci.* **31**:293–322.

28. Franks, L. M., Riddle, P. N., and Seal, P., 1969, Actin-like filaments and cell movement in human ascites tumor cells. An ultrastructural and cine-micrographic study, *Exp. Cell. Res.* **54**:157–162.

29. Volk, T., Geiger, B., and Raz, A., 1984, Motility and adhesive properties of high and low-metastatic murine neoplastic cells, *Cancer Res.* **44**:811–824.

30. Raz, A., and Geiger, B., 1982, Altered organization of cell-substrate contacts and membrane-associated cytoskeleton in tumor cell variants exhibiting different metastatic capabilities, *Cancer Res.* **42**:5183–5190.

31. Kieler, J.v.F., 1984, Invasiveness of transformed bladder epithelium cells, *Cancer Metast. Rev.* **3**:265–296.

32. Babai, F., and Tremblay, G., 1972, Ultrastructural study of liver invasion by Novikoff hepatoma, *Cancer Res.* **32**:2765–2770.

33. Dingemans, K. P., 1974, Invasion of liver tissue by blood-borne mammary carcinoma cells, *J. Natl. Cancer Inst.* **53**:1813–1824.

34. Roos, E., Dingemans, K. P., van de Pavert, I. V., and van de Bergh-Weerman, I. M., 1977, Invasion of lymphosarcoma cells into the perfused mouse liver, *J. Natl. Cancer Inst.* **58**:399–407.

35. Ruoslahti, E., 1984, Fibronectin in cell adhesion and invasion, *Cancer Metab. Rev.* **3**:43–51.

36. Hart, I. R., Raz, A., and Fidler, I. J., 1980, Effect of cytoskeleton-disrupting agents on the metastatic behavior of melanoma cells, *J. Natl. Cancer Inst.* **64**:891–900.
37. Bernacki, R. J., Niedbala, M. J., and Korytnyk, W., 1985, Glycosidases in cancer and invasion, *Cancer Metab. Rev.* **4**:81–102.
38. Dresden, M. H., Heilman, S. A., and Schmidt, J. D., 1972, Collagenolytic enzymes in human neoplasms, *Cancer Res.* **32**:993–996.
39. Strauch, L., 1972, The role of collagenases in tumor invasion, in: *Tissue Interactions in Carcinogenesis* (D. Tarin, ed.), pp. 399–407, Academic, London.
40. Sylven, B., 1968, Lysosomal enzyme activity in the interstitial fluid of solid mouse tumor transplants, *Eur. J. Cancer* **4**:463–474.
41. Jones, P. A., and DeClerck, Y. A., 1982, Extracellular matrix destruction by invasive tumor cells, *Cancer Metab. Rev.* **1**:289–317.
42. Liotta, L. A., 1986, Tumor invasion and metastases—Role of the extracellular matrix: Rhoads memorial award lecture, *Cancer Res.* **46**:1–7.
43. Liotta, L. A., Thorgeirsson, U. P., and Gabrisa, S., 1982, Role of collagenases in tumor cell invasion, *Cancer Metab. Rev.* **1**:277–288.
44. Tarin, D., 1982, Investigations of the mechanisms of metastatic spread of naturally occurring neoplasms, *Cancer Metab. Rev.* **1**:215–225.
45. Woolley, D. E., 1984, Collagenolytic mechanisms in tumor cell invasion, *Cancer Metab. Rev.* **3**:361–372.
46. Bosmann, H. B., and Hall, T. C., 1974, Enzyme activity in invasive tumors of human breast and colon, *Proc. Natl. Acad. Sci. USA* **71**:1833–1837.
47. Honn, K. V., Menter, D. G., Onoda, J. M., Taylor, J. D., and Sloane, B. F., 1984, Role of prostacyclin as a natural deterrent to hematogenous tumor metastasis, in: *Cancer Invasion and Metastasis: Biologic and Therapeutic Aspects* (G. L. Nicolson and L. Milas, eds.), pp. 361–388, Raven, New York.
48. Sloane, B. F., and Honn, K. V., 1984, Cysteine proteinases and metastasis, *Cancer Metab. Rev.* **3**:249–263.
49. Recklies, A. D., Tiltman, K. J., Stoker, T. A. M., and Poole, A. R., 1980, Secretion of proteinases from malignant and nonmalignant human breast tissue, *Cancer Res.* **40**:550–556.
50. Roblin, R. O., 1978, Plasminogen activator production as a possible biological marker for human neoplasia: Some fundamental questions, in: *Biological Markers of Neoplasia: Basic and Applied Aspects* (R. Ruddon, ed.), pp. 421–432, Elsevier, New York.
51. Reich, E., 1973, Tumor-associated fibrinolysis. Abstracted comments, *Fed. Proc.* **32**:2174–2175.
52. Wang, B. S., McLoughlin, G. A., Richie, J. P., and Mannick, J. A., 1980, Correlation of the production of plasminogen activator with tumor metastasis in B16 mouse melanoma cell lines, *Cancer Res.* **40**:288–292.
53. Turley, E. A., 1984, Proteoglycans and cell adhesion: Their putative role during tumorigenesis, *Cancer Metab. Rev.* **3**:325–339.
54. Liotta, L. A., Tryggvason, K., Garbisa, S., Hart, I., Foltz, C. M., and Shafie, S., 1980, Metastatic potential correlates with enzymatic degradation of basement membrane collagen, *Nature (Lond.)* **284**:67–68.
55. Liotta, L. A., Abe, S., Robey, P. G., and Martin, G. R., 1979, Preferential digestion of basement membrane collagen by an enzyme derived from a metastatic murine tumor, *Proc. Natl. Acad. Sci. USA* **76**:2268–2272.
56. Liotta, L. A., Kleinerman, J., Catanzaro, P., and Rynbrandt, D., 1977, Degradation of basement membrane by murine tumor cells, *J. Natl. Cancer Inst.* **58**:1427–1431.
57. Murray, J. C., Liotta, L., Rennard, S. I., and Martin, G. R., 1980, Adhesion characteristics of murine metastatic and nonmetastatic tumor cells *in vitro*, *Cancer Res.* **40**:347–351.
58. Babai, F., 1976, Etude ultrastructurale sur la pathogénie de l'invasion du muscle strié par des tumeurs transplantables, *J. Ultrastruct. Res.* **56**:287–303.
59. del Regato, J. A., 1977, Pathways of metastatic spread of malignant tumors, *Semin. Oncol.* **4**:33–38.
60. Fisher, B., and Fisher, E. R., 1966, The interrelationship of hematogenous and lymphatic tumor cell dissemination, *Surg. Gynecol. Obstet.* **122**:791–798.
61. Zeidman, I., and Buss, J. M., 1954, Experimental studies on the spread of cancer in the lymphatic system. I. Effectiveness of the lymph node as a barrier to the passage of embolic tumor cells, *Cancer Res.* **14**:403–405.
62. Paget, S., 1889, The distribution of secondary growths in cancer of the breast, *Lancet* **1**:571–573.

63. Fisher, E. R., and Fisher, B., 1967, Recent observations on the concept of metastasis, *Arch. Pathol. Lab. Med.* **83:**321–324.

64. del Ragato, J. A., 1978, Physiopathology of metastasis, in: *Pulmonary Metastasis* (L. Weiss and H. A. Gilbert, eds.), pp. 104–113, G. K. Hall, Boston.

65. Lane, M., Goksel, H., Salerno, R. A., and Haagensen, C. D., 1961, Clinicopathologic analysis of the surgical curability of breast cancers: A minimum ten-year study of a personal series, *Ann. Surg.* **153:**483–504.

66. Black, M. M., Freeman, C., Mork, T., Harvei, S. and Cutler, S. J., 1971, Prognostic significance of microscopic structure of gastric carcinomas and their regional lymph nodes, *Cancer* **27:**703–711.

67. Berg, J. W., Huvos, A. G., Axtell, L. M., and Robbins, G. Y., 1973, A new sign of favorable prognosis in mammary cancer: Hyperplastic reactive lymph nodes in the apex of the axilla, *Ann. Surg.* **177:**8–15.

68. Mitchison, N. A., 1954, Passive transfer of transplantation immunity, *Proc. R. Soc. Lond. [B]* **142:**72–87.

69. Billingham, R. E., Brent, L., and Medawar, P. B., 1956, Quantitative studies on tissue transplantation immunity, *Philos. Trans. R. Soc. Lond. [B]* **239:**357–366.

70. Barker, C. F., and Billingham, R. E., 1968, The role of afferent lymphatics in the rejection of skin homografts, *J. Exp. Med.* **128:**197–222.

71. Futrell, J. W., and Myers, G. H., 1972, Role of regional lymphatics in tumor allograft rejection, *Transplantation* **13:**551–557.

72. Crile, G., 1965, Rationale of simple mastectomy without radiation for clinical stage 1 cancer of the breast, *Surg. Gynecol. Obstet.* **120:**975–982.

73. Crile, G., 1969, Possible role of uninvolved regional nodes in preventing metastasis from breast cancer, *Cancer* **24:**1283–1285.

74. Fisher, B., and N. Wolmark, 1975, New concepts in the management of primary breast cancer, *Cancer* **36:**627–632.

75. Fisher, B., Bauer, M. and Margolese, R., 1985, Five-year results of a randomized clinical trial comparing total mastectomy and segmental mastectomy with or without radiation in the treatment of breast cancer, *N. Engl. J. Med.* **312:**665–673.

76. Fisher, B., Redmond, C., Fisher, E., Bauer, M., Wolmark, N., Wickerman, L., Deutsch, M., and Montague, E., 1985, Ten-year results of a randomized clinical trial comparing radical mastectomy and total mastectomy with or without radiation, *N. Engl. J. Med.* **312:**674–681.

77. Fisher, B., Saffer, E. A., and Fisher, E. R., 1974, Studies concerning the regional lymph node in cancer. IV. Tumor inhibition by regional lymph node cells, *Cancer* **33:**631–636.

78. Fisher, B., Wolmark, N., Coyle, J., Saffer, E., and Fisher, E. R., 1985, Studies concerning the regional lymph node in cancer. VIII. Effect of two asynchronous tumor foci on lymph node cell cytotoxicity, *Cancer* **36:**521–527.

79. Pauli, B. U., Schwartz, E. D., Thonar, E. J. M., and Kuttern, K. E., 1983, Tumor invasion and host extracellular matrix, *Cancer Metab. Rev.* **2:**129–153.

80. Brem, H., and Folkman, J., 1975, Inhibition of tumor angiogenesis mediated by cartilage, *J. Exp. Med.* **141:**427–439.

81. Folkman, J., 1984, Angiogenesis: Initiation and modulation, in: *Cancer Invasion and Metastasis: Biologic and Therapeutic Aspects* (G. L. Nicolson, and L. Milas, eds.), pp. 201–208, Raven, New York.

82. Liotta, L. A., Kleinerman, J., and Saidel, G. M., 1974, Quantitative relationships of intravascular tumor cells, tumor vessels and pulmonary metastases following tumor implantation, *Cancer Res.* **34:**997–1004.

83. Liotta, L. A., Kleinerman, J., and Saidel, G. M., 1976, Stochastic model of metastases formation, *Biometrics* **32:**535–550.

84. Salisbury, A. J., 1975, The significance of the circulating cancer cell, *Cancer Treatm. Rev.* **2:**55–72.

85. Fidler, I. J., 1970, Metastasis: Quantitative analysis of distribution and fate of tumor emboli labeled with $^{125}$I-5-iodo-2'-deoxyuridine. *J. Natl. Cancer Inst.* **45:**773–782.

86. Weiss, L., 1977, A pathobiologic overview of metastasis, *Semin. Oncol.* **4:**5–17.

87. Butler, T. P., and Gullino, P., 1975, Quantitation of cell-shedding into efferent blood of mammary adenocarcinoma, *Cancer Res.* **35:**512–517.

88. Gasic, G. J., 1984, Role of plasma, platelets, and endothelial cells in tumor metastasis, *Cancer Metab. Rev.* **3:**99–114.

89. Fidler, I. J., 1973, The relationship of embolic homogeneity, number, size and viability to the incidence of experimental metastasis, *Eur. J. Cancer* **9:**223–227.

90. Liotta, L. A., Kleinerman, J., and Saidel, G., 1976, The significance of hematogenous tumor cell clumps in the metastatic process, *Cancer Res.* **36:**889–894.

91. Poste, G., 1982, Experimental systems for analysis of the malignant phenotype, *Cancer Metab. Rev.* **1:**141–199.

92. Fidler, I. J., and Bucana, C., 1977, Mechanism of tumor cell resistance to lysis by syngeneic lymphocytes, *Cancer Res.* **37:**3945–3956.

93. Warren, B. A., 1973, Environment of the blood-borne tumor embolus adherent to vessel wall, *J. Med. (Basel)* **4:**150–177.

94. Nicolson, G. L., 1982, Metastatic tumor cell attachment and invasion assay utilizing vascular endothelial cell monolayers, *J. Histochem. Cytochem.* **30:**214–220.

95. Mason, R. G., and Saba, H. I., 1978, Normal and abnormal hemostasis—An integrated view, *Am. J. Pathol.* **92:**775–811.

96. Gasic, G. J., Gasic, T. B., Galanti, N., Johnson, T., and Murphy, S., 1973, Platelet-tumor cell interaction in mice. The role of platelets in the spread of malignant disease, *Int. J. Cancer* **11:**704–718.

97. Chew, E. C., Josephson, R. L., and Wallace, A. C., 1976, Morphological aspects of the arrest of circulating cancer cells. in: *Fundamental Aspects of Metastasis* (L. Weiss, ed.), pp. 121–150, North-Holland, Amsterdam.

98. Cliffton, E. E., and Agostino, D., 1965, The effects of fibrin formation and alterations in the clotting mechanism on the development of metastases, *Vascul. Dis.* **2:**43–52.

99. Sindelar, W. F., Tralka, T. S., and Ketcham, A. S., 1975, Electron microscopic observations on formation of pulmonary metastases, *J. Surg. Res.* **18:**137–161.

100. Dvorak, H. F., Senger, D. R., and Dvorak, A. M., 1983, Fibrin as a component of the tumor stroma: Orgins and biological significance, *Cancer Metab. Rev.* **2:**41–73.

101. Cliffton, E. E., and Grossi, C. E., 1974, The rationale of anticoagulants in the treatment of cancer, *J. Med. (Basel)* **5:**107–113.

102. Svanberg, L., 1975, Thromboplastic activity of human ovarian tumours, *Thromb. Res.* **6:**307–313.

103. Gordon, S. G., Franks, J. J., and Lewis, B., 1975, Cancer procoagulant A: A factor X activating procoagulant from malignant tissue, *Thromb. Res.* **6:**127–137.

104. Curatolo, L., Colucci, M., Cambini, A. L., Poggi, A., Morasca, L., Donati, M. B., and Semeraro, N., 1979, Evidence that cells from experimental tumours can activate coagulation factor X, *Br. J. Cancer* **40:**228–233.

105. Hoover, H. C., Ketcham, A. S., Millar, R. C., and Gralnick, H. R., 1978, Osteosarcoma: Improved survival with anticoagulation and amputation, *Cancer* **41:**2475–2480.

106. Ewing, J., 1928, *Neoplastic Diseases*, 6th ed., W. B. Saunders, Philadelphia.

107. Weiss, L., 1980, Cancer cell traffic from the lungs to the liver: An example of metastatic inefficiency, *Int. J. Cancer* **25:**385–392.

108. Calabresi, P., Dexter, D. L. and Heppner, G. H., 1979, Clinical and pharmacological implications of cancer cell differentiation and heterogeneity, *Biochem. Pharmacol.* **28:**1933–1941.

109. Hart, I. R., 1982, "Seed and soil" revisited: Mechanisms of site-specific metastasis, *Cancer Metab. Rev.* **1:**5–16.

110. Nicolson, G. L., 1982, Cancer metastasis organ colonization and the cell surface properties of malignant cells, *Biochim. Biophys. Acta* **695:**113–176.

111. Nicolson, G. L., 1984, Generation of phenotypic diversity and progression in metastatic tumor cells, *Cancer Metab. Rev.* **3:**25–42.

112. Nicolson, G. L., 1984, Tumor progression, oncogenes and the evolution of metastatic phenotypic diversity, *Clin. Exp. Metab.* **2:**85–105.

113. Tarin, D., Vass, A. C. R., Kettlewell, M. G. W., and Price, J. E., 1984, Absence of metastatic sequelae during long term treatment of malignant ascites by peritoneo-venous shunting, *Invasion Metast.* **4:**1–12.

114. Tarin, D., Price, J. E., Kettlewell, M. G. W., Souter, R. G., Vass, A. C. R., and Crossley, B., 1984, Clinicopathological observations on metastasis in man studied in patients treated with peritoneovenous shunts, *Br. Med. J.* **288:**749–751.

115. Tarin, D., Price, J. E., Kettlewell, M. G. W., Souter, R. G., Vass, A. C. R., and Crossley, B., 1984, Mechanisms of human tumor metastasis studied in patients with peritoneovenous shunts, *Cancer Res.* **44:**3584–3592.

116. Fidler, I. J., 1973, Selection of successive tumor lines for metastasis, *Nature (New Biol.)* **242:**148–149.

117. Brunson, K. W., and Nicolson, G. L., 1978, Selection and biologic properties of malignant variants of a murine lymphosarcoma, *J. Natl. Cancer Inst.* **61:**1499–1503.

118. Raz, S., Hanna, N., and Fidler, I. J., 1981, *In vivo* isolation of a metastatic tumor cell variant involving selective and nonadaptive processes, *J. Natl. Cancer Inst.* **66:**183–189.

119. Fidler, I. J., and Nicolson, G. L., 1981, The immunobiology of experimental metastatic melanoma, *Cancer Biol. Rev.* **2:**1–47.

120. Talmadge, J. E., and Fidler, I. J., 1982, Cancer metastasis is selective or random depending on the parent tumour population, *Nature (Lond.)* **297:**593–594.

121. Talmadge, J. E., and Fidler, I. J., 1982, Enhanced metastatic potential of tumor cells harvested from spontaneous metastases of heterogeneous murine tumors, *J. Natl. Cancer Inst.* **69:**975–980.

122. Nicolson, G. L., 1982, Cancer metastasis organ colonization and the cell surface properties of malignant cells, *Biochim. Biophys. Acta* **695:**113–176.

123. Brunson, K. W., and Nicolson, G. L., 1979, Selection of malignant melanoma variant cell lines for ovary colonization, *J. Supramol. Struct.* **11:**517–528.

124. Fidler, I. J., Gersten, D. M., and Budmen, M. B., 1976, Characterization in vivo and in vitro of tumor cells selected for resistance to syngeneic lymphocyte-mediated cytotoxicity, *Cancer Res.* **36:**3160–3165.

125. Frost, P., and Kerbel, R. S., 1981, Immunoselection in vitro of a nonmetastatic variant from a highly metastatic tumor, *Int. J. Cancer* **27:**381–385.

126. Briles, E. B., and Kornfeld, S., 1978, Isolation and metastatic properties of detachment variants of B16 melanoma cells, *J. Natl. Cancer Inst.* **60:**1217–1222.

127. Hart, I. R., 1979, The selection and characterization of an invasive variant of the B16 melanoma, *Am. J. Pathol.* **97:**587–600.

128. Poste, G., Doll, J., Hart, I. R., and Fidler, I. J., 1980, *In vitro* selection of murine B16 melanoma variants with enhanced tissue invasive properties, *Cancer Res.* **40:**1636–1644.

129. Kerbel, R. S., 1979, Immunologic studies of membrane mutants of a highly metastatic murine tumor, *Am. J. Pathol.* **97:**609–622.

130. Reading, C. L., and Hutchins, J. T., 1985, Carbohydrate structure in tumor immunity, *Cancer Metab. Rev.* **4:**221–260.

131. Kerbel, R. S., Dennis, J. W., Lagarde, A. E., and Frost, P., 1982, Tumor progression in metastasis: An experimental approach using lectin resistant tumor variants, *Cancer Metab. Rev.* **1:**99–140.

132. Hanna, N., 1982, Role of natural killer cells in control of cancer metastasis, *Cancer Metab. Rev.* **1:**45–64.

133. Fidler, I. J., and Kripke, M. L., 1977, Metastasis results from preexisting variant cells within a malignant tumor, *Science* **197:**893–895.

134. Kripke, M. L., Gruys, E., and Fidler, I. J., 1978, Metastatic heterogeneity of cells from an ultraviolet light-induced murine fibrosarcoma of recent origin, *Cancer Res.* **38:**2962–2967.

135. Luria, S. E., and Delbruck, M., 1943, Mutations of bacteria from virus sensitivity to virus resistant, *Genetics* **28:**491–511.

136. Fidler, I. J., and Kripke, M. L., 1980, Metastatic heterogeneity of cells from the K-1735 melanoma, in: *Metastatic Tumor Growth*, Cancer Campaign 3 (E. Grundmann, ed.), pp. 71–81, Gustav Fischer Verlag, New York.

137. Fidler, I. J., Gruys, E., Cifone, M. A., Barnes, Z., and Bucana, C., 1981, Demonstration of multiple phenotypic diversity in a murine melanoma of recent origin, *J. Natl. Cancer Inst.* **67:**947–956.

138. Kozlowski, J. M., Hart, I. R., Fidler, I. J., and Hanna, N., 1984, A human melanoma line heterogeneous with respect to metastatic capacity in athymic nude mice, *J. Natl. Cancer Inst.* **72:**913–917.

139. Kozlowski, J. M., Fidler, I. J., Campbell, D., Xu, Z., Kaighn, M. E., and Hart, I. R., 1984, Metastatic behavior of human tumor cell lines grown in the nude mouse, *Cancer Res.* **44:**3522–3529.

140. Giavazzi, R., Campbell, D. E., Jessup, J. M., Cleary, K., and Fidler, I. J., 1986, Metastatic behavior of tumor cells isolated from primary and metastatic human colorectal carcinomas implanted into different sites in nude mice, *Cancer Res.* **46:**1928–1933.

141. Naito, S., von Eschenbach, A. C., Giavazzi, R., and Fidler, I. J., 1986, Growth and metastasis of tumor cells isolated from a human renal cell carcinoma implanted into different organs of nude mice, *Cancer Res.* **46:**4109–4115.

142. Fidler, I. J., 1986, Rationale and methods for the use of nude mice to study the biology and therapy of human cancer metastasis, *Cancer Metab. Rev.* **5:**29–49.

143. Fialkow, P. J., 1970, Genetic marker studies in neoplasia, in: *Genetic Concepts and Neoplasia: A Collection of Papers*, Twenty-third Symposium on Fundamental Cancer Research, M. D. Anderson Hospital and Tumor Institute, 1969, pp. 112–130, Williams & Wilkins, Baltimore.

144. Fialkow, P. J., 1976, Clonal origin of human tumors, *Biochim. Biophys. Acta* **458:**283–321.

145. Ohno, S., 1971, Genetic implication of karyological instability of malignant somatic cells, *Physiol. Rev.* **51:**496–526.

146. Reddy, A. L., and Fialkow, P. J., 1979, Multicellular origin of fibrosarcomas in mice induced by the chemical carcinogen 3-methylcholanthrene, *J. Exp. Med.* **150:**878–887.

147. Deamant, F. D., and Iannaccone, P. M., 1985, Evidence concerning the clonal nature of chemically induced tumors: Phosphoglycerate kinase-1 isozyme patterns in chemically induced fibrosarcomas, *J. Natl. Cancer Inst.* **74:**145–149.

148. Heppner, G. H., and Miller, B. E., 1983, Tumor heterogeneity: Biological implications and therapeutic consequences, *Cancer Metab. Rev.* **2:**5–23.

149. Olsson, L., 1983, Phenotypic diversity in leukemic cell populations, *Cancer Metab. Rev.* **2:**153–163.

150. Miller, F. R., 1982, Intratumor immunologic heterogeneity, *Cancer Metab. Rev.* **1:**319–334.

151. Foulds, L., 1969, *Neoplastic Development,* Vol. 1, Academic, London.

152. Foulds, L., 1975, *Neoplastic Development,* Vol. 2, Academic, London.

153. Prehn, R. T., 1976, Tumor progression and homeostasis, *Adv. Cancer Res.* **23:**203–236.

154. Nowell, P. C., 1976, The clonal evolution of tumor cell populations, *Science* **194:**23–28.

155. Cifone, M. A., and Fidler, I. J., 1982, Increasing metastatic potential is associated with increasing genetic instability of clones isolated from murine neoplasms, *Proc. Natl. Acad. Sci. USA* **78:**6949–6952.

156. Bosslet, K., and Schirrmacher, V., 1982, High frequency generation of new immunoresistant tumor variants during metastasis of a cloned murine tumor line (Esb), *Int. J. Cancer* **29:**195–202.

157. Ling, V., A. F. Chambers, J. F. Harris, and R. P. Hill, 1985, Quantitative genetic analysis of tumor progression, *Cancer Metab. Rev.* **4:**173–194.

158. Hill, R. P., Chambers, A. F., and Ling, V., 1984, Dynamic heterogeneity: Rapid generation of metastatic variants in mouse B16 melanoma cells, *Science* **224:**998–1001.

159. Harris, J. F., Chambers, A. F., Hill, R. P., and Ling, V., 1982, Metastatic variants are generated spontaneously at a high rate in mouse KHT tumor, *Proc. Natl. Acad. Sci. USA* **79:**5547–5551.

160. Lagarde, A. E., 1983, A fluctuation analysis of the rate of reexpression of the metastatic potential in a nonmetastatic mutant of the MDAY-D2 murine tumor, *Invasion Metast.* **3:**52–64.

161. Larizza, L., and Schirrmacher, V., 1984, Somatic cell fusion as a source of genetic rearrangement leading to metastatic variants, *Cancer Metab. Rev.* **3:**193–222.

162. Boon, T., and Kellerman, O., 1977, Rejection by syngeneic mice of cell variants obtained by mutagenesis of a malignant teratocarcinoma cell line, *Proc. Natl. Acad. Sci. USA* **74:**272–275.

163. Boon, T., and Pel, A. V., 1978, Teratocarcinoma cell variants rejected by syngeneic mice: Protection of mice immunized with these variants against other variants and against the original malignant cell line, *Proc. Natl. Acad. Sci. USA* **75:**1519–1523.

164. Boon, T., Snick, J. V., Pel, A. V., Uyttenhove, C., and Marchand, M., 1980, Immunogenic variants obtained by mutagenesis of mouse mastocytoma P815. II. T lymphocyte mediated cytolysis, *J. Exp. Med.* **152:**1184–1193.

165. Fisher, M. S., and Cifone, M. A., 1981, Enhanced metastatic potential of murine fibrosarcomas treated *in vitro* with ultraviolet radiation, *Cancer Res.* **41:**3018–3023.

166. Kerbel, R. S., 1979, Implications of immunological heterogeneity of tumours, *Nature (Lond.)* **280:**358–360.

167. Fidler, I. J., and Hart, I. R., 1981, The origin of metastatic heterogeneity in tumors, *Eur. J. Cancer* **17:**487–494.

168. Miller, B. E., Miller, F. R., and Hepner, G. H., 1981, Interactions between tumor subpopulations affecting their sensitivity to the antineoplastic agents cyclophosphamide and methotrexate, *Cancer Res.* **41:**4378–4381.

169. Poste, G., Doll, J., and Fidler, I. J., 1981, Interactions between clonal subpopulations affect the stability of the metastatic phenotype in polyclonal populations of the B16 melanoma cells, *Proc. Natl. Sci. USA* **78:**6226–6231.

170. Poste, G., Greig, R., Tzeng, J., Koestler, T., and Corwin, S., 1984, Interactions between tumor cell subpopulations in malignant tumors, in: *Cancer Invasion and Metastasis: Biologic and Therapeutic Aspects* (G. L. Nicolson and L. Milas, eds.), pp. 223–243, Raven, New York.

171. Miller, B. E., Miller, F. R., Leith, J., and Heppner, G. H., 1980, Growth interaction *in vivo* between tumor subpopulations derived from a single mouse mammary tumor, *Cancer Res.* **40:**3977–3981.

172. Poste, G., Tzeng, J., Doll, J., Greig, R., Reiman, D., and Zeidman, I., 1982, Evolution of tumor cell heterogeneity during progressive growth of individual lung metastases, *Proc. Natl. Acad. Sci. USA* **79:**6574–6578.

173. Spremulli, E. N., and Dexter, D. L., 1983, Human tumor cell heterogeneity and metastasis, *J. Clin. Oncol.* **1:**496–509.

174. Henderson, J. S., and Rous, P., 1962, The plating of tumor components on the subcutaneous expanses of young mice, *J. Exp. Med.* **115:**1211–1230.

175. Prehn, R. T., 1970, Analysis of antigenic heterogeneity within individual 3-methylcholanthrene-induced mouse sarcomas, *J. Natl. Cancer Inst.* **45**:1039–1044.

176. Raz, A., 1982, Regional emergence of metastatic heterogeneity in a growing tumor, *Cancer Lett.* **17**:153–160.

177. Trope, C., 1982, Different susceptibilities of tumor cell subpopulations to cytotoxic agents, in: *Design of Models for Testing Cancer Chemotherapeutic Agents* (I. J. Fidler and R. J. White, eds.), pp. 64–79, Van Nostrand, New York.

178. Fidler, I. J., and Hart, I. R., 1981, Biological and experimental consequences of the zonal composition of solid tumors, *Cancer Res.* **41**:3266–3267.

179. Talmadge, J. E., Wolman, S. R., and Fidler, I. J., 1982, Evidence for the clonal origin of spontaneous metastases, *Science* **217**:361–363.

180. Poste, G., Tzeng, J., Doll, J., Greig, R., Rieman, D., and Zeidman, I., 1982, Evolution of tumor cell heterogeneity during progressive growth of individual lung metastases, *Proc. Natl. Acad. Sci. USA* **79**:6574–6578.

181. Talmadge, J. E., Benedict, K., Madsen, J., and Fidler, I. J., 1984, The development of biological diversity and susceptibility to chemotherapy in cancer metastases, *Cancer Res.* **44**:3801–3805.

182. Talmadge, J. E., and B. Zbar, 1987, Clonality of pulmonary metastases from the bladder 6 subline of the B16 melanoma studied by Southern hybridization, *J. Natl. Cancer Inst.* **78**:315–320.

183. Baylin, S. B., Weisburger, W. R., Eggleston, J. C., Mendelson, G., Beaven, M. A., Abeloff, M. D., and Ettinger, D. S., 1978, Variable content of histaminase, L-Dopa decarboxylase and calcitonin in small-cell carcinoma of the lung. Biologic and clinical implications, *N. Engl. J. Med.* **299**:105–110.

184. Baylin, S. B., 1982, Clonal selection and heterogeneity of human solid neoplasms, in: *Design of Models for Testing Cancer Therapeutic Agents* (I. J. Fidler and R. J. White, eds.), pp. 50–63, Van Nostrand Reinhold, New York.

185. McCullough, D., 1978, Diagnosis and staging of prostate cancer, in: *Genitourinary Cancer* (D. Skinner and J. deKernion, eds.), pp. 295–309, W. B. Saunders, Philadelphia.

186. Hockey, M. S., Stokes, H. J., Thompson, H., Woodhouse, C. S., Macdonald, F., Fielding, J. W. L., and Ford, C. H. J., 1984, Carcinoembryonic antigen (CEA) expression and heterogeneity in primary and autologous metastatic gastric tumours demonstrated by a monoclonal antibody, *Br. J. Cancer* **49**:129–133.

187. Gold, D. V., Shochat, D., Primus, F. J., Dexter, D. L., Calabresi, P., and Goldenberg, D. M., 1983, Differential expression of tumor-associated antigens in human colon carcinomas xenografted into nude mice, *J. Natl. Cancer Inst.* **71**:117–124.

188. Mareel, M. M., 1983, Invasion *in vitro:* Methods of analysis, *Cancer Metab. Rev.* **2**:201–219.

189. Czerniak, B., Darzynkiewicz, Z., Staiano-Coico, L., Herz, F., and Koss, L. G., 1984, Expression of Ca antigen in relation to the cell cycle in cultured human tumor cells, *Cancer Res.* **44**:4342–4346.

190. Barranco, S. C., Drewinko, B., and Humphrey, R. M., 1973, Differential response by human melanoma cells to 1,3-bis(2-chloroethyl)-1-nitrosourea and bleomycin, *Mutat. Res.* **19**:277–280.

191. Barranco, S. C., Haenelt, B. R., and Gee, E. L., 1978, Differential sensitivities of five rat hepatoma cell lines to anticancer drugs, *Cancer Res.* **38**:656–660.

192. Biorklund, A., Hakansson, L., Stenstam, B., Trope, C., and Akerman, M., 1980, On heterogeneity of non-Hodgkin's lymphomas as regards sensitivity to cytostatic drugs: An in vitro study, *Eur. J. Cancer* **16**:647–654.

193. Tanigawa, N., Mizuno, Y., Hashimura, T., Hondo, K., Satomura, K., Hikasa, Y., Niwa, O., Sugahara, T., Yoshida, O., Kern, D. H., and Morton, D. L., 1984, Comparison of drug sensitivity among tumor cells within a tumor between primary tumor and metastases, and between different metastases in the human tumor colony-forming assay, *Cancer Res.* **44**:2309–2312.

194. Trope, C., Aspergen, K., Kullander, S., and Astredt, B., 1979, Heterogeneous response of disseminated human ovarian cancers to cytostatic *in vitro*. *Acta Obstet. Gynecol. Scand.* **58**:543–546.

195. Trope, C., Hakansson, L., and Dencker, H., 1975, Heterogeneity of human adenocarcinomas of the colon and the stomach as regards sensitivity to cytostatic drugs, *Neoplasma* **22**:423–430.

196. Yung, W. K. A., Shapiro, J. R., and Shapiro, W. R., 1982, Heterogeneous chemosensitivities of subpopulations of human glioma cells in culture, *Cancer Res.* **42**:992–998.

197. Abe, I., Suzuki, M., Hori, K., Saito, S., and Sato, H., 1985, Some aspects of size-dependent differential drug response in primary and metastatic tumors, *Cancer Metab. Rev.* **4**:27–40.

198. Donelli, M. G., Colombo, T., Broggini, M., and Garattinni, S., 1977, Differential distribution of antitumor agents in primary and secondary tumors, *Cancer Treatm. Rep.* **61**:1319–1324.

199. Donelli, M. G., Colombo, T., Dagnino, G., Madonna, M., and Garattinni, S., 1981, Is better drug

availability in secondary neoplasms responsible for better response to chemotherapy?, *Eur. J. Cancer* **17**:201–209.

200. Fugmann, R. A., Anderson, J. C., Stolfi, R., and Martin, D. S., 1977, Comparison of adjuvant chemotherapeutic activity against primary and metastatic spontaneous murine tumors, *Cancer Res.* **37**:496–500.
201. Metcalfe, S. A., Whelan, R. D., Masters, J. R., and Hill, B. T., 1983, *In vitro* responses of human prostate tumour cell lines to a range of antitumour agents, *Int. J. Cancer* **32**:351–358.
202. Schabel, F. M., Griswold, D. P., Corbett, T. H., and Lloyd, H. H., 1977, Quantitative evaluation of anticancer agent activity in experimental animals, *Pharmacol. Ther.* **1**:411–435
203. Smith, K. A., Begg, A, C., and Denckamp, J., 1985, Differences in chemo-sensitivity between subcutaneous and pulmonary tumours, *Eur. J. Cancer Clin. Oncol.* **21**:249–256.
204. Tsuruo, T., and Fidler, I. J., 1981, Differences in drug sensitivity among tumor cells from parental tumors, selected variants, and spontaneous metastases, *Cancer Res.* **41**:3058–3064.
205. Weichselbaum, R. B., Dahlberg, W., and Little, J. B., 1985, Inherently radioresistant cells exist in some human tumors, *Proc. Natl. Acad. Sci. USA* **82**:4732–4735.
206. Welch, D. R., Milas, L., Tomasovic, S. P., and Nicolson, G. L., 1983, Heterogeneous response and clonal drift of sensitivities of metastatic 13762NF mammary adenocarcinoma clones to gamma-radiation *in vitro*, *Cancer Res.* **43**:6–10.
207. Morstyn, G., Russo, A., Carney, D. N., Karawya, E., Wilson, S. H., and Mitchell, J. B., 1984, Heterogeneity in the radiation survival curves and biochemical properties of human lung cancer cell lines, *J. Natl. Cancer Inst.* **73**:801–807.
208. Bradley, E. C., Issell, B. F., and Hellman, R., 1984, The human tumor colony-forming chemosensitivity assay: A biological and clinical review, *Invest. New Drugs* **2**:59–70.
209. Bertelsen, C. A., Sondak, V. K., and Mann, B. D., 1984, Chemosensitivity testing of human solid tumors. A review of 1582 assays with 258 clinical correlations, *Cancer* **53**:1240–1245.
210. Schabel, F. M., Griswold, D. P., Corbett, R. H., Laster, W. R., Mayo, J. G., and Lloyd, M. J., 1979, Testing therapeutic hypothesis in mice and men: Observations on the therapeutic activity against advanced solid tumors of mice treated with anticancer drugs that have demonstrated or have potential clinical utility for treatment of advanced solid tumors of man, *Methods Cancer Res.* **17**:3–49.
211. Rosenberg, S., 1985, Lymphokine-activated killer cells: A new approach to immunotherapy of cancer, *J. Natl. Cancer Inst.* **75**:595–603.
212. Bystryn, J. C., Bernstein, P., Lui, P., and Valentine, F., 1985, Immunophenotype of human melanoma cells in different metastases, *Cancer Res.* **45**:5603–5607.
213. Cillo, C., Mach, J. P., Schreyer, M., and Carrel, S., 1984, Antigenic heterogeneity of clones and subclones from human melanoma cell lines demonstrated by a panel of monoclonal antibodies and flow microfluorometry analysis, *Int. J. Cancer* **34**:11–20.
214. Miller, F. R., 1982, Intratumor immunologic heterogeneity, *Cancer Metab. Rev.* **1**:319–334.
215. Fidler, I. J., Gersten, D. M., and Kripke, M. L., 1979, Influence of immune status on the metastasis of three murine fibrosarcomas of different immunogenicities, *Cancer Res.* **39**:3816–3821.
216. Albino, A. P., Lloyd, K. O., Houghton, A. N., Oettgen, H. F., and Old, L. J., 1981, Heterogeneity in surface antigen and glycoprotein expression of cell lines derived from different melanoma metastases of the same patient, *J. Exp. Med.* **154**:1764–1778.
217. McCune, C. S., Schapira, D. V., and Henshaw, E. C., 1981, Specific immunotherapy of advanced renal carcinoma. Evidence for the polyclonality of metastases, *Cancer* **47**:1984–1987.
218. Natalin, P., Cavaliere, R., Bigotti, A., Nicotra, M. R., Russo, C., Ng, A. K., Giacomini, P., and Ferrone, S., 1983, Antigenic heterogeneity of surgically removed primary and autologous metastatic human melanoma lesions, *J. Immunol.* **130**:1462–1466.
219. Pimm, M. V., Embleton, M. J., and Baldwin, R. W., 1980, Multiple antigenic specificities within primary 3-methylcholanthrene-induced rat sarcomas and metastases, *Int. J. Cancer* **25**:621–629.
220. Wikstrand, C. J., Grahmann, F. C., McComb, R. D., and Bigner, D. D., 1985, Antigenic heterogeneity of human anaplastic gliomas and glioma-derived cell lines defined by monoclonal antibodies, *J. Neuropathol. Exp. Neurol.* **44**:229–241.
221. Olsson, L., and Ebbesen, P., 1979, Natural polyclonality of spontaneous AKR leukemia and its consequence for so-called specific immunotherapy, *J. Natl. Cancer Inst.* **62**:623–627.
222. Kripke, M. L., 1981, Immunologic mechanisms in UV radiation carcinogenesis, *Adv. Cancer Res.* **34**:69–106.
223. Hewitt, H. B., Blake, E. R., and Walder, A. S., 1976, A critique of the evidence for active host defense against cancer, based on personal studies of 27 murine tumours of spontaneous origin, *Br. J. Cancer* **33**:241–259.

224. Frost, P., and Kerbel, R. S., 1983, Immunology of metastasis: Can the immune response cope with disseminated tumor? *Cancer Met. Rev.* **2:**239–256.

225. Frost, P., Liteplo, R. G., Donaghue, T. P., and Kerbel, R. S., 1984, Selection of strongly immunogenic "Tum" variants from tumors at high frequency using 5-azacytine, *J. Exp. Med.* **159:**1491–1501.

226. Kerbel, R. S., Frost, P., Liteplo, R., Carlow, D. A., and Elliot, B. E., 1984, Possible epigenetic mechanisms of tumor progression: Induction of high-frequency heritable but phenotypically unstable changes in the tumorigenic and metastatic properties of tumor cell populations by 5-azacytidine treatment, *J. Cell Physiol. (Suppl.)* **3:**87–97.

227. Fidler, I. J., and Kripke, M. L., 1980, Tumor cell antigenicity, host immunity and cancer metastasis, *Cancer Immunol. Immunother,* **7:**201–205.

228. Fidler, I. J., and Gersten, D. M., 1980, Effect of syngeneic lymphocytes on the vascularity, growth and induced metastasis of the B16 melanoma, in: *Neoplasm Immunity, Experimental and Clinical* (R. G. Crispen, ed.), pp. 3–15, Elsevier North Holland, New York.

229. Kripke, M. L., 1977, Latency, histology, and antigenicity of tumors induced by ultraviolet light in three inbred mouse strains, *Cancer Res.* **37:**1395–1400.

230. Kripke, M. L., 1979, Speculations on the role of ultraviolet radiation in the development of malignant melanoma, *J. Natl. Cancer Inst.* **63:**541–548.

231. Kripke, M. L., and Fisher, M. S., 1976, Immunologic parameters of ultraviolet carcinogenesis, *J. Natl. Cancer Inst.* **57:**211–215.

232. Fisher, M. S., and Kripke, M. L., 1977, Systemic alteration induced in mice by ultraviolet light irradiation and its relationship to ultraviolet carcinogenesis, *Proc. Natl. Acad. Sci. USA* **74:**1688–1692.

233. Fisher, M. S., and Kripke, M. L., 1978, Further studies on the tumor-specific suppressor cells induced by ultraviolet radiation, *J. Immunol.* **121:**1139–1144.

234. Kripke, M. L., and Fidler, I. J., 1980, Enhanced experimental metastasis of ultraviolet light induced fibrosarcomas in ultraviolet light irradiated syngeneic mice, *Cancer Res.* **40:**625–629.

235. Talmadge, J. E., Talmadge, C. B., Zbar, B., McEwen, R., Meeker, A. K., and Tribble, H., 1987, *In vivo* immunologic selection of class I MHC gene deletion variants from the B16-BL6 melanoma, *J. Natl. Cancer Inst.* **78:**1215–1221.

236. Waes, C. V., Urgan, J. L., Rothstein, J. L., Ward, P. L., and Schreiber, H., 1986, Highly malignant tumor variants retain tumor-specific antigens recognized by T helper cells, *J. Exp. Med.* **164:**1547–1565.

237. Dennis, J. W., Laferte, S., Man, M. S., Elliott, B. E., and Kerbel, R. S., 1984, Adoptive immune therapy in mice bearing poorly immunogenic metastases, using T lymphocytes stimulated in vitro against highly immunogenic mutant sublines, *Int. J. Cancer* **34:**709–716.

238. Cheever, M. A., Greenberg, P. D., and Fefer, A., 1984, Potential for specific cancer therapy with immune T lymphocytes, *J. Biol. Resp. Modif.* **3:**113–127.

239. Mule, J. J., Ettinghausen, S. E., Spiess, P. J., Shu, S., and Rosenberg, S. A., 1986, Antitumor efficacy of lymphokine-activated killer cells and recombinant interleukin-2 *in vivo:* Survival benefit and mechanisms of tumor escape in mice undergoing immunotherapy, *Cancer Res.* **46:**676–683.

240. Vollmers, H. P., and Birchmeier, W., 1983, Monoclonal antibodies exhibit the adhesion of mouse B16 melanoma cells *in vitro* and block lung metastasis *in vivo*, *Proc. Natl. Acad. Sci. USA* **80:**3729–3733.

241. Vollmers, H. P., and Birchmeier, W., 1983, Monoclonal antibodies that prevent adhesion of B16 melanoma cells and reduce metastases in mice: Crossreaction with human tumor cells, *Proc. Natl. Acad. Sci. USA* **80:**6863–6867.

242. Oldham, R. K., 1985, Biologicals and biological response modifiers: Design of clinical trials, *J. Biol. Resp. Modif.* **4:**117–128.

243. Oldham, R. K., and Smalley, R. V., 1983, Immunotherapy: The old and the new, *J. Biol. Resp. Modif.* **2:**1–37.

244. Talmadge, J. E., and Herberman, R. B., 1986, The preclinical screening laboratory: Evaluation of immunomodulatory and therapeutic properties of biological response modifiers, *Cancer Treatm. Rep.* **70:**171–182.

# Index

Acquired immunodeficiency syndrome (AIDS), *see* HIV
Adenocarcinomas, 211
Adenylate cyclase system, 312
AFB$_1$-N7-dG-DNA, 65
AFP, 8, 419, 481, 487, 488
*Agrobacterium*
  *radiobacter*, 498, 507
    Agrocin, 507
    pAgK84, 507
    strain K84, 507
  *rhizogenes*, 498
  *rubi*, 498
  *tumefaciens*, 3, 438, 497, 498
α-fetoprotein: *see* AFP
Alterations in biochemical control mechanisms of neoplastic cells, 305–317
  cell-cycle proliferation, 305
  cytoskeletal, 309, 310
    actin-microfilament network, 310
    autocrine growth factors, 310, 538
    cytochalasin B, 310
    pp60$^{src}$ tyrosine kinase, 309, 337
    vinculin, 310
  G proteins, 309, 312, 364, 378, 539, 540
  glycolysis, 308, 309
    aerobic, 308, 310
    Warburg effect, 308
  membrane transport in neoplasia, 306–308
    aminoisobutyrate (AIB), 306
    5-amino-4-imidazolecarboxamide ribotide trans-formylase, 308
    amino acid transport, 307–309
    Ehrlich ascites carcinoma, 306, 308
    G$_1$-S progression, 307
    ionic environment, 307
    methylaminoisobutyrate, 306
    (Na$^+$/K$^+$)ATPase, 306–308
    S phase, 307
    sodium-proton antiport system, 308
    system A, 306, 308, 309
    system ASC, 306

Alterations in biochemical control mechanisms of neoplastic cells (*cont.*)
  membrane transport in neoplasia (*cont.*)
    tropomyosin, 308, 309
    Yoshida ascites hepatoma, 306
  mesenger RNA (mRNA), 305, 423
  mitrochondrial citric acid cycle, 310, 311
    Pasteur effect, 310
  signal transduction, 305, 309, 310, 314, 412
Amine content, amine precursor uptake, amino acid decarboxylation: *see* APUD
Anaplasia, 28, 29
  cytologic, 28
  positional, 29
Anchorage-independent growth, 293, 314
Aneuploid cells, 210, 211
Angiogenesis, 513–525, 533
  factors of, 515–524
    Boyden migration chamber, 515
    chemokinesis, 515
    chemotaxis, 515
    corneal pocket assay, 515
    developing chick chorioallantoic membrane (CAM), 515
    heparin-binding growth factors, 518–524
      basic fibroblast growth factor (bFGF), 520
      cartilage-derived growth factor (CDGF), 520
      chondrosarcoma-derived growth factor (ChDGF), 519, 520
      endothelial cell growth factor (ECGF), 518, 520
      eye-derived growth factor 1 (EDGF-1), 522
      PC12 cells, 523
      retina-derived growth factor (RDGF), 520
  ischemia in angiogenesis, 525
  non-heparin-binding growth factors, 516, 517
    chemotactic factors, 516
    lipids, 516
      prostaglandins E$_1$ and E$_2$ (PGE$_1$ and PGE$_2$), 516, 524
  plasminogen activator, 515
  tumor vasculature, 513–515